Thieme

Surgery for Cochlear and Other Auditory Implants

Mario Sanna, MD, PhD
Professor of Otolaryngology
Department of Head and Neck Surgery
University of Chieti
Chieti, Italy
Director
Gruppo Otologico
Piacenza and Rome, Italy

Paul Merkus, MD, PhD
ENT Surgeon and Neurotologist
Department of Otolaryngology
Section Ear & Hearing
VU University Medical Center & EMGO Institute for Health and Care Research
Amsterdam, The Netherlands

Rolien Free, MD, PhD
ENT Surgeon, Otologist, and Pediatric ENT Surgeon
University Medical Center Groningen
University of Groningen
Director of Cochlear Implant Team Northern Netherlands
Groningen, The Netherlands

Maurizio Falcioni, MD
Otologist and Skull Base Surgeon
Affiliated with the Department of Otolaryngology
University of Parma
Parma, Italy

1200 illustrations

Thieme
Stuttgart · New York · Delhi · Rio de Janeiro

Library of Congress Cataloging-in-Publication Data is available from the publisher.

Important note: Medicine is an ever-changing science undergoing continual development. Research and clinical experience are continually expanding our knowledge, in particular our knowledge of proper treatment and drug therapy. Insofar as this book mentions any dosage or application, readers may rest assured that the authors, editors, and publishers have made every effort to ensure that such references are in accordance with **the state of knowledge at the time of production of the book.**

Nevertheless, this does not involve, imply, or express any guarantee or responsibility on the part of the publishers in respect to any dosage instructions and forms of applications stated in the book. **Every user is requested to examine carefully** the manufacturers' leaflets accompanying each drug and to check, if necessary in consultation with a physician or specialist, whether the dosage schedules mentioned therein or the contraindications stated by the manufacturers differ from the statements made in the present book. Such examination is particularly important with drugs that are either rarely used or have been newly released on the market. Every dosage schedule or every form of application used is entirely at the user's own risk and responsibility. The authors and publishers request every user to report to the publishers any discrepancies or inaccuracies noticed. If errors in this work are found after publication, errata will be posted at www.thieme.com on the product description page.

Some of the product names, patents, and registered designs referred to in this book are in fact registered trademarks or proprietary names even though specific reference to this fact is not always made in the text. Therefore, the appearance of a name without designation as proprietary is not to be construed as a representation by the publisher that it is in the public domain.

Thieme Publishers Stuttgart
Rüdigerstrasse 14, 70469 Stuttgart, Germany
+49 [0]711 8931 421, customerservice@thieme.de

Thieme Publishers New York
333 Seventh Avenue, New York, NY 10001 USA
+1 800 782 3488, customerservice@thieme.com

Thieme Publishers Delhi
A-12, Second Floor, Sector-2, Noida-201301
Uttar Pradesh, India
+91 120 45 566 00, customerservice@thieme.in

Thieme Publishers Rio, Thieme Publicações Ltda.
Edifício Rodolpho de Paoli, 25º andar
Av. Nilo Peçanha, 50 – Sala 2508,
Rio de Janeiro 20020-906 Brasil
Tel: +55 21 3172-2297 / +55 21 3172-1896

Cover design: Thieme Publishing Group
Typesetting by primustype Robert Hurler GmbH, Notzingen, Germany

Printed in Germany by CPI, Leck 5 4 3 2 1

ISBN 978-3-13-176441-6

Also available as an e-book:
eISBN 978-3-13-176451-5

MIX
Papier aus verantwortungsvollen Quellen
FSC® C083411

Contents

Cases

15 Inner Ear Malformations and Implantation

16 Neurofibromatosis Type 2 and Auditory Implantation

17 Implantation in Skull Base and Temporal Bone Lesions

18 Bone Conduction Implants

19 Active Middle Ear Implants: Vibrant Soundbridge

Videos

Preface

Perhaps no other branch in medicine has made such rapid developments in such a short span of time as that of hearing implantology and rehabilitation. In the little more than half a century since the first cochlear implant was devised and placed in the round window by William House in 1961, we have come a long way into the era of auditory brainstem implants and a range of other implantable hearing devices. Giant strides have been made both in the understanding of deafness and in the technology used to treat it. Researchers have published exhaustively on this subject, more so in the last decade. It was in the light of this that we decided to compile this book, and I am extremely pleased to see *Surgery for Cochlear and Other Auditory Implants* come to fruition. It has been the collective effort of my team at the Gruppo Otologico in Piacenza and Rome that has made it possible. Above all, this book is a tribute to the legendary William House—surgeon, inventor, and teacher par excellence. It is due to his pioneering work in the science of implantology, including the cochlear implant and the auditory brainstem implant, that we are what we are. There is a tendency to forget the memory of the giants of the past on whose shoulders we stand today. This book is a reminder to all its readers of the genius and tireless efforts of remarkable physicians and surgeons like William House and many other before and after him.

This book is based on our vast experience of over 20 years with cochlear implants, auditory brainstem implants, and other implantable hearing rehabilitation devices that were developed during that time. The book is targeted at the otological surgeons keen to pursue the discipline of hearing implantology; hence the main focus of the book is on the surgical aspects of hearing implantology and not on electrophysiology and rehabilitation, for which there are other excellent textbooks already available. Having said that, we have left no stone unturned to include all the possible facets relating to surgery, making this book an exhaustive surgical compilation. This includes preoperative protocols, radiology, decision making, intraoperative techniques, difficult surgical situations, complications, and special considerations in implantology. The text describes surgery of all the implantable devices available today including cochlear implants, auditory brainstem implants, active middle ear implants, and bone anchored hearing devices. It also discusses a wide range of surgical situations from routine indications to more challenging ones such as inner ear malformations, congenital absence of the cochlear nerves, implantation in neurofibromatosis (NF) II, implantation in the only hearing ear in solitary vestibular schwannomas, and implantation in chronically discharging ear and in cases with CSF leaks. Special emphasis is given to the radiology of inner ear malformations. The role of subtotal petrosectomy in implantation is discussed in detail. A special chapter is written on single-sided deafness after surgery and its rehabilitation with bone anchored hearing aids and cross hearing. Algorithms have been developed to lay out the decision making process in various situations so as to make it easy for the reader to comprehend. Finally, all this is laid out in a pictorial format with high-quality illustrations that has been popular with the readers of our earlier textbooks and has come to be the hallmark of books from our stable.

The support of Cochlear, Med-El , Advanced Bionics, Neurelec, Oticon Medical, and Sophono has been vital in the making of this book and I thank them. I also thank Paul Merkus and Rolien Free from the Netherlands for their valuable help and coordination with the members of the Gruppo Otologico. I thank Thomas Roland from the United States for participating in this book. Last but not the least I thank my coauthors who worked tirelessly on this book for the last couple of years to produce a very satisfying product.

Mario Sanna, MD, PhD

Contributors

Antonio Caruso, MD
Otologist and Skull Base Surgeon
Gruppo Otologico
Piacenza and Rome, Italy

Giuseppe De Donato, MD
ENT and Skull Base Surgeon
Gruppo Otologico
Piacenza and Rome, Italy

Maurizio Falcioni, MD
Otologist and Skull Base Surgeon
Affiliated with the Department of Otolaryngology
University of Parma
Parma, Italy

Rolien Free, MD, PhD
ENT Surgeon, Otologist, and Pediatric ENT Surgeon
University Medical Center Groningen
University of Groningen
Director of Cochlear Implant Team Northern Netherlands
Groningen, The Netherlands

Anna Lisa Giannuzzi, MD, PhD
Otologist and Skull Base Surgeon
Gruppo Otologico
Piacenza and Rome, Italy

Maurizio Guida, MD
Audiologist
Gruppo Otologico
Piacenza and Rome, Italy

Lorenzo Lauda, MD
ENT and Skull Base Surgeon
Gruppo Otologico
Piacenza and Rome, Italy

Fernando Mancini, MD
ENT and Skull Base Surgeon
Gruppo Otologico
Piacenza and Rome, Italy

Paul Merkus, MD, PhD
ENT Surgeon and Neurotologist
Department of Otolaryngology, Section Ear & Hearing
VU University Medical Center & EMGO Institute for Health and Care Research
Amsterdam, The Netherlands

Enrico Piccirillo, MD
ENT and Skull Base Surgeon
Gruppo Otologico
Piacenza and Rome, Italy

Sampath Chandra Prasad, MS, DNB, FEB-ORLHNS
ENT and Skull Base Surgeon
Gruppo Otologico
Piacenza and Rome, Italy

J. Thomas Roland Jr., MD, FACS
ENT and Skull Base Surgeon
NYU Langone Medical Center and NYU School of Medicine
New York, USA

Alessandra Russo, MD
Otologist and Skull Base Surgeon
Gruppo Otologico
Piacenza and Rome, Italy

Mario Sanna, MD, PhD
Professor of Otolaryngology
Department of Head and Neck Surgery
University of Chieti
Chieti, Italy
Director
Gruppo Otologico
Piacenza and Rome, Italy

Abdelkader Taibah, MD
Neurosurgeon, Otologist, and Skull Base Surgeon
Gruppo Otologico
Piacenza and Rome, Italy

About the Authors

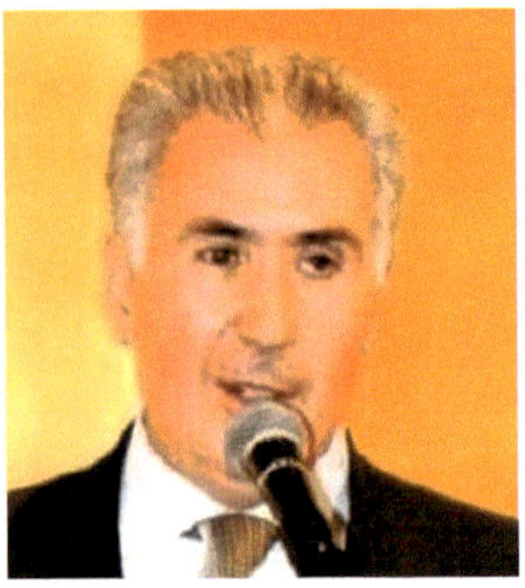

Mario Sanna is Professor and Director of the Otolaryngology Clinic at the University of Cheiti, Italy and the Founder & Director of the Gruppo Otologico (Piacenza-Rome, Italy), an internationally acclaimed center for otology, hearing implantology, and skull base surgeries. Professor Sanna is a master in his field, known across the world for his pioneering work in otology and skull base surgery. He is a founder member of the European Skull Base Society and the Italian Skull Base Society and an honorary member of the French and Spanish otolaryngological societies.

Professor Sanna has authored 15 books and over 375 articles in peer-reviewed journals. His illustrated textbooks are extremely popular and some of them have won international awards. He has been an invited faculty in over 200 conferences and academic meetings. Over 100 fellows and 500 observers have been trained at the Gruppo Otologico. Professor Sanna has contributed tremendously to the knowledge of otology and skull base surgery and is considered by his peers to be one of the pioneers of modern skull base surgery.

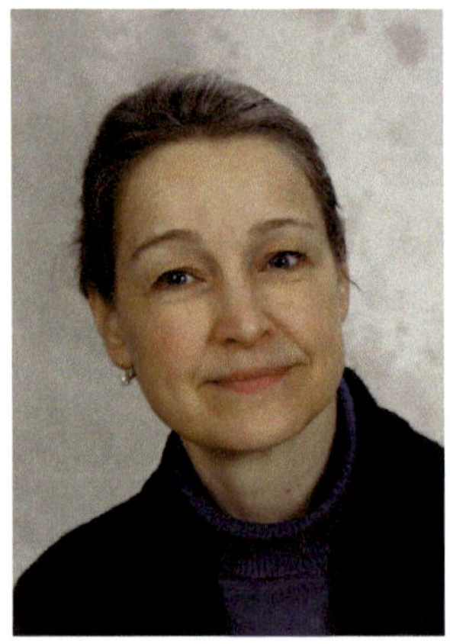

Rolien Free is a Dutch ENT surgeon, who was trained at the University Medical Center Groningen, the Netherlands by Professor Frans Albers. She specialized in otology/neurotology and pediatric ENT surgery and has published several papers on cochlear implantation, otology, and pediatric ENT. Since 2010 she is codirector of the Cochlear Implant Team Northern Netherlands. She has an extensive experience of 10 years in both adult and pediatric cochlear implantation surgery. In 2011 and 2012 she worked as a neuro-otological fellow in Professor Mario Sanna's Gruppo Otologico, Piacenza, Italy. The neuro-otological stipendiums of the Heinsius Houbolt Foundation (Wassenaar, the Netherlands) and the A.I.N.O.T. (Associazione Italiana Neuro-Otologica, Italy) made these fellowships possible. She has tutored several years with Professor Ugo Fisch in his otology and skull base microsurgery courses in Zurich, Switzerland and is tutoring in the cochlear implant and advanced temporal bone dissection course led by Professor Louis Hofmeyr in Pretoria, South Africa. She is currently secretary of CI-ON (National Committee of Dutch Cochlear Implant Teams) and of the Dutch Flemish Society for Pediatric Otorhinolaryngology.

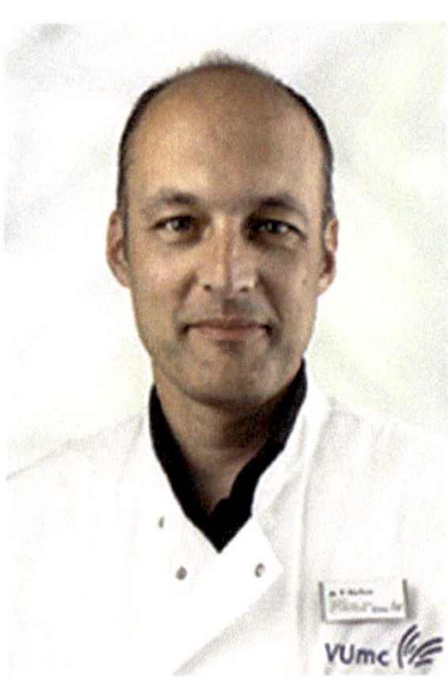

Paul Merkus is a Dutch ENT surgeon (VUmc Amsterdam, the Netherlands) with longstanding experience in adult and pediatric cochlear implant surgery. He has published several papers on cochlear implantation and auditory brainstem surgery and his team is expert in decision making in difficult cases. His knowledge in imaging and ear surgery and his educational talents are well evidenced in this book.

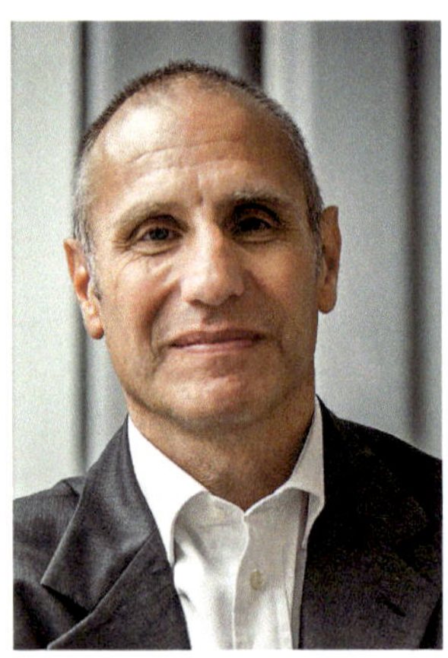

Maurizio Falcioni is an Italian ENT surgeon with more than 20 years' experience in middle ear and skull base surgery. He has published several papers on cochlear implantation and auditory brainstem surgery. His experience is particularly focused on cochlear implantation in difficult cases (concomitant chronic otitis, cochlear ossification, malformation).

1 History of Auditory Implantation

Studying the history of auditory implantation and following the developments that have taken place in only some 50 years is exciting and teaches us about the courage, vision, and endurance of some special individuals in and from different parts of the globe. It also makes us realize that the cochlear implant (CI) has been developed through multidisciplinary efforts and would not have existed if other developments had not paved the way; for example, without the experience with silicone-covered leads in pacemakers, biocompatibility studies, and the existence of antibiotics, this development would not have been possible. The reactions of disbelief and skepticism in the community of auditory professionals, and later the reactions of anxiety and anger in the deaf community to these new developments—which felt like a threat and an offense to their culture and way of living—also demonstrate the sociological impact that the cochlear implant has had and sometimes still has. Finally, this chain of development could not have taken place without serendipity lending a hand, and without some very courageous patients who decided in close consultation with their doctors to become objects of research for this possible new treatment.

Five Eras in the Development of Auditory Implants

- Forerunners
- Pioneers and experimentation: 1957–1960s
- Feasibility studies, safety studies, evaluation of auditory gain: 1970s
- Development of the commercial multielectrode cochlear implant: 1980s
- Development of the auditory brainstem implant: 1990s

1.1 Forerunners

1.1.1 Alessandro Volta (1745–1827) (Fig. 1.1)

Interest in stimulating hearing by use of electricity started in 1790 when Alessandro Volta, an Italian physicist and Count of the region of Lombardia in northern Italy, stimulated his own auditory system by connecting a battery with potential difference of ~50 volts to two metal rods that were inserted into his ears. Apparently he heard a "boom" within his head and then a hissing sound as if "soup was boiling"; he found the experience quite uncomfortable and moreover it lacked tonal quality!

Volta had had an interest in electricity from a very young age and at the age of 18 years was already corresponding with various academics and scientists on the subject. He invented the electrical battery (the voltaic cell; 1800), and also developed an interest in chemistry. He was also the person who discovered methane in a nearby swamp as a gas that could be used as fuel (1778). The son of a family of nine children who was expected to become a priest like five of his siblings, Alessandro Volta contributed significantly as a scientist and became professor in physics at the University of Pavia in 1779 and professor in philosophy at Padova (Padua) in 1815. In his recognition, the unit of potential difference (or "voltage")—the *volt*—has been named after him since 1881.

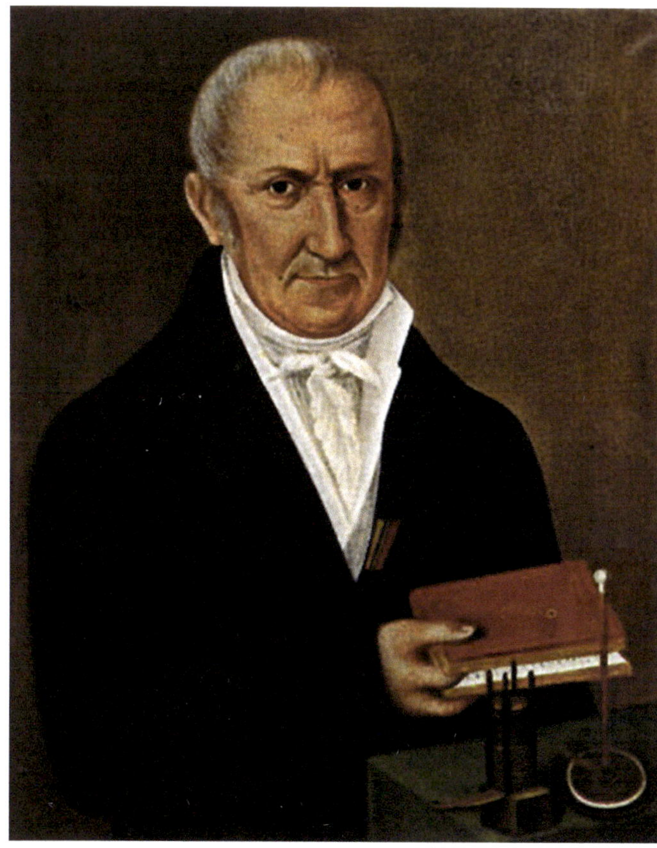

Fig. 1.1 Alessandro Volta with his voltaic cell.

Some other experiments involving electrical stimulation of the auditory system were described in those years, all without tonal quality of sound. In 1855 Duchenne of Boulogne (1806–1875), based in Paris, stimulated the ear with alternating current instead of direct current, leading to a sensation of "the beating of a fly's wings"; still an unsatisfactory outcome.

Several discoveries in the early 20th century (around the 1930s), the era of the development of the telephone, influenced the final development of the auditory implant.[1]

1.1.2 Homer Dudley: the Vocoder

Working as a researcher at the Bell Telephone Laboratories in New York, Dudley described and designed in 1939 a real-time voice synthesizer that produced intelligible speech. The fundamental frequency of speech, the intensity of its spectral components, and its overall power could be extracted using a specially designed circuit. This synthesizer was named the *vocoder* (encoding the voice) and its operating principles formed the basis for the early speech processing schemes in auditory implants.[2]

1.1.3 Wever and Bray: the Cochlear Microphonic

In 1930, Ernest Glen Wever and Charles Bray recorded electrical potentials in the cochlea that reproduced the sound stimulus and described this phenomenon, which was later called the Wever–Bray effect.[3] These experiments were performed on a cat, with an electrode introduced into the auditory nerve. While they thought to record the discharges of the auditory nerve, following the "telephone theory" (signals carried along the cable of the ear, i.e., the auditory nerve), in fact it was the cochlear microphonic that they recorded, produced by the outer hair cells of the cochlea. The telephone theory was later rejected, but Wever and Bray did inspire several CI pioneers.[4]

1.1.4 S.S. Stevens: Electrophonic Hearing

In the 1930s Stanley Smith Stevens and his colleagues described "electrophonic hearing," thought to be the mechanism by which cochlear structures respond to electrical stimulation to produce hearing and therefore only present in intact cochleae. It is now known that electrophonic hearing is a result of the mechanical oscillation of the basilar membrane responding to voltage changes. Before 1957, efforts to stimulate hearing electrically were performed on patients with at least a partially functioning cochlea. The results therefore could have been based on electrophonic hearing instead of on direct stimulation of the auditory nerve. The early pioneers had to prove the effect of their auditory implant as being a result of stimulation of the auditory nerve and not electrophonic hearing.

1.2 Pioneers and Experimentation

1.2.1 In France

Andre Djourno and Charles Eyries (1957)

The first direct electrical stimulation of the auditory nerve was performed in the 1950s by the French-Algerian surgeons Andre Djourno (1904–1996) and Charles Eyries (1908–1996). They each had a different interest and background. Whereas Djourno was a scientist who had studied medicine, and had been interested in medical applications of electricity and nerve stimulation for a long time, Eyries was a trained otolaryngologist and was more of a clinician. He had more interest in the facial nerve embryology and function and ways to restore this function.

Before they worked together, Djourno had already produced a device to continuously measure pulse, had used electroencephalogram to study narcolepsy, and had originated the use of electricity for removal of metal pieces from bones. He also invented some sort of artificial respiration by direct stimulation of the phrenic nerve. With these inventions he showed his deep interest in neural stimulation by the use of prostheses. His next project of interest was the making and testing of "implantable induction coils" (which he called "microbobinages"). He made these coils himself to use for "telestimulation," and tested them in rabbits. The induction coil was placed under the skin and the stimulation was delivered transcutaneously. Subsequently, the rabbit jumped after stimulation of the sciatic nerve. He studied several aspects of telestimulation, among which were electrode biocompatibility, the effect of long-term telestimulation of a nerve, and the effect of stimulus frequency. Because with higher frequency the muscle did not contract and with lower frequency the contraction was painful, he determined that the ideal stimulus frequency was around 450 Hz, finally using his own voice as the telestimulus because it was of the appropriate frequency. This finding might have prepared him for the idea of stimulating the auditory nerve to restore hearing.

A 57-year-old male patient, who presented postoperatively with both bilateral loss of hearing and bilateral loss of facial mobility after bilateral resection of large cholesteatomas, brought Djourno and Eyries together. In the quest for a possible nerve graft, Eyries met Djourno at the laboratories of the medical school in Paris and they decided together with the patient on a surgical procedure with the purpose of restoring facial as well as acoustic nerve function.

This procedure was performed on February 25, 1957, by Eyries, during which the induction coil was placed under the temporal muscle and the active electrode was placed in the stump of the auditory nerve, while at the same time the facial nerve graft was applied. The procedure restored facial nerve function by the graft. The reports on the auditory outcome, also partly tested intraoperatively, showed encouraging responses. After extensive rehabilitation with a speech therapist, auditory sensations were present; discrimination between lower and higher frequencies was detected, but there was no speech perception. Unfortunately, after some weeks the implanted electrode broke down, and a subsequently implanted second device also broke down. Eyries held Djourno responsible for the breakdown of the electrodes and refused to perform a third implantation; this marked the end of their working partnership and communication.

Djourno, however, went on and was approached by a colleague who proposed to organize funding and engineering support for further development of the implant in collaboration with industry, in exchange for exclusivity. A true academician, Djourno refused; he was not interested in profiting from his inventions and detested industry. Out of principle he implanted one more patient together with a different, third surgeon. This implantation was not successful and because of lack of funding Djourno finally stopped working in the field of auditory prostheses.

The activities of Djourno and Eyries were followed up in Paris by Claude-Henri Chouard, a student in Eyries's laboratory. He became instrumental in the development of one of the first functional multichannel implants, the Chorimac-12 (now Neurelec/MXM-Oticon). He considered Charles Eyries as his major source of inspiration. Because of the work and implantation of Djourno and Eyries in 1957, that is seen as the year in which the development of auditory implants started.

1.2.2 Early American Years

The discoveries of Djourno and Eyries did not reach the outside world or the United States quickly: they published their findings in a French medical journal and the connections of Djourno, the scientist rather than the surgeon, with American otolaryngologists were not close. Eyries, the clinician, on the other hand did not show much enthusiasm for the project and that only briefly. William House in California serendipitously was given a translated English summary of the French manuscript via a patient around 1959. The manuscript was very positive on the findings and House became inspired.

William F. House (Fig. 1.2)

At that time, House (1923–2012) was a young dentist-turned-otologist who had completed his residency in 1956 and had just started working in Los Angeles at the Otologic Medical Group, with his half-brother Howard House. Although early in his career, he had already made some significant contributions to the field of otology/neuro-otology by developing the facial recess approach and later he also developed the middle fossa approach. Bill's bar at the fundus of the internal auditory canal, a landmark for the identification of the labyrinthine segment of the facial nerve, carries his (nick) name.

When the manuscript from Paris reached him he was working with John Doyle, a neurosurgeon, on the middle fossa approach. They were working on recording the cochlear nerve response to sound, associated with tinnitus. James Doyle, the brother of John Doyle and an electrical engineer, took charge of the electrical recordings during surgery. Having found success recording sound-induced potentials from the cochlear nerve, they planned on stimulating the nerve to restore hearing.

They first experimented with electrical stimulation to restore hearing during stapes surgery, using promontory or opened oval window stimulation. This was successful: these patients reported that they were able to hear the stimuli. This stimulated the researchers to implant a patient with a device.

The first patient who consented to being implanted was a 40-year-old man with severe deafness due to otosclerosis. Promontory stimulation of the right ear showed responses on January 5, 1961, and 4 days later a gold wire electrode was inserted under local anesthesia via retroauricular approach through the round window into the cochlea. The electrode left the ear via the retroauricular skin. The patient heard electrical stimuli but had poor tolerance of loud noise. After several weeks the implant was removed. A second patient, a woman suffering from congenital syphilis, followed during the same month: she also heard the stimulus. Eventually the wire was removed because of fear of infection. Hoping to be able to produce and study discrimination of the higher frequencies, the first patient was implanted again, this time with a five-wire electrode: the results were not very encouraging and this device also needed to be removed because of risk of infection. This problem with the biocompatibility of the materials used presented a major concern for the follow-up of their experimental procedures.

The thought behind implanting a five-wire electrode was to be able to spread the high-frequency stimuli along spatially separated electrodes; subpopulations of nerve fibers would thus be stimulated, summing to a high-frequency response along the

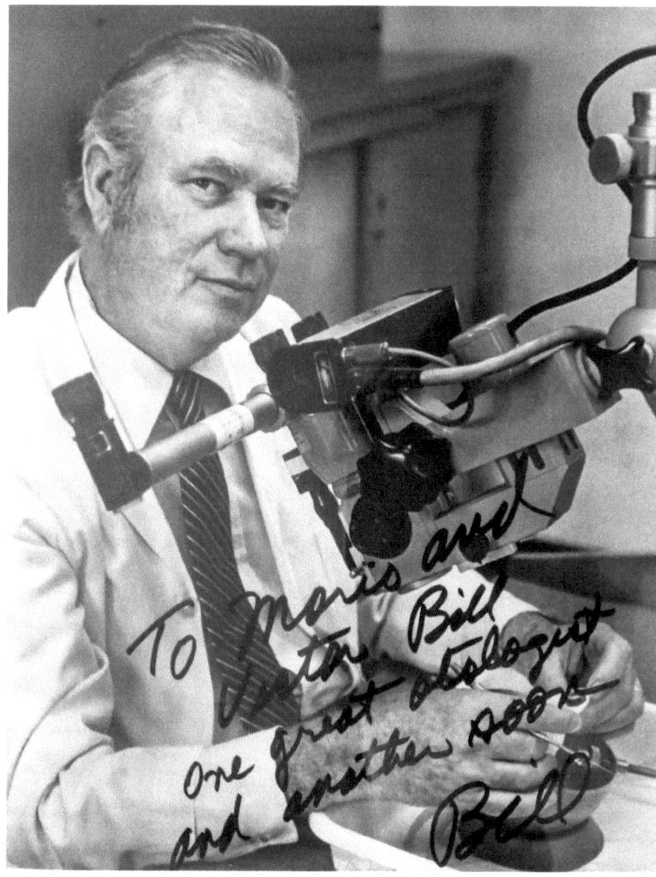

Fig. 1.2 William F. House.

whole nerve. An early patent application for this multielectrode implant was submitted by James Doyle and Earle Ballentyne in 1961. The patent process took time and it was only accepted in 1969. The supporting theory, however, was proven to be wrong because the same signal was applied to all electrodes and thus did not lead to pitch discrimination.

In the meantime the press got hold of the story of these two patients: overenthusiastic articles were printed, leading to deaf patients calling Dr. House and Dr. Doyle for "this cure for their deafness." At the same time, investors became interested in making money from this new medical device. House was worried that these developments were far too optimistic, certainly in the light of the struggles with biocompatibility. Differences in opinion on how to proceed and handle this situation led to a separation between House and the Doyle brothers. The development of the implant became less of a priority to House, who also was running a busy otologic practice, while the Doyle brothers continued with experimenting and implanting, helped by an otologist from Los Angeles, Frederick Turnbull. Although they presented their results optimistically, no systematic analysis was performed. In 1968, James and John Doyle abandoned their research activities due to lack of funding.

F. Blair Simmons at Stanford University

F. Blair Simmons (1930–1998) was the first to stimulate the cochlear nerve in the United States in 1962.

During medical school at Harvard, Simmons worked in the laboratory of S.S. Stevens as a research associate and later also in the Walter Reed Institute before starting his residency in otolaryngology at Stanford University. He became an assistant professor at

Stanford in 1962 and within a month was presented with the chance to stimulate the cochlear nerve during a surgical procedure in an 18-year-old man with a cerebellar ependymoma. This recurrence of tumor presented with a mild hearing loss. An exploratory craniotomy was planned under local anesthesia, giving an opportunity for cochlear nerve stimulation and for receiving feedback from the patient. After the intention was explained, the patient agreed to the intraoperative stimulation and received preoperative training. During the procedure the patient described the bipolar square-wave stimulation directly on the auditory nerve as auditory sensations and was able to discriminate frequencies of stimulation up to 1 kHz. Simmons's first implantation then followed in 1964; the 60-year-old male patient had been deaf on one side and was now losing the hearing in the better-hearing ear, but also suffered from severe loss of sight due to retinitis pigmentosa. He agreed to the procedure wholeheartedly. A six-channel percutaneous device developed by Simmons was implanted via combined retroauricular and transmeatal approach under local anesthesia. A 2-mm cochleostomy and then a 0.1-mm hole in the modiolus gave access to the cochlea and auditory nerve. Testing was performed at Stanford and at Bell Laboratories. The testing was very difficult due to the patient's combination of disabilities, but Simmons proved, by stimulating each electrode separately, that stimulation of the six different parts of the cochlea led to different frequency/pitch perceptions. His implant was a percutaneous device able to stimulate all six electrodes separately, in contrast to the five-wire electrode of House with which all electrodes received the same signal at the same time.

After these experiments and their results, Simmons was pessimistic about the possibility of achieving speech perception and thought that biocompatibility studies first had to be performed before further work on a cochlear implant would be worthwhile.

1.2.3 Later American Years

William House Reengages

Although House had left the field of auditory implant development in frustration and had focused more on clinical practice in the 1960s, with the development of pacemakers and ventriculoperitoneal shunts he sensed that return to the field of cochlear implantation might be possible as the issue of biocompatibility seemed to have been solved. In the 1970s he developed a single-channel device together with engineer Jack Urban. This led in 1972 to the House/3M single-channel device, approved by the U.S. Food and Drug Administration (FDA) in 1984. This was the first implant worldwide to be implanted in a large group of patients.[5]

Robert Michelson

The third implanting surgeon in the field of auditory implants in the United States was Robert Michelson, working in Los Angeles. His preliminary report to the American Academy of Otolaryngology on cochlear implantation using gold wire electrodes in three patients brought a storm of protest; the old-school auditory theories could not explain how electrical stimulation of neural tissue could create cortical auditory perception. The fact that he did not first perform his experiments on animals but operated directly on humans added to the criticism.

Some of his experiments were performed in the Coleman laboratory at the University of California, where he met Francis Sooy.

Implant Team University of California

Around that time in San Francisco, Francis Sooy, the newly appointed head of the ENT department of the university hospital of the University of California–San Francisco (UCSF), was building his own cochlear implant team. His vision was to gather strong individuals of different, multidisciplinary backgrounds and he found and hired Robin Michelson, C. Robert Petit, Mel Bartz (an electrical engineer), and Michael Merzenich (a neurophysiologist) to work together.

In that era there was great skepticism in the audiologic and ENT community and a disbelief in the success of these implants. The lay press had mainly been writing of the miracle, but no analyses were presented for publication in any scientific journals. Robert Petit, a student assistant, joined after meeting Michelson in his laboratory and telling Michelson of his belief in and dream of a multichannel electrode. However, Michelson did not believe that multiple channels were necessary. Nevertheless, they teamed up and worked with a two-channel implant, which was now imbedded in silicone. Merzenich, the neurophysiologist, performed neurophysiologic tests on the cats implanted by Michelson and Petit: one side with normal hearing, the other side with a cochlear implant. Merzenich, at first a skeptic, was convinced that the auditory input from the implant reached the brain of the cat, but it remained difficult to understand what exactly humans heard. Petit searched for new tests; he hired a music professor to create simple tunes with different sound envelopes and different pitches and loudness levels. In carefully controlled and filmed laboratory conditions, one of the newly implanted patients was presented with a song through the implant: it was recorded on film that the patient hummed the melody and tapped the rhythm of the song with a pencil. This movie prompted Francis Sooy to further support the cochlear implant team and was shown at a meeting of otologists in 1972. It finally convinced the professional field that it was indeed possible to stimulate the cochlear nerve and produce auditory cortical perception, although concerns and doubts remained.

1.3 Feasibility, Safety, and Evaluation Studies

1.3.1 The Bilger Report

Francis Sooy was responsible for arranging a meeting in 1974 sponsored by the National Institutes of Health (NIH). It was decided that at this stage cochlear implantation surgery was still experimental, that inclusion criteria needed to be formulated first, and that all further implantation had to cease until a strict and scientific evaluation was performed on hearing outcome and success of the procedure in the patients already implanted.

In 1975, NIH organized this thorough evaluation of the patients that had been implanted thus far in the United States: 13 in total were implanted with single-channel devices by either Robin Michelson (2) or William House (11). The contract to perform this assessment was awarded to a team from the University of Pittsburgh, directed by Robert Bilger. The patients were sent to Pittsburgh for a week for extensive evaluation: psychoacoustic, audiologic, and vestibular tests were performed.

After the study of these 13 patients, three conclusions were drawn: (1) a cochlear implant does give support in lip-reading skills; (2) it improves the quality of life; and (3) (surprisingly) patients also improve in their own speech production after implantation. Overall, the Bilger report concluded that a single-channel device helped deaf people, with minimal risks. This opened finances and funding for research to develop collaboratively a multichannel device. Also, for the time being, the single-channel implant was officially sanctioned.

1.4 Development of a Multichannel Device

1.4.1 United States, Australia, Austria, and France

After the Bilger report and its conclusions, cochlear implant research became more legitimate as did the funding. Questions of the safety and feasibility of electrical stimulation of the auditory nerve in the long term needed to be answered and also the best material for electrical biostimulation needed to be identified. Several groups started working on the development of a multielectrode cochlear implant: among others, the UCSF group led by Francis Sooy, including Merzenich, Michelson, and Robert Schindler, and the Melbourne group led by Graeme Clark. Helped by technological advances in the computer and aerospace industry, they worked on minimizing the receiver device and improving the safety and durability of the electrode array. The physicist Adam Kissiah, working for the NASA/Kennedy Space Center, played an important role: he patented an electronic digital hearing aid in 1977. His design is still used.

Around the same time, work on a multichannel implant was conducted in Vienna, Austria, leading to the implantation of one of the first multichannel devices (3M/Vienna) in December 1977 by Professor Kurt Burian, head of the department of ENT at Vienna University. The implant was developed by Ingeborg and Erwin Hochmair; the later founders of MED-EL in 1989, who before 1988 worked together with the U.S. 3M company, with whom they teamed up during a stay at Stanford University.

In France, Claude-Henri Chouard together with Patrick MacLeod also worked on a multichannel implant. As early as 1976 a French paper was published by Pialoux, Chouard, and MacLeod detailing experiences with a multichannel (8- and 12-channel) device, the Chouard–Bertin device (also called the Chorimac-8 and Chorimac-12).[6] In 1977 a patent was filed for this multichannel device and its electrophysiologic technique. With the help of the French government this group developed its implant system further, which later became known as the Neurelec/MXM (now Neurelec/Oticon) implant system (there is no FDA approval at the time of writing in 2014).

William House, however, continued working on his, now approved, single-channel device and, together with Jack Urban, refined the House 3M single-channel implant, which was the first FDA-approved implant. More than 1,000 were implanted from 1972 to 1985, after which the age criteria of the FDA began to be lowered (see the timeline box in the next column).

The activities in Australia (Melbourne group) and separately in the United States (UCSF) led eventually to the introduction of the Cochlear Nucleus device from Australia and the Advanced Bionics Clarion device from the United States. They were introduced from 1984 onward and overtook the single-channel devices because of better spectral perception and speech recognition abilities as demonstrated in large clinical studies with adults. In 1985 first FDA approval was granted for adults (Cochlear Nucleus), and in 1990 for children from the age of 2 years onward (Cochlear Nucleus).

FDA Approval Timeline

- 1984: single-channel electrode array in adults (House/3M)
- 1985: multichannel electrode array in adults (Cochlear Nucleus 22)
- 1985: first implantation in children (5 and 10 years)
- 1990: multichannel implantation from 2 years onward (Cochlear Nucleus)
- 1996: approval of the Clarion device in adults (Advanced Bionics)
- 1997: approval of the Clarion device in children (Advanced Bionics)
- 1998: multichannel implantation from 18 months onward (Cochlear Nucleus)
- 2000: multichannel implantation from 12 months onward (Cochlear Nucleus)
- 2000: multichannel ABI approval (Cochlear Nucleus)
- 2001: approval of the Combi 40+ Med-el device

Given that with the FDA approvals safety was no longer a major research question, attention was directed to other questions: speech processing was one of these items; earlier implantation in congenitally deaf children was another.

Combined work in universal neonatal hearing screening programs, earlier diagnosis of deafness and a team approach, education and rehabilitation of implantees, and a growing acceptance of the deaf community followed.

1.4.2 Graeme Clark, Melbourne University Australia (1935)

On the other side of the globe, Graeme Clark, an otolaryngologist, grew up with a deaf father who was a pharmacist. From a very young age he witnessed the difficulties his father had with communication and this energized him in his future goals. As a medical student he read the work of Blair Simmons and his discovery of the tonotopy of the cochlea and was impressed. In 1969 he studied single and multichannel devices in experimental animal studies at the University of Sydney and documented in his thesis that single-channel devices had limited utility. He searched for a systemic scientific approach to develop a multichannel device, looking at speech processing strategies, electrode array design, and development of a reliable implantable receiver. His efforts led to one of the first multichannel devices, implanted in 1978, and funded by what was to become Cochlear Company, the University of Melbourne, and the Australian government.

Some of the important findings of Clark and his group were the round window insertion resulting in less trauma, and the use of platinum electrodes for safest long-term stimulation. In 1981 he showed that without use of lip reading some open set speech understanding with the multichannel implant was possible.[7]

1.4.3 Anxiety and Hostility in Deaf Communities

Whereas at the start and during the earlier development of cochlear implants the professionals—who, limited at that time by their concepts and knowledge of the auditory system, did not believe the reports that were being put forward—were the resistant group, later it was the deaf community itself that raised objections. Protests were organized at conferences and meetings concerning cochlear implantation in the late 1980s and early 1990s. The professionals working at that time on cochlear implants found very strong and active opposition. In particular the decision to implant congenitally deafen children at a very young age without their own consent, implying the concept of disability, was offensive. The term "cultural genocide" was even used to express the threatened feelings within the deaf community, which mainly consisted of prelingually deafened people using sign language. Critics from the deaf culture argued that the cochlear implantation and the rehabilitation focusing on mastery of hearing and speech production would lead to a poor self-image by the child as a "disabled" person rather than a proud deaf person using sign language. In New York and the United Kingdom these revolts turned into battles.

Nowadays cochlear implants are more mainstream and many congenitally deaf, early-implanted children attend mainstream education instead of deaf schools or schools for the hearing deprived.

1.5 Development of the Auditory Brainstem Implant

1.5.1 Auditory Brainstem Implant

Although during the pioneering years several surgeons had already stimulated the cochlear nerve directly at the modiolus or at the cerebellopontine angle, or stimulated the inferior colliculus,[8] the development of the auditory brainstem implant (ABI) started in 1979. In that year, a female patient with neurofibromatosis type 2 (NF2) asked for placement of a single-channel electrode on her brain in a quest for hearing restoration. Although the outcome was thought to be very doubtful, her perseverance led to the first auditory brainstem implantation in 1979 by William House and the neurosurgeon William Hitselberger at the House Ear Institute.[9,10] A single ball-type electrode was placed within the cochlear nucleus complex and led to hearing sensations. However, probably due to a shift of the electrode, these effects were lost and a new design of electrode, better situated to the anatomy, was developed, resulting in a Dacron mesh/platinum ribbon two-electrode array (in collaboration with the Huntington Medical Research Institute). Around 25 patients were implanted with this system and their outcomes proved to be comparable to the results of the single-channel cochlear implant (sound awareness and support of lip-reading skills). When the number of electrodes in the ABI was increased to three it became clear that the auditory outcome and especially pitch might vary according to electrode location, showing tonotopy to be present in the cochlear nucleus also. The first multichannel brainstem implant used was presented in 1991[11] and was slightly modified in 1993.[12] This led to better speech perception performance and sound quality. Clinical multicenter trials started in 1994 with a multichannel brainstem implant (Nucleus Multichannel ABI, Cochlear). The implant was approved by the FDA as an investigational device in June 1994, but this device was eventually a hearing solution for NF2 patients. Whereas the ABI used in the United States started out with 2, 3, and later 8 electrodes, the current unified ABI of Cochlear is the former European ABI with 21 electrodes developed in 1991–1993.

Nowadays, around 1,000 ABIs have been placed, with around 100 in congenitally deaf children. As well as NF2 patients, non-NF2 patients with congenital cochlear malformations, cochlear nerve aplasia, cochlear aperture stenosis, and extensive cochlear ossification have also been implanted with an ABI. Final FDA approval was granted in 2000 for adults (18 years and older) and NF2 only, but is now granted for NF2 patients of 12 years or older with "reasonable expectations." In Europe and Asia at least 144 ABIs have been implanted in children and adults for other indications besides NF2.[13]

A remaining problem with the current ABI is the fact that the surface electrodes do not reach the cochlear nucleus and its tonotopy as well as does the cochlear implant. The higher frequencies, located below the surface of the nucleus, in particular are difficult to reach. To address this, a Penetrating ABI (PABI) was designed (House Ear Institute, Cochlear, and Huntington Institute; 2008), with a 10-microelectrode array to penetrate 1–2 mm into the cochlear nucleus (which is 2 × 8 mm) in addition to the 12 surface electrodes on a separate array. Although thresholds were lower, activation of higher pitches, and more selective stimulation were attained, the overall speech understanding was not significantly better than with a normal ABI.[14]

Additionally, for patients with damage of the cochlear nucleus or brainstem (mostly due to NF2) the auditory midbrain implant (AMI; 2015) or inferior colliculus implant (ICI) was designed. Around six patients have been implanted and showed disappointing results, although sound awareness and limited support of lip-reading skills are found to be comparable to the early ABI results in NF2 patients.[15,16]

1.5.2 Summary of Discoveries and Developments

The development of auditory implants has truly been a multidisciplinary, international endeavor. Alongside the development of the auditory implant, knowledge of the function and physiology of the cochlea and the auditory pathway grew; greater knowledge of the process of speech perception went hand in hand with advances in material and electrical technology. A summary of the most significant discoveries and most important professionals is presented in the timeline in **Fig. 1.3**.

1.5.3 New Developments and Future

Developments in auditory implants have not come to a standstill. Since hearing preservation and electroacoustical stimulation are already becoming mainstream, the next horizons will be the total implantable cochlear implant (TICI), enlargement of the experience with ABI in non-NF2 patients, regulation of the vast number of patients all needing regular service, improvement of the per-

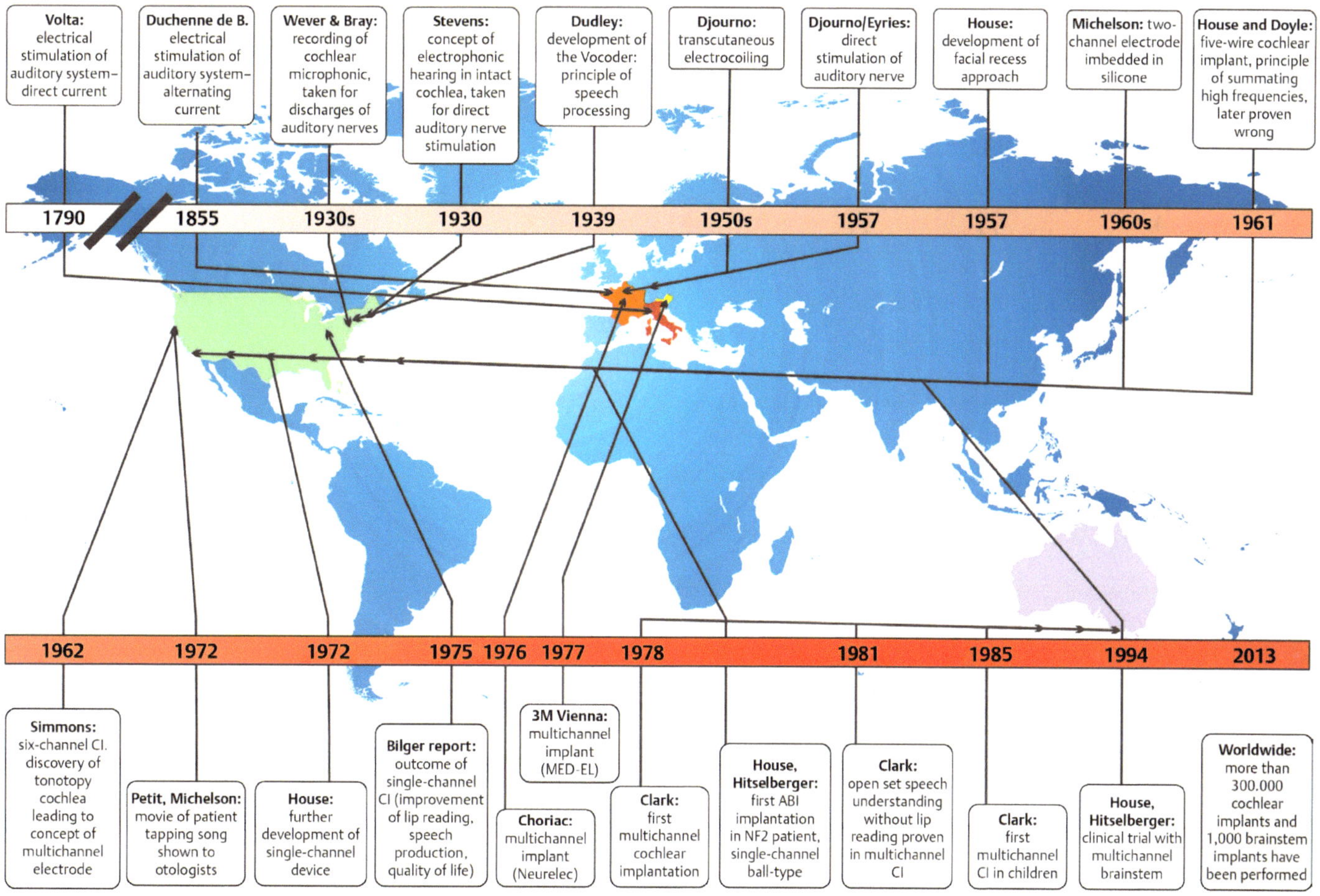

Fig. 1.3 Developments in auditory implantation on a timeline and world map.

ception of music with cochlear implants, and widening the availability of hearing rehabilitation in the developing countries as well.

Today more than 300,000 cochlear implants have been inserted, around 1,000 auditory brainstem implants have been surgically placed, and in the Western world bilateral implantation in children is becoming standard practice because better incidental learning conditions at school and better environmental hearing are proven benefits. The development in the field of auditory implantation over the past 50 years has truly been remarkable and has led to a profound change in the daily life, working conditions, and quality of life of the deaf or hearing-deprived patient.

References

1. Eisen MD. The history of cochlear implants. In: Niparko JK, ed. Cochlear Implants: Principles & Practices. 2nd ed. Philadelphia: Lippincott Williams & Wilkins, Wolters Kluwer; 2009
2. Dudley H. The automatic synthesis of speech. Proc Natl Acad Sci U S A 1939;25(7):377–383
3. Wever EG, Bray CW. Action currents in the auditory nerve in response to acoustical stimulation. Proc Natl Acad Sci U S A 1930;16(5):344–350
4. Hallpike CS, Rawdon-Smith AF. The origin of the Wever and Bray phenomenon. J Physiol 1934;83(2):243–254
5. House WF. Cochlear implants. Ann Otol Rhinol Laryngol 1976; 85(3Pt2, suppl 27):1–93
6. Pialoux P, Chouard CH, MacLeod P. Physiological and clinical aspects of the rehabilitation of total deafness by implantation of multiple intracochlear electrodes. Acta Otolaryngol 1976;81(5-6):436–441
7. Clark GM, Tong YC, Martin LFA, Busby PA. A multiple-channel cochlear implant. An evaluation using an open-set word test. Acta Otolaryngol 1981;91(3-4):173–175
8. Simmons FB, Mongeon CJ, Lewis WR, Huntington DA. Electrical stimulation of acoustical nerve and inferior colliculus (results in man). Arch Otolaryngol 1964;79:559–568
9. Edgerton BJ, House WF, Hitselberger W. Hearing by cochlear nucleus stimulation in humans. Ann Otol Rhinol Laryngol Suppl 1982;91(2 Pt 3):117–124
10. Hitselberger WE, House WF, Edgerton BJ, Whitaker S. Cochlear nucleus implants. Otolaryngol Head Neck Surg 1984;92(1):52–54
11. Laszig R, Kuzma J, Seifert V, Lehnhardt E. The Hannover auditory brainstem implant: a multiple-electrode prosthesis. Eur Arch Otorhinolaryngol 1991;248(7):420–421
12. Laszig R, Sollmann WP, Marangos N. The restoration of hearing in neurofibromatosis type 2. J Laryngol Otol 1995;109(5):385–389
13. Merkus P, Di Lella F, Di Trapani G, et al. Indications and contraindications of auditory brainstem implants: systematic review and illustrative cases. Eur Arch Otorhinolaryngol 2014;271(1):3–13. doi: 10.1007/s00405-013-2378-3. Epub 2013
14. Otto SR, Shannon RV, Wilkinson EP, et al. Audiologic outcomes with the penetrating electrode auditory brainstem implant. Otol Neurotol 2008;29(8):1147–1154
15. Lenarz T, Lim HH, Reuter G, Patrick JF, Lenarz M. The auditory midbrain implant: a new auditory prosthesis for neural deafness—concept and device description. Otol Neurotol 2006;27(6):838–843
16. Lim HH, Lenarz T. Auditory midbrain implant: Research and development towards a second clinical trial. Hear Res. 2015. doi: 10.1016/j.heares.2015.01.006. [Epub ahead of print]

Further Reading

Berliner KI. The controversial beginnings of neurotology: William F. House's struggles as a medical innovator. Otol Neurotol 2011;32(9):1399–1406

Blume SS. Histories of cochlear implantation. Soc Sci Med 1999;49(9):1257–1268

Clark G. Cochlear Implants: Fundamentals & Applications. New York: Springer-Verlag; 2003

Colletti L, Shannon R, Colletti V. Auditory brainstem implants for neurofibromatosis type 2. Curr Opin Otolaryngol Head Neck Surg 2012;20(5):353–3570

Djourno A, Eyries C, Vallancien P. [Preliminary attempts of electrical excitation of the auditory nerve in man, by permanently inserted micro-apparatus]. Bull Acad Natl Med 1957;141(21-23):481–483

Eisen MD. History of Cochlear Implants. In: Waltzman SB, Roland JT, eds. Cochlear Implants. 2nd ed. Stuttgart: Thieme; 2006

House WF, Urban J. Long term results of electrode implantation and electronic stimulation of the cochlea in man. Ann Otol Rhinol Laryngol 1973;82(4):504–517

Michel J, Verain A. [Sound sensations produced by electric stimulation of the structures of the middle ear and the tympanic chord]. Ann Otolaryngol Chir Cervicofac 1975;92(1-2):33–60

Möller AR. History of cochlear implants and auditory brainstem implants. In: Möller AR, ed. Cochlear and Brainstem Implants. Basel: Karger; 2006:1–10

Möller AR. Physiological basis for cochlear and auditory brainstem implants. In: Möller AR, ed. Cochlear and Brainstem Implants. Basel: Karger; 2006:206–223

Otto SR, Brackmann DE, Hitselberger WE, Shannon RV, Kuchta J. Multichannel auditory brainstem implant: update on performance in 61 patients. J Neurosurg 2002;96(6):1063–1071

Rubinstein JT. How cochlear implants encode speech. Curr Opin Otolaryngol Head Neck Surg 2004;12(5):444–448

Shannon RV. Advances in auditory prostheses. Curr Opin Neurol 2012;25(1):61–66

Wilson BS, Dorman MF. Cochlear implants: a remarkable past and a brilliant future. Hear Res 2008;242(1-2):3–21

Wilson BS, Lawson DT, Müller JM, Tyler RS, Kiefer J. Cochlear implants: some likely next steps. Annu Rev Biomed Eng 2003;5:207–249

2 Surgical Anatomy in Auditory Implantation

Auditory implantation requires good knowledge of the anatomical structures that may be encountered during middle ear implant surgery, cochlear implant (CI) surgery, or auditory brainstem implant (ABI) surgery. Because the 3D anatomy of the middle ear, temporal bone, cochlea, cerebellopontine angle, and the brainstem is complicated, it is difficult to learn the anatomical composition only from a book. Intensive work in a temporal bone dissection laboratory and study of temporal bone instructional DVDs are mandatory to gain better insight into these anatomical relations. The dissections shown in this chapter have been performed especially to give appreciation of the anatomical relationship of the structures needed in auditory implantation.

2.1 Anatomy of the Middle Ear and Mastoid

2.1.1 The Mastoid (Fig. 2.1)

The usually well-aerated cells of mastoid and antrum are a perfect route for access to the middle ear and epitympanum. The landmarks for opening up the mastoid cavity are, posteriorly, the sigmoid sinus and, posterior fossa dura; superiorly, the middle cranial fossa dura; and, anteriorly, the posterior wall of the external ear canal. For easiest access to the facial recess, the posterior wall of the external ear canal needs to be thinned well. The digastric ridge is the most caudal landmark in the mastoid cavity, defining the facial nerve leaving the mastoid via the stylomastoid foramen, situated just anterior-medially to this ridge.

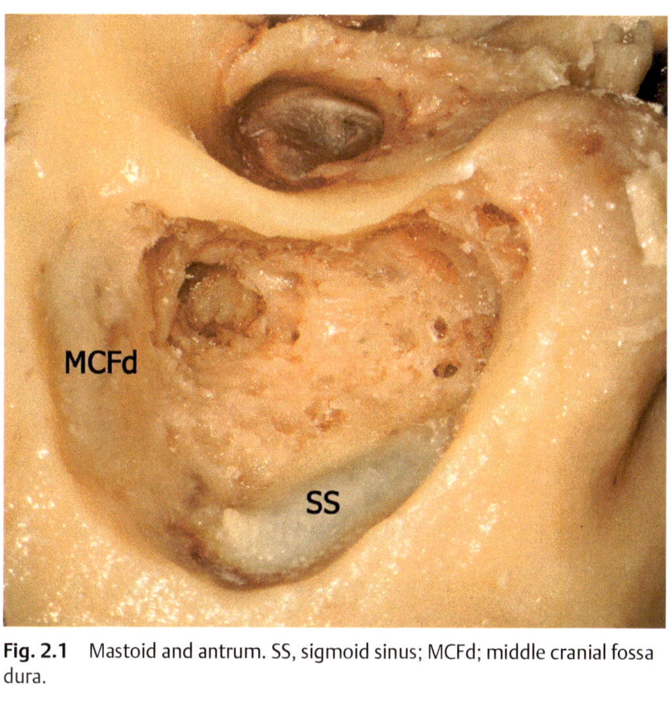

Fig. 2.1 Mastoid and antrum. SS, sigmoid sinus; MCFd; middle cranial fossa dura.

In case of a well-aerated cavity without pathology, a limited mastoidectomy with proper access will suffice for cochlear implantation. In case of pathology in the mastoid, all pathology needs to be removed meticulously.

2.1.2 The Antrum (Fig. 2.1)

The antrum is the largest mastoidal cell and connects the mastoid air cells with the tympanic cavity via the aditus ad antrum ("the entrance of the antrum"). It is located just posteriorly to the epitympanum, inferiorly to the middle fossa plate, and posterior-lateral to the labyrinth. Since the antrum is very consistent and there is no important structure lateral to it, it serves as one of the most important landmarks in the initial stage of mastoidectomy. On the medial wall of the antrum is found the prominence of the lateral semicircular canal: one of the most important landmarks for identification of the facial nerve and the incus. The prominence of the lateral canal, together with the digastric ridge, defines the vertical segment of the facial nerve. Both structures can be used to identify the facial nerve before starting to drill the posterior tympanotomy.

2.1.3 The Tympanic Cavity

The mesotympanum is the middle portion of the tympanic cavity located just medial to the tympanic membrane (**Fig. 2.2**). It is bordered superiorly by the epitympanum (attic), which hosts the corpora of malleus and incus, and inferiorly by the hypotympanum, which starts inferior-laterally from the inferior border of the round window. The mesotympanum and epitympanum are separated by the tympanic segment of the facial nerve. The protympanum, located in the anterior part of the tympanic cavity, harbors the tympanic orifice of the eustachian tube, just inferior to the semicanal of the tensor tympani muscle and lateral to the genu of the carotid artery. The anterior epitympanum can be found anterior from James's cog, a bony eminence at the roof of the epitympanum. The cog is sometimes also regarded as a landmark for the facial nerve; it points at the facial nerve.

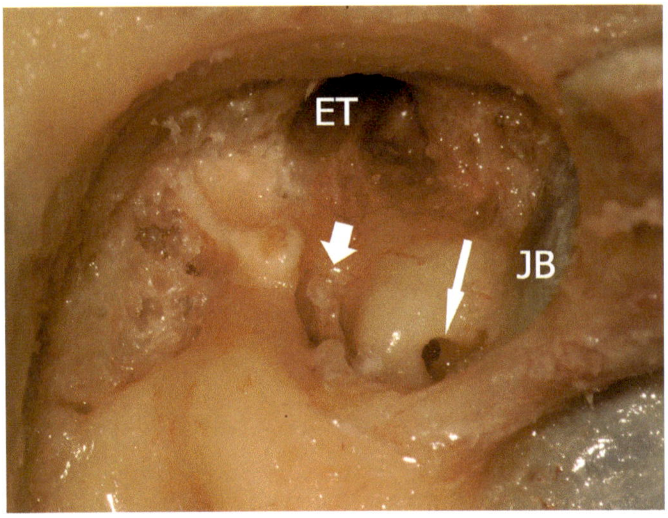

Fig. 2.2 An overview of the middle ear cavity after removal of the posterior canal wall. The oval window niche (*short arrow*) and round window niche (*long arrow*), access to the eustachian tube (ET), and relation to the jugular bulb (JB) are clearly visible.

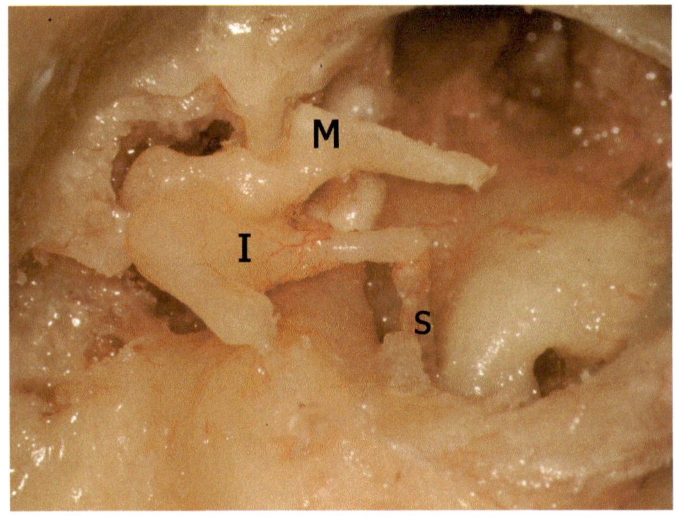

Fig. 2.3 The ossicles in a canal wall down cavity. M, malleus; I, incus; S, stapes.

2.1.4 The Ossicles

The Malleus

The malleus is the most lateral of the ossicles and is only a minor landmark in auditory implantation (**Fig. 2.3**). The tendon of the tensor tympani muscle is attached to the neck of the malleus and originates from the cochleariform process, which is an important landmark in the middle ear for identification of the horizontal part of the facial nerve. The tensor tympani muscle is located in the semicanal anterior to the cochleariform process, on the medial wall of the anterior epitympanum.

The Incus

The short process of the incus projects posteriorly and is lodged in the fossa incudis located just anterior-laterally to the eminence of the lateral semicircular canal. This is an important landmark for drilling the posterior tympanotomy at the facial recess. The long process projects into the tympanic cavity, and forms an articulation with the stapes at its lenticular process (**Fig. 2.3**). The incus is also supported by the malleus anteriorly at the malleoincudal articulation and by the posterior incudal ligament posteriorly.

The Stapes and Stapedius Muscle

The smallest bone in the human body is located in the oval window. It has two crura, the anterior crus and posterior crus, on top of the stapes footplate. The footplate is accommodated in the oval window. The connective tissue lying between the footplate and the edge of the oval window is called the annular ligament. The stapedius muscle inserts onto the head and the posterior crus of the stapes and originates from the eminentia pyramidalis on the posterior mesotympanic wall, where this muscle is hidden in the bone, anterior-medial to the facial nerve. Its length can vary. To improve the access to the round window during the drilling of the posterior tympanotomy, this muscle must sometimes be skeletonized or even be uncovered.

A contraction of the stapedius muscle tilts the stapes and its footplate, and the resulting tension in the annular ligament limits sound transmission into the inner ear, to some extent protecting the inner ear from noise trauma. This contraction is seen when the cochlea and cochlear nerve endings are stimulated at a signal that mimics 80–100 dB. This is the physiologic function of the stapedius reflex; moreover, the stapedius reflex can also be used to test the correct position of the electrode in the cochlea during CI surgery: the electrical stapedius reflex (see Chapter 4).

2.1.5 The Oval Window

The oval window is located at the bottom of a deep depression surrounded by eminences: the promontory inferiorly, the fallopian canal superiorly with the tympanic segment of the facial nerve, the cochleariform process anterior-superiorly, and the pyramidal eminence (eminentia pyramidalis) with stapedius tendon posteriorly (**Fig. 2.4**). The tympanic segment of the facial nerve runs just superior to the oval window and near the posterior edge of it, the nerve turns inferiorly toward its vertical segment. The oval window and the stapes (if still present) are landmarks for the round window. The stapes and oval window can be seen through the facial recess, whereas the round window is not always as easily visible. The round window is more medial and

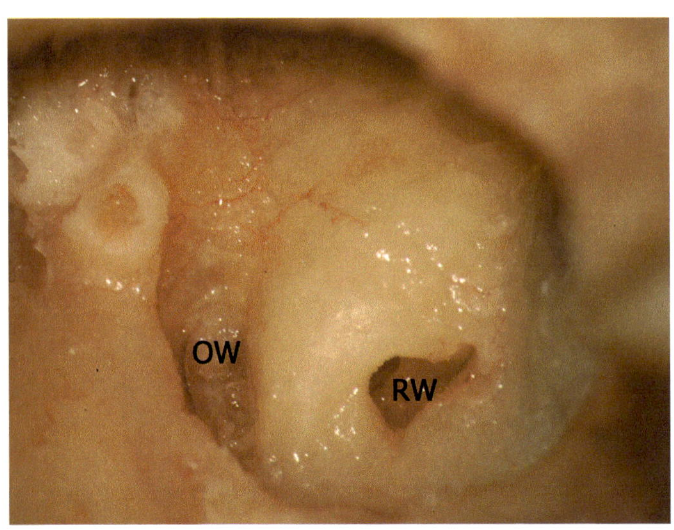

Fig. 2.4 The oval (OW) and round window (RW) niches in close up.

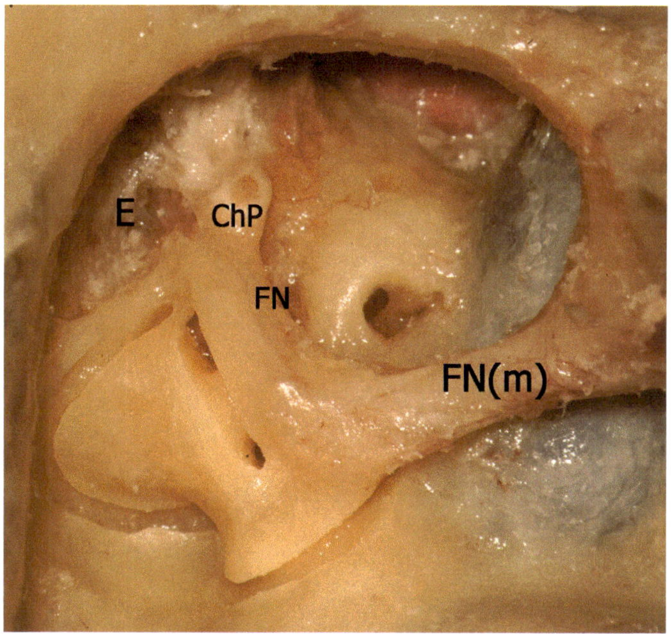

Fig. 2.5 The course of the facial nerve through the middle ear, separating the epitympanum (E) from the mesotympanum. ChP, cochleariform process; FN, tympanic portion of the facial nerve; FN(m), mastoid portion of the facial nerve.

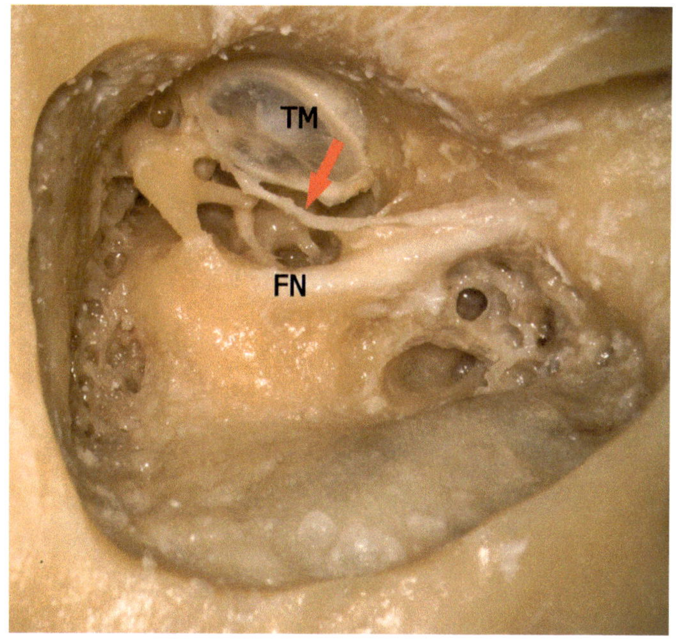

Fig. 2.6 Anatomical relations of the posterior tympanotomy. Posterior as well as inferior tympanotomy have been created in this specimen. Note the close relation between annulus of the tympanic membrane and chorda tympani (*arrow*). TM, tympanic membrane; FN, facial nerve.

caudal to the oval window and mostly perpendicular in orientation. Especially in ossification of the round window, the oval window, stapes, and promontory become the most important landmarks to perform a drill-out procedure of the basal turn of the cochlea (see Chapter 11).

2.1.6 The Facial Nerve

The tympanic segment of the facial nerve courses obliquely in the medial wall of the tympanic cavity separating the epitympanum from the mesotympanum (**Fig. 2.5**). The tympanic segment of the facial nerve starts at the first genu at the geniculate ganglion just superior to the cochleariform process and the tensor tympani tendon and then runs superior-laterally to the oval window. Around the posterior edge of the oval window, the nerve follows a gentle curve, the second genu, coursing inferior-laterally, changing its location from the medial wall of the tympanic cavity to the posterior wall of the mesotympanum. At this curved section, the nerve is positioned inferior-medially to the lateral semicircular canal, and courses almost parallel to it. The short process of the incus lies laterally to the nerve and to the lateral semicircular canal. This position should be kept in mind at the start of the posterior tympanotomy. Note that the vertical segment of the facial nerve, immediately after the second genu of the facial nerve, can vary in anatomy, not only in malformations or syndromic patients. A more aberrant position of the nerve located inferiorly to the oval window or divided into branches can also be found. Coronal CT images can provide valuable preoperative information on the individual anatomy and course of the facial nerve (see Chapter 3).

Landmarks for Identification of the Facial Nerve

- Cochleariform process
- Incus
- Lateral semicircular canal
- Posterior semicircular canal
- Digastric ridge

2.1.7 The Chorda Tympani (Fig. 2.6)

The chorda tympani, a branch of the facial nerve, courses lateral to the long process of the incus and medially to the manubrium of the malleus after emerging from the posterior wall of the middle ear at the posterior spine. This nerve contains sensory fibers for taste and secretory fibers innervating the submandibular and sublingual glands. The chorda tympani can branch off the mastoid segment of the facial nerve at a variable level, either just above the stylomastoid foramen or at a more superior or even more inferior level.

The size of the posterior tympanotomy (a surgical entity) is defined by the angle between the chorda tympani and facial nerve as explained later in the text.

2.1.8 The Cochleariform Process and Tensor Tympani Muscle (Fig. 2.7 and Fig. 2.8)

The tensor tympani muscle lies in its semicanal, which runs superior and parallel to the eustachian tube toward the cochleariform process. At this bony process, the tendon of the tensor tympani muscle makes a right angle and directs laterally to attach to the neck of the malleus. The cochleariform process is the posterior end of the semicanal of the tensor tympani muscle. It is located

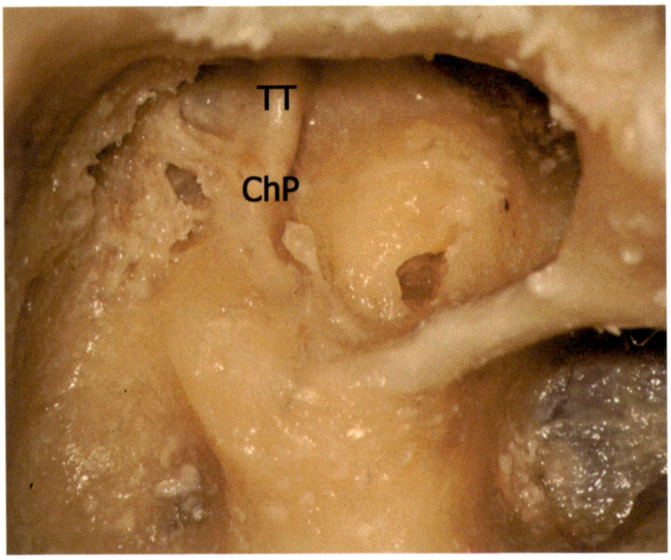

Fig. 2.7 The cochleariform process (ChP) and the semicanal of the tensor tympani muscle (TT).

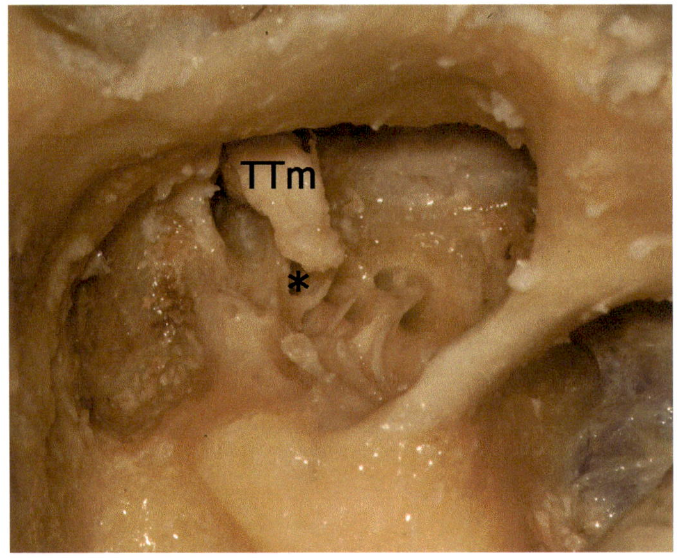

Fig. 2.8 The tensor tympani muscle (TTm) freed from its semicanal. The muscle can now be deflected and used to close off the eustachian tube. Note also the apical turn (*) in relation to the cochleariform process.

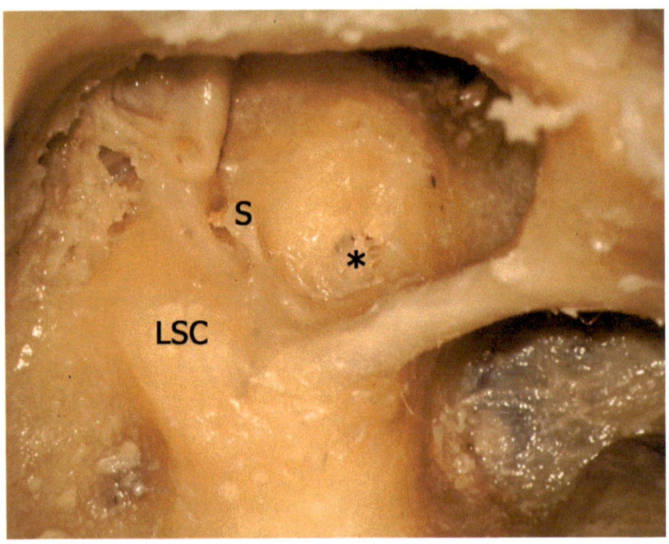

Fig. 2.9 A pseudomembrane (*) covers the round window niche. LSC, lateral semicircular canal; S, stapes.

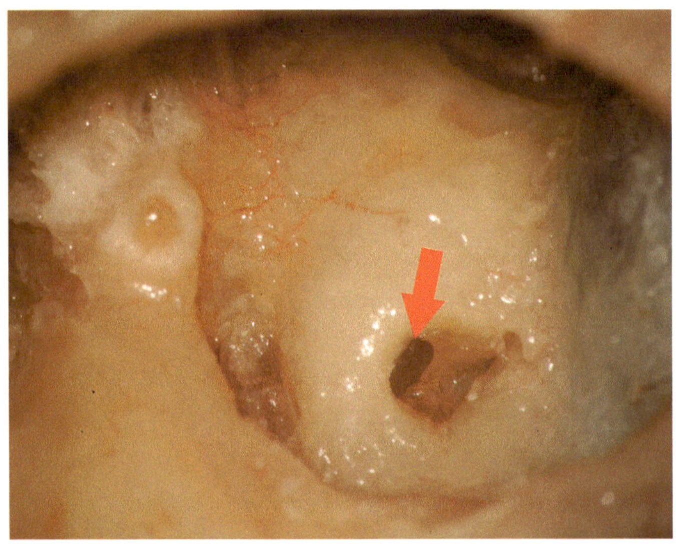

Fig. 2.10 After removal of the pseudomembrane, the true round window membrane becomes visible. Note the dark gray color of the membrane (*arrow*).

just anterior-superior to the oval window, and just inferior-lateral to the tympanic segment and first genu of the facial nerve. It remains an important landmark in the temporal bone, especially when the ossicles are not present, because it defines the position of the tympanic portion of the facial nerve. When performing a surgical drill-out in an ossified cochlea, the cochleariform process is the main landmark to find the apical turn of the cochlea, which is located directly medially. Also James's cog can be used as a landmark when the cochleariform process is eroded: this is a bony process attached to the roof of the epitympanum and is positioned in the same plane as the cochleariform process.[1–3]

2.1.9 The Round Window (Fig. 2.9 and Fig. 2.10)

The round window is located in the round window niche, inferiorly to the oval window. The round window is covered superiorly by a bony overhang, especially superior-posteriorly, creating the round window niche. It lies in a mostly horizontal plane, slightly tilted anteriorly. A bony projection ("lip") can also be found at the anterior-inferior margin of the round window niche. Both overhangs make it usually difficult to see the round window membrane directly and more extensive exposure to appreciate the complete round window is regularly needed.[4] A pseudomembrane consisting of a mucosal layer closing off the round window niche is frequently present, recognizable by a whitish color (**Fig. 2.9**) instead of the normal dark gray color of the true membrane (**Fig. 2.10**). The round window is situated in the inferior-posterior wall of the basal turn, parallel to the direction of the basal turn, more or less like a "side entrance" (**Fig. 2.16**).

To appreciate the angle of the round window, one has to imagine that a 0° view would be a perfect perpendicular view at the round window, equivalent to the inferior and superior border of the window both at equal distances from the vertical segment of the facial nerve.[5] The round window angle (in adults) is tilted, with the inferior border ~48° (±9°) turned more anterior.[5] The size of the round window is ~1.35 mm^2, but varies from 0.8 to 1.75 mm^2.[4,6]

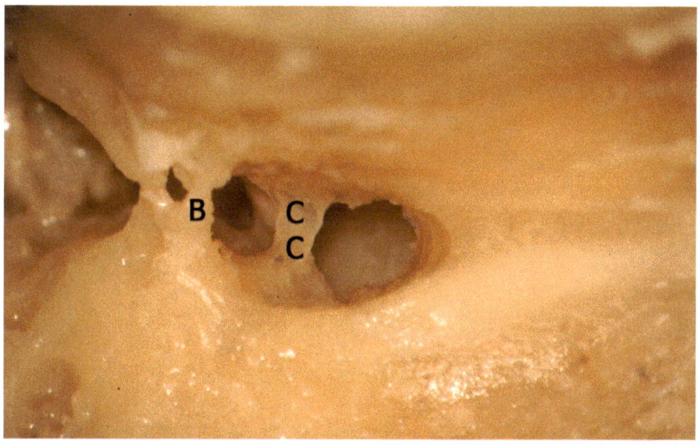

Fig. 2.11 The chordal crest (CC). The buttress (B) can also be appreciated.

Relations of the Round Window

A few important relations need to be kept in mind when drilling at the round window edges:

- To view the complete round window, the overhang superiorly and the inferior bony projection should be removed.
- The superior border of the round window is closest to the basilar membrane and osseous spiral lamina.[7,8]
- The opening of the cochlear aqueduct may lie within 0.5 mm of the edge of the round window membrane; where the cochlear aqueduct ends inferiorly in the scala tympani.[4]
- The intracochlear inferior border of the round window, often called the crista fenestrae, is not closely related to the spiral ligament, the basilar membrane, or the osseous spiral lamina, while the anterior and anterior-inferior border are.[8,9]

2.1.10 The Facial Recess and the Posterior Tympanotomy (Fig. 2.11 and Fig. 2.12)

The posterior mesotympanum contains deep recesses. The facial nerve running in the middle divides them into the tympanic sinus medially and the facial recess laterally. The facial recess is bordered by the bony tympanic annulus laterally and the vertical segment of the facial canal medially. It is subdivided into two segments by a bony bridge called the chordal crest that connects the pyramidal eminence and the emergence of the chorda tympani called the chordal eminence (**Fig. 2.11**). During surgery one could encounter this crest as a last lateral-medially oriented layer within the posterior tympanotomy before entering the tympanic cavity. The inferior extension of the facial recess is to the hypotympanum and is not related to the position where the chorda tympani branches off the facial nerve.

By performing a posterior tympanotomy, the facial recess is opened, giving access from mastoid cavity to the tympanic cavity. Care must be taken not to damage the tympanic annulus in this procedure, which lies just few millimeters lateral from the chorda tympani (**Fig. 2.6** and **Fig. 2.12**). An inferior tympanotomy reaches the hypotympanum, opening up the facial recess usually inferior from the chorda tympani.

The borders of the posterior tympanotomy are:

- Superior: short process of the incus
- Posterior-medial: vertical section of the facial nerve
- Inferior: chorda tympani–facial nerve angle
- Anterior-lateral: chorda tympani

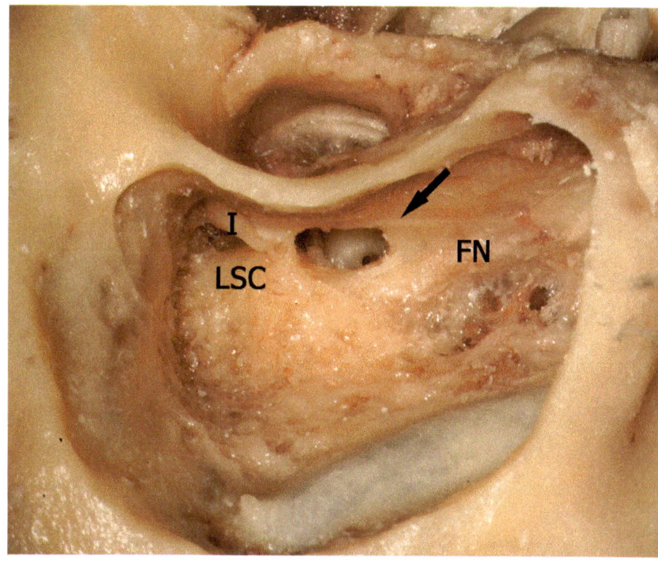

Fig. 2.12 The posterior tympanotomy, giving access to the round window niche. FN, facial nerve; I, incus; LSC, lateral semicircular canal; *arrow*, chorda tympani.

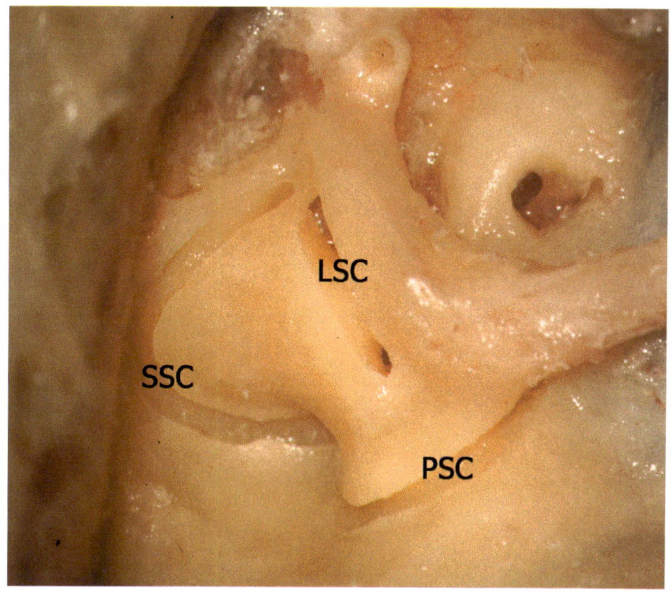

Fig. 2.13 The semicircular canals have been opened in this specimen. LSC, lateral semicircular canal; PSC, posterior semicircular canal; SSC, superior semicircular canal.

Proceeding, the chorda tympani is found running from inferior-posteriorly toward superior-anteriorly, creating an angulation, a V-shape, with the facial nerve. After removal of the chordal crest generally the tympanic cavity can be seen and the stapes and the promontory can be visualized. The angle between the facial nerve and the round window is very variable.[10] To create a clear view of the round window and to obtain the best angle of electrode insertion during cochlear implantation, the facial nerve usually has to be skeletonized.[11]

2.1.11 The Labyrinth

Semicircular Canals (Fig. 2.13)

The prominence of the lateral semicircular canal in the medial wall of the antrum slopes ~30° from a true horizontal line/surgical view, running from anterior-superiorly to posterior-inferiorly. At the anterior end of the lateral semicircular canal it widens to form the lateral ampulla that accommodates sensory cells and opens to the utricle. It is located in the medial wall of the posterior attic.

The other two semicircular canals are located nearly perpendicularly to the lateral semicircular canal. The posterior semicircular canal lies just posterior to the lateral semicircular canal, and the posterior edge of the lateral semicircular canal points almost to the center of the posterior semicircular canal (Donaldson's line, an imaginary line bisecting the lateral semicircular canal, will separate the posterior semicircular canal into equal superior and inferior parts). The posterior semicircular canal is located nearly parallel to the posterior fossa dura. Its ampulla is located at its inferior end, just medial to the mastoid segment of the facial nerve. The superior end of the posterior semicircular canal joins the superior semicircular canal, forming the common crus.

The superior semicircular canal is located just beneath the middle cranial fossa plate. Its ampulla is at the anterior end, just superior-medial to the ampulla of the lateral semicircular canal. The subarcuate artery can be found centrally in the plain of the superior semicircular canal and is a branch of the internal auditory artery, supplying the labyrinth.

The Vestibule (Fig. 2.14)

The vestibule is the hollow space within the petrous bone medial to the second genu of the facial nerve, containing the utricle and saccule. It lies anterior-medially to the semicircular canals, medial to the oval window, lateral to the fundus of the internal auditory canal, and posterior to the cochlea. Its posterior-lateral surface receives five openings from the semicircular canals. There is no connection between the vestibule and the scala tympani, while the vestibule is anteriorly in continuation with the scala vestibuli.

The Cochlea and Promontory (Fig. 2.15)

The promontory is the prominent eminence located anterior-inferiorly to the oval window, and anteriorly to the round window. It corresponds to the basal turn of the cochlea. The Jacobson nerve, a branch of the glossopharyngeal nerve (CN IX), can be found crossing the promontory.

The cochlea is located on the medial surface of the middle ear and can be found by the promontory, the oval window niche, and the round window niche as the most important landmarks. The cochlea is situated tilted forward and superiorly with its apex (**Fig. 2.16** and **Fig. 2.17**). The 2.5 turns of the cochlea curve around a central cone of bone, the modiolus, arising from the fundus of the internal auditory canal and containing the fibers of the cochlear nerve and the spiral ganglion cells. From the modiolus, a shelflike bony projection, the osseous spiral lamina extends halfway into the cavity of the cochlear turns. The basilar membrane and subsequently the membranous spiral ligament connect the edge of the osseous spiral lamina to the lateral surface of the cochlear turns, dividing into the scala vestibuli and the scala tympani. The membranous structure, in the middle between the two scalae, is called the scala media and is located laterally to the osseous spiral lamina. This is the scala where the organ of Corti is located. In addition, the round window corresponds to the scala tympani, and the oval window corresponds to the scala vestibuli (**Fig. 2.18**).

The cochlea is anteriorly in close proximity to the carotid artery, so performing a cochlear drill-out procedure of the basal turn could lead to damage of the carotid artery. The middle turn of the cochlea can be found 3 to 4 mm anteriorly from the stapes footplate, while the apical turn is situated medial to the cochleariform process. Removal of the tensor tympani muscle gives better access to the apical turn (**Fig. 2.8**). The intracochlear anatomy is visible in **Fig. 2.16** and subsequent figures.

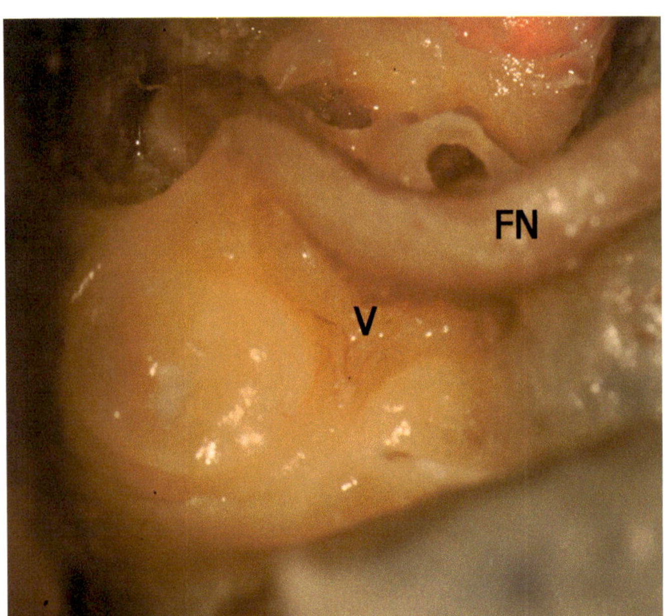

Fig. 2.14 In addition to the semicircular canals, now the vestibule (V) is also opened. FN, facial nerve.

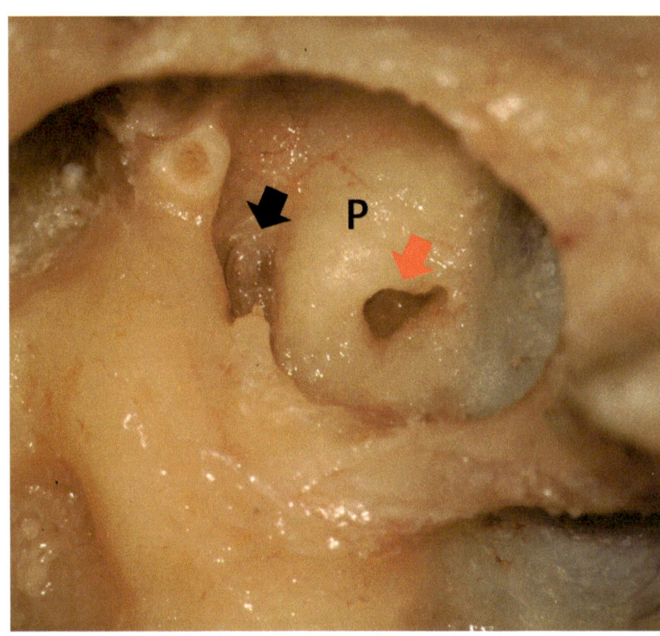

Fig. 2.15 The promontory (P) is located anterior-inferiorly to the oval window (*black arrow*) and anteriorly to the round window (*red arrow*).

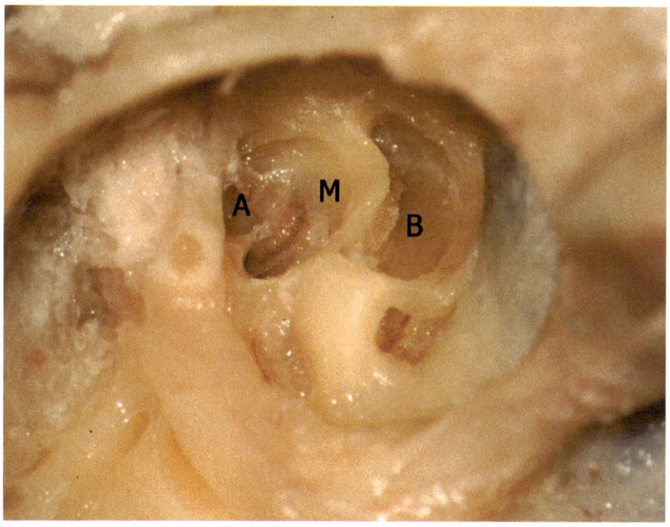

Fig. 2.16 The basal (B), middle (M), and apical (A) turns are drilled open in this specimen.

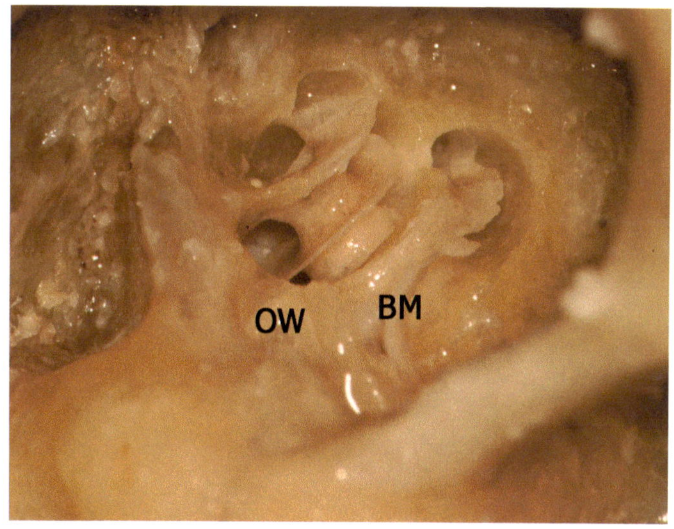

Fig. 2.17 Note the position of the basilar membrane (BM) in the basal turn. Also note the close relationship between the oval window (OW) and middle turn.

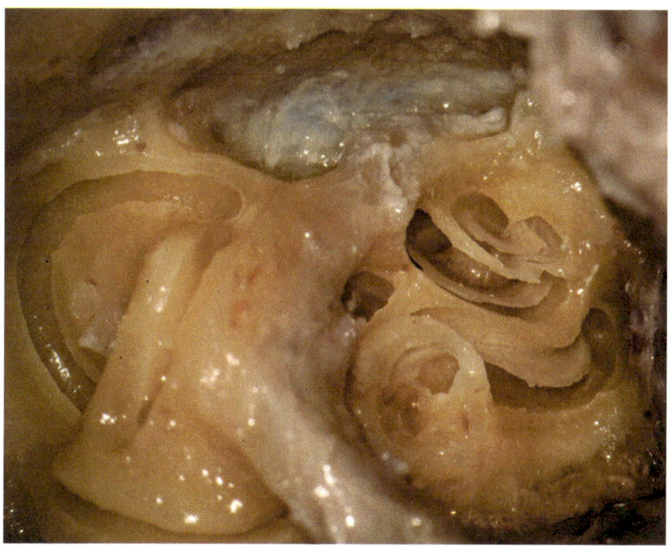

Fig. 2.18 The cochlea has been drilled out; the basal, middle, and apical turns can be appreciated. Intracochlearly the osseous spiral lamina is clearly visible separating the scala vestibuli and scala tympani. Also the change in position (from anterior-posterior to superior-inferior) of the osseous spiral lamina just behind the round window and lower in the basal turn can be seen.

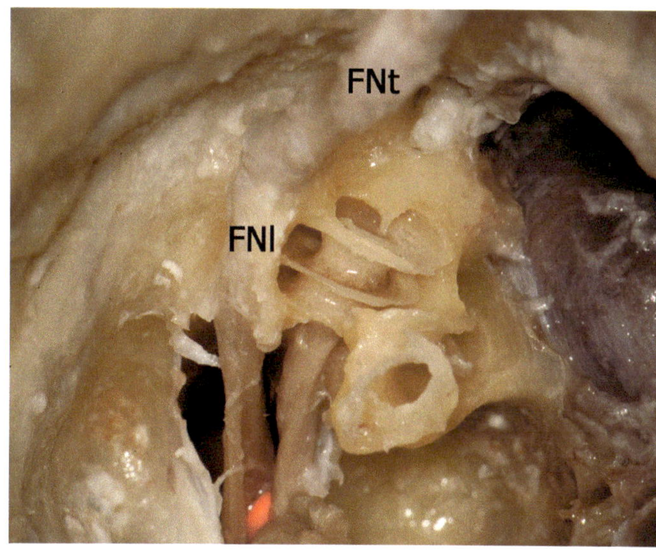

Fig. 2.19 This figure shows a drilled-out cochlea of the right ear in relation to the internal auditory canal. The tympanic segment of the facial nerve (FNt) is detached and reflected anteriorly, in line with the labyrinthine segment of the facial nerve (FNl), to allow closer dissection of the cochlear aperture. Note the anterior-superior tilting of the cochlea.

Cochlear Turns (Fig. 2.16–Fig. 2.22)

Inside the cochlea the spiral ligament and the stria vascularis are located along the lateral wall. In the basal turn the location of the basilar membrane turns from a position parallel and very close to the round window to a superior-inferior plane halfway the basal turn. Following this change in plane of the basilar membrane, the scala tympani also changes position within the basal turn. Close to the round window the scala tympani is situated as the most posterior scala, but at the level of the basal turn it is the medial-inferior scala. This anatomy has consequences for cochlear implantation surgery. Opening of the round window should be performed anterior-inferiorly, away from the basilar membrane, which is directly behind the superior part of the round window (**Fig. 2.17**). The direction of insertion of the cochlear electrode should be anterior-inferiorly also, as not to puncture the basilar membrane or damage the spiral osseous ligament (see **Fig. 2.20** and **Fig. 2.21**).

2.1.12 The Sigmoid Sinus and Jugular Bulb (Fig. 2.23)

The sigmoid sinus connects the transverse sinus with the jugular bulb and is situated between the inner and outer layers of the dura. It receives the superior petrosal sinus and connects via the emissary vein with the posterior auricular vein. The emissary vein is sometimes encountered during cochlear implant surgery while preparing for the receiver well. The jugular bulb is located in the jugular foramen, connecting the sigmoid sinus and the internal jugular vein. The jugular bulb is located medial to the mastoid segment of the facial nerve, and inferior to the semicircular canals and cochlea. The distance between the facial nerve and the jugular bulb varies, as well as the position of the bulb in the hypotympanum (**Fig. 2.22**). Sometimes the jugular bulb reaches the inferior border of the cochlea (high-riding bulb). In some cases, the jugular bulb is dehiscent in the hypotympanum. It should be remembered that the lower cranial nerves IX to XI

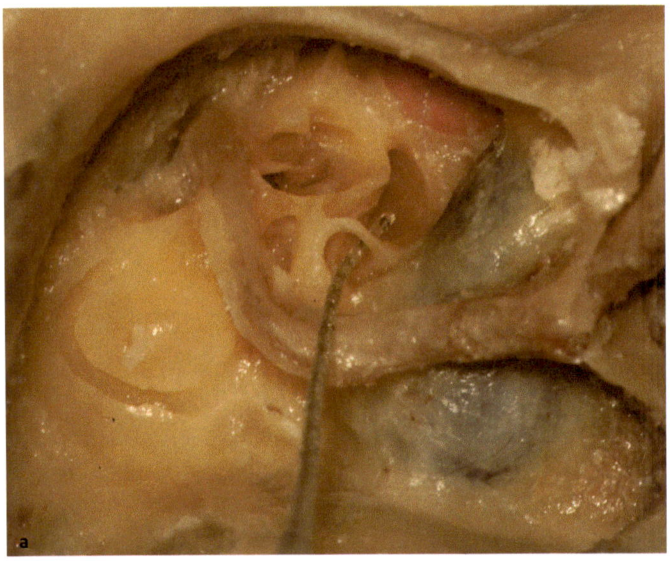

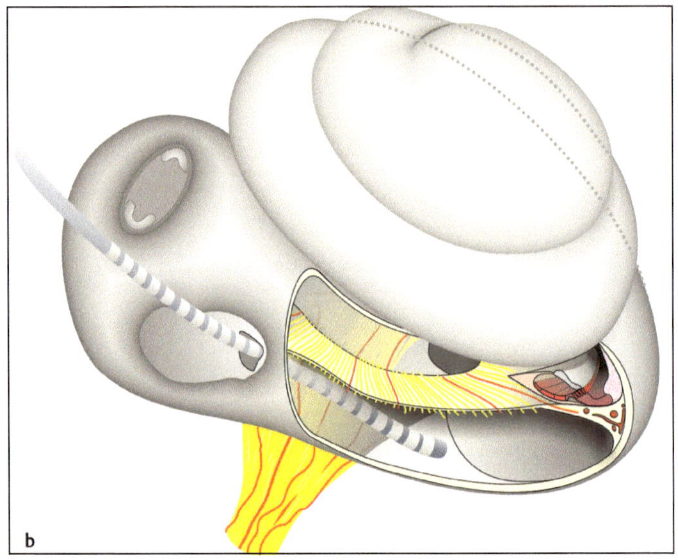

Fig. 2.20a,b

a Insertion of an electrode array into the scala tympani of the basal turn, following the right axis of introduction. The direction is anterior-inferiorly, to lessen the chance of damage to the basilar membrane as much as possible.

b Schematic drawing.

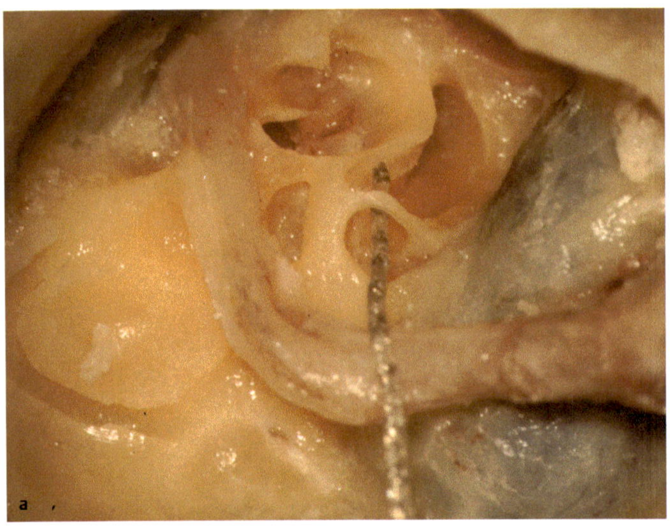

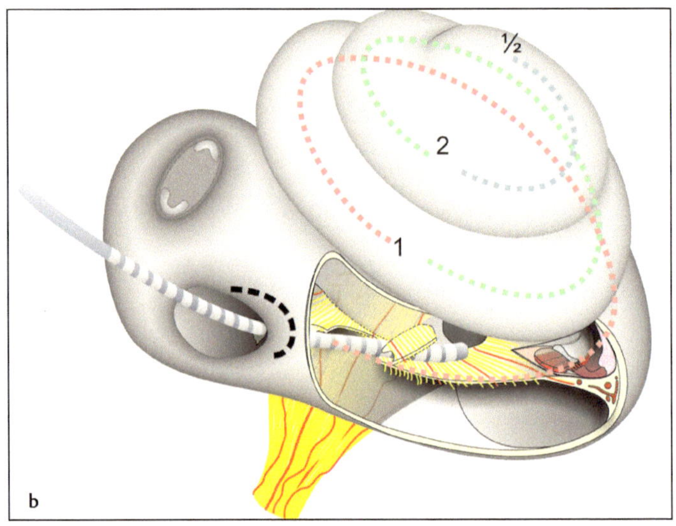

Fig. 2.21a, b

a In this example the electrode array is directed too much anteriorly and superiorly, and is making contact with or damaging the basilar membrane (not visible in the figure), the spiral osseous ligament, and the modiolus.

b Schematic drawing.

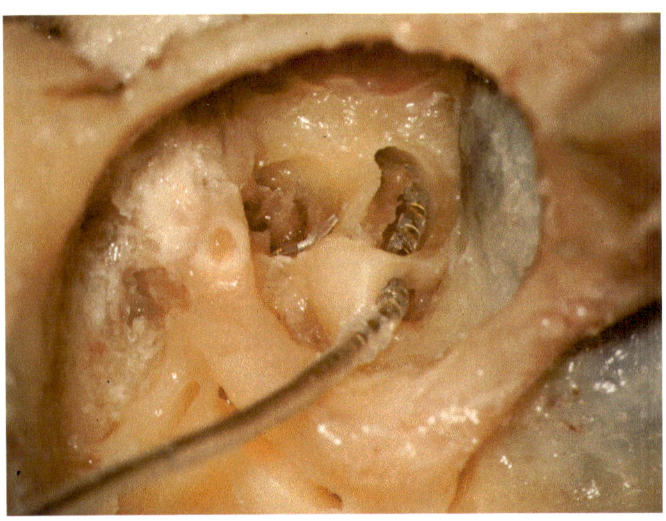

Fig. 2.22 In this example too little of the superior bony overhang of the round window niche is removed, making the electrode array kink in the round window cochleostomy; the array could become damaged.

pass the skull base through the jugular foramen medial to the jugular bulb.

The superior petrosal sinus connects with the cavernous sinus and drains inferior cerebral and cerebellar veins as well as veins from the tympanic cavity. It runs in an attached margin of the tentorium cerebelli, in a groove called the superior petrosal sulcus.

Also the inferior petrosal sinus drains to the jugular bulb and connects with the cavernous sinus. It drains the veins from the internal auditory canal, the pons and medulla oblongata, and the inferior surface of the cerebellum.

2.1.13 The Carotid Artery (Fig. 2.23)

The carotid artery enters the temporal bone through the carotid foramen. It ascends vertically in the area just anterior-inferior to the cochlea. It then turns anterior-medially with nearly a 90° angle toward the petrous apex, forming its horizontal segment just inferior-medially to the eustachian tube. The horizontal segment of the carotid artery then crosses underneath (inferiorly to) the eustachian tube and proceeds to the foramen lacerum, entering the intracranium. In 2% of cases, the bony shell separating the carotid artery and the eustachian tube is absent.[12,13] The distance between the cochlea and the carotid artery ranges from 1 mm to several millimeters. The location of the carotid artery should be well known in cochlear drill-out procedures, in subtotal petrosectomy approach, and in other more extensive procedures (**Fig. 2.20, Fig. 2.22,** and **Fig. 2.23**).

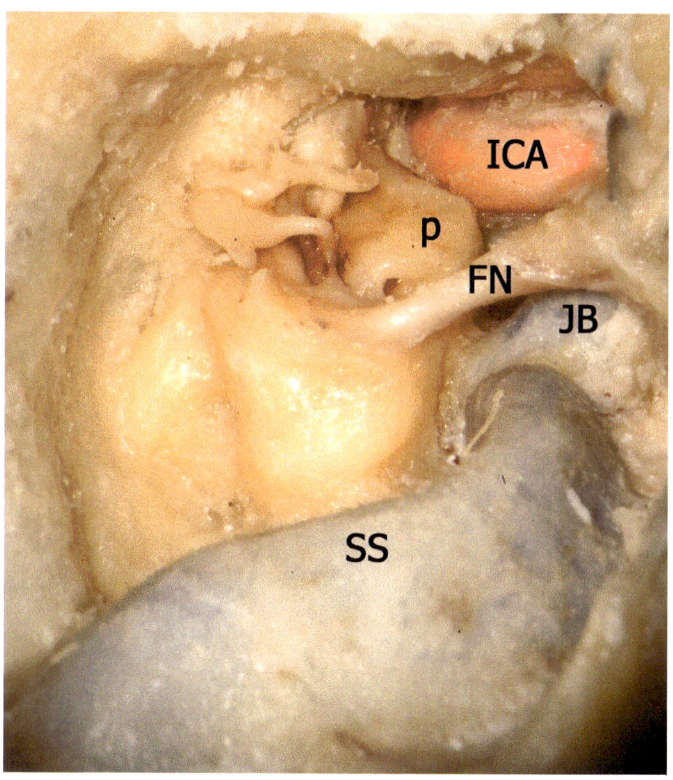

Fig. 2.23 In this extended canal wall down cavity the sigmoid sinus (SS) and ascending portion of the internal carotid artery (ICA) are skeletonized and clearly visible. The relationship of both structures with the promontory (p) can be appreciated. Note also the relationship of the jugular bulb (JB) with the mastoid segment of the facial nerve (FN).

2.1.14 Facial Recess versus Subtotal Petrosectomy

Exposure of the round window is usually achieved through a facial recess approach (**Fig. 2.24**). When required, a subtotal petrosectomy may offer a wider approach with improved control of the anatomical structures (**Fig. 2.25**).

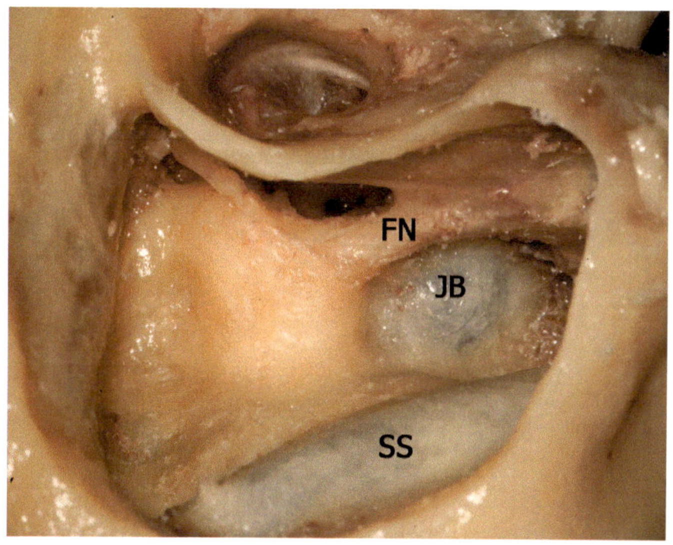

Fig. 2.24 This figure shows the access to the round window niche through a posterior tympanotomy approach. FN, facial nerve; SS, sigmoid sinus; JB, jugular bulb.

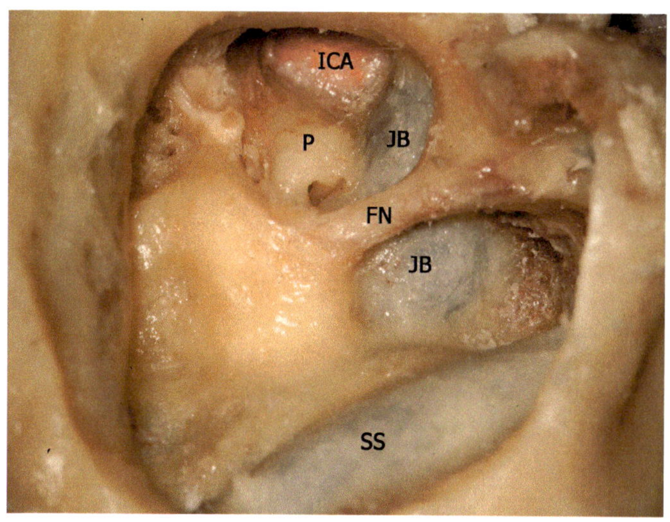

Fig. 2.25 The posterior canal wall has been removed as in a combined cochlear implantation and subtotal petrosectomy approach: access and visibility into middle ear and cochlea are better. Note the internal carotid artery (ICA), the high jugular bulb (JB) anterior and posterior to the facial nerve (FN), and their relationship with the promontory (P). SS, sigmoid sinus.

2.2 Anatomical Dissection of Left Temporal Bone for Cochlear Implantation (Fig. 2.26–Fig. 2.36)

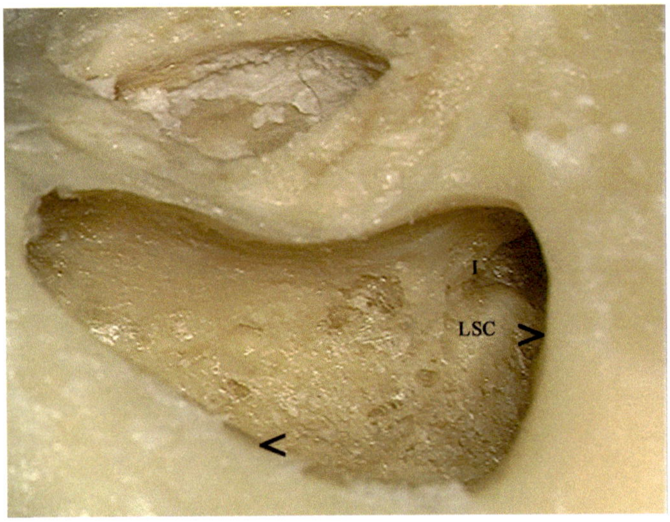

Fig. 2.26 Mastoidectomy for cochlear implantation has been completed. Since the surgery is not intended to eradicate pathologic tissue, a limited mastoidectomy will be sufficient. Also, externalization of the cavity is not necessary, as square edges (>,<) will hold the electrode arrays situated in the cavity. The posterior canal wall is thinned. Two landmarks of the facial nerve are identified: the lateral semicircular canal (LSC) and the short process of the incus (I). Atticotomy is not required but can be performed for better light and visibility. The facial nerve is seen in the almost transparent skeletonized bone (*arrows*).

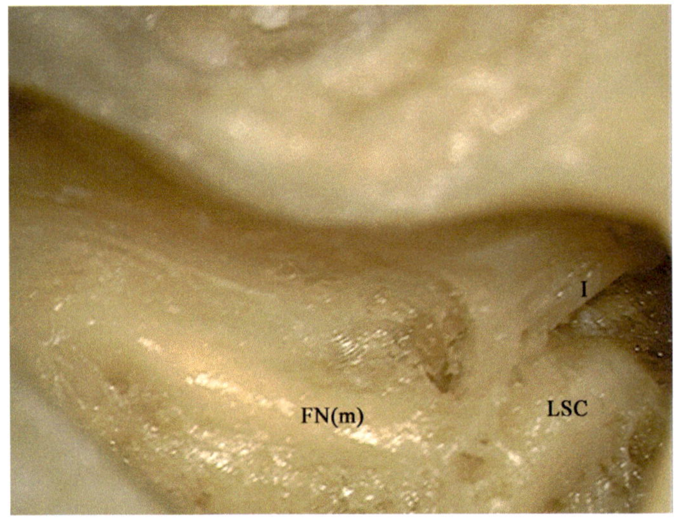

Fig. 2.27 The posterior tympanotomy is conducted in the area just inferior to the short process of the incus and lateral to the facial nerve. The direction of the drilling, in this area, should be parallel to the facial nerve, with liberal rinsing to protect the facial nerve from damage by heating. I, incus; LSC, lateral semicircular canal; FN(m), facial nerve, mastoid segment.

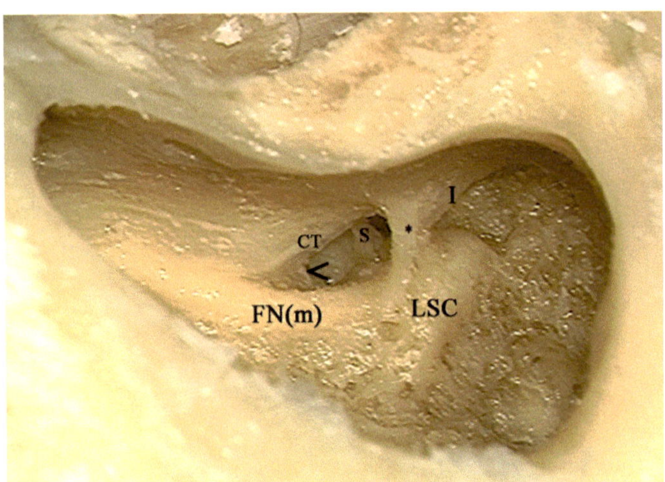

Fig. 2.28 Posterior tympanotomy in progress. A small bony bridge posterior to the incus called the buttress (∗) can be left. Laterally to the facial nerve the chorda tympani nerve is seen (CT). In some cases with a narrow posterior tympanotomy, the chorda tympani nerve should be sacrificed to obtain sufficient access for safe surgery. There is wide variability in the branching off of the chorda tympani from the facial nerve (<). Care must be taken not to drill too far anterior-laterally along the posterior ear canal with risk of injury to the tympanic annulus. I, incus; LSC, lateral semicircular canal; FN(m), mastoid segment of the facial nerve; S, stapes.

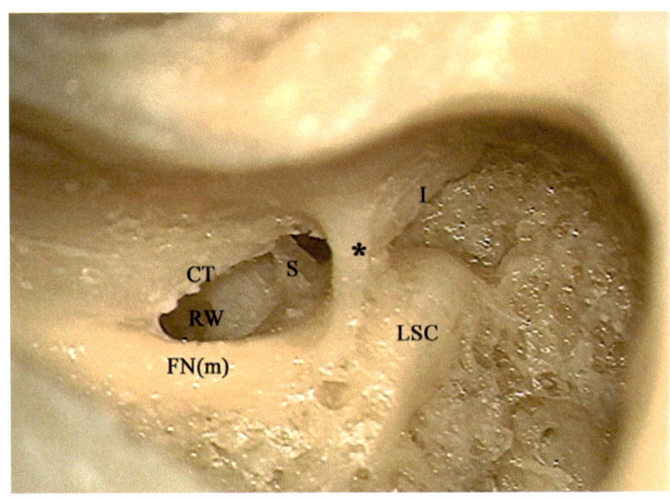

Fig. 2.29 The posterior tympanotomy is extended inferiorly for access to the round window niche (RW). The stapes (S) is seen superiorly to the round window niche. ∗, buttress; I, incus; CT, chorda tympani; LSC, lateral semicircular canal; FN(m), mastoid segment of the facial nerve.

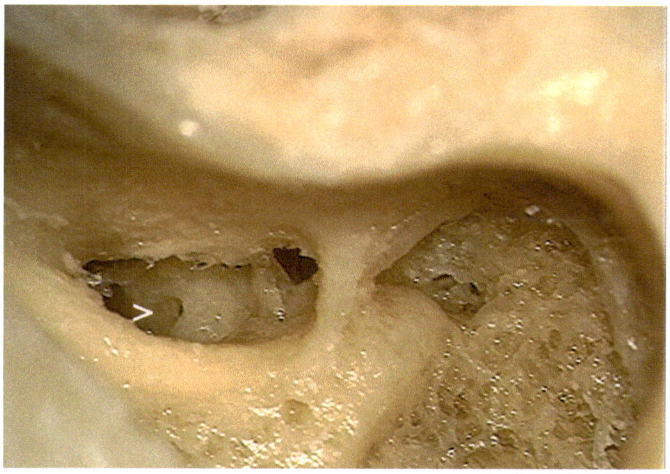

Fig. 2.30 In larger magnification, the round window niche (>) and the stapes are clearly seen. Note that the visibility of and the access to the round window membrane is hampered by a bony overhang at the superior-posterior edge of the round window niche. Inferiorly a hypotympanic cell is visible; it resembles the round window niche and is sometimes taken for the round window, leading to a false route for insertion of the cochlear electrode.

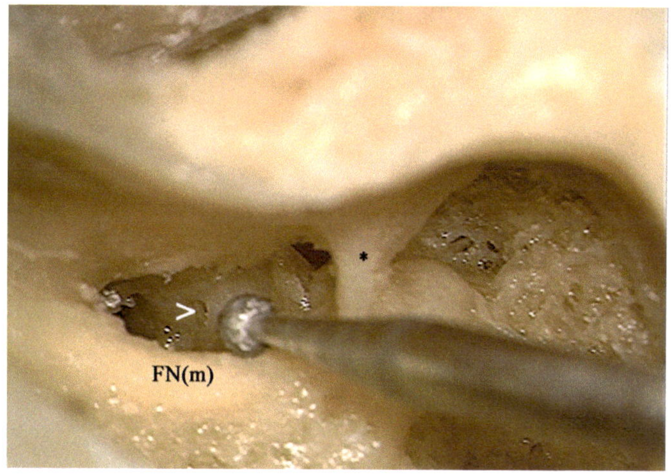

Fig. 2.31 The bony overhang covering the round window membrane is removed with a small diamond bur. Care must be taken not to damage the stapes and the round window itself. The chorda tympani nerve is sacrificed in this specimen for teaching purposes. Contact between the rotating shaft of the drill and the facial nerve should be avoided. Even without direct trauma, heat injury may occur. ∗, buttress; FN(m), mastoid segment of the facial nerve; >, round window.

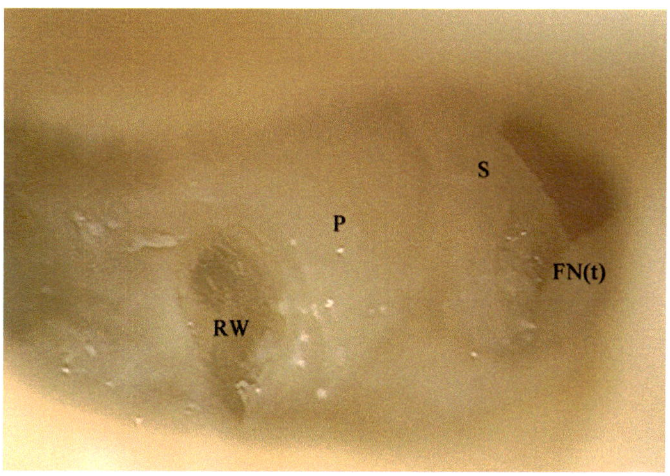

Fig. 2.32 The round window membrane is now clearly visible. It has a dark gray color. In the presence of a pseudomembrane (not visible on this image) a white membrane is visible, which can be peeled off, uncovering the true round window membrane. RW, round window; P, promontory; FN(t), tympanic segment of the facial nerve; S, stapes.

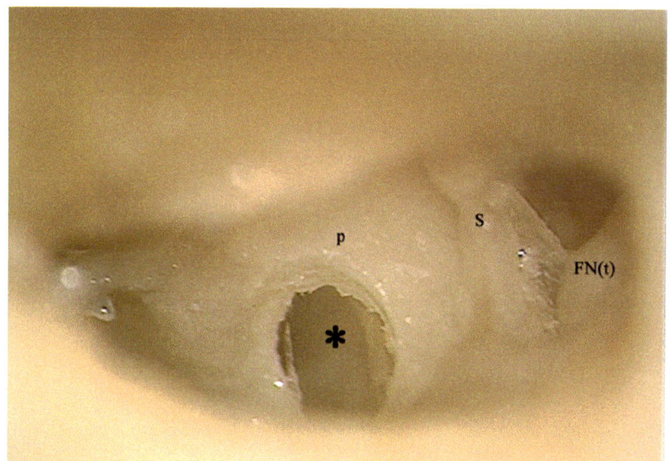

Fig. 2.33 The round window membrane is opened with a small hook with a gentle movement, the membrane is reflected, and the scala tympani (∗) is opened. P, promontory; S, stapes; FN(t), tympanic segment of the facial nerve.

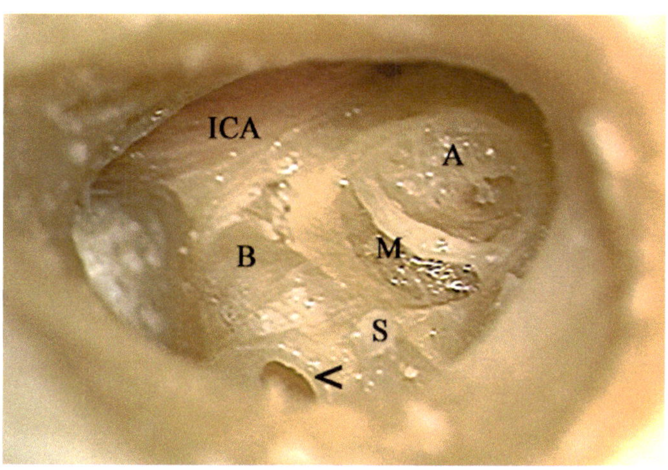

Fig. 2.34 After removal of the tympanic membrane and ossicles, the basal turn of the cochlea is skeletonized and the middle and apical turns are opened. The vertical portion of the internal carotid artery is skeletonized as well. Since the basal turn courses inferior-anteriorly from the round window, when opening the cochlea through a promontory cochleostomy, drilling should be performed more inferiorly to the round window to avoid damage of the spiral ligament and the stria vascularis. ICA, carotid artery; B, basal turn; M, middle turn; A, apical turn; S, stapes; <, round window.

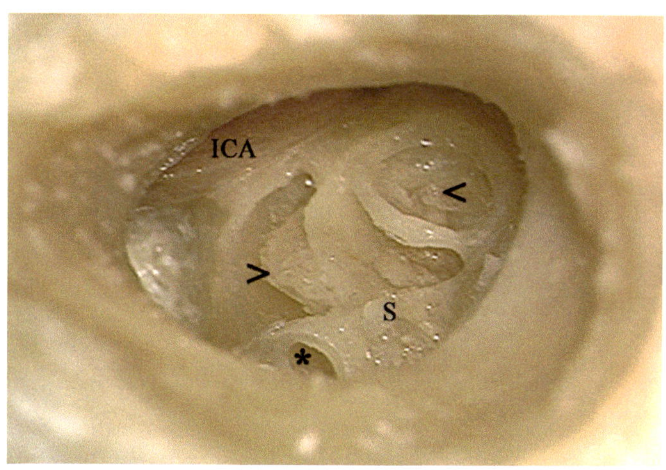

Fig. 2.35 The intracochlear anatomy is shown after removal of the lateral wall. Each turn comprises the scala tympani and the scala vestibuli. These two compartments are separated by an osseous structure called the spiral lamina (>) and a membranous structure, the scala media, located laterally to the spiral lamina (already removed in this image). The round window corresponds to the scala tympani, and the oval window corresponds to the scala vestibuli. ICA, carotid artery; S, stapes; <, apex of the modiolus; ∗, round window.

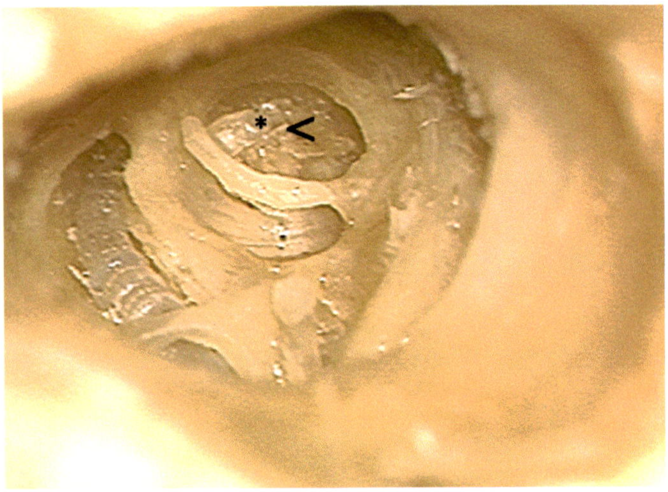

Fig. 2.36 The array of the cochlear implant has been inserted, hugging the modiolus and reaching the middle turn. *, tip of the array; <, tip of the modiolus.

2.3 Anatomy of the Lateral Skull Base, Brainstem, and Cochlear Nucleus

2.3.1 Internal Auditory Canal

The internal auditory canal is a bony channel with a length of almost 1 cm running in a lateral direction from the cerebellopontine angle (CPA) to the vestibule through the petrous bone. The long axis of the internal auditory canal lies in line with the long axis of the external auditory canal. Its orifice, the porus, can be studied from the intracranial side of the petrous bone. Its posterior border has a sharp angle, while its anterior border is wider. The dura of the posterior cranial fossa continues into the internal auditory canal, lining the whole length, and ends by merging with the contained nerves as they enter their corresponding foramina (**Fig. 2.37**). Also the internal auditory artery and vein and sometimes a loop of the anterior inferior cerebellar artery (AICA) are present in the internal auditory canal.

At the fundus, the most lateral part of the internal auditory canal, the crista falciformis, also called the horizontal crest, separates the entire canal into a superior and an inferior half. The inferior half hosts the cochlear nerve anteriorly and the inferior vestibular nerve posteriorly (**Fig. 2.38**). A vertical crest, called Bill's bar, divides the superior half into a posterior part containing the superior vestibular nerve and an anterior part hosting the facial nerve (**Fig. 2.39** and **Fig. 2.40**). The singular nerve is located posterior-inferiorly to the inferior vestibular nerve and leaves the inferior vestibular nerve before reaching the fundus. It reaches the ampulla of the posterior canal through a separate canal that can be found more medially in the posterior-inferior wall of the internal auditory canal.

2.3.2 Anatomy of the Posterior Fossa Related to ABI Surgery

The anatomy and structures important for auditory brainstem implantation will be concentrated on the cranial nerves and nuclei V–XII, the flocculus and the choroid plexus, the Luschka foramen, and the lateral recess and the vessels that supply and drain this area (**Fig. 2.41**–**Fig. 2.48**).

Cerebellopontine Angle and Brainstem

The cerebellopontine angle is the area of the posterior cranial fossa limited laterally by the posterior surface of petrous bone, anteriorly by the prepontine cistern, and posterior-medially by the cerebellum, the middle and inferior cerebellar peduncle, the pons, and the medulla oblongata. The last four structures seem to be "enwrapped" by the cerebellum.[14] The same area is also described as the cerebellomedullary or the cerebellopontine fissure. It has a triangular shape in anterior-posterior view.

Superiorly its conventional limit is considered a horizontal plane crossing through the trigeminal nerve (V). Inferiorly its conventional limit is a horizontal plane crossing through the glossopharyngeal nerve (IX). The cranial nerves X–XII lie below the cerebellopontine angle (CPA) (**Fig. 2.43**), while the trochlear nerve (IV) lies above, closely related to the superior cerebellar artery (SCA) (**Fig. 2.42**).

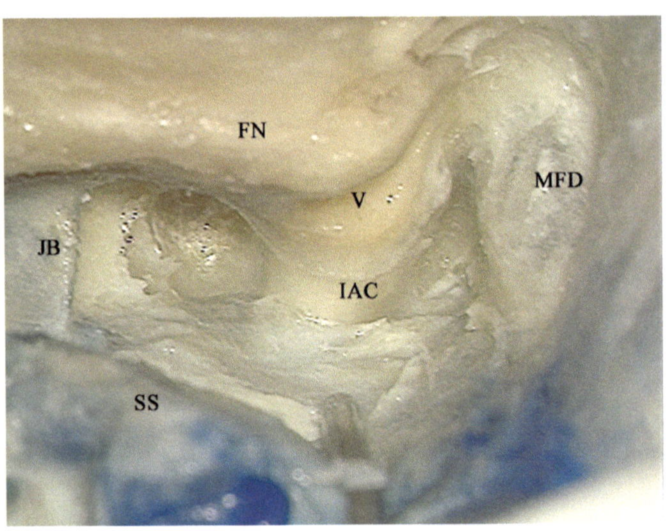

Fig. 2.37 (*Left ear*) Adequately skeletonized internal auditory canal (IAC). V, vestibule; FN, facial nerve; MFD, middle fossa dura; JB, jugular bulb; SS, sigmoid sinus.

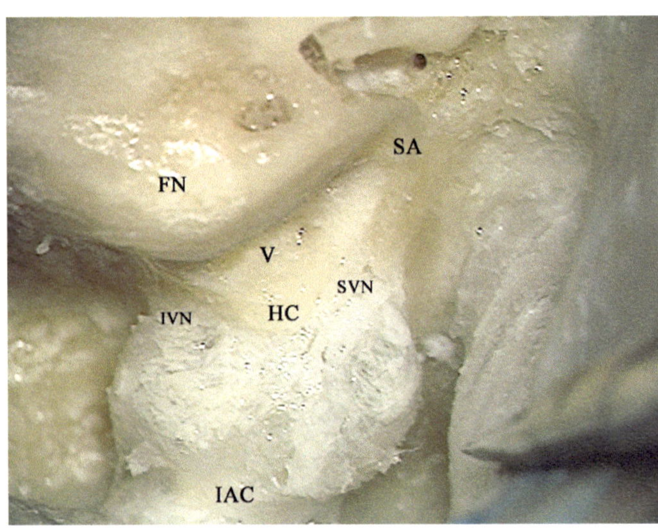

Fig. 2.38 (*Left ear*) Fully exposed internal auditory canal (IAC). V, vestibule; HC, horizontal crest; SVN, superior vestibular nerve; IVN, inferior vestibular nerve; SA, superior ampulla; FN, facial nerve.

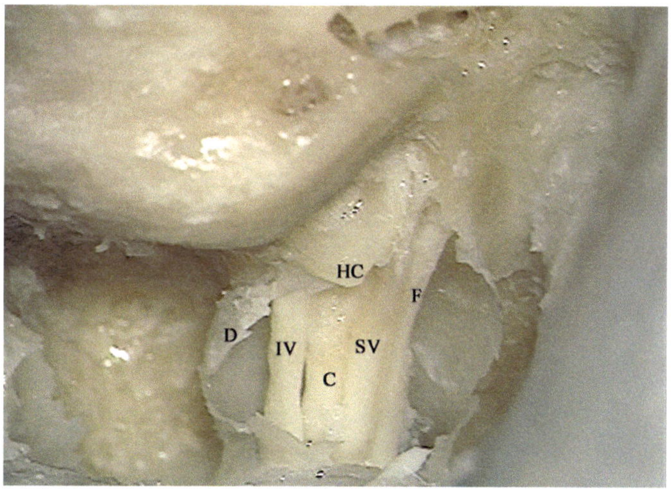

Fig. 2.39 (*Left ear*) Contents of the internal auditory canal after opening the dura. F, facial nerve; SV, superior vestibular nerve; C, cochlear nerve, IV, inferior vestibular nerve; D, dura; HC, horizontal crest.

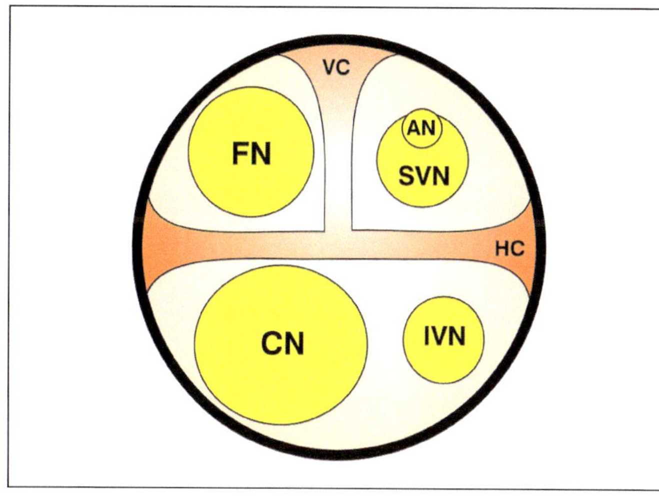

Fig. 2.40 (*Right ear*) Diagram of the internal auditory canal near the fundus, in cross section. The superior ampullary nerve (AN) is shown overlapping the superior vestibular nerve (SVN). CN, cochlear nerve; FN, facial nerve; HC, horizontal crest; IVN, inferior vestibular nerve; VC, vertical crest (Bill's bar).

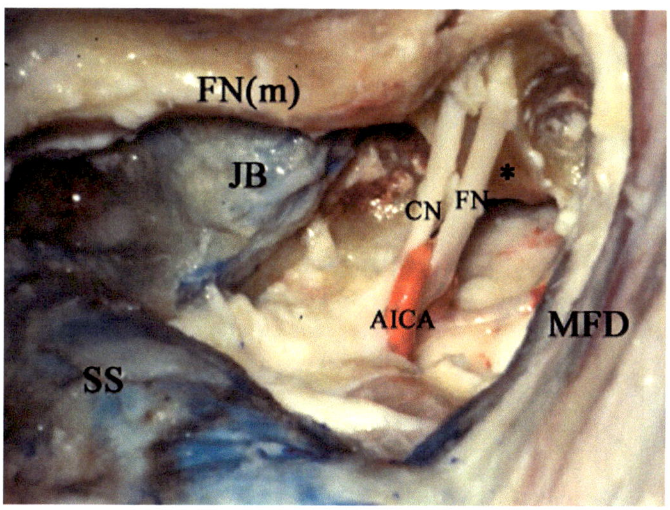

Fig. 2.41 (*Left ear*) Cadaveric dissection through a translabyrinthine approach showing the intracanalicular structures. Note that the AICA runs between the facial nerve and the cochlear nerve in this specimen. FN(m), mastoid segment of facial nerve; JB, jugular bulbus; SS, sigmoid sinus; MFD, middle fossa dura; AICA, anterior inferior cerebellar artery; CN, cochlear nerve; FN, intracanalicular facial nerve; *asterisk*, anterior wall of the internal auditory canal.

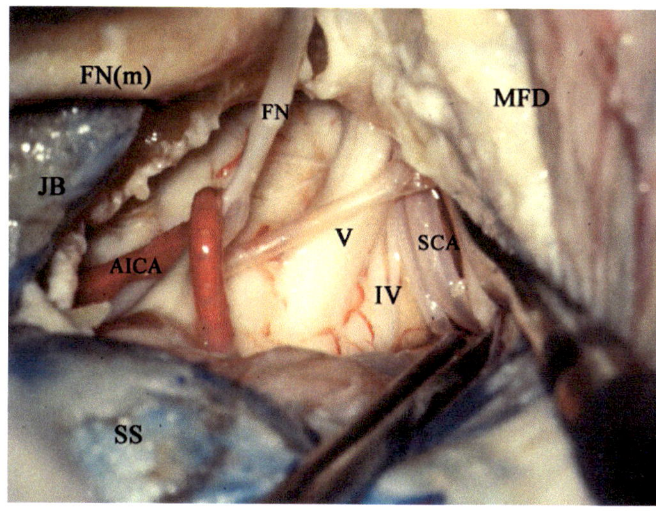

Fig. 2.42 (*Left ear*) Superior surgical view of the CPA through a translabyrinthine approach. The trochlear nerve (IV) and superior cerebellar artery (SCA) can be observed. AICA, anterior inferior cerebellar artery; FN, facial nerve; FN(m), mastoid segment of facial nerve; JB, jugular bulb; SS, sigmoid sinus; V, trigeminal nerve; MFD, middle fossa dura.

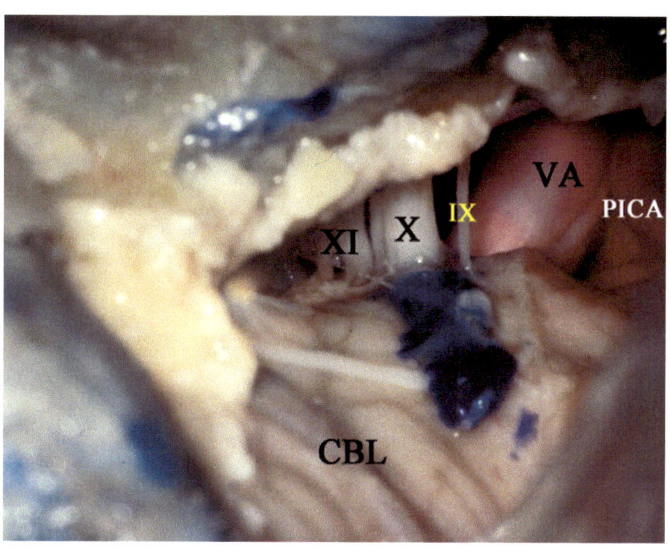

Fig. 2.43 (*Left ear*) Inferior surgical view of the CPA through a translabyrinthine approach. The glossopharyngeal nerve (IX), vagus nerve (X), accessory nerve (XI), posterior inferior cerebellar artery (PICA), and vertebral artery (VA) can be seen. CBL, cerebellum.

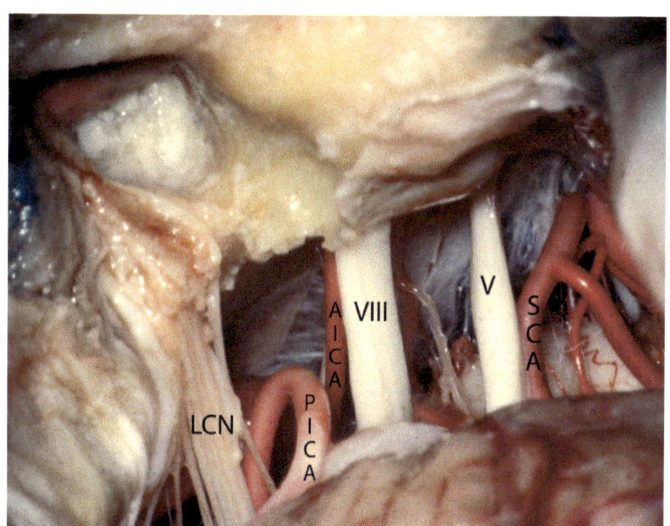

Fig. 2.44 General view of the CPA, left ear; showing the three main cerebellar arteries and their relation to the cranial nerves. LCN, lower cranial nerves; PICA, posterior inferior cerebellar artery; AICA, anterior inferior cerebellar artery; VIII, vestibulocochlear nerve; V, trigeminal nerve; SCA, superior cerebellar artery.

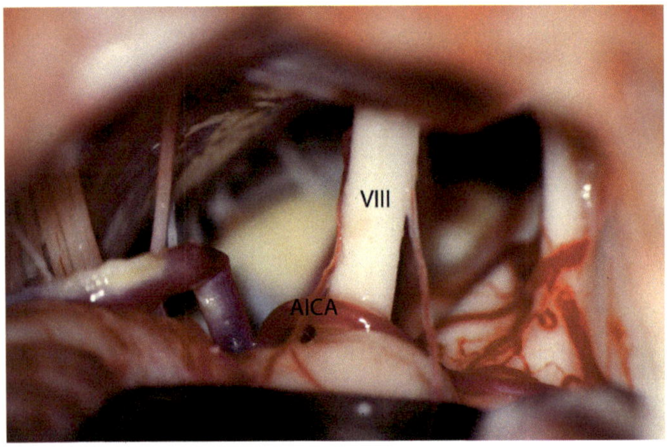

Fig. 2.45 Loop of the anterior inferior cerebellar artery (AICA) around the vestibulocochlear-facial bundle (VIII).

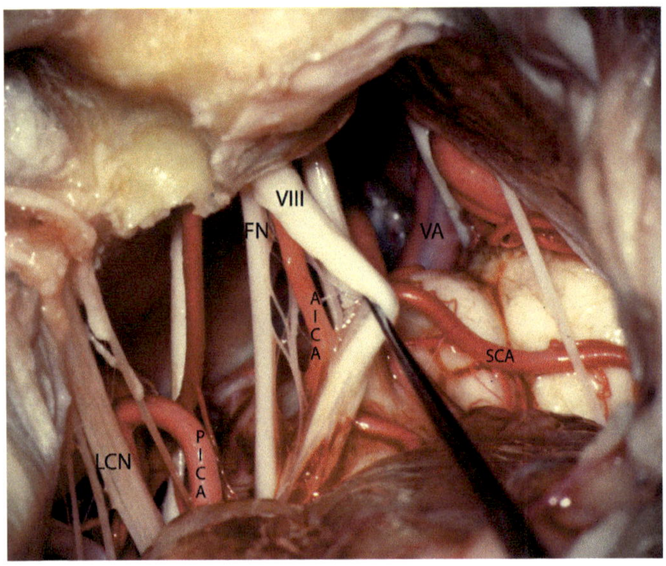

Fig. 2.46 Position of the facial nerve anterior-medially with respect to the vestibulocochlear nerve. The anterior inferior cerebellar artery may run in between the two nerves. LCN, lower cranial nerves; PICA, posterior inferior cerebellar artery; FN, facial nerve; AICA, anterior inferior cerebellar artery; VIII, vestibulocochlear nerve; VA, vertebral artery; SCA, superior cerebellar artery.

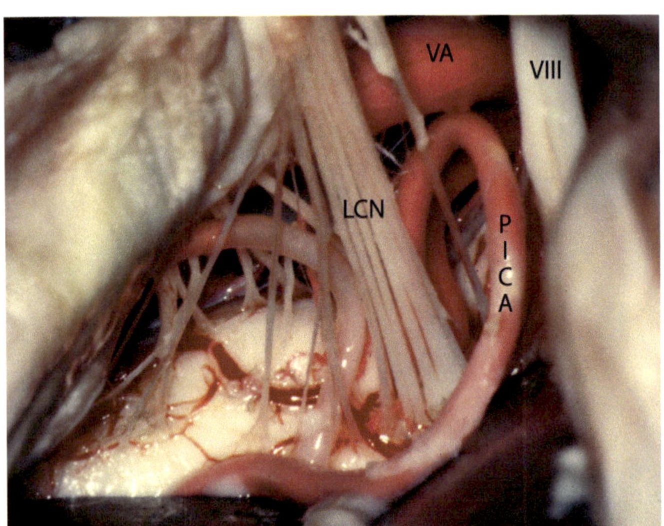

Fig. 2.47 Inferiorly, the posterior inferior cerebellar artery originates from the vertebral artery. Note the close relationship between the artery and the lower cranial nerves. LCN, lower cranial nerves; PICA, posterior inferior cerebellar artery; VIII, vestibulocochlear nerve; VA, vertebral artery.

Nerves and Nuclei

(**Fig. 2.42–Fig. 2.49**. *The course of the nerves and location of the nuclei are described unilaterally for clarity.*)

The **trigeminal nerve** (V) originates from different nuclei in the mesencephalon, pons, and medulla. It is the largest cranial nerve in diameter and leaves the mid-pons on the lateral-anterior side, coursing anteriorly. It then enters the gasserian ganglion located in the Meckel cave, where it splits into its three components.

The **abducens nerve** (VI) is a small nerve and can be found leaving the pontomedullary sulcus at the anterior side; it runs superiorly and anteriorly, crosses the prepontine cistern, and enters the Dorello canal toward the cavernous sinus, where it is located lateral from the carotid artery. The nucleus of the abducens nerve is found in the lower part of the pons, on the same level as the facial nucleus, but more anteriorly, and superior from the cochlear nucleus, just posterior to the mid level of the fourth ventricle.

The **facial nerve** (VII) exits its nucleus, which is situated superior-medial-posteriorly to the cochlear nucleus in the medial-central part of the pons and leaves the pons anterior-laterally via the pontomedullary sulcus medial from where the vestibulocochlear nerves exit the sulcus.

The **vestibulocochlear nerve** (VIII) exits the brainstem also at the pontomedullary junction as a bundle. The facial and vestibulocochlear nerves exit from the brainstem obliquely; the nerves run slightly superiorly.[15] Both nerves course through the CPA cistern and enter the porus acusticus of the internal auditory canal as two separate structures: the facial nerve and the vestibulocochlear bundle. The vestibular and cochlear components of the eighth nerve enter the meatus together and divide in separately identifiable nerves within the internal auditory canal in the most lateral 3–4 mm of the canal; this varies among individuals.

The cochlear nucleus is found on the posterior-lateral surface of the pons close to the pontomedullary junction; the vestibular nuclei (four on each side) can be found medially and superiorly to the cochlear nucleus, also on the anterior side of the lateral recess.

The nuclei of the **glossopharyngeal** (IX) and **vagal** (X) **nerves** are located in the medulla oblongata along the dorsal surface close to the fourth ventricle. They emerge out of the posterior-lateral or postolivary sulcus of the medulla oblongata, just inferior to the pontomedullary junction. The glossopharyngeal nerve consists usually of one rootlet, very rarely of two, and is positioned superiorly to the vagal nerve, which can be recognized by its many rootlets (seven or more). The **accessory nerve** (XI) has a nucleus in the medulla oblongata giving the cranial root, which is the smaller root consisting of four or five delicate rootlets. It is positioned just inferior to the vagal nerve rootlets. The larger spinal part of the accessory nerve originates from the cervical spinal cord up to C5 and has multiple roots. The spinal root runs upward, passing the vertebral artery posteriorly, passes the foramen magnum, joins the medullary root just superior to or in the jugular foramen, and then leaves through the jugular foramen (**Fig. 2.48**). The accessory nerve has communications with the dorsal roots of the upper cervical nerves; the communications with the first cervical nerve is largest.[16] Between these three lower cranial nerves (IX, X, XI) there is exchange of fibers and function.

The nuclei of the **hypoglossal nerve** (XII) are located centrally-dorsally in the medulla oblongata. The hypoglossal nerve exits more anteriorly than the other three nerves via the anterolateral, preolivary sulcus, coursing laterally, passing behind the vertebral artery toward the hypoglossal foramen. It consists in the majority of cases of two main trunks, superior and inferior, with separate dural orifices, but teamed up before leaving the skull base once entering the hypoglossal canal. These two roots of the hypoglossal nerve are separated by the posterior inferior cerebellar artery (PICA) that runs between them (**Fig. 2.49**). The hypoglossal canal is located 5 mm above the occipital condyle; it courses anterior-laterally and exits anteriorly superior of the occipital condyle, medial to the jugular foramen.

The direction of all lower cranial nerves (IX, X, XI, XII) is lateral-anterior-superiorly running up to enter the jugular foramen, where they pierce the dura over the jugular foramen. They then make a turn inferiorly and course more or less vertically along the medial wall of the jugular fossa. In the jugular fossa they are situated in separate dural sheaths.

Finally, an important structure in relation to ABI is the **solitary nucleus** located from the level of the cochlear nucleus in the lower pons running inferiorly to the medulla oblongata. It harbors the visceral sensory parts of cranial nerves VII, IX, and X. As it relates closely to the cochlear nucleus, this structure can be stimulated during evoked auditory brainstem response (EABR) measurements in ABI. The vagal component is especially important because of the risk of cardiac arrest during stimulation and this is one of the reasons ABI fitting has to be performed in an intensive care ward.

Arteries

The arterial supply to the brainstem, CPA, and cerebellum is by the vertebrobasilar system. The intradural segments of the vertebral arteries, originating from the subclavian arteries, enter the skull base through the foramen magnum and run upward along the clivus. At the level of the pontomedullary junction the vertebral arteries unite and form the basilar artery that runs in the midline along the anterior surface of the brainstem. The vertebrobasilar system is very variable and tortuous vessels with loops are often encountered.[16] It gives off three pairs of cerebellar arteries (**Fig. 2.44**). The AICA and PICA are the important arteries in ABI surgery because they may be found around the Luschka foramen, while the vertebral and basilar artery are only sometimes encountered here.[14] The SCA is located more superiorly, relating to the trigeminal nerve, and supplies the posterior surface of the cerebellum.

The anterior inferior cerebellar artery (AICA) arises at the pontine level. It is the most important vascular structure within the CPA and gives off the internal auditory artery (labyrinthine artery). Near its origin from the basilar artery it is related to the abducens nerve (VI), then it courses posteriorly, and it might loop around or through the vestibulocochlear-facial bundle (**Fig. 2.41** and **Fig. 2.42**) or enter the internal auditory canal with a loop. It ends by reaching the surface of the middle cerebellopontine fissure, where it supplies the petrosal surface of the cerebellum.

The posterior inferior cerebellar artery (PICA) arises from the vertebral artery and is related to the lower cranial nerves. It terminates by supplying the suboccipital surface of the cerebellum (**Fig. 2.47–Fig. 2.49**). Usually the PICA and AICA are related in size: if the PICA is large, then the AICA is small and vice versa.

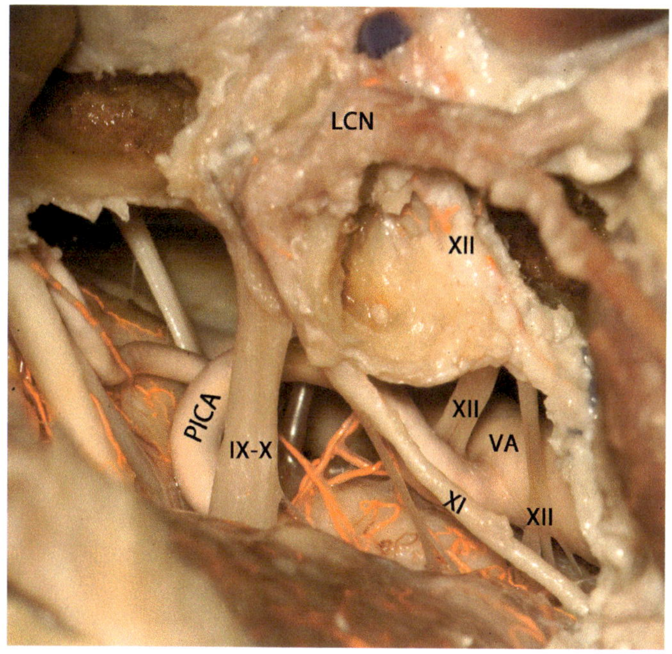

Fig. 2.48 The lower cranial nerve and PICA are visualized. Note the spinal part of the accessory nerve (XI). The two roots of the hypoglossal nerve join into the hypoglossal foramen. IX, glossopharyngeal nerve; X, vagus nerve; LCN, lower cranial nerves; XII, hypoglossal nerve; PICA, posterior inferior cerebellar artery; VA, vertebral artery.

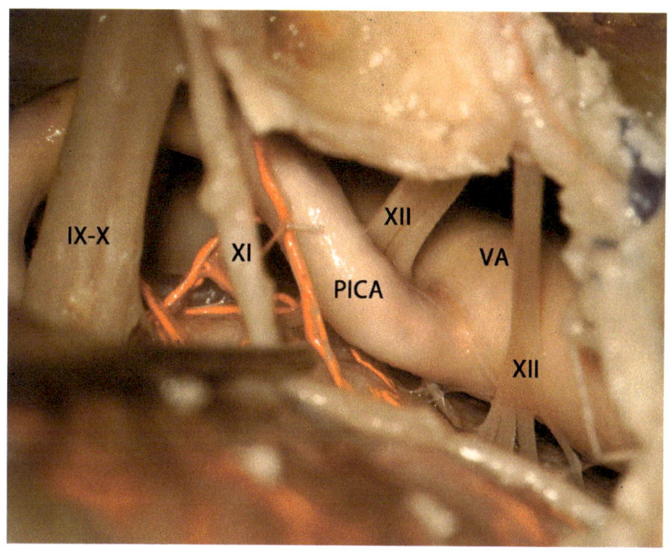

Fig. 2.49 In this detail the PICA leaving the vertebral artery is visible. Also both parts of the hypoglossal nerve (XII) can be seen, running toward the hypoglossal foramen (not visible). IX, glossopharyngeal nerve; X, vagus nerve; XI, accessory nerve; XII, hypoglossal nerve; PICA, posterior inferior cerebellar artery; VA, vertebral artery.

Veins

There are also veins that can be encountered during ABI surgery. In general their course is more variable than the course of the arteries and they can obstruct access to the Luschka foramen. Whereas arteries can distort and compress the structures in the CPA, veins mainly obstruct. The vein of the cerebellomedullary fissure is the largest; also veins of the middle cerebellar peduncle, pontomedullary sulcus, and inferior petrosal bridging veins can cross and obstruct.[17]

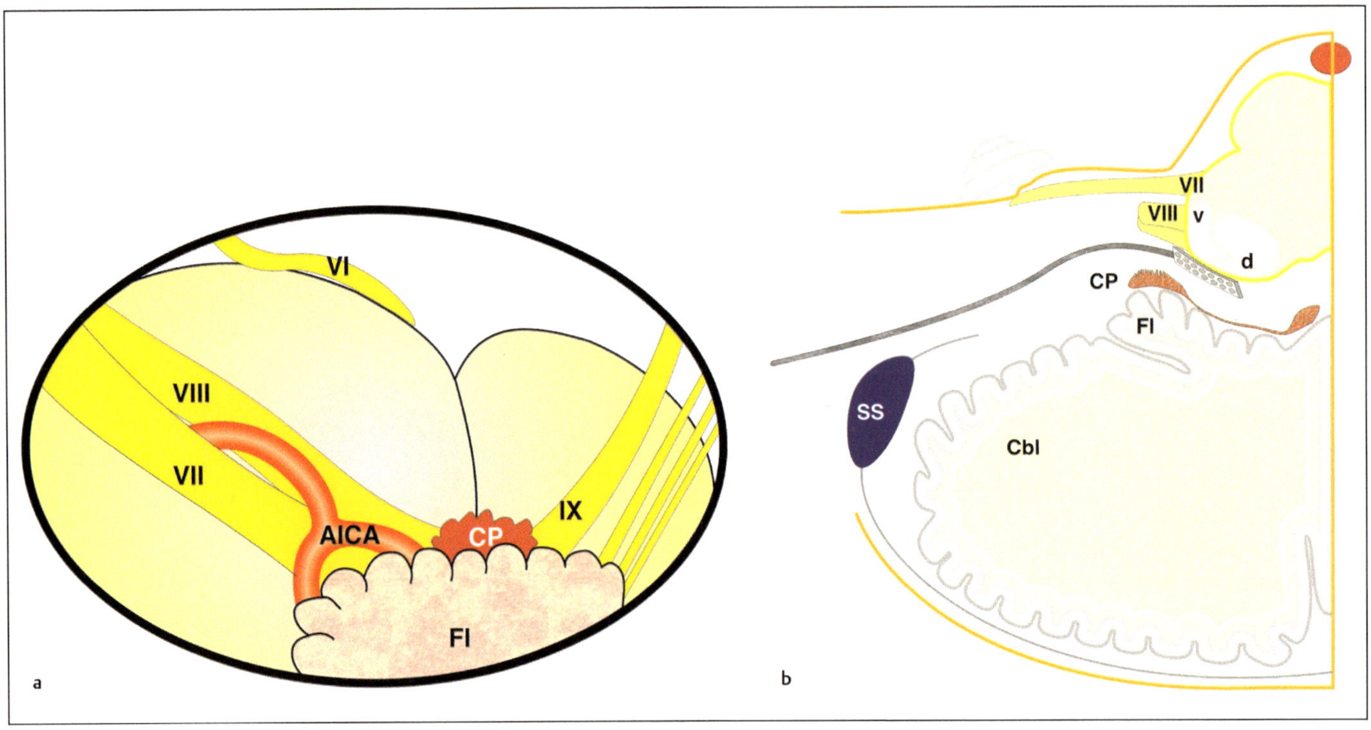

Fig. 2.50a, b

a Landmarks for identifying the foramen of Luschka. The choroid plexus (CP) exits the foramen. AICA, anterior inferior cerebellar artery; Fl, flocculus; VI, abducens nerve; VII, facial nerve; VIII, vestibulocochlear nerve; IX, glossopharyngeal nerve.

b Anatomy of the fourth ventricle and the lateral recess and the location of the cochlear nucleus. This illustration shows an ideal placement of an array of electrodes. Cbl, cerebellum; CP, choroid plexus; d, dorsal cochlear nucleus; Fl, flocculus; SS, sigmoid sinus; v, ventral cochlear nucleus; VII, facial nerve; VIII, stump of the vestibulocochlear nerve.

The Choroid Plexus, Luschka Foramen, and Lateral Recess of the Fourth Ventricle

Both the choroid plexus and Luschka foramen are important landmarks for access to the lateral recess of the fourth ventricle and to the ventral and dorsal cochlear nucleus. The choroid plexus and Luschka foramen can be found at the base of the vestibulocochlear and glossopharyngeal nerves (**Fig. 2.50–Fig. 2.53**), located just posteriorly. Identification of the flocculus of the cerebellum leads to the choroid plexus, which projects from the fourth ventricle and exits through the Luschka foramen. The choroid plexus, present in all ventricles in the brain, is highly vascularized tissue producing cerebrospinal fluid (CSF) filtered out of blood. It also has a filtering function to clean the CSF of metabolic waste material, excess of neurotransmitters, and foreign substances and thus has a function in maintaining the delicate extracellular environment of the CSF. The lateral recess with the Luschka foramina (on both sides), together with the foramen of Magendie, form the only connection of the fourth ventricle with the subarachnoid space, which needs to be open to make circulation of CSF possible.[14]

Retracting the choroid plexus posterior-laterally will open up the foramen of Luschka some more, giving access to the lateral recess of the fourth ventricle.

On the inferior-lateral side of the Luschka foramen, a sheetlike structure is visible: the rhomboid lip, which forms an extension of the choroid plexus and is part of the taenia choroidea extending further superior-medially. The rhomboid lip, forming a pouch on the anterior-lateral side of the Luschka foramen, sometimes needs to be cut to provide access to the foramen. The taenia choroidea forms a small visible ridge of tissue on the posterior-lateral surface of the pons and is considered the line of separation between the intraventricular and extraventricular parts of the ventral cochlear nucleus.[16–19]

Compression of these anatomical structures by a vestibular schwannoma or another tumor can distort the anatomy and make recognition more difficult. Additional confirmation of the right location can be acquired by the anesthesiologist performing the Valsalva maneuver in the patient; this will show CSF coming from the Luschka foramen.

Landmarks of the Lateral Recess

- Origin of the vestibulocochlear and glossopharyngeal nerve
- The flocculus of the cerebellum
- The choroid plexus exiting the foramen of Luschka

The lateral recess is a curved pouch formed by the union of the "roof" (posterior) and the "floor" (anterior) of the fourth ventricle. It varies in size in between individuals. The anterior surface consists of the medial and inferior cerebellar peduncle connecting the pons and medulla with the cerebellum; the posterior surface of the lateral recess is formed by the cerebellum; medially it is the fourth ventricle.

Obtaining access to the lateral recess is easier in the translabyrinthine approach: a gentle retraction of the flocculus is enough to expose the root entry zone of the eighth cranial nerve and the choroid plexus. In contrast, access in the retrosigmoidal approach necessitates significantly more retraction of the cerebellum and flocculus, because the approach to the CPA is from more posteriorly.

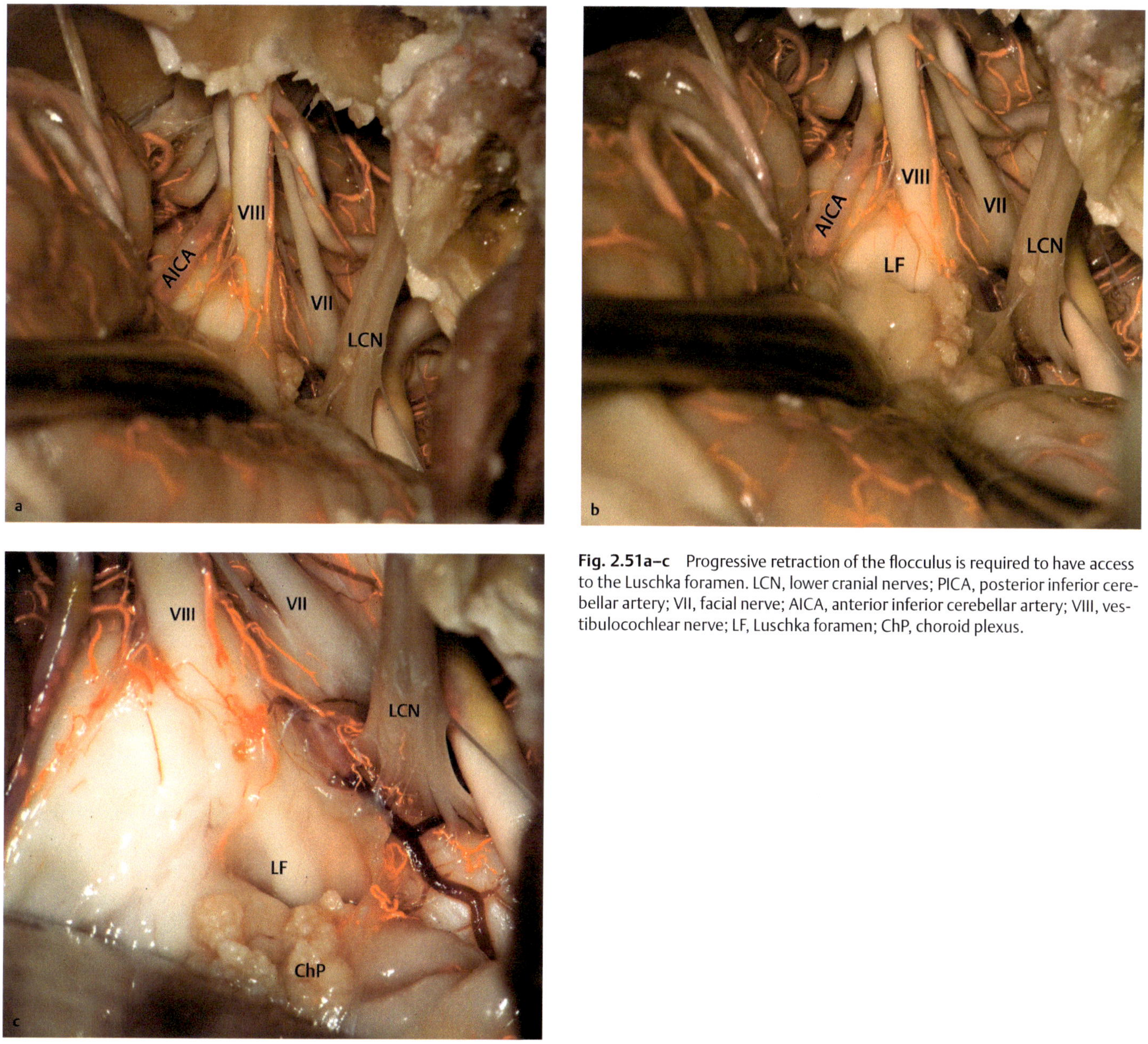

Fig. 2.51a–c Progressive retraction of the flocculus is required to have access to the Luschka foramen. LCN, lower cranial nerves; PICA, posterior inferior cerebellar artery; VII, facial nerve; AICA, anterior inferior cerebellar artery; VIII, vestibulocochlear nerve; LF, Luschka foramen; ChP, choroid plexus.

The Ventral and Dorsal Cochlear Nuclei

The cochlear nucleus extends from the root entry zone of the vestibulocochlear nerve at the posterior-lateral surface of the brainstem to the anterior wall ("floor") of the lateral recess of the fourth ventricle medially.

The **ventral cochlear nucleus** is positioned on the posterior-lateral surface of the inferior cerebellar peduncle of the brainstem. It is situated partly outside the lateral recess (extraventricular) and partly inside the lateral recess (intraventricular); the taenia choroidea separates the two. The ventral cochlear nucleus is difficult to visualize and can be partially hidden by the rhomboid lip, choroid plexus, and flocculus. The ventral cochlear nucleus might be affected in tumors affecting the CPA or Luschka foramen.[17] In case of tumor removal with sectioning of the cochlear nerve, accelerated degeneration of the proximal parts of the cochlear nerve will also include the extraventricular part of the ventral cochlear nucleus, as this structure consists mainly of axons of the cochlear spiral ganglion cells. This area is also known as the root entry zone.[15,18]

The **dorsal cochlear nucleus** is situated in the anterior wall of the lateral recess of the fourth ventricle (the "floor") on the posterior surface of the inferior cerebellar peduncle. It can be clearly seen as a prominence, called the auditory tubercle. Its position is lateral to the hypoglossal nucleus and the vestibular area. Tumors affecting the lateral recess or anterior-inferior part of the lateral recess will influence the dorsal cochlear nucleus.

Surgical Positioning of the ABI

There is controversy whether the ABI should be in contact with the ventral cochlear nucleus (giving better tonotopical representation and better access to the higher auditory pathways[15,20] but being more difficult to reach with less opportunity for fixation and having nuclei and tracts in the vicinity that could give nonauditory side effects) or with the dorsal cochlear nucleus (which is clearly visible as a prominence, gives better opportunities for fixation of the electrode carrier, and can be better stimulated because it is more superficially positioned in the pons). It must also be considered that the ventral cochlear nucleus, especially

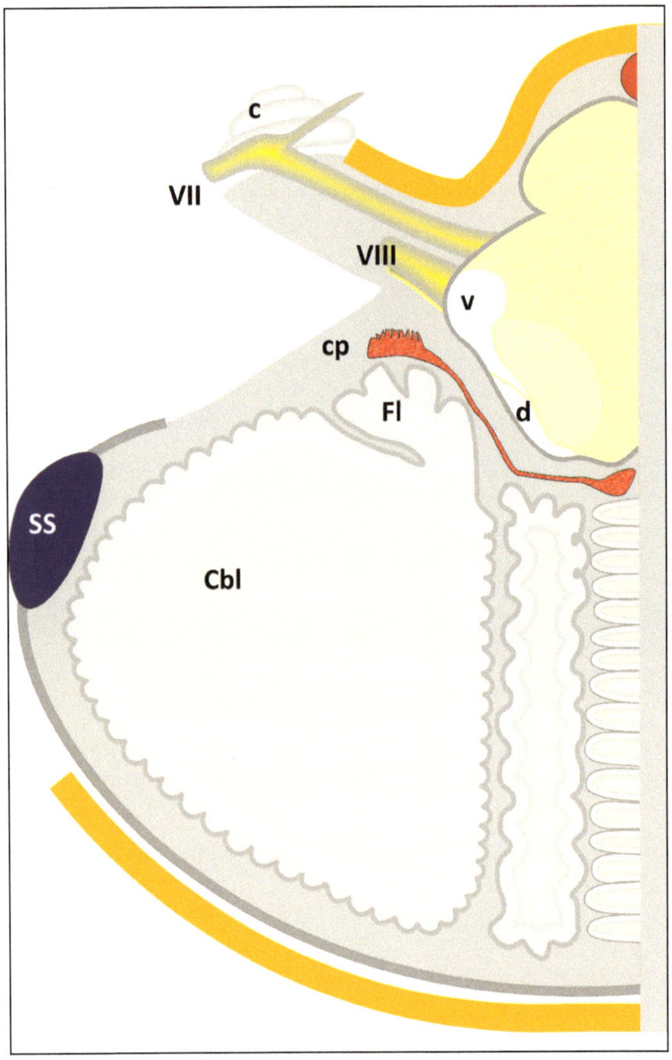

Fig. 2.52 Schematic drawing of the position of the cochlear nuclei. The flocculus (Fl) obstructs the opening of the Luschka foramen and the entrance of the lateral recess. Within the lateral recess the choroid plexus (CP) is the most prominent structure and is the best landmark for the Luschka foramen and the lateral recess. The facial nerve (VII) is more ventrally (anteriorly) located; dorsally (posterior), the cochleovestibular nerve (VIII). The positions of the ventral and dorsal cochlear nuclei (v and d) are schematically indicated. SS, sigmoid sinus; Cbl, cerebellum; C, cochlea.

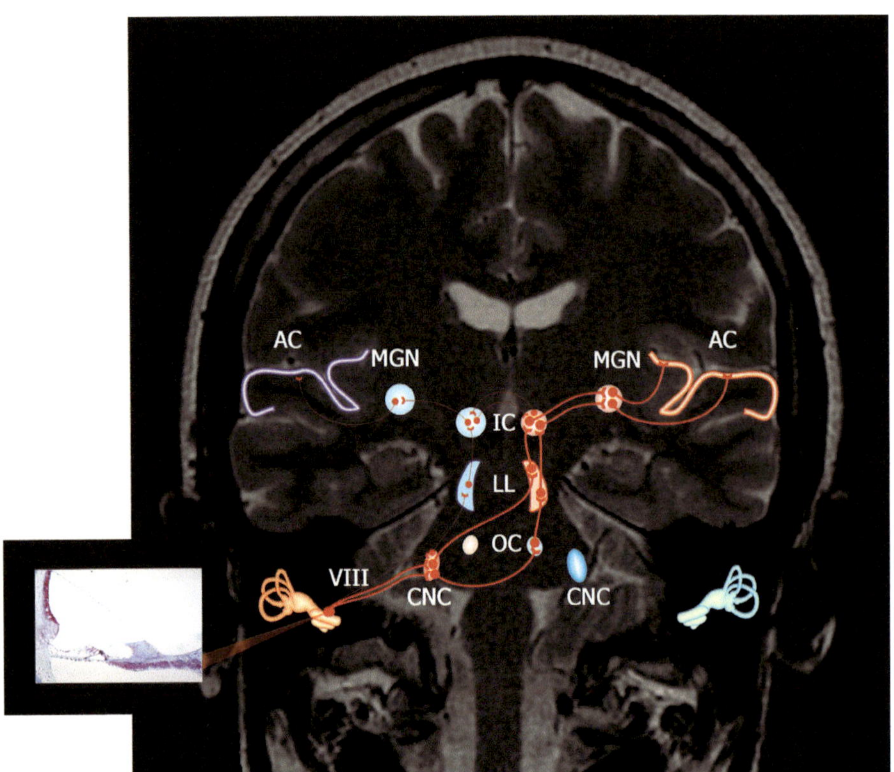

Fig. 2.53 Schematic representation of ascending auditory pathways. VIII, cochlear nerve; CNC, cochlear nucleus complex; OC, superior olivary complex; LL, tract and nuclei of the lateral lemniscus; IC, inferior colliculus; MGN, medial geniculate body; AC, auditory cortex.

the extraventricular part, is more often affected by compression or degeneration of neural axons. Brackmann et al, as well as Terr et al, recommended placement entirely within the lateral recess, stimulating the dorsal cochlear nucleus as well as the intraventricular part of the ventral cochlear nucleus to give low stimulation thresholds and good speech audiometric performance with minimal nonauditory effects.[15,17,20]

The surface of the electrode carrier of the ABI should face anterior-medially for best contact with the posterior-lateral surface of the brainstem, the position of the cochlear nucleus.

It should make a 140° degree angulation superiorly toward the axis of the vestibulocochlear nerve[17] and also be pointed posterior-medially for best contact with the cochlear nucleus, while the electrodes should face anterior-medially. An easier way to remember this is, for the right ear, to position the electrode carrier to the 1 o'clock position in relation to the 12 o'clock position being the position of the exit of the vestibulocochlear nerve, while for the left ear it should be the 11 o'clock position.

Information on the correct positioning of the electrode carrier with optimal contact with the cochlear nucleus can best be measured during surgery: EABR will give guidance in the position of the ABI and will make possible small adjustments in position for better auditory stimulation.[19] During ABI stimulation, non-auditory effects can also arise due to activation of other cranial nerve nuclei or tracts in the region of the cochlear nucleus and lateral recess. In order of frequency of occurrence, this can be related to the location of the nuclei and tracts: vestibular, vagal (cardiac arrest), hypoglossal, glossopharyngeal, and facial nerve. Monitoring of the cranial nerves V, VII, IX, and X is therefore advised as well as the EABR recordings.

References

1. Sanna M. Anatomy of the posterior mesotympanum. In: Zini C. Sheehy J, Sanna M, eds. Microsurgery of Cholesteatoma of the Middle Ear. Milan: Ghedini; 1980:69–73
2. Gacek RR. Surgical landmark for the facial nerve in the epitympanum. Ann Otol Rhinol Laryngol 1980;89(3 Pt 1):249–250
3. Schuknecht HF, Gulya AJ. Anatomy of the Temporal Bone with Surgical Implications. Philadelphia: Lea & Febiger; 1986
4. Roland PS, Wright CG, Isaacson B. Cochlear implant electrode insertion: the round window revisited. Laryngoscope 2007;117(8):1397–1402
5. Shapira Y, Eshraghi AA, Balkany TJ. The perceived angle of the round window affects electrode insertion trauma in round window insertion—an anatomical study. Acta Otolaryngol 2011;131(3):284–289
6. Okuno H, Sando I. Anatomy of the round window. A histopathological study with a graphic reconstruction method. Acta Otolaryngol 1988;106(1-2):55–63
7. Franz BKH, Clark GM, Bloom DM. Surgical anatomy of the round window with special reference to cochlear implantation. J Laryngol Otol 1987;101(2):97–102
8. Briggs RJS, Tykocinski M, Stidham K, Roberson JB. Cochleostomy site: implications for electrode placement and hearing preservation. Acta Otolaryngol 2005;125(8):870–876
9. Adunka OF, Radeloff A, Gstoettner WK, Pillsbury HC, Buchman CA. Scala tympani cochleostomy II: topography and histology. Laryngoscope 2007;117(12):2195–2200
10. Hamamoto M, Murakami G, Kataura A. Topographical relationships among the facial nerve, chorda tympani nerve and round window with special reference to the approach route for cochlear implant surgery. Clin Anat 2000;13(4):251–256
11. Meshik X, Holden TA, Chole RA, Hullar TE. Optimal cochlear implant insertion vectors. Otol Neurotol 2010;31(1):58–63
12. Sanna M, Sunose H, Mancini F, Russo A, Taibah A. Middle Ear and Mastoid Microsurgery. 2nd ed. Stuttgart: Thieme; 2012
13. Sekhar LN, Estonillo R. Transtemporal approach to the skull base: an anatomical study. Neurosurgery 1986;19(5):799–808
14. Sharifi M, Ungier E, Ciszek B, Krajewski P. Microsurgical anatomy of the foramen of Luschka in the cerebellopontine angle, and its vascular supply. Surg Radiol Anat 2009;31(6):431–437
15. Terr LI, Fayad J, Hitselberger WE, Zakhary R. Cochlear nucleus anatomy related to central electroauditory prosthesis implantation. Otolaryngol Head Neck Surg 1990;102(6):717–721
16. Wen HT, Rhoton AL Jr, Katsuta T, de Oliveira E. Microsurgical anatomy of the transcondylar, supracondylar, and paracondylar extensions of the far-lateral approach. J Neurosurg 1997;87(4):555–585
17. Abe H, Rhoton AL Jr. Microsurgical anatomy of the cochlear nuclei. Neurosurgery 2006;58(4):728–739, discussion 728–739
18. Quester R, Schröder R. Topographic anatomy of the cochlear nuclear region at the floor of the fourth ventricle in humans. J Neurosurg 1999;91(3):466–476
19. Nevison B. A guide to the positioning of brainstem implants using intraoperative electrical auditory brainstem responses. Adv Otorhinolgaryngol 2006;64:154–166
20. Brackmann DE, Hitselberger WE, Nelson RA, et al. Auditory brainstem implant: I. Issues in surgical implantation. Otolaryngol Head Neck Surg 1993;108(6):624–633

Further Reading

Adunka O, Gstoettner W, Hambek M, Unkelbach MH, Radeloff A, Kiefer J. Preservation of basal inner ear structures in cochlear implantation. ORL J Otorhinolaryngol Relat Spec 2004;66(6):306–312

Bielamowicz SA, Coker NJ, Jenkins HA, Igarashi M. Surgical dimensions of the facial recess in adults and children. Arch Otolaryngol Head Neck Surg 1988;114(5):534–537

Briggs RJS, Tykocinski M, Xu J, et al. Comparison of round window and cochleostomy approaches with a prototype hearing preservation electrode. Audiol Neurootol 2006;11(Suppl 1):42–48

Eby TL, Nadol JB Jr. Postnatal growth of the human temporal bone. Implications for cochlear implants in children. Ann Otol Rhinol Laryngol 1986;95(4 Pt 1):356–364

Sanna M, Khrais T, Falcioni M, Russo A, Taibah A. The Temporal Bone, a Manual for Dissection and Surgical Approaches. Stuttgart: Thieme; 2006

Sanna M, Mancini F, Russo A, Taibah A, Falcioni M. , Di Trapani G. Atlas of Acoustic Neurinoma Microsurgery. 2nd ed. Stuttgart: Thieme; 2011

Sanna M, Saleh E, Khrais T, et al. Atlas of Microsurgery of the Lateral Skull Base. 2nd ed. Stuttgart: Thieme; 2008

Schwartz MS, Otto SR, Shannon RV, Hitselberger WE, Brackmann DE. Auditory brainstem implants. Neurotherapeutics 2008;5(1):128–136

3 Radiology in Auditory Implantation

Imaging is only a part of the work-up in cochlear and auditory brainstem implantation as these patients are thoroughly evaluated by a multidisciplinary team before the decision for implantation is made (see Chapter 5). Nevertheless, imaging remains indispensable in this process for judging the feasibility of surgery and may influence the side of implantation, the surgical approach, the type of device, and the type of electrode; at the same time it might give information on the cause of hearing loss.

Contraindications for cochlear implantation can result in no intervention, a staged procedure, or an indication for implantation of an auditory brainstem implant (ABI). It might additionally alter the counseling of the patient or parents regarding the outcomes of implantation, the possible alternative surgical strategies, and the additional risks of surgery. Sometimes it might be necessary to refer to another, more experienced cochlear implant team.

Appropriate training for systematically judging and interpreting the different structures on the CT and MRI scans is necessary in the work-up for implantation. We advise that you develop your own standard routine and review all structures: this is the best form of training. In our experience, blind confidence in radiology reports is unwise; it is especially the combination of surgical and anatomical knowledge with radiologic information wherein lies the additional value of the ENT surgeon. Nonetheless, proper collaboration or consultation with an experienced (neuro-)radiologist is deemed essential.

In this chapter the general radiology of the temporal bone and the cerebellopontine angle is discussed, with a special focus on radiologic evaluation prior to auditory implantation. Particular radiologic topics (such as meningitis or otosclerosis) are addressed in the special indications section of this book (see Chapters 12 to 17).

3.1 General Radiology of the Temporal Bone

Otologists and neurotologists have to be familiar with the advantages and drawbacks of both CT and MRI scanning modalities and should be able to choose the appropriate one according to the nature of the pathology and of course to the planned surgery.

3.1.1 Computed Tomography

Multislice high-resolution CT allows precise demonstration of fine middle ear structures such as the ossicular chain and the inner ear, with thin slices of less than 1 mm, in limited scanning time. The preferred direction of axial scanning or reconstruction should be at the plane of the lateral semicircular canal.

Preoperative identification of the ossicular chain, the labyrinth, the middle and posterior fossa dura with sigmoid sinus, the facial nerve canal, and the pneumatization of the mastoid helps to plan a surgical strategy and to reduce surgical risks. A CT scan can be seen as a geographical map guiding one toward the cochlea. It also gives the surgeon a chance to recognize anatomical variations such as a low middle cranial fossa dura, an anterior sigmoid sinus, a high jugular bulb, or a poorly pneumatized mastoid. **Table 3.1** gives an overview of the important structures to be checked prior to cochlear implant (CI) surgery.

3.1.2 Magnetic Resonance Imaging

In contrast to a CT scan, MRI excels in distinguishing different soft tissues without showing the bony anatomical margins. The different types of sequences in MRI, with and without contrast, make MRI extremely helpful in the assessment of the patency of the cochlea, the nerves in the internal auditory canal (especially in the sagittal plane), pathology in the cerebellopontine angle (CPA), and intracranial pathology including the auditory pathway.

These two modalities, CT and MRI, are complementary, and preferably both should be employed in implant surgery. CT imaging, however, represents the geographical map and is of overriding importance. The accessibility and cost of MRI can be of con-

Table 3.1 Checklist for preoperative CT examination for cochlear implantation

Location	Check
Mastoid	Pneumatization
	Position of the facial nerve
	Position of the middle cranial fossa dura Anterior or lateral position of the sigmoid sinus
	Mastoid–round window axis: how is the access and angle to the basal turn?
Middle ear	High/dehiscent jugular bulb
	Aberrant /dehiscent carotid artery
	Persistent stapedial artery
	Aberrant facial nerve presence of ossicles
	Other
Cochlea	
ossification	See Chapter 11: ossification
otosclerosis	see Chapter 13: otosclerosis
morphology	See Chapter 15: malformations
Internal auditory canal and vestibular aqueduct	See Chapter 15: malformations
Presence of pathology	See Chapters 10, 14, and 17 (fracture, tumors, infection, etc.)

Source: adapted from Lo 1998.[2]

Table 3.2 Radiologic differential diagnosis of cochlear, labyrinthine, and IAC lesions

Lesion	CT	MRI T1W	MRI T2W (heavily weighted)	MRI T1C+	Special features
Cochlea and labyrinth					
Obliteration/fibrosis	Not visible	→	↓	– (passive) + (active)	Enhancement depending on stage of inflammation
Ossification	Calcification (mostly in basal turn of scala tympani)	→	↓	–	Seen in end stage of inflammation
Inflammation/labyrinthitis	Not visible	→	→ ↓	+	Due to meningitis, infection, trauma, autoimmune
Hemorrhage	Not visible	↑	→ ↑	→ +	hyperintensity T1W without contrast most important
Intracochlear schwannoma	Normal cochlea, bony erosion rare	→ ↑	Focal defect	+ (focal enhancement)	
Cochlear otosclerosis	Bone hypodensity around the labyrinth	→ Ring visible	→, Rarely ↑ foci	+ Foci	CT most important Starts anteriorly to the vestibule, fissura ante fenestram
Malformation	All labyrinth malformations visible	–	Malformation best visible	–	Classification according to dysformity
Internal auditory canal (IAC)					
IAC	Bony IAC	→	↑	→	Diameter best seen on CT
Cranial nerve hypoplasia/aplasia	Not visible	–	Best visible	–	Sagittal imaging through the IAC gives most information
Vestibular schwannoma	Not visible	↓ →	→ ↑	+	IAC involved; acute bone tumor angle; often cystic
Meningioma	Sometimes permeative-sclerotic changes	↓ →	→ ↑	+	Dural tail, obtuse bone-tumor angle

cern, but MRI is necessary when there is doubt about cochlear patency or cochlear nerve integrity or to evaluate possible intracranial lesions, see **Table 3.2**. Some surgeons report having made MRI the preferred modality in preoperative imaging for cochlear implantation.[1]

Indications for MRI in CI Surgery

- Uncertainty about ossification or patency of the cochlea, especially in the acute phase of disease (in meningitis, otosclerosis, autoimmune inner ear disease, or trauma cases).
- Uncertainty about the presence of cochlear nerve aplasia, hypoplasia (in unilateral or bilateral congenital sensorineural hearing loss, cochleovestibular malformations, or a narrow internal auditory canal or in auditory neuropathy).
- Uncertainty about the presence of a CPA or petrous apex lesion.
- Suspicion of an intracranial lesion or to rule out intracranial lesions after meningitis, cytomegalovirus infection, and other pathologies.

3.2 Radiology in Cochlear Implantation

In standard cochlear implantation the cochlear implant (CI) electrode is introduced through the transmastoid posterior tympanotomy, inserted through or near the round window, and advanced in the scala tympani of the basal turn toward the apical turn. Hence, the radiologic anatomy of the mastoid cavity, the facial recess, the tympanic cavity, the course of the facial nerve in all segments, the chorda tympani, the cochlea, the round window niche, the scalae, and the internal auditory canal with its nerves must be carefully evaluated by preoperative imaging. A radiology checklist prior to CI surgery can be seen in **Table 3.1** Malformations or other causes of hearing loss can also be revealed. Also other possible pathology must be excluded. Cochlear and internal auditory canal (IAC) examination is particularly important and a helpful overview of the distinguishing features of different cochlear and IAC pathologies is given in **Table 3.2**.

3.3 Radiology in Auditory Brainstem Implantation

In auditory brainstem implantation the route toward the brainstem can be either via an enlarged translabyrinthine approach or via a retrosigmoid approach. Both approaches require sufficient knowledge of the CPA and brainstem, and of the translabyrinthine or retrosigmoidal region.

In addition to knowledge of the radiologic anatomy, for cochlear implantation information is needed on the labyrinth, the jugular bulb, the cochlear aqueduct, the width of the fourth ventricle, and access to the Luschka foramen. Knowledge of the other cranial nerves and vessels is also necessary.

3.4 Axial and Coronal CT Sections

Abbreviations

The following abbreviations are used in the images presented in the following pages.

A: antrum
Ad: aditus ad antrum
ALC: ampulla of lateral semicircular canal
APC: ampulla of posterior semicircular canal
ASC: ampulla of superior semicircular canal
C: cochlea
COA: cochlear aperture
C2: second turn of cochlea
Ca: apical turn of the cochlea
Cb: basal turn of the cochlea
Cm: middle turn of the cochlea
CA: carotid artery
CAq: cochlear aqueduct
CC: common crus
CP: cochleariform process
CT: chorda tympani
EV: emissary vein
EAC: external auditory canal
FL: flocculus
FN: facial nerve
FP: footplate of stapes
FR: foramen rotundum
GG: geniculate ganglion
GSP: great superficial petrosal nerve
HC: horizontal crest (falciform crest)
Hyc: hypoglossal canal
I: incus
ISJ: incudostapedial joint
IAC: internal auditory canal
JB: jugular bulb
KS: Körner septum
LF: Luschka foramen
LP: lenticular process of incus
LR: lateral recess of the fourth ventricle
LS: labyrinthine segment of facial nerve
LSC: lateral semicircular canal
M: malleus
P: promontory
PE: pyramidal eminence
PSC posterior semicircular canal
RW: round window
RWN: round window niche
S: stapes
SA: subarcuate artery
SH: head of stapes
SM: stapedius muscle
SN: canal for singular nerve
SS: sigmoid sinus
SSC: superior semicircular canal
SSL: superior suspensory ligament
TMJ: temporomandibular joint
TTm: tensor tympani muscle
TTt: tendon of tensor tympani muscle
Ty: tympanic membrane
V: vestibule
VA: vestibular aqueduct
VC: vertical crest (Bill's bar)

3.4.1 CT Mastoid Axial Images (Fig. 3.1–Fig. 3.9)

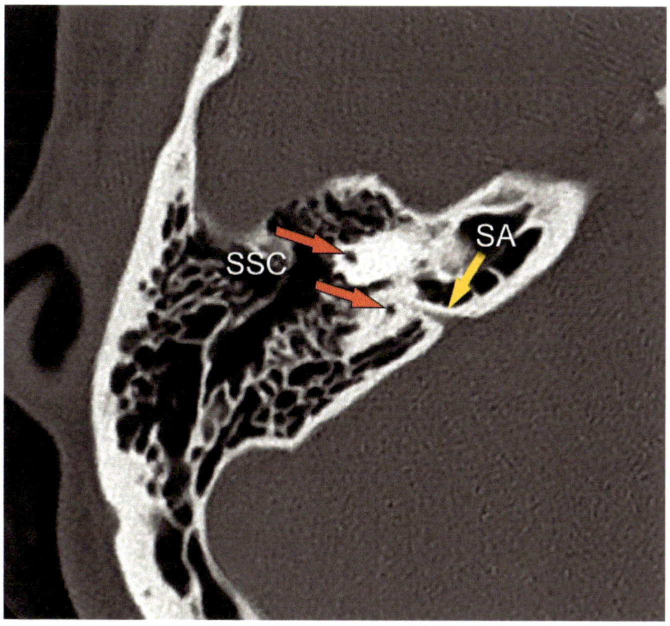

Fig. 3.1 A CT scan is best viewed in a standardized routine as part of a structured approach to diminish the chance of overlooking pathology. Both sequences, axial and coronal, need to be viewed, either from superior to inferior and subsequently anterior to posterior or vice versa. Pneumatization and aeration of the mastoid, the position of the subarcuate artery (SA, *yellow arrow*) and the superior semicircular canal (SSC, *red arrows*), which is cut twice in this image, can be appreciated.

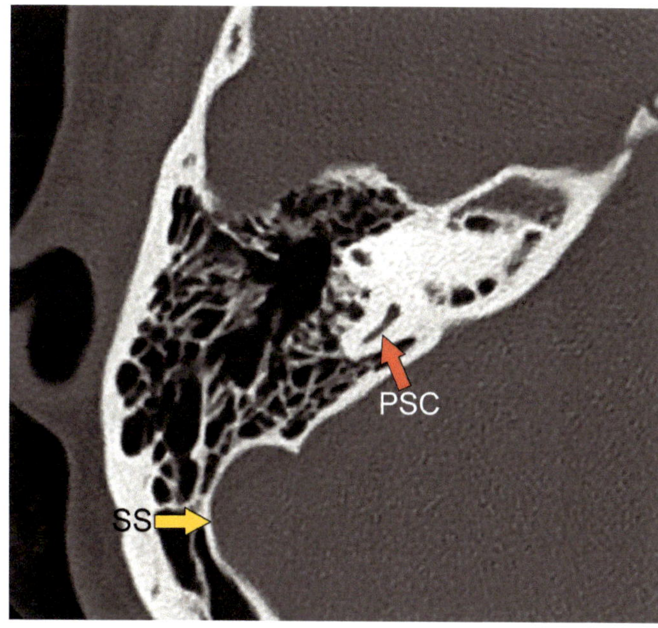

Fig. 3.2 The posterior semicircular canal (PSC) is perpendicular to the direction of the SSC and runs parallel to the posterior cranial fossa. The posterior cranial fossa is bordered laterally by the sigmoid sinus (SS). In this case the sigmoid sinus is not obstructing the access and the view into the middle ear in case of a transmastoidal approach.

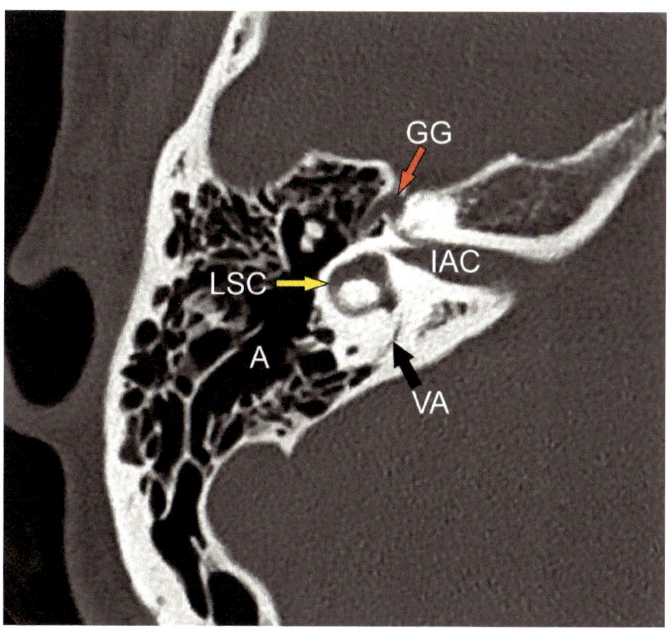

Fig. 3.3 The lateral semicircular canal (LSC) and its surroundings. In this image, a well pneumatized mastoid is present; the largest mastoidal cell, the antrum (A), can be clearly seen. The internal auditory canal (IAC), with the labyrinthine part of the facial nerve is just splitting off the IAC in this picture. The first genu of the nerve at the ganglion geniculi (GG, *red arrow*) and the start of the tympanic part of the facial nerve can also be seen here. The vestibular aqueduct (VA) is normal in size and should not exceed 1.5 mm (see Chapter 15 on malformations). Note that the apex of the petrous bone is filled with bone marrow.

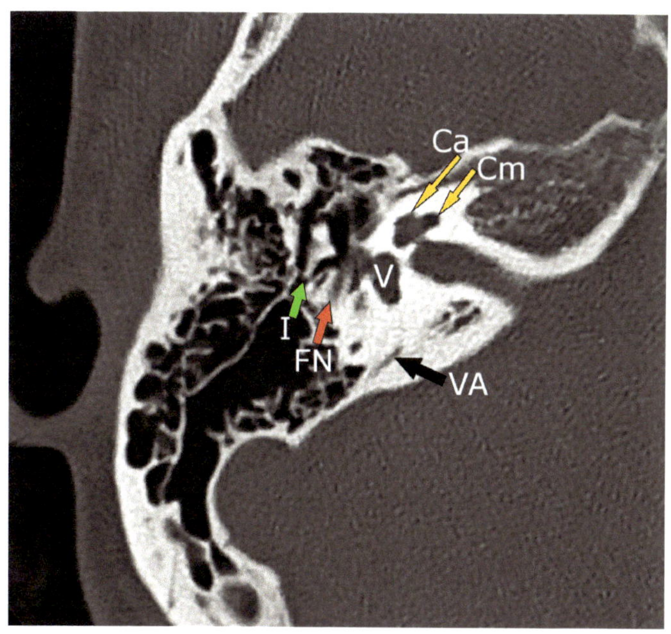

Fig. 3.4 The apical (Ca) and middle turn (Cm) are now visible, situated anterior-medially to the vestibule (V) of the labyrinth. Furthermore, the short process of the incus (I, *green arrow*) is visible, which runs directly parallel to the tympanic part of the facial nerve (FN, *red arrow*) just anterior to the second genu. The facial nerve turns at the second genu from the horizontal tympanic section to the more vertical mastoidal section.

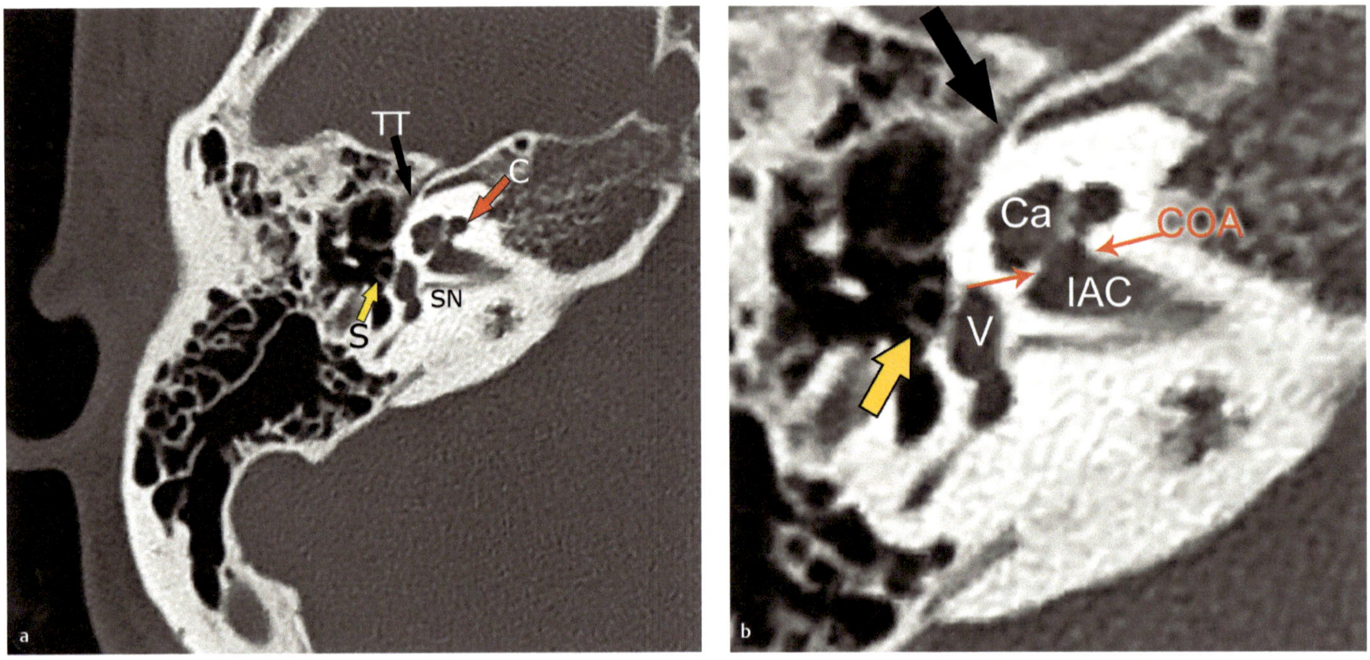

Fig. 3.5 a, b The axial view at the level of the stapes (*yellow arrow*). Both crurae of the stapes are visible just lateral to the vestibule (V). Situated in the junction of the posterior semicircular canal and the vestibule is the singular nerve canal (SN) also called the posterior ampullary nerve canal. In this image also the tensor tympani tendon (TTt) and muscle (TTm) are seen (*black arrows*). The cochlea (C) is connected with the internal auditory canal through the cochlear aperture (COA, opening between the *red arrows* in the enlargement. Note the septum between the middle turn and apical turn (Ca) along the anterior-medial border of the cochlea, making both turns visible. This is an important structure in differentiating from an incomplete partition type II (see Chapter 15, malformations).

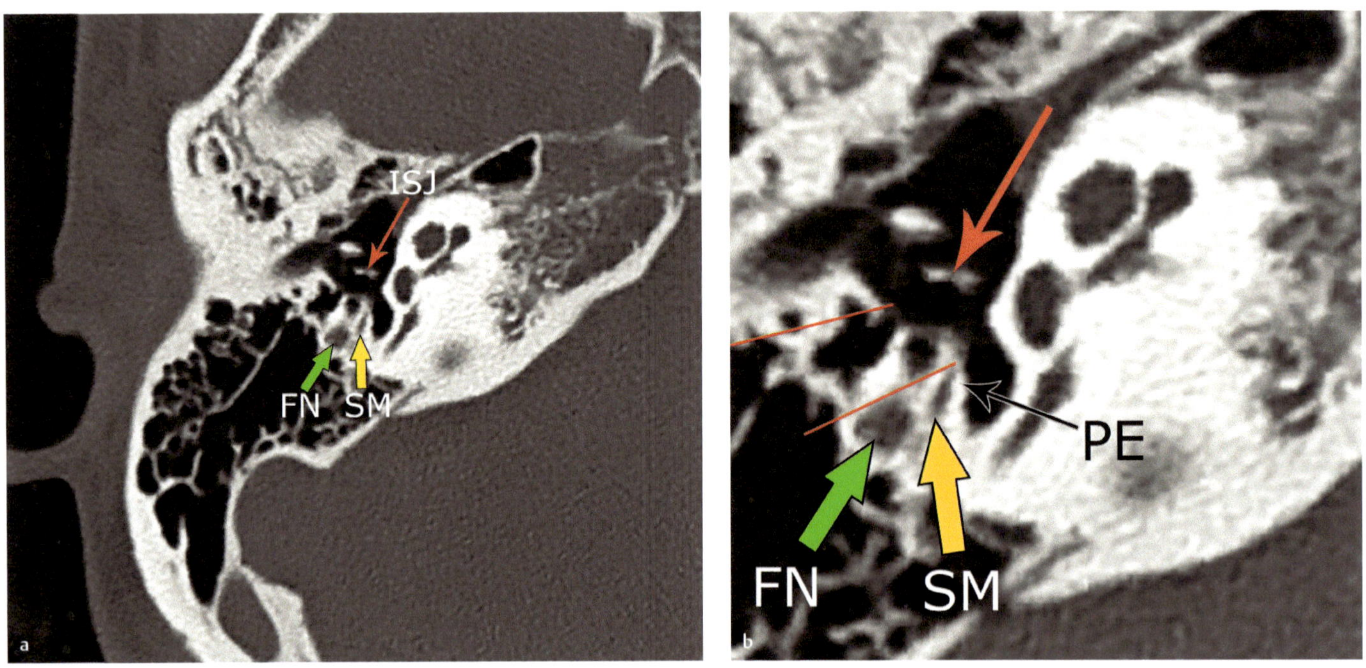

Fig. 3.6 a, b In this image the facial nerve is cut in its vertical position (FN, *green arrow*) and directly medial to it is the tendon of the stapedius muscle (SM, *yellow arrow*), which exits from a triangular shaped process: the pyramidal eminence (PE, enlargement **b**). The head of the stapes and the lenticular process of the incus are marked with a *red arrow* at the incudostapedial joint (ISJ, *red arrow*). This joint is visible through a posterior tympanotomy and to create a good exposure of the round window area first some bone covering the facial nerve and stapedius muscle should be removed. The *red lines* (in insert) represent the direction and opening of the posterior tympanotomy.

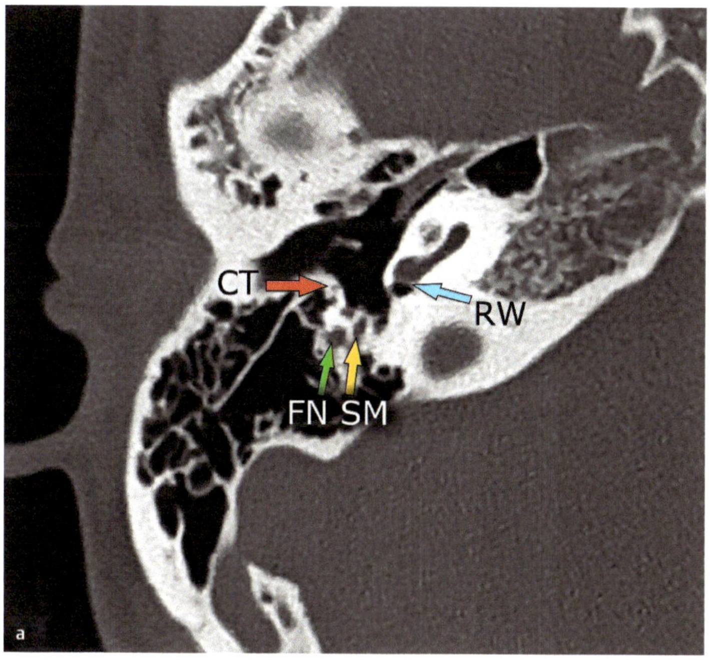

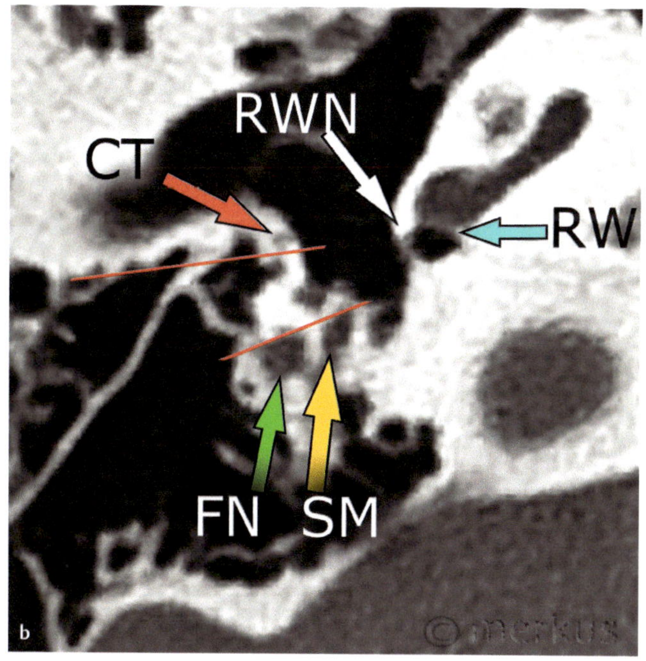

Fig. 3.7 a, b Axial CT scan at the level of the round window (RW, *blue arrow*): At the posterior end of the basal turn the round window and the round window niche (RWN, *white arrow*) can be appreciated. This image provides the surgeon with information about the amount of drilling needed to create a clear view at the round window. Furthermore, the posterior tympanotomy (two *red lines*) can be planned. In this particular case, the lateral area of the posterior tympanotomy is well pneumatized, but more medially still much bone is covering the facial nerve (FN) and the stapedius muscle (SM). The most lateral border of the posterior tympanotomy is the chorda tympani (CT), which can be found in many CT scans if attention is paid to it.

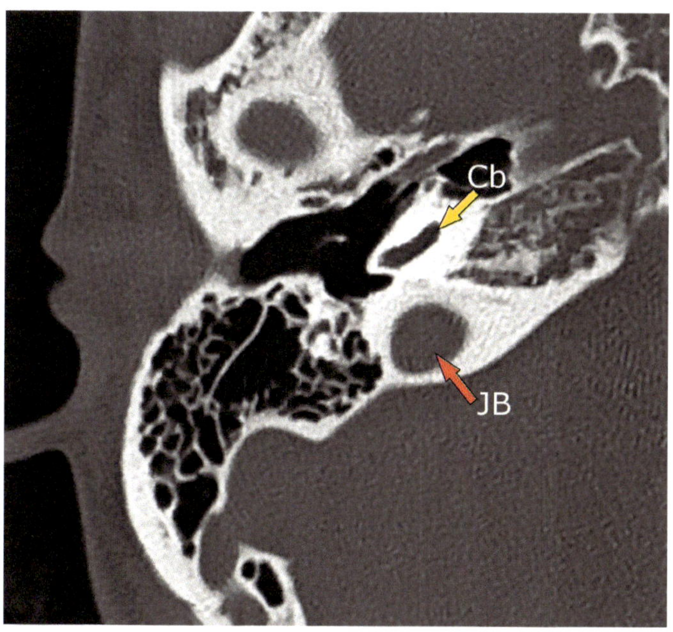

Fig. 3.8 In this image the first part of the basal turn of the cochlea (Cb) is fully visible. This region is mostly affected in ossification cases, so it is important to know its normal appearance. The jugular bulb (JB) can also be seen at this level.

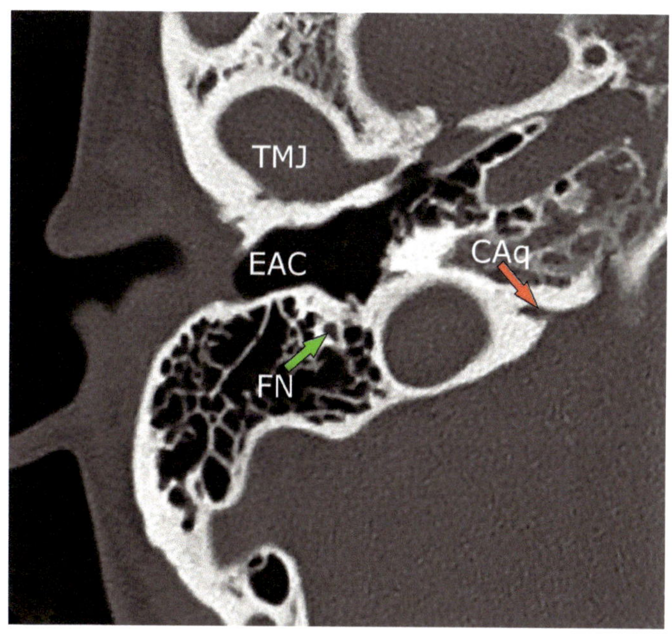

Fig. 3.9 On this axial image in the plane just below the cochlea the horizontal part of the carotid artery and the superior part of the temporomandibular joint (TMJ) become visible. The bony shell of the TMJ is also the anterior border of the external auditory canal (EAC). The posterior ear canal is the anterior border of the mastoid. At this level in the mastoid the facial nerve (FN, *green arrow*) runs in its vertical section. Also the bony canal of the cochlear aqueduct (CAq, *red arrow*) is now well seen, contrary to the more lateral part of the aqueduct. The lateral part of the aqueduct is often hardly visible as the diameter tapers down, running toward the scala tympani of the cochlear basal turn.

3.4.2 CT Mastoid Coronal Images (Fig. 3.10–Fig. 3.14)

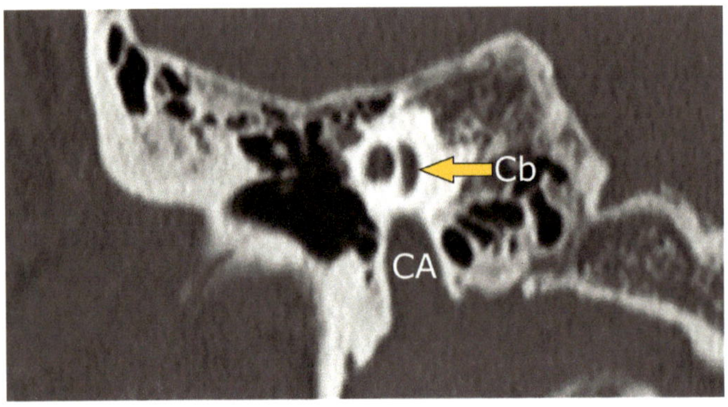

Fig. 3.10 In this most anterior coronal image the cochlear basal turn (Cb, *yellow arrow*) is seen, as well as the carotid artery (CA) directly inferior to the cochlea in this view.

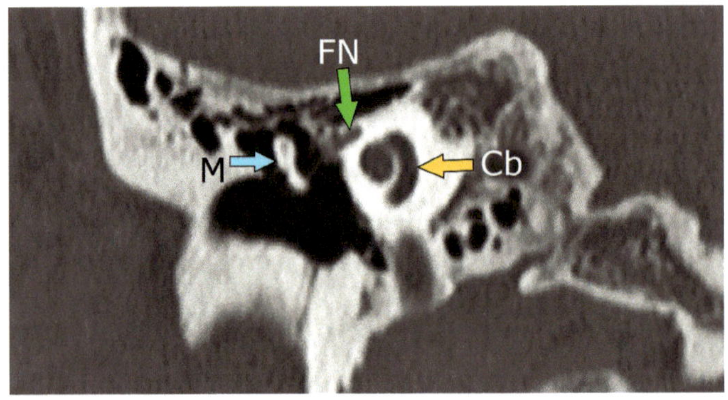

Fig. 3.11 Next to the cochlear basal turn (Cb, *yellow arrow*), the geniculate ganglion of the facial nerve (FN, *green arrow*) and the head of the malleus (M, *blue arrow*) are also visible.

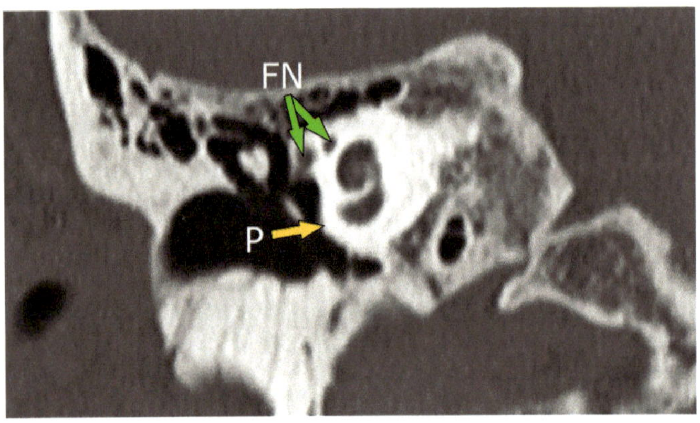

Fig. 3.12 The facial nerve (FN, *green arrows*) is seen in this image in two parts. Closest to the cochlea is the labyrinthine part and more in contact with the middle ear is the tympanic part. More anterior of this image the ganglion geniculi of the facial nerve is located. The bulging bony part within the middle ear is the promontory (P, *yellow arrow*), which is the outer wall of the cochlea.

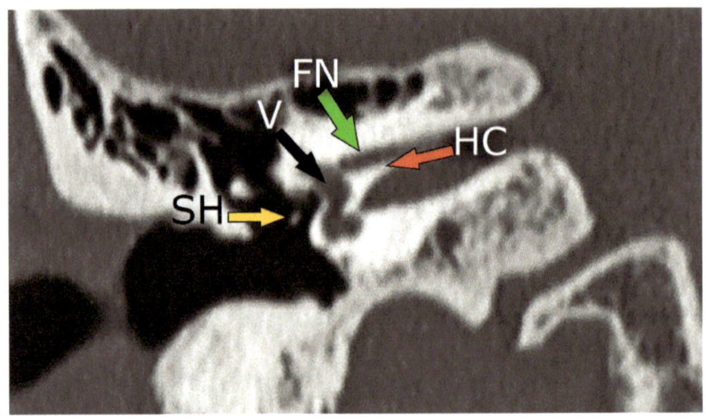

Fig. 3.13 This image, more posterior than the image above, shows the labyrinthine segment of the facial nerve (FN, *green arrow*), the vestibule (V, *black arrow*), and the head of the stapes (SH, *yellow arrow*). The horizontal crest, dividing the fundus of the IAC into a superior half and an inferior half, may also be appreciated (*red arrow*).

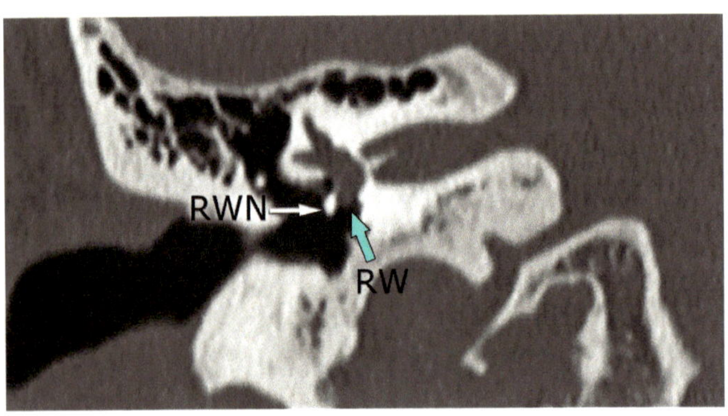

Fig. 3.14 This coronal image is important for an overview of the round window area. The bony overhang of the round window niche (RWN, *white arrow*) and the round window (RW, *blue arrow*) itself can be appreciated.

3.5 Magnetic Resonance Imaging

The MRI sequences for imaging of the CPA/temporal bone can be difficult to distinguish when they are not used regularly. The differences are explained in the overview here. In general, bony structures and air are black and not visible on MRI.

The following mnemonic can be used as a reminder in distinguishing between the different sequences:
"ONE nose and TWO watery eyes"

On T1-weighted (T1W) images *with contrast*, the hyperintense nasal mucosa will stand out, whereas the fluid within the eyes will be hyperintense on T2-weighted (T2W) images.

A T1W image *without contrast* usually has less hyperintense parts and will mainly be valuable in combination with the contrast-enhanced T1W images.

(See **Fig. 3.15–Fig. 3.19**.)

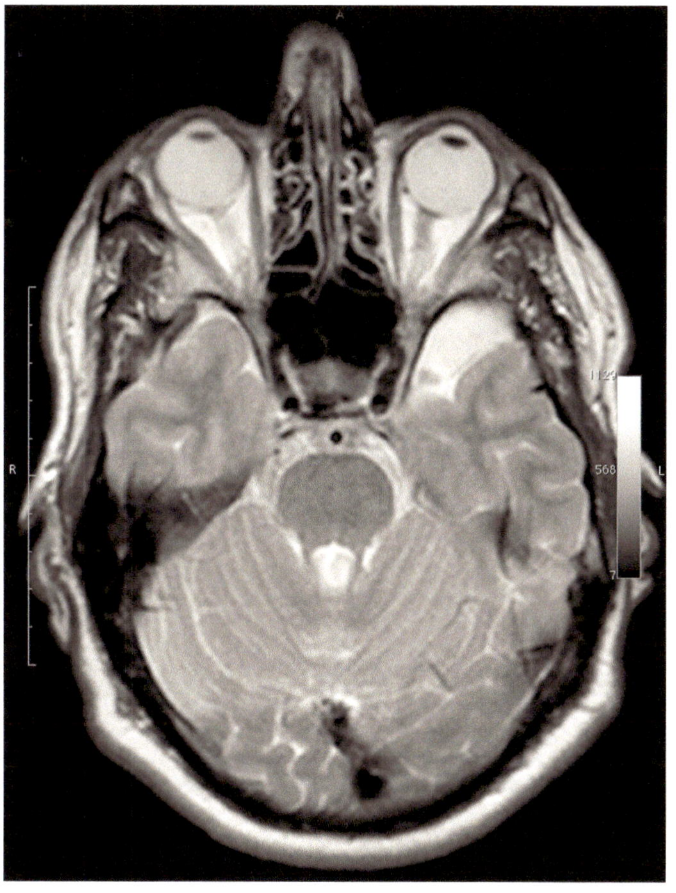

Fig. 3.15 T2W MR image.
Brain: gray/isointense;
CSF: **white/hyperintense**;
Nasal mucosa: gray/isointense;
Eyes: **hyperintense.**

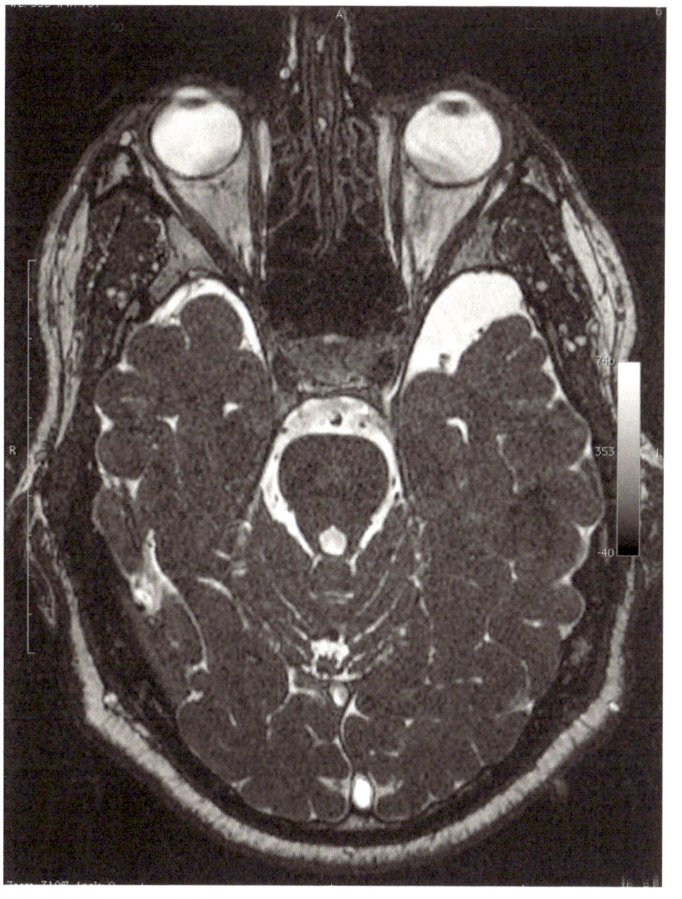

Fig. 3.16 Heavily T2W.
Brain: gray/isointense;
CSF: **white/hyperintense**;
Nasal mucosa: gray/isointense;
Eyes: **hyperintense ("TWO eyes").**

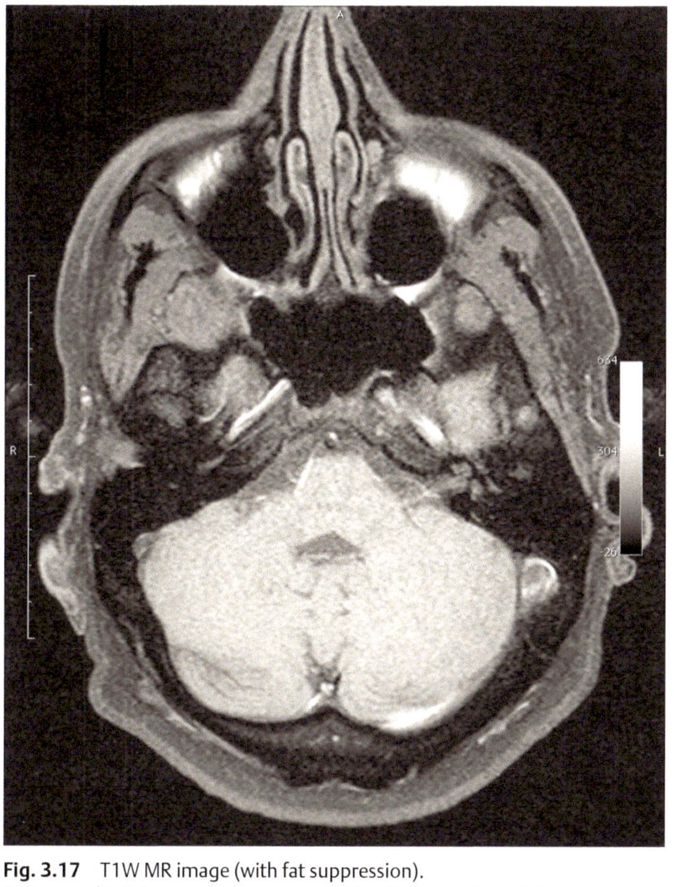

Fig. 3.17 T1W MR image (with fat suppression).
Brain: gray/isointense;
CSF: black/hypointense;
Inflammation: hypointense;
Nasal mucosa: **hypointense**;
Eyes: gray/isointense;
Fat: hypointense.

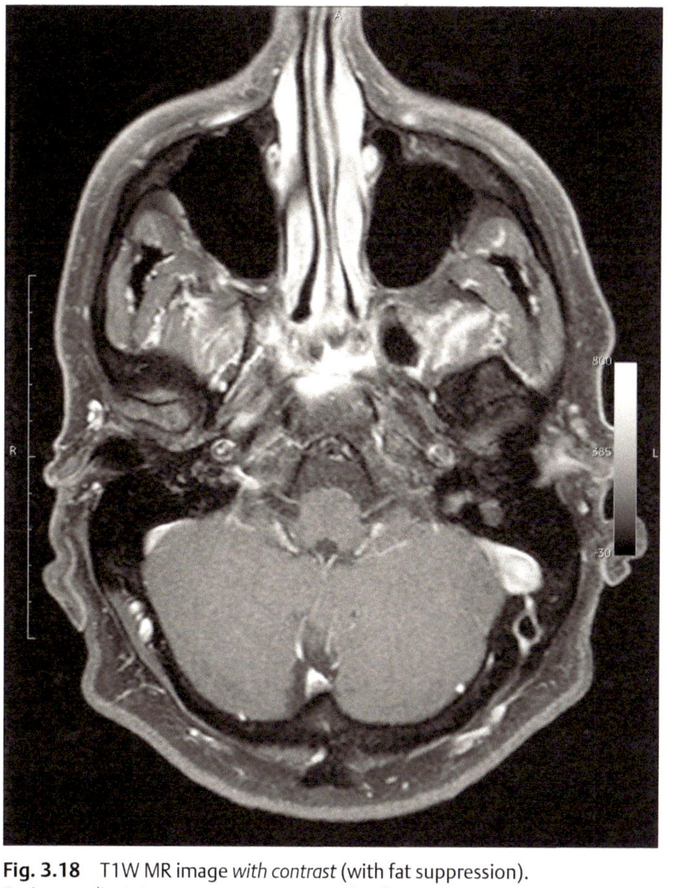

Fig. 3.18 T1W MR image *with contrast* (with fat suppression).
Brain: gray/isointense;
CSF: black/hypointense;
Inflammation: hyperintense;
Nasal mucosa:
hyperintense ("ONE nose");
Eyes: gray/isointense;
Fat: hypointense.

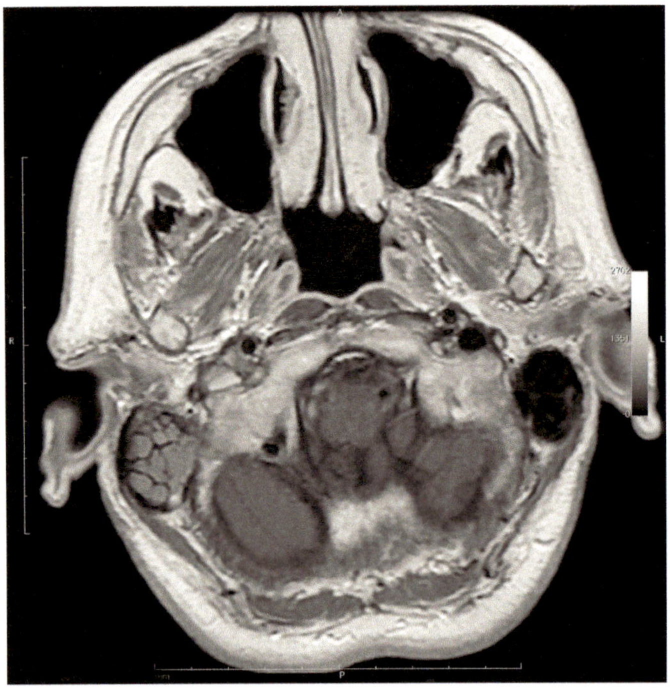

Fig. 3.19 T1W MR image without fat suppression. Same as **Fig. 3.18** except fat: **hyperintense**.

In the following, the radiologic anatomy is shown in T2W CISS (constructive interference into steady state) sequence.[3] This sequence is comparable to the FIESTA or DRIVE sequences and gives a heavily weighted T2W image. In heavily weighted T2W images the CSF and the intracochlear fluids are hyperintense compared with brain tissue.

(See **Fig. 3.20–Fig. 3.39.**)

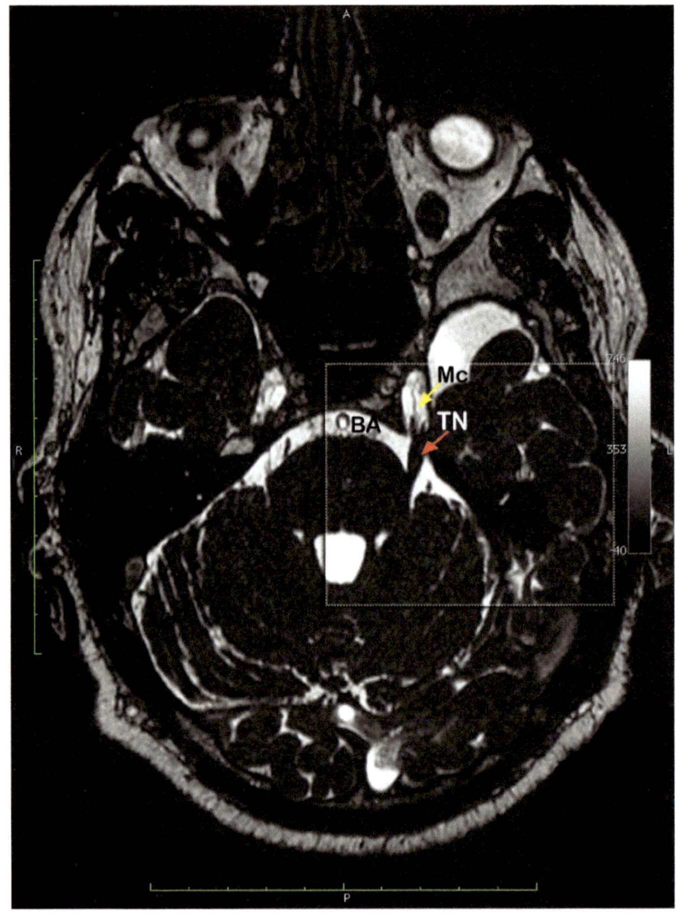

Fig. 3.20 The trigeminal nerve (TN, *red arrow*), large in diameter, is often well seen on MRI. It runs from the lateral side of the mid-pons toward the Meckel cave (Mc). The basilar artery (BA) can also be appreciated and is located anterior to the brainstem in the prepontine cistern. Enlargements of slices in the rectangular area indicated are shown in **Fig. 3.21–Fig. 3.34** and **Fig. 3.37**.

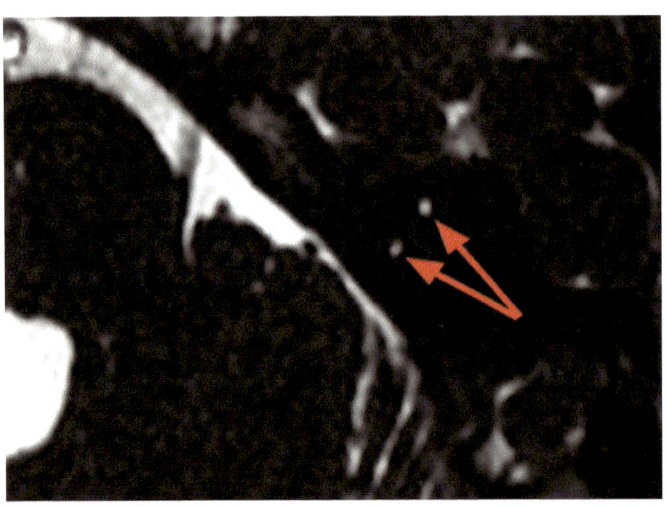

Fig. 3.21 In this image the superior semicircular canal (SSC) is seen as two dots (*two red arrows*).

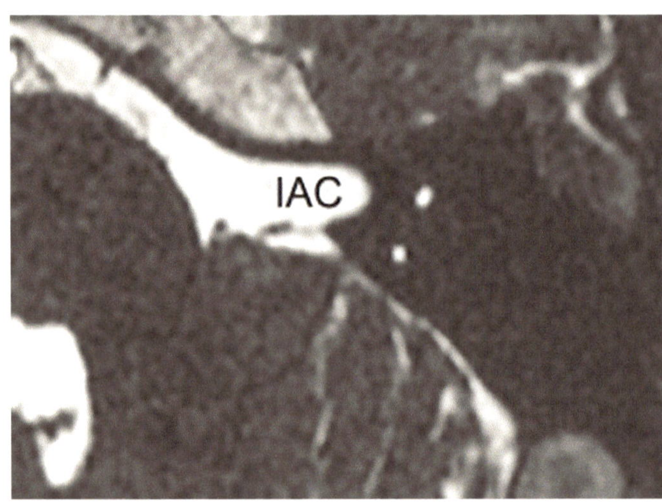

Fig. 3.22 From the cerebellopontine angle the internal auditory canal (IAC) can be followed laterally, extending to its fundus. It is filled with CSF as the dura extends up to the cochlea and labyrinth.

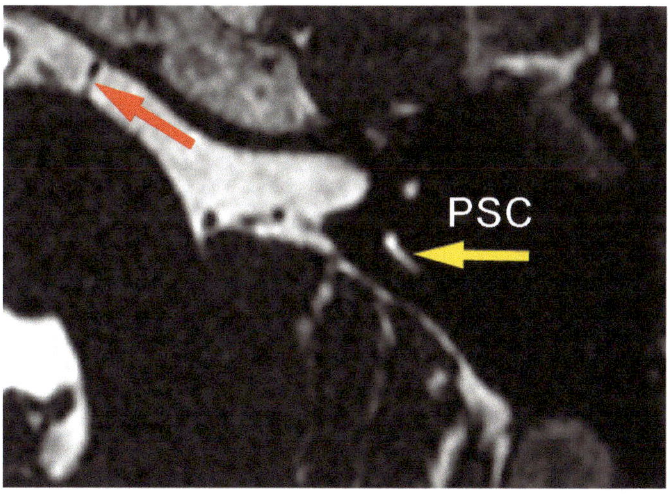

Fig. 3.23 Proceeding from superior to inferior, the posterior semicircular canal (PSC, *yellow arrow*) is the next structure to be seen on MRI. Note that it runs parallel to the posterior fossa dura. The sixth cranial nerve (*red arrow*) is also seen in this image.

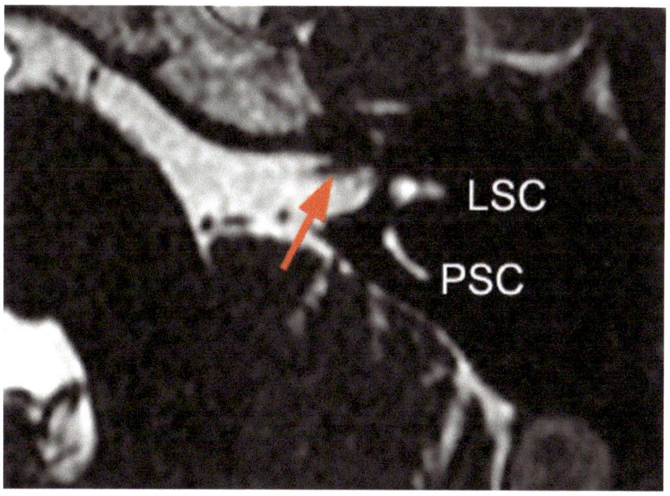

Fig. 3.24 The facial nerve (*red arrow*) is seen first at the fundus of the IAC. Also the anterior part of the lateral semicircular canal (LSC) can be appreciated in this image.

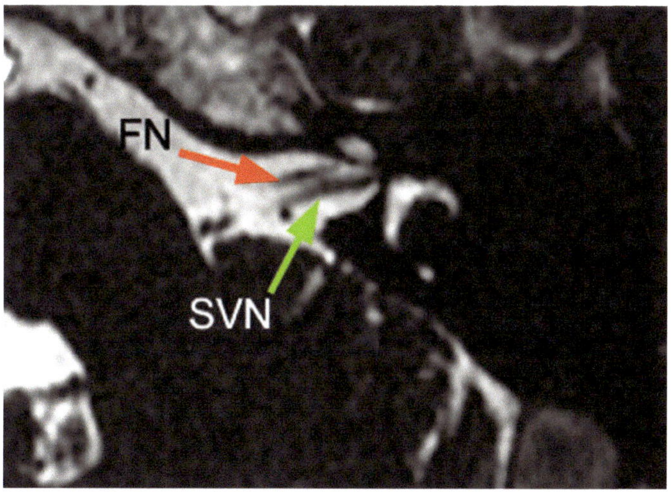

Fig. 3.25 The superior vestibular nerve (SVN, *green arrow*) then becomes visible posterior to the facial nerve. In this image and the more inferior images it runs parallel to the facial nerve (FN, *red arrow*) (like a "'tram line").

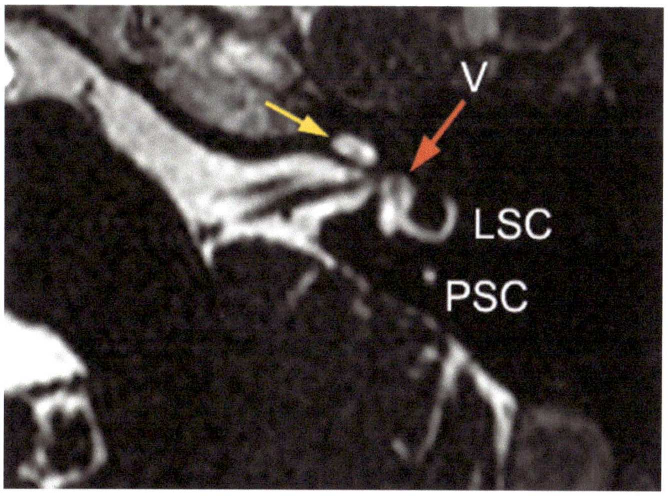

Fig. 3.26 The superior half of the middle turn of the cochlea is visible. In clear images the separation (by the basilar membrane/spiral ligament) of the middle turn into the scala tympani (medially, and close to the IAC) and scala vestibuli (laterally) can be appreciated (*yellow arrow*). Almost the complete lateral semicircular canal (LSC) and the vestibule (V, *red arrow*) can be seen in this image.

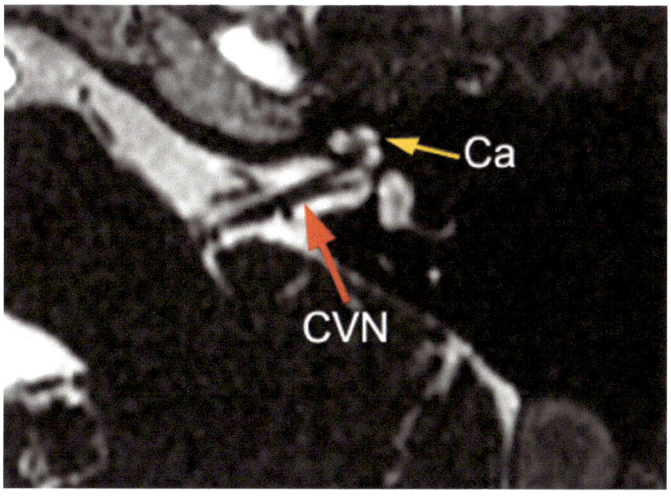

Fig. 3.27 In the IAC a dividing nerve can be seen (*red arrow*). This is the level of the vestibulocochlear nerve (CVN) where it divides into the cochlear nerve and the inferior vestibular nerve. It should not be mistaken for the superior vestibular nerve, which divides from the same common vestibulocochlear nerve but runs in a more superior plane and therefore differs from it by only one level (see green arrow in **Fig. 3.25**) The apical turn of the cochlea is also visible (Ca, *yellow arrow*).

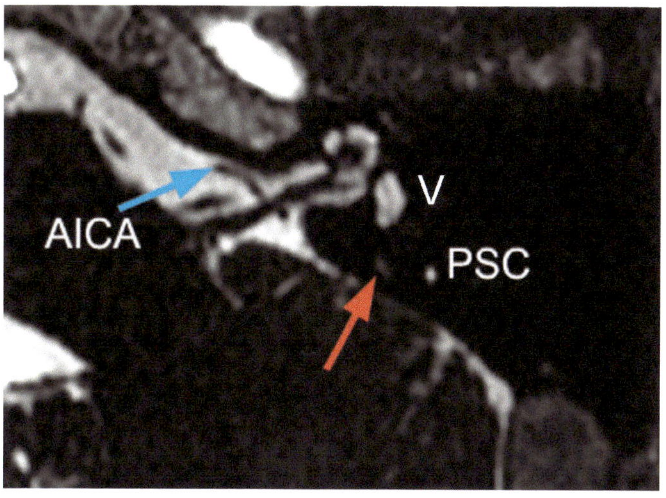

Fig. 3.28 In the IAC, or close to it, the anterior inferior cerebellar artery (AICA, *blue arrow*) often runs in a loop. Many variations in the position of this structure can be seen. The vestibular aqueduct (*red arrow*) can hardly be seen on most MR images. The contrast between the tiny duct and it surroundings is only clearly visible when the duct is larger than normal (see Chapter 15 on malformations). The vestibule is indicated with V.

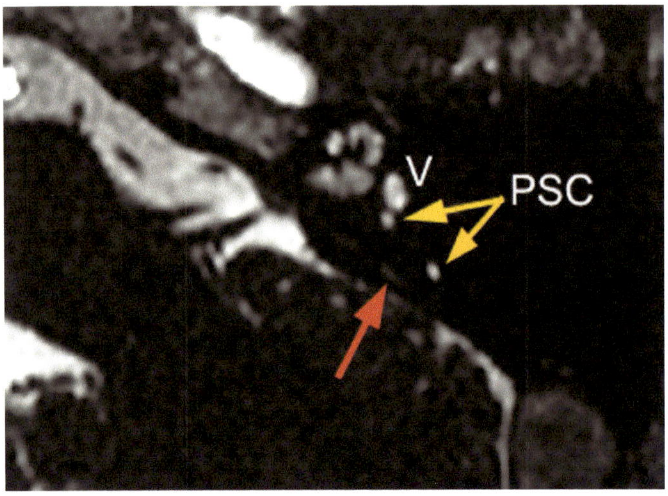

Fig. 3.29 Within the cochlea the first and second turns can be seen, and the vestibule (V) is also visible. In this image the root entry zone of the vestibulocochlear nerve at the brainstem is visible. The vestibular aqueduct (*red arrow*) runs almost parallel to the posterior semicircular canal (PSC, *yellow arrows*).

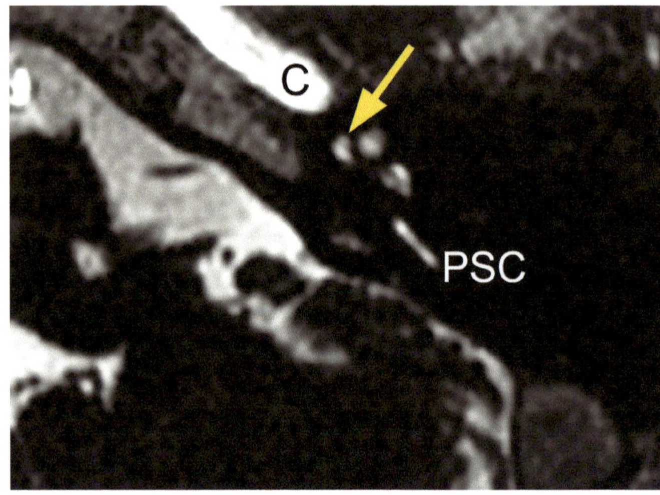

Fig. 3.30 The inferior part of the posterior semicircular canal (PSC) can be appreciated in this image. Also the horizontal section of the carotid artery (C) is clearly visible and its close distance to the first turn of the cochlea (*yellow arrow*) is well visualized.

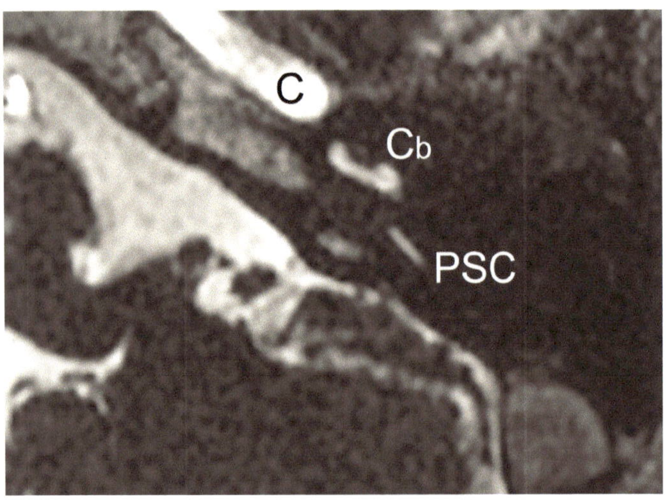

Fig. 3.31 The basal turn of the cochlea (Cb) is almost fully visible. The scala tympani is visible; the scala vestibuli is only partly visible. The horizontal part of the carotid artery (C) and the inferior part of the PSC are also visible.

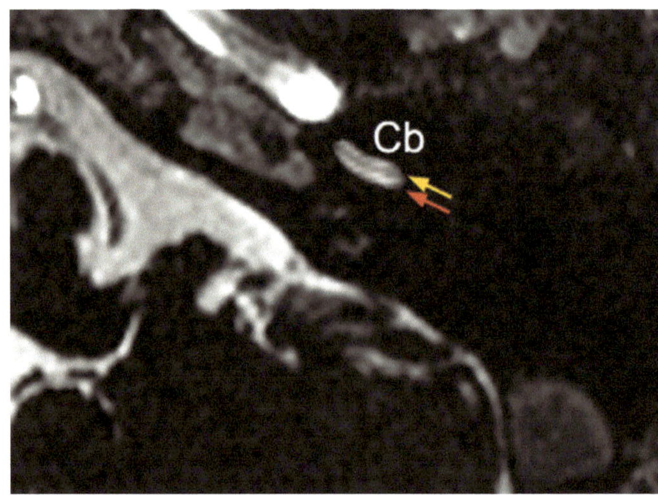

Fig. 3.32 The basal turn (Cb) is completely in view. Both scalae (scala tympani, *red arrow*; scala vestibuli, *yellow arrow*) are visible and are fluid filled. This is one of the most important images for checking the patency of the basal turn in case of possible ossification or fibrosis.

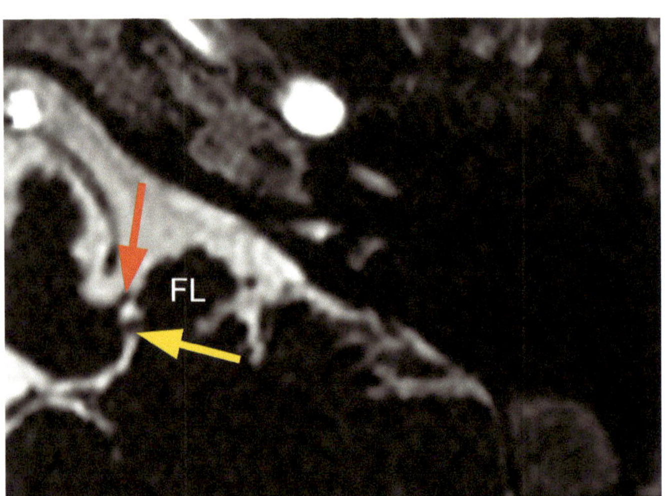

Fig. 3.33 The flocculus (FL) is visible as a "cauliflower" within the CSF. Medial to the flocculus, the pons, the facial nerve (CN VII, *red arrow*), and the vestibulocochlear nerve (CN VIII, *yellow arrow*) can be appreciated.

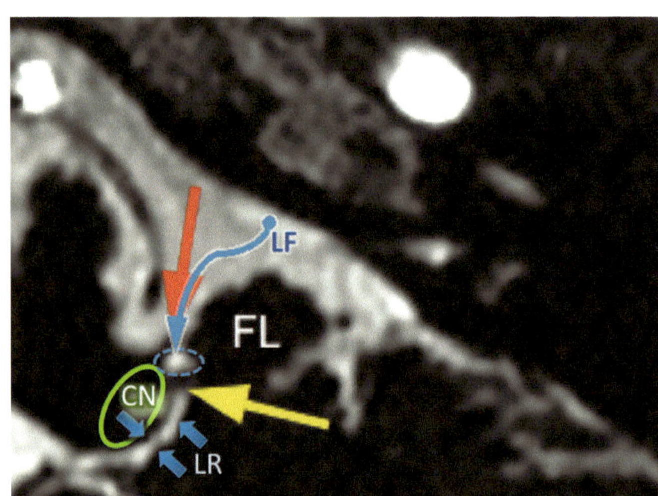

Fig. 3.34 On this enlargement further structures are indicated to clarify the fine anatomy. The flocculus can be retracted posteriorly, the opening found medially is the Luschka foramen (LF, *dotted blue circle*). This gives access to the lateral recess (LR, *small blue arrows*) of the fourth ventricle. The facial nerve (*red arrow*) is more ventrally (anteriorly) located; the dorsal (posterior) nerve is the vestibulocochlear nerve (*yellow arrow*). The cochlear nucleus (CN, *green oval*) is not distinguishable on MRI images, but the location is shown schematically here.

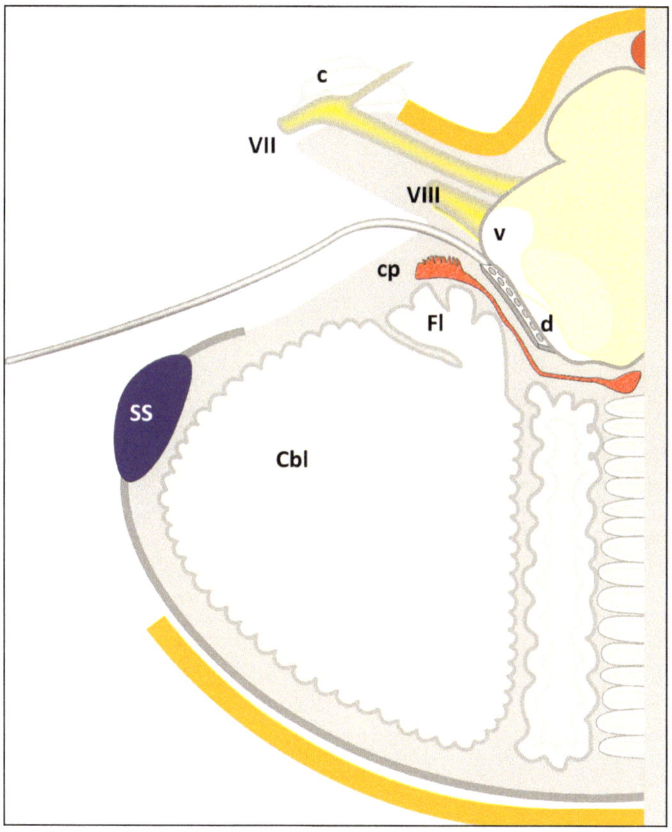

Fig. 3.35 The position of the ABI in the lateral recess is shown in this schematic drawing. The flocculus (Fl) can be retracted posteriorly, to open the Luschka foramen and the entrance of the lateral recess. Within the lateral recess the choroid plexus (cp) is the most prominent structure and is the best landmark for the Luschka foramen and the lateral recess. The facial nerve (VII) is more ventrally (anteriorly) located; dorsally (posteriorly) is the vestibulocochlear nerve (VIII). The positions of the ventral and dorsal cochlear nuclei (v and d) are shown schematically. SS, sigmoid sinus; Cbl, cerebellum.

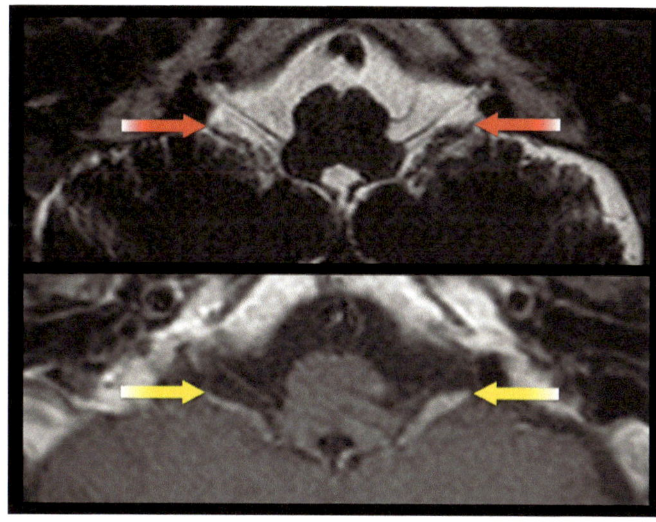

Fig. 3.36 Two images of the lateral recess in the same patient. The top image is the heavily T2W image with the *red arrows* pointing to the area of the flocculus and choroid plexus. In the lower image, a contrast-enhanced T1W image, the *yellow arrows* point at the same area, but with better differentiation. The lower contrast-enhanced T1W image clearly shows the choroid plexus as an enhancing structure in contrast to the flocculus.

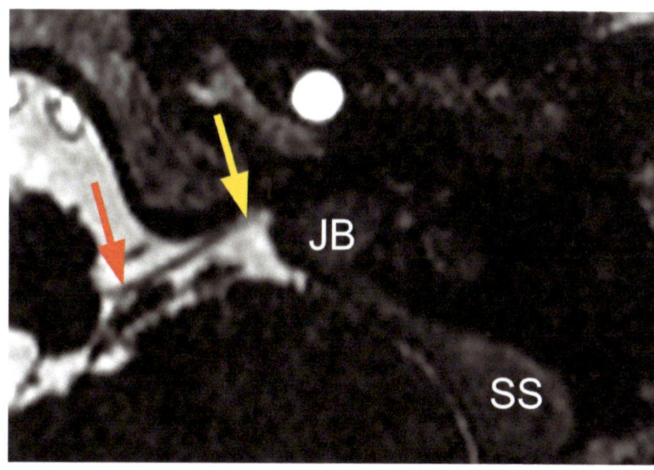

Fig. 3.37 The glossopharyngeal (CN IX) nerve is shown here, running from the medulla oblongata (*red arrow*) toward the jugular foramen (*yellow arrow*), close to the jugular bulb (JB). The sigmoid sinus (SS) is also visible.

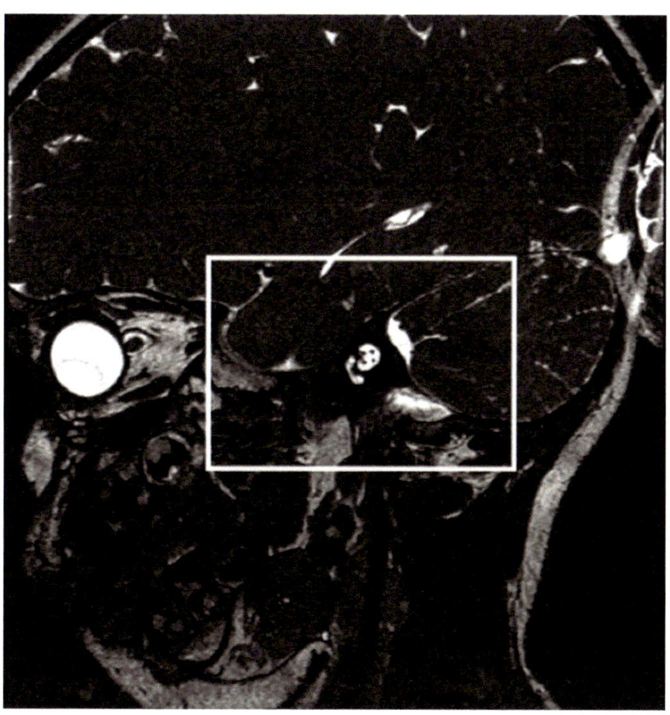

Fig. 3.38 The presence of the nerves within the IAC can be judged best in sagittal view. This additional imaging is important in the work-up of patients with congenital deafness in whom hypoplasia or aplasia of the cochlear nerve needs to be investigated. The other nerves in the internal auditory canal can also be assessed. This image and the next represent a sagittal view of the lateral part of the internal auditory canal, where all nerves are separate entities, in contrast to more medially where the vestibulocochlear bundle is present as one structure and the facial nerve as a separate structure.

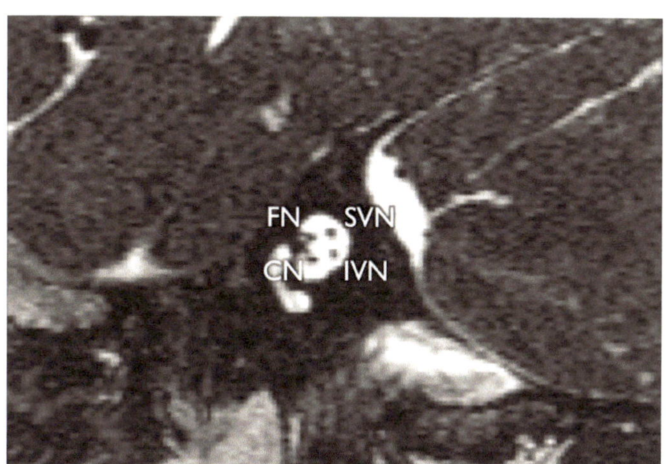

Fig. 3.39 The cochlea is seen anterior-inferiorly from the IAC, on the lower left side in this image, and is the easiest landmark for orientation in this sagittal image of a left ear. The cochlea is closest to the cochlear nerve (CN) (anterior-inferiorly). The facial nerve (FN) is located, anterior-superiorly, while posterior-superiorly the superior vestibular nerve (SVN) and posterior-inferiorly the inferior vestibular nerve (IVN) can be seen. *Reminder:* "7-up, Coke down": the seventh cranial nerve is up (superior), the cochlear nerve is down (inferior).

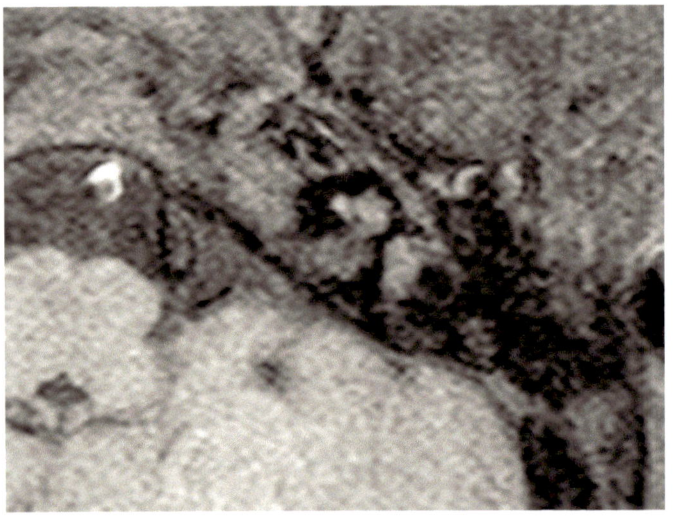

Fig. 3.40 T1W MR image without contrast. If the intensity of the fluid compartment in the cochlea or labyrinth is increased on a T1W image, compared with the normal intensity, they could contain (fibrous) tissue. On this image the cochlea and labyrinth are hardly visible. The cochlea and the labyrinth should be equally intense as the CSF. CSF is less intense than brain tissue on a T1W image without contrast. (Fresh) Hemorrhage and some pathologies such as cholesterol granuloma appear hyperintense on a T1W image without contrast.

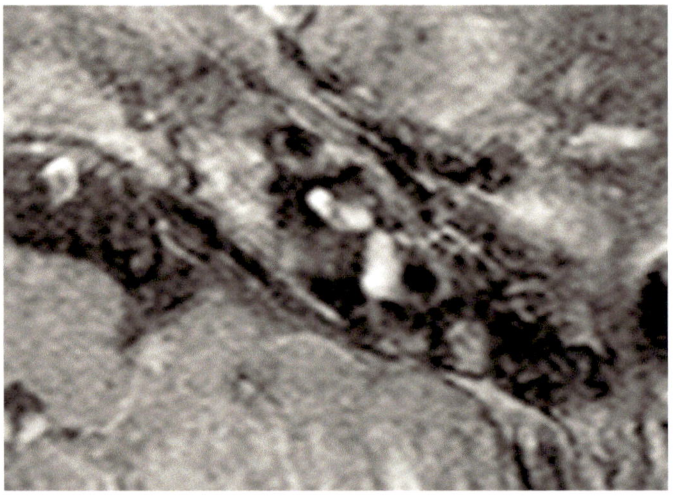

Fig. 3.41 T1W MR image with contrast. Enhancement means increased perfusion/increased contrast uptake in the location of the enhancement. In this case an active postmeningitis inflammation of the cochlea and labyrinth is present. Enhancement can also be seen in tumors such as vestibular schwannoma or in intracochlear hemorrhage.

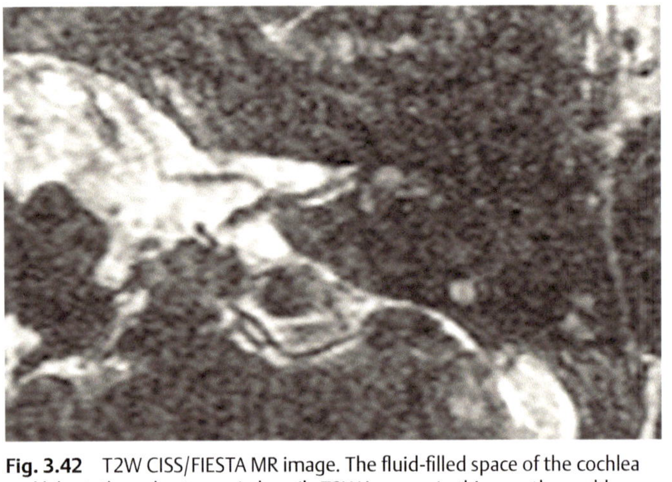

Fig. 3.42 T2W CISS/FIESTA MR image. The fluid-filled space of the cochlea and labyrinth are best seen in heavily T2W images. In this case the cochlea and labyrinth are hardly visible, whereas the CSF in the IAC is clearly seen. The labyrinth is almost fully obliterated with fibrous tissue or is totally ossified. The vestibule can still be distinguished.

Enlargements of the three **most commonly used MRI sequences** in patients with hearing loss are shown in **Fig. 3.40–Fig. 3.42**. Scans of a patient with acute hearing loss following bacterial meningitis are presented to demonstrate the advantage of each sequence.

Other radiologic cases are illustrated and discussed in the chapters on special indications, Chapters 12 to 17.

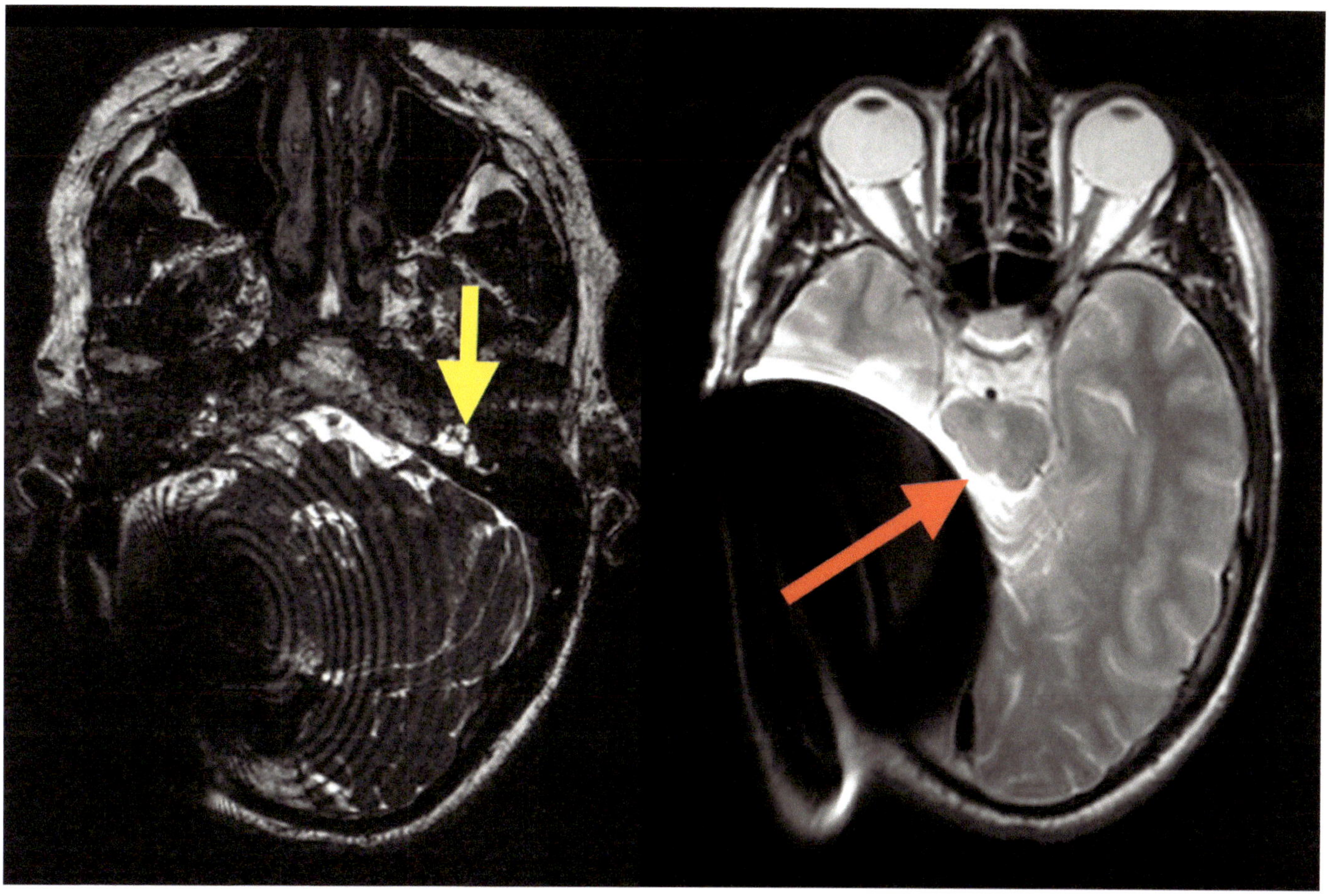

Fig. 3.43 1.5 T images with right-side cochlear implant and with receiver-stimulator magnet in place. Note that the CPA and inner ear structures are only well visualized at the contralateral side (*yellow arrow*). An artifact of around 8 cm is seen (*red arrow*).

3.5.1 Artifact of Cochlear and Auditory Brainstem Implant on MRI

The magnet of the receiver-stimulator creates an artifact on the image if the magnet is kept in place. Guidelines must be followed in preparing the patient for scanning when a MRI scanner up to 1.5 T field strength is used. The guideline or protocol, provided by the implant manufacturer, mostly describes a firm headbandage during scanning. One should consult the guidelines applicable to each specific brand of cochlear/auditory brainstem implant for further information. MRI investigation with a 3 T scanner without removing the magnet is not advised.

The images shown in **Fig. 3.43** and **Fig. 3.44** can be expected with a 1.5 T MRI machine.

Indications for MRI in ABI Surgery

- Uncertainty about ossification or patency of the cochlea, especially in the acute phase of disease (in meningitis, otosclerosis, autoimmune inner ear disease, or trauma cases).
- Uncertainty about presence of cochlear nerve aplasia, hypoplasia (in uni- or bilateral congenital sensorineural hearing loss (SNHL), cochleovestibular malformations, a narrow internal auditory canal, or in auditory neuropathy).
- Uncertainty about the presence of a CPA or petrous apex lesion.
- Suspicion on an intracranial lesion or to rule out intracranial lesions after meningitis, cytomegalovirus infection, and other infections.

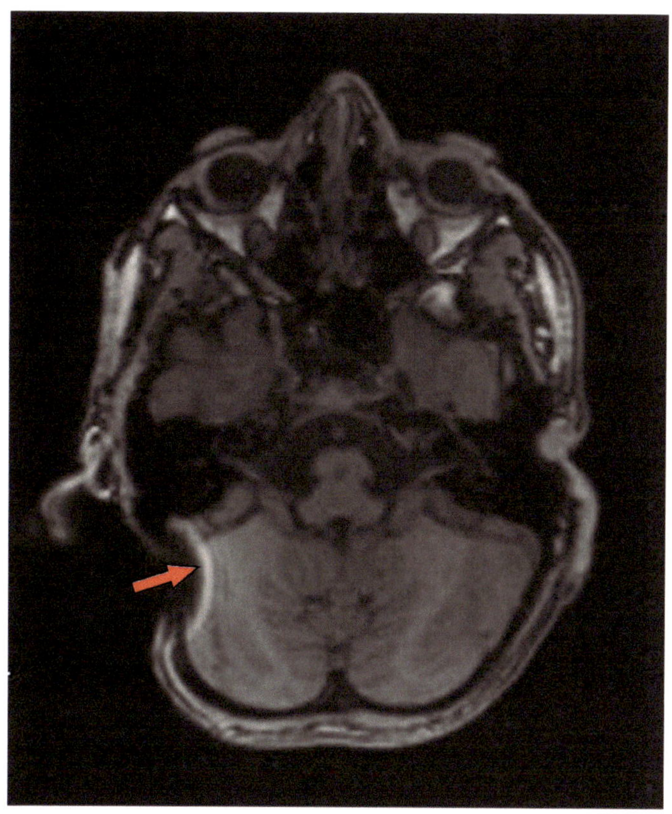

Fig. 3.44 1.5 T image with right-side cochlear implant in place but with magnet removed. The CPA and inner ear on both sides can still be investigated. The artifact is around 3 cm in size.

- Prior to (translabyrinthine) ABI surgery, radiologic and anatomical knowledge is needed of the labyrinth, the jugular bulb, the cochlear aqueduct, the width of the fourth ventricle, and access to the Luschka foramen. Knowledge of the other cranial nerves and vessels is necessary, especially in the CPA.

Pearls and Pitfalls in Radiology

- High-quality imaging is essential in cochlear or auditory brainstem implantation.
- CT without contrast is like a roadmap for the surgeon; the surgery should be planned according to the CT scan.
- Special attention preoperatively should be addressed to the position of the middle fossa dura, sigmoid sinus, and facial nerve. Furthermore, attention should be paid to the facial nerve in relation to the chorda tympani, the stapedius muscle, and the round window.
- The round window should be examined on CT scan in the axial as well as the coronal plane: the bony overhang, the window itself, and the patency of the basal turn are essential in the preoperative planning.
- In malformations and prior to drill-out procedures all details need to be examined, as complications are more frequent.
- In MRI basic knowledge of the different sequences is essential to be able understand the different images and to differentiate among different types of pathology.
- The best sequence to learn or with which to start the evaluation of a MR image of the CPA/temporal bone is the heavily weighted T2W sequence.
- Heavily weighted T2W images resemble the CT images and will show the normal anatomy of the labyrinth and cranial nerves most adequately.
- Heavily weighted T2W images show the normally fluid-filled scalae of the cochlea and should therefore be used to analyze obliteration of the cochlea. The lack of fluid can be caused by fibrosis with or without ossification. A CT scan will show the extent of the ossification.
- MRI is advised for evaluating patients who have possible obliteration intracochlearly, as in postmeningitis, posttraumatic situations, otosclerosis, autoimmune, and (possible) postinfectious cases.

References

1. Mackeith S, Joy R, Robinson P, Hajioff D. Pre-operative imaging for cochlear implantation: magnetic resonance imaging, computed tomography, or both? Cochlear Implants Int 2012;13(3):133–136
2. Lo WW. Imaging of cochlear and auditory brain stem implantation. AJNR Am J Neuroradiol 1998;19(6):1147–1154
3. Casselman J, Kuhweide R, Deimling M, et al. Contructive interference in steady state-3DFT MR imaging of the inner ear and cerebellopontine angle. AJNR Am J Neuroradiol 1993;14(1):47–57

Further Reading

Harnsberger HR, et al. Diagnostic Imaging. Head and Neck. 2nd ed. Salt Lake City: Amirsys Inc.; 2004

Lemmerling M, Kollias SS. Radiology of the Petrous Bone. Berlin: Springer; 2003

4 Instruments and Implants

4.1 Cochlear Implantation: Instruments, Monitoring, and Implants

4.1.1 Instruments for Cochlear Implant (CI) Surgery

The number of instruments should be limited but has to be sufficient for adaptation to the surgery when alternative surgical steps are needed. The instruments should always be arranged on the instrument table in the same order to facilitate easiest management by the scrub nurse.

Operating Table Setup for Mastoid/CI Surgery (Fig. 4.1)

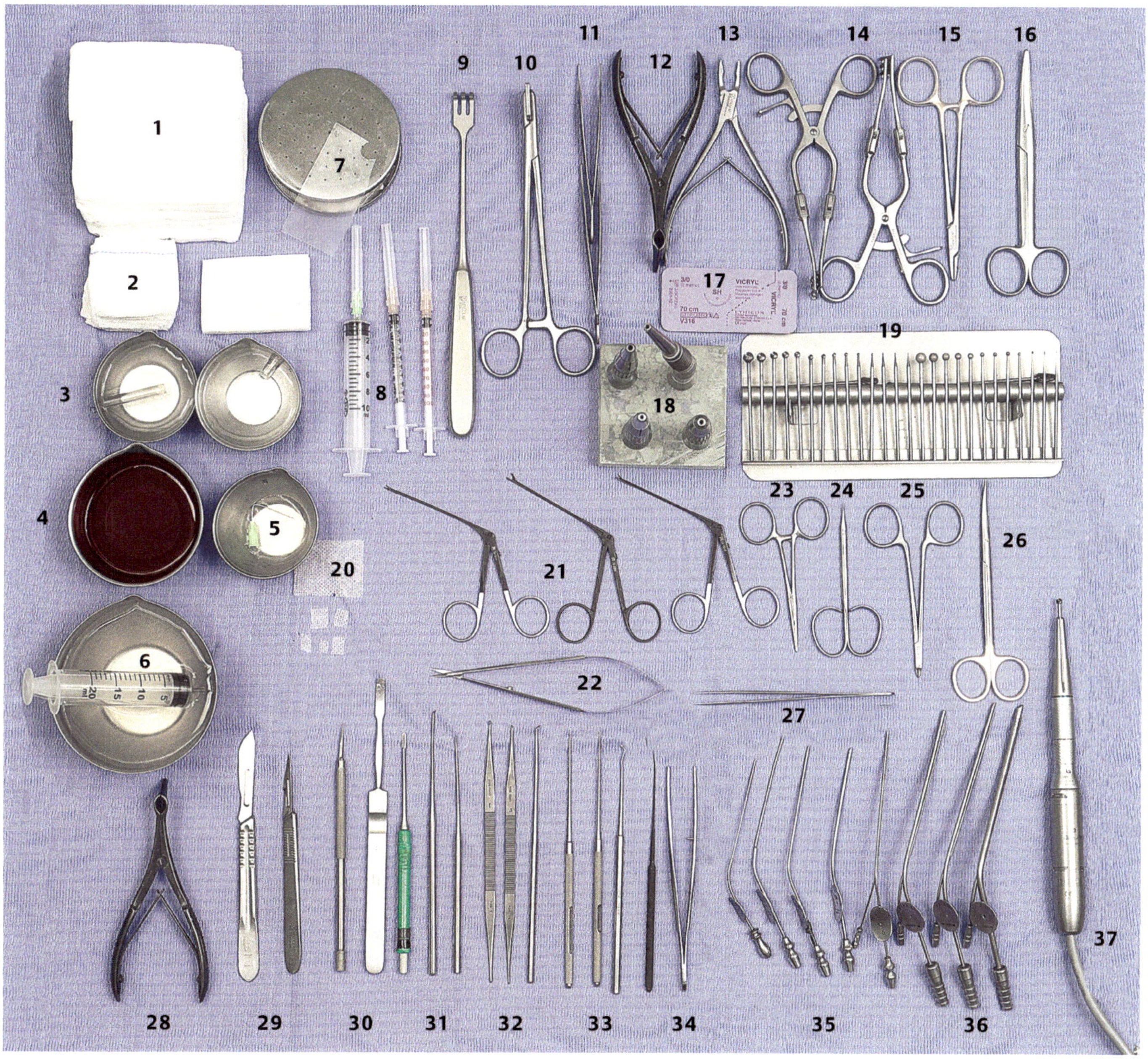

Fig. 4.1 The picture shown is of a table setup for regular mastoid surgery. Some instruments are not used in standard CI surgery. If a conversion to a more extended approach is needed (subtotal petrosectomy) this setup is still sufficient. Special CI instruments provided by the CI companies can be used in addition, to facilitate the placement of the implant. Preparation of pictures of each instrument table used may be helpful. A badly organized instrument table will frequently disturb the process of surgery and the surgeon's concentration. We generally prefer straight instruments to angled ones, including the handpieces of drills, to ensure delicate manipulation. **1**, folded gauze (large); **2**, folded gauze (small); **3–6**, metal cups with physiologic saline solution, antiseptic solution, and local anesthetic; **7**, Silastic sheeting; **8**, injectors; **9**, skin retractor; **10**, fascia pressure forceps; **11**, forceps (uncinated); **12**, nasal speculum; **13**, rongeur; **14**, self-retaining retractor; **15**, needle holder; **16**, scissors; **17**, Vicryl (surgical thread); **18**, handpieces for drills, straight and angled; **19**, tungsten carbide and diamond burs; **20**, cottonoid; **21**, microforceps and microscissors; **22**, spring scissors; **23**, forceps (for incus); **24**, scissors; **25**, malleus nipper; **26**, scissors; **27**, forceps (fine tip); **28**, nasal speculum; **29**, scalpels; **30**, Lempert periosteum elevator; **31**, microdissectors; **32**, curettes; **33**, hooks and needle; **34**, forceps with teeth; **35**, suction tubes; **36**, suction irrigators; **37**, electrosurgical motor with hand drill.

Special Instruments for CI Surgery Provided by the Supplying Companies

Advanced Bionics Instruments (Fig. 4.2–Fig. 4.12)

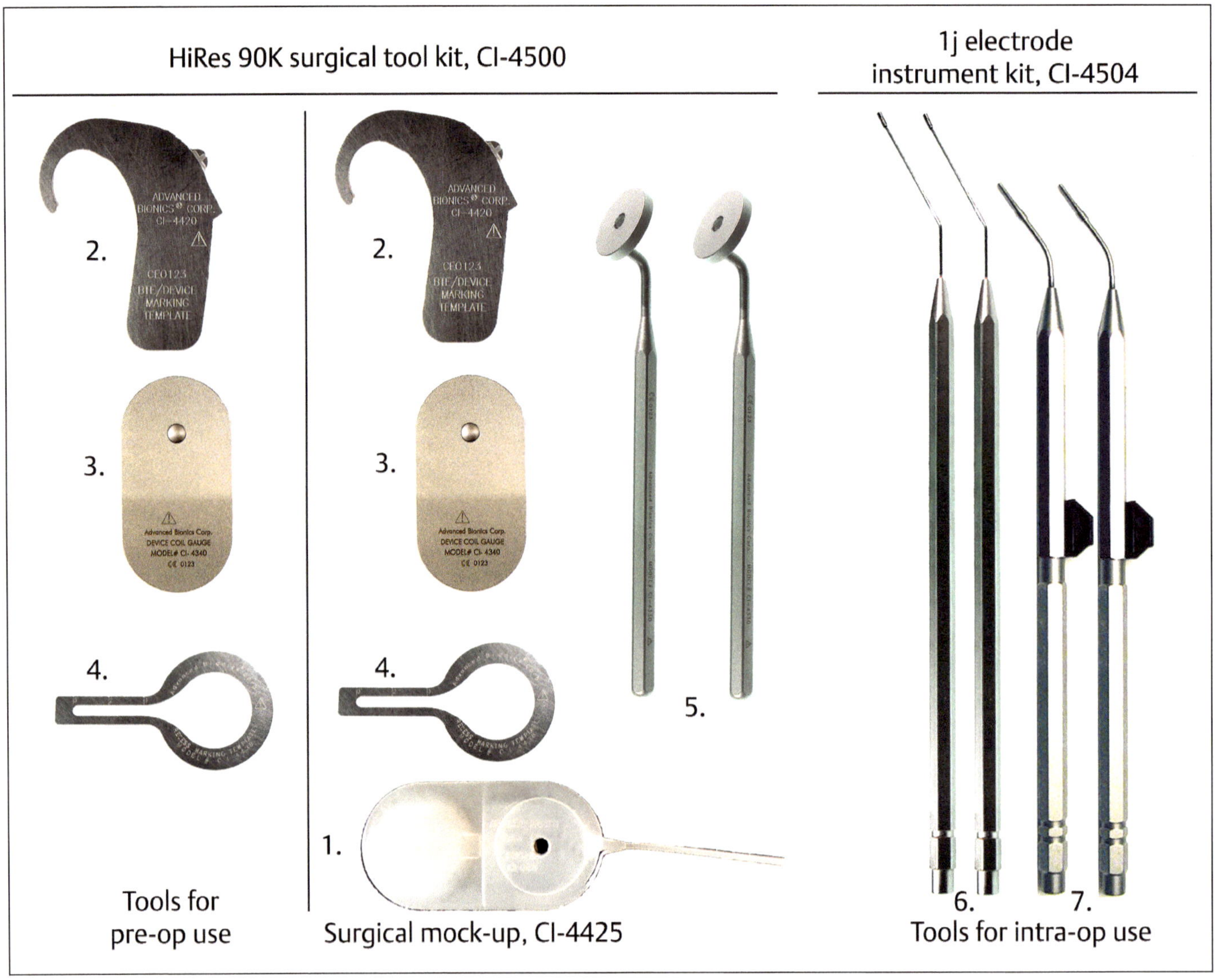

Fig. 4.2 Surgical kit for the Advanced Bionics HiRes 90K implant. **1**, surgical silicone mock-up; **2**, processor marking template; **3**, device coil gauge model; **4**, recess marking template; **5**, recess template; **6**, cochleostomy sizing gauge (for FDA markets); **7**, insertion tool for the 1j electrode.

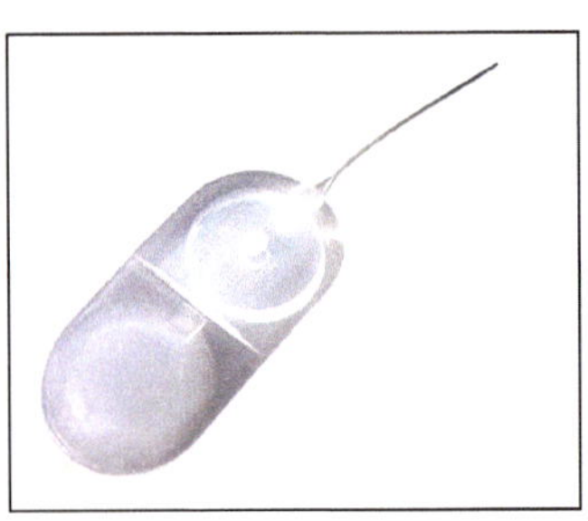

Fig. 4.3 HIRES90K silicone surgical mock-up.

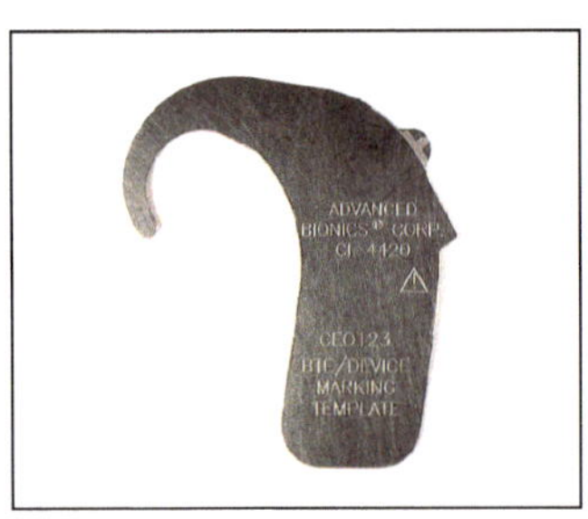

Fig. 4.4 Behind the ear (BTE) processor template.

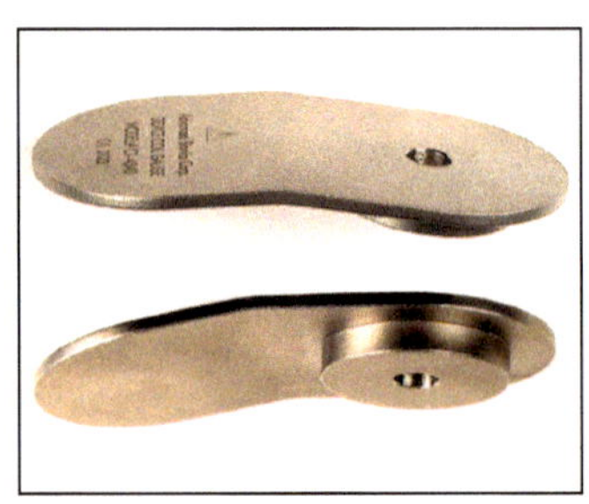

Fig. 4.5 Receiver-stimulator template HIRES90K implant.

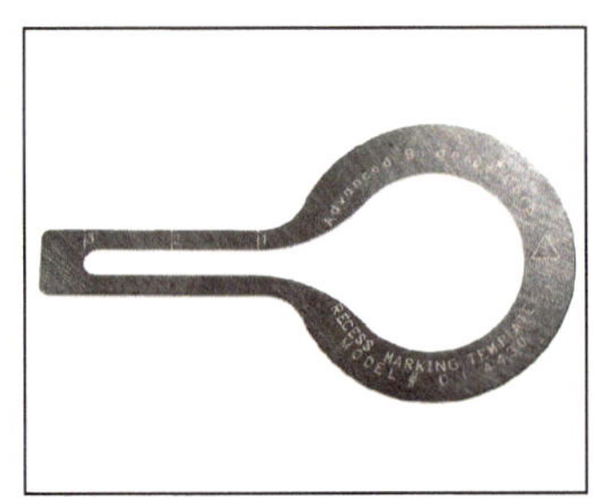

Fig. 4.6 Recess marking template.

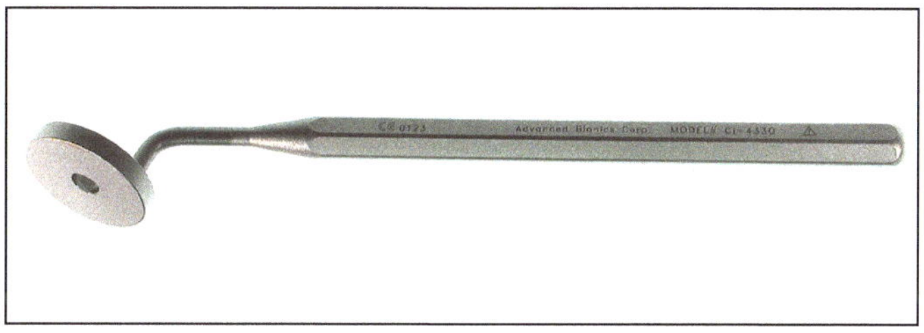

Fig. 4.7 Recess gauge.

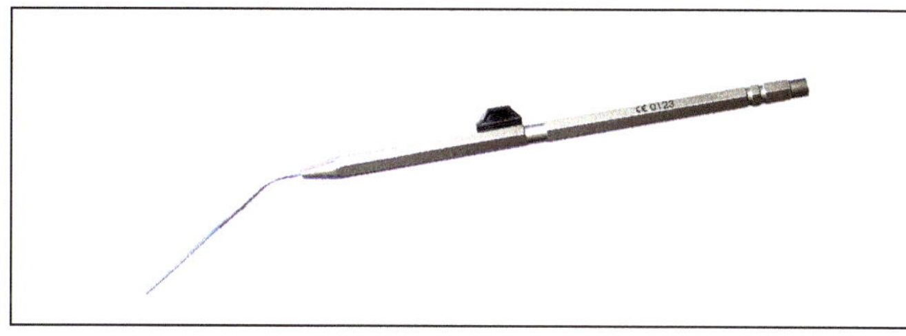

Fig. 4.8 HiFocus 1j electrode insertion tool and tube.

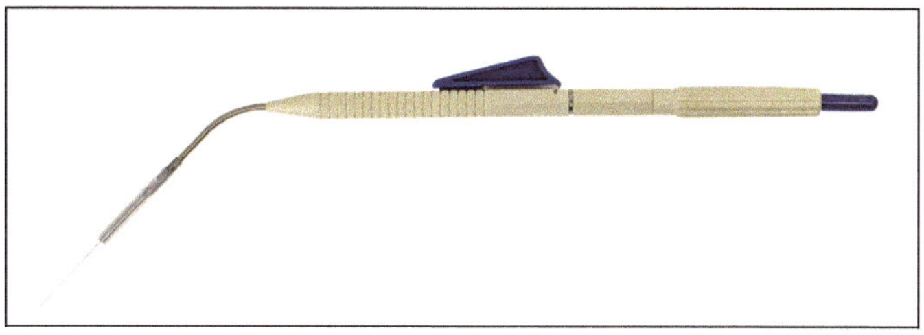

Fig. 4.9 HiFocus mid-scala insertion tool.

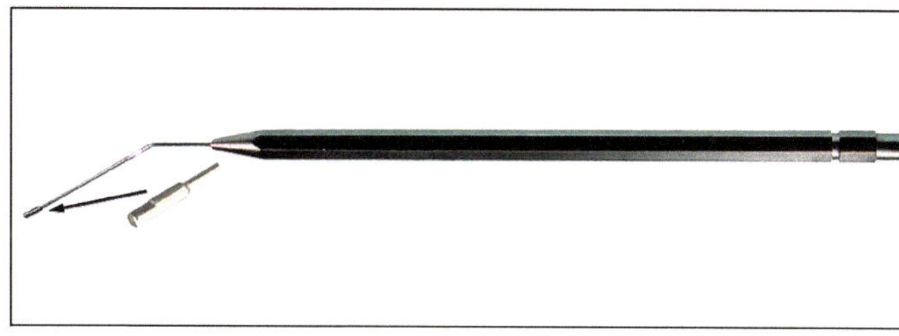

Fig. 4.10 Helix cochleostomy sizing gauge.

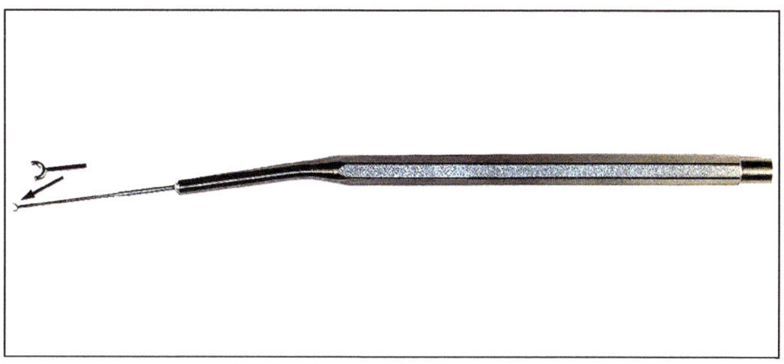

Fig. 4.11 Claw tool.

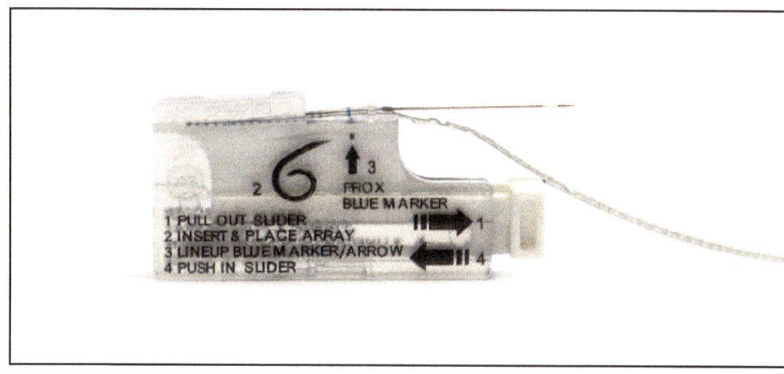

Fig. 4.12 Electrode reloading tool.

Cochlear Instruments (Fig. 4.13)

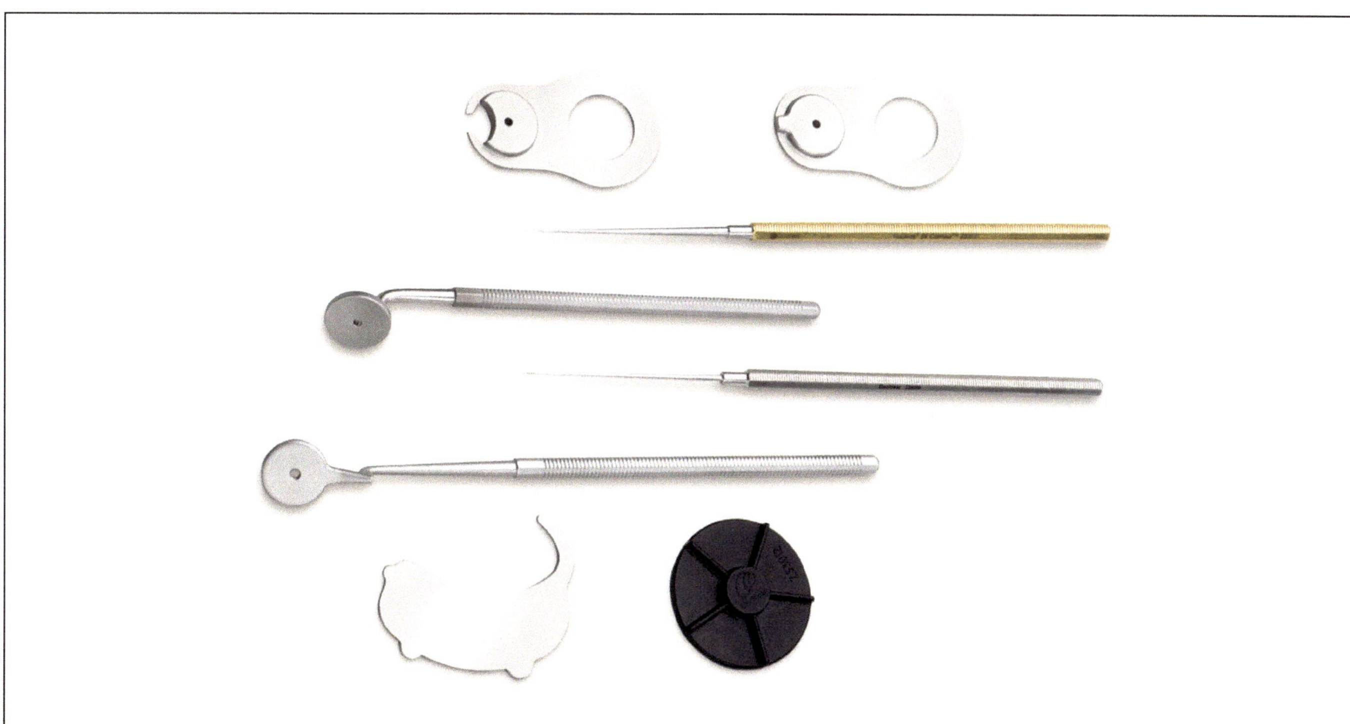

Fig. 4.13 From left to right: two implant templates; two contour electrode claws (gold and silver); two recess gauges (with and without electrode channel); one processor (BTE) template; one spacer for intraoperative testing (black). Not shown is an advanced off-stylet forceps.

MED-EL Instruments (Fig. 4.14–Fig. 4.20)

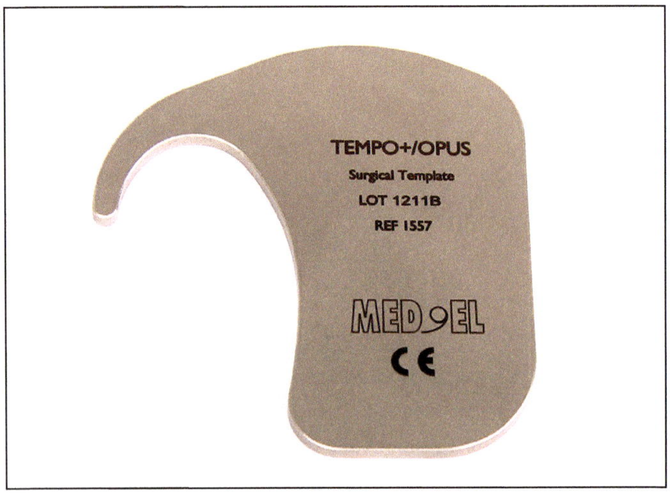

Fig. 4.14 Processor template.

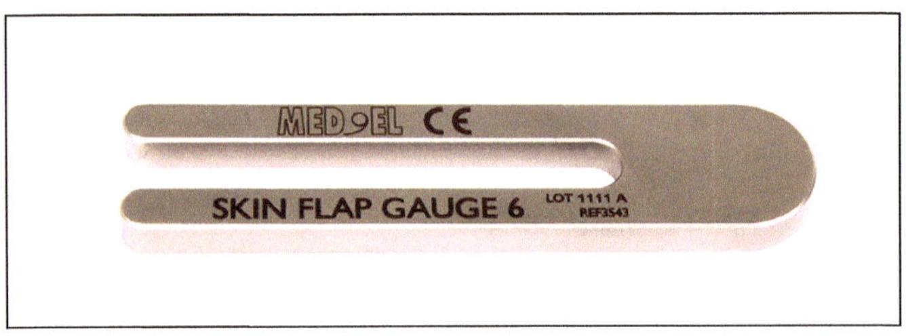

Fig. 4.15 Skin flap gauge.

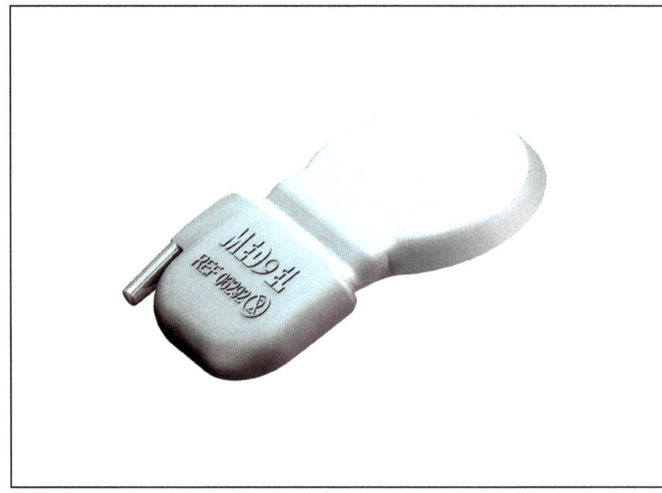

Fig. 4.16 MED-EL implant silicone template.

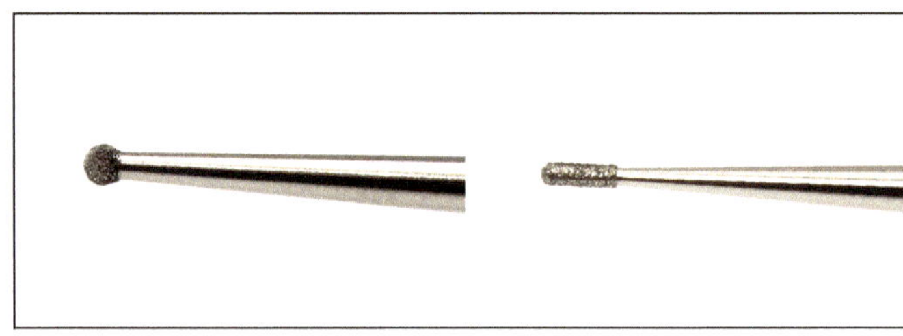

Fig. 4.17 Diamond burs. The bur heads are shown in detail. The rounded bur (left) is 1.2 mm and the other (right) is 0.6 mm in diameter.

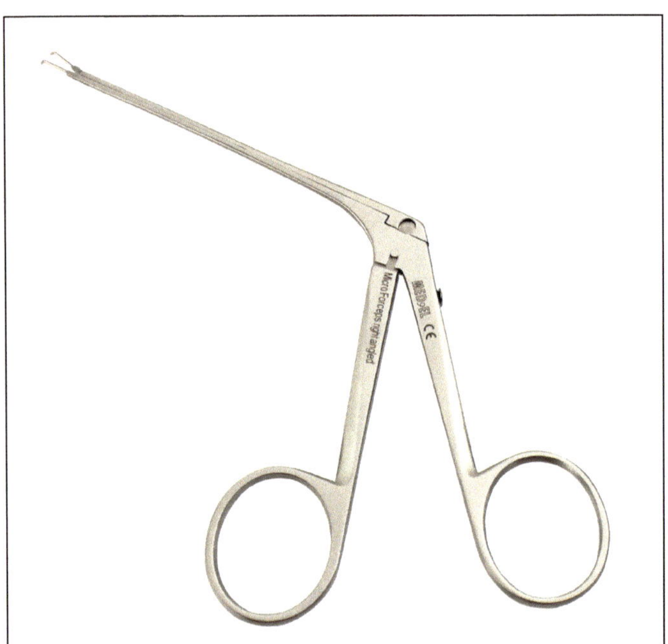

Fig. 4.18 Angled microforceps for insertion. The right-sided version is shown. This type of forceps is also available angled to the other side.

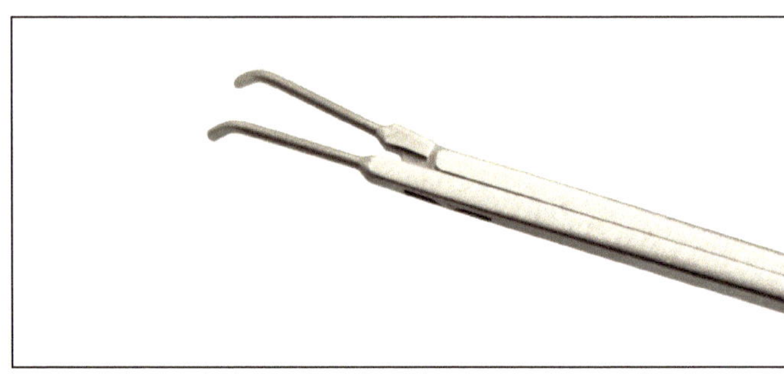

Fig. 4.19 Angled microforceps tip (angled tips right are shown here).

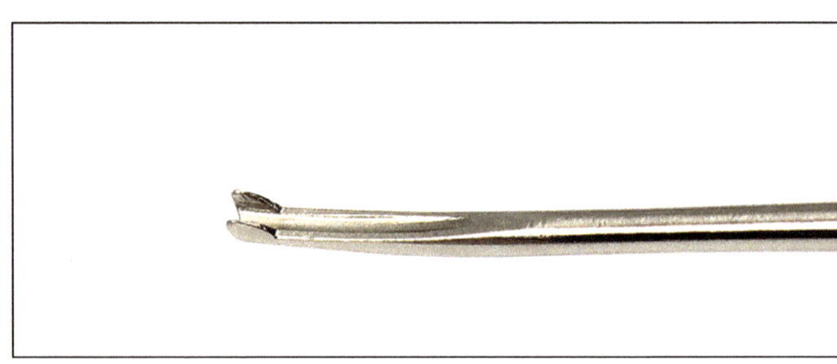

Fig. 4.20 Surgical claw (detail).

Neurelec Instruments

The Neurelec implants are fixed with screws. Their instruments are designed for this technique. See **Fig. 4.21–Fig. 4.25.**

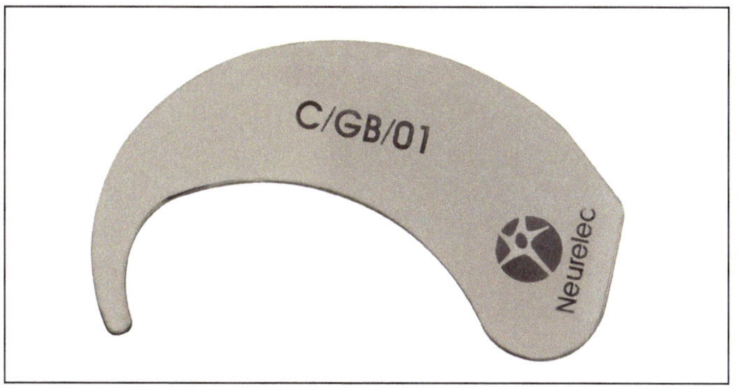

Fig. 4.21 Processor dummy.

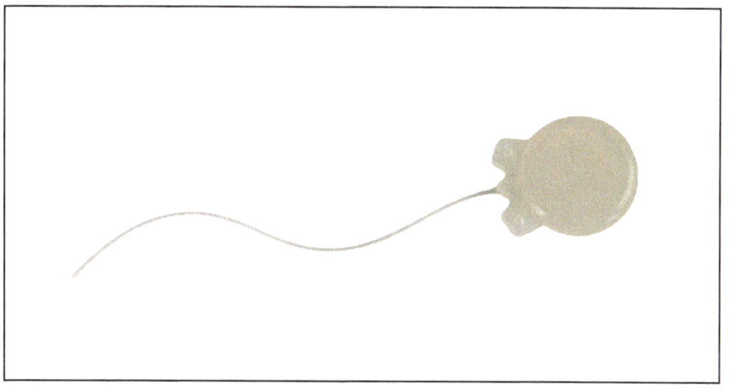

Fig. 4.22 Implant dummy.

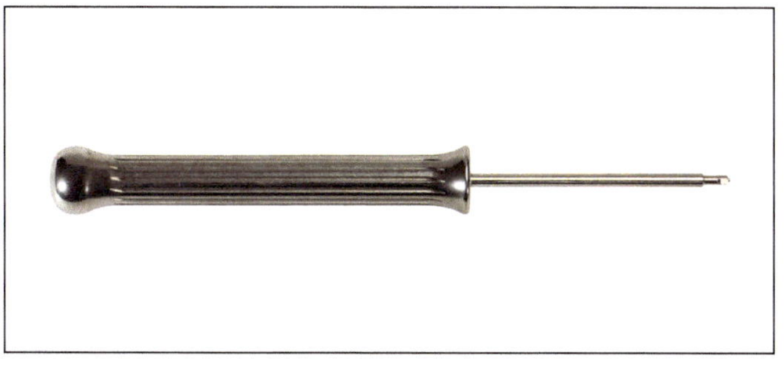

Fig. 4.23 Screwdriver.

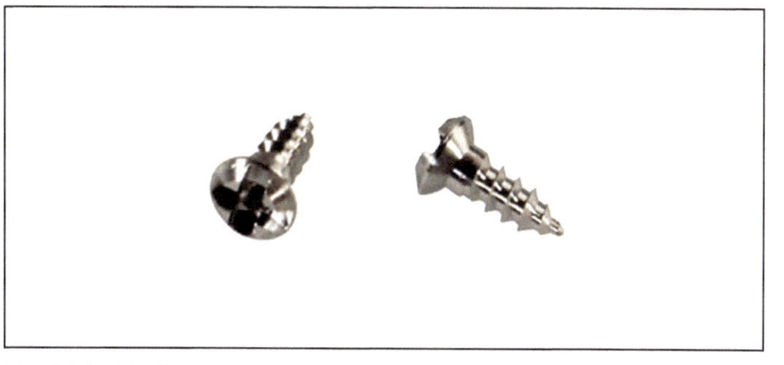

Fig. 4.24 Fixation screws.

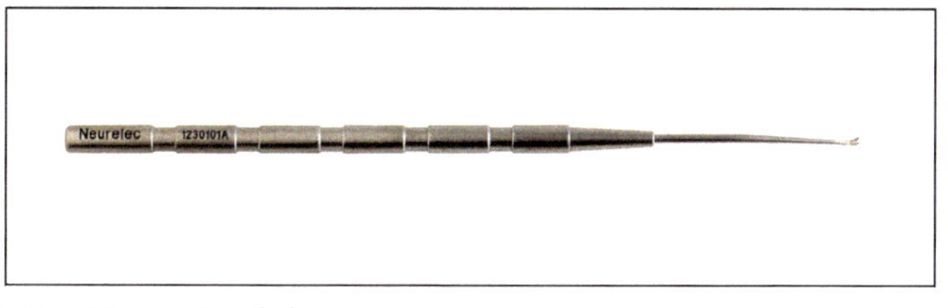

Fig. 4.25 Insertion fork.

4.1.2 Perioperative Medication in CI Surgery

Antibiotics and Infection Prevention

In general, antibiotics are not needed in tympanic and mastoid surgery. Of course many exceptions and preferences exist and CI surgery is one of the surgeries in which antibiotic coverage is preferred. There is no evidence-based protocol, but a number of considerations can help avoid infection, as described here.

Bacterial Concerns

In the literature, the most common bacteria to cause a fulminant infection in combination with a cochlear implant are *Pseudomonas aeruginosa* and *Staphylococcus aureus* species.[1,2] Device-related infections may be difficult to eradicate because these two species can develop biofilms on the implant. As these biofilms are more resistant to antibiotic treatment, they are involved in a higher rate of implant extrusion and the subsequent need to explant.[3,4]

The perioperative antibiotic regime should therefore cover at least these two species. An example of a peroperative intravenous regime is:

In adults 24 hours, starting 45 minute prior to incision:
- Clindamycin 600 mg 3 times a day for 1 day
- Ceftazidime 2 g 3 times a day for 1 day

In children 24 hours, starting 45 minute prior to incision:
- Clindamycin 40 mg/kg/day in 3–4 doses (max. 1.8 g)
- Ceftazidime 100–150 mg/kg/day in 3–4 doses (max. 6 g)

Outpatient Concerns

Does the patient have a history of many ear infections? Is there a recent culture of the external ear canal? Is there a predominant anatomical/medical factor predisposing to development of ear infections, such as cleft palate or diabetes? Has there been any previous ear surgery? Is there a cholesteatoma, atelectasis, or radical cavity (see Chapters 12 and 14)?

A preventive policy would be to culture the external ear canal in all CI candidates, and in case of a positive culture to treat the patient a week prior to the implantation using local eardrops according to the culture. As described in the section on complications in cochlear implantation (Chapter 7, Case 7.4), a patient with a history of *Pseudomonas aeruginosa* infections of the ear canal had a slowly progressive intracochlear infection with *Pseudomonas*. This was probably due to iatrogenic bacterial transmission at implantation. From that case onward, we have included a preoperative culture and possible local antibiotics in the work-up of each CI patient.

Preoperative Concerns

The duration of the procedure, presence of diabetes or systemic disease, an adequate (prophylactic) antibiotic regime, appropriate dosage (related to weight!) in a child, and proper sterilization of the implant tools are all of concern.

Perioperative Concerns

The start of the antibiotic infusion must be at least 30 minutes before incision. The following should also be properly considered: hair shaving, which should be done just before incision; adequate cleaning and skin sterilization; changing of surgical gloves before insertion; use of clean tools for implant handling; reduction of the chances of hematoma development; and reduction of operation room door movements.

Postoperative Concerns

A proper head bandage will reduce the chances of a hematoma. Postoperative antibiotics can be prolonged (therapeutic regime). Duration of stay of sutures, awareness of other health care professionals, and accessibility and continuation of specialized care (especially during evening hours and weekends) must all be considered.

Hyaluronic Acid

Hyaluronic acid (e.g., Healon; Abbott, Illinois, USA) is a viscous fluid that is often used in ophthalmologic surgery and is sold in a ready-to-use syringe with a fine needle. It can be used at insertion to decrease insertion forces and prevent bone dust and blood from entering the cochlea.[5] Another preventive technique is to position a small Silastic sheet in the posterior tympanotomy to avoid debris, blood, or bone dust from attaching to the electrode at insertion. Forceful insertion should be avoided, and insertion should stop when the point of first resistance is reached. We have found that a viscous fluid combined with corticosteroids can be additionally helpful in hearing preservation.

Corticosteroids

The use of corticosteroids in cochlear implantation is discussed extensively in Chapter 9 on electroacoustic stimulation. The idea of adding corticosteroids during implantation, or even prolonged use, has been considered since patients with residual hearing have been considered as CI candidates. Corticosteroids can be considered to avoid an immune reaction within the cochlea and consequent negative intracochlear effects. Systemic, local (middle ear/round window), and even intracochlear administration has been investigated.[6,7] It appears that corticosteroid application improves the chances of residual hearing preservation. On the other hand, the overall immune reaction within a CI candidate can play a role,[8] several dosing regimens are proposed,[6,7] and several application routes are investigated, all of which make it difficult to give clear advice.[9]

4.1.3 Monitoring and Electrophysiologic Testing during CI Surgery

Facial Nerve Monitoring

Facial nerve monitoring is an additional security system, but not a substitute for knowledge on the anatomy of the facial nerve. We consider that too much reliance on the system may even carry risks, especially for beginners. If surgeon believes they are safe with the monitor, they may damage the nerve in one rough move before being warned. Especially in CI and auditory brainstem implant (ABI) surgery the facial nerve is always in the surgical field. Good knowledge of the system is required to be able to work with it as an extra tool during surgery and not get agitated by it. In malformations of the labyrinth there is often an associated abnormal course of the facial nerve.[10] The surgeon should be prepared to skeletonize the facial nerve canal, and the use of the facial nerve monitor and stimulator can be very helpful in these cases. During surgery, the use of facial nerve monitoring and stimulation precludes the use of muscle relaxants. During intraoperative electrophysiologic tests, monitoring may show facial nerve stimulation by one or more electrodes, allowing the surgeon and/or the audiologist to try to solve the problem in the same stage. Extensive explanation of facial nerve monitoring is given in Section 4.2.

Coagulation

Bipolar coagulation should be used around delicate middle ear and mastoid structures such as the facial nerve, the sigmoid sinus, and the middle or posterior fossa dura since the equipment allows precise coagulation with minimal risk of spreading current and heat to surrounding structures. Monopolar coagulation can cause facial nerve damage, rupture of the sigmoid sinus, or CSF leakage. To avoid any mistakes some surgeons use only bipolar coagulation during middle ear and mastoid surgery as bipolar coagulation is sufficient and the use of monopolar can easily be dispensed with. Once the implant is in place all coagulation should be avoided and preferably the coagulation device should be switched off to prevent artifacts in the neural response measurements. If coagulation is absolutely necessary then only bipolar coagulation with a low current should be used. The management of bleeding is described extensively in Section 4.2.

Electrophysiologic Testing

At the time of the actual insertion, the audiologist has to be called into the operation room; few surgeons do the testing without an audiologist in the room.[11] Every company has its own software for performing intraoperative measurement, and different names are given to these measurements depending with the particular software. However, overall, the intraoperative measurements are comparable between the different brands.

Several types of measurements can be made; each is briefly explained below. The impact on the surgeon of these measurements is debatable. Malfunctioning electrodes or a completely malfunctioning device (out-of-the-box) are very rare occurrences, as are misplacement or kinking. Although the audiologic measurements can support proper insertion, in case of doubt radiologic imaging is preferred.[12]

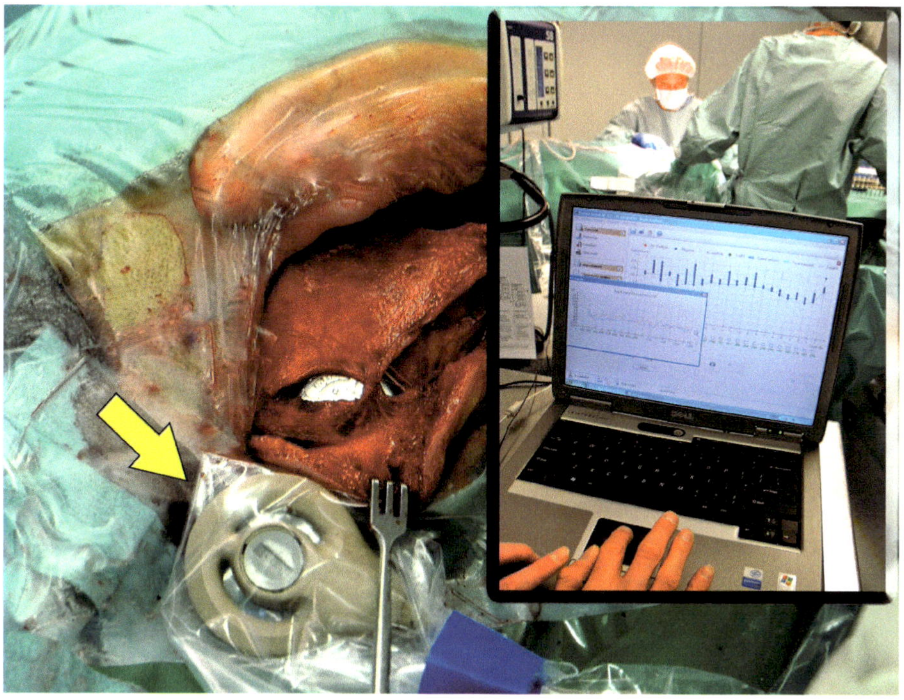

Fig. 4.26 Neural response measurements. Before closure of the wound the neural responses are measured. An audiologist can perform the measurements and stimulates the electrode at the different "channels." The magnet coil (*yellow arrow*) is inserted in a sterile pouch, positioned on top of the implant magnet and at the other side connected to the computer (see insert). This is more important in children than in adults because, during the first fitting of young CI recipients, stimulation can be started just below the T levels (threshold levels) found in peroperative measurements. Impedance and stapedial reflex measurements are also (often) performed intraoperatively.

Impedance Measurement

Correct placement of the ground electrode(s) is often necessary to get proper impedance. Impedance measurement confirms the integrity of the electrodes on the electrode array in the cochlea and it provides information on individual electrode integrity, such as short or open circuits. High impedance can be due to a bubble of air in the cochlea, improper placement of the electrode (not in a "fluid-rich" environment), or improper placement of the ground electrode.

Electrically Evoked Stapedial Reflex Threshold (ESRT) Measurement

The stapedial reflexes can be measured by suitable stimulation of CN VIII (afferent) followed by a visible contraction of the stapedial muscle and tendon innervated via CN VII (efferent). This measurement can be done for the different electrodes. In some alternative surgical approaches a clear view of the tendon is impossible and therefore measurement of the ESRT is impossible.

Neural Response/Electrically Evoked Compound Action Potential (ECAP) Measurement

This measurement confirms the reaction of the auditory nerve. It is rapid, it is not degraded by motion artifacts, and it is unaffected by type or depth of anesthesia, making the neural measurements feasible in both the operating room and in the outpatient clinic. Absence of intraoperative neural responses is rare; however, when they are absent it does not indicate a lack of stimulation or a dysfunctional device.[13]

Spread of Excitation (SOE)

Spread of excitation measurements provide information regarding the selectivity of neural excitation fields around each electrode; when these overlap it may suggest presence of a tip fold-over.[14] Although they are very rare, when using an alternative cochlear implantation technique (suprameatal technique) fold-overs can be more common and present in up to 5% of cases.[15] See **Fig. 4.26–Fig. 4.28**.

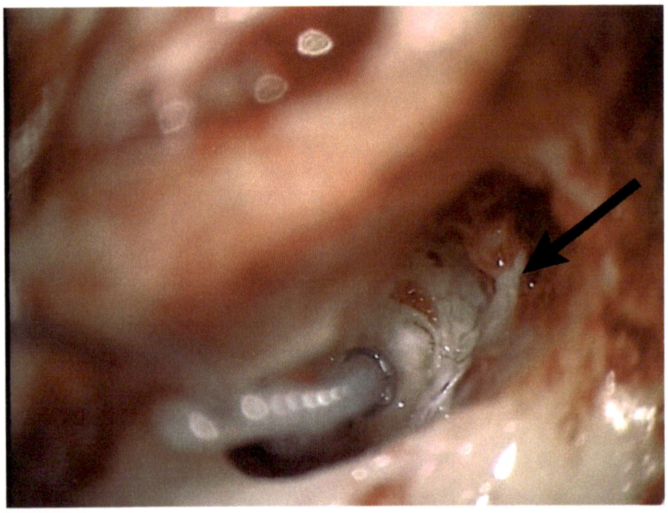

Fig. 4.27 Stapedial reflex measurement. With the electrode array inserted and the cochleostomy covered with periosteal pieces, impedance and stapedial reflex measurements can be performed. The *black arrow* points at the stapedial tendon, which contracts when the cochlear nerve is well stimulated.

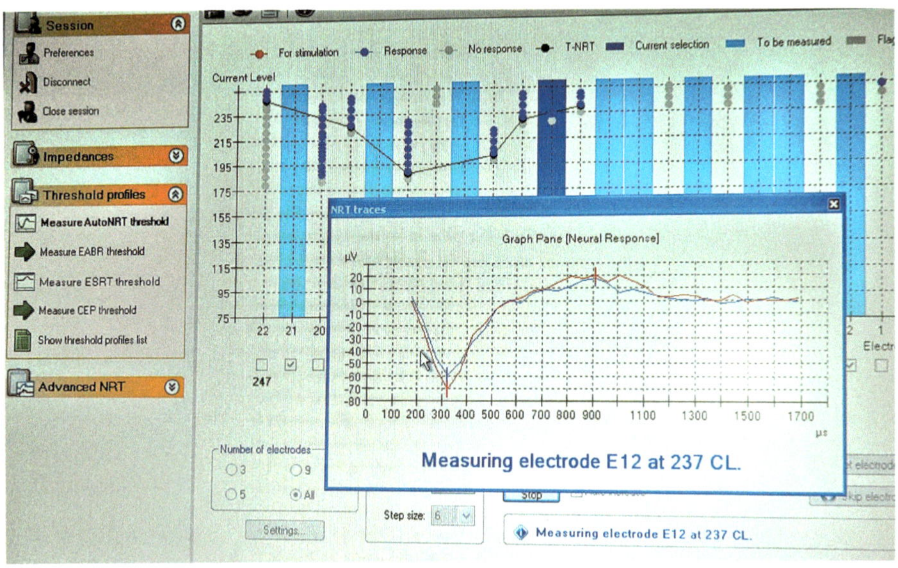

Fig. 4.28 Neural response measurements. An example of the display of intraoperative neural response measurements from different electrodes. If the outcomes are satisfactory, the wound can be closed.

4.1.4 Cochlear Implants and Electrodes Currently Available

(**Note:** Companies are listed in alphabetical order. The information is provided by the named companies and is liable to regional differences and changes over time, presented images of 2014.)

Advanced Bionics Cochlear Implant (Fig. 4.29–Fig. 4.32)

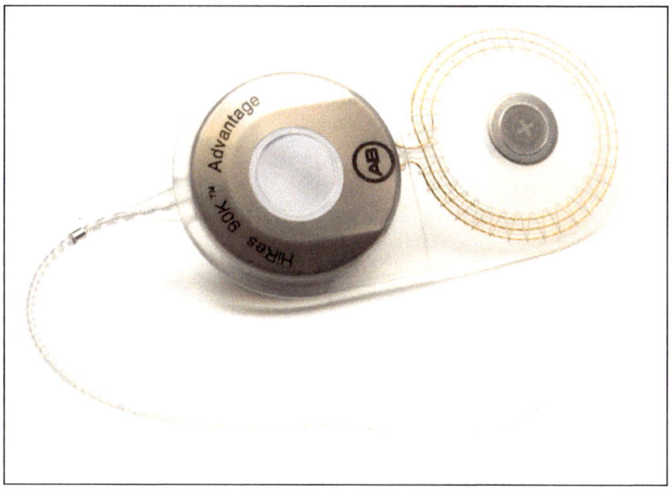

Fig. 4.29 The Advanced Bionics HiRes 90K Advantage implant, shown with a 1j electrode.

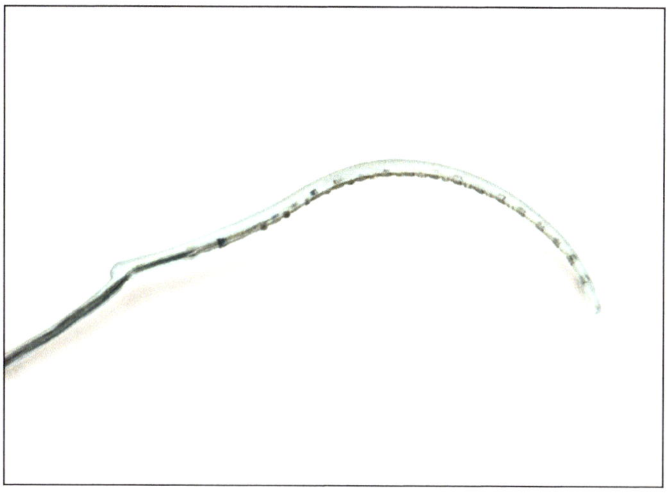

Fig. 4.30 The lateral wall HiFocus 1j electrode. Precurved electrode; number of electrodes, 16; length, 25 mm; diameter at base, 0.8 mm; diameter at tip, 0.4 mm.

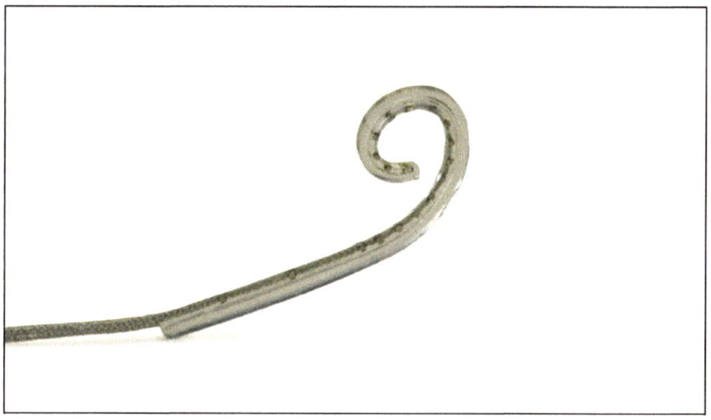

Fig. 4.31 The precurved HiFocus Helix electrode; stylet is removed. Lateral wall electrode; number of electrodes, 16; length, 24.5 mm; diameter at base, 1.1 mm; diameter at tip, 0.6 mm.

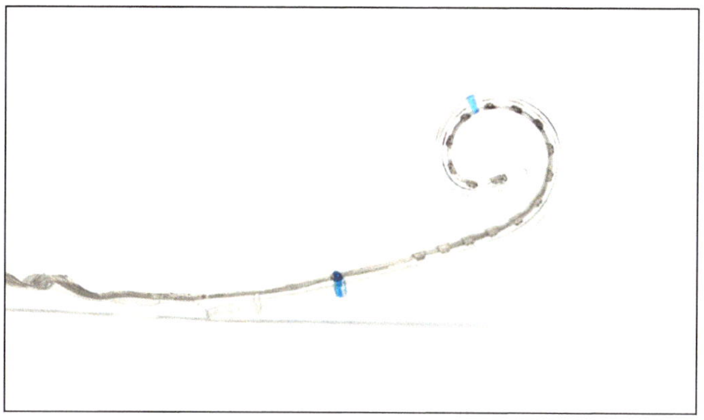

Fig. 4.32 The HiFocus Mid-Scala electrode. Mid-scala electrode; number of electrodes, 16; length, 18.5 mm; diameter at base, 0.7 mm; diameter at tip, 0.5 mm.

Cochlear Nucleus Cochlear Implant (Fig. 4.33–Fig. 4.40)

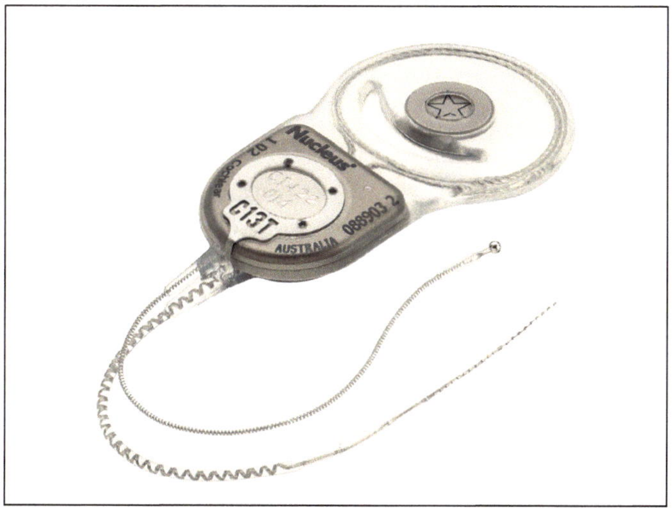

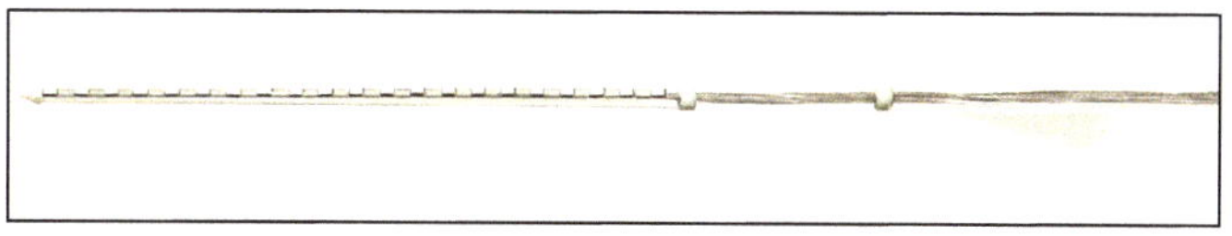

Fig. 4.34 Cochlear Nucleus CI422. Electrode enlargement; lateral wall electrode; number of electrodes, 22; length, 25 mm; diameter at base, 0.6 mm; diameter at tip, 0.3 mm.

Fig. 4.33 Nucleus Cochlear CI422 implant.

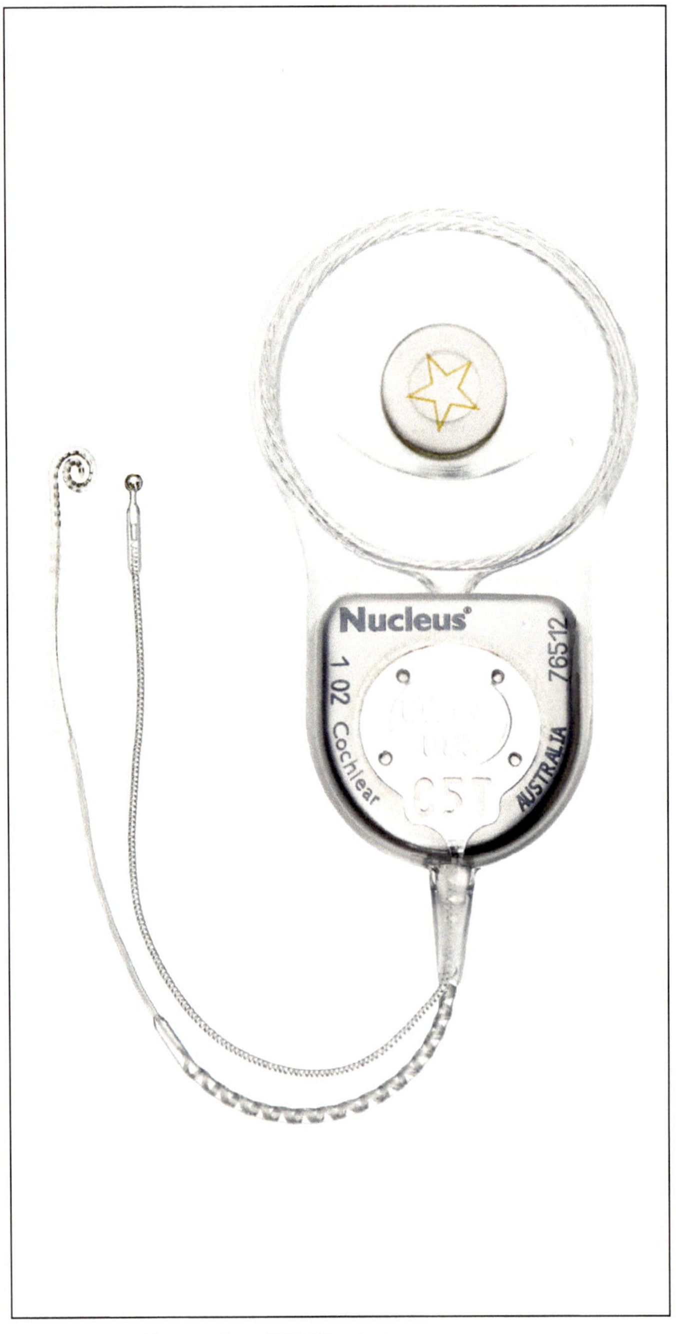

Fig. 4.35 Cochlear Nucleus CI24RE implant.

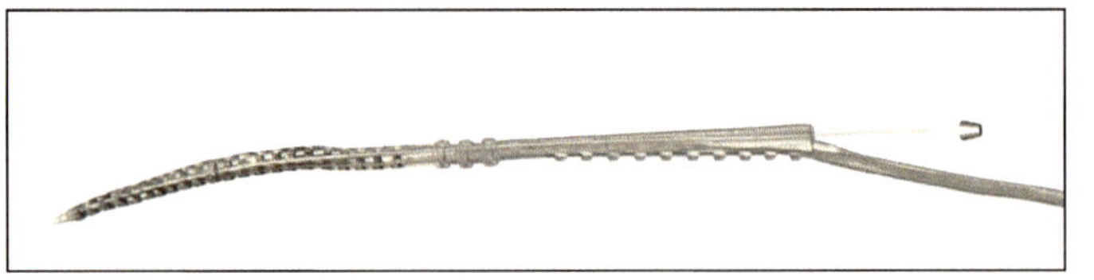

Fig. 4.36 Cochlear Contour Advance electrode with stylet. Precurved half-band electrode; number of electrodes, 22; length, 19 mm; diameter at base, 0.8 mm; diameter at tip, 0.5 mm.

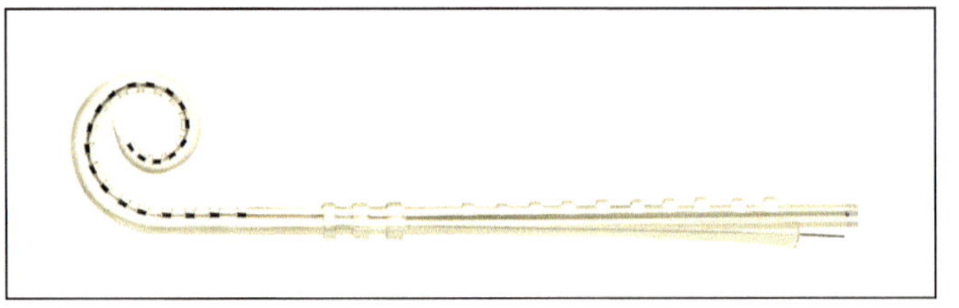

Fig. 4.37 Cochlear Contour Advance electrode after removal of stylet.

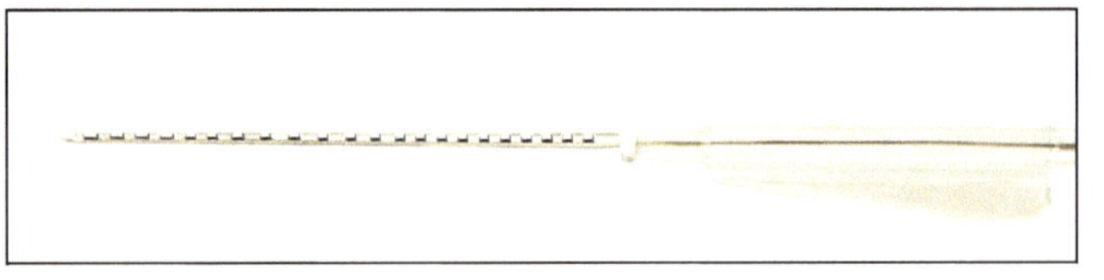

Fig. 4.38 Cochlear Hybrid electrode. Lateral wall electrode; number of electrodes, 22; length, 16 mm; diameter at base, 0.4 mm; diameter at tip, 0.25 mm.

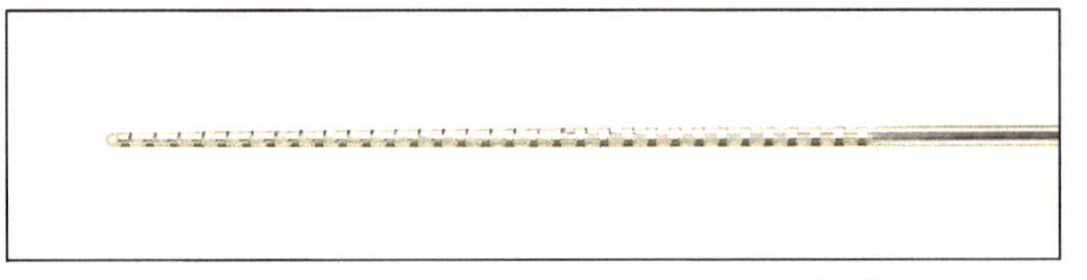

Fig. 4.39 Cochlear Freedom straight electrode. Lateral wall full-band electrode; number of electrodes, 22; length, 23.9 mm; diameter at base, 0.6 mm; diameter at tip, 0.4 mm.

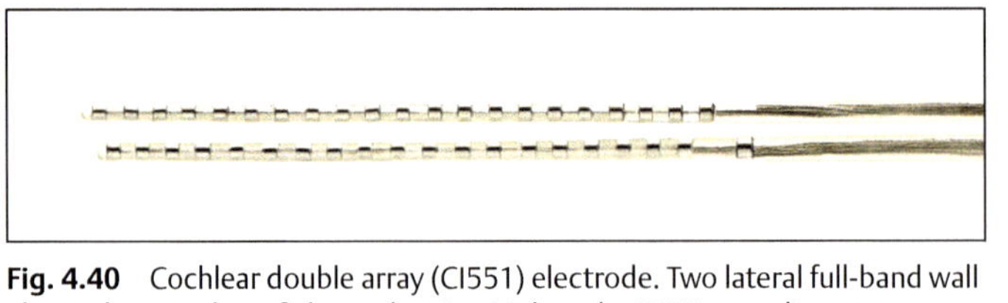

Fig. 4.40 Cochlear double array (CI551) electrode. Two lateral full-band wall electrodes; number of electrodes, 2 × 11; length, 15.75 mm; diameter at base, 0.6 mm; diameter at tip, 0.4 mm.

MED-EL Cochlear Implant (Fig. 4.41–Fig. 4.49)

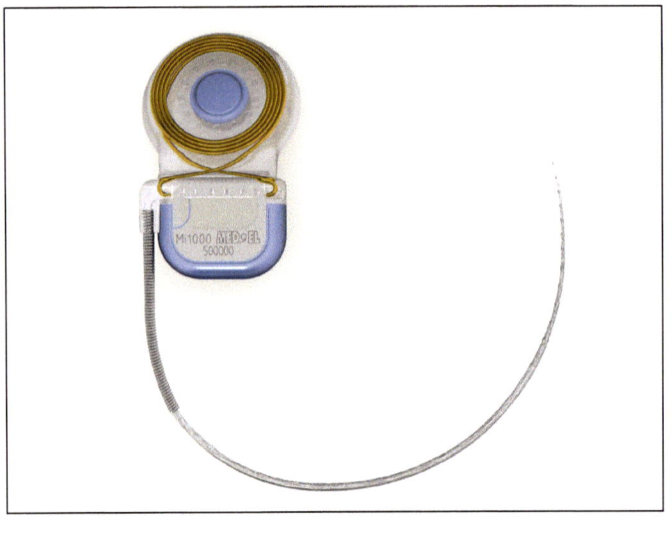

Fig. 4.41 The MED-EL Concerto implant.

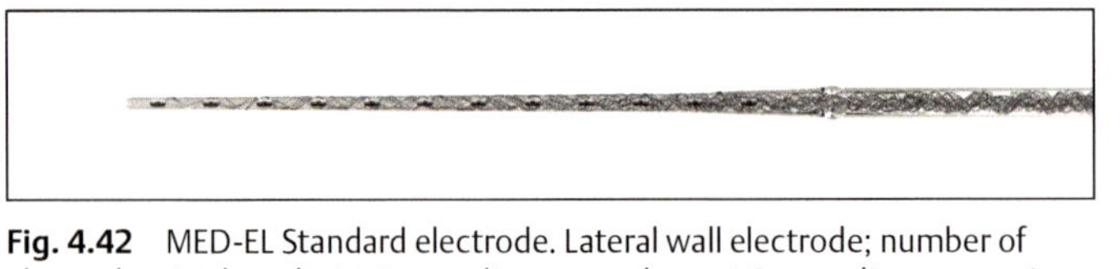

Fig. 4.42 MED-EL Standard electrode. Lateral wall electrode; number of electrodes, 24; length, 31.5 mm; diameter at base, 1.3 mm; diameter at tip, 0.5 mm.

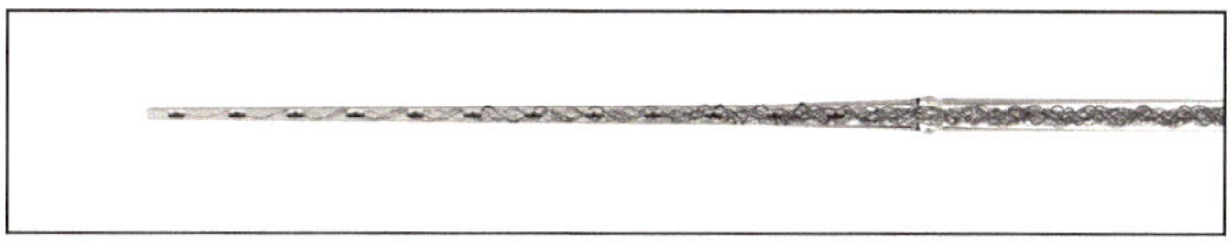

Fig. 4.43 MED-EL FlexSoft electrode. Lateral wall electrode; number of electrodes, 19; length, 31.5 mm; diameter at base, 1.3 mm; diameter at tip, 0.4 mm.

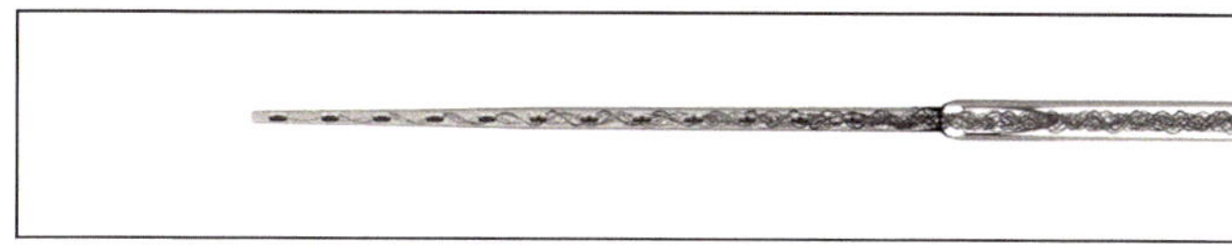

Fig. 4.44 MED-EL FLEX 28 electrode. Lateral wall electrode; number of electrodes, 19; length, 28 mm; diameter at base, 0.8 mm; diameter at tip, 0.4 mm.

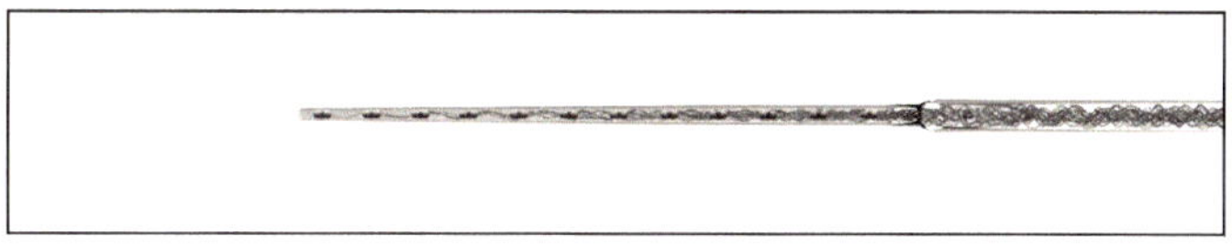

Fig. 4.45 MED-EL FLEX 24 (FLEX EAS) electrode. Lateral wall electrode; number of electrodes, 19; length, 24 mm; diameter at base, 0.8 mm; diameter at tip, 0.3 mm.

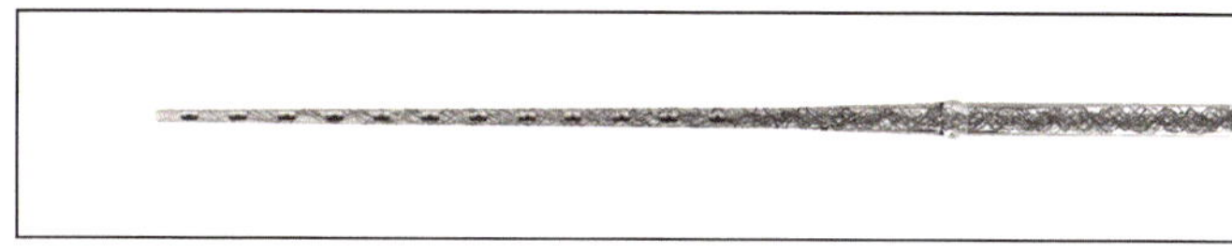

Fig. 4.46 MED-EL Medium electrode. Lateral wall electrode; number of electrodes, 24; length, 24 mm; diameter at base, 0.8 mm; diameter at tip, 0.5 mm.

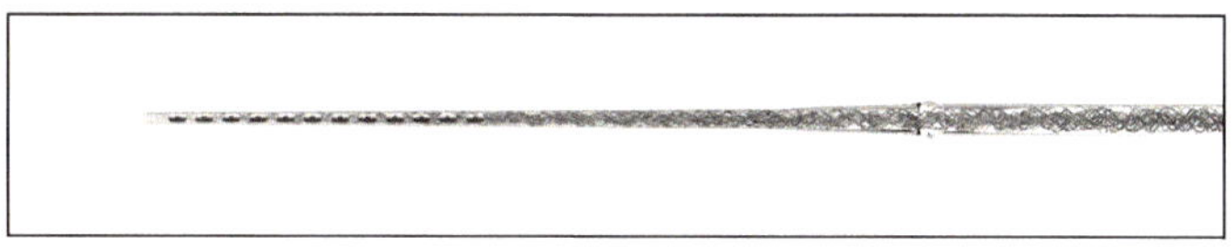

Fig. 4.47 MED-EL Compressed electrode. Lateral wall electrode; number of electrodes, 24; length, 15 mm; diameter at base, 0.7 mm; diameter at tip, 0.5 mm.

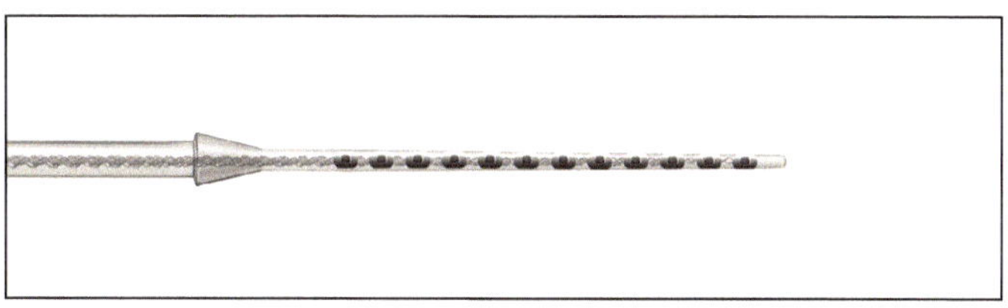

Fig. 4.49 The cork-stopper–like FORM electrode by MED-EL designed especially for malformed cochleae. Lateral wall electrode; number of electrodes, 24; length, 19 or 24 mm; diameter stopper, 1.9 mm; diameter at base, 0.8 mm; diameter at tip, 0.5 mm.

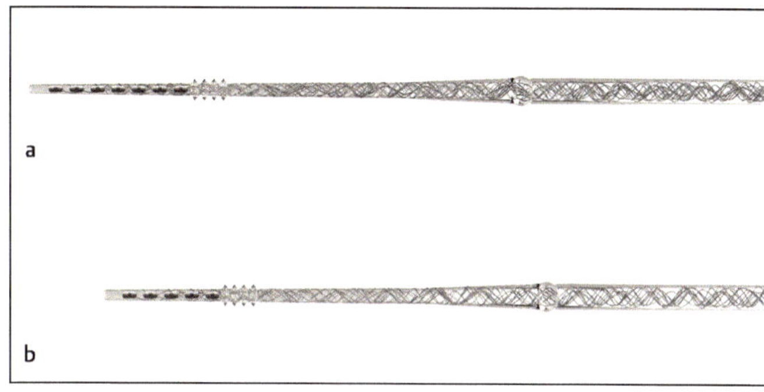

Fig. 4.48a, b

- **a** MED-EL Split electrode. Split large electrode; number of electrodes, 14; length, 9.6 mm; diameter at base, 1.0 mm; diameter at tip, 0.6 mm.
- **b** Split small electrode; number of electrodes, 10; length, 7.4 mm; diameter at base, 1.0 mm; diameter at tip, 0.6 mm.

Neurelec Digisonic SP Cochlear Implant (Fig. 4.50–Fig. 4.54)

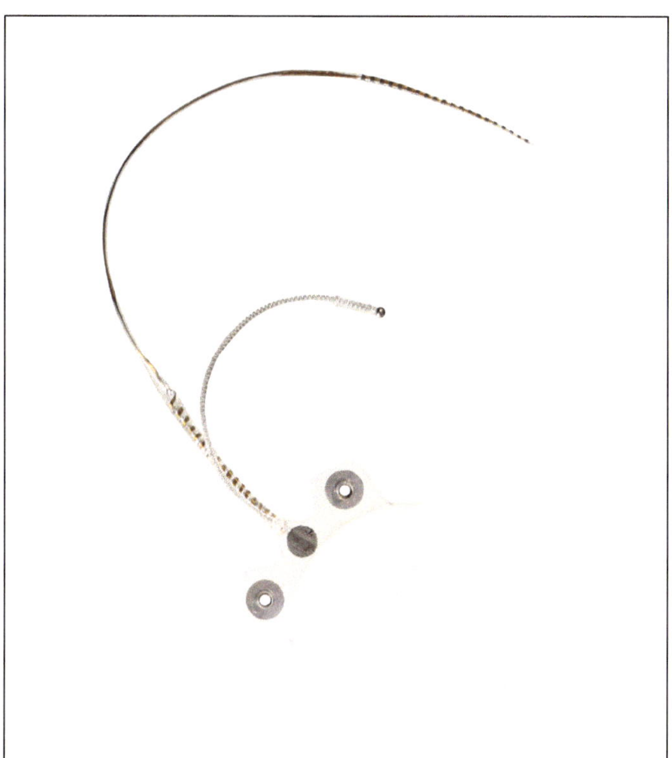

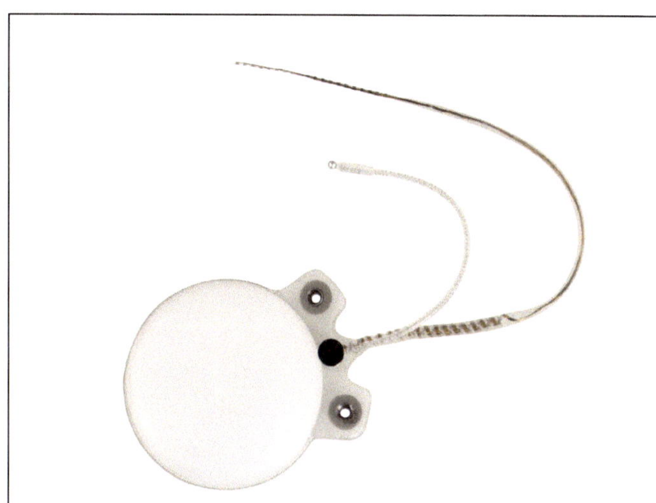

Fig. 4.51 The Neurelec Digisonic SP EVO cochlear implant with a smaller straight electrode for atraumatic insertion.

Fig. 4.50 The Neurelec Digisonic SP implant with a titanium base encapsulated in a ceramic-silicone casing.

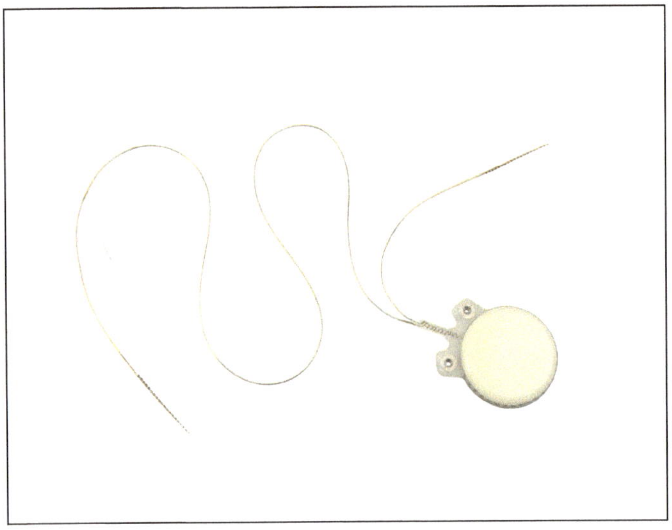

Fig. 4.52 Neurelec Digisonic SP Binaural implant with two electrodes at one implant. Two lateral wall electrodes; number of electrodes, 2 × 12; length, 17 mm; diameter at base, 1.0 mm; diameter at tip, 0.5 mm.

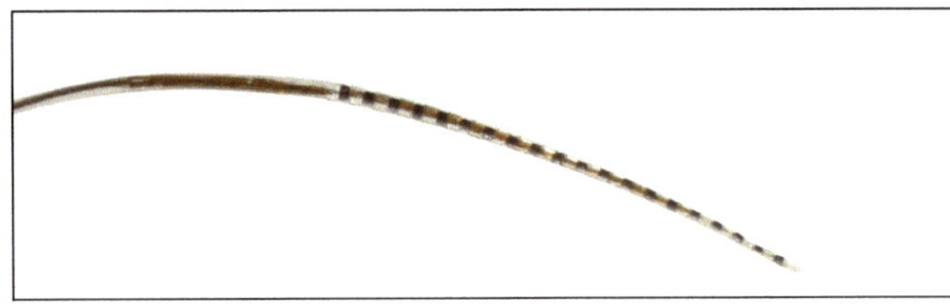

Fig. 4.53 Neurelec Digisonic SP electrode. Lateral wall electrode; number of electrodes, 20; length, 26 mm; diameter at base, 1.1 mm; diameter at tip, 0.5 mm.

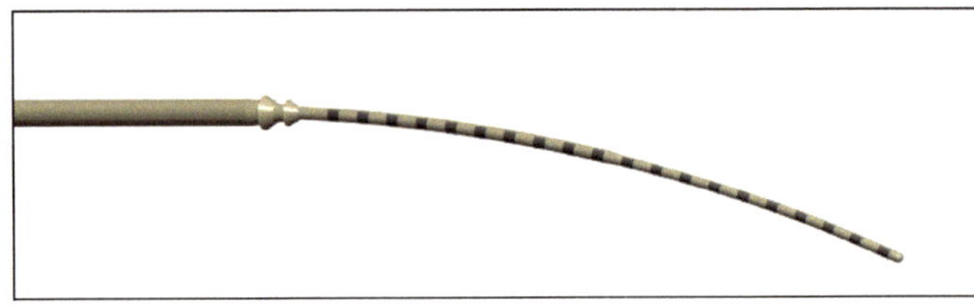

Fig. 4.54 Neurelec Digisonic SP EVO electrode. Lateral wall electrode; number of electrodes, 20; length, 25 mm; diameter at base, 0.5 mm; diameter at tip, 0.4 mm.

4.2 Auditory Brainstem Implantation: Instruments, Monitoring, and Implants

4.2.1 Surgical Instruments in ABI Surgery (Fig. 4.55)

Suction Irrigation

Suction irrigators of different sizes with finger control are used throughout surgery. The channel for irrigation is connected to an infusion set and the rate of infusion is controlled by the scrub nurse. Brackmann suction irrigation tips (**Fig. 4.56**) are specially equipped with side holes near the blunt tip and are used for intradural work or during manipulation of fine, delicate structures. Traditional suction tips can be very dangerous when used near delicate neurovascular structures. The side holes of the Brackmann type distribute the suction power and hence provide effective but indirect suctioning without endangering the fine structures lying near the tip.

Molecular Resonance Generator

In our practice we prefer the use of the Vesalius machine (molecular resonance generator, **Fig. 4.57**), which delivers quanta of energy that are calibrated for human tissue and thus match the bond energy of the target "human cell bonds." In this way, all the energy will be used to break these molecular bonds, avoiding an increase in the kinetic energy and consequently not producing a rise in temperature.

This scalpel produces an alternating current characterized by high-frequency waves combined in a particular way (CSS method); the fundamental wave is at 4 MHz, and the subsequent harmonics are at 8, 12, and 16 MHz, amplitude decreasing with increasing frequency.

The Vesalius machine can be used in several modes:

- Cutting only (seldom used)
- Combined cutting and coagulating
- Coagulation only

Cutting

Cutting is caused by the breaking of the cellular structure through the energy supplied from the tip of the electronic scalpel. For the reasons mentioned above, the cutting is cold, precise, and with variable thickness. From a clinical point of view, this means that the percentage of secondary necrosis is minimal and that the recovery will be of primary intention with reduced edema and postoperative pain.

Coagulation

Coagulation is obtained through the denaturation of "fibrinogen protein." In other words, the coagulation functionality alters the quaternary structure of the protein, triggering the physiologic cascade of coagulation. This reaction is induced by a particular electrical wave, and at a temperature of ~63°C. This procedure avoids the creation of a necrotic plug, which needs thousands of volts and exposes the patient to dangerous voltages and to large areas of secondary necrosis.

Advantages of the Vesalius Machine

We have noted the following advantages in using the Vesalius machine:

- Inflammatory reaction and postoperative pain are reduced.
- The biological tissues around the operated area suffer less thermal damage, resulting in fewer complications, greater preservation of nervous tissues both anatomically and functionally, and more rapid recovery.
- Cutting is clear and precise, thus there is no damage or alteration of tissue taken for biopsy.
- Effective and reliable coagulation of vascular structures helps immensely in achieving a bloodless operating field.

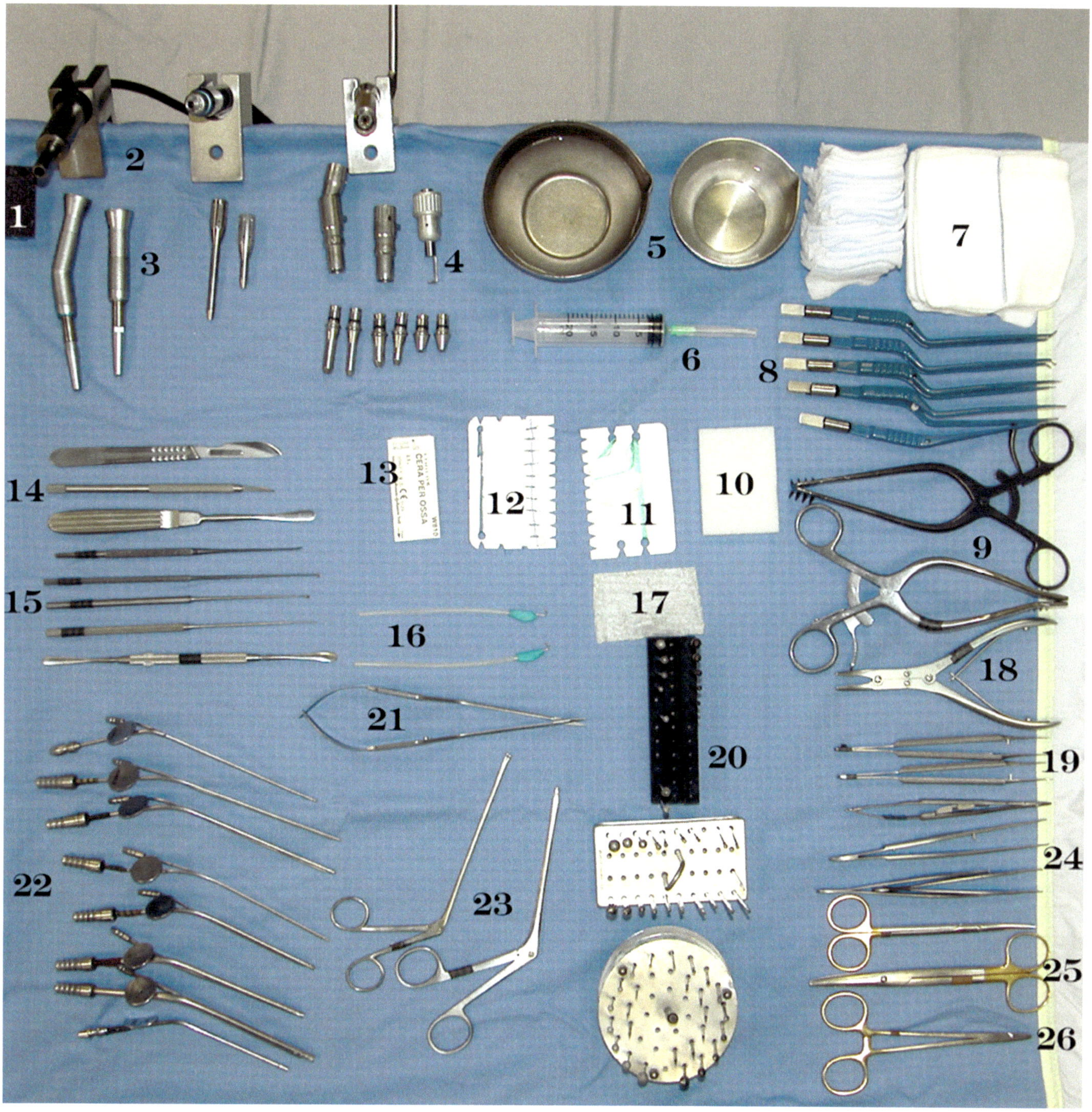

Fig. 4.55 Operating table setup for ABI/skull base surgery. **1**, scratch pad; **2**, micromotors; **3**, handpieces; **4**, craniotome tips; **5**, metal cups for saline and abdominal fat placement; **6**, 20-mL syringe; **7**, gauze; **8**, bipolar forceps; **9**, self-retaining retractors; **10**, Gelfoam; **11**, Merocel; **12**, tampons; **13**, bone wax; **14**, surgical knives; **15**, dissectors and elevators; **16**, hooks for flap retraction; **17**, Surgicel; **18**, rongeur; **19**, microforceps and needle holder; **20**, burs arranged on their racks; **21**, microscissors; **22**, suction-irrigation tubes, both Brackmann and regular tips; **23**, Weill forceps; **24**, toothed and nontoothed forceps; **25**, scissors; **26**, needle holder.

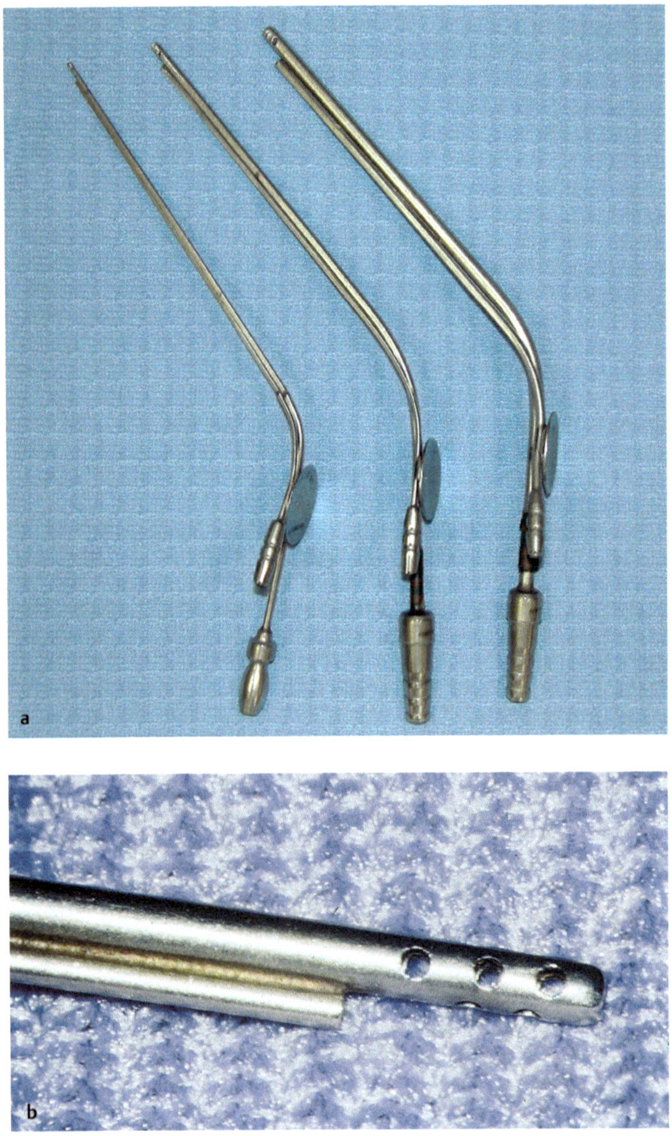

Fig. 4.56a, b Brackmann suction irrigator.
a Different sizes of the suction irrigators.
b The side holes at the tip are clearly visible.

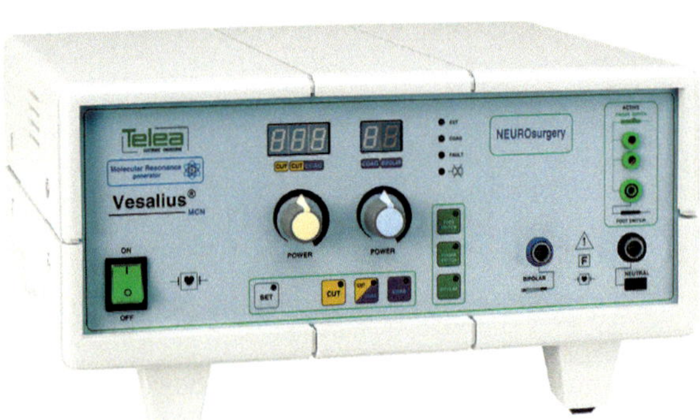

Fig. 4.57 Vesalius bipolar coagulation/cutting machine.

Microinstruments

The minimum number of instruments should be used. An overcrowded instrument table with numerous useless items is like a disturbing nightmare for the scrub nurse in these lengthy procedures. The scrub nurse should organize the instrument table in the same order to facilitate handling and proper and prompt management. See **Fig. 4.55** and **Fig. 4.58–Fig. 4.63**.

4.2.2 Management of Bleeding in ABI Surgery

Monopolar Coagulation

Monopolar coagulation is used to achieve hemostasis while making the initial incisions of the skin and musculoperiosteal tissue. After insertion of the auditory brainstem implant (ABI) (or cochlear implant), only bipolar coagulation should be used.

Bipolar Coagulation

Bipolar coagulation is an essential tool in skull base surgery. Tips of different sizes should be available (**Fig. 4.64**):

- Fine tips (0.3 mm) are used in the most delicate work for coagulating fine vessels intracranially.
- Large tips (1 and 1.3 mm) are used for debulking and coagulation of the tumor and tumor capsule.

Copious irrigation while using bipolar coagulation is important to prevent the tips from sticking to the structure coagulated. Sticking may cause rebleeding or tearing and further injury. Black deposits formed on the tips make the bipolar coagulator less efficient and may cause sticking. Such deposits should be cleaned by the nurse using a scratch pad. The use of a scalpel for such a task should be discouraged as it causes scratching and irregularity of the tip surface. The Vesalius system as described above has the advantage that it does not stick to the structure being coagulated.

Small tears of the sigmoid sinus can be managed by the judicious use of bipolar coagulation. For such cases, the bipolar coagulator is adjusted to a low setting, continuous irrigation is used, and the tips of the bipolar coagulator are used to approximate the tear edges while performing coagulation. In contrast, the bipolar coagulator should never be used to manage bleeding from small tears of the jugular bulb, as more bleeding usually occurs.

Bleeding from Bony Surfaces

Bleeding from bony surfaces is controlled using diamond burs without irrigation. The heat generated by the diamond bur is usually sufficient to stop such minor bleeding. Significant bleeding from bony surfaces can be stopped using bone wax. A small piece of bone wax is applied and is pressed firmly with the thumb. When the bleeding surface is deeply located in the operative field, a small piece of bone wax shaped like a sphere is applied using a septal dissector and is compressed using cottonoids.

Gelatin Sponge

Gelatin sponge (Spongostan, Ferrosan, Italy; or Gelfoam, Johnson & Johnson, New Brunswick, New Jersey, USA) has an enormous capacity to absorb blood. The pressure exerted by the weight of the blood-soaked gelatin sponge in contact with an oozing surface

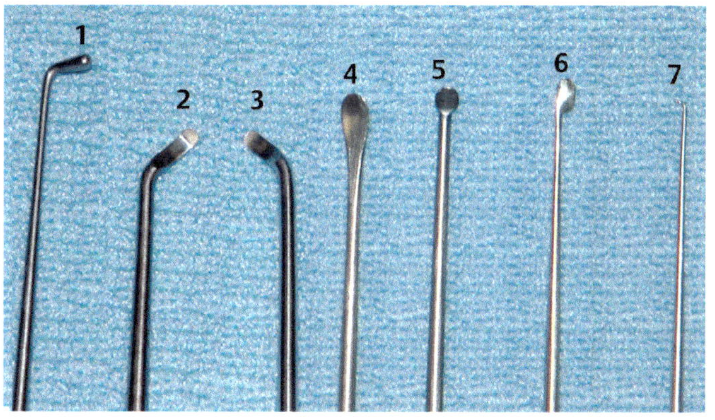

Fig. 4.58 Close-up view of tips of the microinstruments: **1**, blunt-tip right-angled hook; **2**, double curved raspatory (right-sided); **3**, double curved raspatory (left-sided); **4**, straight microdissector; **5**, round dissector 45°; **6**, vertical dissector; **7**, 90° angled sharp hook.

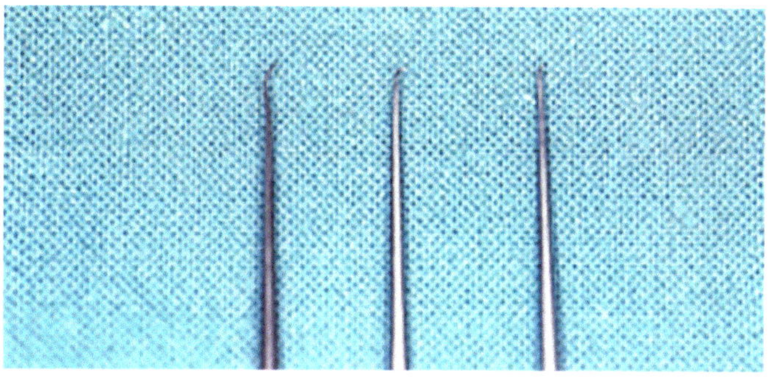

Fig. 4.59 Close-up view of curved needle, 90° hook, and sharp curved hook from the left.

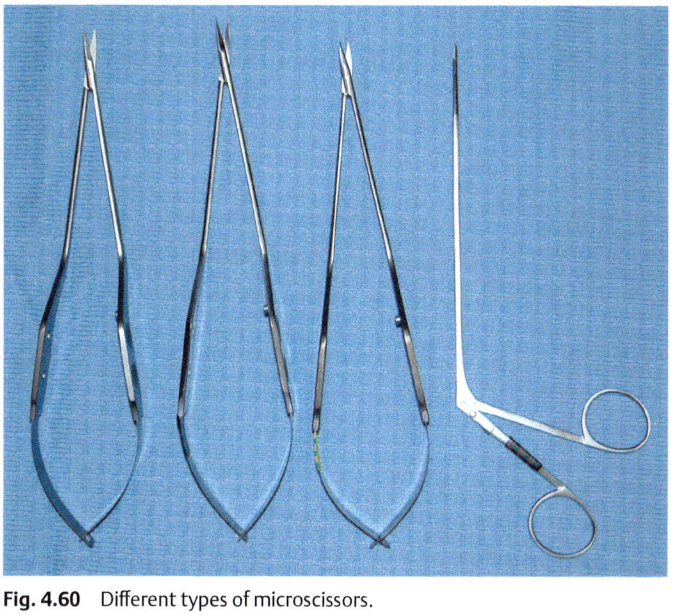

Fig. 4.60 Different types of microscissors.

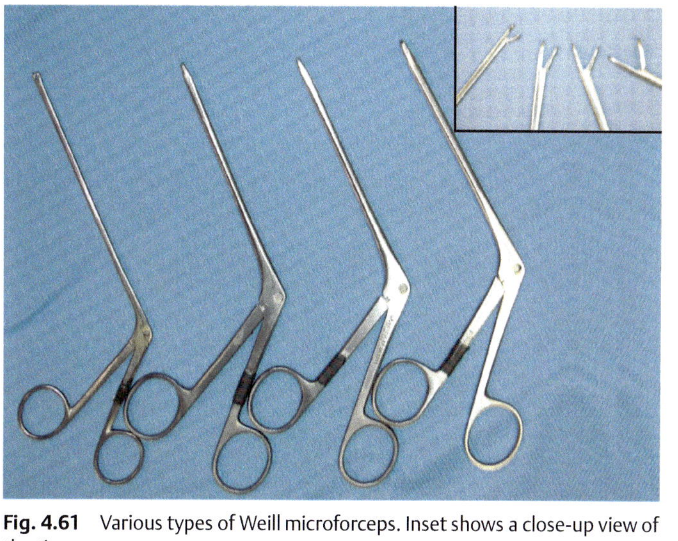

Fig. 4.61 Various types of Weill microforceps. Inset shows a close-up view of the tips.

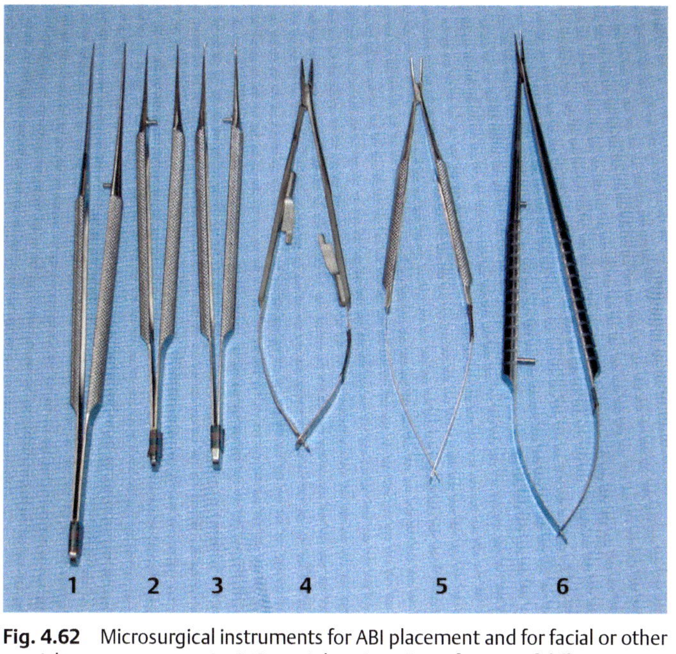

Fig. 4.62 Microsurgical instruments for ABI placement and for facial or other cranial nerve anastomosis: **1**, **2**, straight micro tissue forceps of different lengths; **3**, curved micro tissue forceps; **4**, microsurgery needle holder; **5**, microscissors; **6**, micro suturing forceps.

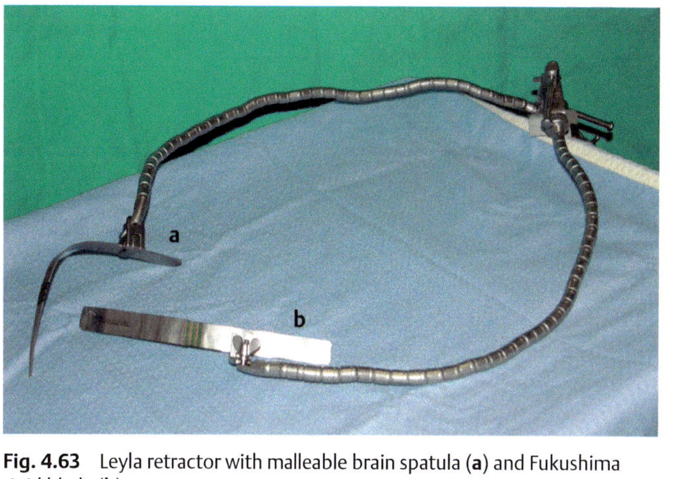

Fig. 4.63 Leyla retractor with malleable brain spatula (**a**) and Fukushima rigid blade (**b**).

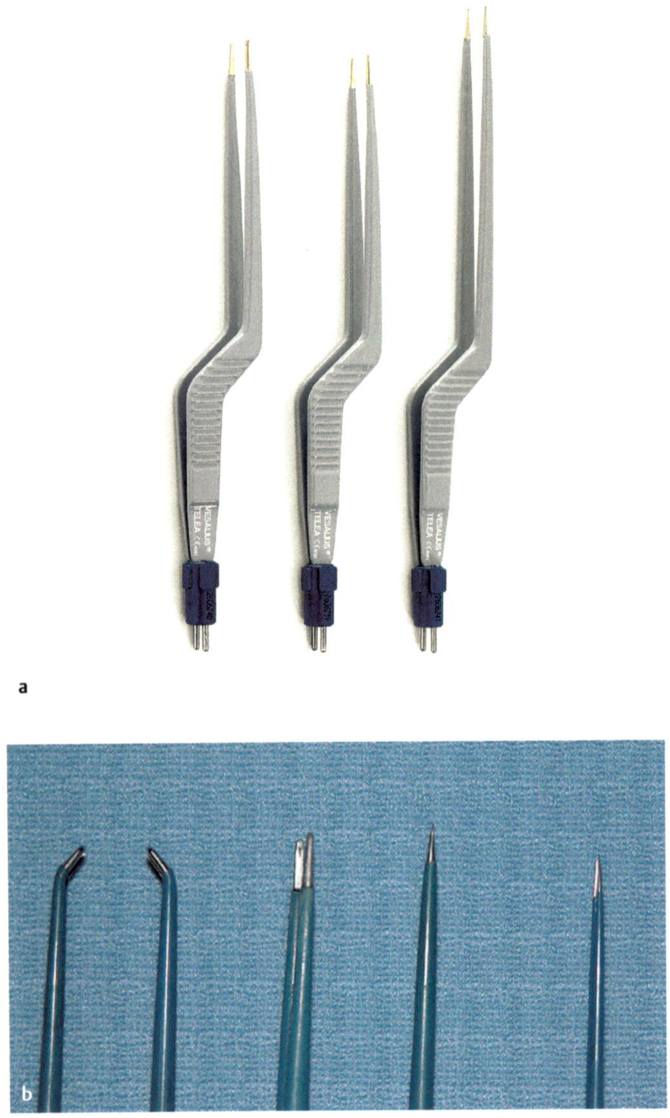

Fig. 4.64a, b Different types of bipolar forceps. (**a**) Angled forceps and bayonet forceps with straight tips and angled tips. (**b**) Close-up of the tips we use with cautery.

assists in hemostasis. The advantage of this material is that it can be left in place to be absorbed over 20 to 45 days. It is used for the control of capillary ooze and bleeding from small arterioles, particularly in those locations where bipolar coagulation can be injurious (e.g., bleeding from vessels over the facial nerve).

Oxidized Regenerated Cellulose

Oxidized regenerated cellulose (Surgicel, Johnson & Johnson, New Brunswick, New Jersey, USA) acts as an organic acid and hence behaves like a caustic agent that reacts with blood to produce a reddish-brown mass functioning as an artificial clot. Additionally, this agent has proved to have a potent bactericidal action.

Surgicel is mainly used to stop capillary ooze. This is particularly useful at the level of the cerebellum in the presence of diffuse venous bleeding. Use of this agent is also especially important at the brainstem to stop bleeding because use of bipolar coagulation is not possible. It can also be used for intraluminal packing of venous sinuses in case of inadvertent injury or intentional transection as a part of the approach.

Because of its tissue reaction, excessive Surgicel left in the cerebellopontine angle may lead to postoperative fever. As this agent swells when in contact with blood, it should be used carefully in confined spaces so as not to cause pressure neuropathy of adjacent nerves.

Hemostatic Matrix

A thrombin solution called Floseal (Baxter International Inc., Deerfield, Illinois, USA) is indicated in surgical procedures as an adjunct to hemostasis when control of bleeding by ligature or conventional procedures is ineffective or impractical. Floseal is not intended as a substitute for meticulous surgical technique and the proper application of ligatures or other conventional procedures for hemostasis. It stops bleeding 97% of the time within 6 to 10 minutes and is a good alternative for controlling bleeding from oozing to spurting. One should know that Floseal should not be used in the closure of skin incisions, must not be injected into blood vessels, and should not be used in the absence of active bleeding. Excess of the material (material not incorporated in the hemostatic clot) should always be removed from the site of application by gentle irrigation.

4.2.3 Monitoring of Facial and Cochlear Nerves in ABI (or CI) Surgery

When the aim is preservation of hearing, an ipsilateral ear stimulator is applied and electrodes are placed to monitor evoked auditory brainstem responses (ABR) and/or direct cochlear nerve action potential (CNAP). Of course, this situation is extremely rare in ABI or CI surgery cases. See **Fig. 4.65**.

Facial Nerve Monitoring

Intraoperative facial nerve monitoring (IFNM) has become established as an integral part of skull base and otologic surgery. It helps to identify the facial nerve accurately, thereby enhancing preservation of it. This is particularly important when tumors or anatomical variations place the nerve at a higher risk.

The Avalanche T neuromonitor (Langer Medical GmbH, Waldkirch, Germany) has been especially developed for intraoperative use in surgery. The neuromonitor allows surgeons to easily stimulate and identify nerves and to subject them to an integrity check independently of the application or medical field in which it is used. The upgradable modular system enables the use of up to 8 channels for electromyography and 4 channels for evoked potentials (sensory, motor, and auditory evoked potentials).

Patients are routinely monitored using the nerve integrity monitor (NIM) (**Fig. 4.66**). The monitor displays simultaneously in the 2-/4-channel neuro-otology surgery mode the activity of the orbicularis oculi muscle and the orbicularis oris muscle. To avoid interferences and artifacts, this machine is supplied with a "muting probe" that is connected around the output cable of equipment such as the bipolar cautery or other external devices that generate interfering signals. The muting performance can be scheduled on four muting probe jack positions according to the intensity of the electrocautery equipment, to reduce artifacts.

Recording Electrodes

To detect the electromyographic responses, we use EEG-type needle silver chloride monopolar electrodes with a diameter of 1.2 mm and a length of 1 cm. There are also surface electrodes available, but the EEG-type needle electrodes are more stable during surgery and more sensitive in recording the facial muscle activity.

Patient Interface Box

The patient interface box is a device that acts as a connection between the electrodes and the NIM pulse. This device has sites for the recording electrode inputs and for the stimulating electrodes:

- Thirteen sites for the following electrode
- Two sites for the orbicularis oris muscle
- Two sites for the orbicularis oculi muscle
- Four additional sites for monitoring other nerves
- Two sites for the monopolar stimulating electrode
- Two sites for the bipolar stimulating electrode
- One green input jack for the EEG ground electrode

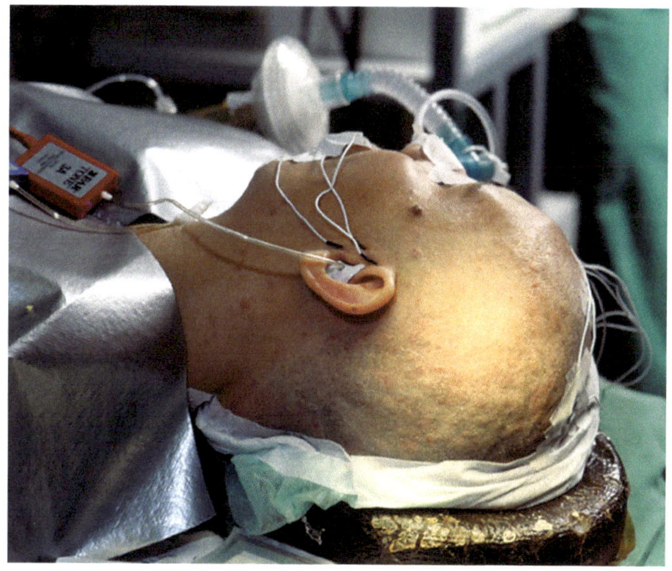

Fig. 4.65 A patient prepared for surgery in a hearing-preservation procedure. Note the electrodes and the microphone placed in the ear for eighth-nerve monitoring.

Electromyographic (EMG) responses are essentially unaffected by the commonly used anesthetics. An important exception is muscle relaxants, which inhibit the transmission of action potentials across the neuromuscular junction and interfere with IFNM. Therefore, after endotracheal intubation, no muscle relaxants should be used during operations in which IFNM is required.

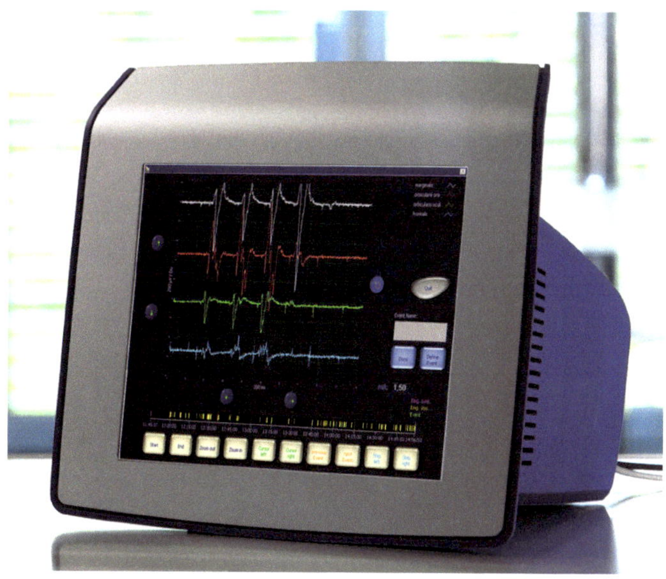

Fig. 4.66 The Avalanche nerve integrity monitor.

Positioning of the Electrodes

Preparation of the patient starts after general anesthesia. Location of the recording electrodes has to be done by the medical staff who will be present in the operating theater for the surgical procedure and if possible by the electrophysiologist. Proper location of electrodes before draping is crucial because it is almost impossible to change their positions once the operation has started (**Fig. 4.67**).

After insertion of the needle electrodes, each electrode is fixed to the skin using adhesive tape; then the wires of the four electrodes of the two channels together with the ground electrode wire are grouped together and passed away from the field and fixed together with an adhesive tab.

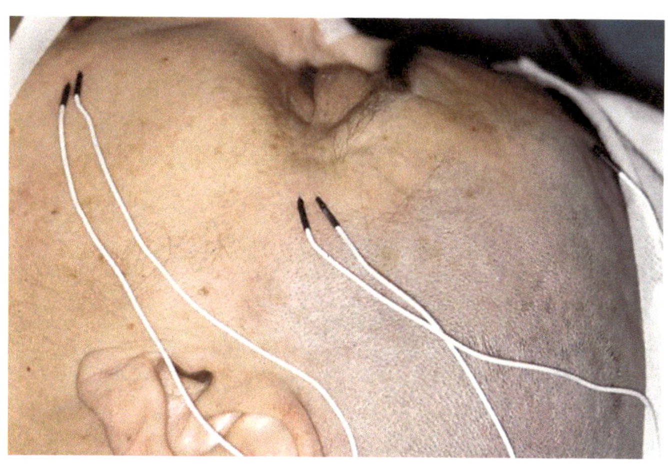

Fig. 4.67 Electrodes are properly positioned in the orbicularis oculi and orbicularis oris muscles.

Localization of the Facial Nerve (Mapping)

Monopolar or bipolar stimulation can be useful in early localization and identification of the facial nerve during surgery for vestibular schwannoma and other cerebellopontine angle (CPA) tumors. For example, in cases of medium-to-large tumors, the facial nerve is frequently displaced and stretched, and identification of the nerve can be very difficult. Thus electrical stimulation is used to probe the tumor mass or the surrounding structures and to localize the course of the facial nerve. For this purpose, monopolar stimulation is recommended because it ensures a larger area of stimulation than does bipolar.

- We generally start to stimulate with an intensity of 0.05 mA and progressively increase the stimulus in steps of 0.02 mA until EMG responses are induced. The range of mapping stimulation that we use is from 0.05 mA to 0.4 mA. The stimulus is delivered with square-wave pulses of 0.1 or 0.2 milliseconds duration at a rate of four to six per second.

- We usually do not perform mapping of the facial nerve in the temporal bone for the mastoid portion and the second genu because anatomical identification is generally preferred. Stimulation between 0.5 mA and 1 mA can be used to confirm the precise course of the facial nerve and the thickness of bone covering the facial nerve course in the temporal bone.
- A current of 1 mA corresponds to ~1 mm of bone thickness.

Technique

Electrical stimulation is commonly used to distinguish the facial nerve from the vestibulocochlear nerve, the other cranial nerves, and the soft tissues. The range of stimulus intensity we routinely use for identification of the facial nerve in the CPA is 0.05 to 0.20 mA. The stimulator is generally set to a constant current stimulus with a rate of 4 pulses per second and stimulus duration of 100 milliseconds.

Facial Nerve Monitoring Considerations

The specialized personnel dedicated to IFNM need good knowledge of neurophysiology and skull base anatomy. It is of paramount importance to evaluate electrophysiologic data in association with the anatomy to correlate the EMG potentials with the surgical steps. Only in this way is it possible to achieve significant information and results by this technique. IFNM assures better postoperative facial nerve results, but surgeons should always keep in mind that it cannot substitute for their own surgical experience.

4.2.4 Intraoperative Cochlear Nerve Monitoring (ABR and CNAP)

Introduction

With increased availability of MRI scanning, we have more occasions to see a patient with a small vestibular schwannoma (VS) and with still serviceable hearing. The role of hearing-preservation surgery is thus becoming more significant. If hearing preservation is intended, we perform either the middle cranial fossa (MCF) approach or the combined retrosigmoid–retrolabyrinthine (RS-RL) approach under intraoperative cochlear nerve monitoring.

With this, preservation of the cochlear nerve integrity is of significance in vestibular schwannoma surgery in deaf patients (often NF2). If the cochlear nerve is sacrificed during tumor removal, a cochlear implant is not feasible in this ear. If the integrity of the nerve is preserved, an attempt at cochlear implantation can be made. Currently, a device to stimulate the cochlea during surgery, in combination with electrically evoked auditory brainstem response (EABR) recordings, is being developed. With positive recordings during stimulation, CI placement would be beneficial; with no EABR reaction, CI function—or in some cases placement—is doubtful. An enlarged translabyrinthine approach is performed for removal of the VS if there is no serviceable hearing. This gives the advantage that both the cochlea and the CPA are easy accessible, within the same procedure.

For intraoperative cochlear nerve monitoring (ICNM) the cochlear nerve action potential (CNAP) is used in addition to the evoked auditory brainstem response (ABR). Recording auditory evoked potentials directly from the eighth cranial nerve (CNAP) is believed to have an advantage over recording ABR, since it is "real-time" monitoring and its potentials are larger in amplitude and accordingly more sensitive than those recorded from electrodes placed at a long distance (ABR). CNAP is currently more popular for monitoring the function of the cochlear nerve, but is not more reliable

The responses obtained in ICNM depend not only on the integrity of the nerve but also on the blood supply of the nerve and the cochlea. It should be kept in mind that the use of electrocautery and surgical maneuvers can affect the intraoperative responses and may lead to misinterpretation. It is also emphasized that an anatomically intact cochlear nerve after surgical removal does not necessarily imply a viable cochlear nerve (see Chapter 17).

Evoked Auditory Brainstem Response

Modifications in the ABR stimulation, the so-called fast auditory brainstem response technique, may be helpful for obtaining an interpretable waveform more rapidly. Since the changes in the waveform result from the surgical manipulation, they should be immediately reported to the surgeon. Otherwise, one cannot know which manipulation caused these unfavorable changes.

- After induction of general anesthesia, which usually does not affect recording, the ear canal is inspected and sterilized with alcohol.
- A soft ear mold with an attached 30-cm plastic tube that terminates at a small transducer is placed inside the external canal (**Fig. 4.68**) and is secured with silicone paste (**Fig. 4.69**). This prevents water from entering the ear canal and avoids dislodgement of the transducer during surgery.
- Needle electrodes are inserted at the following sites. The active electrode (+) is inserted in the scalp at vertex and the ground electrode is located at the vertex 3 cm anterior to the active electrode. The third electrode (−) is inserted in the pretragal area for the MCF approach, or in the mastoid tip area for the RS-RL approach (**Fig. 4.70** and **Fig. 4.71**).
- The stimuli used are clicks, presented at a rate of 31 to 51 pulses per second (pps). The intensity of the stimuli is 130 dB SPL (sound pressure level). The system we currently use is shown in **Fig. 4.72**.
- Once the proper placement of the electrode is accomplished, baseline ABR traces are recorded and will be used as a reference during the operation (**Fig. 4.73**).
- In standard far-field ABR recordings, 1,500 sweeps are required to produce an interpretable waveform. This takes a few minutes. In our setup we use an analog filter combined with a digital filter (WF 25 and WF 50),[16] which permits us to obtain an interpretable wave V with the number of sweeps ranging between 50 and 200. This process usually takes less than 5 seconds. All the parameters are shown in **Table 4.1**. During the critical steps of the surgery continuous recording is feasible for detecting potential trauma as soon as possible (**Fig. 4.74**).
- The surgeon is usually informed when the delay of the latency of wave V is more than 0.5 milliseconds or when either there is disappearance of any of the waves or gross changes are observed in the traces. In those situations the operation is

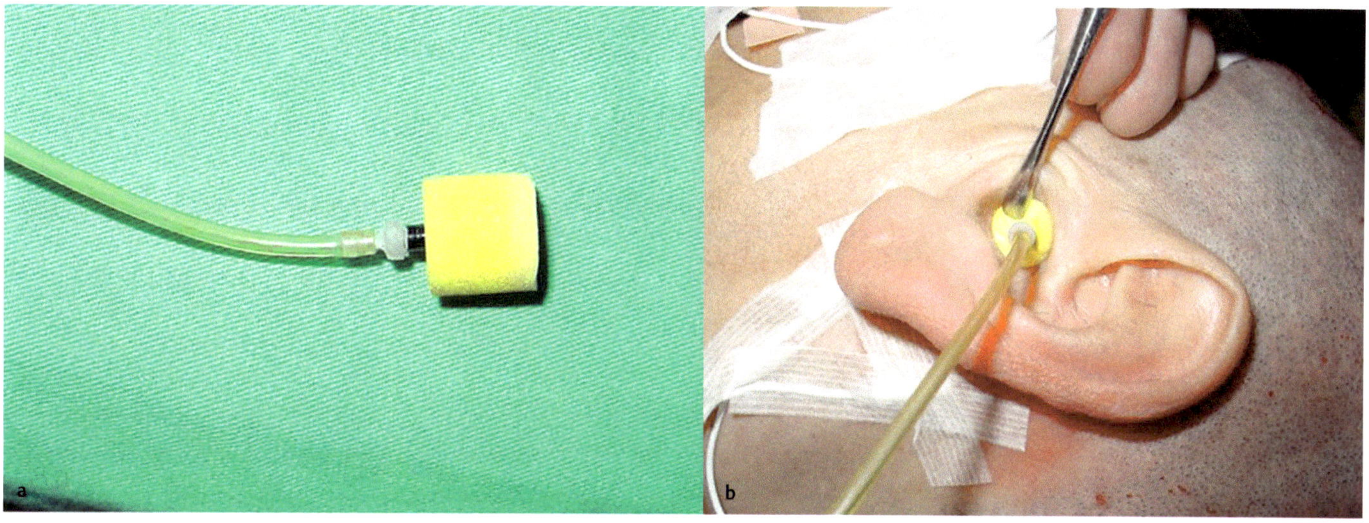

Fig. 4.68a, b

a Ear mold, which contains a small transducer providing stimulation, with a 30-cm plastic tube.

b The ear mold is inserted into the external ear canal.

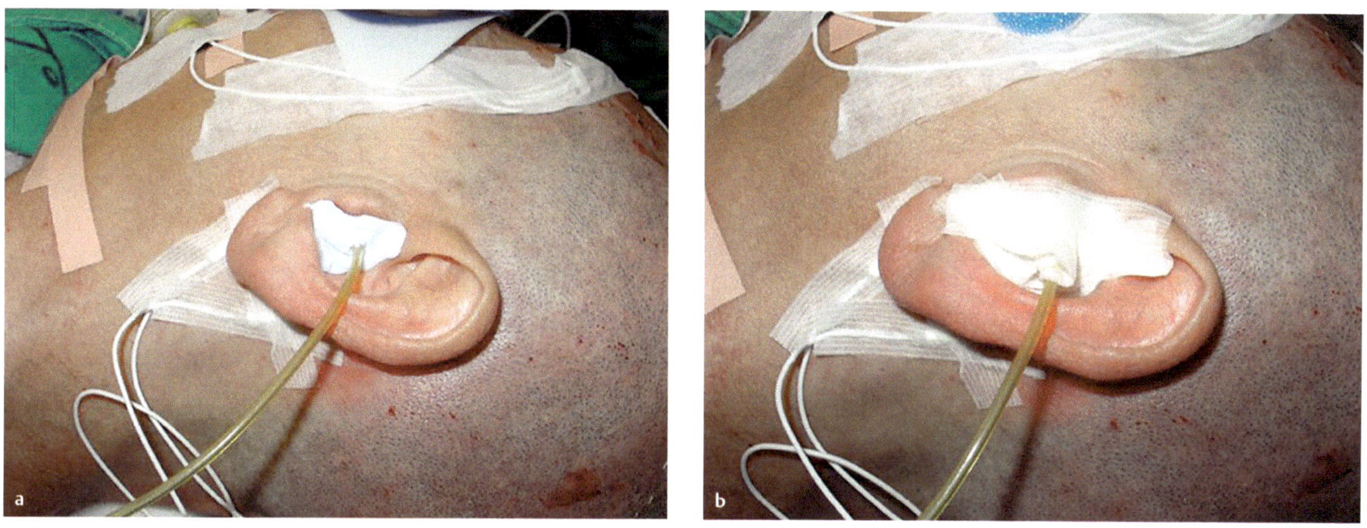

Fig. 4.69a, b

a The ear mold is secured with silicone paste. This avoids dislodgement of the transducer.

b The transducer is further secured with adhesive tape.

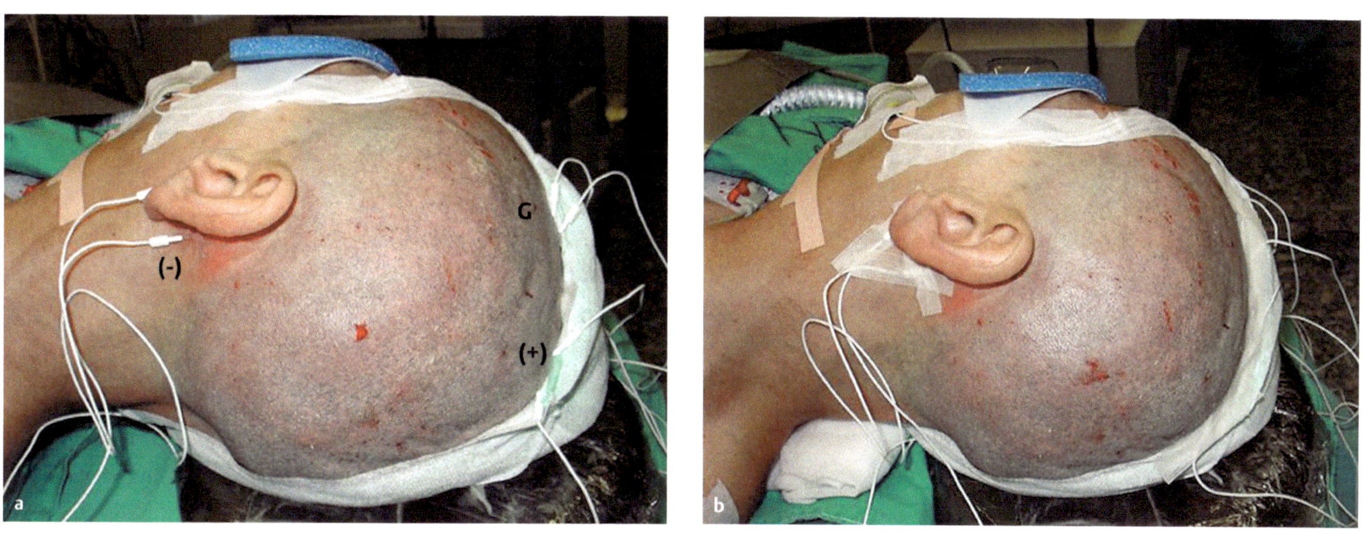

Fig. 4.70a, b

a Insertion of the needle electrodes. G, ground electrode; (+), positive electrode; (−), negative electrode.

b Securing of the needle electrodes with adhesive tape.

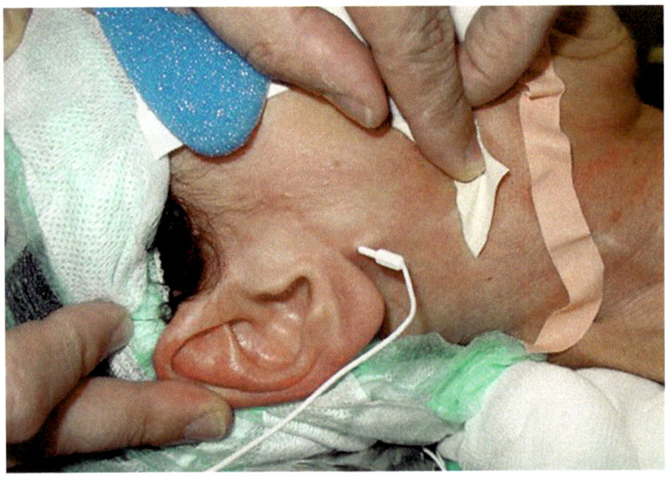

Fig. 4.71 Another needle electrode is inserted in the contralateral mastoid tip area as the negative for CNAP.

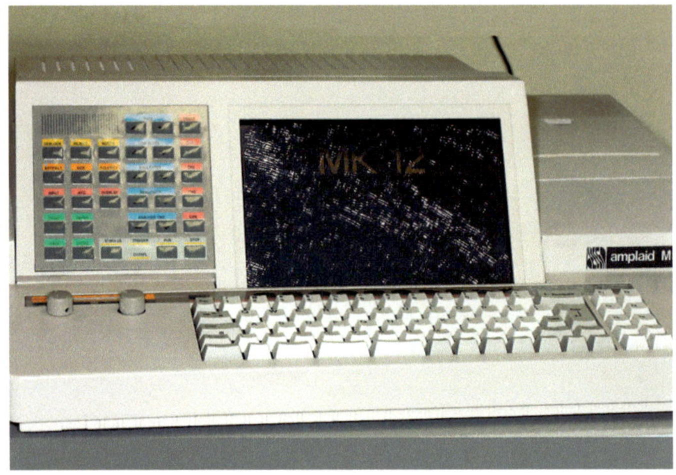

Fig. 4.72 The system we currently use to monitor the ABR.

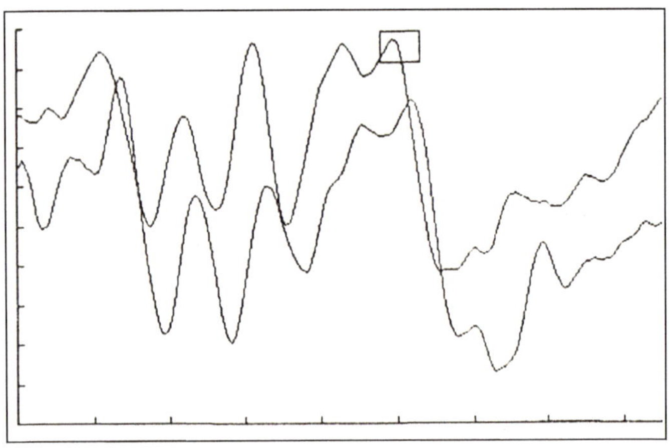

Fig. 4.73 Intraoperative ABR typically showing the baseline at the beginning of the surgery and the final recording. Note the mild additional delay of the V wave produced by surgery.

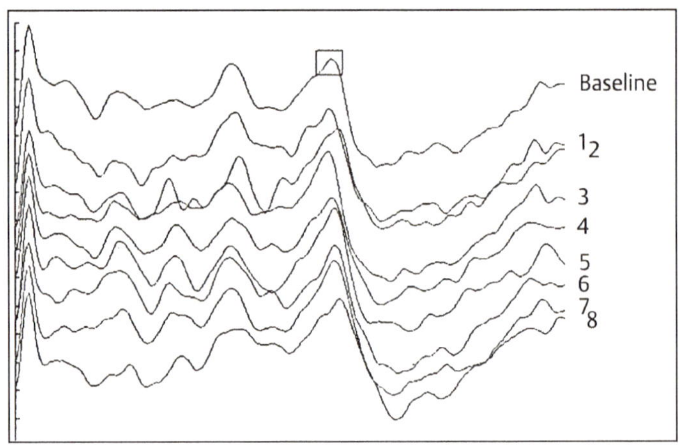

Fig. 4.74 Another example of intraoperative recording, showing a continuous recording during the critical steps of the surgery.

Table 4.1 Parameters of intraoperative fast-ABR

Parameter	Value
Low filter	100 Hz
High filter	2500 Hz
Amplifier sensitivity	2.5 μV/div
Average sensitivity	100 nV/div
Stimulus	Click
Rate	31/s–51/s
Polarity	Alternating
Masking	Off
Intensity	130 dB SPL

Table 4.2 Parameters of intraoperative CNAP

Parameter	Value
Low filter	100 Hz
High filter	2500 Hz
Amplifier sensitivity	1 μV/div
Average sensitivity	1 μV/div
Stimulus	Click
Rate	31/s
Polarity	Alternating
Averaging	50
Intensity	130 dB SPL
Sweep time	10 milliseconds

paused for a while to see whether the traces will recover. We usually do not give any vasodilating agent either locally or systemically.

Direct Cochlear Nerve Action Potential

Compound action potentials can be recorded from the intracranial portion of the eighth cranial nerve in operations in which this nerve becomes exposed (**Table 4.2**). These potentials can then be used for ICNM and can inform us of the viability of the cochlear nerve in real time. A multithreaded silver wire electrode is used to record the cochlear nerve potentials. The tip of the electrode is devoid of Teflon coating but is covered with a cotton pledget. This electrode is placed directly on the cochlear nerve proximal to the tumor.

- The negative electrode is inserted in the contralateral mastoid tip area and the ground electrode is inserted at the vertex (**Fig. 4.71**).
- Once the cochlear nerve is identified, the silver wire electrode should be placed. Gelfoam is usually applied to the electrode to keep the cotton pledget in contact with the eighth cranial nerve (**Fig. 4.75**).

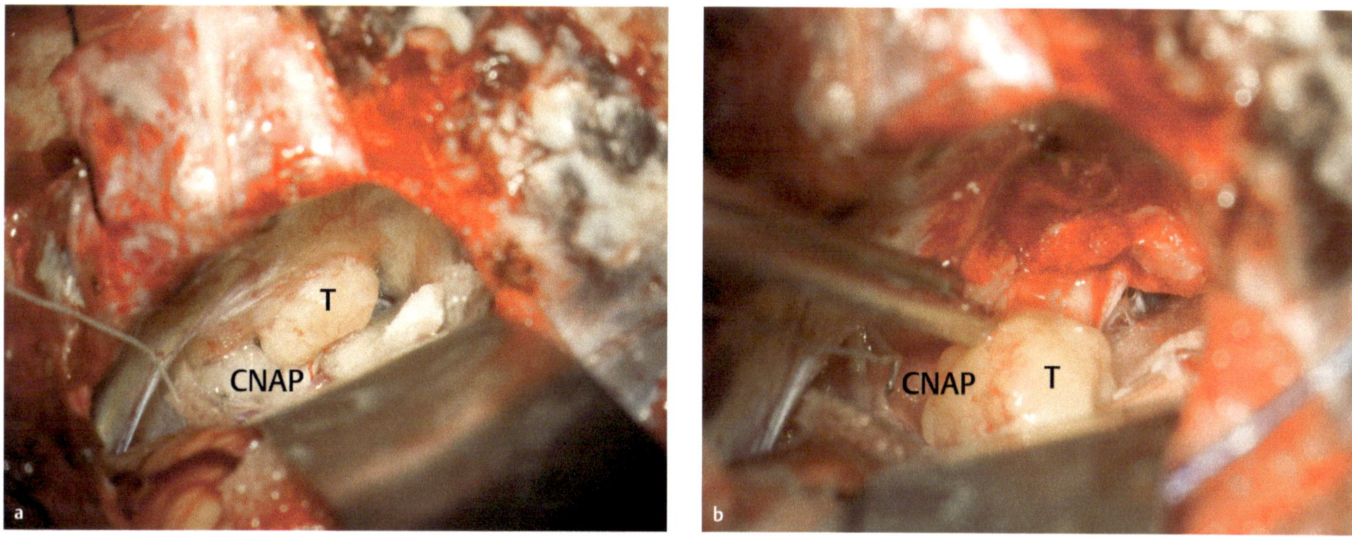

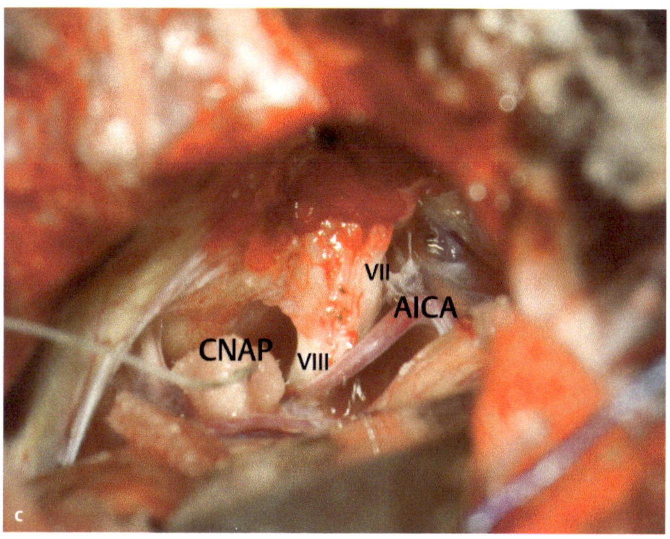

Fig. 4.75a–c Retrosigmoid-retrolabyrinthine approach for the removal of left-sided vestibular schwannoma. The CNAP is monitored during the operation.

a Placement of the electrode on the proximal part of the eighth nerve to the tumor (T).

b During tumor removal.

c After the tumor has been totally removed.
AICA, anterior inferior cerebellar artery; CNAP, cochlear nerve action potential probe; VII, facial nerve; VIII, vestibulocochlear nerve.

- Additionally we fix the electrode with a suture (Vicryl 4–0) onto the dura to avoid or reduce its the movement during surgical maneuvers that may affect the interpretation.
- The electrode should never obstruct the view of the surgeon.

Cochlear Nerve Monitoring Considerations

- **Hearing preservation.** ICNM is generally applied to surgery in which hearing preservation is aimed for. CNAP is currently used to monitor the cochlear nerve function in addition to ABR. Specialized personnel who are familiar with the neurophysiologic background of ABR and CNAP should also observe ICNM. Since the effectiveness of ICNM is still a matter of debate, surgeons should know that it cannot overcome the difficulty in preserving hearing in removal of the vestibular schwannoma.
- **Deafened patients (CI or ABI after tumor removal).** A reliable system to assure a functional cochlear nerve after tumor removal is not available at the time of writing. The microscopically intact cochlear nerve is the first step, but this will not provide any information about the functionality of the nerve. An intraoperative electrode device delivering electrical stimuli within the cochlea during ABR recordings (electrically evoked ABR) to actually mimic the functionality, and therefore the possibility of a CI, is currently under investigation.

ABR during ABI Electrode Array Placement

At the time of electrode array placement, proper positioning is confirmed via electrically evoked ABR (EABR). Stimulation is administered via electrodes at the four corners of the array, and the presence or absence of EABR at each location is used to guide any repositioning that may be necessary. Attention should be paid as this could be a time-consuming task and requires an experienced electrophysiologist, who provides feedback to the surgeon; EABRs typically comprise one, two, or three visible waves as shown in **Fig. 4.76**.

A strategy of a “cross-sectional check” for peaks was applied in which first four electrodes were measured and subsequently adjacent electrodes. Continuous feedback to the surgeon was given, mostly by means of a simple schematic drawing **Fig. 4.77**. Monitoring of the facial nerve can be performed simultaneously, to detect undesirable stimulation. As soon as most of the electrodes have a clear EABR, closure of the translabyrinthine approach can performed.

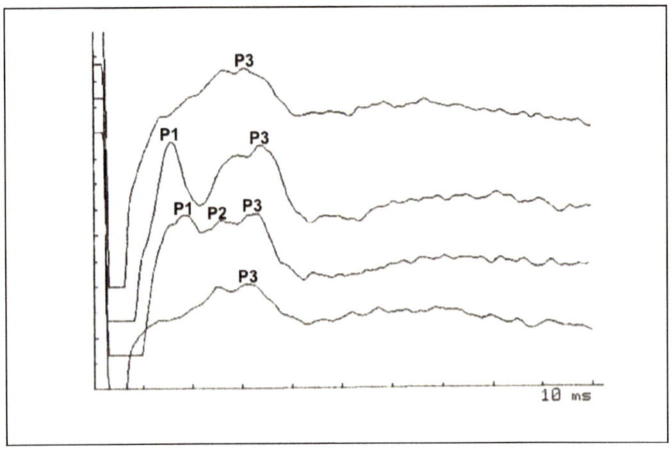

Fig. 4.76 Intraoperative BAERs typically comprise one, two, or three visible waves from an acoustic ABR. The three wave responses represent wave III (P1), wave IV (P2), and wave V (P3).

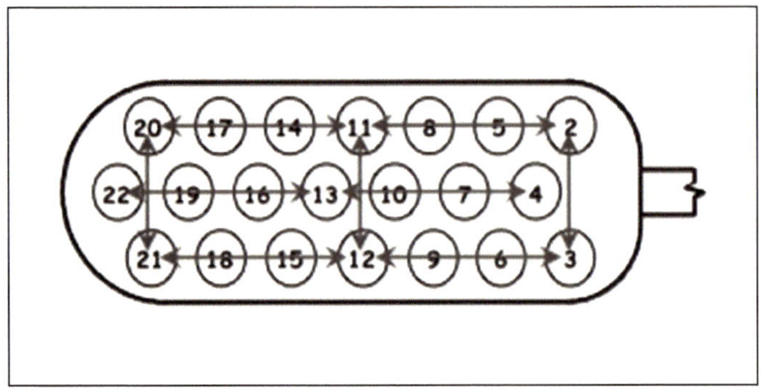

Fig. 4.77 ABI electrode cross-sectional testing: a drawing of the electrode testing intraoperatively, showing the scheme of bipolar stimulation of the different electrodes to establish correct positioning of the array. The first electrodes tested are 13 toward 22; then 13 toward 4; then 11 toward 20; and finally 11 toward 2. The other electrodes are tested subsequently. (The example illustrated here is for the assessment of the 21 electrodes of the Nucleus 24M ABI.)

4.2.5 Perioperative Medication and Care in ABI Surgery

Postoperative Management after ABI

At the end of the procedure, the wound is dressed in the usual manner and a crepe bandage is applied (Fig. 4.27). This dressing is usually kept in place undisturbed for 5 days. As always in intradural procedures, no drains are inserted. Extubation is performed on the operating table. We do not recommend prolonged intubation as a routine postoperative procedure since it can interfere with monitoring of the patient for complications.

The patient is then transferred to the intensive care unit and is monitored for pulse rate, respiratory rate, arterial oxygen saturation, and electrocardiogram tracing. The blood pressure monitor takes recordings at different intervals. In addition, the level of consciousness of the patient, pupillary reflexes, and motor responses are also checked. All these parameters are recorded every 15 minutes for the first 6 hours postoperatively and then half-hourly for 12 to 18 hours.

After 24 hours, the patient is transferred to the ward. Observation of the vital signs and level of consciousness continues every 2 hours in the first day in the ward and then 4-hourly thereafter until discharge. The indwelling urinary catheter and the nasogastric tube are removed after transfer to the ward. Oral fluids are usually started at that time. Early ambulation is encouraged after the first 24 hours to minimize the risk of pulmonary embolism.

Medication

- **Antibiotics:** Intravenous administration of piperacillin, 2 g every 4 hours, is continued for 48 hours. If there is suspicion of infection, it may be further continued.
- **Corticoids:** Dexamethasone, 4 mg either intramuscularly or intravenously, is given in the case of a large tumor for which manipulation of the brainstem and cerebellum has been needed.
- **Other:** Neither narcotics nor sedatives are used for at least the first 48 hours postoperatively, because these may interfere with the assessment of patient's consciousness. Ketoprofen, 160 mg intravenously once or twice a day, is administered.

Discharge

After 5 days, the dressing is removed and the wound is checked. The dressing is then reapplied for an additional 5 days. All sutures are removed 12 to 14 days postoperatively. The majority of patients are discharged on the 5th or 6th day.

4.2.6 Implants for Brainstem Implantation

Auditory Brainstem Implants and Their Electrode Arrays Currently Available

(**Note:** Companies are listed in alphabetical order. The information is provided by the named companies and is liable to regional differences and changes over time, presented images of 2014.)

See **Fig. 4.78–Fig. 4.83**.

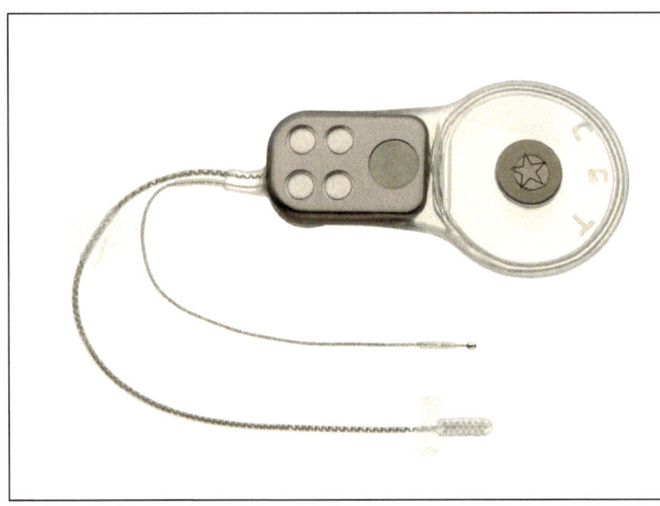

Fig. 4.78 Cochlear Nucleus ABI implant ABI24 with removable magnet and a titanium and silicone case.

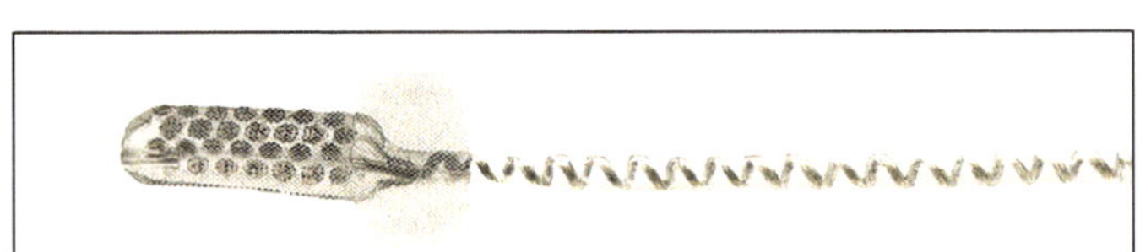

Fig. 4.79 Cochlear ABI implant electrode array; surface electrodes, 21; dimensions, 3 mm × 8.5 mm.

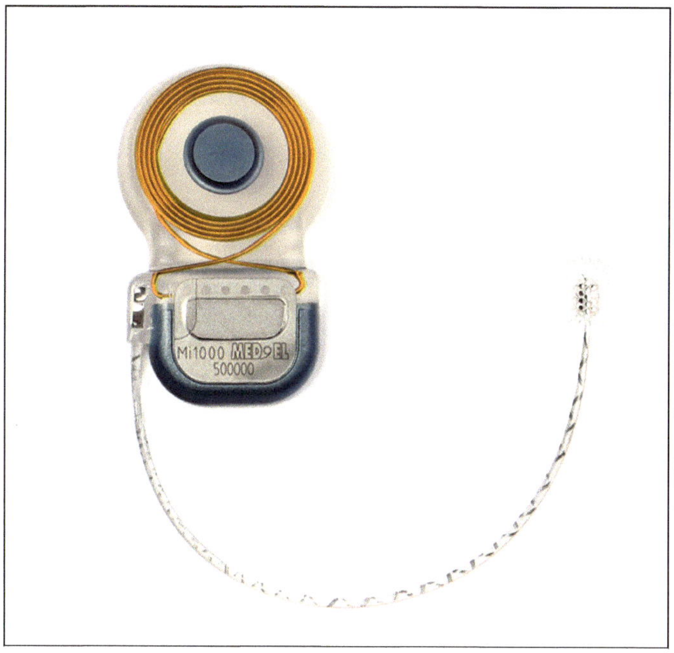

Fig. 4.80 MED-EL ABI implant.

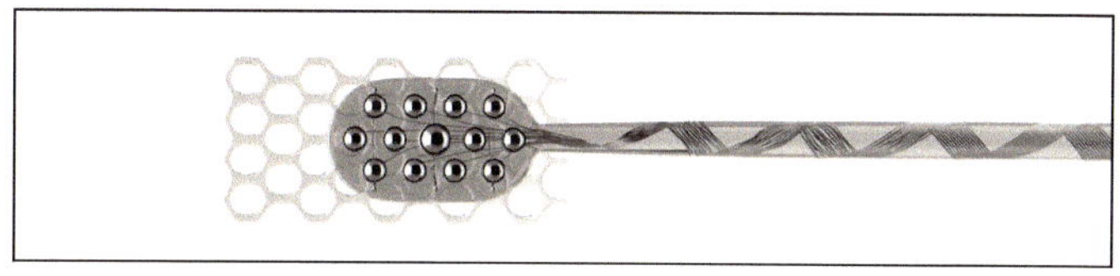

Fig. 4.81 MED-EL ABI implant electrode array; surface electrodes, 12.

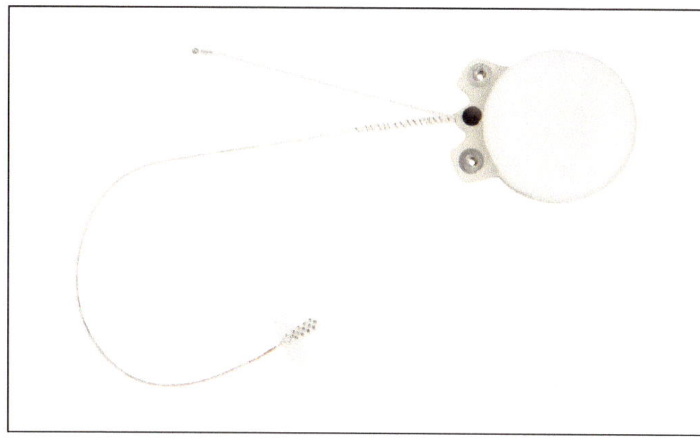

Fig. 4.82 Neurelec Digisonic SP ABI implant with a nonremovable magnet and a ceramic case.

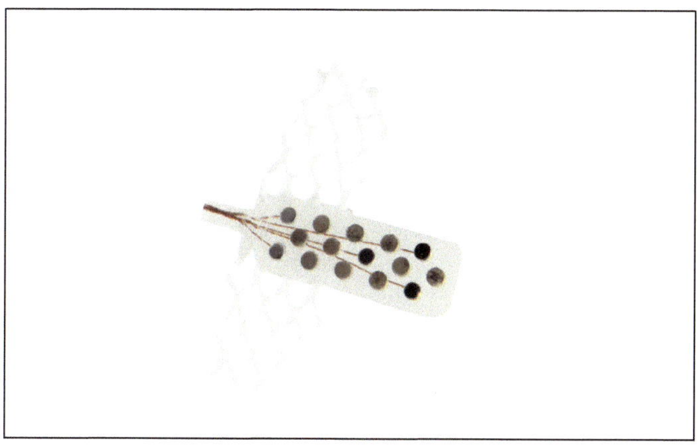

Fig. 4.83 Neurelec Digisonic SP ABI implant electrode array; surface electrodes, 15; dimensions, 7.8 mm × 3 mm.

References

1. Antonelli PJ, Ojano-Dirain CP. Microbial flora of cochlear implants by gene pyrosequencing. Otol Neurotol 2013;34(7):e65–71
2. Ciorba A, Bovo R, Trevisi P, et al. Postoperative complications in cochlear implants: a retrospective analysis of 438 consecutive cases. Eur Arch Otorhinolaryngol 2012;269(6):1599–1603
3. Antonelli PJ, Lee JC, Burne RA. Bacterial biofilms may contribute to persistent cochlear implant infection. Otol Neurotol 2004;25(6):953–957
4. Vlastarakos PV, Nikolopoulos TP, Maragoudakis P, Tzagaroulakis A, Ferekidis E. Biofilms in ear, nose, and throat infections: how important are they? Laryngoscope 2007;117(4):668–673
5. Laszig R, Ridder GJ, Fradis M. Intracochlear insertion of electrodes using hyaluronic acid in cochlear implant surgery. J Laryngol Otol 2002;116(5):371–372
6. Maini S, Lisnichuk H, Eastwood H, et al. Targeted therapy of the inner ear. Audiol Neurootol 2009;14(6):402–410
7. Chang A, Eastwood H, Sly D, James D, Richardson R, O'Leary S. Factors influencing the efficacy of round window dexamethasone protection of residual hearing post-cochlear implant surgery. Hear Res 2009;255(1-2):67–72
8. Souter M, Eastwood H, Marovic P, et al. Systemic immunity influences hearing preservation in cochlear implantation. Otol Neurotol 2012;33(4):532–538
9. Barriat S, Poirrier A, Malgrange B, Lefebvre P. Hearing preservation in cochlear implantation and drug treatment. Adv Otorhinolaryngol 2010;67:6–13
10. Song JJ, Park JH, Jang JH, et al. Facial nerve aberrations encountered during cochlear implantation. Acta Otolaryngol 2012;132(7):788–794
11. Shapiro WH, Bradham TS. Cochlear implant programming. Otolaryngol Clin North Am 2012;45(1):111–127
12. Cosetti MK, Troob SH, Latzman JM, et al. An evidence-based algorithm for intraoperative monitoring during cochlear implantation. Otol Neurotol 2012;33(2):169–176
13. Cosetti MK, Shapiro WH, Green JE, et al. Intraoperative neural response telemetry as a predictor of performance. Otol Neurotol 2010;31(7):1095–1099
14. Cohen LT, Saunders E, Richardson LM. Spatial spread of neural excitation: comparison of compound action potential and forward-masking data in cochlear implant recipients. Int J Audiol 2004;43(6):346–355
15. Grolman W, Maat A, Verdam F, et al. Spread of excitation measurements for the detection of electrode array foldovers: a prospective study comparing 3-dimensional rotational x-ray and intraoperative spread of excitation measurements. Otol Neurotol 2009;30(1):27–33
16. Moller AR. Use of zero-phase digital filters to enhance brain-stem auditory evoked potentials (BAEPs). Electroencephalogr Clin Neurophisiol 1988;71:226–232

5 Cochlear Implantation

Cochlear implantation is a technique that fundamentally changed the therapeutic possibilities for patients with a profound to severe congenital or acquired sensorineural hearing loss.

With the insertion of an electrode into the cochlea (the cochlear implant, CI), the cochlear nerve is stimulated electrically instead of acoustically. This leads to a different kind of sound perception. CI patients therefore have to learn to listen to and interpret these new sounds and will need extensive rehabilitation with a speech-language therapist and preferably a training partner at home. Many cochlear implant patients will only reach their fullest performances after months to years.

The procedure for selecting the right candidates for cochlear implantation is a multifactorial process usually implemented in a multidisciplinary team consisting of

- ENT surgeon (surgical feasibility and medical history)
- Audiometrist (audiometric indication)
- Speech-language therapist (speech intelligibility rate, lip-reading skills, learning ability)
- Psychologist (learning ability, resistance to changes) or remedial teacher (developmental possibilities of a child, contact skills, need for communication)
- Social worker (social network, training partner, home situation)

Each discipline takes different factors into account, all of which may influence the decision to implant and the successful outcome of cochlear implantation.

The outcomes of cochlear implant surgery remain variable, depending on many patient-related factors and some implant-related factors. It is therefore necessary to counsel candidates about the variability of outcomes, incorporating the experience of the different disciplines in the advice provided.

In candidates with a possibly less favorable outcome—such as, following meningitis, those with severe inner ear malformation, or congenitally deafened children with cerebral damage (cytomegalovirus)—it is wise to counsel about the expected less favorable outcome. Patients and parents need to have enough understanding of the advantages and disadvantages to be able to choose or reject implantation. Being transparent about the expected results will also prevent expectations running too high.

Counseling can describe the following levels of outcome: I, signal function (awareness of sounds); II, support of lip-reading skills; III, open set speech understanding. Only some of the patients in this last category can use the telephone for longer conversations.

5.1 Cochlear Implant Candidates

In general we can identify three groups of candidates:

1. Postlingually deafened children and adults
2. Prelingually deafened children
3. Early pre- and perilingually deafened adults and adolescents

Postlingually deafened patients with acquired hearing loss are good CI candidates, as long as the cochlear nerve has kept its integrity and the cochlea is accessible.

Infants with congenital (prelingual) hearing loss are often good CI candidates with very good linguistic development after implantation. Their outcome depends on the age of implantation, the etiology of the hearing loss, and on their additional disabilities and cognitive status. It is important for this group to be implanted at an early age, because the development of their auditory pathways and concomitant speech-language development will depend on the input received from the cochlear implant. Currently, the preferred age of implantation is around 6 to 10 months.

Early deafened adults and adolescents are also possible CI candidates, although the results in this group are very variable. The outcome is related to the amount of development of the auditory pathways in earlier years and its concomitant speech-language development. Better hearing at a younger age for a longer period of time or auditory stimulation of residual hearing using hearing aids for a prolonged period of time will lead to better outcome with the cochlear implant. Careful selection of the individuals in this group of candidates is therefore necessary and their speech intelligibility score, language development, type of education, and lip-reading skills are factors to be taken into account. The speech therapist plays an essential role in this decision-making process.

5.2 Etiology of Hearing Loss

The etiology of the patient's congenital or acquired sensorineural hearing loss can influence the work-up and timing of implantation.

In adults the most common causes are presbycusis, otosclerosis, Meniere disease, autosomal dominant mid- or late-onset deafness, and hearing loss caused by infection or surgery of the middle ear or mastoid. Less common but well-known causes of severe hearing loss or acute deafness are bacterial meningitis, autoimmune inner ear diseases, and skull base lesions, including fractures of the otic capsule.

In children with congenital hearing loss the most common cause is genetic hearing loss, with more than 60% being autosomal recessive in origin and around 30% syndromic.[1] Other important causes of hearing loss in children are congenital or acquired cytomegalovirus infection, malformations of the inner ear, aplasia or hypoplasia of the cochlear nerve, and bacterial meningitis.

Some of these indications need a different work-up and decision-making process, as well as a different surgical technique. These entities are discussed in separate chapters in the book (see Chapters 12 to 17).

In this chapter we discuss standard cochlear implantation in adults. Special surgical approaches and their indications, such as electroacoustic stimulation, subtotal petrosectomy approach combined with cochlear implantation, and implantation in cochlear ossification, are presented in Chapters 9 to 11.

5.3 Current Indications for Cochlear Implantation

The indications mentioned below are not rigid limits but criteria that many implant teams use. Each patient is assessed individually and the decision is based on many factors. Audiometric evaluation is one of them.

The *basic* audiometric indication is:

- Severe to profound bilateral sensorineural hearing loss with little or insufficient benefit from conventional hearing aids.
- In *adults* with postlingual hearing loss:
  - Speech audiometry tested with hearing aids in a free field setting at 65–75 dB sound pressure level with a score of ≤ 50%.
- In *congenitally deaf children* or (young) children with prelingual hearing loss:
  - Auditory brainstem response audiometry (ABR) with no responses or responses at 80 dB or more.
  - Free field test with hearing aids after trial of at least 3 months, with responses only above 60 dB or no responses at all (up to 100–120 dB stimulation).
- In *early deafened adults and adolescents*:
  - Speech audiometry tested with hearing aids in a free field setting at 65–75 dB sound pressure level with a score of ≤ 50% + additional evaluation of speech intelligibility and lip-reading skills.

5.3.1 Contraindications for Cochlear Implantation

Contraindications

- Cochlear nerve aplasia, confirmed by appropriate testing
- Cochlear aplasia, Michel deformity
- Deafness of central origin

Relative contraindications

- Cochlear nerve hypoplasia
- Bilateral cochlear ossification, confirmed on MRI and not accessible via drill-out procedure
- Psychiatric pathology

The general medical and psychological condition of the patient has to be in a state that allows elective surgery. The patient needs to be able to participate in speech-language therapy. A social support system is important around the time of implantation.

5.3.2 Special Indications, Differential Work-up, and Special Surgical Techniques

- For the technique of electroacoustic stimulation, see Chapter 9.
- For the technique of subtotal petrosectomy combined with cochlear implantation (see Chapter 10):
  - Chronic otitis media/cholesteatoma (see Chapters 10 and 14)
  - Presence of a radical cavity (see Chapters 10 and 14)
  - Cochlear ossification/obliteration (see Chapters 10 and 11)
  - Inner ear malformations (see Chapters 10 and 15)
  - Fracture of the labyrinth (see Chapters 10 and 17)
  - Unfavorable anatomical conditions (see Chapter 10)
  - Revision surgery (see Chapter 10)
- For techniques in cochlear ossification (see Chapter 11):
  - Meningitis (see Chapters 11 and 12)
  - Otosclerosis (see Chapters 11 and 13)
  - Otomastoiditis/labyrinthitis (see Chapters 11 and 14)
  - Trauma (see Chapters 11 and 17)
- For technique in selected skull base lesions (see Chapters 10, 16, and 17)

5.4 Surgical Steps

The surgery requires proper positioning for mastoidectomy, hair shaving, and facial nerve monitoring. The use of antibiotics, the required instruments, monitoring, and other perioperative management are discussed in Chapter 4.

Surgical Steps in Cochlear Implantation

- Skin incision
- Musculoperiosteal layer
- Mastoidectomy
- Posterior tympanotomy
- Exposure of the round window
- Drilling out of the receiver well
- Fixation of the implant
- Insertion of the cochlear electrode
- Electrophysiologic testing
- Fixation of the electrode
- Closure

5.4.1 Skin Incision

Different skin incisions are used for cochlear implant surgery, the choice depending largely on the preference of the surgeon. The rationale behind most skin incisions is to prevent extrusion of the array and to create adequate coverage of the implant. It is important that enough space for the speech processor behind the auricle is available, without creating pressure points on the skin lateral to the subcutaneous receiver-stimulator (being stuck between speech processor and receiver-stimulator). For this reason the

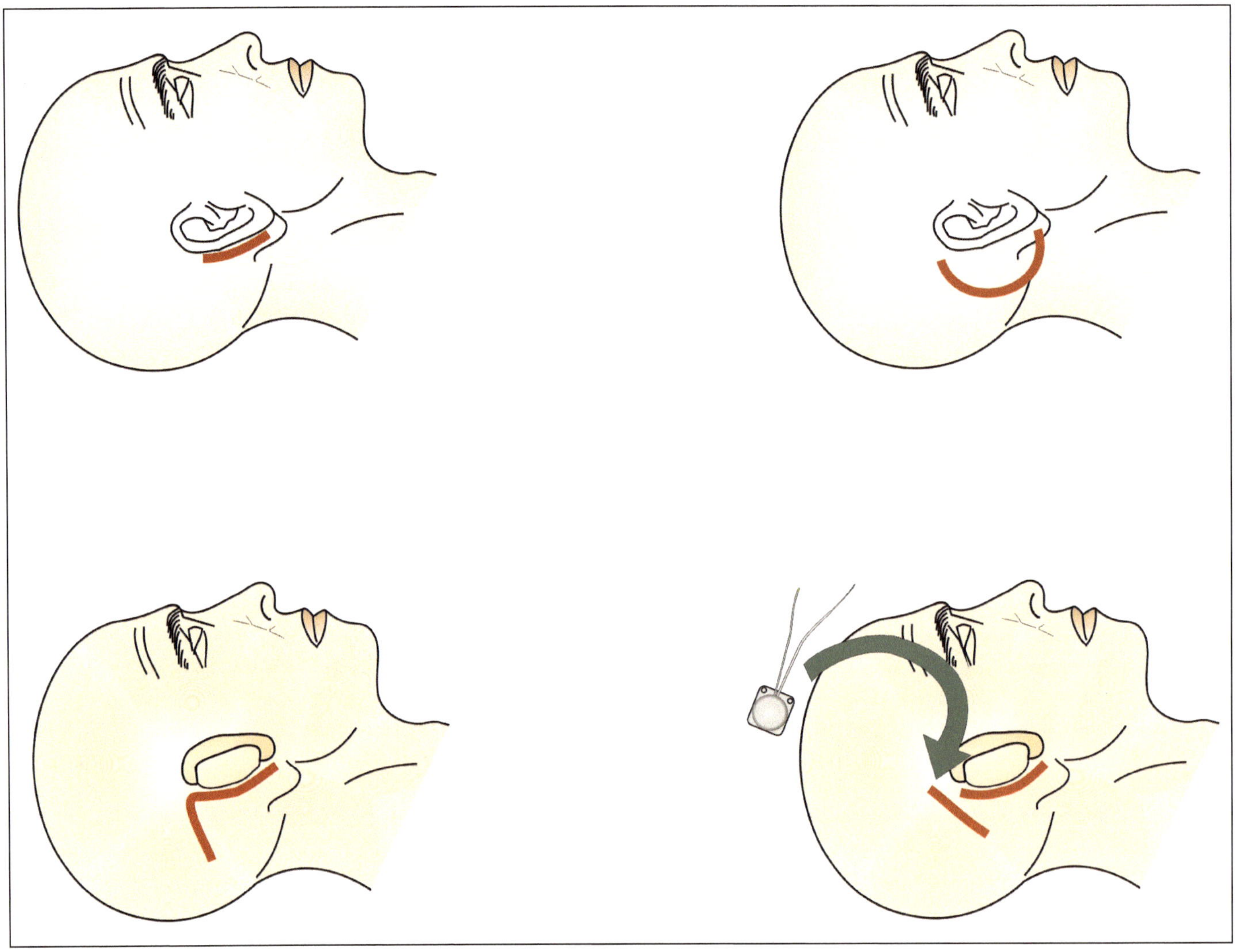

Fig. 5.1 Four types of skin incisions.

receiver-stimulator should not be positioned too far anteriorly. Preferably the skin incision is situated anterior-inferior to the location of the receiver-stimulator and not crossing it, protecting the receiver-stimulator maximally by covering with skin and temporal muscle.

When there has been previous surgery, effort must be made to use the previous (scarred) incision, because vascularization of small islands of skin created by several incisions close together can become problematic, with skin necrosis and resulting defects.

Four types of skin incisions are frequently used (see **Fig. 5.1**):

- Normal retroauricular incision
- Wide C shaped retroauricular incision
- Lazy S incision
- Minimal access incision

When previous surgery has been performed, it is best to use the same normal retroauricular incision. When a new incision needs to be made, the templates that the implant companies provide can be used to ensure that the incision line is situated just behind the position of the speech processor.

The wide C shaped retroauricular incision is especially useful in well-aerated mastoids with a lot of temporal bone drilling or in surgery where more access might be necessary, as in subtotal petrosectomy approach. However, the use of this type of incision creates a wound and a scar over the location of the receiver-stimulator; this is not a favorable situation.

Using the lazy S incision in adults gives proper coverage of the implant and also good access for drilling out the receiver well. In children care must be taken to avoid the mastoid tip when using this incision, because of the more lateral position of the facial nerve at the mastoid tip.

Minimal access incisions can be used, but severe stretching of the skin for introduction of the implant or getting access to the middle ear and cochlea creates more problematic scarring of the skin. In minimal access surgery two incisions are sometimes used: one for getting access to the mastoid and middle ear, the other for placement of the receiver-stimulator. This creates extra risks of skin flap–related problems and infections.

5.4.2 Musculoperiosteal Layer

It is necessary to create a musculoperiosteal flap or periosteal flaps that adequately cover the cochlear implant and electrode arrays postoperatively. Some surgeons create alternating flaps in relation to the skin incision, so as to get the best coverage and protection of the implant.[2] Care must be taken not to create too large a pocket underneath the temporal muscle, or between temporal muscle, the periosteal flaps, and the skin: this can lead to a void filled with hematoma and to risk of infection.

5.4.3 Mastoidectomy and Posterior Tympanotomy

The mastoidectomy can be limited when no pathology is present. An internal rim of cortical bone can be left along the cavity to hold the electrode array. Visualization of the horizontal, tympanic part of the facial nerve, the short process of the incus, the lateral semicircular canal, and sometimes also the digastric ridge is helpful for assessment of the position of the vertical, mastoidal segment of the facial nerve.

These landmarks are also essential for drilling the posterior tympanotomy. The chorda tympani can be explored more inferiorly, leading to the chordal crest, which can be removed for better access. The posterior tympanotomy is then created; it has the shape of a triangle. Widening the posterior tympanotomy improves the visibility of the cochlea and round window niche and improves the working space, and it also increases the illumination by the microscope.

Some surgeons prefer to identify the facial nerve before drilling the posterior tympanotomy.

Inexperienced CI surgeons tend to drill not medially enough (the facial nerve is then not properly skeletonized) when starting the posterior tympanotomy: during drilling anteriorly and laterally care must be taken not to damage the tympanic annulus, which can be found just lateral to the chorda tympani (see Chapter 2, **Fig. 2.12**).

The buttress can be left for protection of the short process of the incus, and this will give better fixation of the cochlear electrode if fixation within the posterior tympanotomy is used.

Variations of the normal anatomy make the round window niche more or less visible through the posterior tympanotomy (**Fig. 5.2a–c**). Even a superior extension of the pneumatization of the hypotympanum can mask the real position of the niche (**Fig. 5.2d**).

5.4.4 Exposure of the Round Window

The round window can usually only be seen in a restricted view, covered by a bony overhang superiorly and a bony projection inferiorly creating the round window niche. Frequently, a pseudomembrane is present, a mucosal layer covering the niche. The overhang and inferior bony projection need to be removed to visualize the complete round window. In particular, the superior part needs to be removed to enable one to reach the scala tympani at the right axial line for insertion. This would be from a posterior-superior toward anterior-inferior position. See **Fig. 5.3–Fig. 5.5**.

The color of the true round window is dark gray. The pseudo-membrane has a whitish aspect. In cases with fibrosis or ossification of the cochlea a white aspect of the round window can also be seen.

5.4.5 Drill-out of the Receiver Well

For some implants a receiver-stimulator well has to be drilled out; templates of the implants are used, provided by the supplier. For others only a pocket needs to be created or the implant can be fixated with screws. See **Fig. 5.6–Fig. 5.9**.

In children and adults with a thin cortical bone of the skull, drilling of the receiver well with removal of the most external circle of the tabula interna creates an island of bone that can be pushed medially. This offers the possibility of producing an adequate fit even in a shallow cortical bone.

5.4.6 Fixation of the Implant

Fixation of the implant is advisable; MRI examination may be necessary at a later time and fixation of the implant is mandatory for this.

Two small bony canals, superior and inferior of the receiver well, are created for fixation of the implant using a nonresorbable tie-down suture. In children the skull can be too thin for these bony canals, but tight suturing of the temporal muscle over the implant is necessary. Care must be taken not to place the fixating suture over the fragile electrodes, which could result in damage to the electrode. Damage to the dura or the emissary vein must also be avoided as a subperiosteal or even subdural hematoma can occur.[3] See **Fig. 5.10–Fig. 5.13**.

Some implants can be fixated by drilling a canal from the receiver well to the mastoid cavity for the electrode arrays to run through. This fixates the implant and also protects the most vulnerable part of the electrode, just where it exits the receiver-stimulator.

Mobilization of the skin and temporal muscle to create access for the receiver-stimulator gives opportunity for developing a hematoma, with subsequent risk of infection. For this reason the skin and muscle should be mobilized as little as possible, preferably not further than a tight pocket, and a firm bandage for 24 to 48 hours is mandatory.

Just before the actual insertion of the electrode array into the cochlea, the implant is placed in its receiver pocket or well and fixated.

5.4.7 Cochleostomy

The insertion of the electrode into the cochlea is usually performed in the widest and easiest accessible scala, the scala tympani. The scala tympani approach can be performed through the round window, with or without widening of the entrance, or through a separate bony cochleostomy created inferiorly to the round window.

The round window approach gives safe and easy access to the scala tympani, with a minimum amount of drilling on the cochlea, good chances of saving the residual hearing, and the smallest likelihood of vestibular complaints postoperatively.[4]

The landmarks of the round window are discussed in Chapter 2. The round window membrane is opened using a small hooked instrument as atraumatically as possible. The direction of the hooked instrument should be anterior-inferiorly. Care must be taken not to open the superior region, because the basilar membrane is situated immediately behind the round window.

The crista fenestrae, on the inferior inside border of the round window, also called the "hook" region, forms the narrowest anatomical point to the scala tympani. It may represent a sharp obstacle during the insertion of the electrode array, with the possibility of damaging the array. In some patients this needs to be

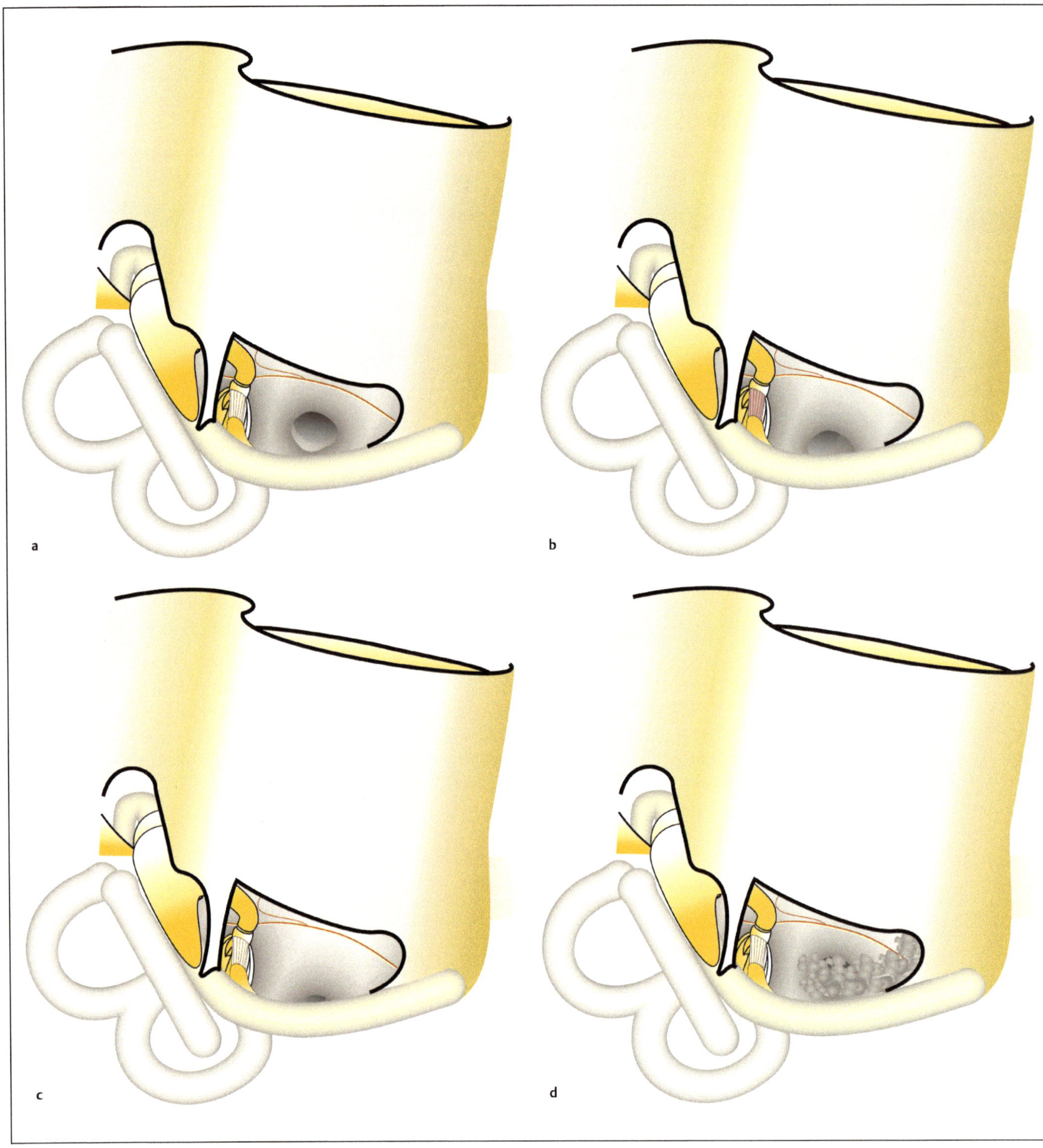

Fig. 5.2a–d
a–c Different degrees of visibility of the round window niche.
d Superior extension of hypotympanic pneumatization.

opened up more to gain proper access to the scala tympani ("margin cochleostomy").

Some surgeons prefer a separate cochleostomy, or in some cases a separate cochleostomy is necessary when the anatomical conditions make round window insertion impossible. This cochleostomy is created inferiorly from the round window, giving access also to the scala tympani (see Chapter 2 for the best position). This procedure can be performed using gentle drilling until the endocochlear lining becomes visible, and opening the lining with a small hooked instrument to get access to the scala tympani.

5.4.8 Insertion of the Cochlear Electrode

An important consideration in cochlear implantation is the prevention of blood and bone dust from entering the cochlea after cochleostomy. Hyaluronic acid solution can be used for this purpose. Some surgeons also use hyaluronic acid solution as a lubricant during insertion.

Slow and smooth introduction of the cochlear electrode is important, avoiding intracochlear trauma or misplacement of the electrode array while using the correct insertion angle toward the scala tympani (see Chapter 2).

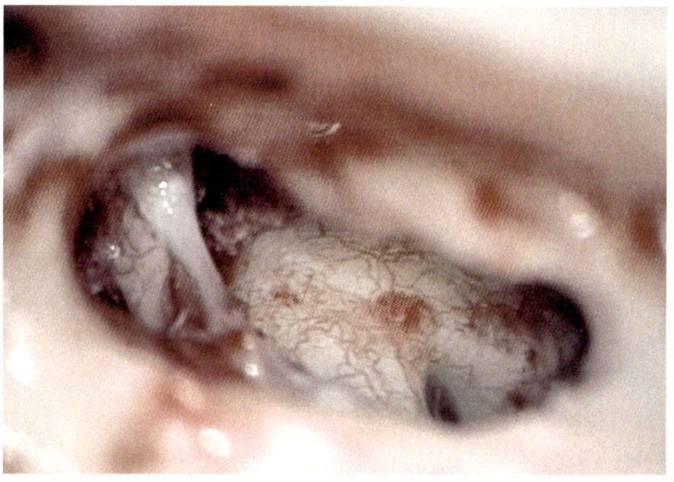

Fig. 5.3 Round window blocked. The round window niche with superior overhang still present. The stapedial tendon is clearly visible.

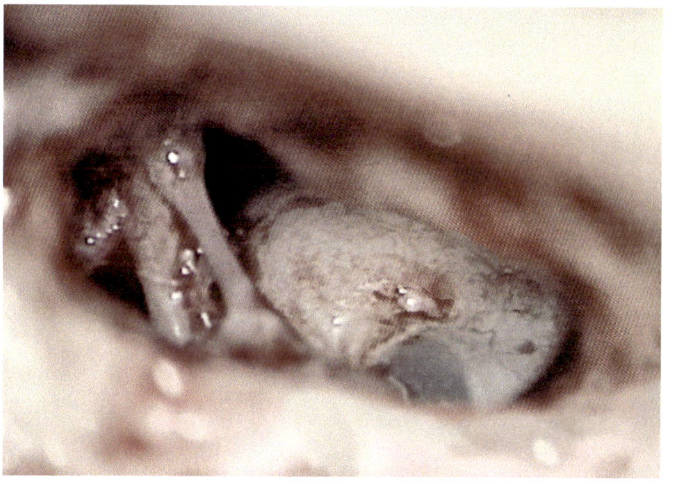

Fig. 5.4 Round window view. After removal of the superior bony overhang, the round window can be better appreciated.

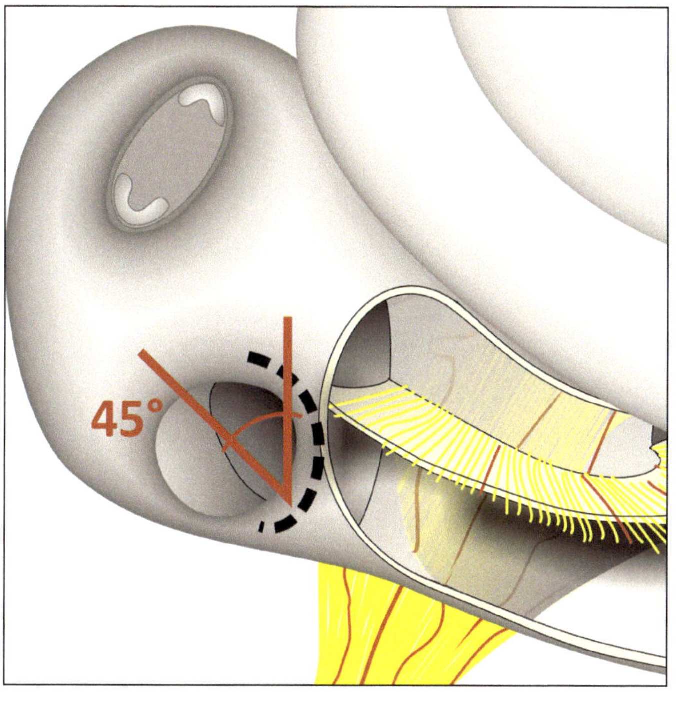

Fig. 5.5 Schematic drawing of the round window niche showing the angulation of the round window membrane.

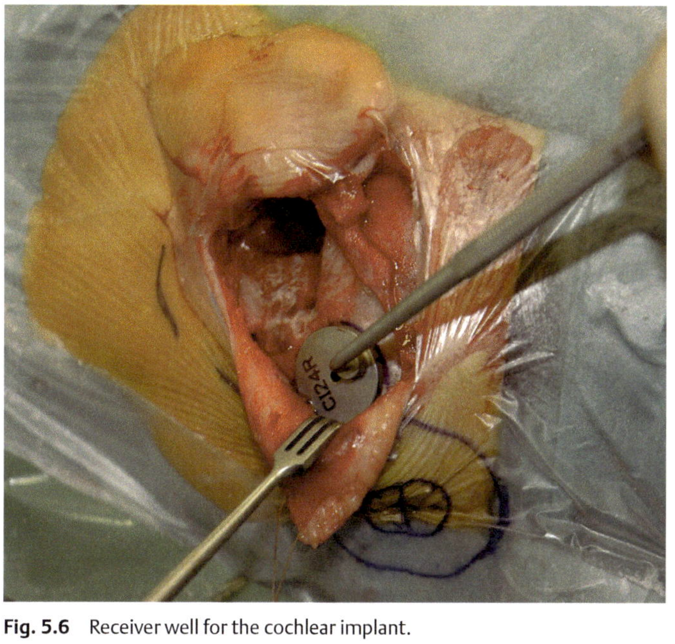

Fig. 5.6 Receiver well for the cochlear implant.

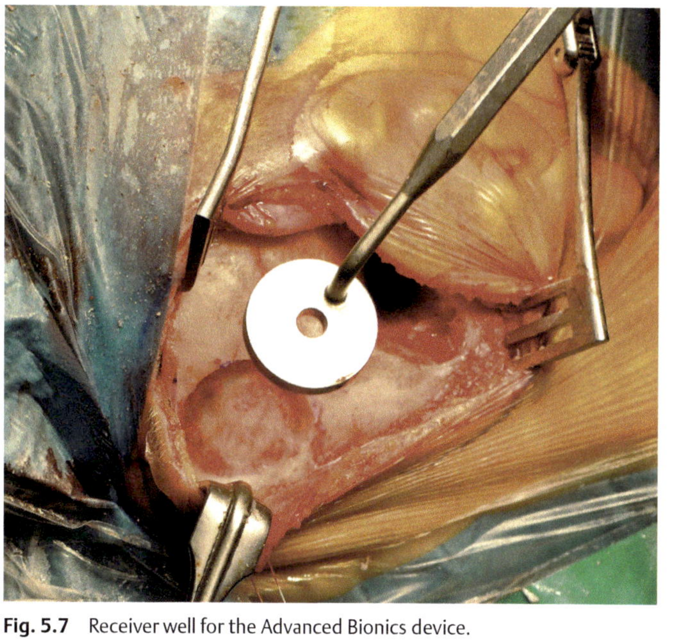

Fig. 5.7 Receiver well for the Advanced Bionics device.

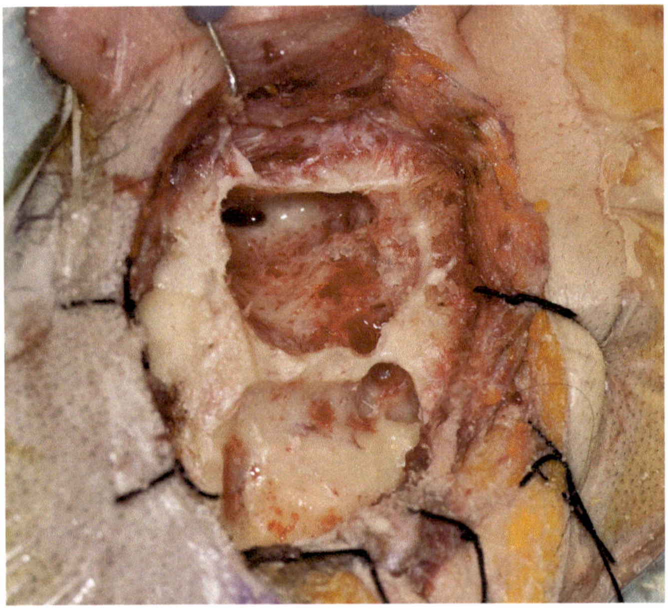

Fig. 5.8 Receiver well for the MED-EL implant.

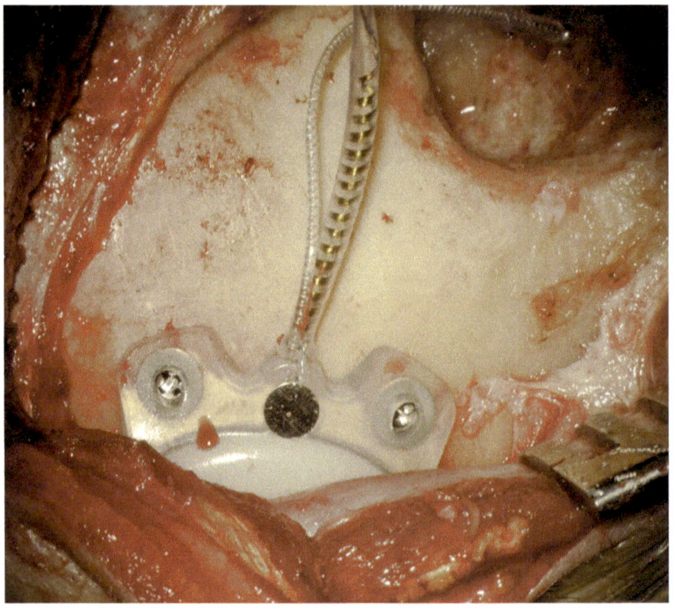

Fig. 5.9 Fixation of the Neurelec implant with screws.

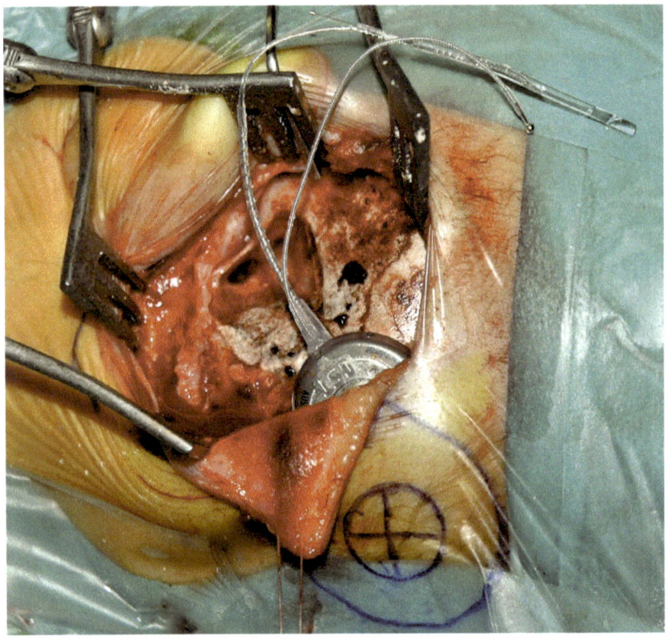

Fig. 5.10 Fixation only using a pocket, without sutures or screws. A tight subperiosteal pocket is advisable, and suturing of the musculoperiosteal flap also needs to be tight. In case there will be postoperative MR imaging, the use of sutures or screws is advised.

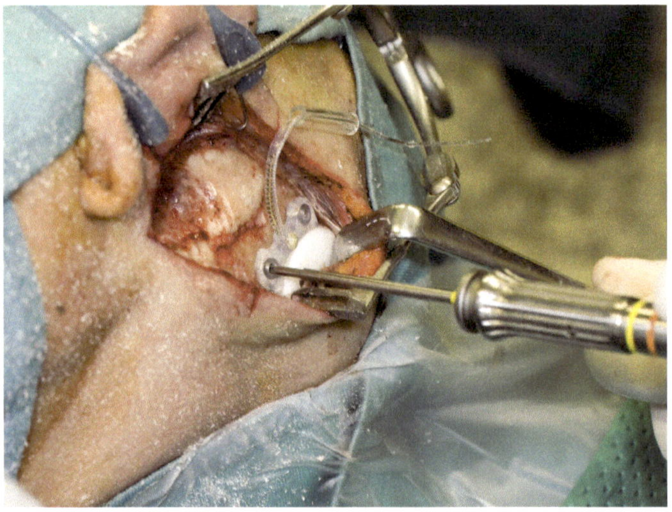

Fig. 5.11 Fixation with screws.

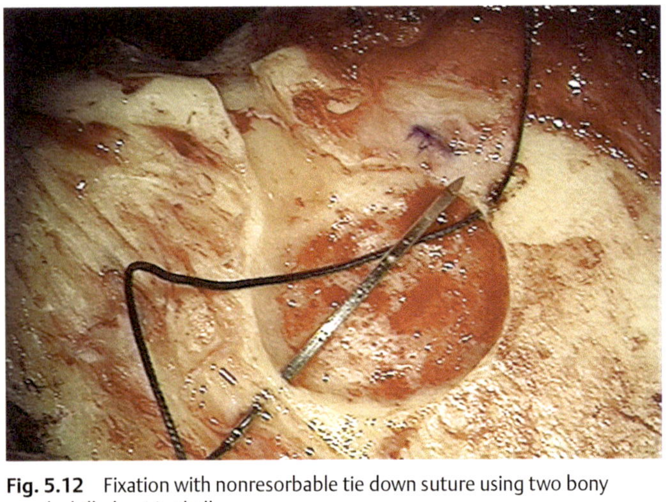

Fig. 5.12 Fixation with nonresorbable tie down suture using two bony canals drilled out in skull.

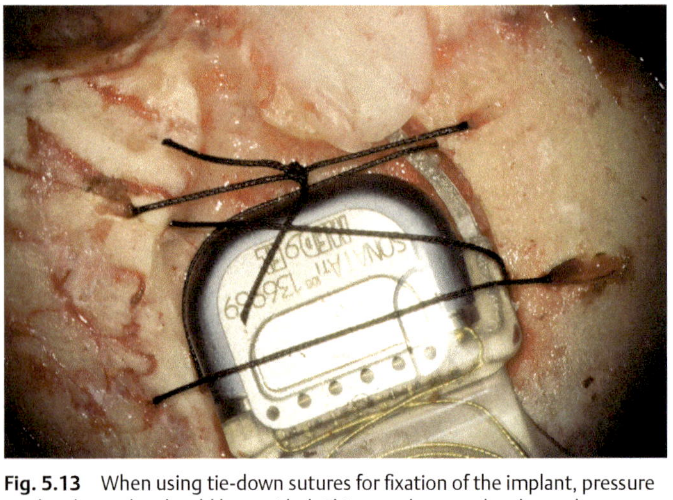

Fig. 5.13 When using tie-down sutures for fixation of the implant, pressure on the electrodes should be avoided. This may damage the electrode array, as is visible in this picture.

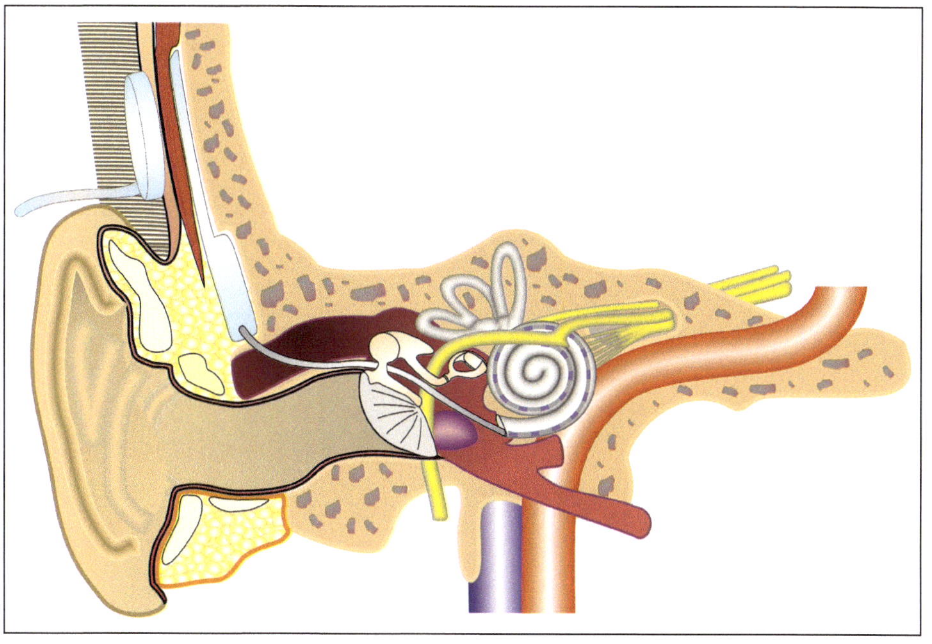

Fig. 5.14 A schematic drawing showing the implant in place at the end of the surgical procedure.

With a precurved implant an "advanced-off stylet" technique should be used: after insertion of the first part of the electrode array (usually there is a mark on the array), the last part is gently pushed off the stylet, while the stylet is kept in a stable position. In the insertion of a lateral wall electrode, a friction-free implantation without kinking of the electrode is attempted. In midmodiolar electrode insertion also a forceless introduction without kinking is desirable.

Once resistance is met, the electrode array needs to be drawn back slightly and after a gentle rotatory movement the procedure can be repeated.

Although they are used particularly in EAS (electroacoustic stimulation, see Chapter 9), these soft surgery techniques are useful also in conventional cochlear implantation because (1) their uniform use will lead to a standardized technique for all CI patients; (2) they give optimal opportunities to save the intracochlear structures and possibly also the residual hearing during conventional cochlear implantation; and (3) they lead to fewer complaints of postoperative dizziness.[4]

5.4.9 Electrophysiologic Testing

Before the cochlear electrode is fixated, preoperative electrophysiologic testing has to be performed. Impedance, stapedius reflex, and neural response measurements give information on the correct functioning and position of the electrode. Threshold levels can also be obtained. These measurements are described in Chapter 4.

5.4.10 Fixation of the Implant

Fixation of the implant in the cochleostomy is performed with small rectangular pieces of fascia harvested from the temporal muscle. Fixation in the posterior tympanotomy can also be achieved using a small piece of muscle. Fibrin glue can be used additionally in both locations.

5.4.11 Closure (Fig. 5.14)

Subsequently, the musculoperiosteal flaps and skin are closed in 2 or 3 layers. In young children the skin can be sutured using an intracutaneous, absorbable suture.

A tight circular bandage remains for 24 to 48 hours. Especially in children care needs to be taken for proper fixation of the head bandage. In the postoperative period additional protection of the implant and wound can be useful, for example, by the wearing of a hat, cap, or loose-fitting head bandage especially in children who are unstable and tumble often.

Case 5.1 Surgical Steps

Standard Cochlear Implantation (Left Ear) (Fig. 5.1.1–Fig. 5.1.21)

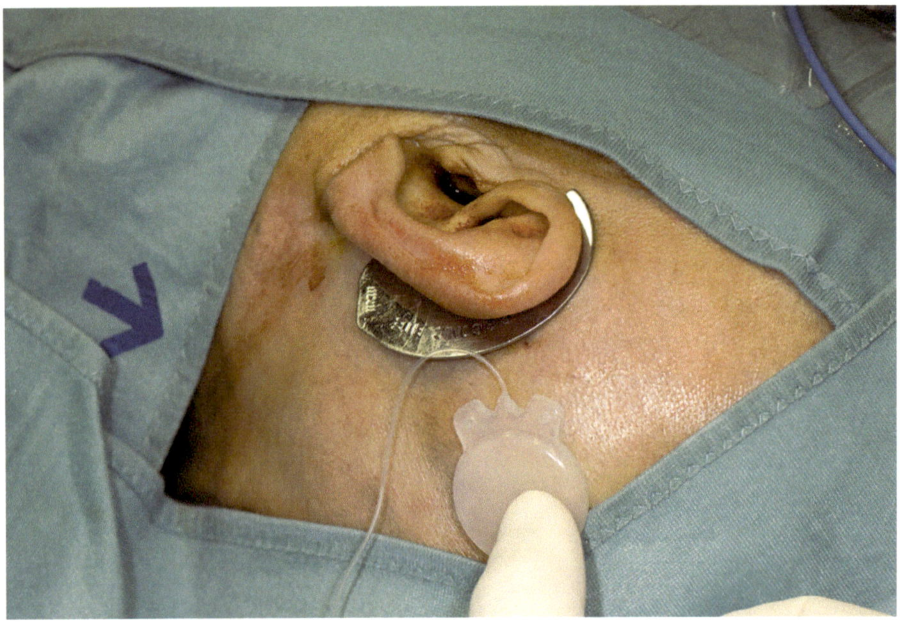

Fig. 5.1.1 Before surgery, the patient's hair is removed as in lateral skull base surgery. The electrodes for facial nerve monitoring are installed. Dummies of the internal unit and the behind-the-ear speech processor are placed before the incision is made to provide an idea of the correct positioning of the implant. Adequate distance should be maintained between the auricle and implant to enable the speech processor to be worn without causing pressure points.

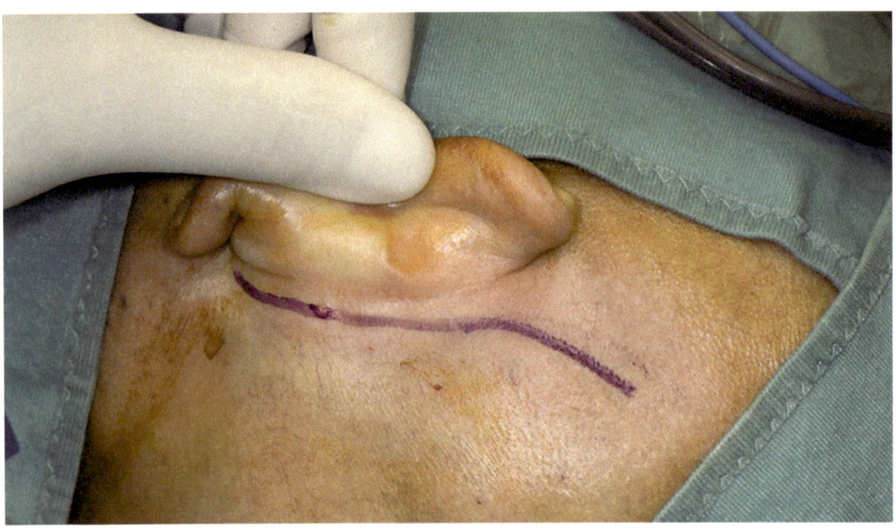

Fig. 5.1.2 The retroauricular skin incision is extended superiorly to expose sufficient area of the skull for placement of an internal unit (lazy S incision).

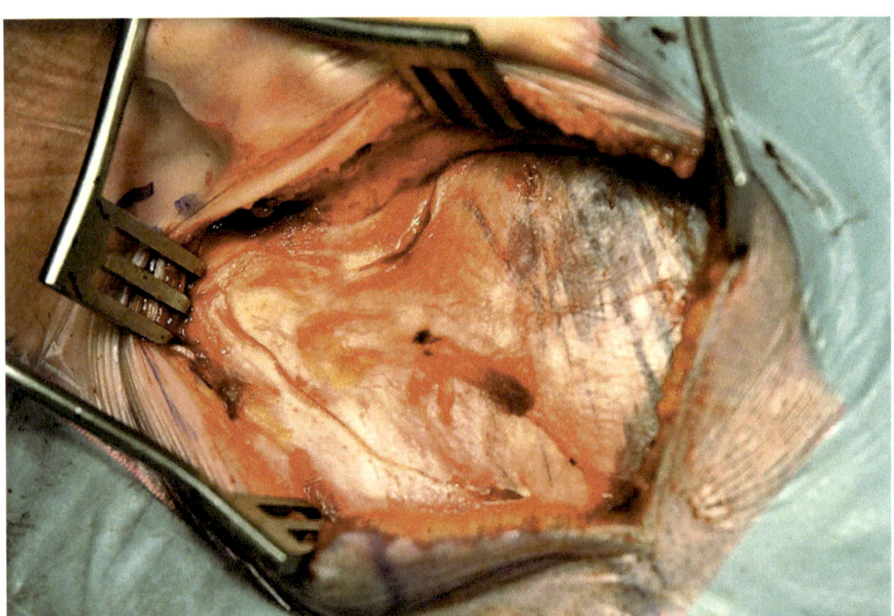

Fig. 5.1.3 The skin and subcutis are opened to the level of the fascia of the temporal muscle. In the same plane the periosteal layer over the mastoid tip and external auditory canal is identified.

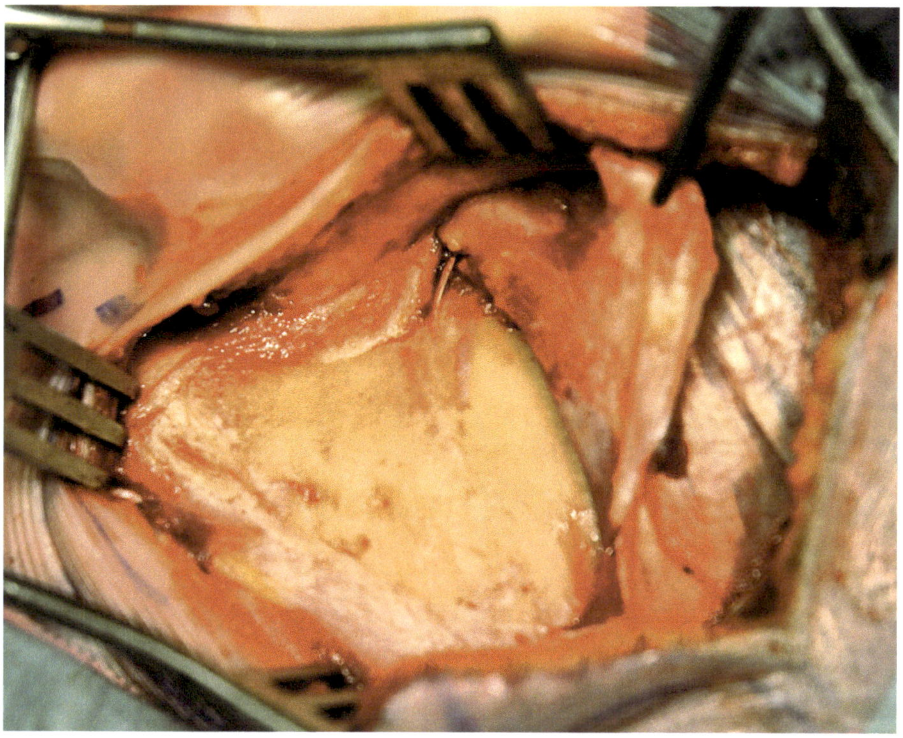

Fig. 5.1.4 After the skin is opened, the periosteum is detached from the skull, taking care not to tear it. Exposure of not only the squamous portion of the temporal bone but also the posteroinferior part of the parietal bone by passing the squamous suture line is required for accommodating the implant and creation of the receiver well. In this image the cranial-based flap is shown, which gives good exposure and a secure closing layer.

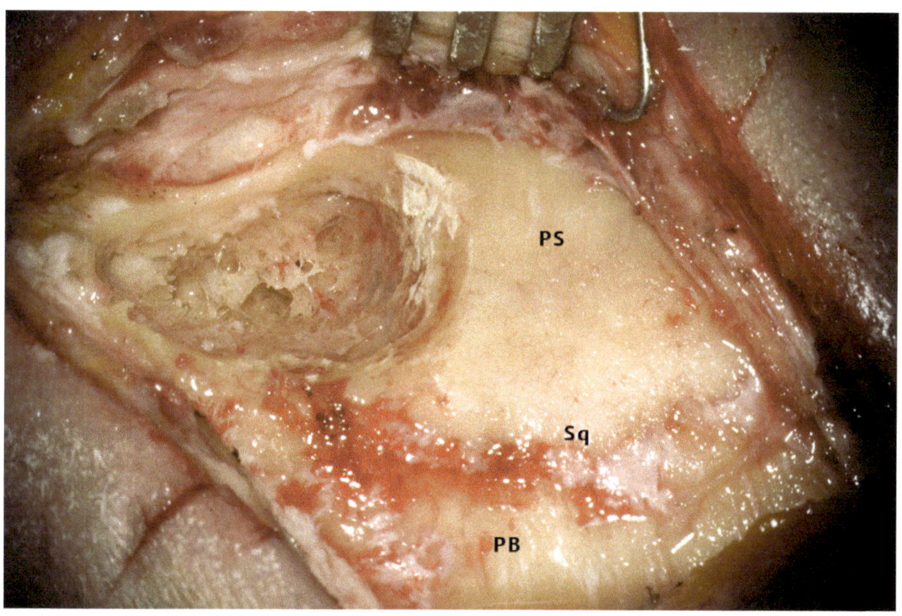

Fig. 5.1.5 The lateral surface of the skull is widely exposed and a limited mastoidectomy is performed. The mastoidectomy should be wide enough to allow the posterior tympanotomy to performed safely, but the posterior edge of the cavity should be preserved as much as possible to accommodate the internal unit. The posterior wall of the external auditory canal should be sufficiently thinned for easy access to the posterior tympanotomy. PB, parietal bone; PS, squamous part of temporal bone; Sq, squamous suture.

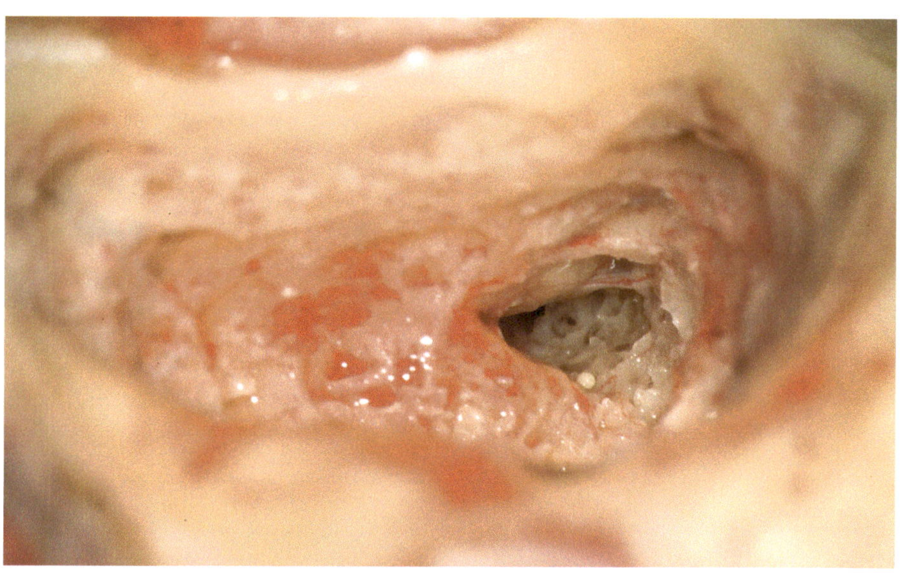

Fig. 5.1.6 To be able conduct a mastoidectomy and posterior tympanotomy safely, it is important to identify the important landmarks in the mastoid. The incus and the lateral semicircular canal should be visualized even though posterior epitympanotomy is not necessary.

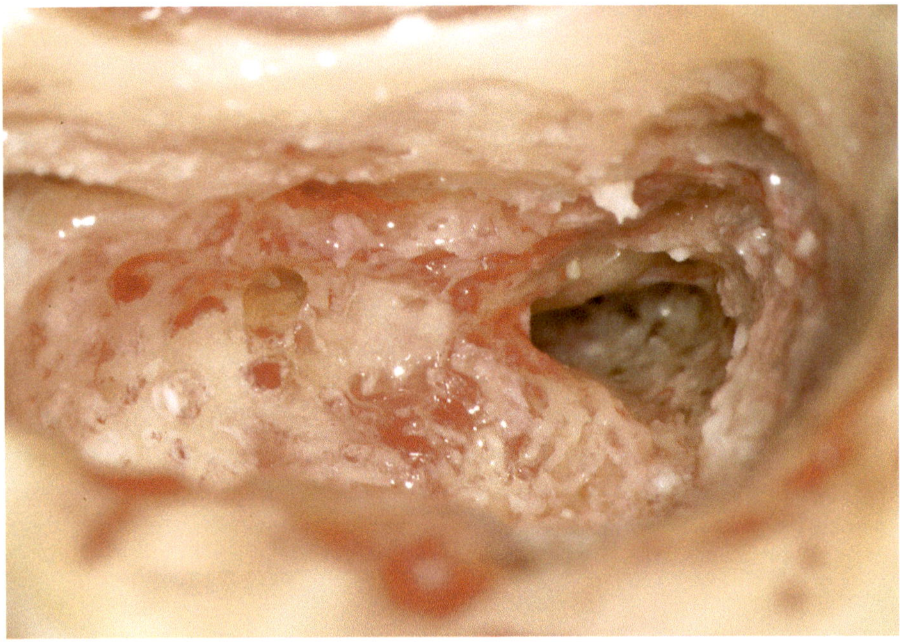

Fig. 5.1.7 The area just inferior to the short process of the incus is drilled, starting the posterior tympanotomy.

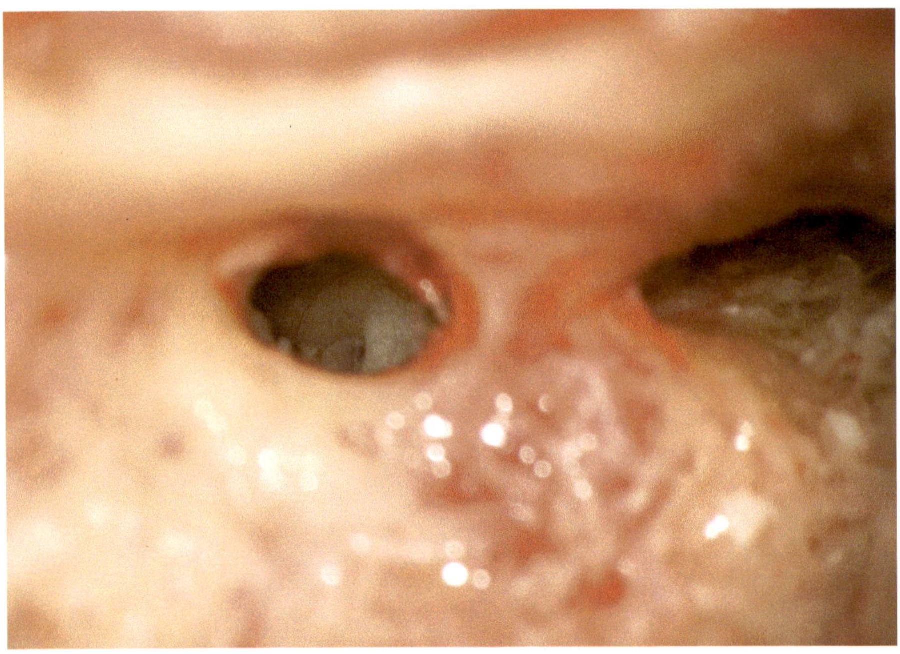

Fig. 5.1.8 The initial opening of the posterior tympanotomy is shown. Through the posterior tympanotomy, the superior edge of the round window niche covering the round window membrane is seen. Since the posterior tympanotomy is small, care should be taken not to damage the facial nerve located just medial to the posterior tympanotomy. The direction of the drilling should always be parallel to the nerve with maximum rinsing.

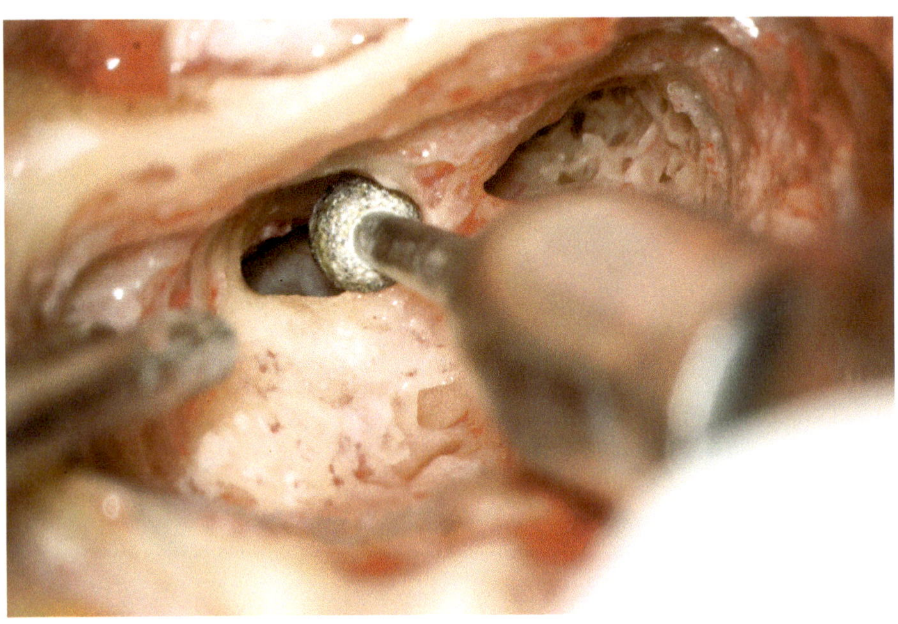

Fig. 5.1.9 The posterior tympanotomy is enlarged using a large diamond bur. Since an electrode is inserted through the round window, the posterior tympanotomy should have sufficient inferior extension to expose the round window niche. Both the round window membrane and the stapes should be visualized for safe surgery.

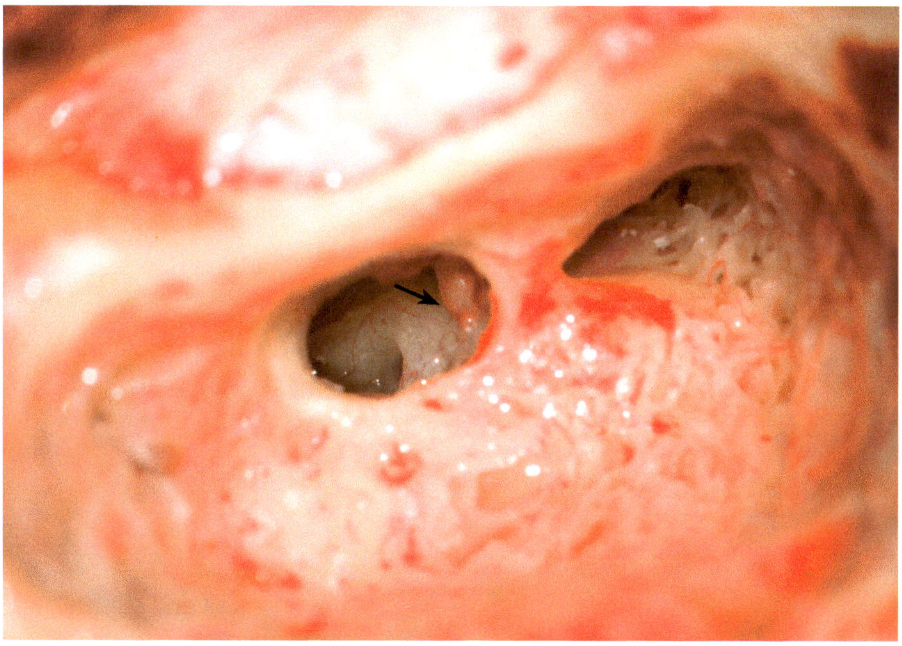

Fig. 5.1.10 The posterior tympanotomy is completed. The round window niche and the incudostapedial joint *(arrow)* can be seen simultaneously.

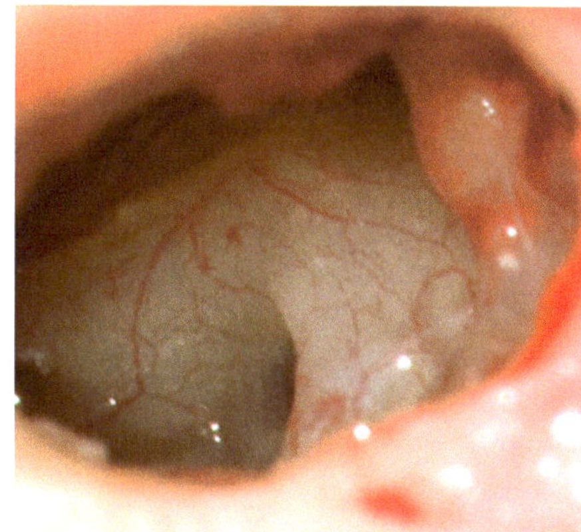

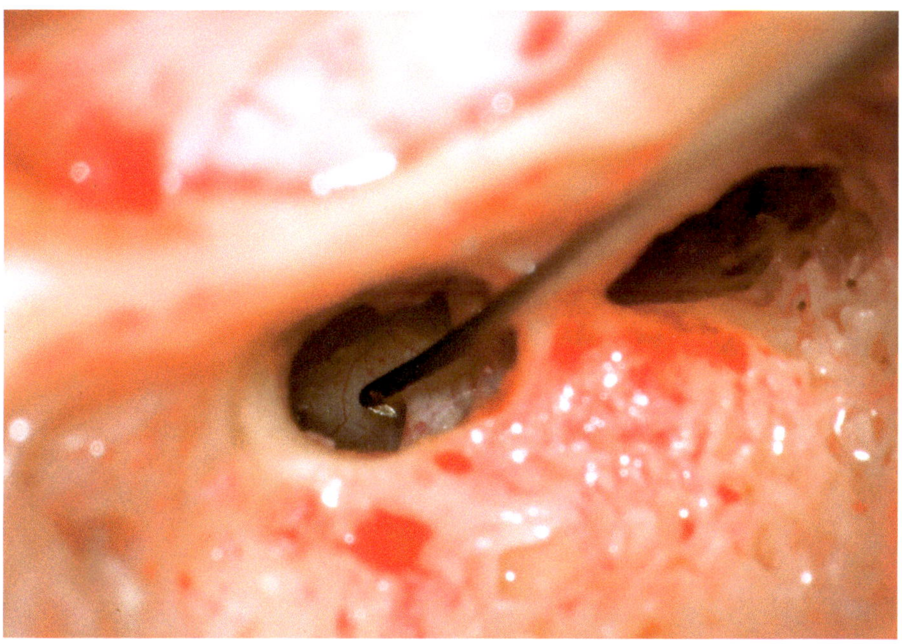

Fig. 5.1.11 A hook is introduced to show the depth of the bony overhang covering the round window membrane.

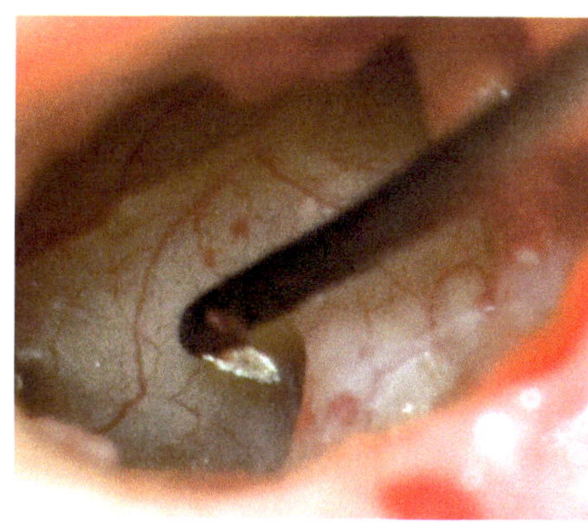

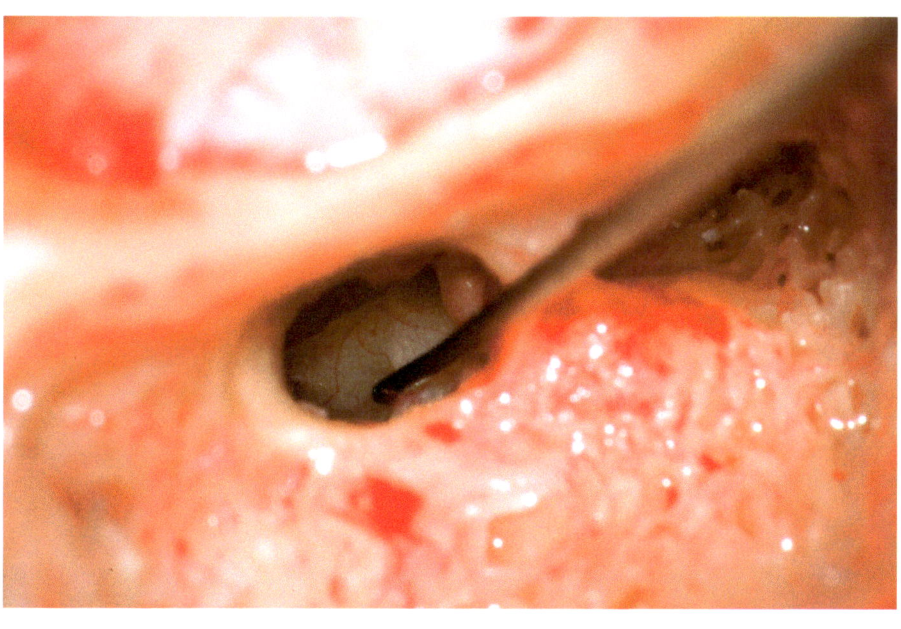

Fig. 5.1.12 Note that the tip of the instrument is much shorter than the bony overhang.

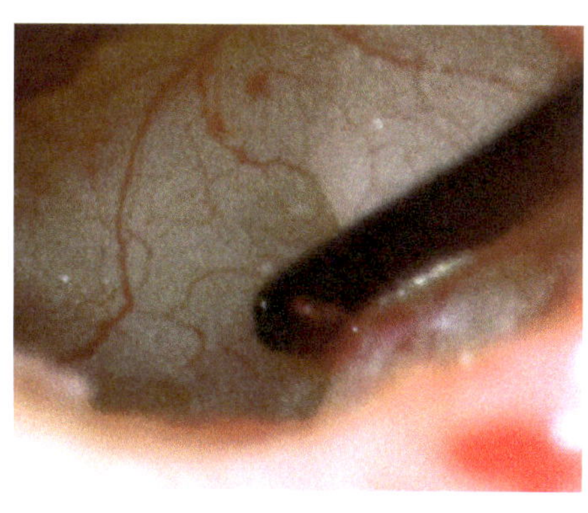

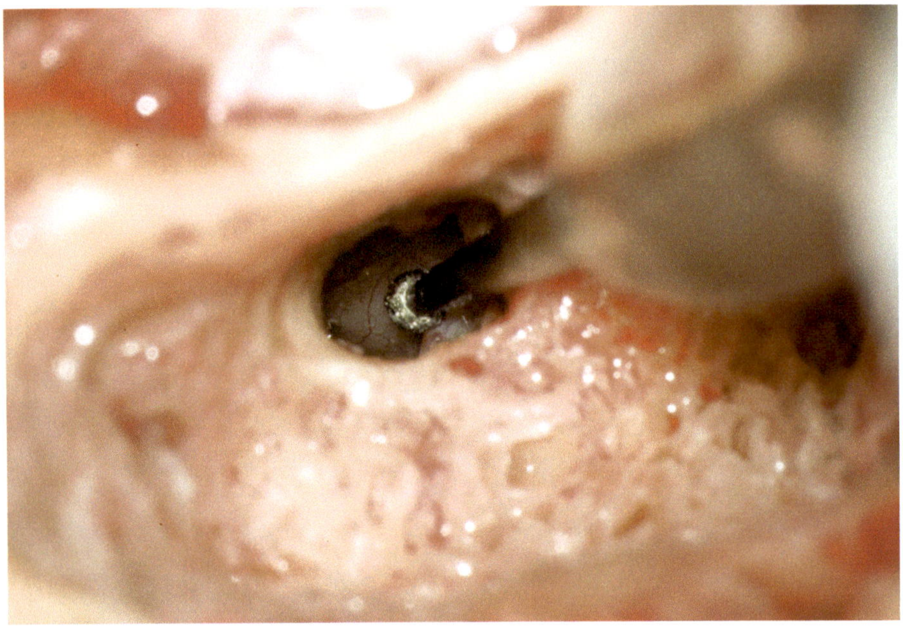

Fig. 5.1.13 The bony overhang covering the round window membrane is removed with a small diamond bur of adequate shaft length. Care must be taken while drilling the overhang not to injure the facial nerve with the shaft or by the heating due to the drilling.

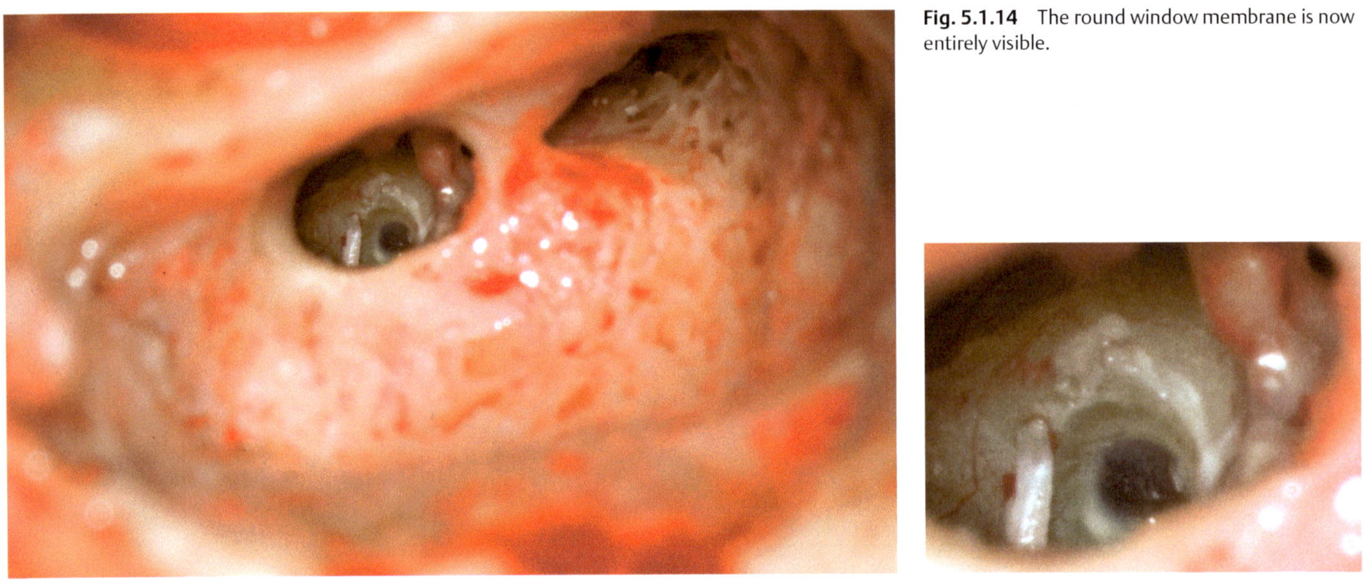

Fig. 5.1.14 The round window membrane is now entirely visible.

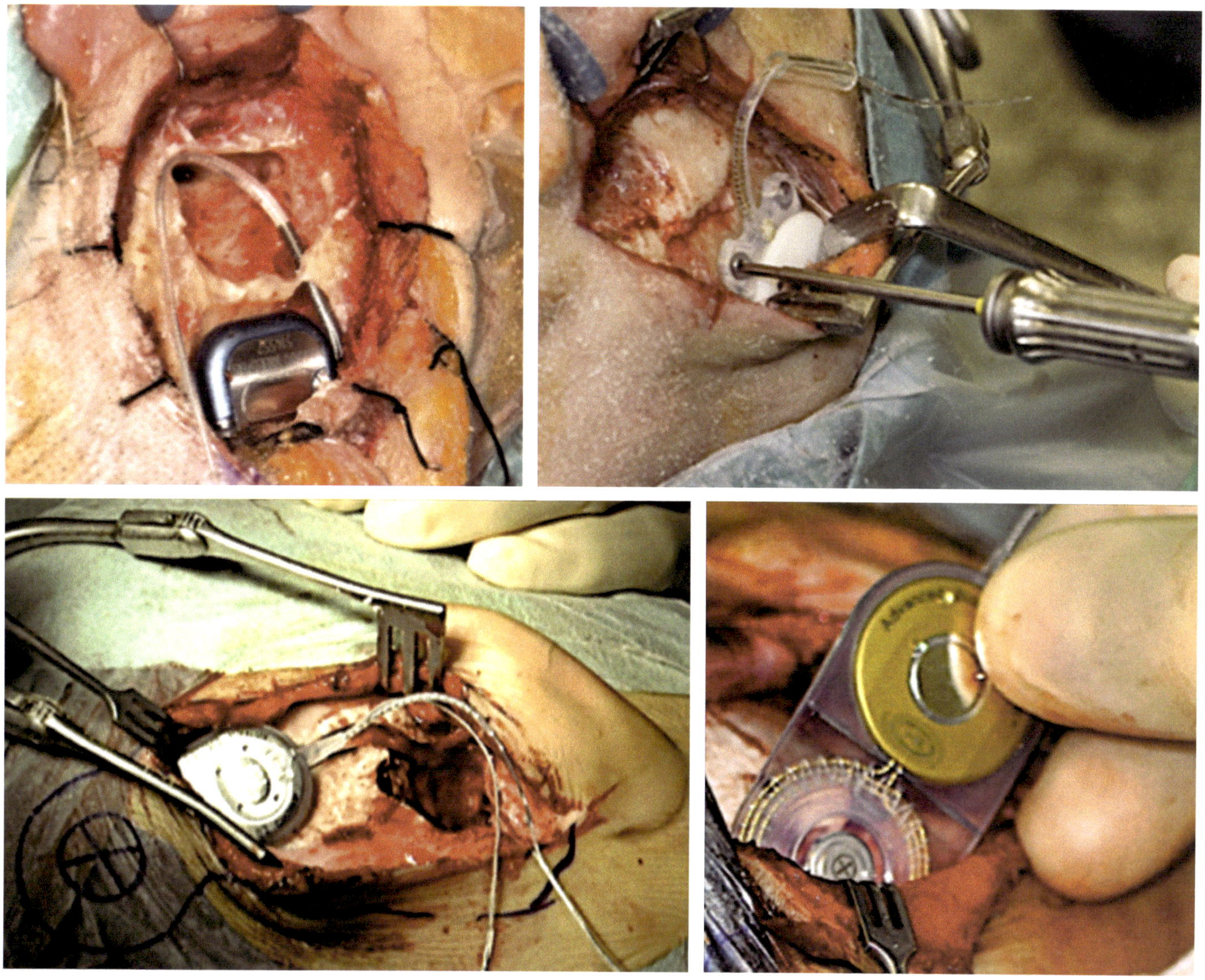

Fig. 5.1.15 After the posterior tympanotomy is completed and the well and pocket have been prepared, the cochlear implant is inserted and fixated to the skull. All implants are fixated differently: an example of each brand of implant is shown here. An overview of all CI brands and electrodes is given in Chapter 4.

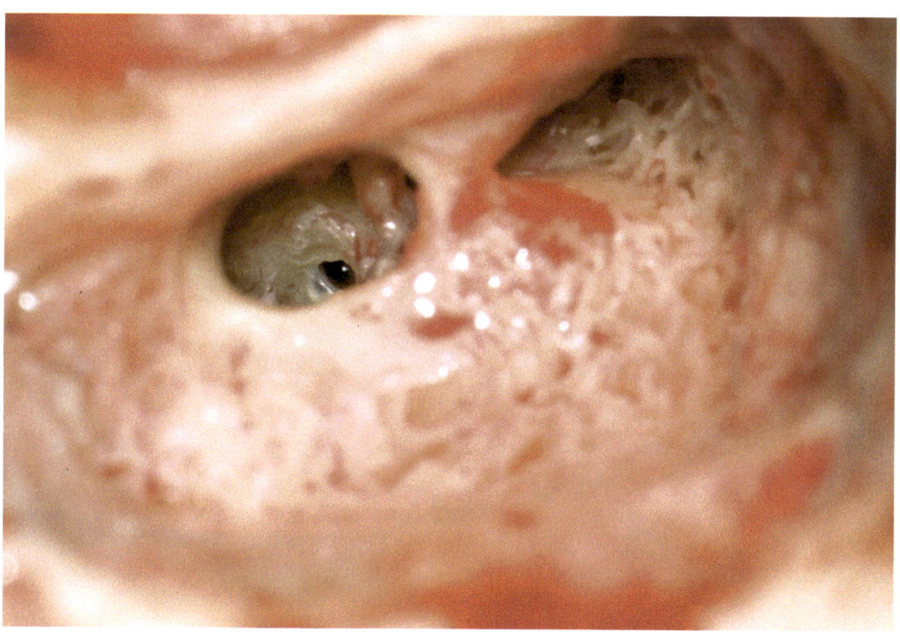

Fig. 5.1.16 The round window is opened carefully, detaching the anterior inferior edge of the round window membrane and reflecting it medially using a small hook. For a better chance of maintenance of residual hearing, no suction is applied to the perilymph in the round window.

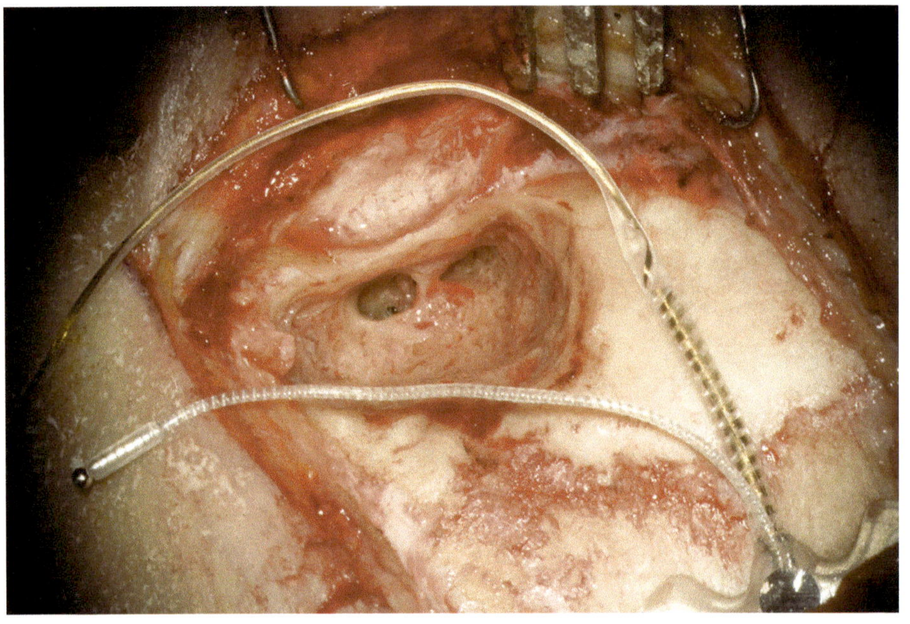

Fig. 5.1.17 The cavity with posterior tympanotomy and the electrodes are shown. Bone dust has been removed by rinsing before opening the round window.

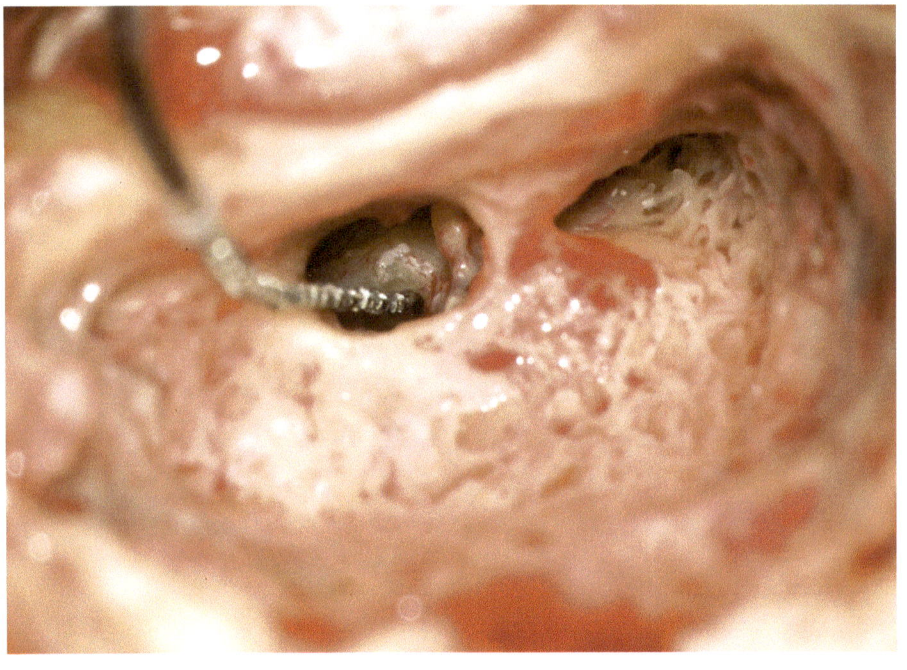

Fig. 5.1.18 The tip of the electrode array is inserted through the opened round window using a nontoothed straight forceps. The cochlear electrode is slowly and gently inserted into the cochlea.

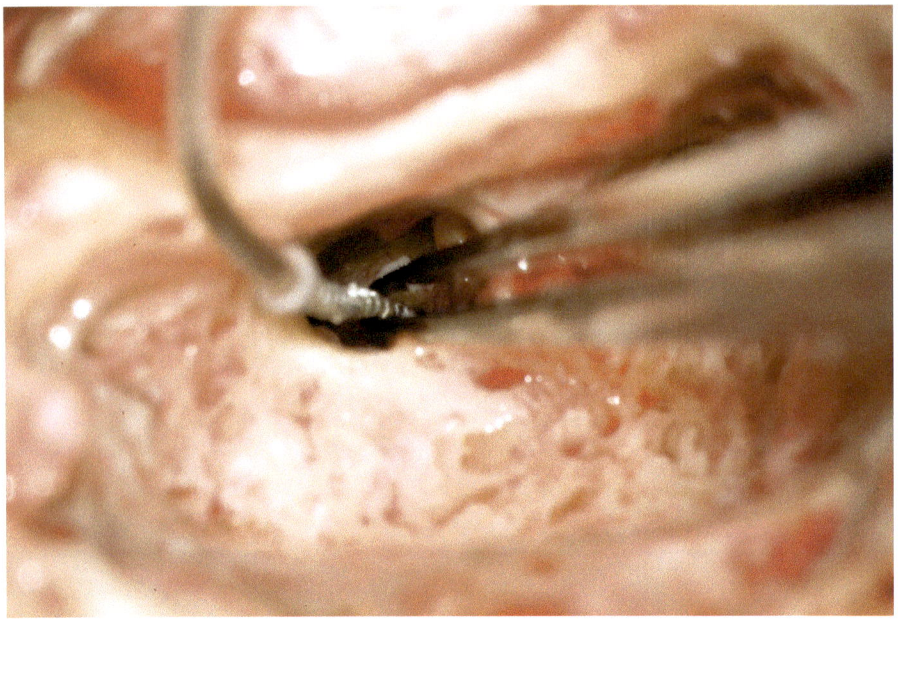

Fig. 5.1.19 The electrode array is advanced gently with a watchmaker's forceps. If some resistance is experienced, insertion must be stopped; the electrode must be slightly withdrawn and can be inserted again very gently after a small rotatory movement. If it is not possible to introduce all electrodes, some of them may remain outside and will have to be turned off by the audiologist in a later stage of the revalidation.

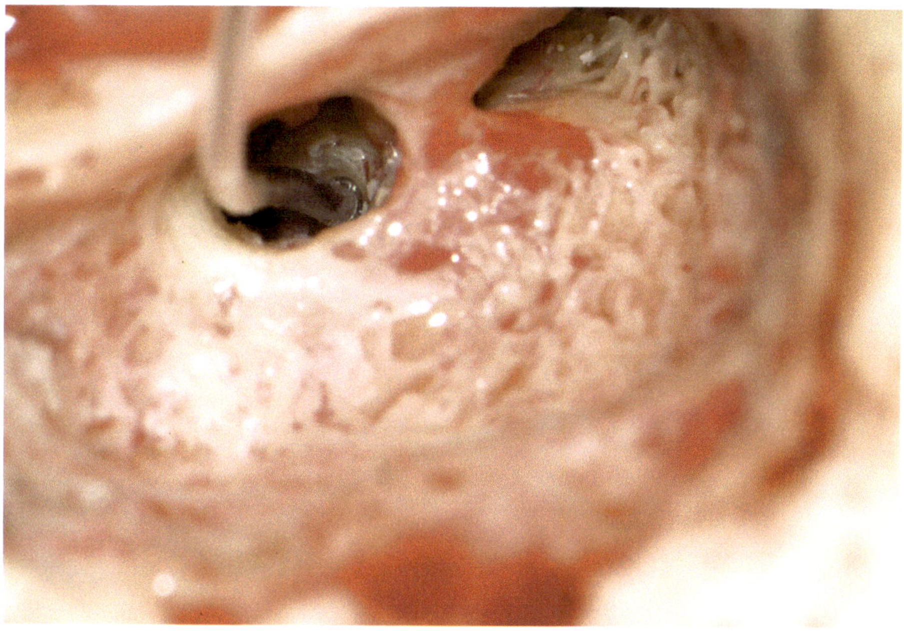

Fig. 5.1.20 The insertion is completed; a full insertion has been performed.

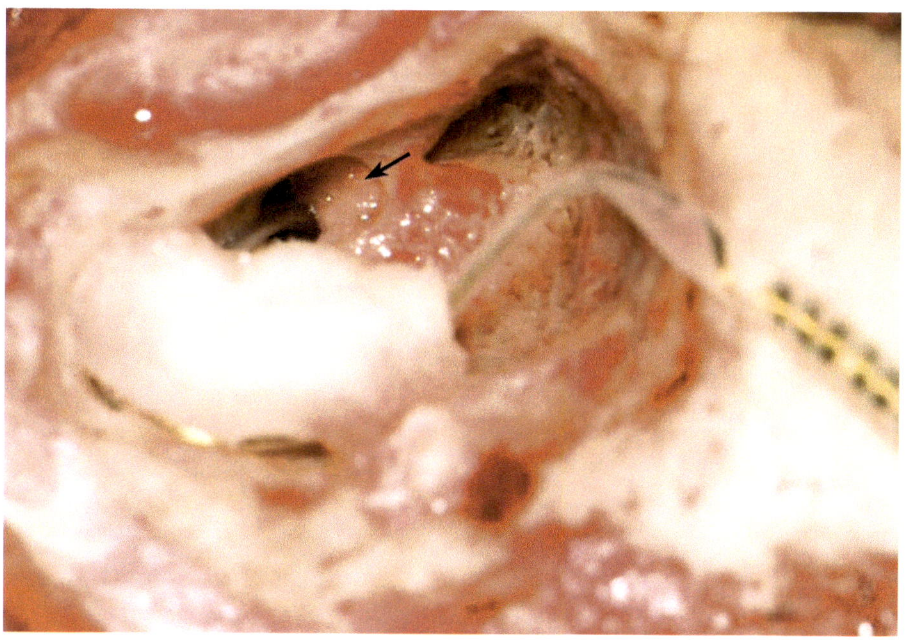

Fig. 5.1.21 The cochlear electrode is fixated in the round window with small pieces of muscle or fascia, and fibrin glue is applied over it. The electrode is secured in the posterior tympanotomy with a piece of temporal muscle.

Case 5.2 Surgical Steps

Standard Cochlear Implantation (Left Ear) (Fig. 5.2.1–Fig. 5.2.20)

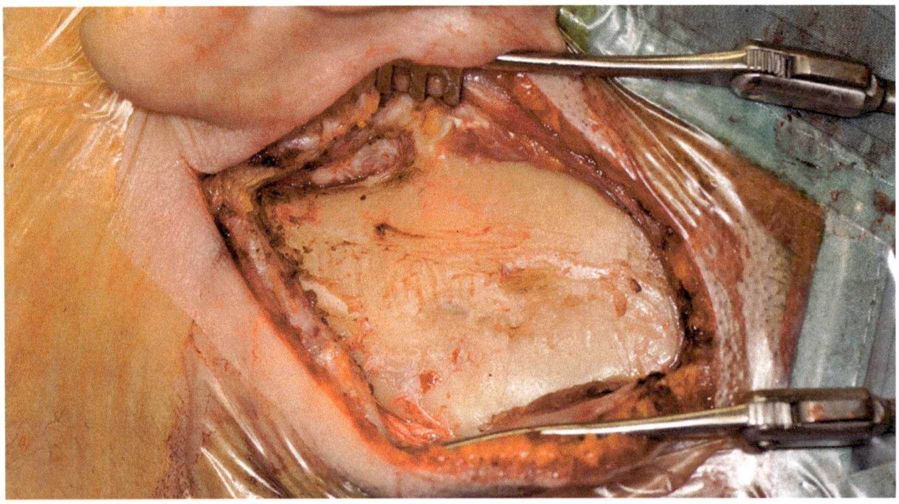

Fig. 5.2.1 Opening of the skin and subcutis via a lazy S incision. The planum mastoideum is widely accessible.

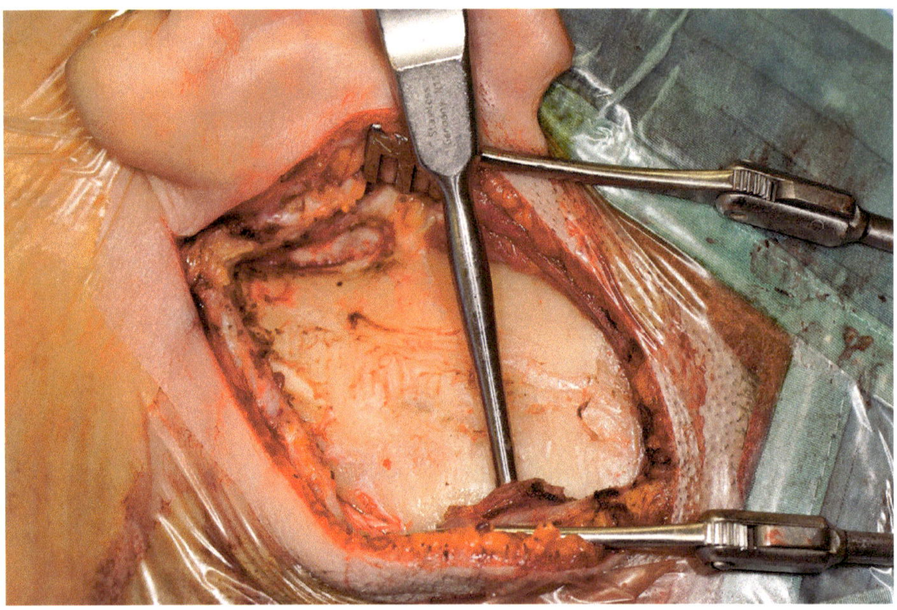

Fig. 5.2.2 A pocket for the receiver stimulator is created using raspatory.

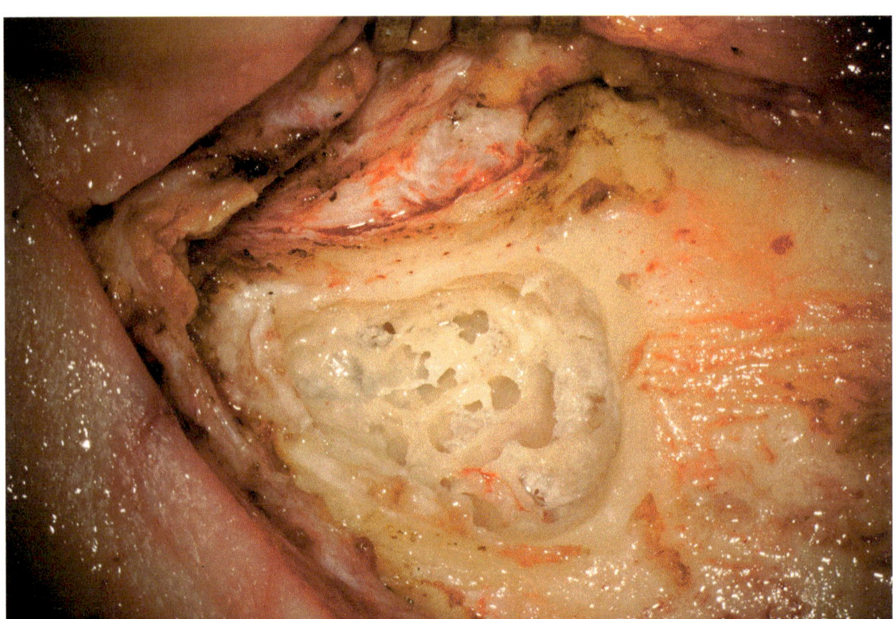

Fig. 5.2.3 Beginning of the mastoidectomy.

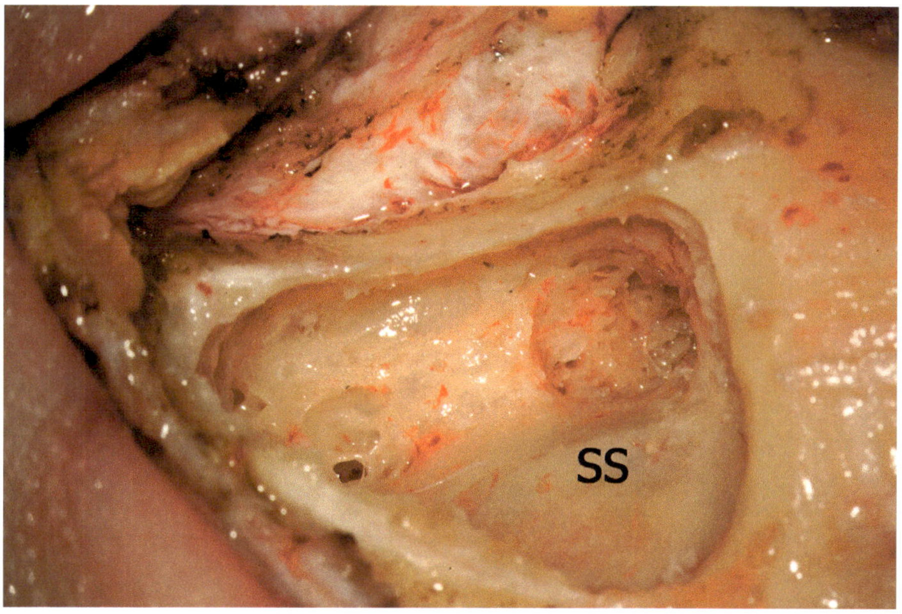

Fig. 5.2.4 The sigmoid sinus (SS) is now skeletonized and the antrum is opened.

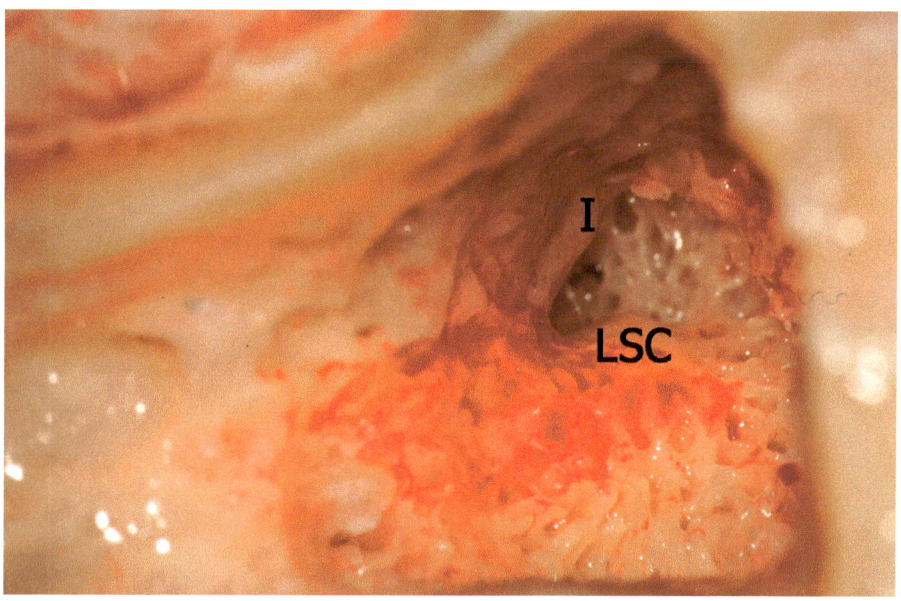

Fig. 5.2.5 After opening the epitympanum, the short process of the incus (I) can be identified. The lateral semicircular canal (LSC) is also visible.

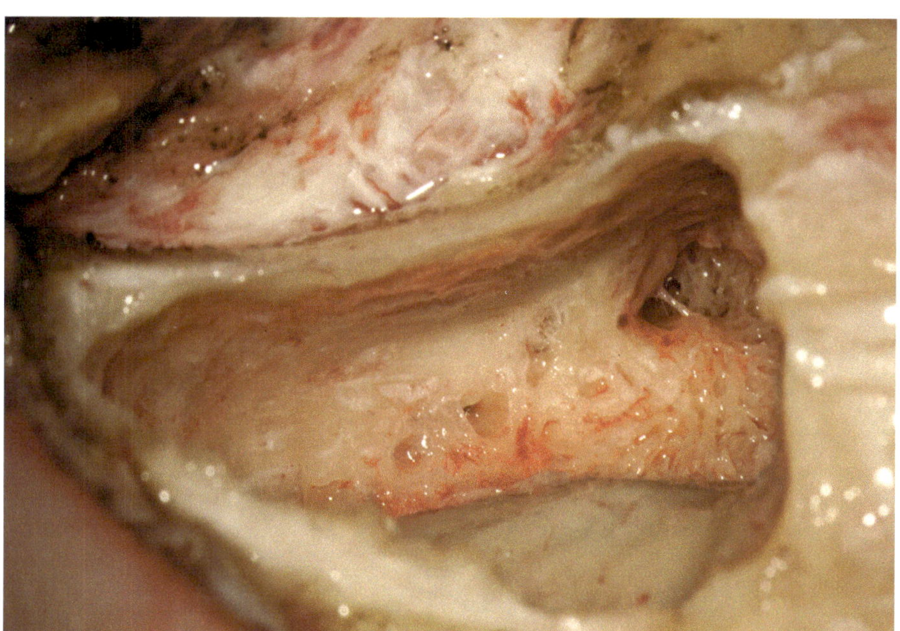

Fig. 5.2.6 The posterior external ear canal is skeletonized in preparation for the posterior tympanotomy.

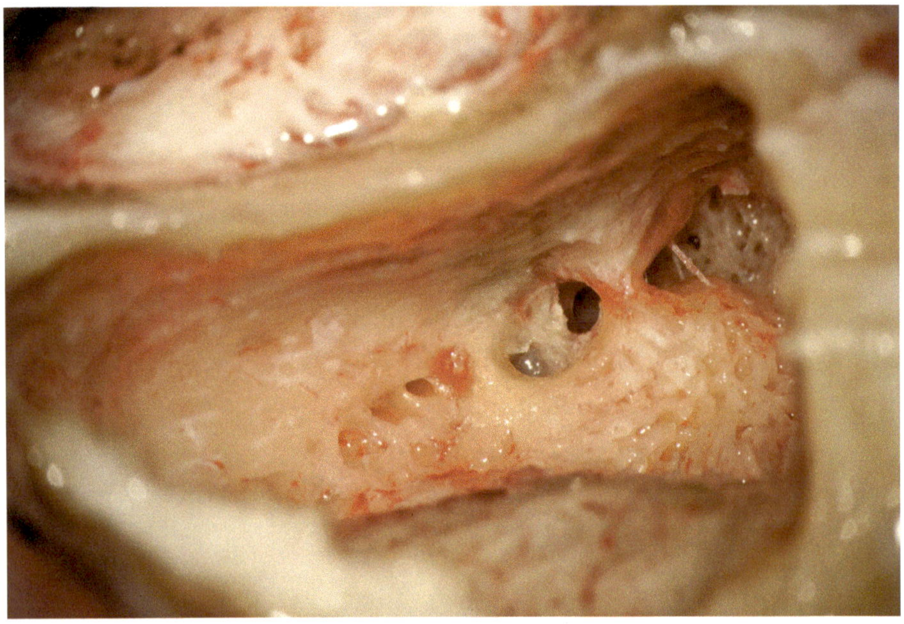

Fig. 5.2.7 With the lateral semicircular canal, incus, and horizontal part of the facial nerve as the most important landmarks, the posterior tympanotomy is now opened. Note that the posterior tympanotomy usually (as in this patient) contains aerated cells.

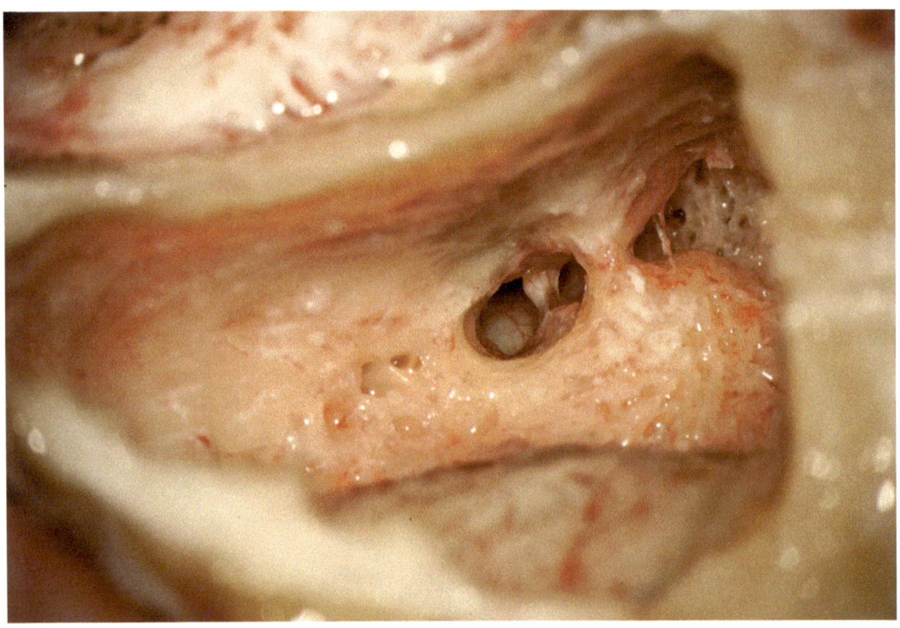

Fig. 5.2.8 The triangle between the vertical part of the facial nerve and chorda tympani is drilled out. The eminentia pyramidalis with stapedius tendon becomes visible. Also a small part of the promontory can already be seen, but the round window niche is not visible yet.

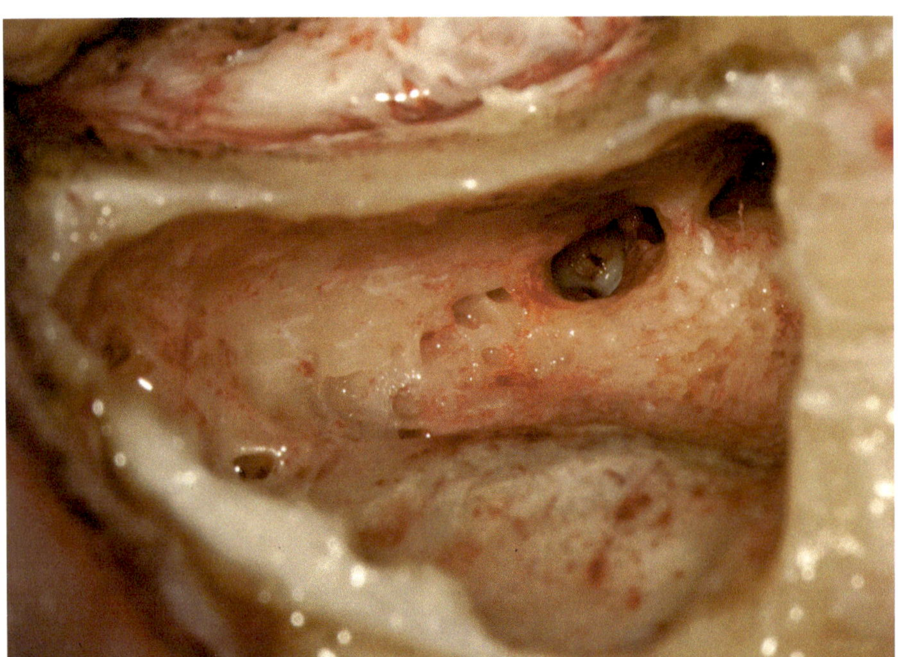

Fig. 5.2.9 After opening up of the posterior tympanotomy more caudally, the promontory and entire round window niche can be seen.

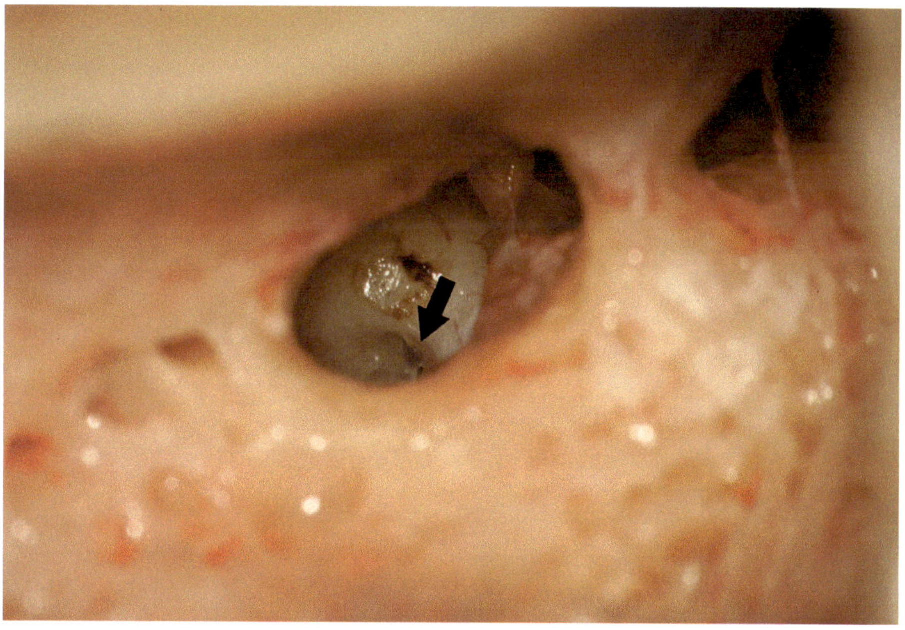

Fig. 5.2.10 Close-up: the promontory and entire round window niche (*arrow*) can now be seen.

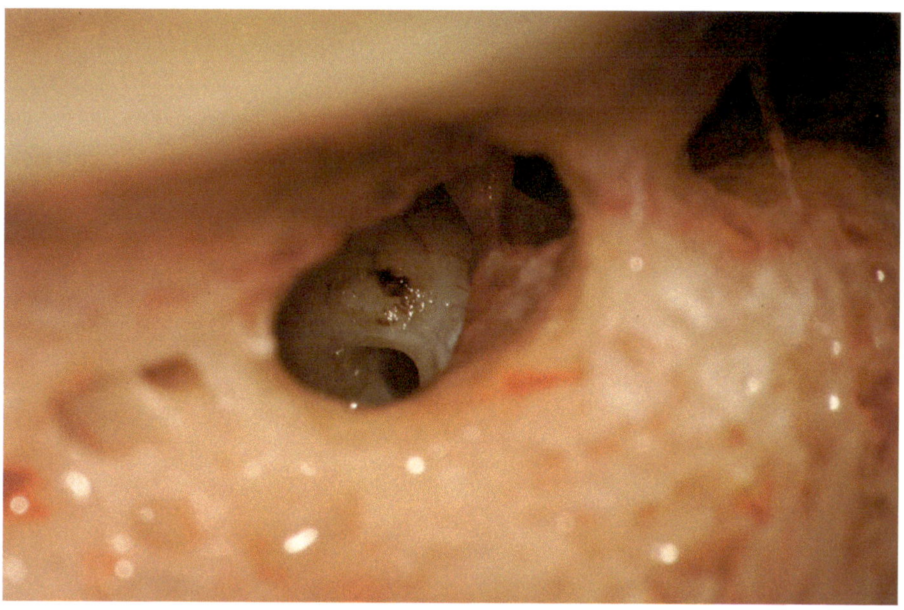

Fig. 5.2.11 The superior bony overhang over the round window can be appreciated.

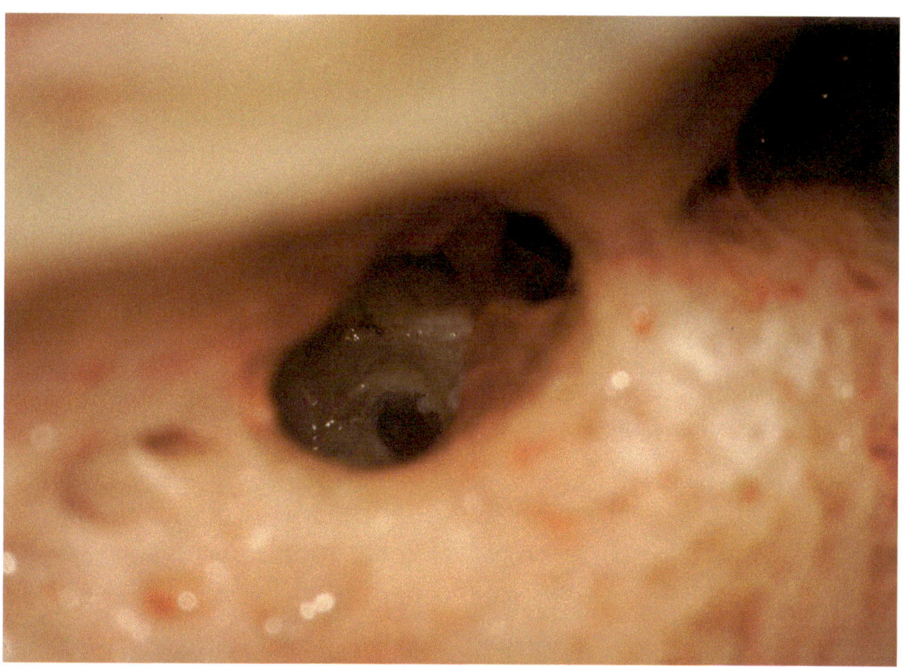

Fig. 5.2.12 The superior bony overhang has been removed by drilling with a small diamond drill: the entire membrane of the round window can now be seen.

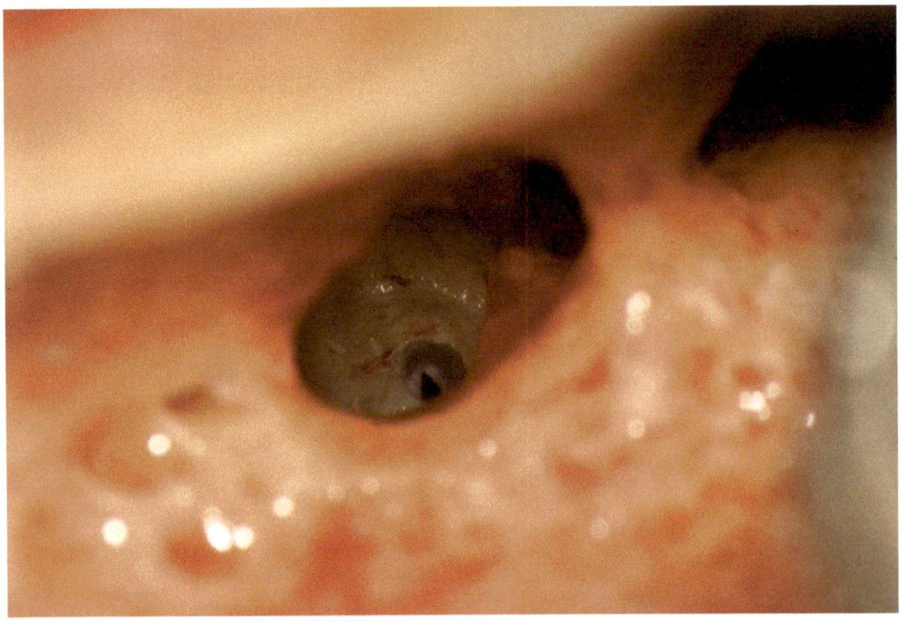

Fig. 5.2.13 The round window is opened anteri-or-inferiorly with a small instrument. This is done only after the receiver well has been created and after all other drilling has been finalized to prevent bone dust and blood from entering the cochlea.

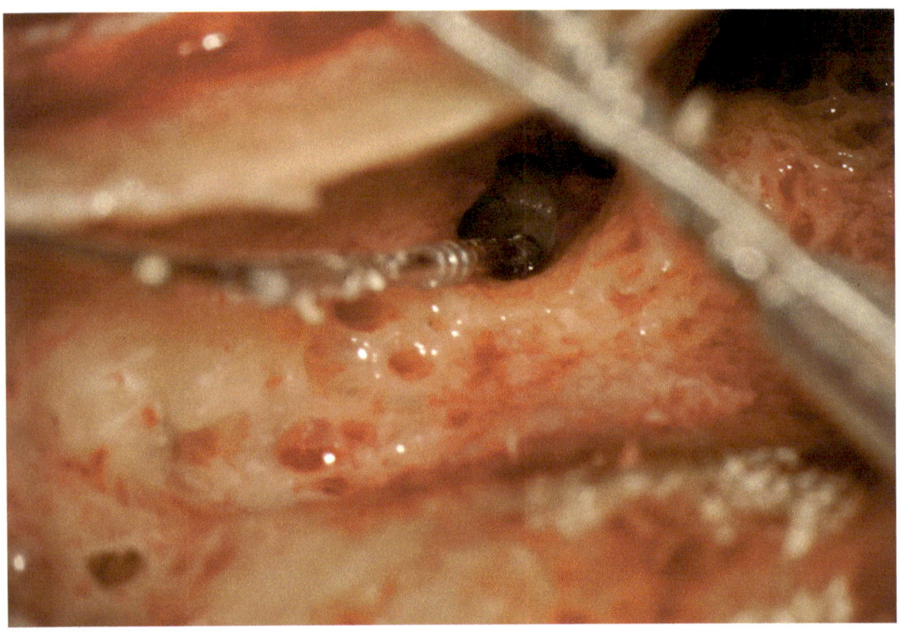

Fig. 5.2.14 The cochlear electrode array can now be inserted: with a gentle, fluid movement the electrode is brought into the scala tympani of the basal turn. The direction of insertion should be superior-posterior to anterior-inferior; in line with the axis of the basal turn.

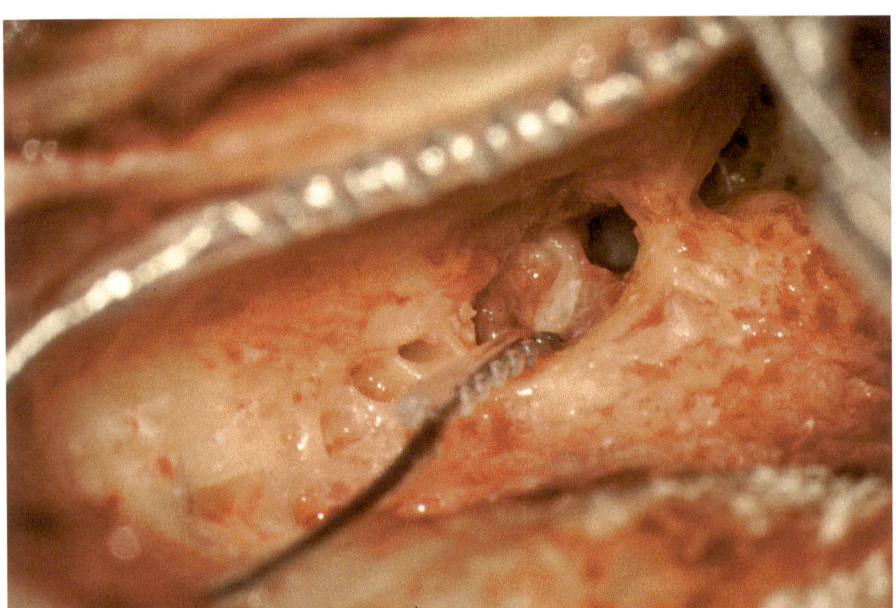

Fig. 5.2.15 The electrode array is fixated at the round window with small pieces of fascia around the electrode. In the posterior tympanotomy the electrode can be fixated with a piece of muscle harvested from the retroauricular muscle.

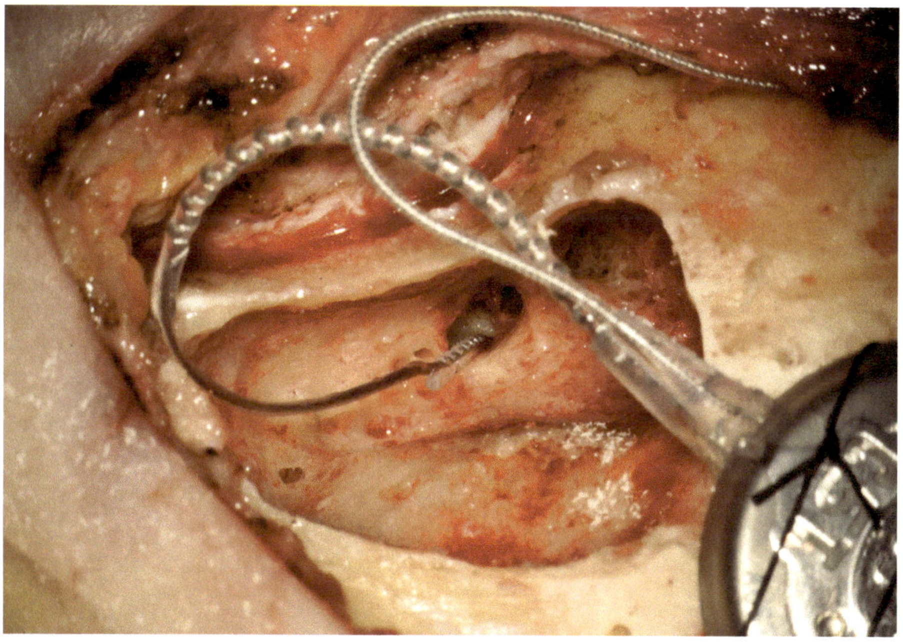

Fig. 5.2.16 The surplus of the electrode array can best be kept in the mastoid cavity. The ground electrode of this implant type is positioned anteriorly under the temporal muscle.

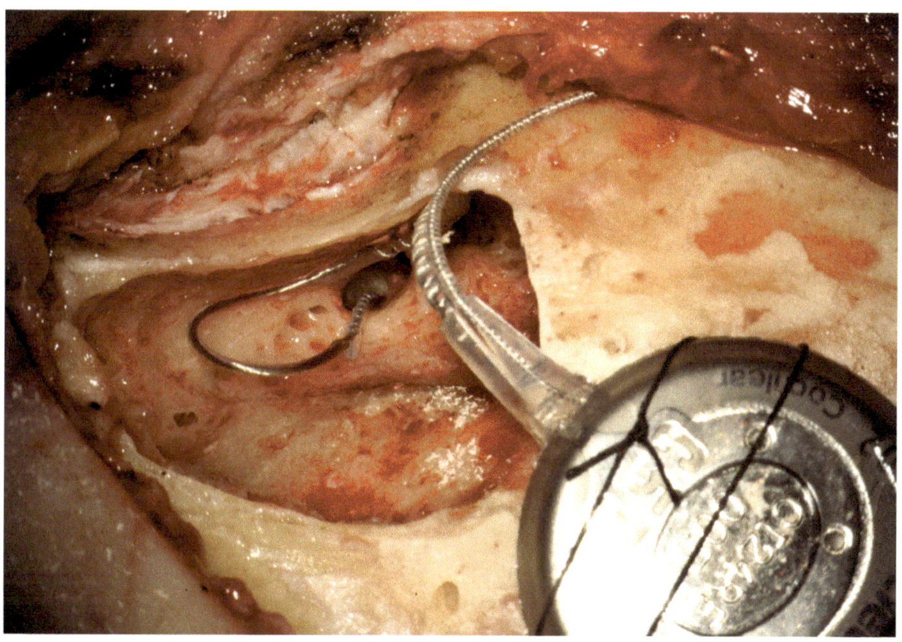

Fig. 5.2.17 The electrode arrays are best protected in the mastoid cavity.

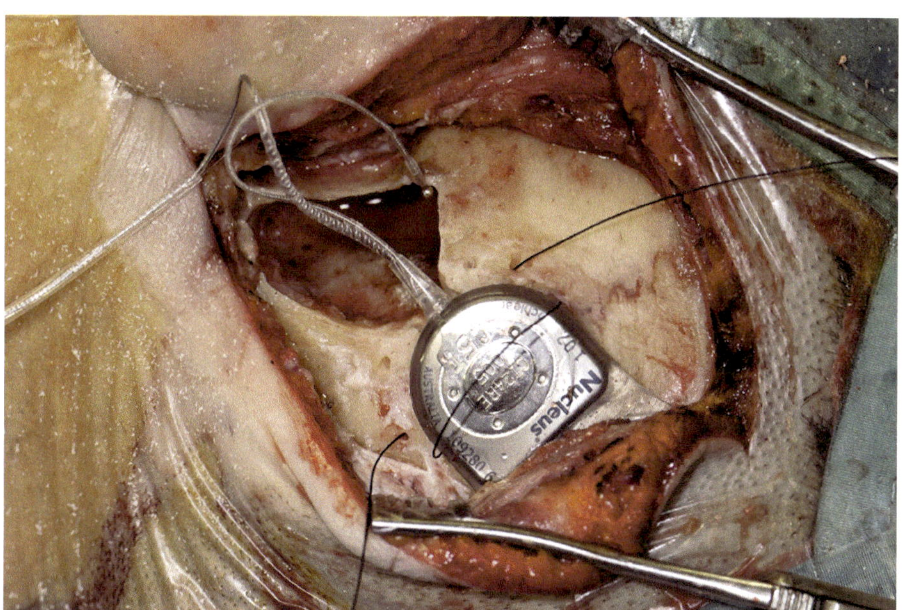

Fig. 5.2.18 Before the cochlea is opened the receiver well has to be drilled. In this example two small canals are drilled on either side of the receiver well to fixate the implant.

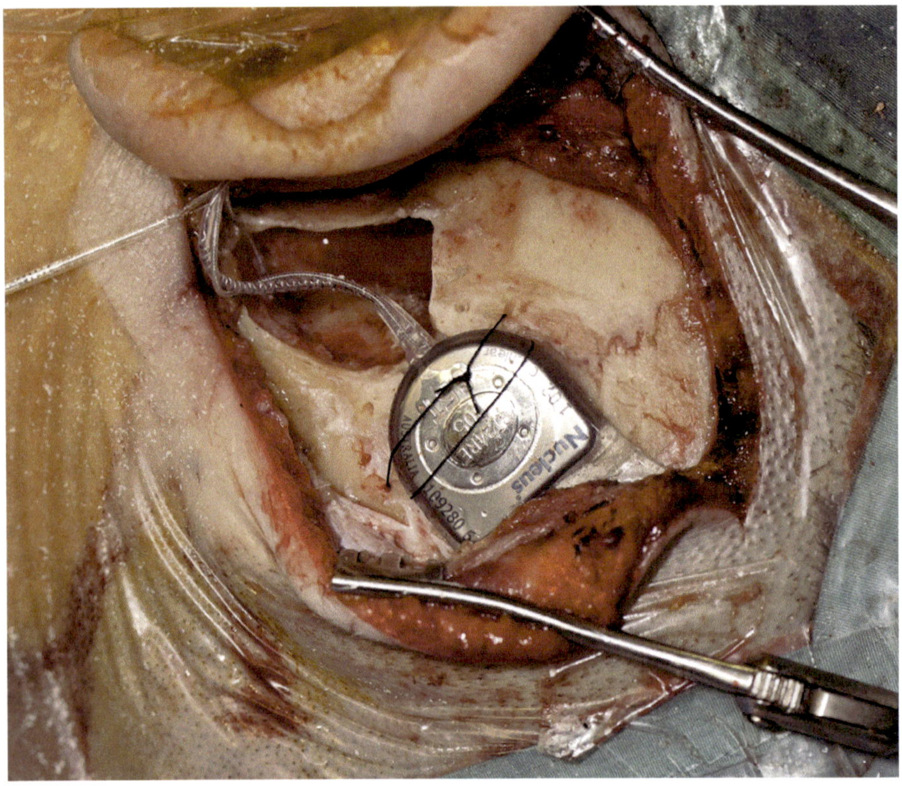

Fig. 5.2.19 The receiver stimulator is fixated in the receiver well using nonresorbable sutures.

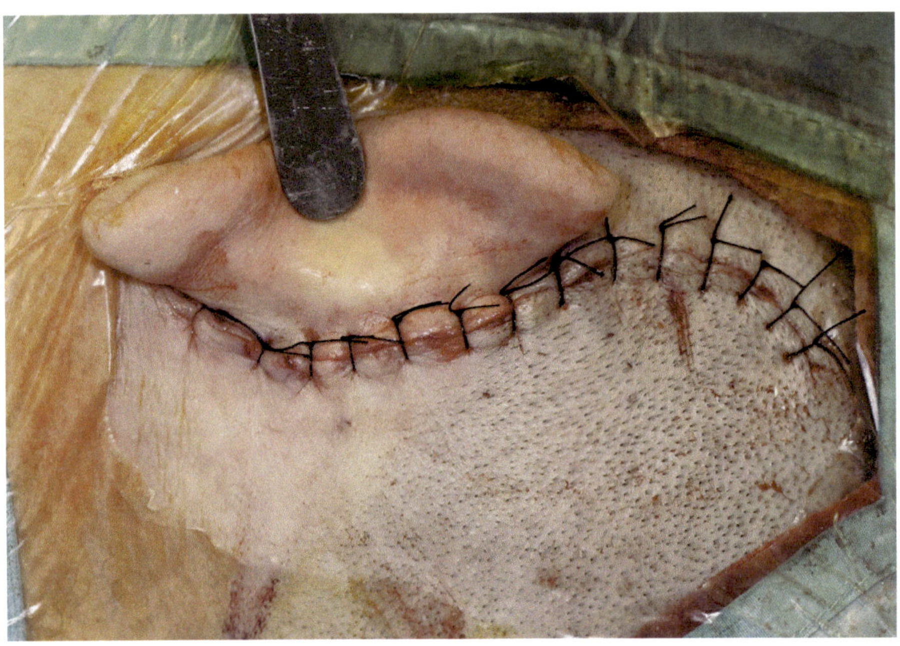

Fig. 5.2.20 The retroauricular wound is closed in two or three layers. As the caudal part of the incision is behind the pinna and the cranial part within the hairline, this is cosmetically not a problem.

5.5 Risks and Complications of Cochlear Implantation

Risks and complications of cochlear implantation in adults (as well as in children) are discussed in Chapter 7.

Pearls and Pitfalls in Cochlear Implantation

- The surgery is usually performed through a narrow window. Even though there is no pathology in the middle ear, the posterior tympanotomy should be sufficiently large to obtain complete control of the round window. In some cases, it is necessary to sacrifice the chorda tympani for better visualization.
- Facial nerve monitoring should be used. The round window is the most natural route for electrode array insertion, giving simple access to the scala tympani.
- The technique of creating a separate cochleostomy is more difficult with a higher risk of damage to the stria vascularis, the basilar membrane, and the osseous spiral ligament.
- The round window is often covered and not directly visible. The bony overhang and inferior lip covering the round window should be removed by drilling. Insertion is easiest when the complete membrane of the round window is visible. Before the round window membrane is opened, the implant must be secured to the skull and be ready to be inserted.
- The round window membrane should be opened with great care. Do not use suction over the opened window. Also bone dust or blood should be prevented from entering the cochlea.
- Insertion of the cochlear electrode array must be performed gently. If there is any resistance, stop the insertion, pull the array back slightly, and gently insert again. Some rotatory movement may help.

Reference Videos

See Video 5.1, Video 5.2, and Video 5.3.

References

1. De Leenheer EM, Janssens S, Padalko E, Loose D, Leroy BP, Dhooge IJ. Etiological diagnosis in the hearing impaired newborn: proposal of a flow chart. Int J Pediatr Otorhinolaryngol 2011;75(1):27–32
2. Boscolo-Rizzo P, Muzzi E, Barillari MR, Trabalzini F. Non-sutured fixation of the internal receiver-stimulator in cochlear implantation. Eur Arch Otorhinolaryngol 2011;268(7):961–965
3. Sunkaraneni VS, Banerjee A, Gray RF. Subdural haematoma: a complication of cochlear implantation. J Laryngol Otol 2004;118(12):980–982
4. Todt I, Basta D, Ernst A. Does the surgical approach in cochlear implantation influence the occurrence of postoperative vertigo? Otolaryngol Head Neck Surg 2008;138(1):8–12

Further Reading

Addams-Williams J, Munaweera L, Coleman B, Shepherd R, Backhouse S. Cochlear implant electrode insertion: in defence of cochleostomy and factors against the round window membrane approach. Cochlear Implants Int 2011 Aug;12 Suppl 2:S36–S39. doi: 10.1179/146701011X13074645127478

Adunka OF, Pillsbury HC, Buchman CA. Minimizing intracochlear trauma during cochlear implantation. Adv Otorhinolaryngol 2010;67:96–107. doi: 10.1159/000262601. Epub 2009

Atturo F, Barbara M, Rask-Andersen H. On the anatomy of the 'hook' region of the human cochlea and how it relates to cochlear implantation. Audiol Neurootol 2014;19(6):378–385. doi: 10.1159/000365585. Epub 2014

Briggs RJ, Tykocinski M, Stidham K, Roberson JB. Cochleostomy site: implications for electrode placement and hearing preservation. Acta Otolaryngol 2005 Aug;125(8):870–876

Havenith S, Lammers MJ, Tange RA. Hearing preservation surgery: cochleostomy or round window approach? A systematic review. Otol Neurotol 2013 Jun;34(4):667–674. doi: 10.1097/MAO.0b013e318288643e

Leong AC, Jiang D, Agger A, Fitzgerald-O'Connor A. Evaluation of round window accessibility to cochlear implant insertion. Eur Arch Otorhinolaryngol 2013 Mar;270(4):1237–1242. doi: 10.1007/s00405-012-2106-4. Epub 2012

Li PM, Wang H, Northrop C, Merchant SN, Nadol JB Jr. Anatomy of the round window and hook region of the cochlea with implications for cochlear implantation and other endocochlear surgical procedures. Otol Neurotol 2007 Aug;28(5):641–648

Mangus B, Rivas A, Tsai BS, Haynes DS, Roland JT Jr. Surgical techniques in cochlear implants. Otolaryngol Clin North Am 2012 Feb;45(1):69–80. doi: 10.1016/j.otc.2011.08.017

Santa Maria PL, Gluth MB, Yuan Y, Atlas MD, Blevins NH. Hearing preservation surgery for cochlear implantation: a meta-analysis. Otol Neurotol 2014 Dec;35(10):e256–e269. doi: 10.1097/MAO.0000000000000561

Seyyedi M, Nadol JB Jr. Intracochlear inflammatory response to cochlear implant electrodes in humans. Otol Neurotol 2014 Oct;35(9):1545–1551. doi: 10.1097/MAO.0000000000000540

6 Special Considerations in Pediatric Cochlear Implantation

Cochlear implantation seems similar in children and adults, but especially in young children the anatomical differences, the growth of the mastoid, and the physiology will modify the surgery. Special considerations in pediatric cochlear implantation are explained in the following pages.

Factors Contributing to the Differences in Pediatric Cochlear Implantation

Pediatric Temporal Bone Anatomy

- The position of the facial recess and position of the round window (electrode insertion issues)
- The growth of the temporal bone (position of the facial nerve at the stylomastoid foramen and the position of the electrode array in the mastoid)
- The presence of bone marrow (control of blood loss)
- The thickness of the cortical bone (creation of a bony island in the skull and fixation of the implant)

Anesthesiologic Issues in Young Children

- There are differences in the induction, the positioning, and the temperature control and also volumetric differences.

Bilateral Pediatric Cochlear Implantation and Anesthesiologic Factors

- Duration of surgery
- Symmetric positioning of the receiver-stimulator
- The use of a temporary drain in the first procedure in simultaneous implantation

6.1 Position of the Facial Nerve

The facial nerve exits the temporal bone at the stylomastoid foramen; however, the position of this foramen is different in children. As the mastoid tip is not yet developed, the foramen is situated slightly inferior, but almost posterior, to the bony external auditory canal. To avoid injury to the facial nerve the cutaneous incision in children up to the age of 2 years should be positioned more posteriorly and should leave the immature mastoid tip untouched.[1,2] Another approach can be to lift the cutaneous layer at the end of a superiorly located incision, before lengthening the incision over the mastoid tip. See surgical steps at the end of this chapter (see also **Fig. 6.6** and **Fig. 6.7**).

6.2 The Anatomical Relations between the Facial Recess, the Round Window, and the Basal Turn in Children

In children the cochlea is already at mature size at birth[3] and the facial recess dimensions are not different than in adults.[4,5] Still, the differences between adult and pediatric cochlear implantation are more than simply anecdotal.

Two main differences in the anatomy of children compared with adults will alter the surgical orientation and could make the approach to the basal turn of the cochlea more difficult. First, the external ear canal has a steeper angle to the vertical section of the facial nerve and also to the plane perpendicular to the round window membrane. This results in a narrower view of the posterior tympanotomy and the round window in the pediatric population.[6] Second, the angle of the facial recess is more tilted. Both the scala tympani of the basal turn and the round window are therefore more difficult to see than in adults.[6]

6.3 Growth of the Temporal Bone

The size of the labyrinth and the tympanic cavity are already of mature size at birth. The rest of the temporal bone, however, will develop over time (**Fig. 6.1**). The pneumatization of the temporal bone will increase and in particular the mastoid tip will expand, giving the facial nerve at the stylomastoid foramen more protective coverage. Also the length of the ear canal will increase. The distance between the cortical bone and the labyrinth will increase in the first 18 years of life as it reaches an adult size.[3,7] The distance of the mastoid tip from the sinodural angle, and most likely the receiver-stimulator well, will increase during development, approximately 3 cm or more, whereas the fossa incudis and facial recess distance toward the round window will remain the same length.[3,7] As a result of this, the positioning of the electrode array in young children should not be in the caudal mastoid but more cranially.[8]

6.4 Bone Marrow and Blood Loss

In young children the bone marrow can bleed easily and continuously. Bipolar coagulation will not easily stem the bleeding as it comes from the bony mastoid cells; a nonirrigated diamond bur or bone wax will stop the bleeding.

6.5 Fixation of the Receiver-Stimulator

Tie-down sutures are not always necessary for good fixation of the implant.[9,10] Good fixation depends on the incision, the musculoperiosteal closure, fixation in a bony well, the thickness of the bone and skin, and the health status of the patient. In young patients the cortical bone is thin and the placement of an implant could require deepening of the receiver-stimulator well onto the dura. A small bony island can be created to give an adequate depth of the well. In the set-up of the position of the receiver-stimulator

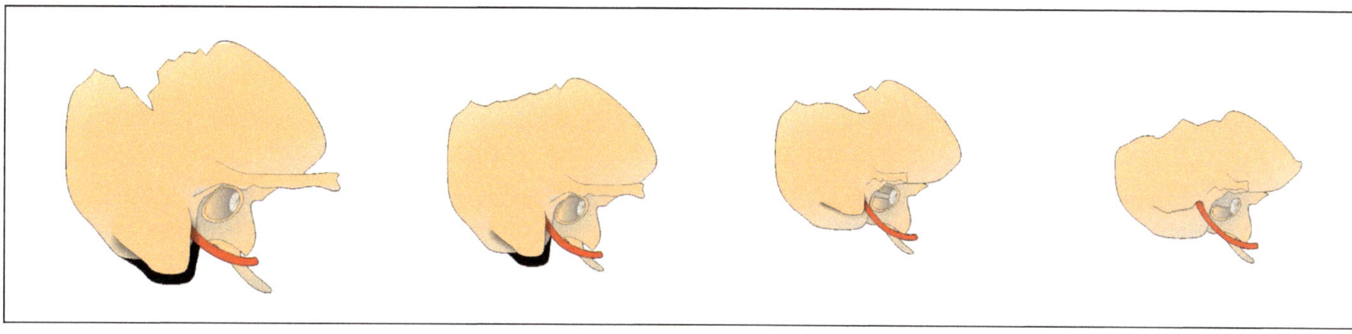

Fig. 6.1 In this figure the position of the facial nerve in correlation to the external auditory canal is clearly visible. As the mastoid tip develops, the nerve is situated inferior-posterior to the bony ear canal at a superficial, lateral position and will, during growth, become positioned more inferiorly and will be protected by the mastoid tip.

one should remember that the implant should not be closer to the pinna than the size of a normal external processor, even in small patients. Pressure of the external processor on the skin over the implant can be painful and can even cause a pressure point or a skin lesion.

6.6 Anesthesiologic Technique

In young children up to 12 months of age, the anesthesiologic risks of surgery are higher than the risks of the surgery itself.[11] The pediatric anesthesiologist plays a crucial role in ensuring safe surgery. Patients younger than 12 months of age have specific physiologic characteristics that increase the anesthesiologic risks. Precautions should therefore be taken in induction, in positioning, and with temperature control and blood loss.

Parental presence is highly desirable during **induction** of anesthesia: it reduces separation anxiety significantly and has been shown to decrease the numbers of distressed children during induction.[12] The choice of anesthetic agents, gaseous or intravenous, for induction should be based on minimizing postoperative nausea and vomiting and minimizing the intraoperative bleeding.

Because of the length of the procedure special care must be taken in the **positioning** of the child. The neck and cervical spine are very flexible and luxation of the cervical vertebrae is reported.[13] Folds or wiring underneath the child can cause skin injury during the operation. If the implantation is bilateral, the alternating position of the head should be anticipated. Furthermore, the pediatric trachea is of a shorter length, which makes the infant patient more prone to accidental extubation with head movement. Because of this the anesthesiologist or ENT surgeon should manually secure the tube while moving the head. During surgery, just as in adults, the use of facial nerve monitoring and stimulation precludes the use of long-acting muscle relaxants.

Infants are particularly vulnerable to **hypothermia** because of both large body-surface-to-weight ratio and limited ability to cope with cold. It is important to minimize heat loss, and therefore to preheat the operation room, apply a temperature control blanket, and monitor body temperature perioperatively.

Due to the small circulating blood volume, young infants are vulnerable to cardiovascular compromise, and hemostasis is of the utmost importance. **Hypovolemic effects** can occur when blood loss exceeds 10% of the total blood volume,[14] which corresponds to 65 mL of blood loss in a baby of 6 months (of ~8 kg). Therefore, blood loss needs to be measured and gauzes used need to be weighed.

6.7 Electrophysiologic Measurements

Before closure of the wound, the neural response is measured. This is more important in children than in adults, as during the first CI fitting session of the young recipient the CI levels can be set at levels just below the lowest neural response levels found during preoperative measurements.

Impedance and stapedial reflex measurements are also (often) performed. See Chapter 4 for further description and explanation.

6.8 Bilateral Pediatric Cochlear Implantation

A recent European consensus report states the indications for and concerns about bilateral cochlear implantation.[15]

There is no evidence to date to suggest that children undergoing sequential procedures with short interimplant delays of less than 1 year perform any differently from children receiving simultaneous implants. However, a single surgical procedure for simultaneous implantation reduces the cumulative costs of two surgical procedures without increasing the surgical hazard, maximizes auditory experience, and represents the optimal rehabilitation of the profoundly deaf child.

It is stated that "the infant or child with unambiguous cochlear implant candidacy should receive bilateral cochlear implants simultaneously as soon as possible after definitive diagnosis of deafness to permit optimal auditory development." Children with complex etiologies, progressive hearing loss, or significant residual hearing in one or both ears should *not* be implanted as soon as possible, but require behavioral testing to determine implant candidacy.[16] Similarly to unilateral pediatric cochlear implantation, it is recommended to use an atraumatic surgical technique designed to preserve cochlear function and minimize cochlear damage so as to allow a possible re-implantation in future.

6.8.1 Surgical Considerations in Bilateral Implantation (Fig. 6.2–Fig. 6.22)

The height of the coil of the implant is directly related to the position of the receiver-stimulator. In bilateral implantation the symmetry of the two coils on the skull can be important to the parents and the patient. An easy method to assure a symmetrical position is to draw a paper blueprint of the implant position on the first side as shown in the surgical photographs later (see **Fig. 6.24–Fig. 6.28**).

Another tip in bilateral surgery is for avoidance of a hematoma at the first implant side. A temporary drain can be placed on top of the musculoperiosteal layer before turning the head for the second-side surgery. This drain should be removed when the head bandage is applied.

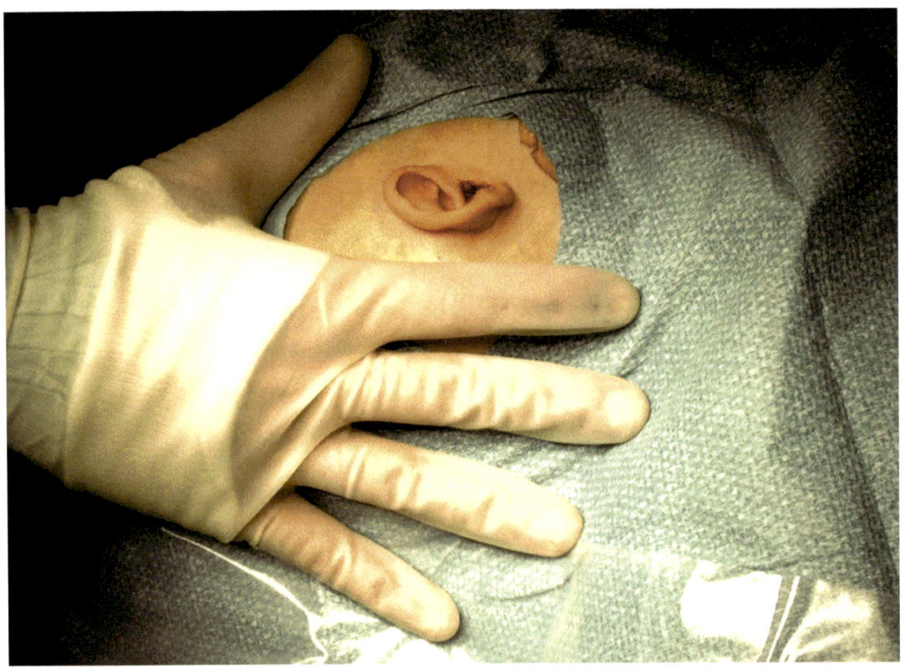

Fig. 6.2 Dimensions in a pediatric skull. The skin, the bone, the vessels, and the nerves of a pediatric patient are of smaller dimensions and are more flexible and therefore more fragile. The surgical technique and approach should be more delicate and adjusted to the anatomical proportions and physiologic properties.

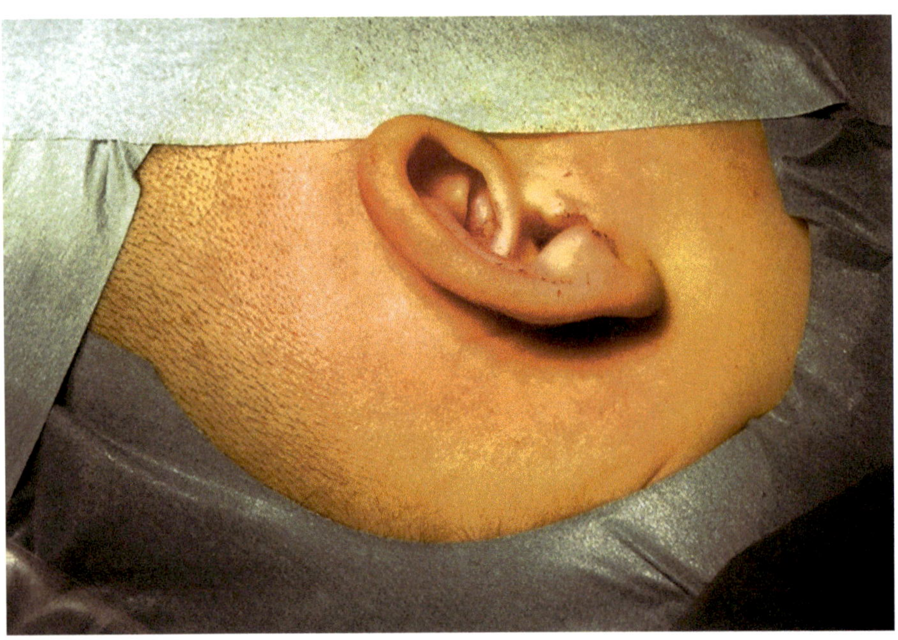

Fig. 6.3 Preparation 1. In the preparation of the surgery, smaller instruments: smaller drills, knife 15, and intracutaneous sutures should be available. Although a smaller mastoid is expected, the actual field of surgery should not be reduced as the implant and processor dimensions are adult size.

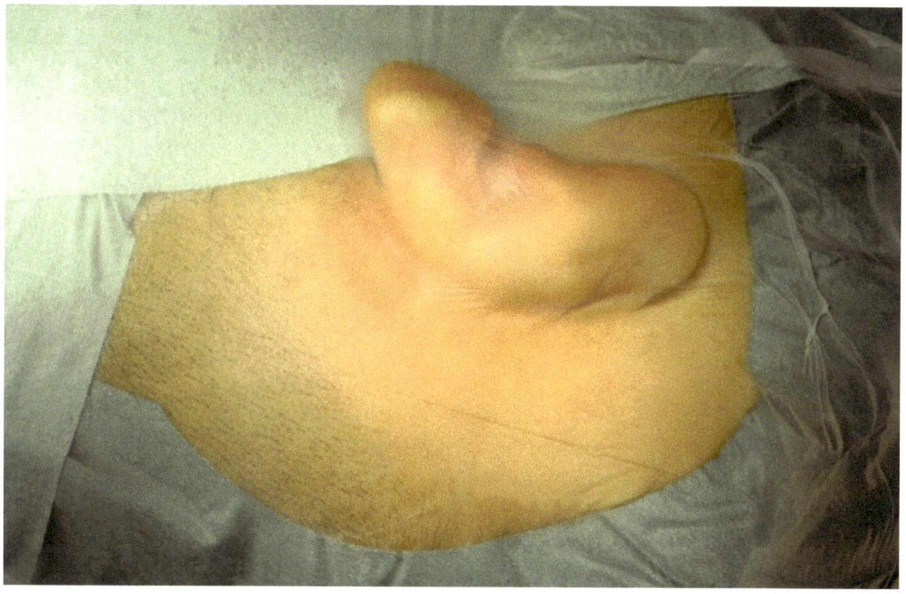

Fig. 6.4 Preparation 2. It is helpful for the surgery to fixate the reflected pinna with transparent plastic adhesive drape. It is also useful to draw the position of the implant, the processor, the mastoid tip, and the incision.

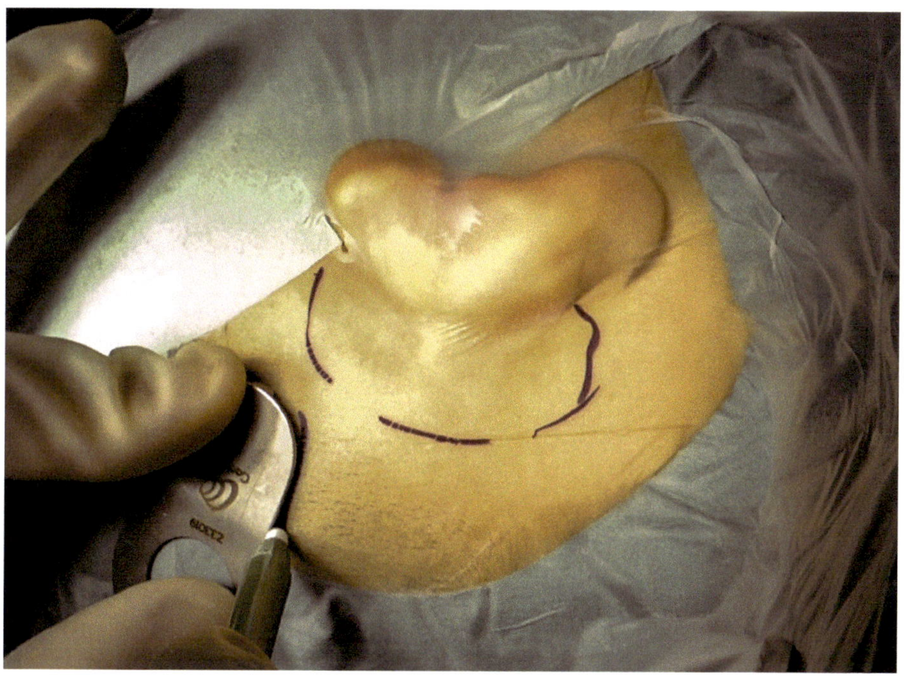

Fig. 6.5 Preparation 3. When the position of the implant is planned it should be on a fairly "flat" surface to ensure easy insertion into the created pocket and well. The esthetically acceptable positioning of the magnet coil can also be important for the patient and the parents. Furthermore, the implant should not be closer to the pinna than the processor line (in this picture the curved discontinuous line). Pressure of the external processor on the skin over the implant can be painful and can even cause a pressure point or a skin lesion.

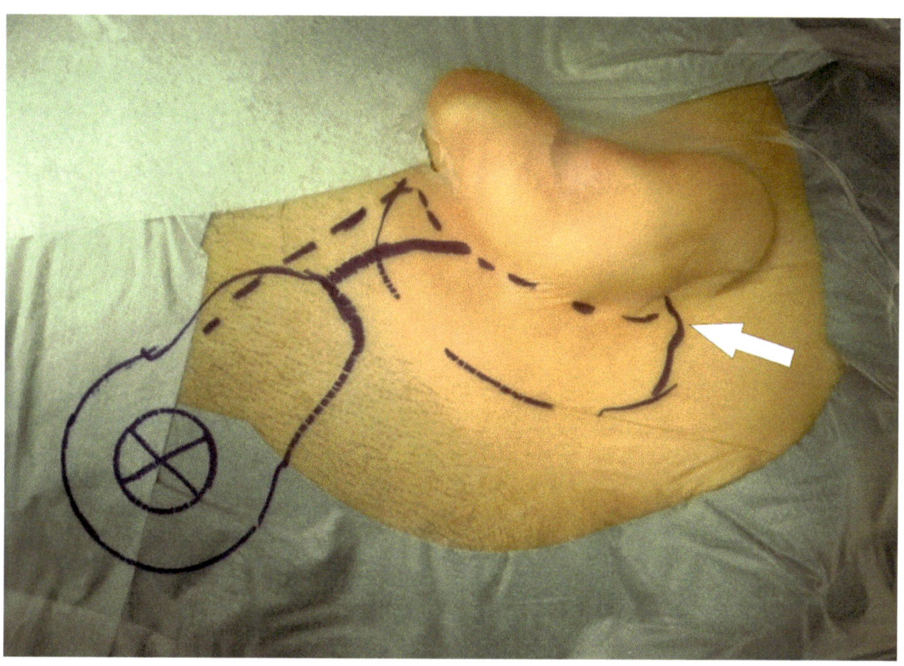

Fig. 6.6 Incision line. Several incision lines are possible as explained earlier. The dotted line shown here is a lazy S incision with the beginning and end close to the mastoid tip and halfway to the implant. The mastoid tip in this case is exactly in the same line as the caudal border of the drawing of the external processor (*arrow*). If a longer incision is preferred, the cutaneous layer must be lifted at the end of a superiorly located incision, before lengthening the incision over the mastoid tip (and the superficially located facial nerve).

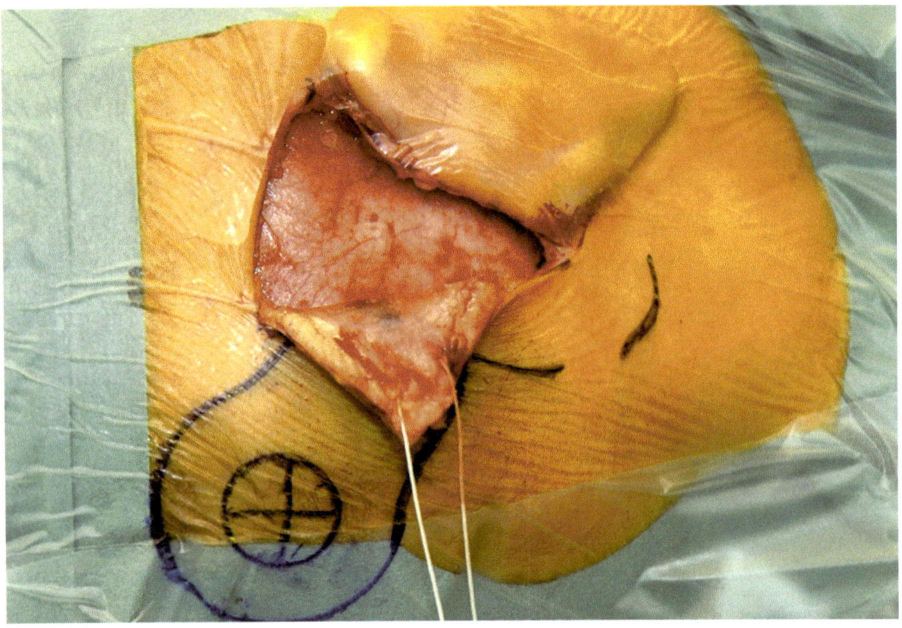

Fig. 6.7 Incision. The incision is made toward the mastoid tip. At each point of the incision care must be taken not to incise too deeply (knife 15) to avoid injury to the musculoperiosteal layer beneath it. At the mastoid tip the skin is elevated before incising.

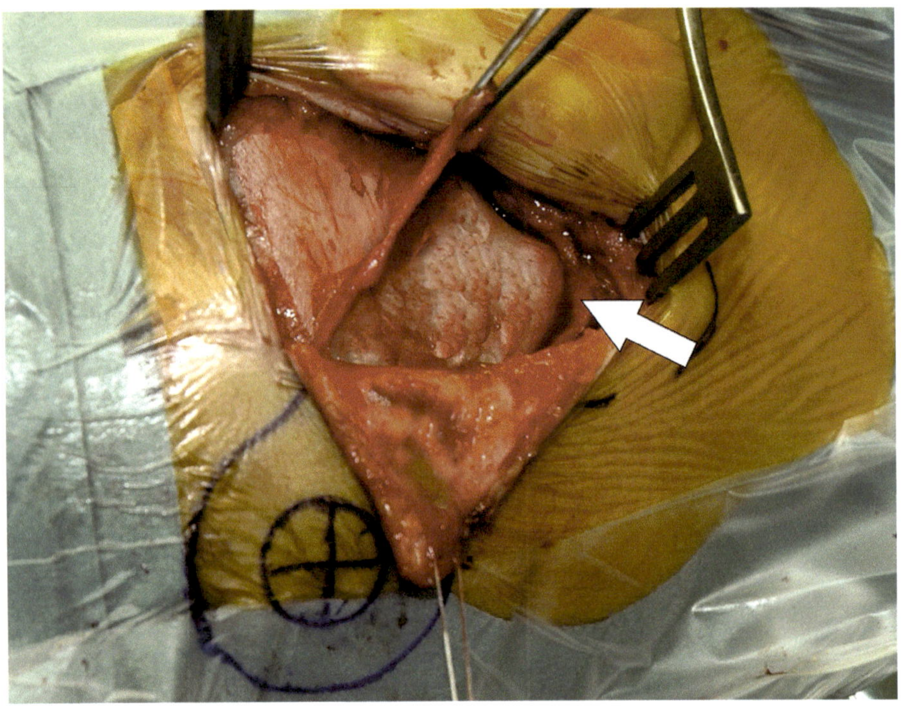

Fig. 6.8 Muscle flap. To create a good layer under which the implant and the electrodes can be securely fixed, the thin muscle must be handled with care. In this case a cranially based flap is used to easily cover the electrode lead and have the (sub)cutaneous and musculoperiosteal suture lines perpendicular, and not directly on top of each other. Note the underdeveloped mastoid tip (*white arrow*).

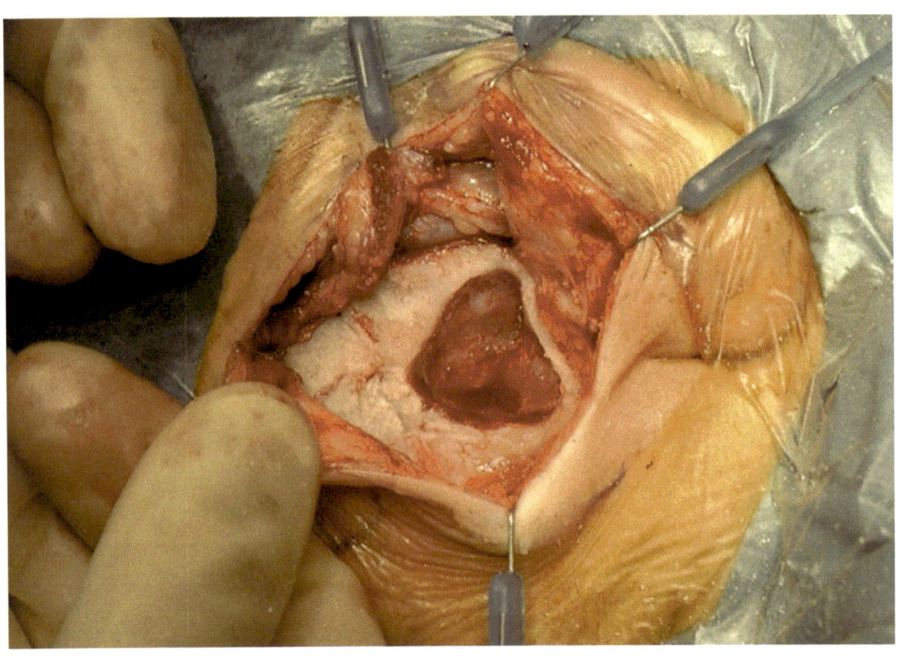

Fig. 6.9 Mastoidectomy and bone marrow. The borders of the mastoidectomy are often easily found, as the bone is softer than in adults and the dimensions are smaller. The cavity is shallow and sometimes the only cell encountered is the antrum. In young children the bone marrow can bleed easily and continuously. Bipolar coagulation will not easily stem the bleeding as it comes from the mastoid cells; a nonirrigated diamond bur or bone wax will stop the bleeding.

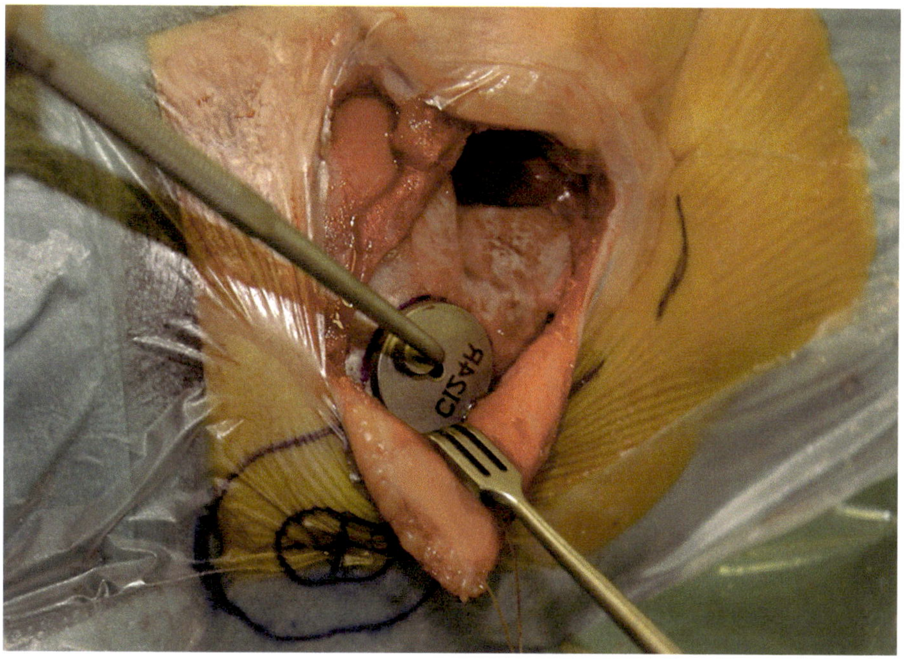

Fig. 6.10 Creating the receiver-stimulator well. In some implants the receiver-stimulator is designed to be fixated in a bony well. With the use of templates the well can be marked on the bone before it is drilled.

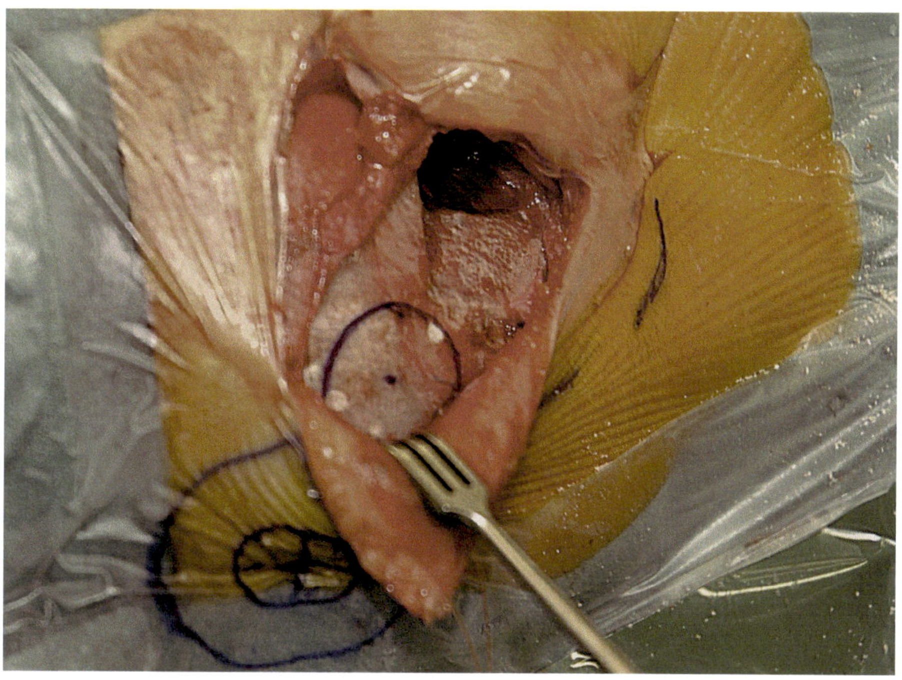

Fig. 6.11 Creating the receiver-stimulator well. The well in young children often consists of a cortical layer, a bone marrow layer, and then a thin cortical layer (tabula interna) before the middle cranial fossa dura is exposed. The size of the well can be verified with a template.

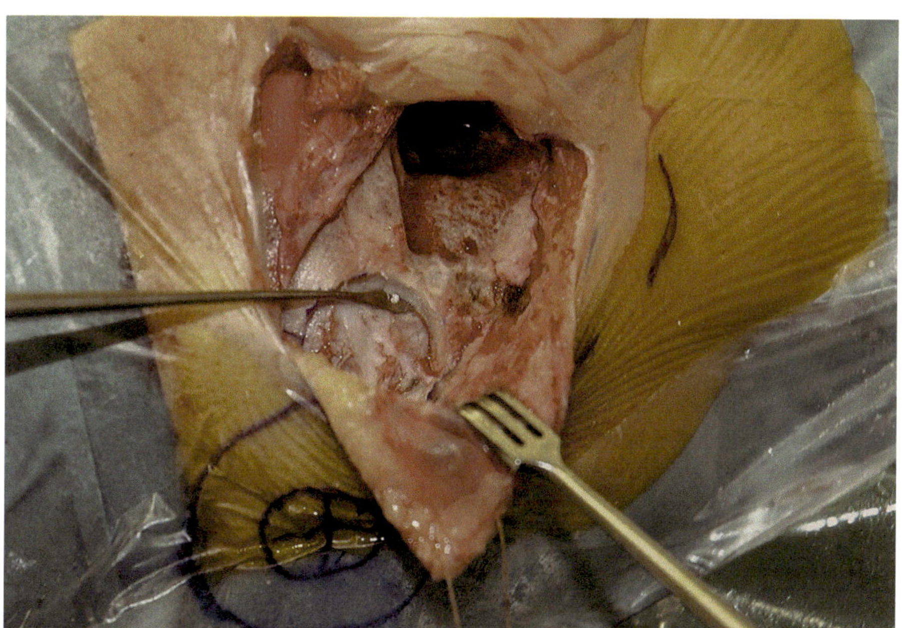

Fig. 6.12 Creating the receiver-stimulator well on the dura. Once the dura is in sight, the borders of the well are drilled upon the dura. If the bone well is very shallow, the dura can be gently mobilized circumferentially, which allows the implant to be fixated in the well without the dura pushing the implant out. The middle part of the well is still covered with a thin layer of bone. This is called "the bony island."[8]

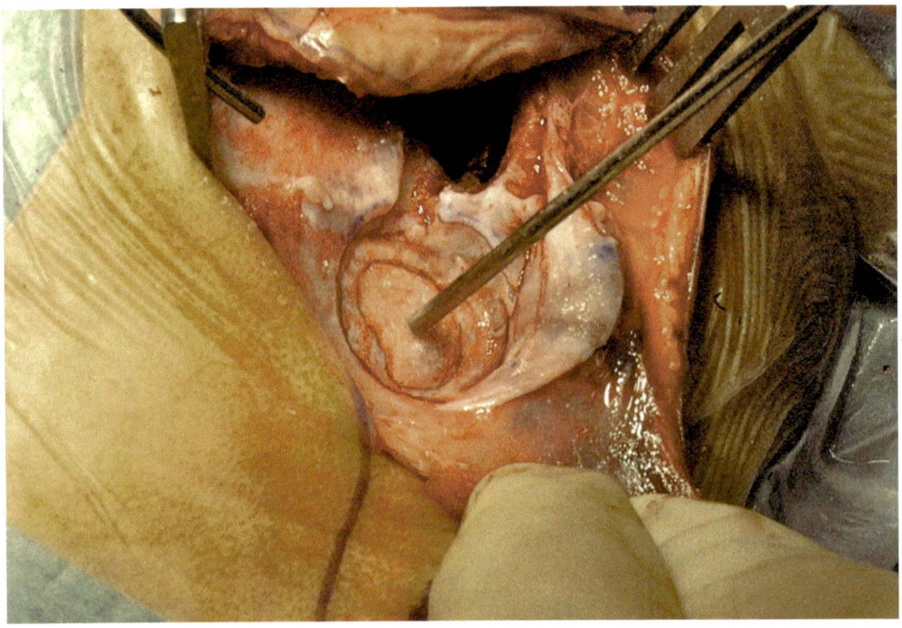

Fig. 6.13 A close-up of the bony island in the receiver-stimulator well. The mobility of the island can be checked with a blunt instrument.

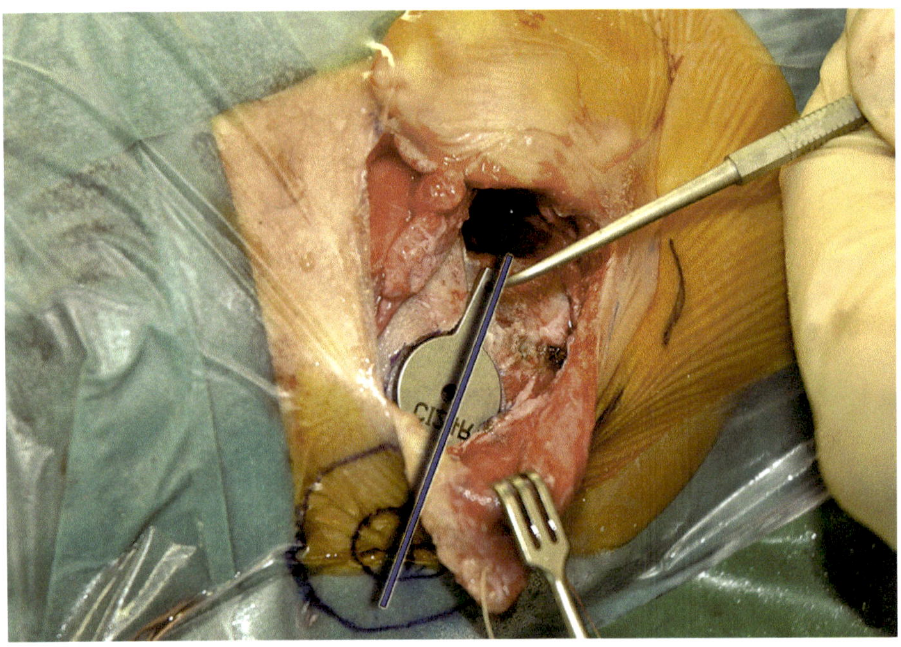

Fig. 6.14 The electrode lead canal. The position of the electrode lead canal depends on the planned position of the receiver-stimulator magnet coil. The canal should be drilled in a straight line from the planned position of the coil (marked on the patient with ⊗). Although tempting, it is not always the shortest line to the antrum. The imaginary line is drawn in this picture in blue.

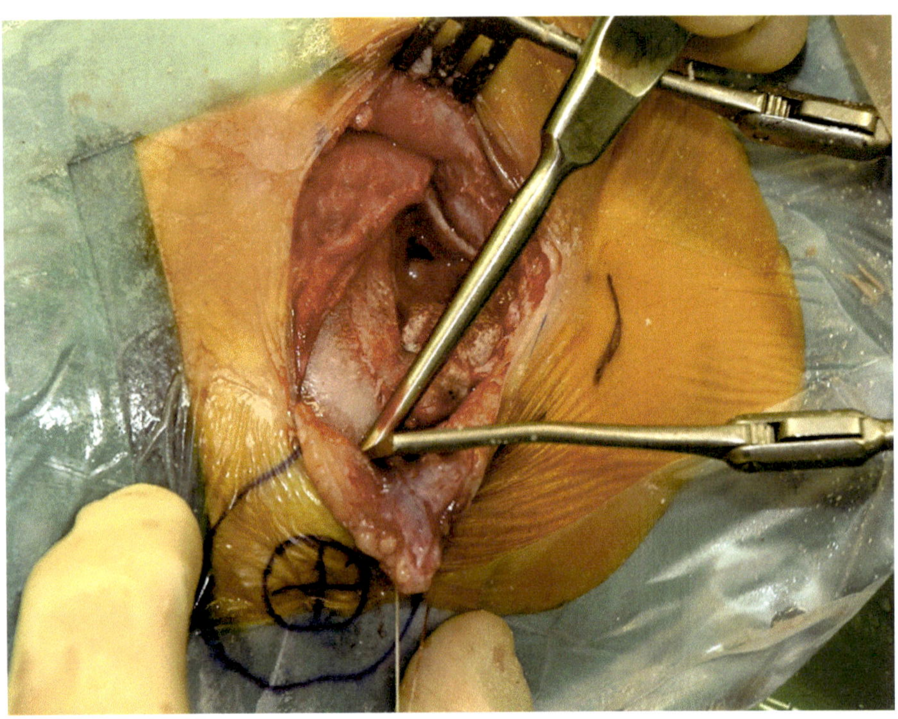

Fig. 6.15 The subperiosteal pocket for the receiver-stimulator. A tight subperiosteal pocket can be created for the receiver-stimulator with a raspatory, holding the borders of the planned pocket down with two fingers. Tie-down sutures are not used in this case with a tight pocket.

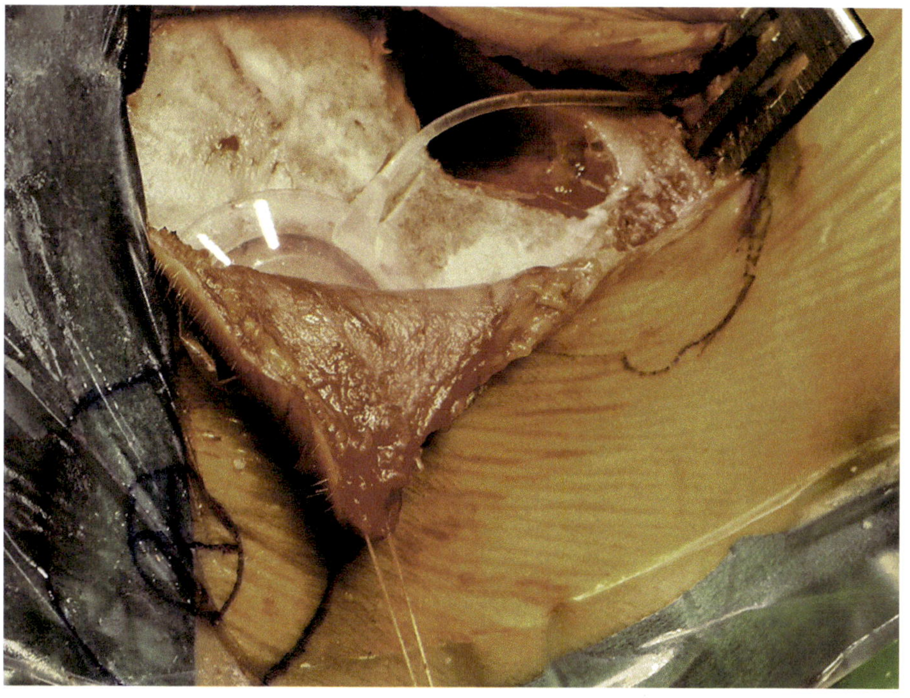

Fig. 6.16 The subperiosteal pocket for the receiver-stimulator. Some implants have a disposable silicone dummy with which to test the pocket subsequently.

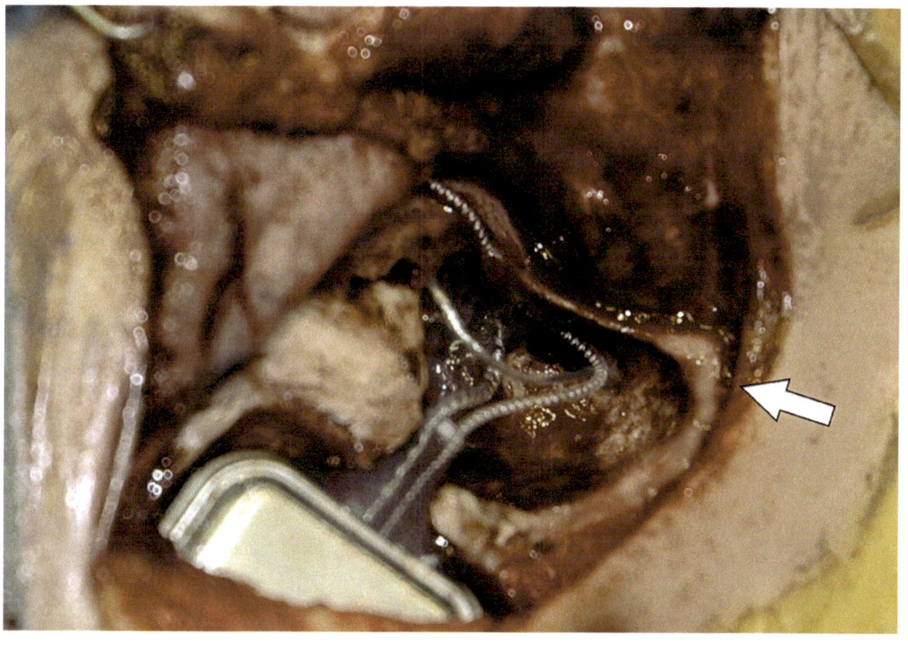

Fig. 6.17 Placement of the electrodes in the mastoid. Placement or fixation of the electrode lead more superiorly is preferred, as the mastoid tip (*white arrow*) shows the most prominent growth over time. Although not known exactly, growth could influence the position of the electrode in the cochlea. See the graph in **Fig. 6.1**. The lead should be gently folded in the cranial part of the mastoid cavity.

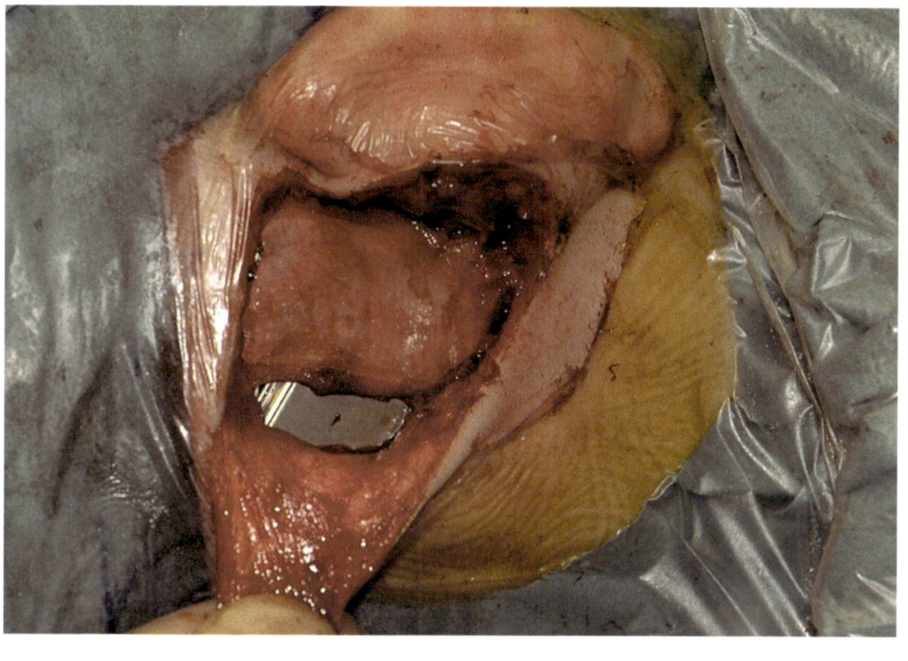

Fig. 6.18 Tight closure of the muscular layer. The cranial-based flap is sutured over the implant and electrodes. First the caudal border, then the anterior and posterior border. Care must be taken not to damage the electrode (not to entrap it in a suture) or to damage the receiver-stimulator (puncture it with the needle).

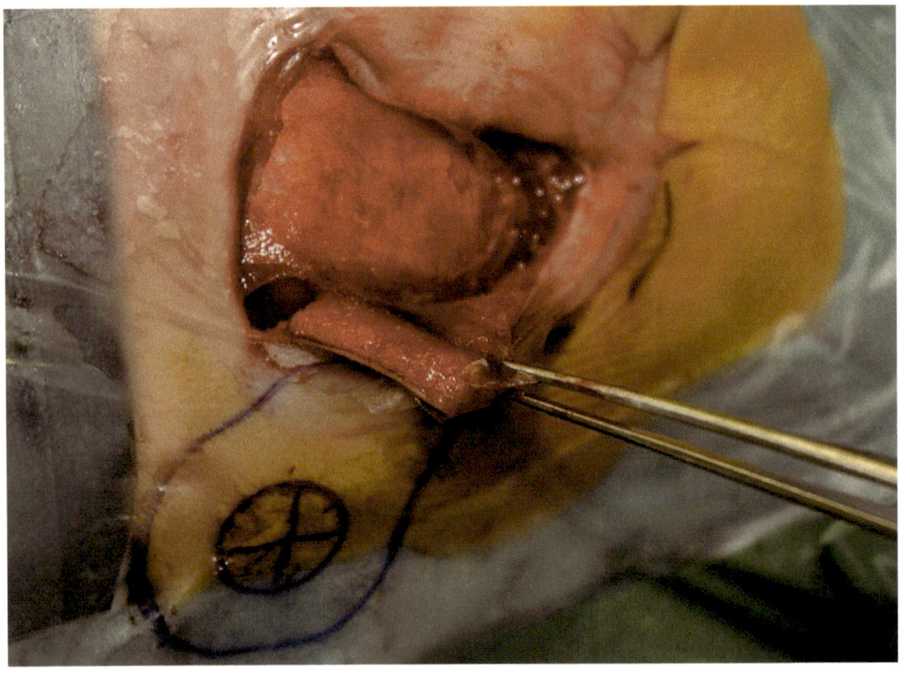

Fig. 6.19 Tight closure of the muscular layer. Once the musculoperiosteal layer is closed the implant is completely covered. If a subcutaneous hematoma developed, it would not be directly in contact with the implant.

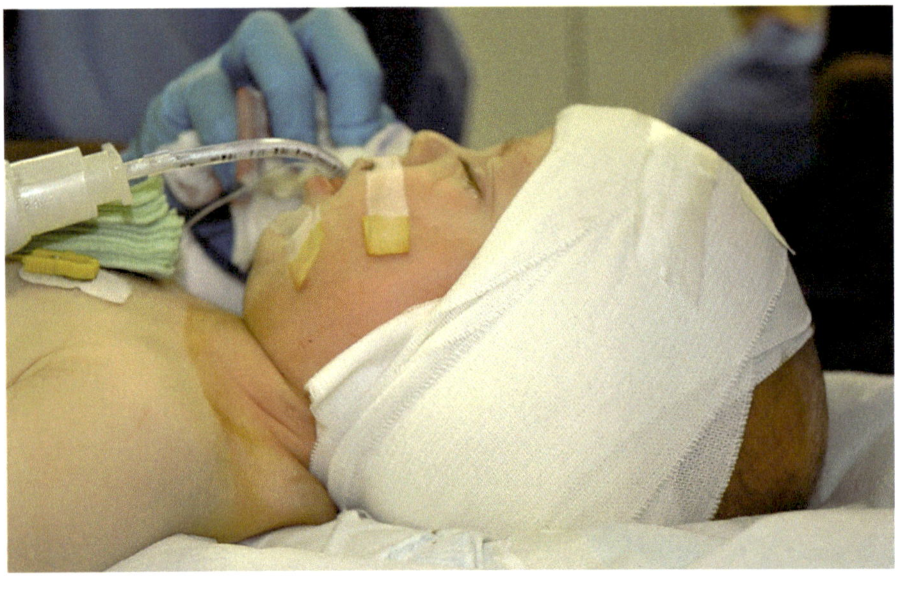

Fig. 6.20 End of the surgery. After a pediatric cochlear implantation the parents are often called to inform them about the course of the procedure. If the parents are near the child when the child is waking up it will reduce anxiety and distress.

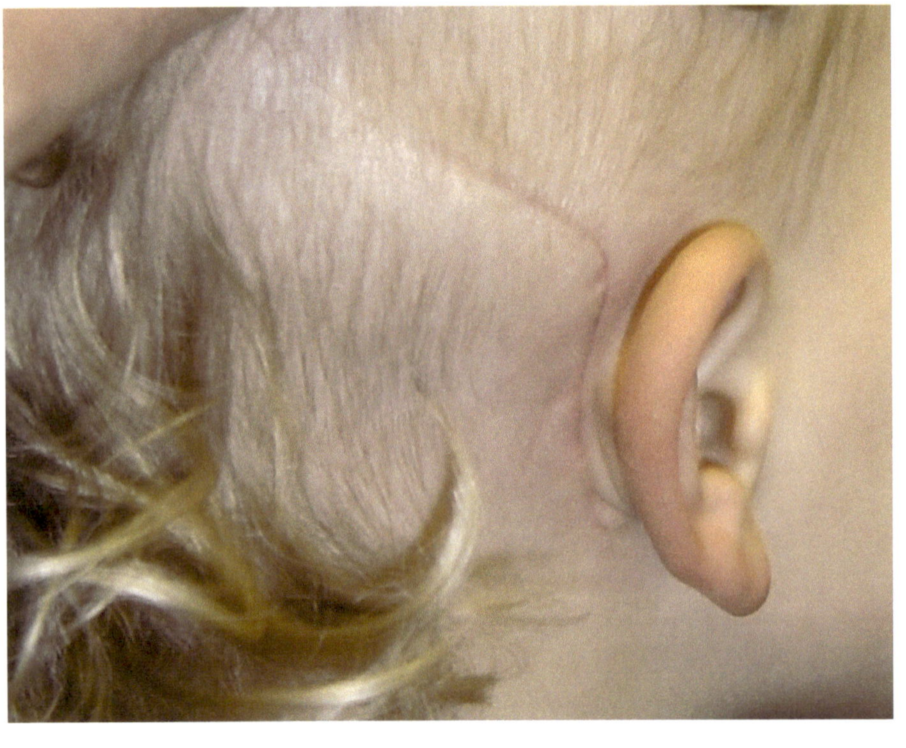

Fig. 6.21 Postoperative scar. Three weeks after surgery the incision is a tiny line. The hair is growing back and rehabilitation can start shortly.

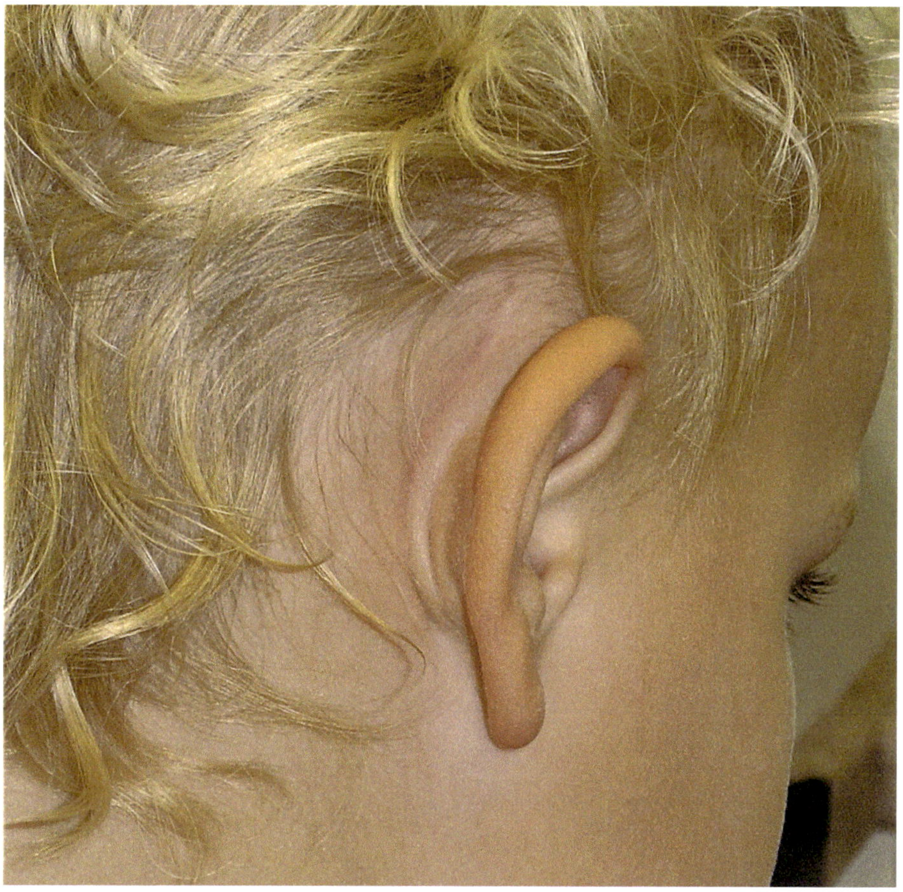

Fig. 6.22 Postoperative scar. One year later the incision is scarcely visible.

6.8.2 Special Steps in Bilateral Implantation (Figs. 6.23–Fig. 6.34)

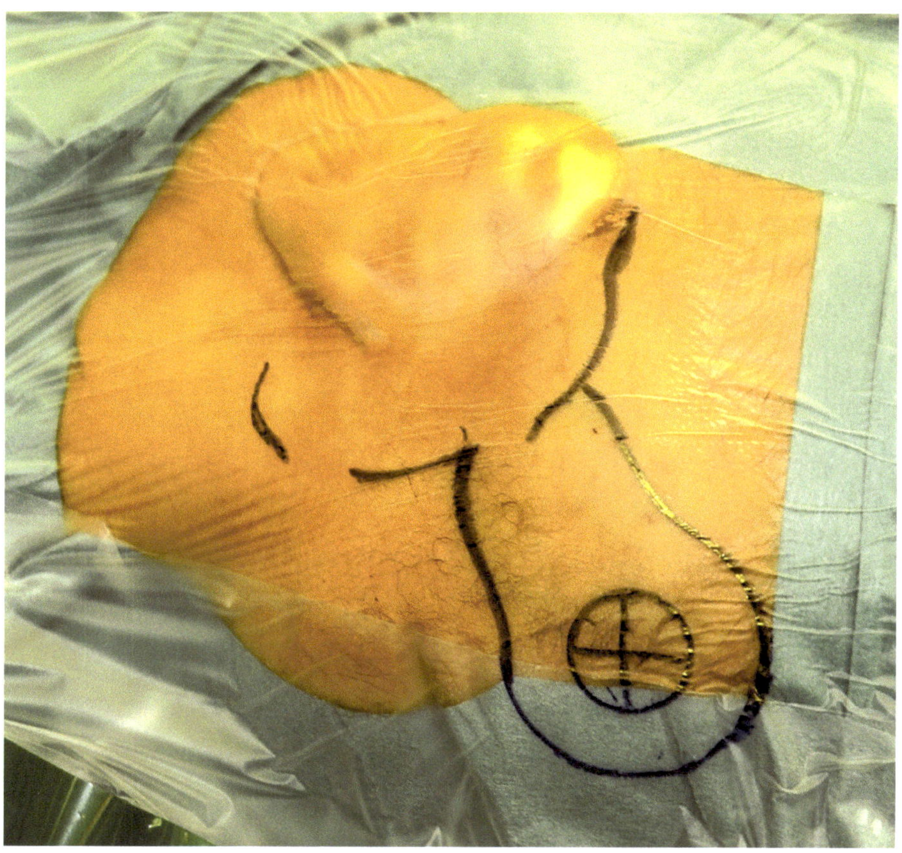

Fig. 6.23 Positioning the blueprint for bilateral implantation. The first side of implantation can be used to set the position of the receiver-stimulator and ultimately the symmetrical height of the two external coils. This can be done using simply a sterile piece of paper and a permanent marker.

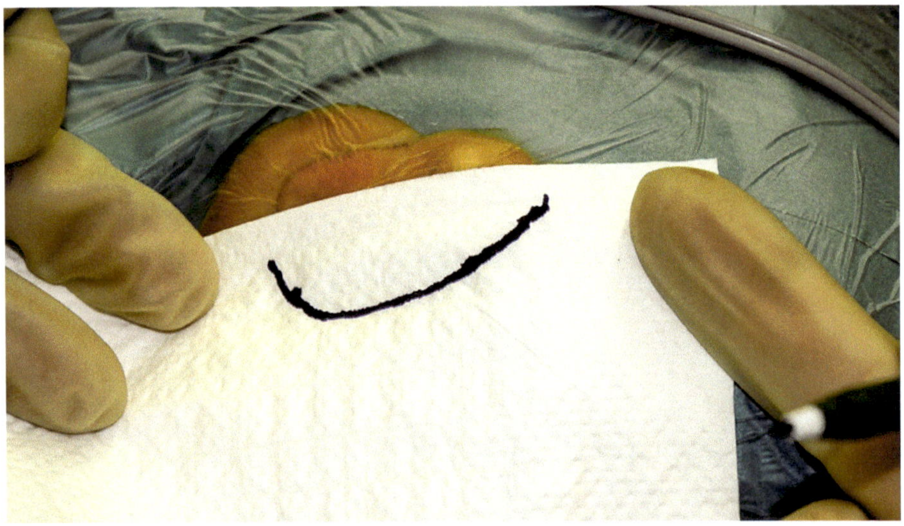

Fig. 6.24 Once the position of the receiver-stimulator has been planned and marked, the paper is brought to the posterior edge of the reflected pinna. The curve of this rim is precisely marked on the paper.

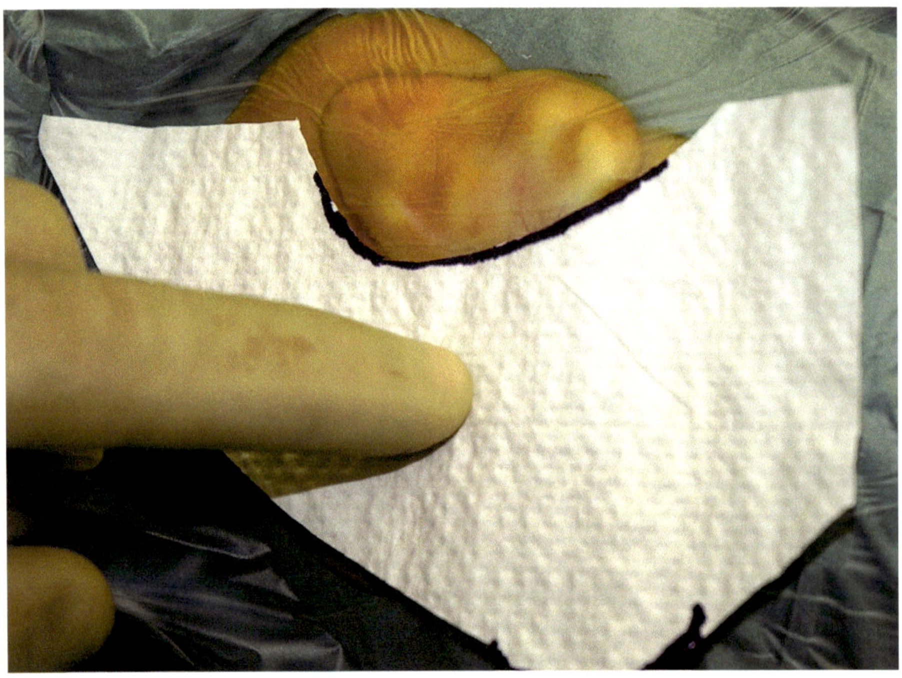

Fig. 6.25 Positioning the blueprint for bilateral implantation. The paper blueprint now fits the posterior rim of the reflected pinna, with the superior and inferior border exactly at the beginning and end of the retroauricular sulcus. The position of the receiver-stimulator can now be drawn on the same blueprint and then cut at the border of the coil position.

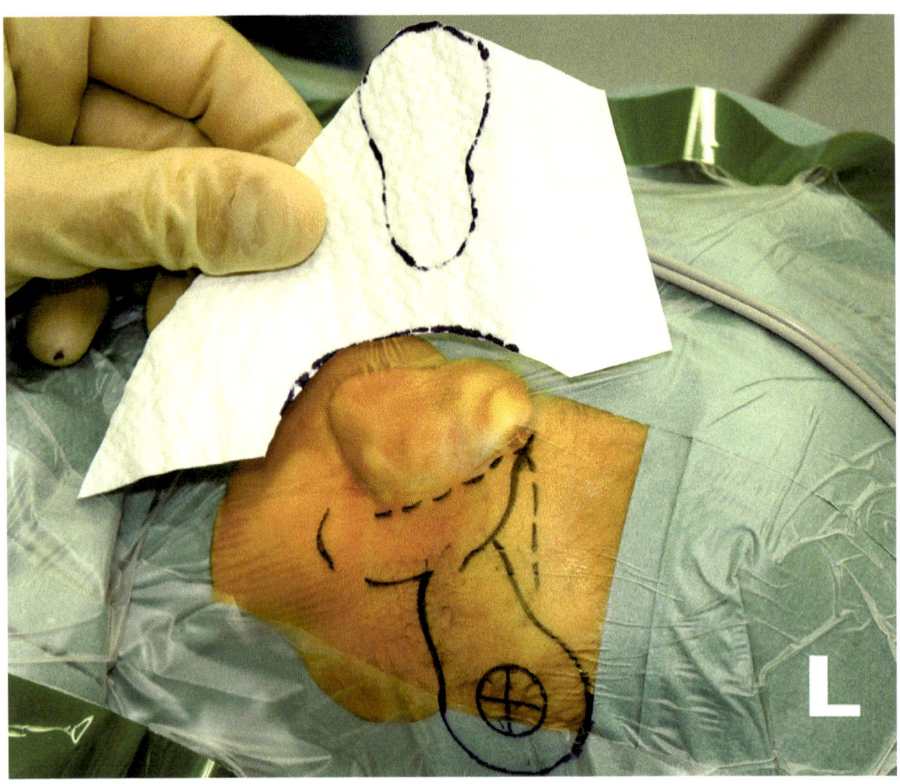

Fig. 6.26 Positioning the blueprint for bilateral implantation. The position of the receiver-stimulator can now be drawn completely on the same blueprint so that when reflecting the paper blueprint of this ear it forms a blueprint for the contralateral ear. The blueprint must be kept sterile for the surgery of the second side.

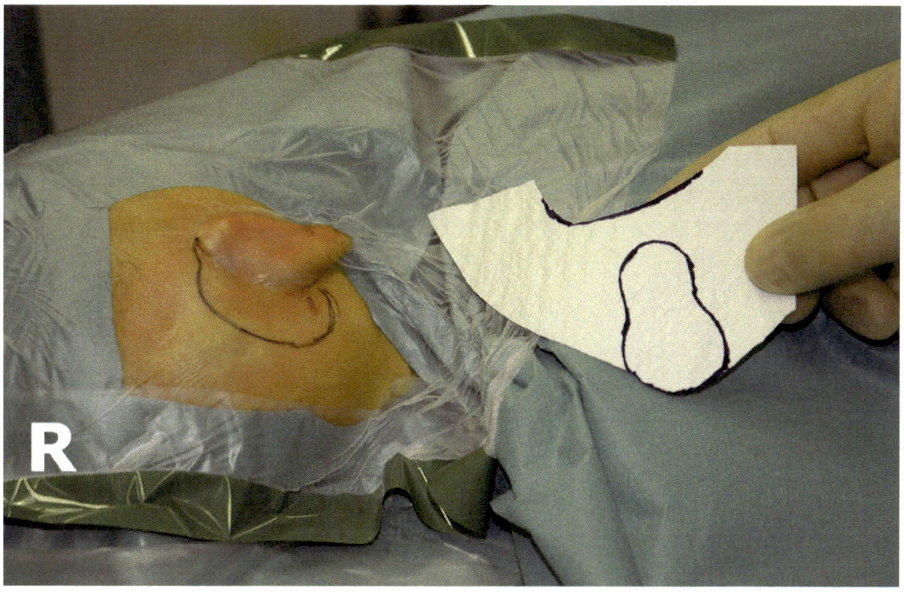

Fig. 6.27 Use of the blueprint at the contralateral side. At the beginning of the second side procedure, the blueprint is used to plan the position of the second implant so as to obtain symmetrical positioning.

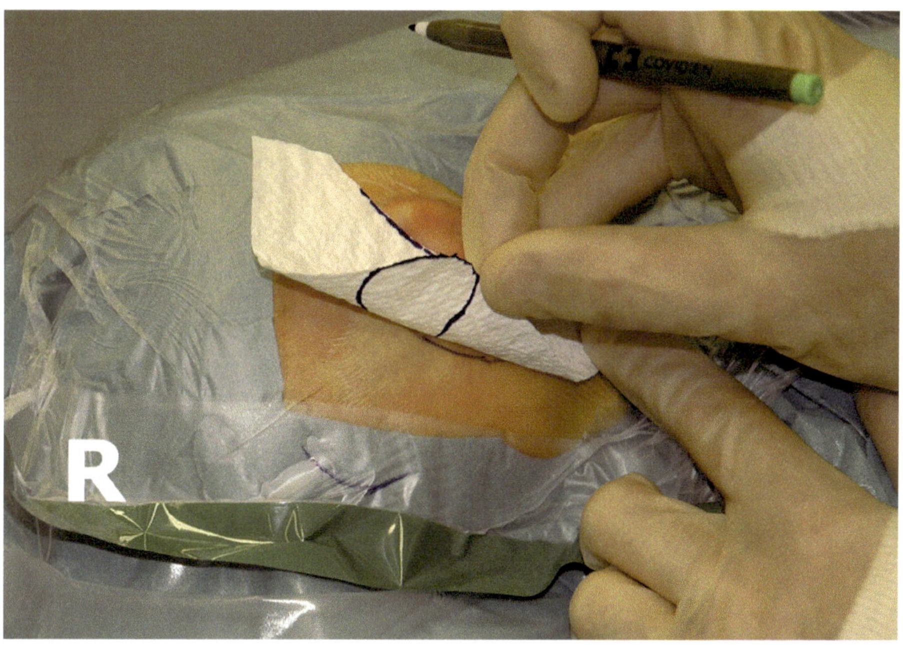

Fig. 6.28 Positioning the blueprint in bilateral implantation. The blueprint is placed at the contralateral (reflected) pinna in the opposite orientation. The border of the implant coil is marked on the adhesive drape. The symmetrical position of the implant coil is now marked. The drawing is completed and the second side surgery can begin.

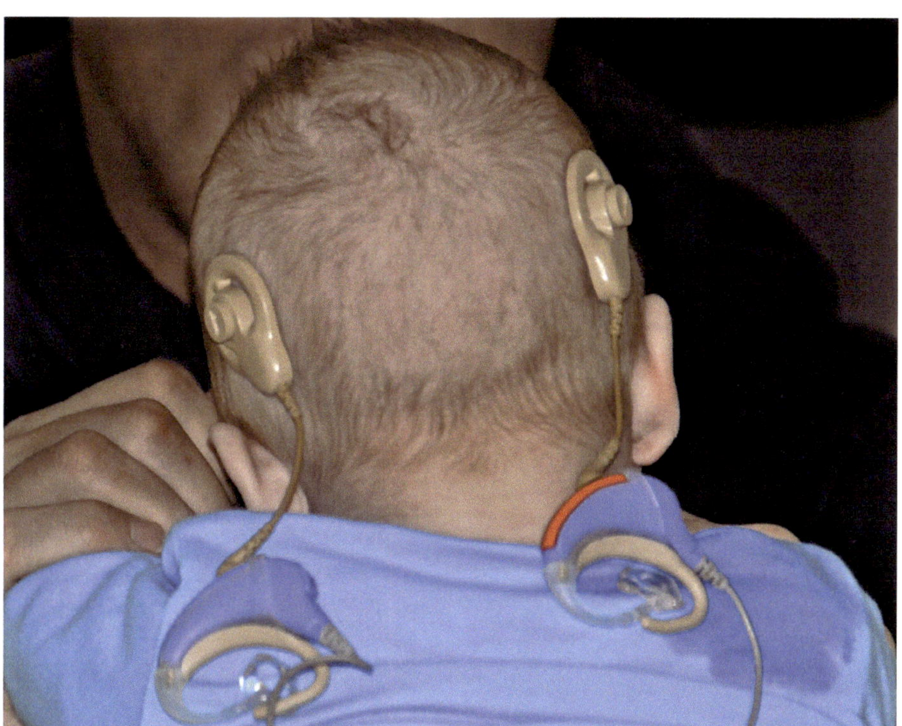

Fig. 6.29 Positioning the blueprint in bilateral implantation. The symmetrical position of the implants can be appreciated, especially in young children without hair.

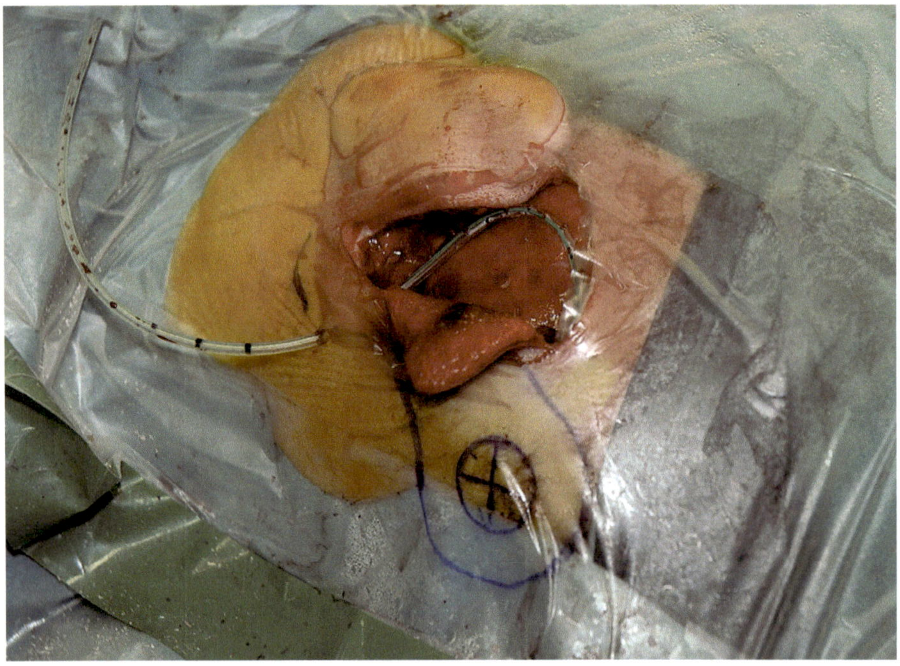

Fig. 6.30 Temporary drain in bilateral CI placement. In simultaneous bilateral cochlear implantation the chance of a hematoma on the side operated first can be reduced by use of a temporary drain, which is removed just before or during placement of the head bandage. A complete closure of the musculoperiosteal layer on top of the implant is necessary to place this drain without any risk to the implant during removal of the drain.

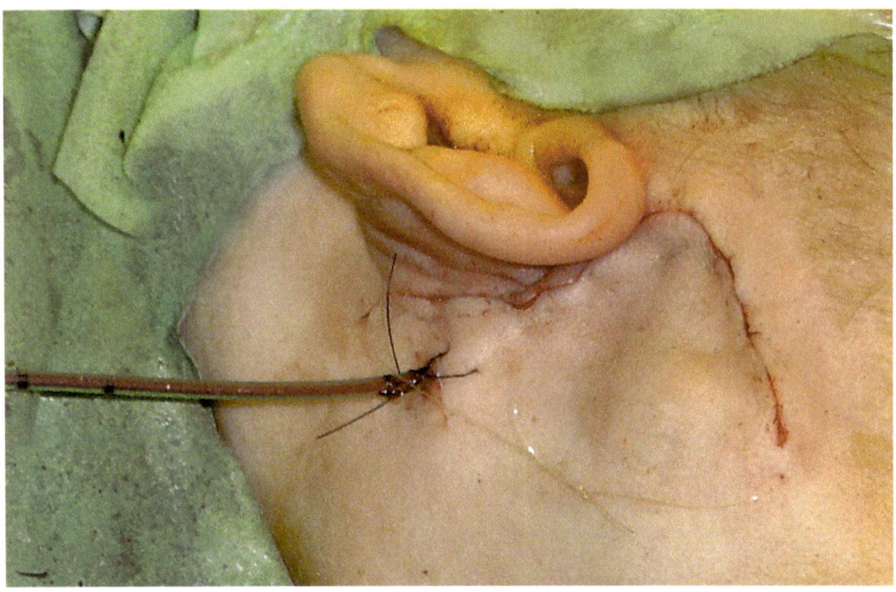

Fig. 6.31 Temporary drain in bilateral CI placement. The drain is secured by a simple suture that is removed just before the placement of the head bandage covering both implanted ears.

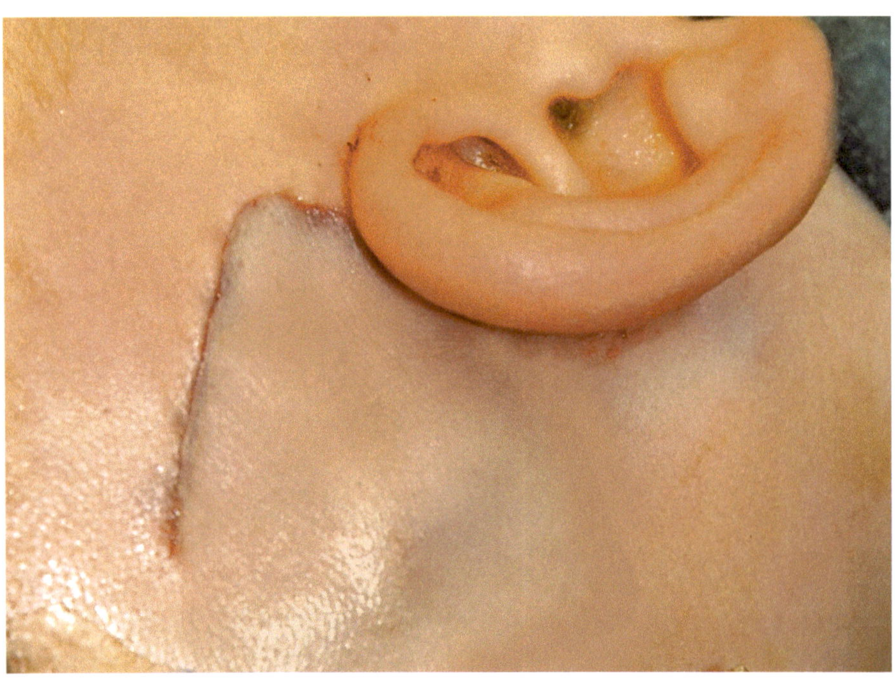

Fig. 6.32 Wound closure. The second side is implanted and closed in the same fashion as the first side. In small children intracutaneous sutures are preferred to avoid difficulty in removing the sutures. In addition, parental satisfaction is greater with an aesthetically pleasing outcome. No drain is used on this side.

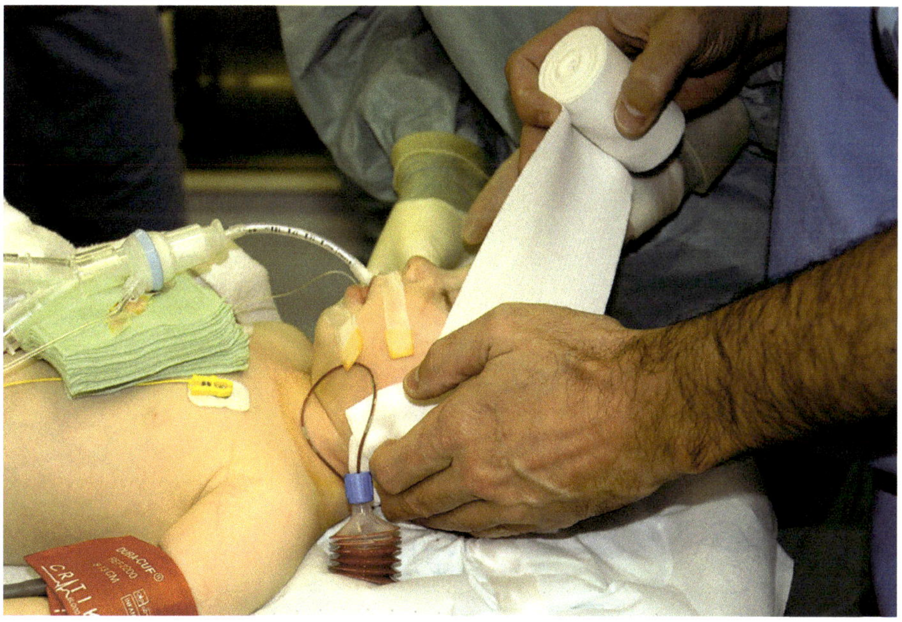

Fig. 6.33 Head bandage. The stich at the drain is cut and then a firm head bandage is applied to both implanted ears. It should remain for at least 24 hours to provide adequate hemostatic effect. In young children slight edema can appear at the uncovered top of the head, but this will subside as soon as the head bandage is removed.

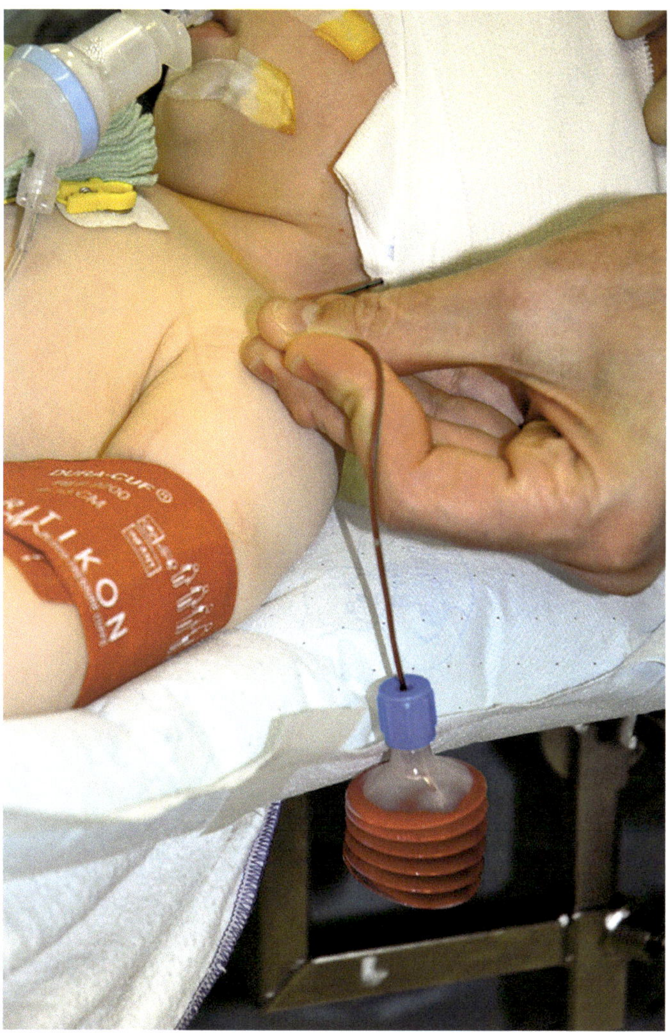

Fig. 6.34 Removal of the drain once the head bandage is in position. It should be easy to remove the drain once the head bandage is in place.

Pearls and Pitfalls in Pediatric Cochlear Implantation

- Be aware of the small anatomy of the temporal bone.
- Make sure that the anesthesiologist has (sufficient) pediatric experience.
- Make a drawing of the position of the (adult size) implant on the skin or on a transparent plastic adhesive drape.
- In bilateral implantation: make a duplicate or blueprint of this position on a paper, to use as blueprint in the second ear.
- Avoid the mastoid tip in the incision line, to avoid injury to the superficially located facial nerve.
- Be gentle with the skin and the subcutaneous and musculoperiosteal layer, as they are all needed for a good closure.
- Be aware of the different angle toward the round window in pediatric cochlear implantation in comparison to adult cochlear implantation.
- Make the well for the receiver-stimulator sufficiently deep. In a thin bony skull the well has to be onto the dura. A bony island can be created.
- Avoid fixture of the electrode in the mastoid tip of a young patient.
- Save the neural response measurements, as they can be helpful in the fitting of young patients.
- In bilateral implantation, use a temporary drain to avoid a hematoma.

References

1. Bayazit YA, Goksu N, Ozbilen S. Mini-incision for pediatric cochlear implantation with a MED-EL device. ORL J Otorhinolaryngol Relat Spec 2007;69(5):311–315
2. James AL, Papsin BC. Cochlear implant surgery at 12 months of age or younger. Laryngoscope 2004;114(12):2191–2195
3. Eby TL, Nadol JB Jr. Postnatal growth of the human temporal bone. Implications for cochlear implants in children. Ann Otol Rhinol Laryngol 1986;95(4 Pt 1):356–364
4. Bielamowicz SA, Coker NJ, Jenkins HA, Igarashi M. Surgical dimensions of the facial recess in adults and children. Arch Otolaryngol Head Neck Surg 1988;114(5):534–537
5. Eby TL. Development of the facial recess: implications for cochlear implantation. Laryngoscope 1996;106 (5 Pt 2, Suppl 80)1–7

6. McRackan TR, Reda FA, Rivas A, et al. Comparison of cochlear implant relevant anatomy in children versus adults. Otol Neurotol 2012;33(3):328–334
7. Dahm MC, Shepherd RK, Clark GM. The postnatal growth of the temporal bone and its implications for cochlear implantation in children. Acta Otolaryngol Suppl 1993;505:1–39
8. Roukema BY, Van Loon MC, Smits C, et al. Cochlear implantation after bacterial meningitis in infants younger than 9 months. Int J Otolaryngol 2011;2011:845–879
9. Boscolo-Rizzo P, Muzzi E, Barillari MR, Trabalzini F. Non-sutured fixation of the internal receiver-stimulator in cochlear implantation. Eur Arch Otorhinolaryngol 2011;268(7):961–965
10. Alexander NS, Caron E, Woolley AL. Fixation methods in pediatric cochlear implants: retrospective review of an evolution of 3 techniques. Otolaryngol Head Neck Surg 2011;144(3):427–430
11. Jöhr M, Ho A, Wagner CS, Linder T. Ear surgery in infants under one year of age: its risks and implications for cochlear implant surgery. Otol Neurotol 2008;29(3):310–313
12. Hannallah RS. Who benefits when parents are present during anaesthesia induction in their children? Can J Anaesth 1994;41(4):271–275
13. Kim SY, Choi JW, Choi BY, Koo JW. Atlantoaxial rotary subluxation after tympanoplasty. Otol Neurotol 2011;32(7):1108–1110
14. Battersby EF. Paediatric anaesthesia. In: Adams DA, Cinnamond MJ, eds. Scott-Brown's Otolaryngology. Oxford:Butterworth-Heinemann; 1997:6–24
15. Ramsden JD, Gordon K, Aschendorff A, et al. European Bilateral Pediatric Cochlear Implant Forum consensus statement. Otol Neurotol 2012;33(4):561–565
16. Leigh J, Dettman S, Dowell R, Sarant J. Evidence-based approach for making cochlear implant recommendations for infants with residual hearing. Ear Hear 2011;32(3):313–322

7 Complications and Revision Surgery in Cochlear Implantation

The complication rate in cochlear implant surgery as reported in the literature is 4 to 15%.[1–6] Most of these studies distinguish between major and minor complications, as first described by Cohen et al.[7] The complications that necessitate revision surgery (the major complications) have a mean incidence of around 4 to 5%,[3,5] but the range is between 2.3 and 13.3%.[8,9]

7.1 Major Complications

Definition

Major complications are complications requiring explantation of the device, surgical re-exploration, facial paresis or paralysis, or other serious complications with continuous discomfort or dysfunction.[7]

Major Complications in CI Surgery

- Meningitis
- Cerebrospinal fluid (CSF) leakage
- Facial nerve paresis or paralysis
- Severe facial nerve stimulation, requiring explantation
- Hematoma or abscess, requiring surgical intervention
- Mastoiditis/middle ear infections with granulation tissue
- Cholesteatoma
- Skin necrosis and exposed implant
- Extrusion of the electrode/receiver-stimulator
- Tinnitus or vertigo, resulting in nonuse or re-implantation
- Dislocation/incorrect position of the electrode, requiring surgical intervention
- Device failure (see Device Failure Complications section)

7.2 Minor Complications

Definition

In minor complications, minimal or no intervention is needed as most of these complications will resolve by themselves, or can be overcome by minor medical or audiologic management.

It is suggested that minor complications should cause little distress to the patient.[4,10]

Minor Complications in CI Surgery

- Chorda tympani lesions (reversible or irreversible)
- Transient facial palsy
- Anterior swelling/hemifacial swelling
- Retroauricular emphysema
- Minor wound problem/wound infection
- Otitis media
- Pain/headache
- Vertigo
- Tinnitus
- Ear drum perforation

7.3 Device Failure Complications

Device failures range from 0.8 to 26.7%[1,11] but depend on the scale of the implant center, the time of follow-up, and the brands and types of implants used. In the decade up to the time of writing (2015) the overall device failure rate has improved.[12] Failure modes are most commonly related to trauma, electronic dysfunction, or CSF leakage. After device failure, explantation and re-implantation is a safe and acceptable treatment option.

Definition

The device exhibits characteristics outside the manufacturer's specification, resulting in a loss of clinical benefit or failure to attain benefit.[13,14]

Other definitions concerning device function are:

- **Functioning device:** The device has no evidence of any device-related malfunction or no deficiency can be observed from the available test results.
- **Characteristics decrement:** A device has measured characteristics outside the manufacturer's specification, but still of benefit to the patient.
- **Performance decrement:** Unexplained but documented decrement in performance or a device that causes nonauditory sensations necessitating explantation.
- **Loss to follow-up:** Those implanted patients who have been lost to clinical surveillance.

In a consensus paper, specialists and cochlear implant companies have agreed on the uniform reporting of these failures.[13,14] With this uniform reporting, the cumulative survival rate (CSR) per implant type can be calculated. The CSR can be split into rates for adults and children, if needed.[12]

Device failure can also be split into "hard" device failures and "soft" device failures.[15]

7.3.1 Hard Device Failure

Definition

The absence of auditory input or electronic lock between external and internal components. In a short: *a proven malfunctioning device.*

Although the failure rates have decreased over the years with newer implants, the most common reason for re-implantation is hard device failure.[3]

7.3.2 Soft Device Failure

Definition

A soft device failure is considered a malfunction of the implant but without any proof with available in vivo methods of testing. In short: *a suspected device failure without any proof.*

The proposed work-up of a soft failure includes of four items of evaluation[16]:

1. **Symptoms:** take careful history and write down an exact description of the symptoms (auditory and nonauditory).
2. **Medical evaluation:** evaluate history, physical examination, and imaging to assess electrode position; evaluate central nervous system pathology; and rule out intracochlear ossification or infection.
3. **Audiologic evaluation:** assess speech performance and mapping to evaluate a drop in performance, a failure to achieve expected benefit, or a change in sensitivity to stimulation.
4. **Device assessment:** evaluate the function of the hardware using device integrity testing, programming, and troubleshooting.

Soft device failure is an uncommon occurrence. Before this diagnosis is established, two steps must have been taken: First, a thorough evaluation of the function of the implant by the manufacturer and the implant team in cooperation with the patient has to be performed (steps as described above). Second, the suspected implant should be removed, examined, and the technical failure should be identified. Often a soft device failure is a working diagnosis and initially a conservative approach must be taken to attempt to solve the problem. If there is a proven malfunction of the device, it is considered a hard failure.

Device Failures

- **Hard failure:** proven device failure:
  - Failure from impact
  - Sealing failure
  - Electronic failure
  - Electrode problem
  - Others
  - No specific cause
- **Soft failure:** suspicion of device failure

7.4 Pediatric vs. Adult Complication Rate

The overall revision rate in cochlear implant surgery is estimated to be 5 to 8%,[1,3] but when comparing the pediatric and adult revision rates a difference is apparent. Adult revisions are estimated to be less than 5%,[15] whereas some pediatric studies show a 13% revision rate.[17] The reason for this difference could be the vulnerability of children to infection as well as to trauma. This is often associated with a hard device failure. Another suggested reason for failure could be the more complex surgical anatomy in young children, especially in congenital malformation cases or in relation to their cause of deafness (meningitis, local infection).[3] Although often seen, this difference in re-implantation rate between children and adults was not found in all centers.[3]

7.5 Bilateral vs. Unilateral Implant Complication Rates

Although there are not many reports on this aspect, the overall impression is that patients who received a cochlear implant bilaterally do *not* have twice the risk of a complication.[3] Nevertheless, vestibular effects and bilateral chorda tympani injury could be a concern.[18]

7.6 Therapeutic Options for Several Complications

7.6.1 Flap Infection/Subcutaneous Hematoma or Seroma

Most cochlear implant centers use perioperative antibiotics. In the postoperative period antibiotic treatment can be prolonged, especially when an infection is suspected (redness, swelling, and pain over the implant). When a hematoma or seroma is present, infection prevention should be aggressive.[3] Care must be taken when a *Pseudomonas aeruginosa* or a methicillin-resistant *Staphylococcus aureus* (MRSA) infection is suspected and readmission should be considered for administration of intravenous antibiotics.[19] This may seem rather radical, but an infection around the implant can eventually cause extrusion, or an unmanageable infection resulting in explantation.[19] In cases with suspicion of a low-grade infection, nuclear scanning can be helpful.[19] The formation of a bacterial biofilm around the implant has also been described[20] and can only be treated with explantation.

7.6.2 Receiver-Stimulator or Electrode Extrusion (Fig. 7.1)

Occasionally, the receiver-stimulator extrudes through the skin even years after the surgery. Various factors can be of influence in the occurrence of extrusion. To avoid extrusion, particular attention should be paid to the skin incision, flap development, choice of sutures, fixation of the receiver-stimulator, position of the receiver-stimulator, and sometimes the choice of side for implantation. These points are explained step by step in Chapter 5 (p. 67–69). The surgical history, social history, and general medical condition are important factors to be aware of prior to surgery. These may affect wound healing, when local blood supply is compromised due to previous ear surgery, diabetes mellitus, or smoking, or may affect the risk of infection according to the dermatologic or infectious history.[5] Most array extrusions can be dealt

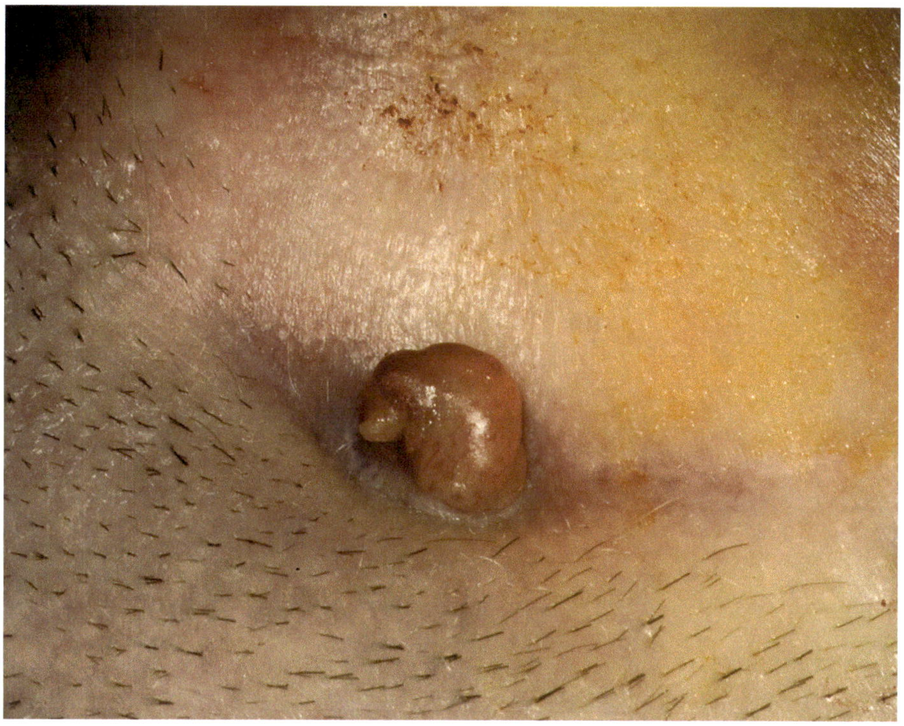

Fig. 7.1 Granulation tissue located in the retroauricular scar, as a result of the electrode array beneath it. This lesion was treated with local excision and undermining of the skin and subcutaneous layer without damaging the electrode. Tensionless closure in two layers followed.

with locally but it is still advisable to perform the surgery under general anesthesia, as the patient should not move during delicate handling of the electrode. Cutting, damaging, or sudden extraction of the electrode array should be avoided throughout the procedure. Furthermore, the repositioning of the electrode is often a matter of creating a covering flap, which normally exceeds the bounds of local anesthesia.

7.6.3 Facial Nerve Stimulation

Postoperative facial nerve stimulation is a more common complication in otosclerosis and osteogenesis imperfecta.[21] Precurved electrodes have their contact endings facing the modiolus and this could reduce the problem. If the problem remains, then reprogramming the electrodes can be of help. Usually, the electrodes in the superior part of the cochlea stimulate the facial nerve just superiorly (see Chapter 3 on radiology). These electrodes can then be switched off one by one and the side effect should subside (for additional information see Chapter 13 on otosclerosis and implantation). In some very severe cases it can be challenging to program the implant so that no facial nerve stimulation occurs; even re-implantation has been suggested for this.[15,22]

7.6.4 Facial Nerve Injury

In the surgical approach using the posterior tympanotomy, the facial nerve can be well identified and injury can easily be avoided. Facial nerve monitoring will also be of great help but it does not replace proper knowledge of the anatomy and accurate training in performing a posterior tympanotomy. In malformations, the chance of an anomalous facial nerve increases (see Chapter 15). Accurate imaging and interpretation are necessary for proper surgical planning. In these cases, in which the course of the facial nerve is uncertain or interfering with a normal approach, one might think of a subtotal petrosectomy. A subtotal petrosectomy (see Chapter 10) provides a wide access and visibility and diminishes the chance of iatrogenic injury and postoperative infection. In this way, a subtotal petrosectomy protects the facial nerve if it is dehiscent in the course of the electrode.

If a slight facial nerve injury does occur, a high dose of prednisone will diminish swelling and further damage, but it might still take weeks before recovery of the facial nerve function. If there is a severe injury or total interruption of the facial nerve, direct anastomosis or a graft should be considered. It is important to remember that the best results are seen with a facial nerve graft performed within the first months after the injury. After 6 to 12 months the results are much worse.[23]

7.6.5 Electrode Placement

Sometimes the electrode insertion, although gentle, forceless, and well directed, does not follow smoothly when inserting the last few millimeters of the electrode array. Malpositioning or kinking of the electrode can be the result; the electrode can end up in the wrong position, that is, within the hypotympanum, in an otospongiotic double ring (see Chapter 13, Case 13.6), in the semicircular canal (as shown in **Fig. 7.2**), or even in the carotid artery (see Case 7.3). Examples of this are shown here and at the end of this chapter. Audiologic testing (see Chapter 4), radiography, or CT scan during surgery may be used in difficult cases or when malpositioning is suspected. Further diagnostic assessment postoperatively may also be needed. A displaced electrode can be readjusted immediately or at a later stage.

7.6.6 CSF Gusher/CSF leakage

A CSF gusher, which is CSF coming from the internal auditory canal through an opening in the cochlea into the tympanic cavity, should be anticipated during preoperative imaging. Cases most

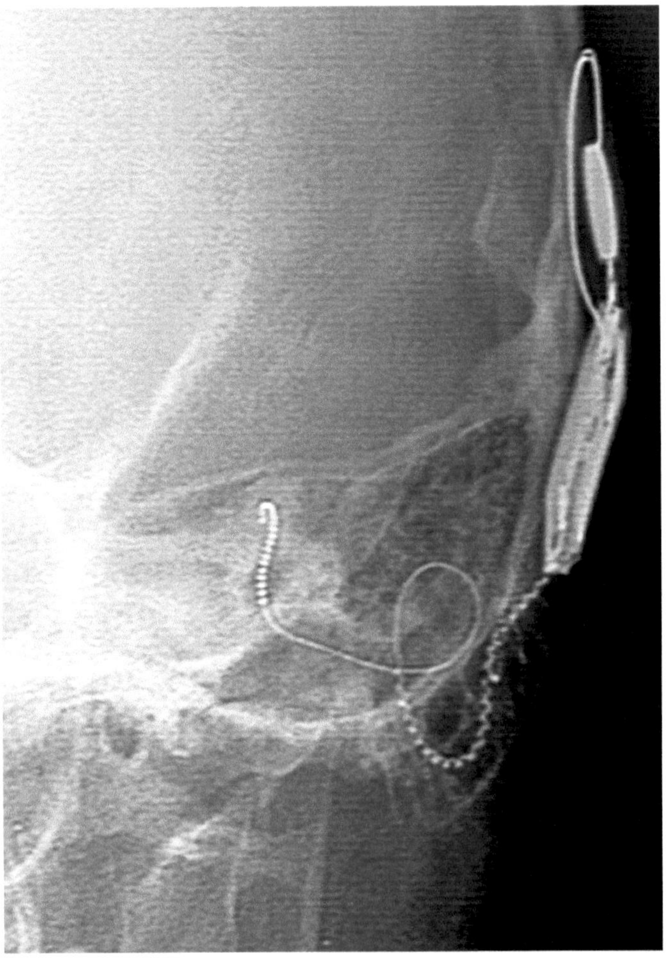

Fig. 7.2 Placement of the electrode in the superior canal. The patient experienced vertigo directly after surgery. On the postoperative image the electrode was in the superior semicircular canal.

often associated with a gusher are an incomplete partition type 1, a common cavity, or an enlarged cochlear aperture as in incomplete partition type 3. A gusher can usually be controlled by waiting for the flow to subside (10–15 minutes) and firmly packing the cochleostomy with soft tissue such as fascia, periosteum, or muscle. A CSF leak could also occur during cochlear implantation, in association with (previous) cholesteatoma, fractures, tumors, or other pathology. To avoid meningitis as a direct or late complication of a CSF leak, the best approach, next to the proper sealing of the leak, would be a subtotal petrosectomy (see Chapter 10 on subtotal petrosectomy). A lumbar CSF drain increases the risk of meningitis and is not needed in combination with a subtotal petrosectomy.

7.6.7 Revision Surgery/Re-implantation

In most re-implantation cases the hearing typically remains the same, but worsening of the hearing is possible. Revision surgery can be harmful to the patient or to the implant and has to conform with the expectations of the patient and/or the guardian(s). It is wise to be conservative regarding expectations postoperatively as in revision surgery the outcome is unpredictable, and preoperative counseling of the expectations should be managed accordingly.[3]

Case 7.1 Extrusion of the Electrode Array (Left Ear) (Fig. 7.1.1–Fig. 7.1.4)

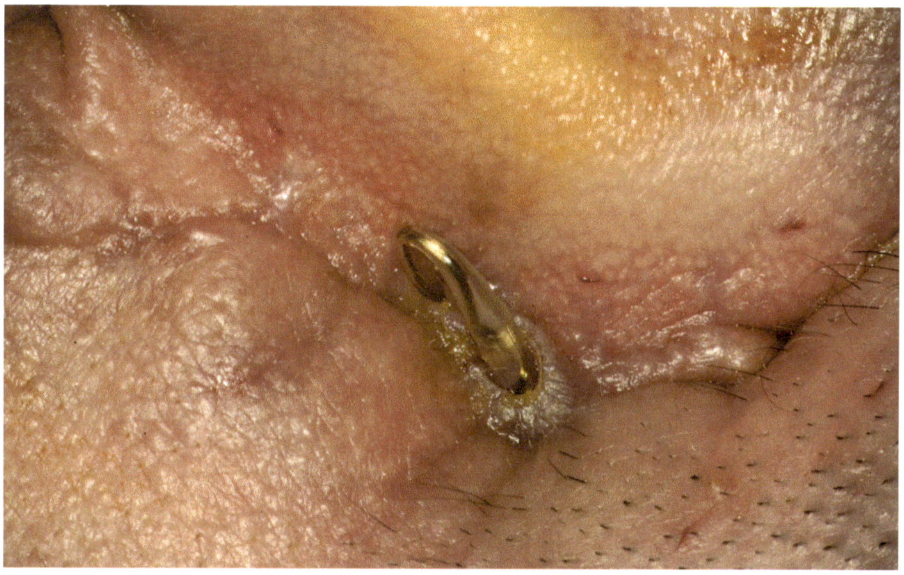

Fig. 7.1.1 A 42-year-old man received a CI because of progressive bilateral hearing loss since childhood. After 2 years he experienced extrusion of the electrode array through the retroauricular scar, as shown here.

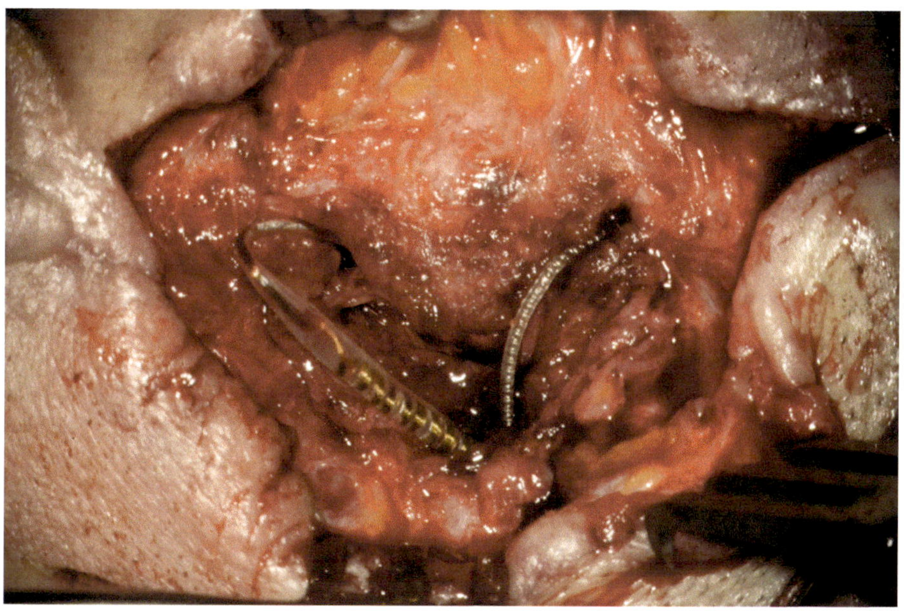

Fig. 7.1.2 The scar was opened, scar tissue was removed, and the cavity was gently opened without damage to the electrode or receiver-stimulator.

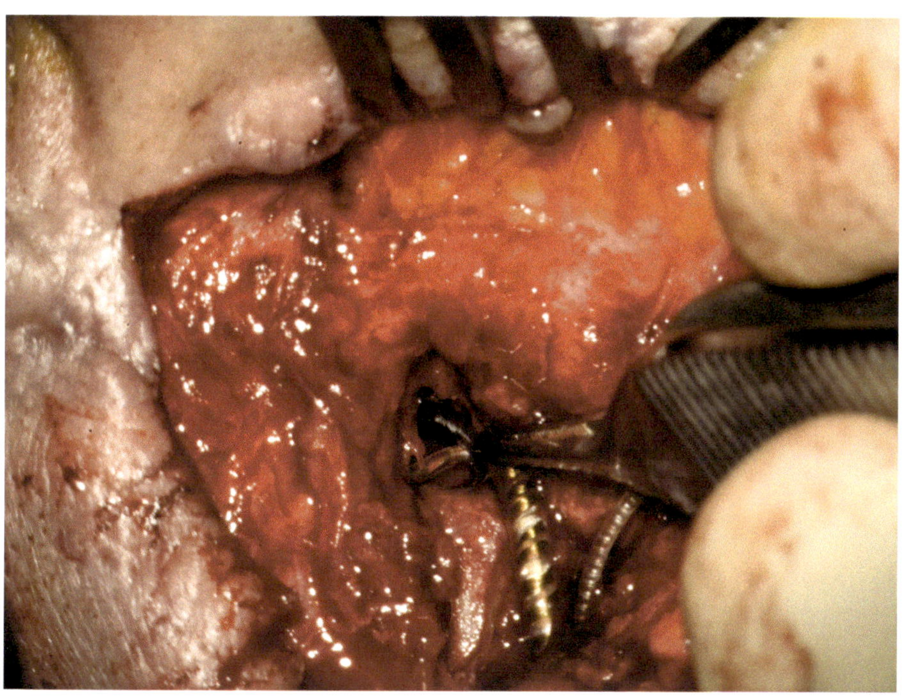

Fig. 7.1.3 The electrode and receiver stimulator were left in place and the position of the electrode array was readjusted.

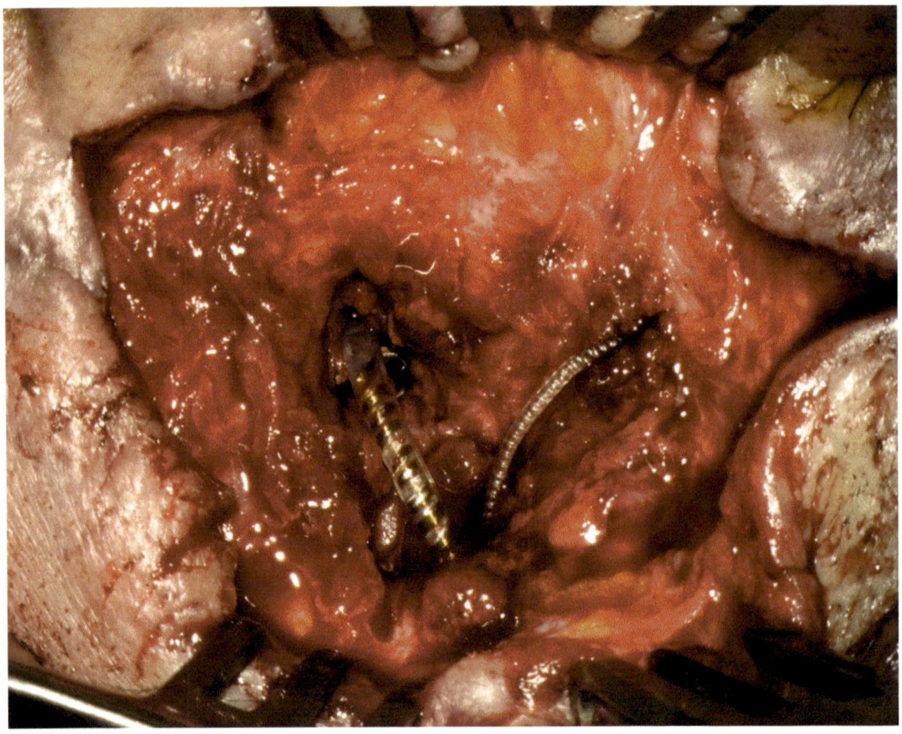

Fig. 7.1.4 Once the electrode array was positioned in the cavity and remained in that position without any force, the subcutaneous layer and the skin were closed.

Comment

The position of the electrode should not be immediately beneath the incision line. Furthermore, the opening should be in at least two layers with different incision lines.

Case 7.2 Revision Surgery after Placement of Electrode in the Carotid Canal (Right Ear) (Fig. 7.2.1–Fig. 7.2.9)

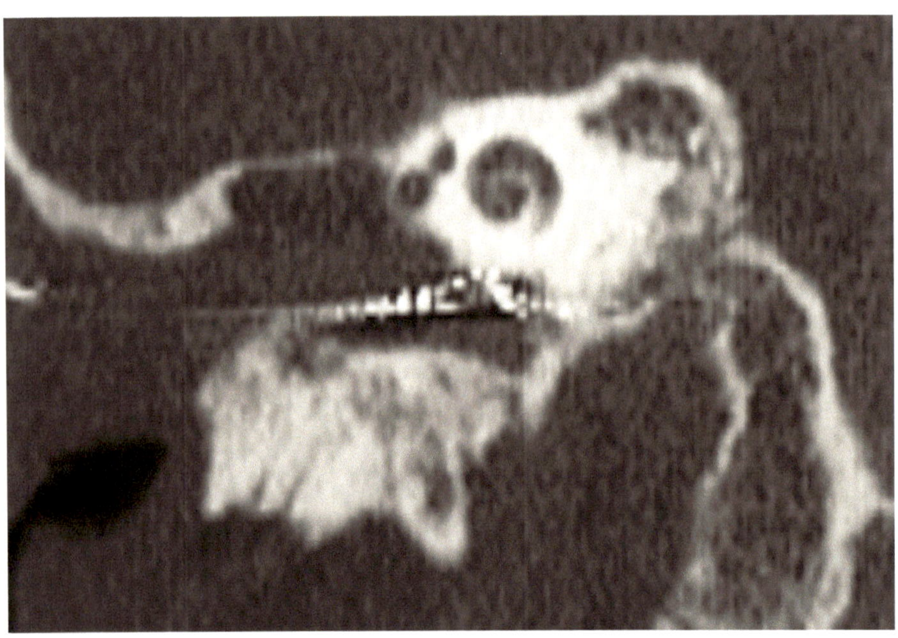

Fig. 7.2.1 A 39-year-old man had used hearing aids since childhood, probably because of post-meningitis hearing loss. After deterioration of the hearing, cochlear implantation was attempted in another department, without success. During the second attempt the electrode was not inserted into the cochlear lumen.

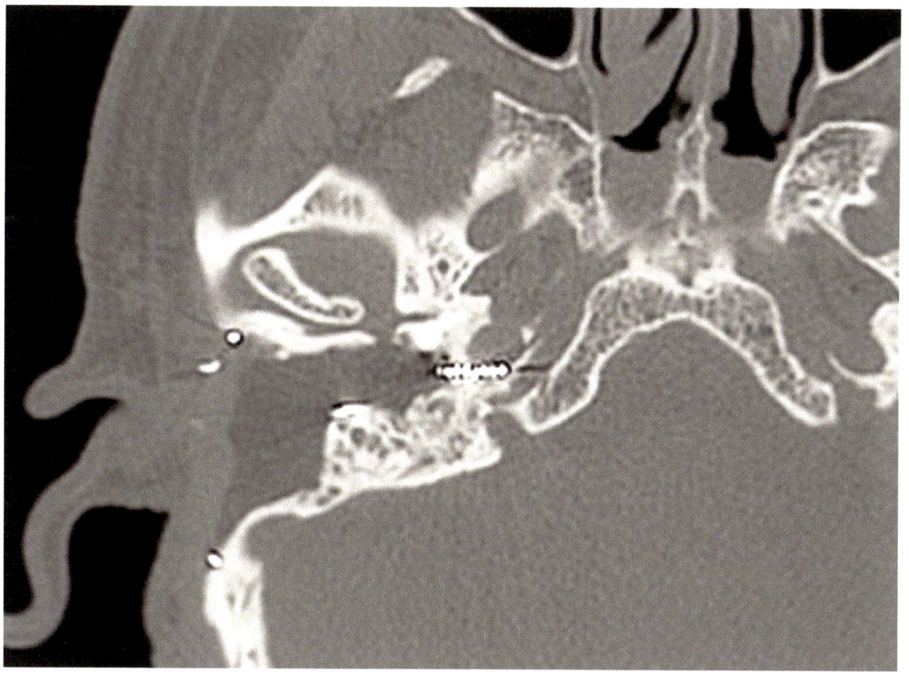

Fig. 7.2.2 On axial scan the electrode is visible at the medial border of the vertical part of the internal carotid canal.

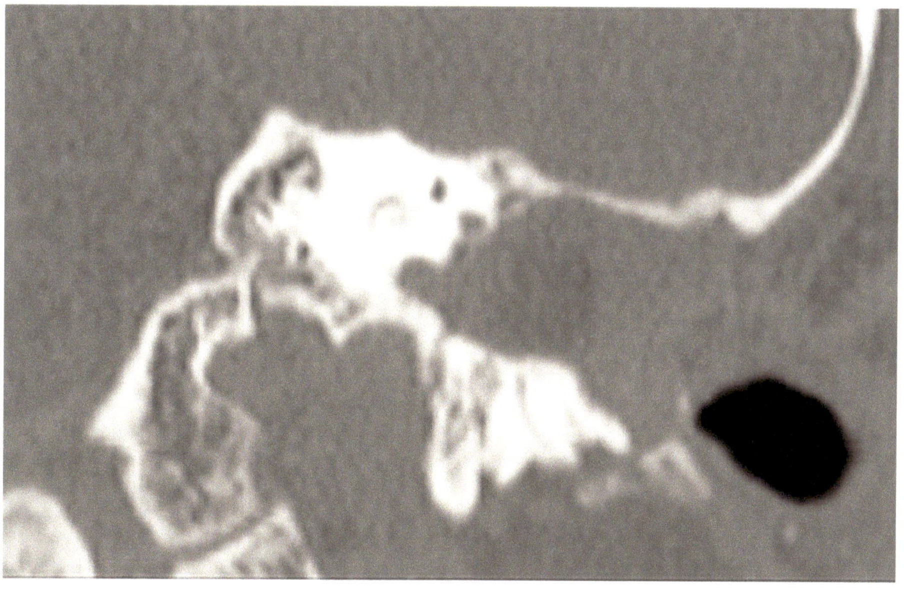

Fig. 7.2.3 There was no option to implant the contralateral side as this side showed severe cochlear ossification. The patient was counseled for revision surgery on the right side with partial removal of the first CI and an attempt to insert a new one.

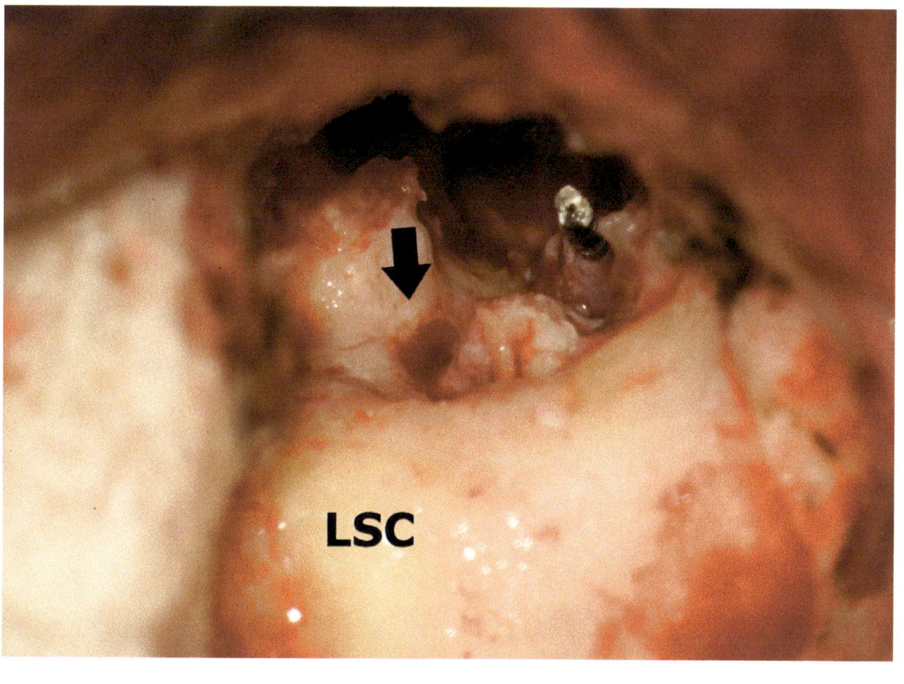

Fig. 7.2.4 The patient had already been treated with a subtotal petrosectomy. On reopening of the cavity the round window niche was filled with scar tissue (*black arrow*). The electrode array was cut near the carotid canal and its tip was left in place to minimize risk to the internal carotid artery. LSC, lateral semicircular canal.

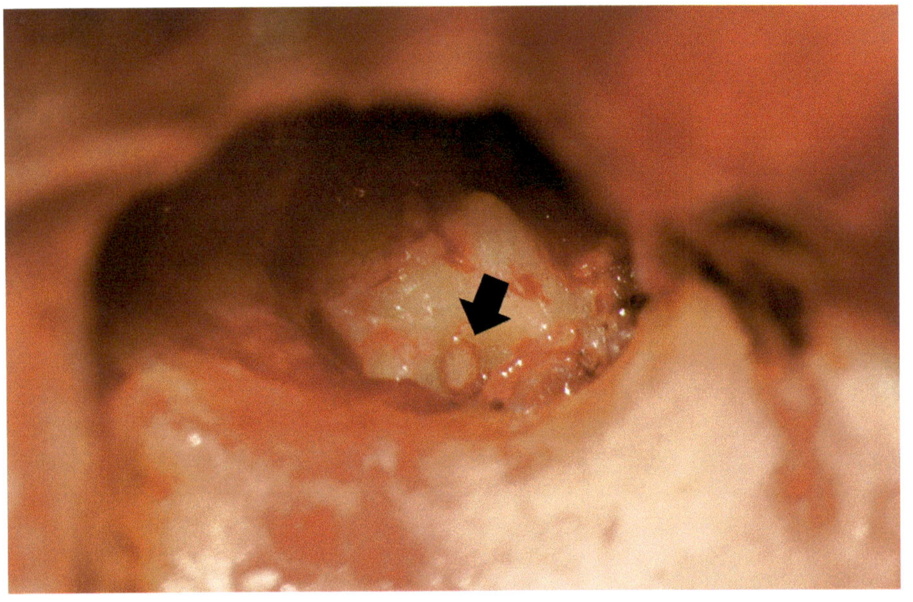

Fig. 7.2.5 The part of the electrode array still extending into the tympanic cavity was cut, but the tip was left in place. Removal of the scar tissue exposed the whitish round window (*arrow*).

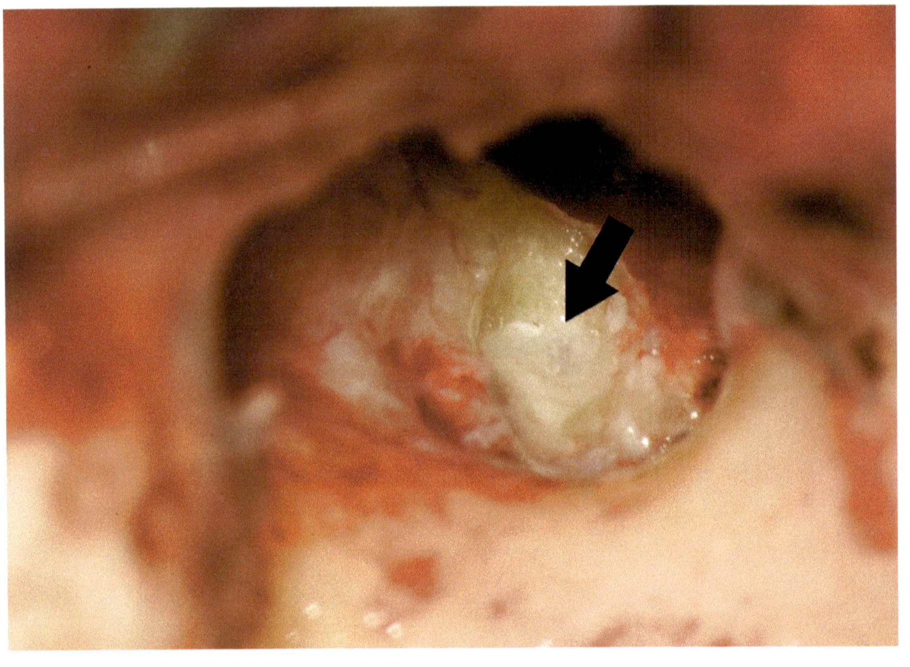

Fig. 7.2.6 The promontory anterior-inferior to the round window was drilled. Ossification filling the basal turn is shown (*arrow*).

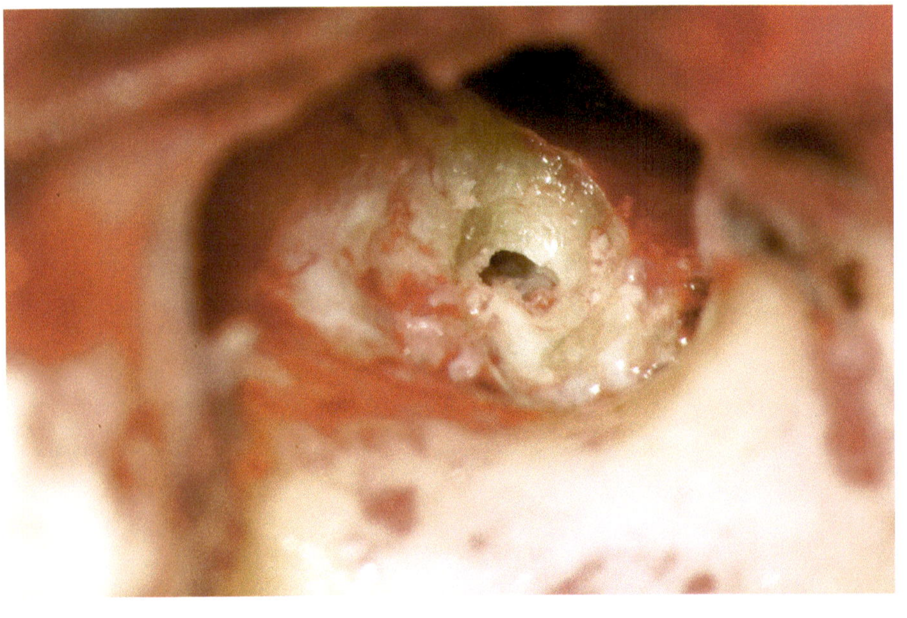

Fig. 7.2.7 The ossification was limited to the area near the round window; a lumen without ossification was easily reached. The opening of the basal turn is shown.

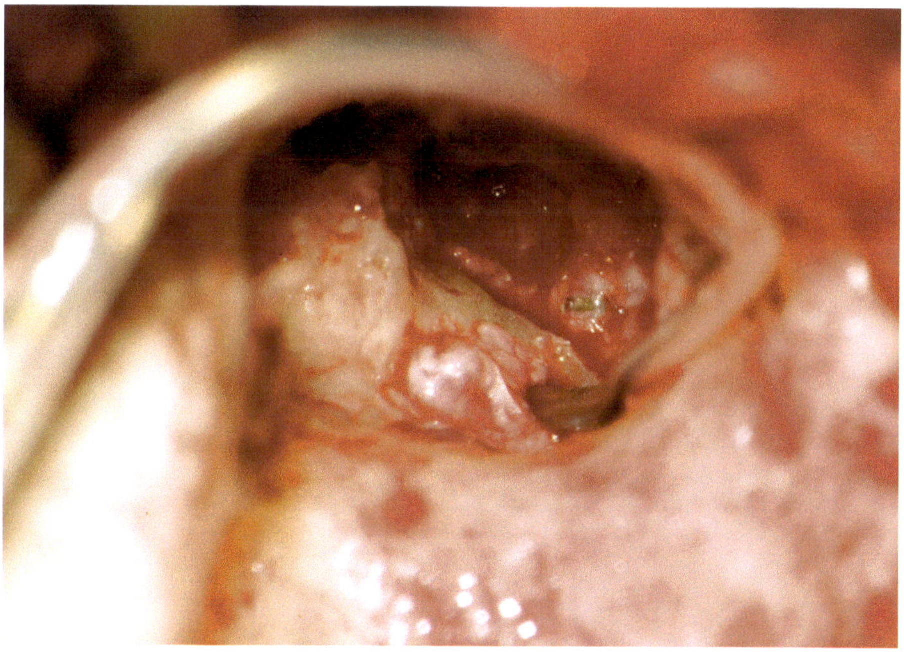

Fig. 7.2.8 An electrode array was inserted, and the opening was closed off using periosteum. The cavity was closed off with abdominal fat.

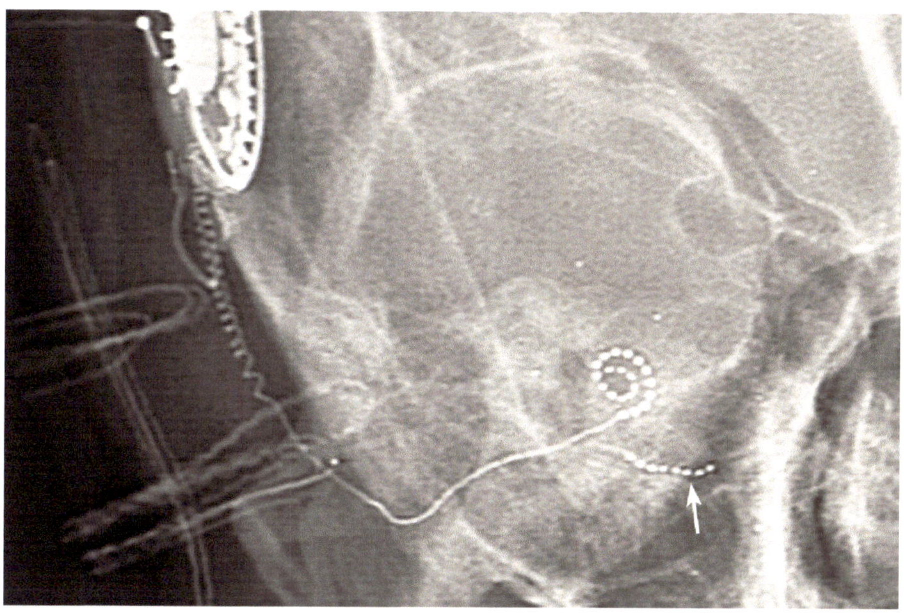

Fig. 7.2.9 Postoperative radiograph. The tip of the electrode array previously inserted into the carotid canal is still visible, next to the new intracochlear electrode (*arrow*). After 36 months of follow-up the patient has 85% open-set speech perception.

Comment

In a difficult case, as in postmeningitis ossification of the basal turn, the decision to perform an open approach (in a subtotal petrosectomy procedure) is easily taken when the electrode is prone to misplacement.

Case 7.3 Cholesteatoma and Kinking of the Electrode (Fig. 7.3.1–Fig. 7.3.9)

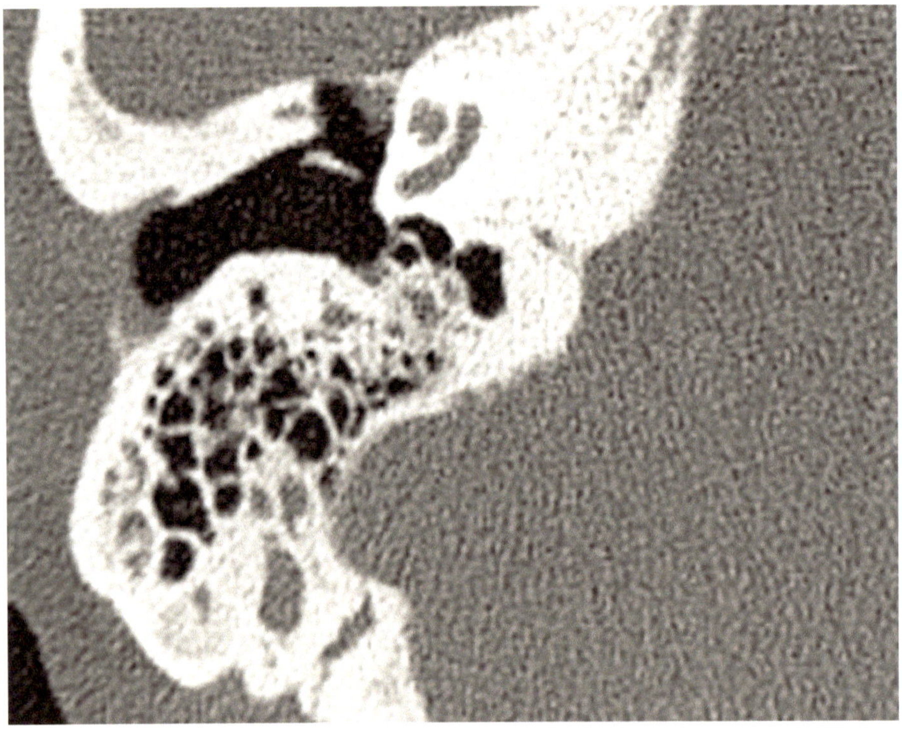

Fig. 7.3.1 A 61-year-old woman with hereditary hearing loss was evaluated for cochlear implantation. She had some benefit of her hearing aid on the left ear. Both cochleae were patent (right cochlea shown here). Some mastoid cells are opacified, but no active otitis was present. In childhood, the patient had had some episodes of otitis media. Because of her residual hearing in the left ear she was scheduled for a CI on the right side.

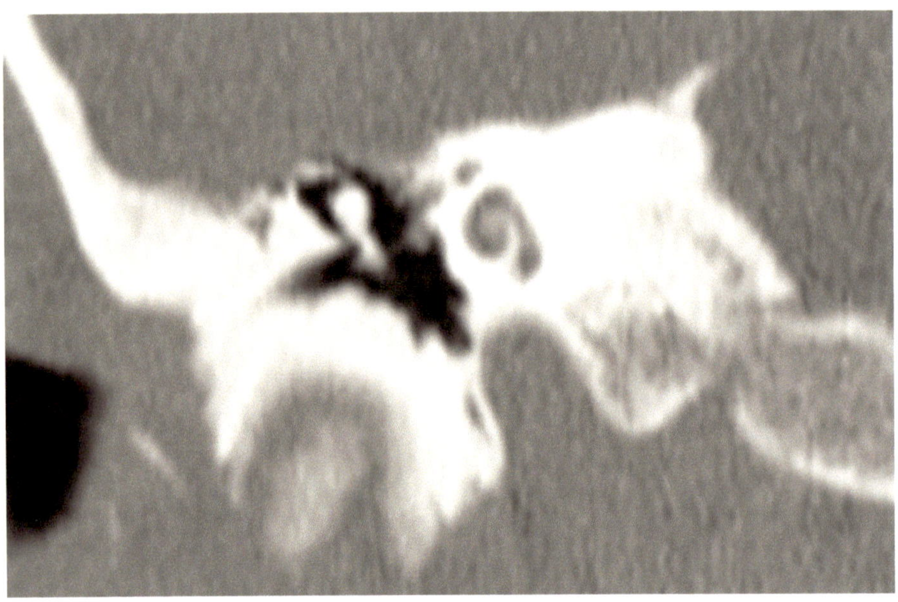

Fig. 7.3.2 The attic and scutum were without any abnormalities.

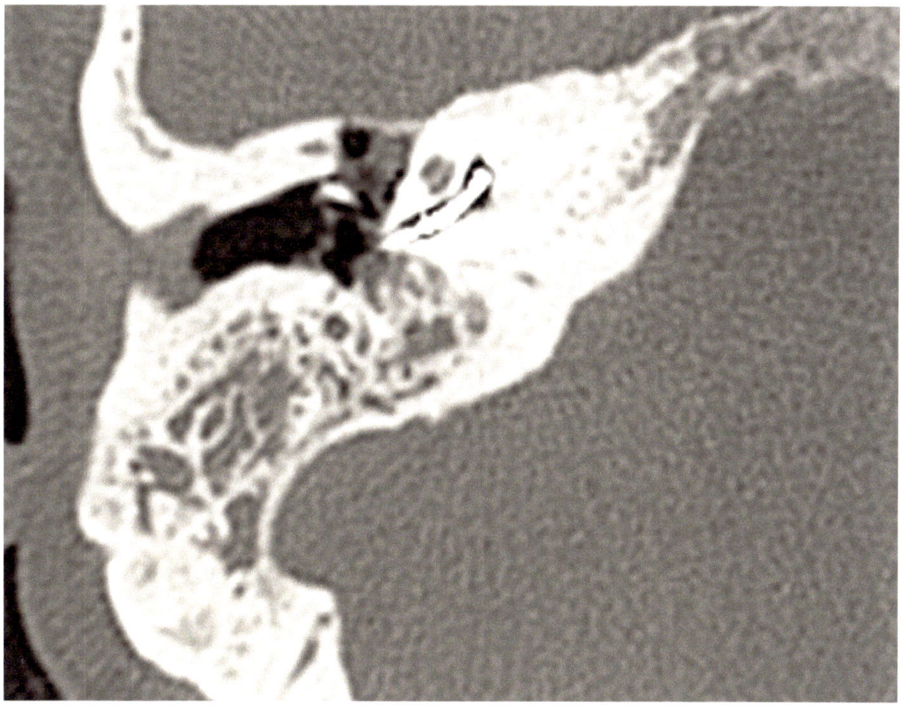

Fig. 7.3.3 The patient had a successful implantation and rehabilitation. After 2 years she returned with ear pain. At otoscopy a cholesteatoma was seen at Shrapnell. CT images showed opacification of the mastoid. The implant functioning was acceptable, with a speech discrimination score (SDS) of 100%.

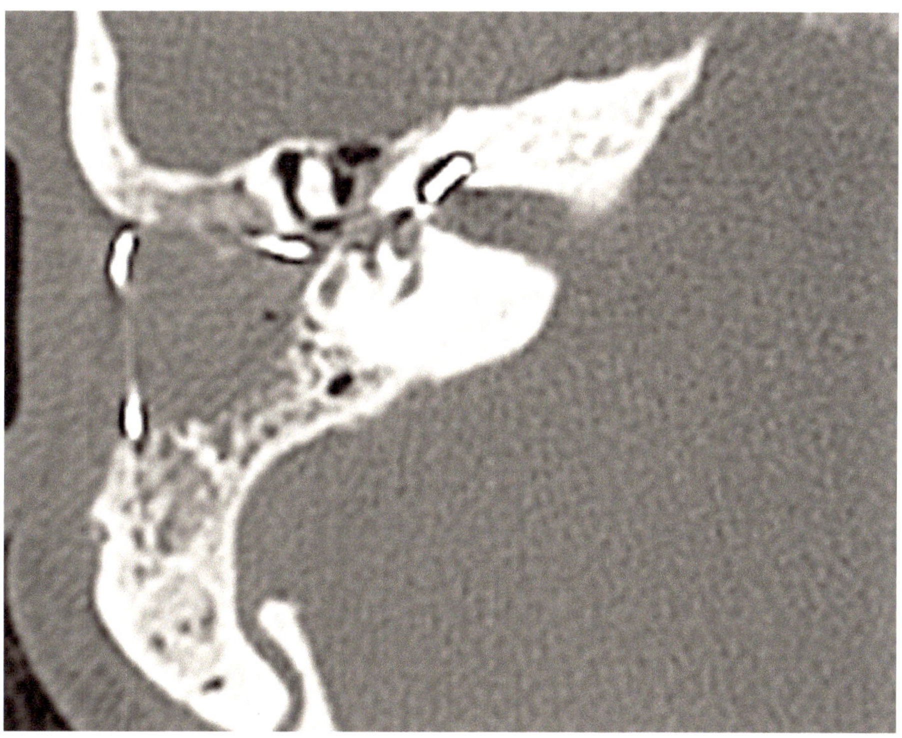

Fig. 7.3.4 The mastoid cavity was almost completely opacified.

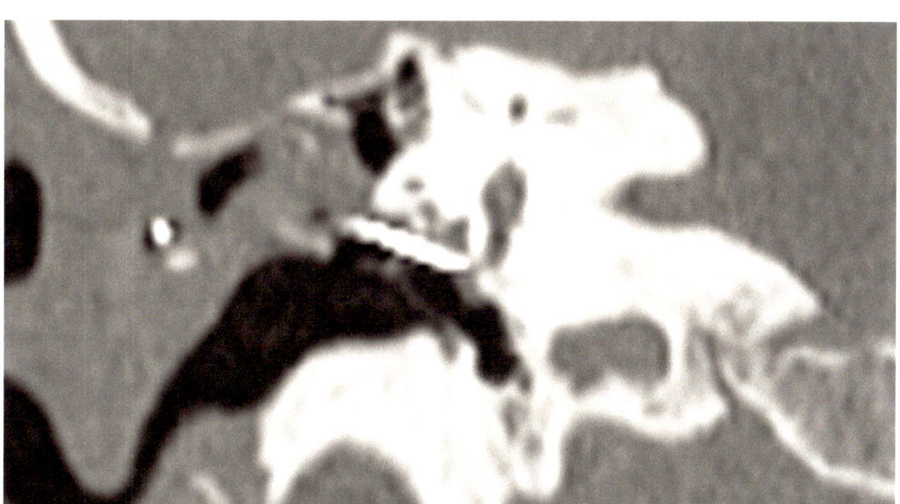

Fig. 7.3.5 An opacification around the electrode was seen, which was most likely the cholesteatoma. The patient was scheduled for explanation and eradication of the cholesteatoma.

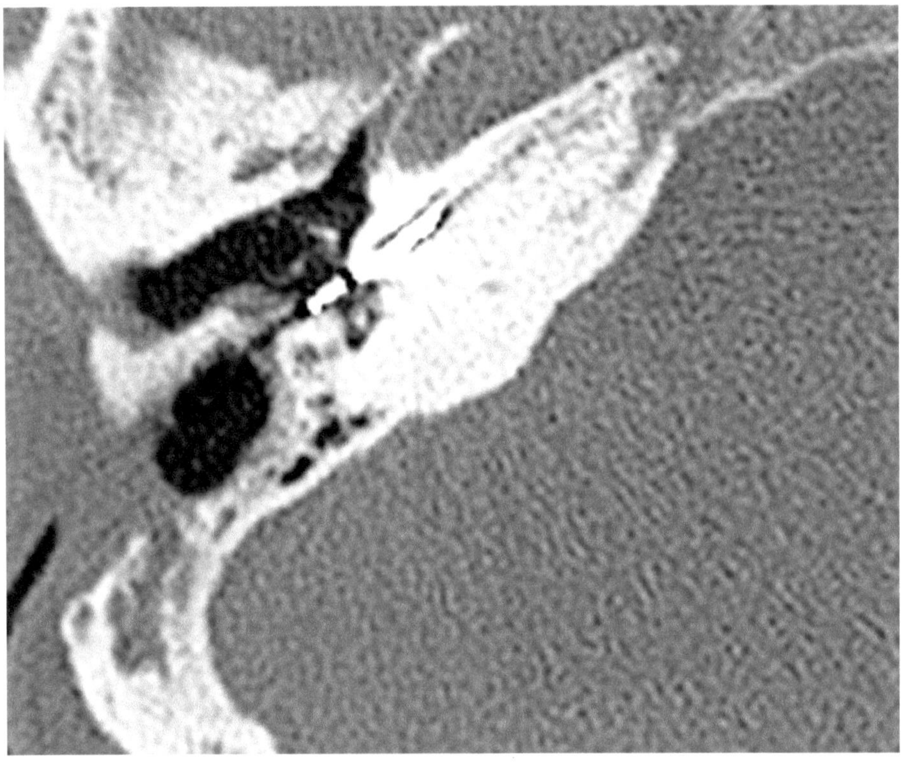

Fig. 7.3.6 The electrode was cut at the posterior tympanotomy and left in the cochlea, to keep the lumen patent. In a canal wall up procedure the cavity was cleared of cholesteatoma. Eight months later she was seen without any complaints except for her hearing deprivation. A CT scan revealed the remaining intracochlear part of the electrode and no signs of residual cholesteatoma.

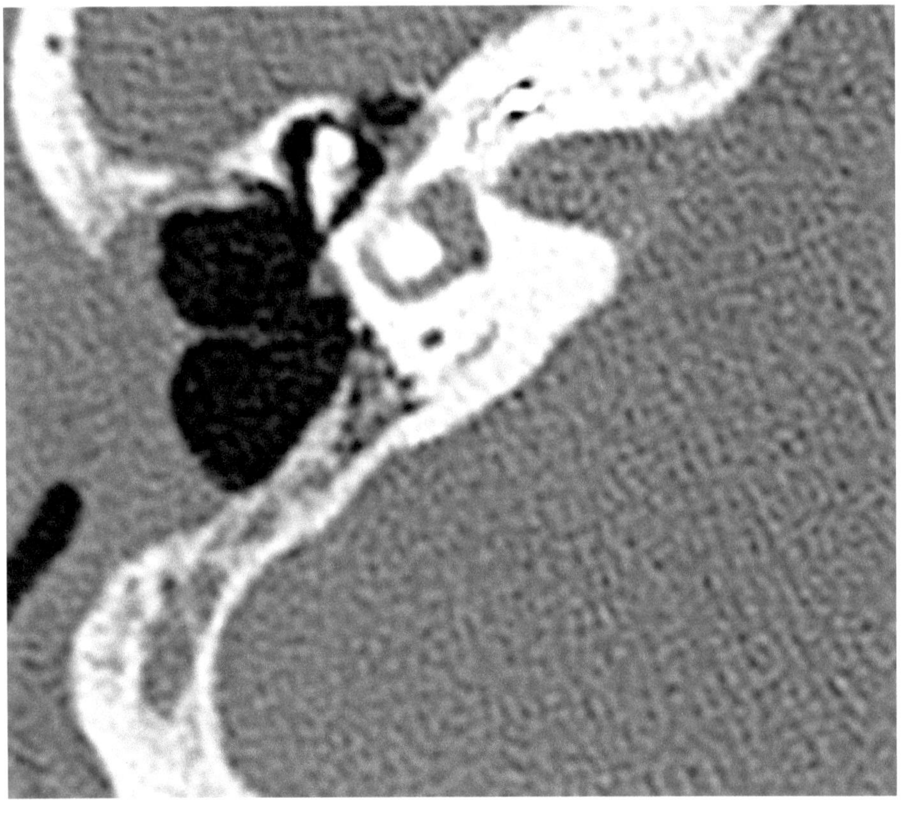

Fig. 7.3.7 The mastoid was free of any cholesteatoma.

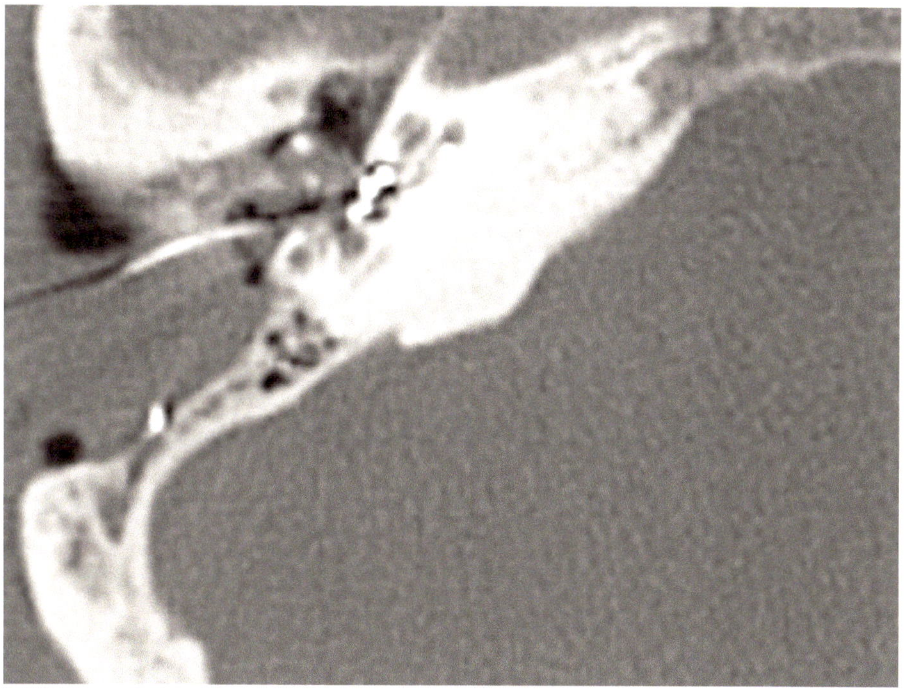

Fig. 7.3.8 The intracochlear electrode was removed and a similar precurved electrode was smoothly inserted. After insertion of 14 (of 20) electrodes during the advanced off-stylet technique, the electrode array could not be moved forward. Even after gentle rotational movement and slight pulling back of the electrode, the electrode could not be inserted completely. The electrode kinked at the round window and it was decided not to revise the implant immediately.

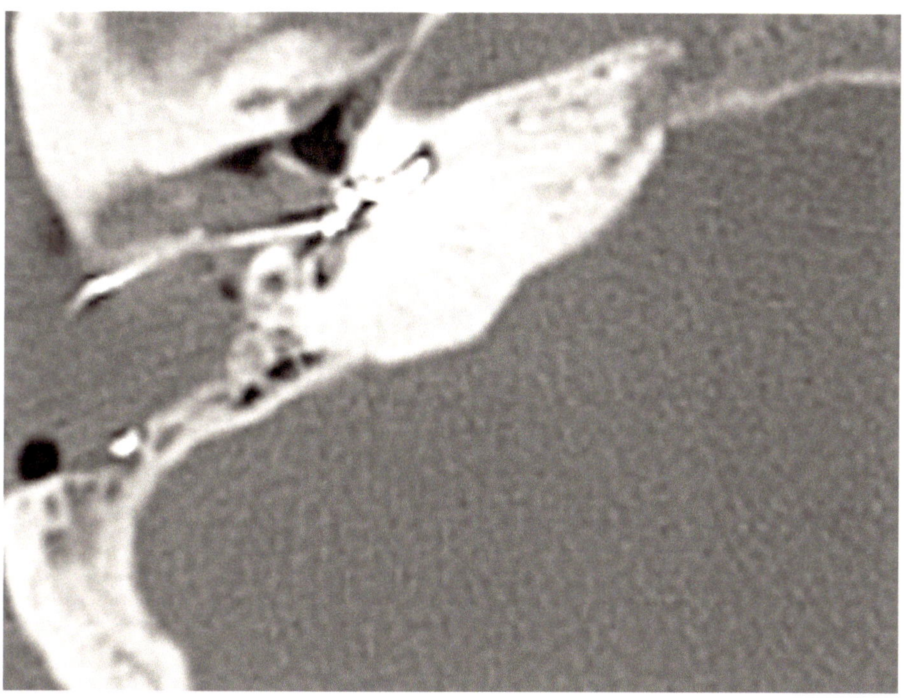

Fig. 7.3.9 The patient was well-informed postoperatively and she did not favor revision surgery but started rehabilitation with the 14 intracochlear electrodes. Her speech discrimination score did not reach the old level (SDS 40%). Still, the patient does not contemplate a revision surgery or a CI on the contralateral side.

Comment

Re-implantation is almost always easily possible according to the literature, but beware that in real practice it is not always smooth and easy.

Case 7.4 Infection of the Cochlea, 6 Months after Cochlear Electrode Insertion (Fig. 7.4.1–Fig. 7.4.10)

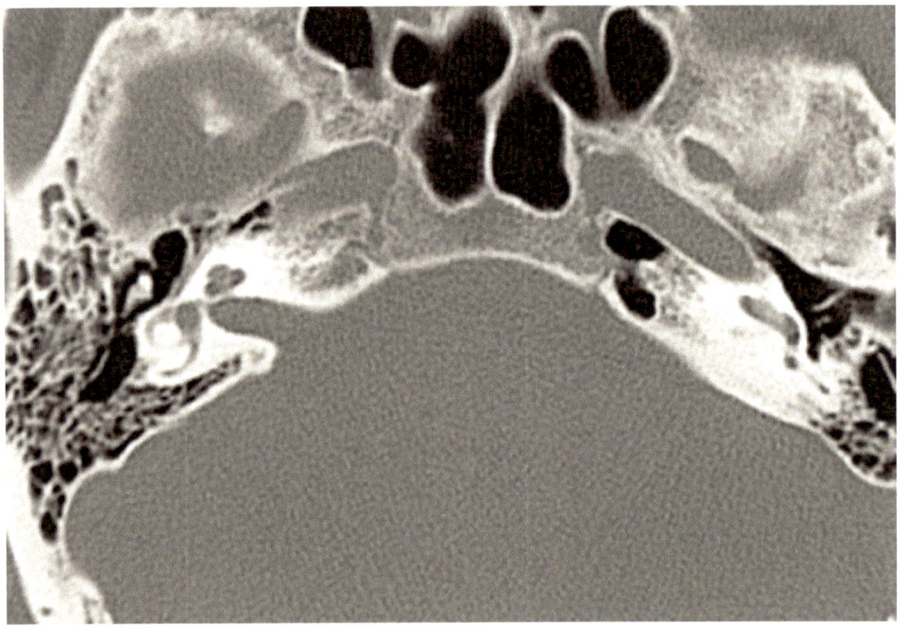

Fig. 7.4.1 As previously reported,[19,21] a 60-year-old woman was assessed for cochlear implantation because of profound hereditary hearing loss. Shown here is her preoperative CT scan: both cochlea are open and accessible for cochlear implantation.

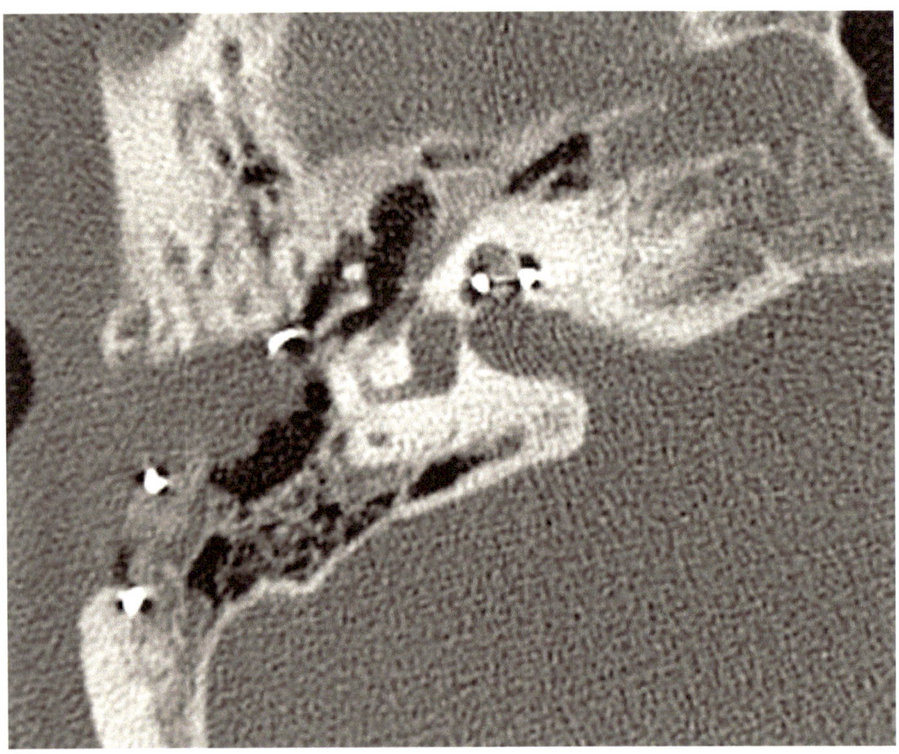

Fig. 7.4.2 Six months after a successful implantation in the right ear, a CT scan was performed because of complaints of pain. No abnormalities in blood tests or cochlear implant audiometric testing were found. The CT scan showed a normal electrode placement and no signs of infection. Around the electrode array black "airlike" artifacts can be seen.

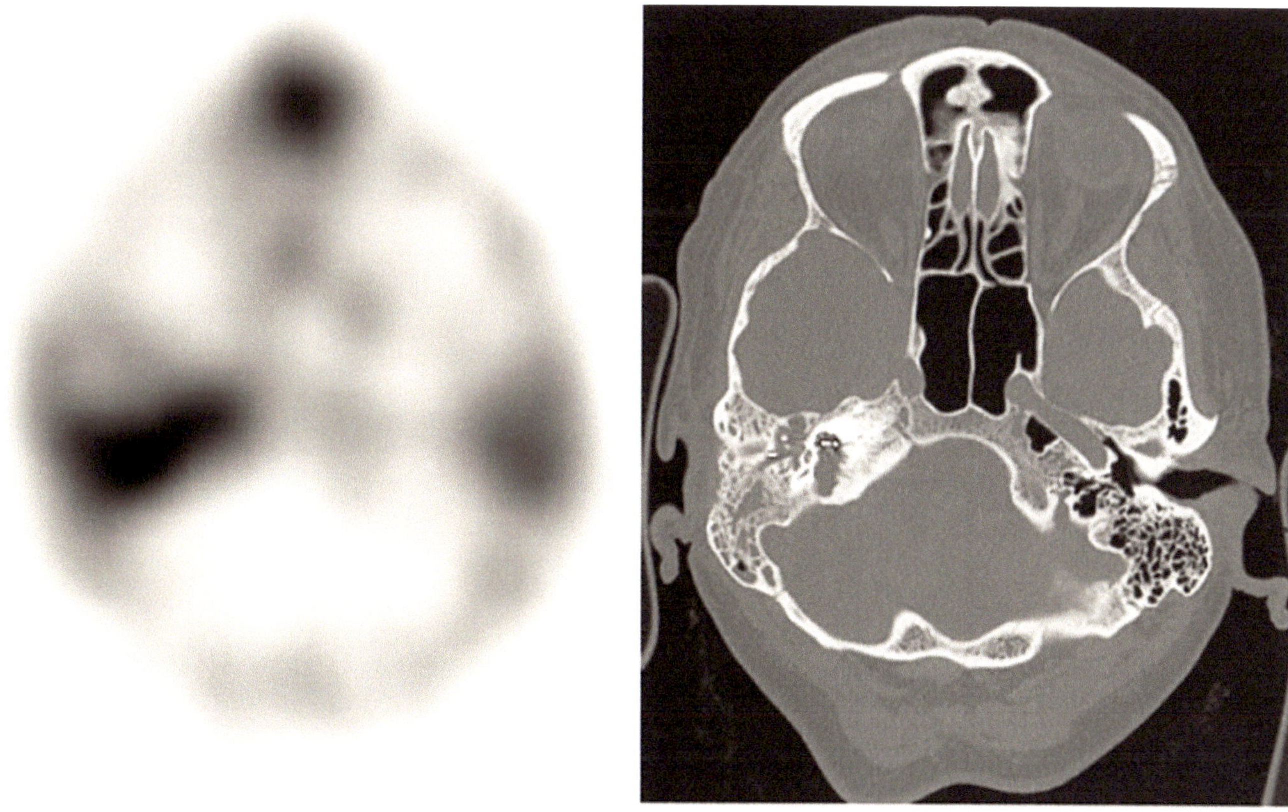

Fig. 7.4.3 Nuclear gallium SPECT scan. In the following months there was a persistent complaint of pain, some improvement of her pain on antibiotics, and changes in the impedances of the CI, with decreasing CI performance. A nuclear scan was performed, which showed an increased uptake in the medial and apical temporal bone. On otoscopy no signs of infection were seen.

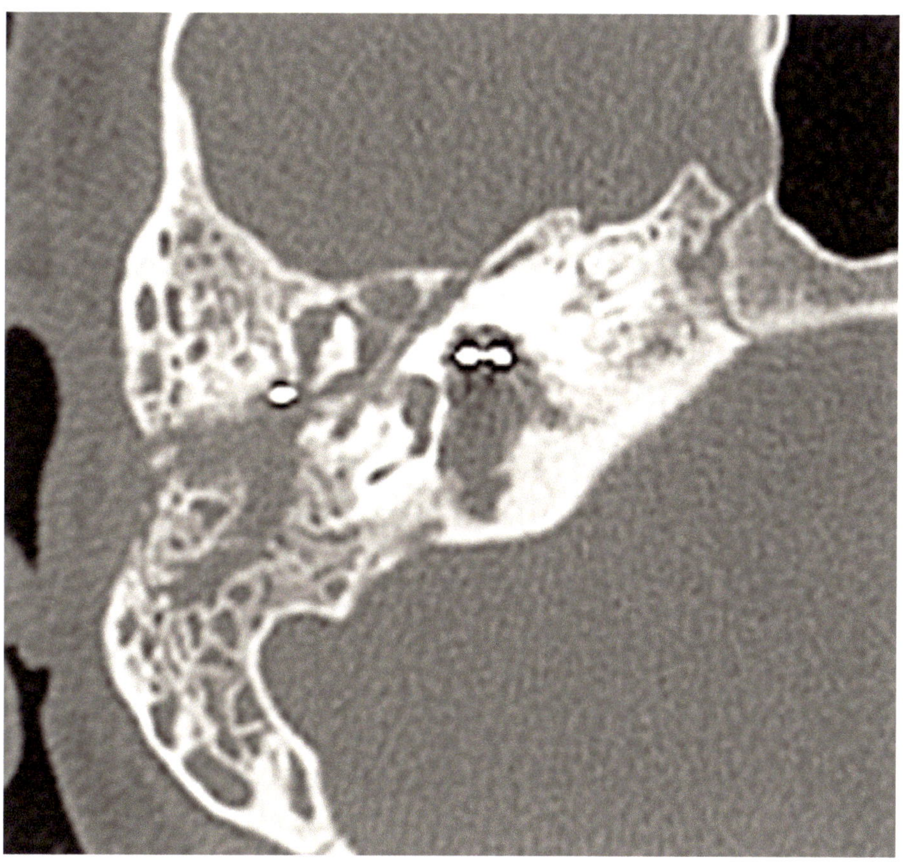

Fig. 7.4.4 A second CT scan was performed, which now showed bone resorption around the cochlea. The implant was no longer used because of improper functioning and lack of auditory improvement. Broad-spectrum antibiotics were administrated intravenously as middle ear culture, during placement of a ventilation tube, had not shown any bacterial growth. Explantation of the complete CI was planned.

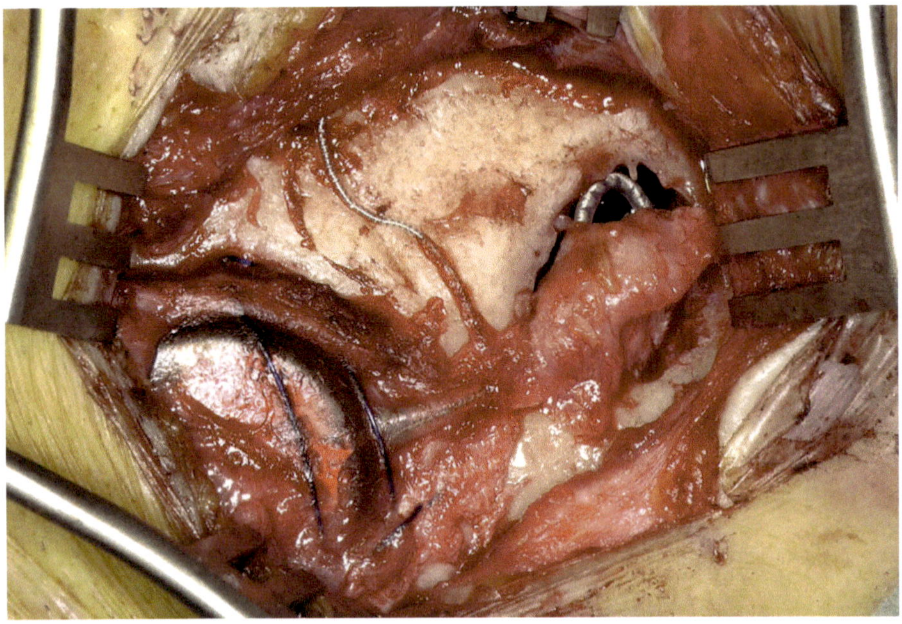

Fig. 7.4.5 The mastoid cavity was not infected and only scar tissue was found.

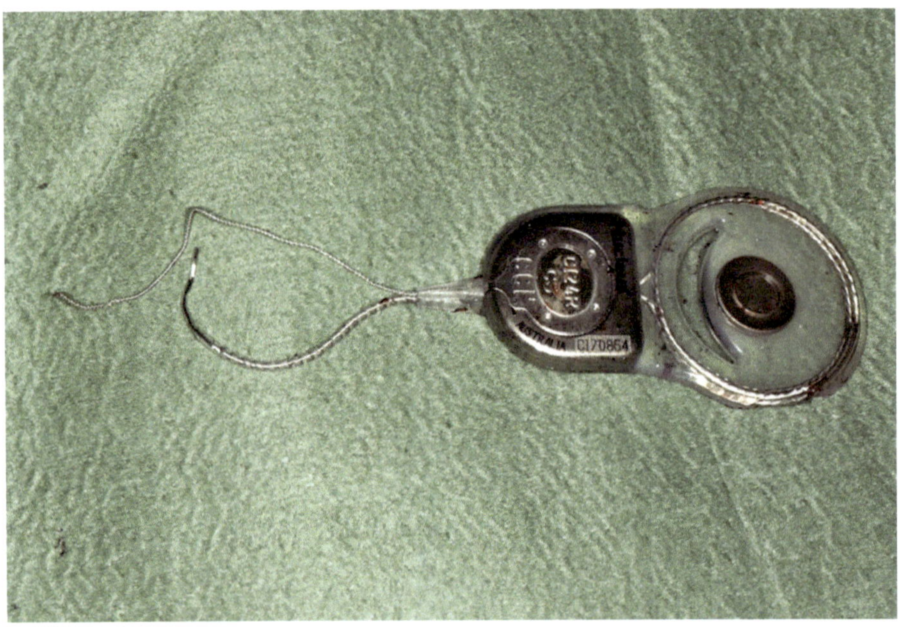

Fig. 7.4.6 The electrode tip and the ball electrode were cut for removal of most of the implant.

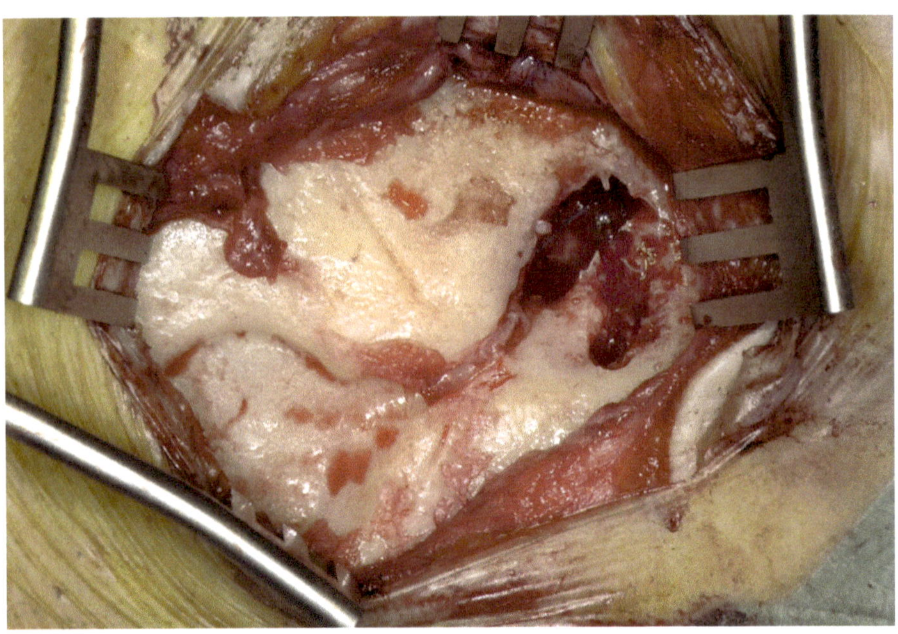

Fig. 7.4.7 The implant bed was not infected and the mastoid was rinsed with antibiotics.

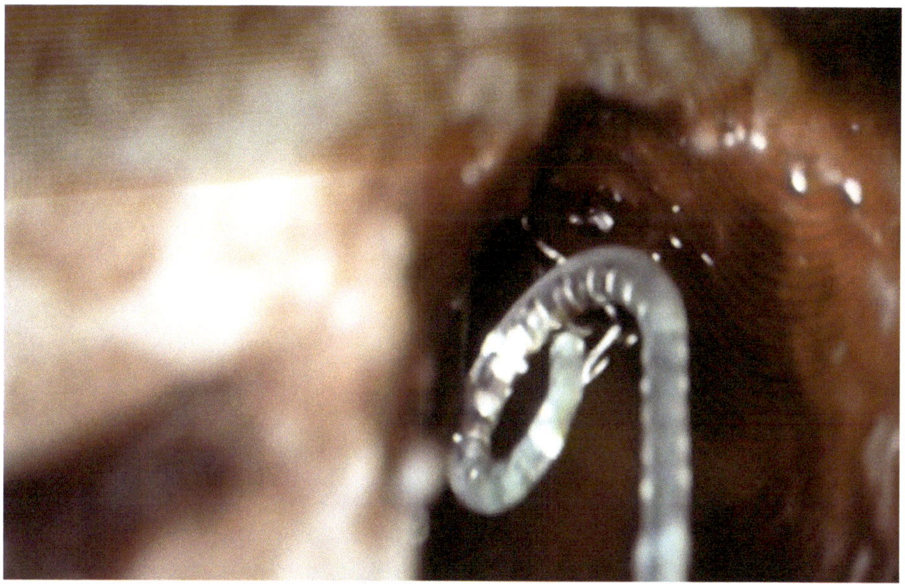

Fig. 7.4.8 The electrode was removed and cultured: *Pseudomonas aeruginosa* was found. The patient was treated for 3 months with an appropriate intravenous antibiotic regime. The gallium SPECT scan was repeated for therapy evaluation.

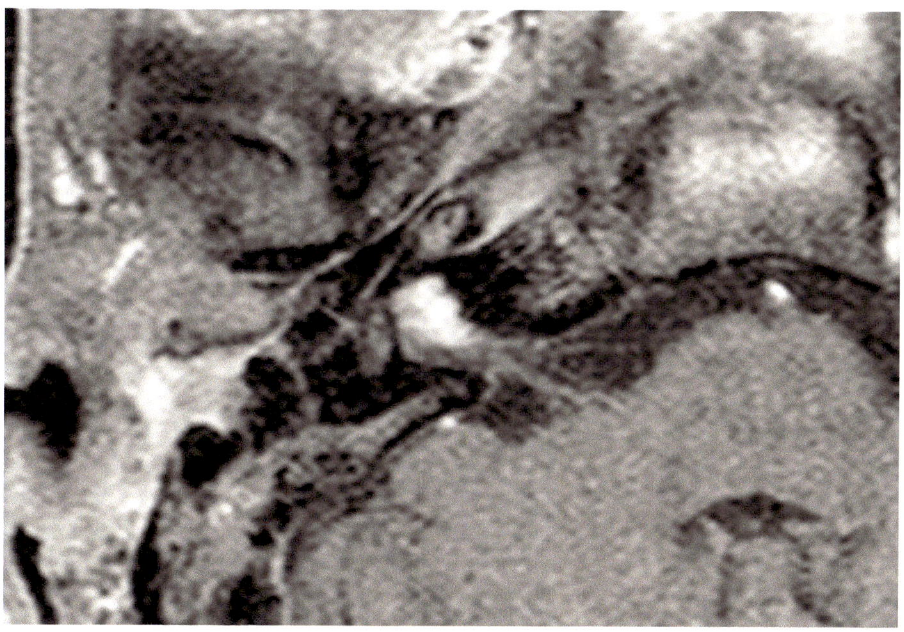

Fig. 7.4.9 Several months later, contrast-enhanced T1W MR images showed a still enhancing cochlear region with no fine structure of the cochlea visible.

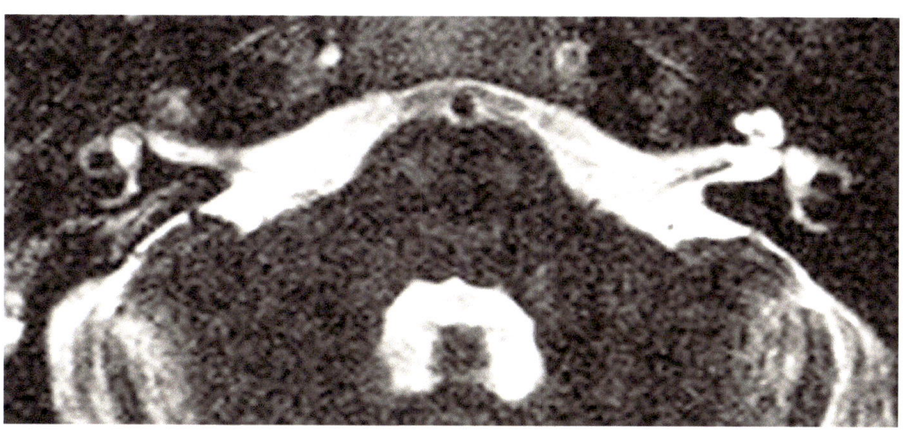

Fig. 7.4.10 The morphology of the cochlea on this T2W CISS MR image is no longer visible on the right side. The left side is normal and was implanted 1 year after explantation of the right ear. In retrospect it was found that a pseudomonad was cultured from the ear canal in another hospital several years before CI placement. Could this have been an iatrogenic infection?

Comment

To avoid iatrogenic infection in CI patients, we now perform a culture of the ear canal some weeks prior to surgery, as hearing aid users are more prone to bacterial or yeast accumulation in the ear canal. Eardrops are prescribed in case of a positive culture for 1 week prior surgery to lower the bacterial/yeast load during surgery.

Case 7.5 Mastoiditis after Cochlear Implantation (Fig. 7.5.1–Fig. 7.5.10)

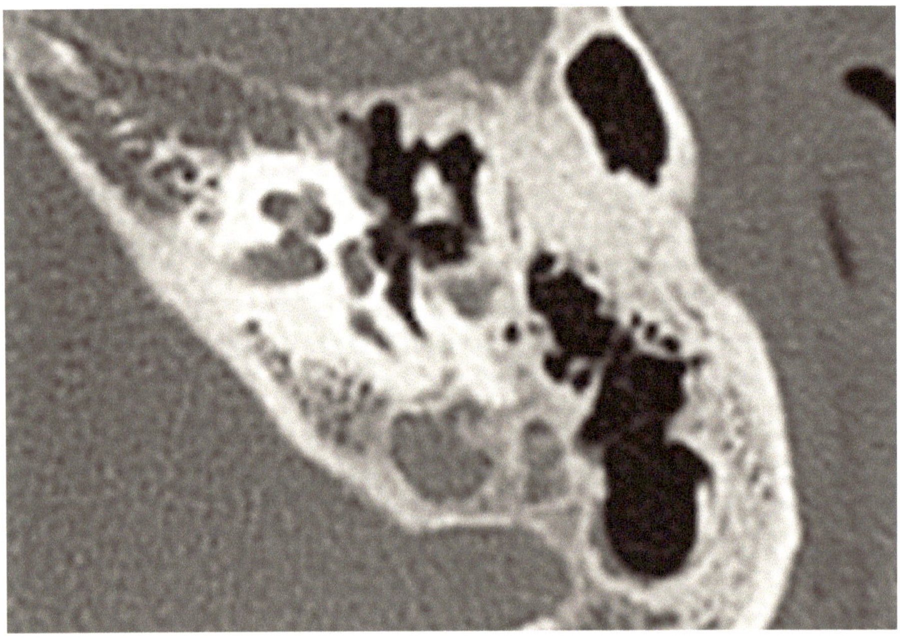

Fig. 7.5.1 A 55-year-old woman had suffered ear infections during childhood. The preoperative CT scan showed a normal cochlear anatomy but the mastoid had a thickened cortical layer and a sclerotic anatomy. A few cells were opacified, but overall the mastoid was aerated.

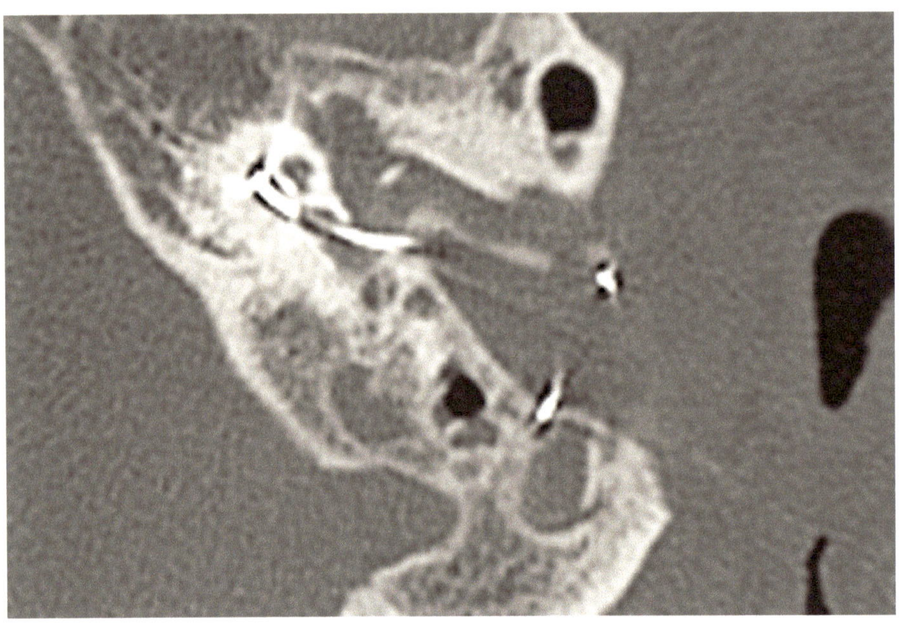

Fig. 7.5.2 Immediately after implantation the patient developed mastoiditis. She was admitted and a CT scan was performed. The complete mastoid was opacified, as shown here. She was treated with intravenous antibiotics.

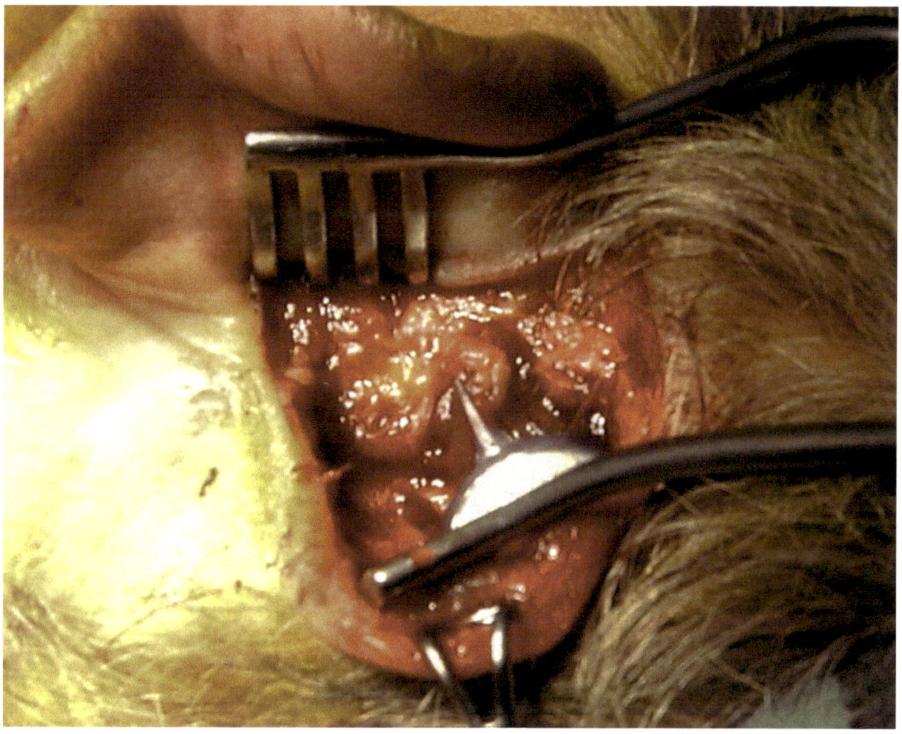

Fig. 7.5.3 The infection did not subside, so a cleaning and local antibiotic rinsing procedure was carried out. The opening and the granulation and fibrous tissue that completely filled the cavity can be seen here.

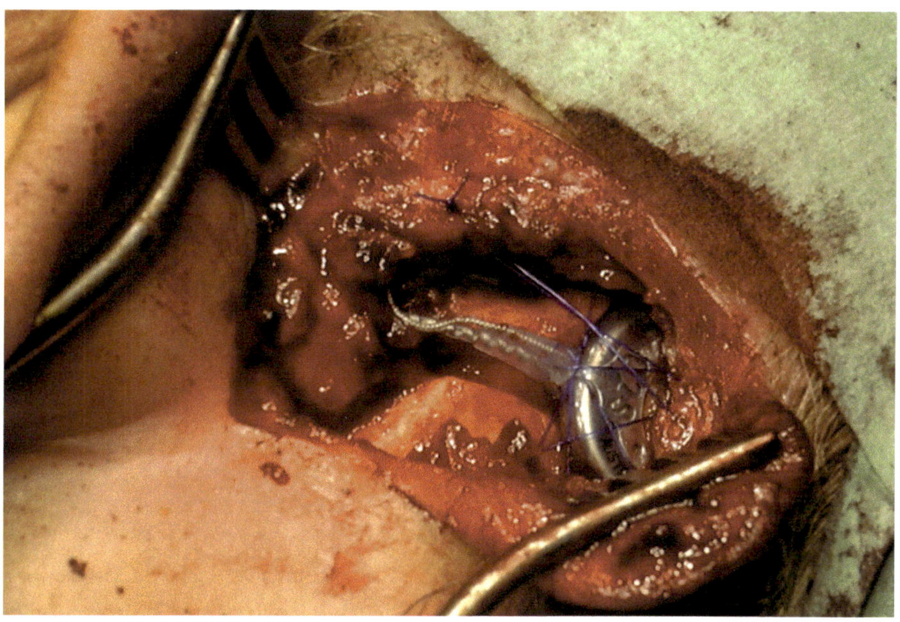

Fig. 7.5.4 The implant was not properly fixated in its receiver-stimulator well due to the extensive fibrous tissue, which was pushing the implant out of its well. As much tissue as possible was removed and then the implant was secured with sutures for good fixation.

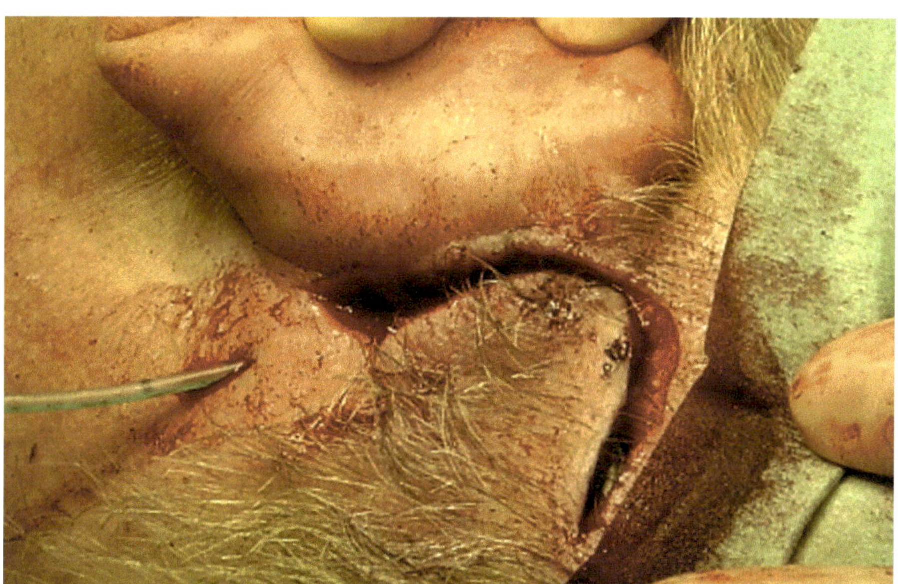

Fig. 7.5.5 The CI site was cleaned, a culture was taken, the implant was rinsed in antibiotics, and most of the granulation tissue was removed. A drain was applied. The drain was removed after a couple of days.

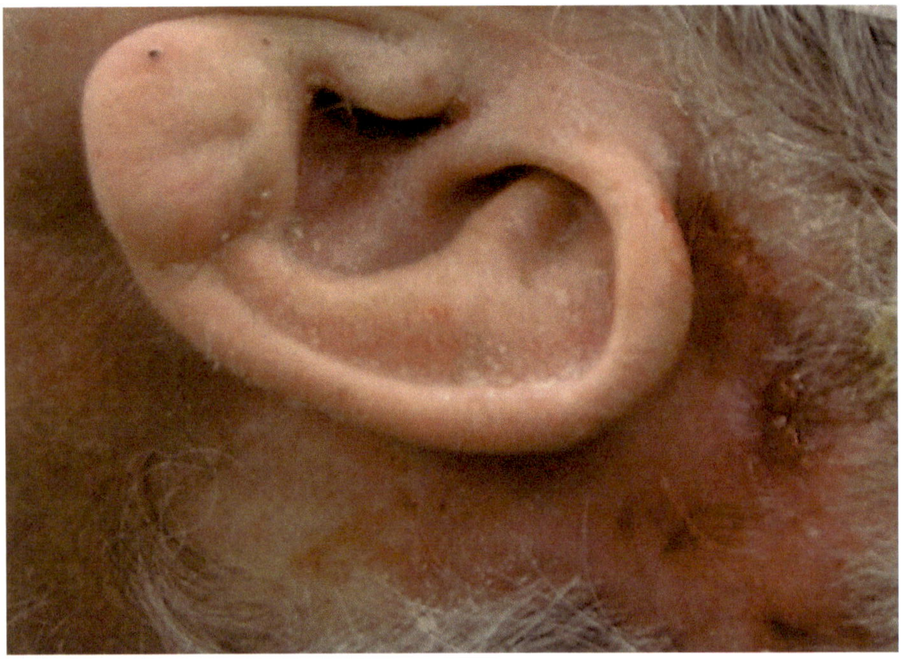

Fig. 7.5.6 After several weeks of antibiotics the successful therapy was stopped and the implant was still in use. The success was only of short duration as the infection returned rapidly. Explantation was planned.

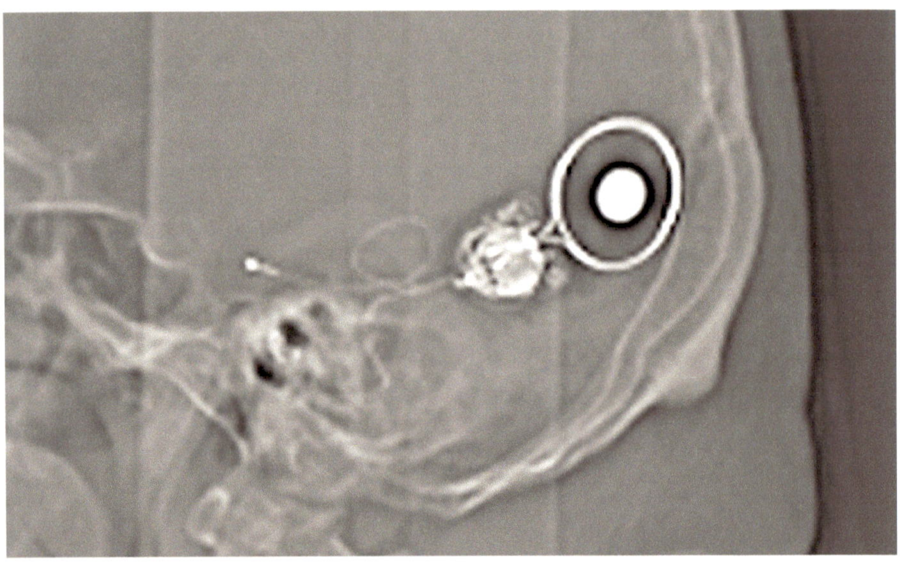

Fig. 7.5.7 Topogram. The topogram of a CT scan or a plain lateral radiograph can be used to see the position of the reference electrode and where to find it on the temporal bone cortex. Sometimes it is located very anteriorly, which is important for the incision.

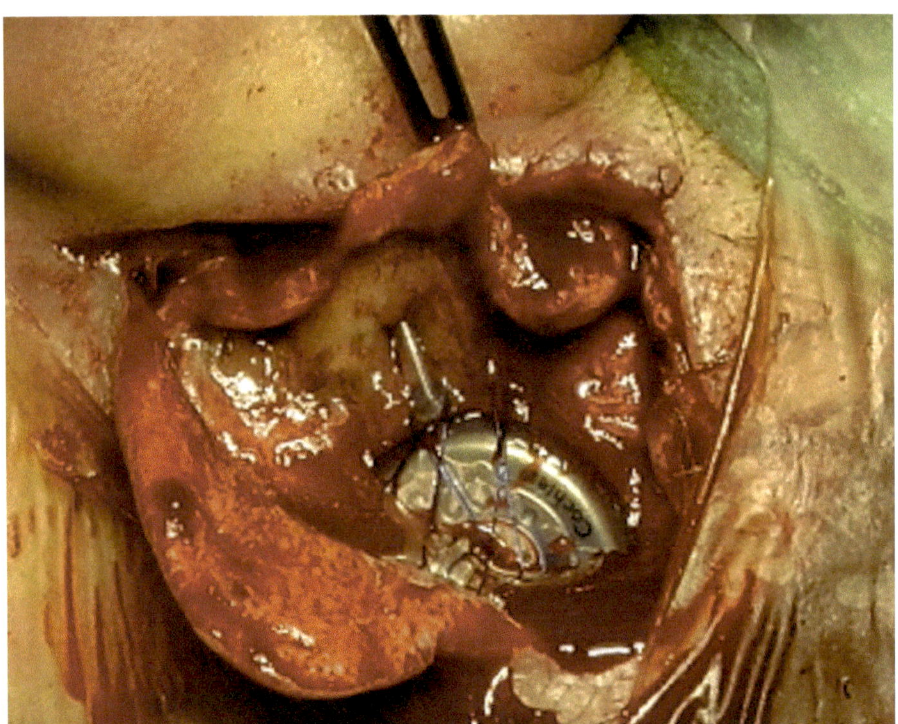

Fig. 7.5.8 The implant was found situated in a mass of mucosal granulation with a lot of debris.

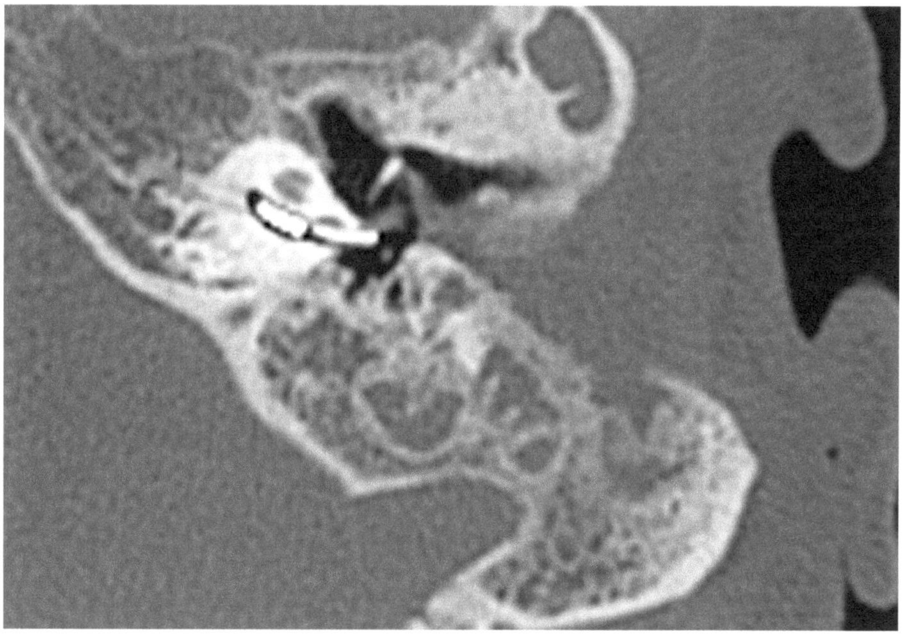

Fig. 7.5.9 The cochlear electrode array was cut in the middle ear just outside the cochlea. The antibiotic regime was prolonged for 6 weeks. The sinus pathology was also treated medically and was monitored.

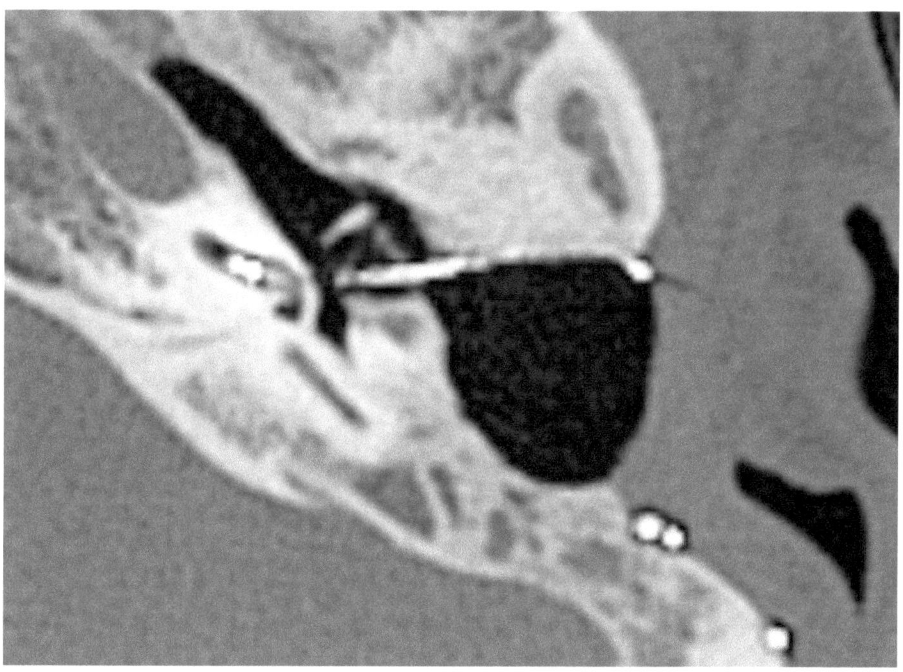

Fig. 7.5.10 Six months later no signs of infection were found during scanning, laboratory tests, and physical examination. She was scheduled for renewed CI placement. During the perioperative period the patient received antibiotic prophylaxis. A standard cochlear implantation was performed, after removal of the cut electrode. In retrospect, a combined subtotal petrosectomy with cochlear implantation was indicated in this case.

Comment

In a patient with recurrent otitis and sinusitis the best way to avoid postoperative infection is to culture prior to surgery, administer (at least) 1 week of antibiotics starting 1 day before surgery, and consider a subtotal petrosectomy with removal of all mucosal lining.

Case 7.6 Cochlear Implantation Revision Surgery Due to Device Failure (Fig. 7.6.1–Fig. 7.6.7)

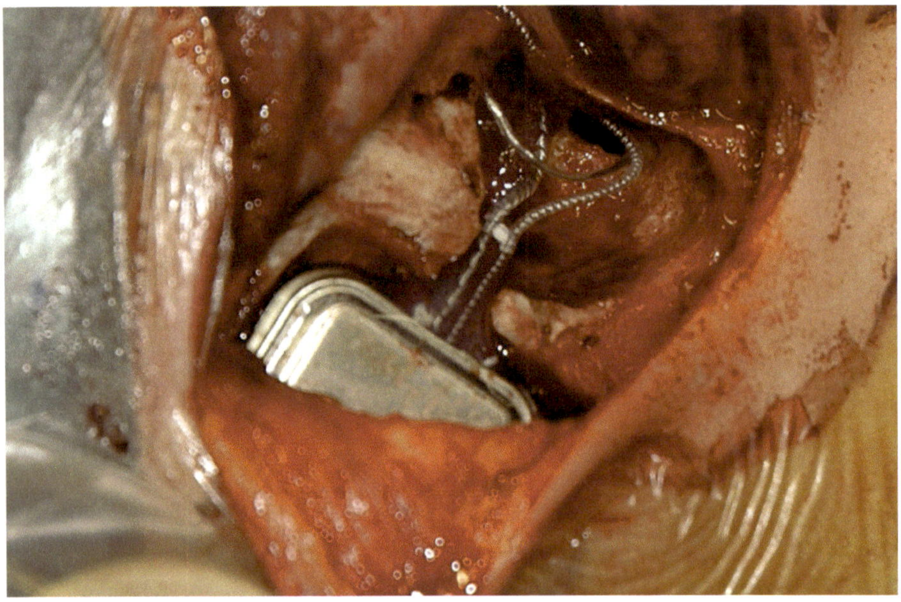

Fig. 7.6.1 An 8-month-old boy was implanted bilaterally directly after discovery of bacterial meningitis, before any fibrosis was visible on MRI (see Chapter 12). A standard straightforward implantation was performed as shown. He recovered well and had a good start with his rehabilitation.

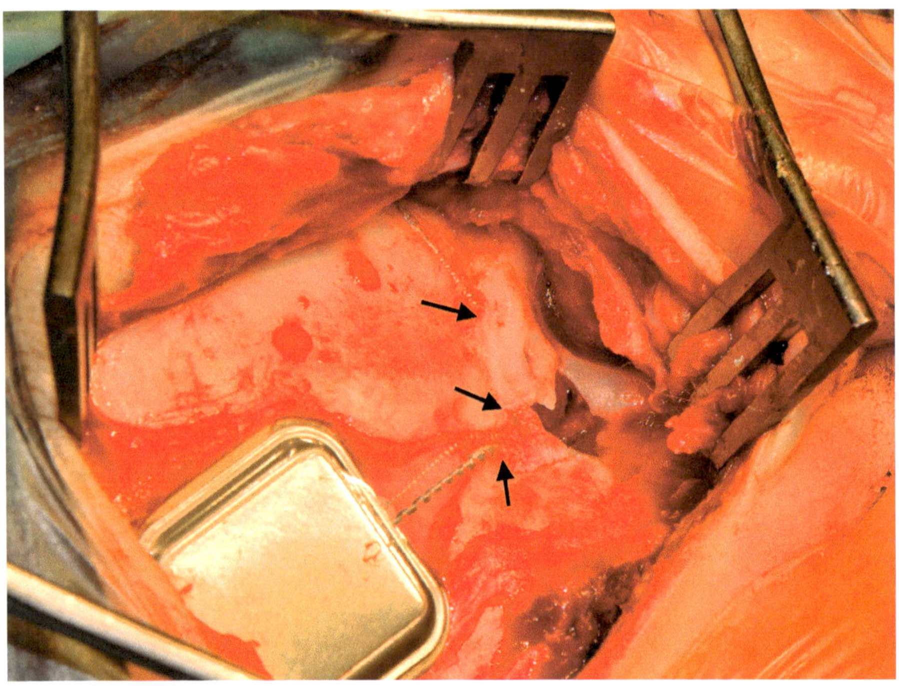

Fig. 7.6.2 Due to a hard device failure with sudden loss of functionality, the implant on the right side had to be replaced. New bone formation can cover the electrodes in as little as 6 months, as shown here (*arrows*). This makes removal of the implant without any damage to the electrodes or implant more difficult; careful drilling avoiding harm to the electrodes is necessary. Especially when the cause of device failure is unknown, it is important to keep the implant with electrodes intact so as to be able to perform postoperative testing.

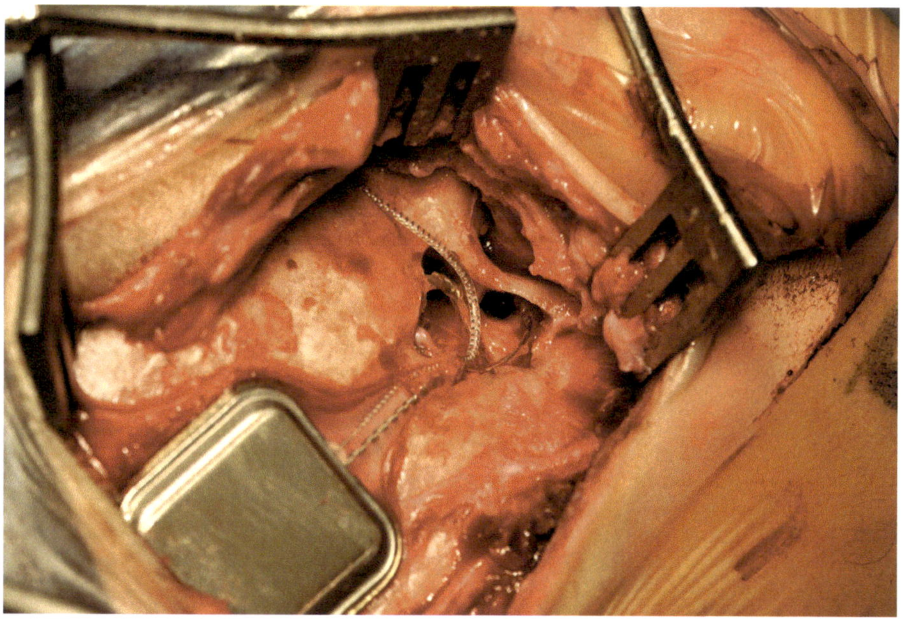

Fig. 7.6.3 On careful removal of the newly formed bone, the electrodes become visible. The reference electrode can sometimes be fully engulfed by bone and absolutely should not be retrieved. On the other hand, the cochlear electrode array is preferably cut at the posterior tympanotomy to make feasible removal of the intracochlear electrode during direct view of the cochlea at high magnification.

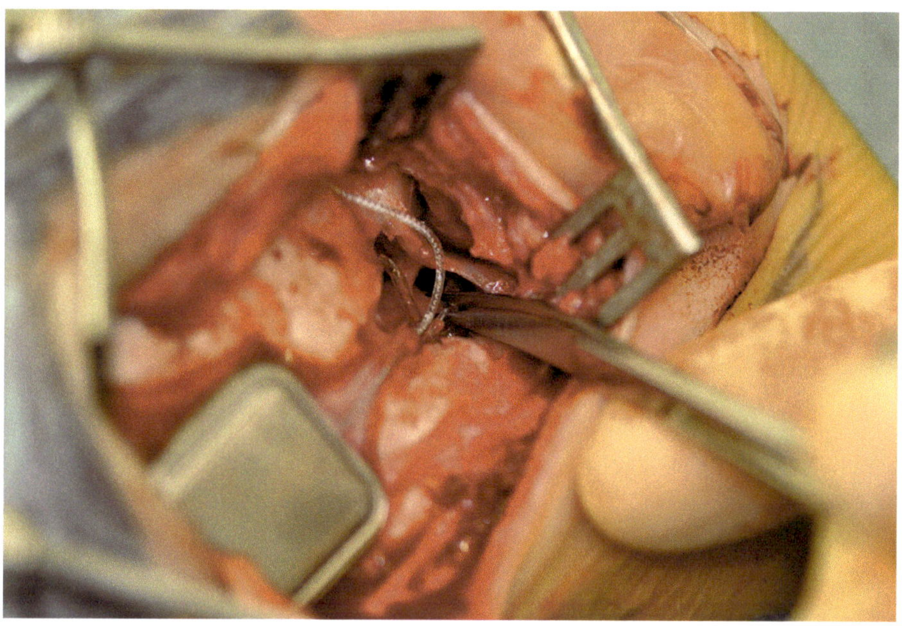

Fig. 7.6.4 A device failure of unknown cause makes explanation and re-implantation, preferably during the same procedure, inevitable. The electrode was cut at the posterior tympanotomy with angled surgical scissors (no microinstrument) as illustrated. The distal end in the cochlea can then be removed after preparation of the new implant well and during direct view of the cochleostomy/round window.

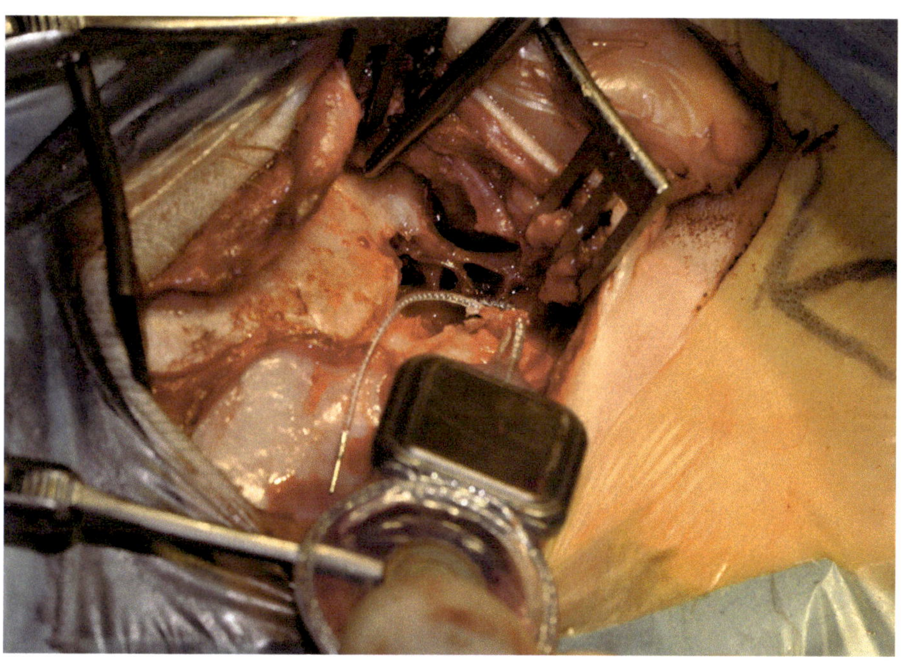

Fig. 7.6.5 The implant can now be removed and scar tissue taken off the implant before sending it to the manufacturer for investigation. As an alternative, it is possible to rotate the "old" device anteriorly and provisionally fixate it and subsequently remove the complete implant after preparation of the new implant well and introduction of the new implant receiver-stimulator.

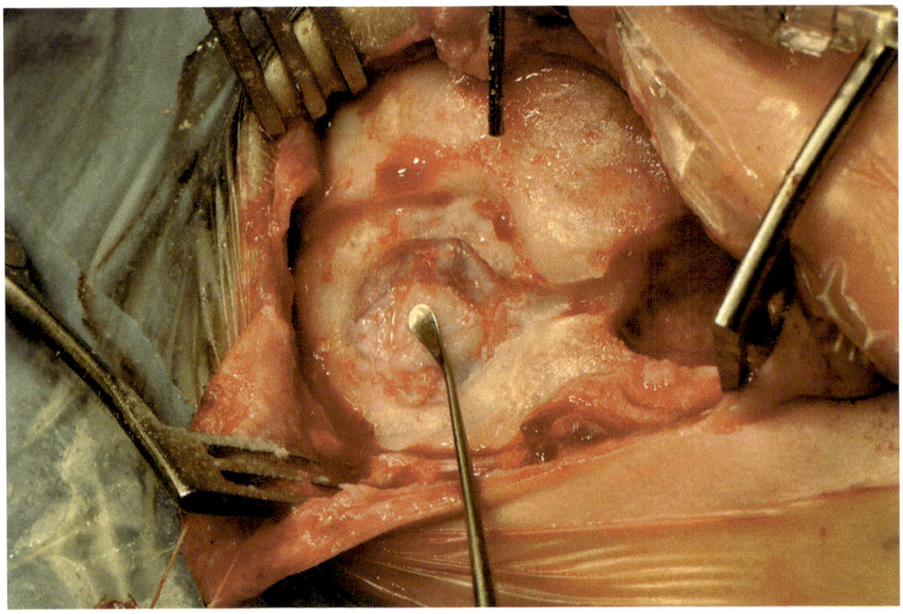

Fig. 7.6.6 The implant well is prepared on the dura with a "bony island" (see Chapter 6) and the previous electrode canal is adjusted.

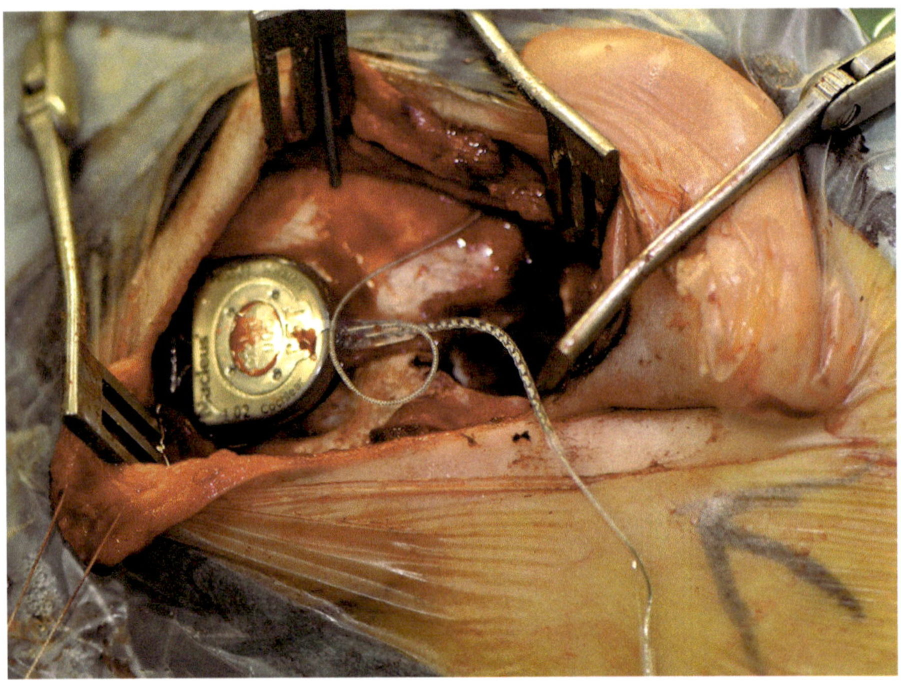

Fig. 7.6.7 A new implant is placed and just before insertion the cut distal electrode array is removed. A silicone dummy "test array" can be used to provide information on the intracochlear lumen. The removed electrode array portion is collected in the same return container as the rest of the "old" implant. In a very short time the re-implantation in this case restored to the child the same reactions as before, which improved markedly over time.

Comment

Removal of a device without damaging the implant is difficult and takes more time than expected. New bone formation can be present even within 6 months after first implantation.

Case 7.7 Implant Displacement (Fig. 7.7.1–Fig. 7.7.3)

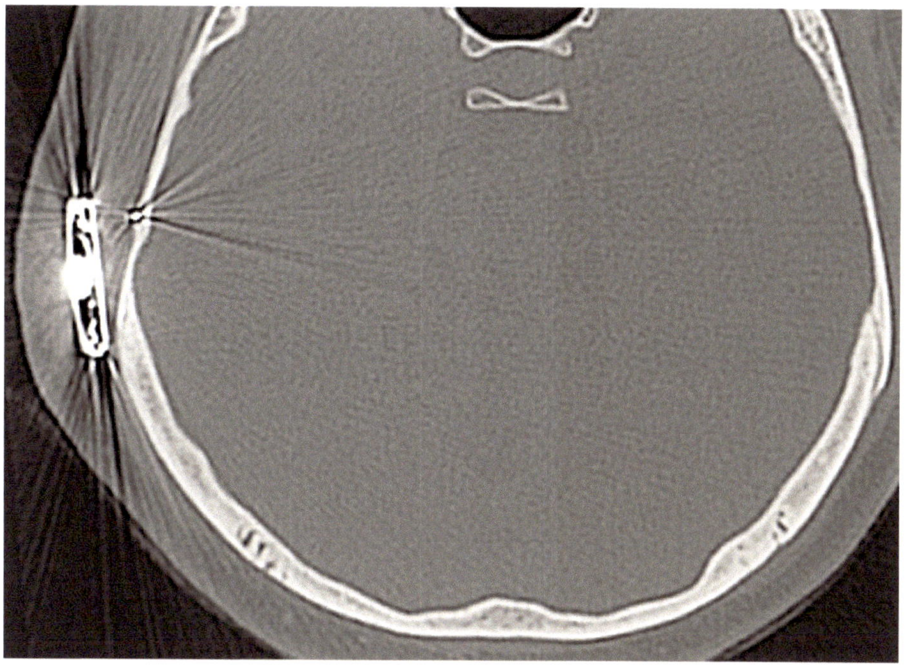

Fig. 7.7.1 In this patient the cochlear implant had been displaced by trauma. The screw is still in the correct position, as shown on this CT scan, and the implant is detached from the skull.

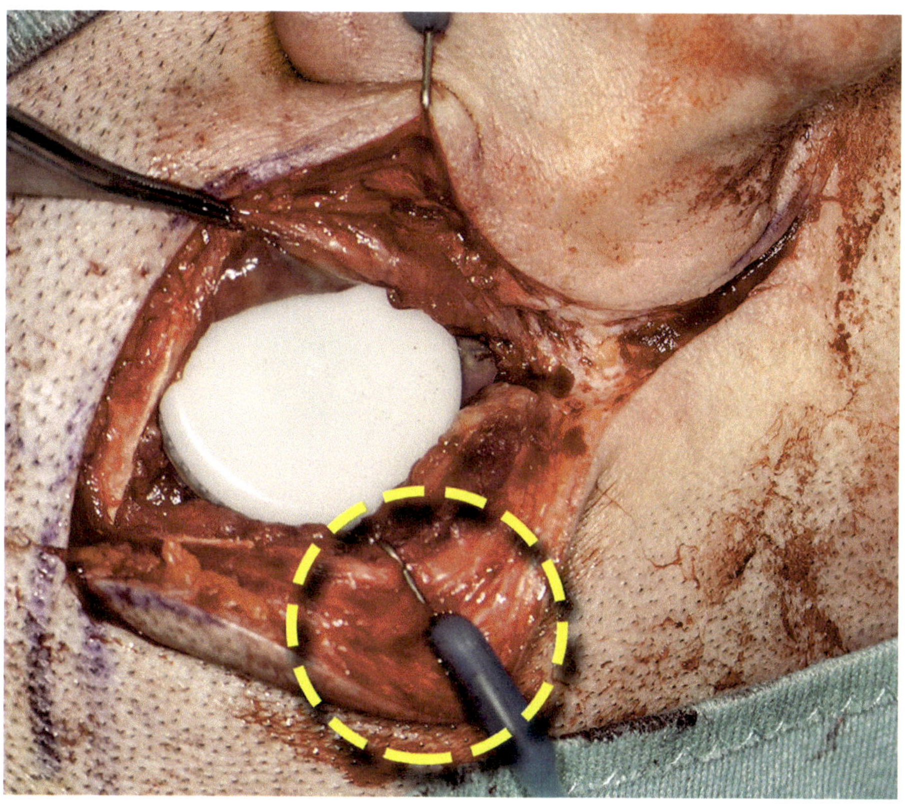

Fig. 7.7.2 The implant was delicately uncovered and an anterior displacement was seen. The original position was more posterior, indicated here by the yellow dashed circle.

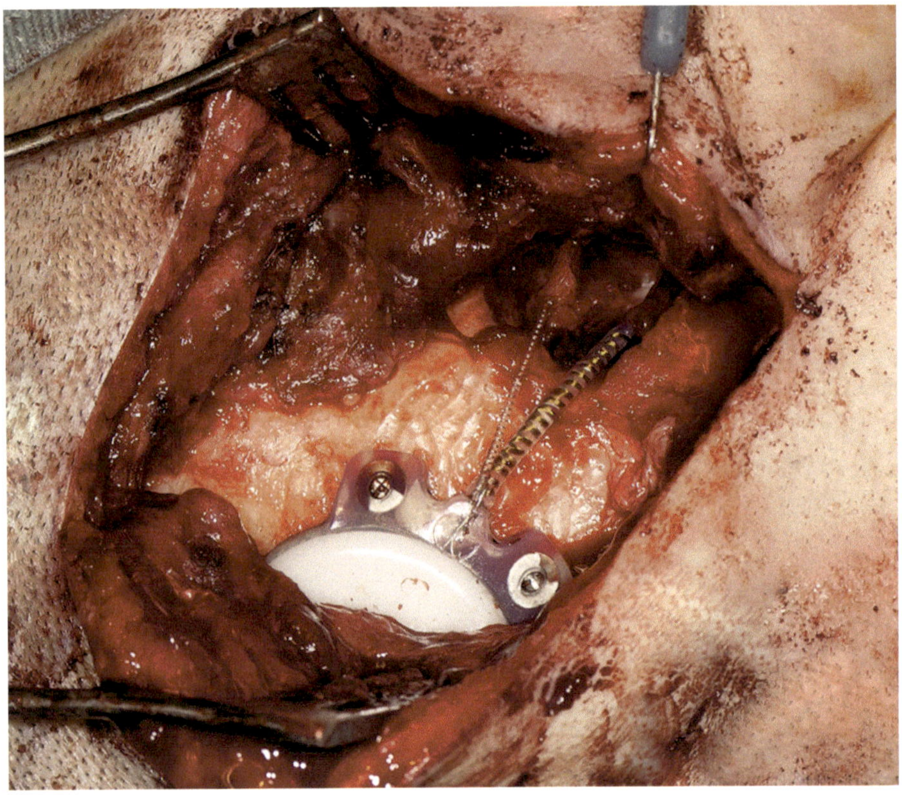

Fig. 7.7.3 The bone at the original position was exposed and prepared for new fixation, making sure that the implant was completely in contact with the bone, without any tilting. The screws have best grip if they are precisely perpendicular to the skull bone. A close look at the implant and electrode is also necessary to rule out any damage that could cause failure again in the future.

Comment

Proper positioning with or without screws is necessary to avoid displacement. In case of screws, make sure that they have accurate grip during tightening and are not directly placed at a bony cleft or at a locally uneven location.

Case 7.8 Implant Displacement (Figs. 7.8.1 and 7.8.2)

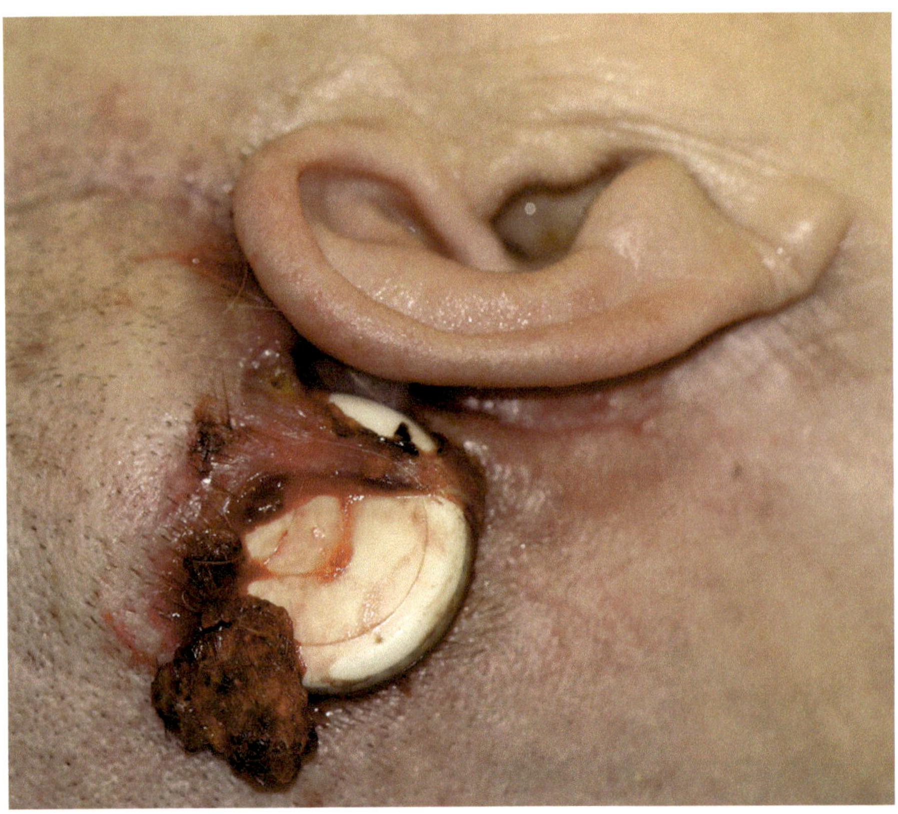

Fig. 7.8.1 This patient experienced implant extrusion within the first year after placement. In a second surgery the skin was readjusted over the implant, but after a while the extrusion and retraction of the skin occurred again. The patient was referred to our center and the situation was found to be severe. The skin was retracted, the subcutaneous layer was infected, and the implant was more on than underneath the skin. It seemed doubtful that there was enough healthy skin, muscle, and local regenerative support to undertake re-implantation on this side.

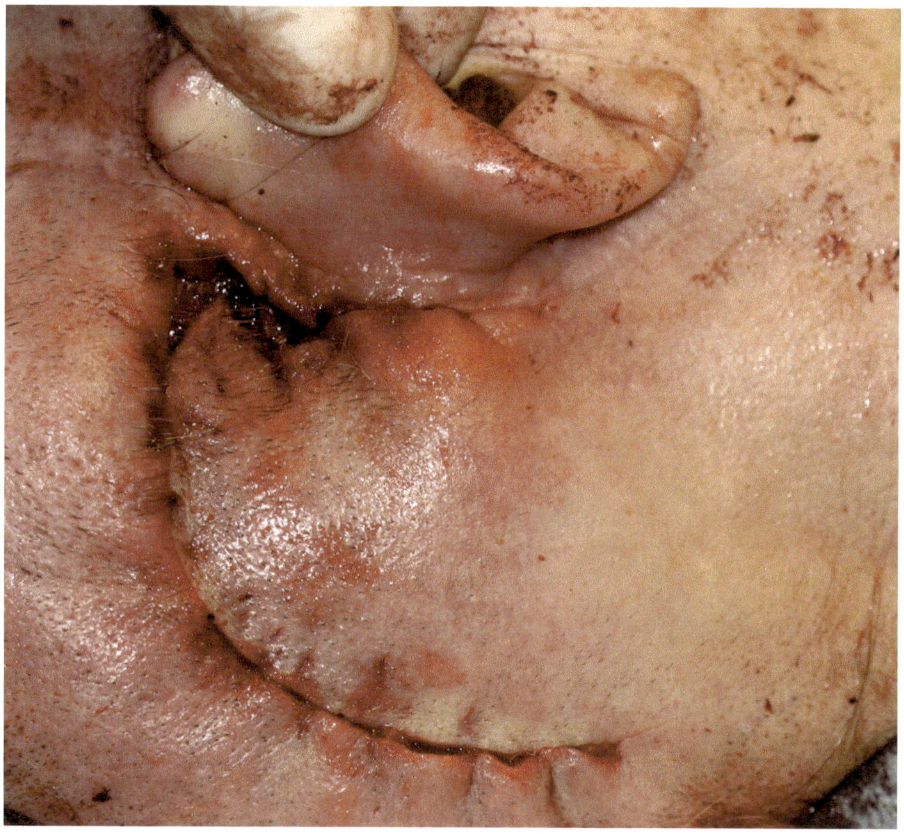

Fig. 7.8.2 After consultation with the patient it was decided to remove the implant on this side and implant a new CI on the contralateral side. The wound was closed primarily and resolved satisfactorily. Contralateral re-implantation was successful.

Comment

Closure in several tensionless layers, with differently orientated incision lines, can be suggested to assure good blood supply, appropriate fixation, and minimal risk of extrusion through the incision lines. Care must be taken to keep the skin layer and temporal muscle layer as thick as possible.

Case 7.9 Infection in the Operative Cavity at Implantation (Fig. 7.9.1–7.9.6)

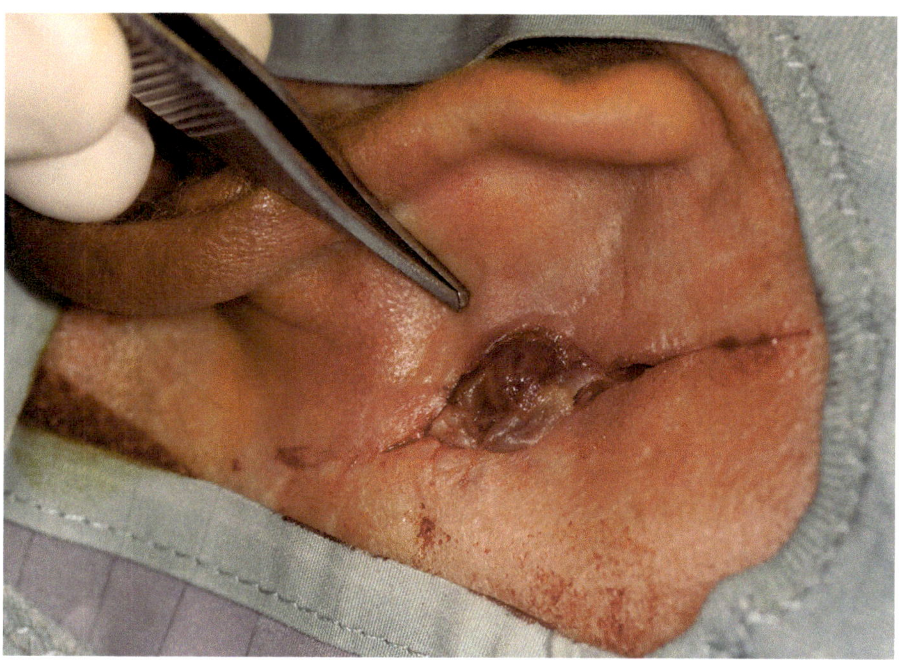

Fig. 7.9.1 A 42-year-old man had a subtotal petrosectomy and implantation. After 1 year the patient complained of retroauricular pain. During revision surgery the cavity was filled with granulation tissue. It was decided to explant the CI, treat him with intravenous antibiotics for 1 week, and re-implant. Because of the strong infection it was preferred not to leave the array in the cochlea.

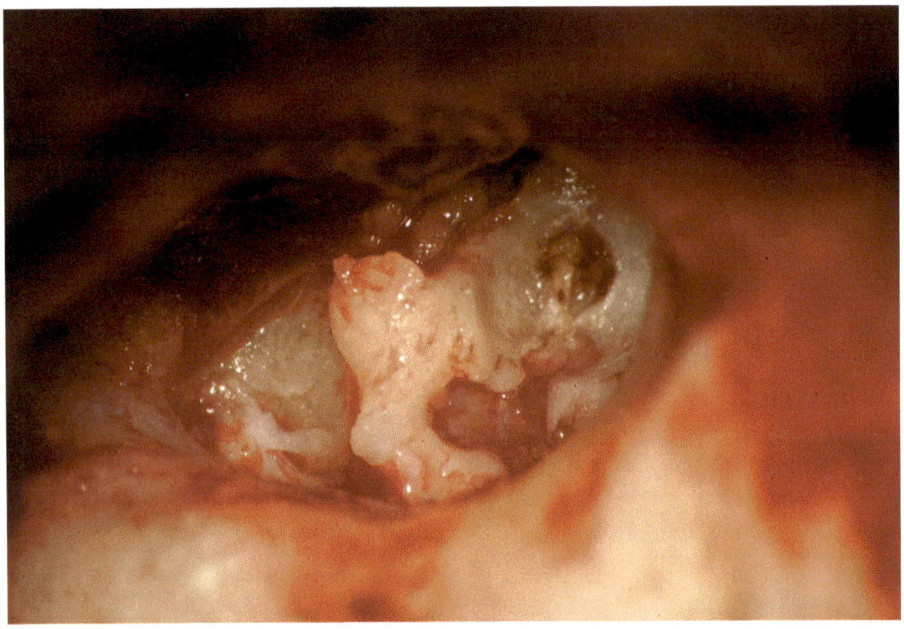

Fig. 7.9.2 At re-implantation a strange bone neoformation was found in the area of the round window niche. Now the anatomy was clearer than at explantation, which was difficult due to granulation tissue and profuse bleeding.

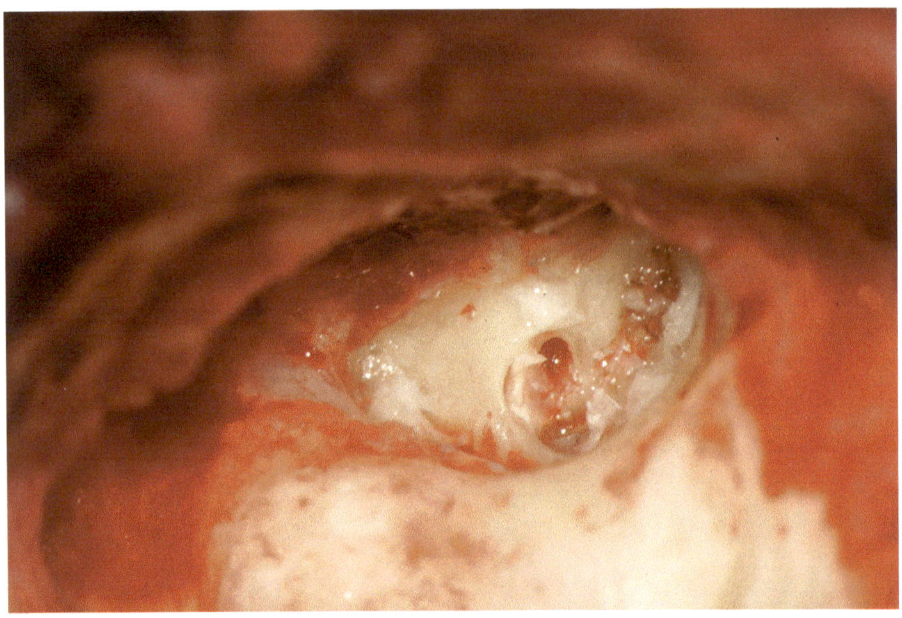

Fig. 7.9.3 The bone neoformation in the area of the round window niche was removed and the round window was opened. This bone neoformation/calcification must have developed after removal of the electrode array. Luckily, it was only at the round window.

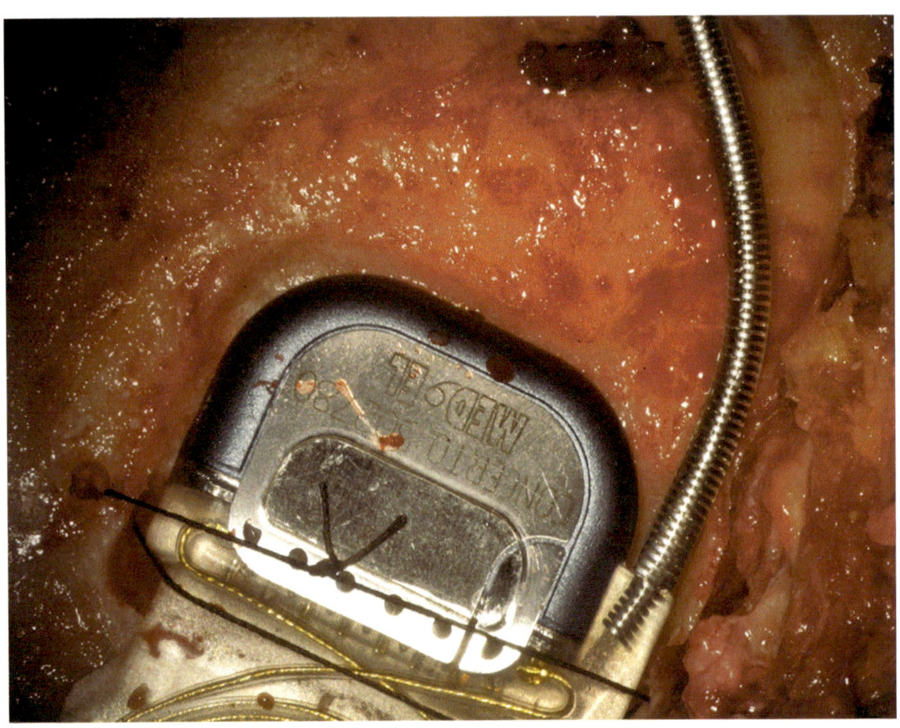

Fig. 7.9.4 A new implant was inserted in its well and fixated with a suture.

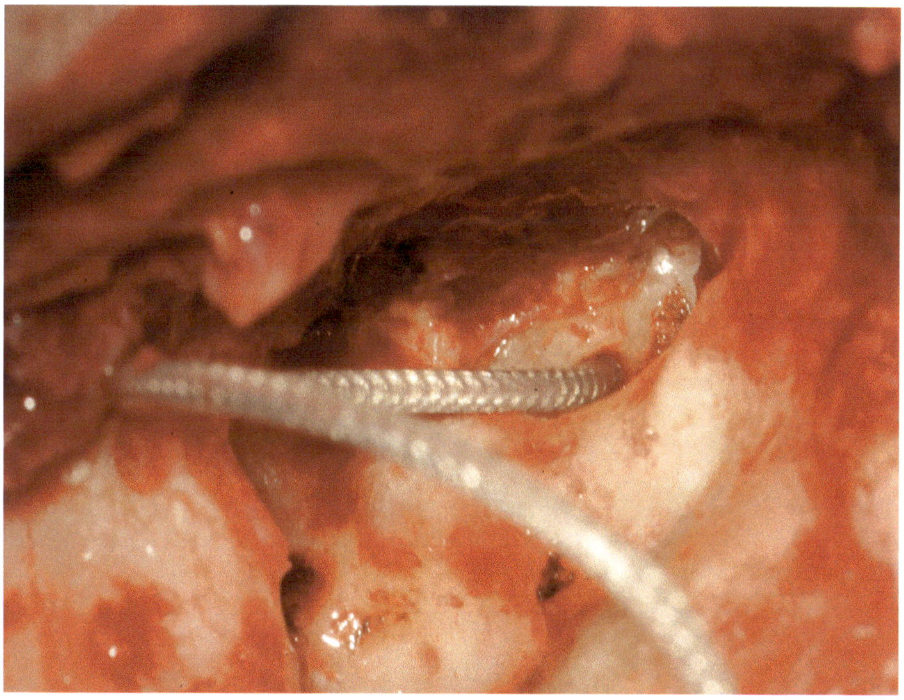

Fig. 7.9.5 The electrode was inserted and good neural response measurement achieved during surgery.

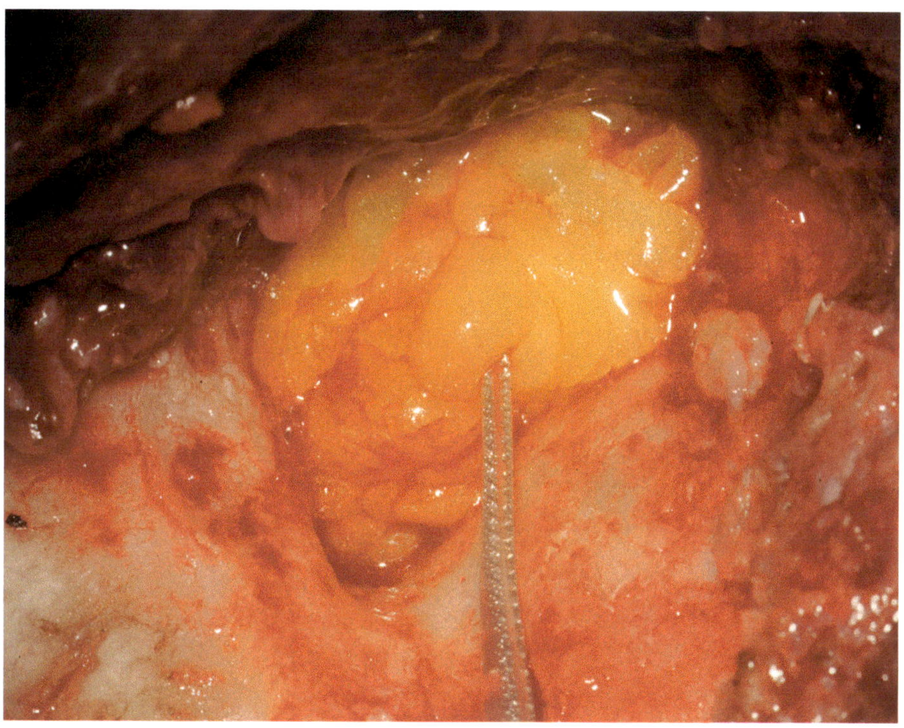

Fig. 7.9.6 The cavity was once again obliterated with fat. The postoperative course was uneventful.

Comment

A stepwise explantation and implantation is perfectly feasible and sometimes necessary in case of a fulminant infection. If possible, keep an intracochlear electrode array in place at explantation, as new bone formation can hamper re-implantation .

Case 7.10 CI Explantation and Simultaneous Re-implantation (Fig. 7.10.1–Fig. 7.10.7)

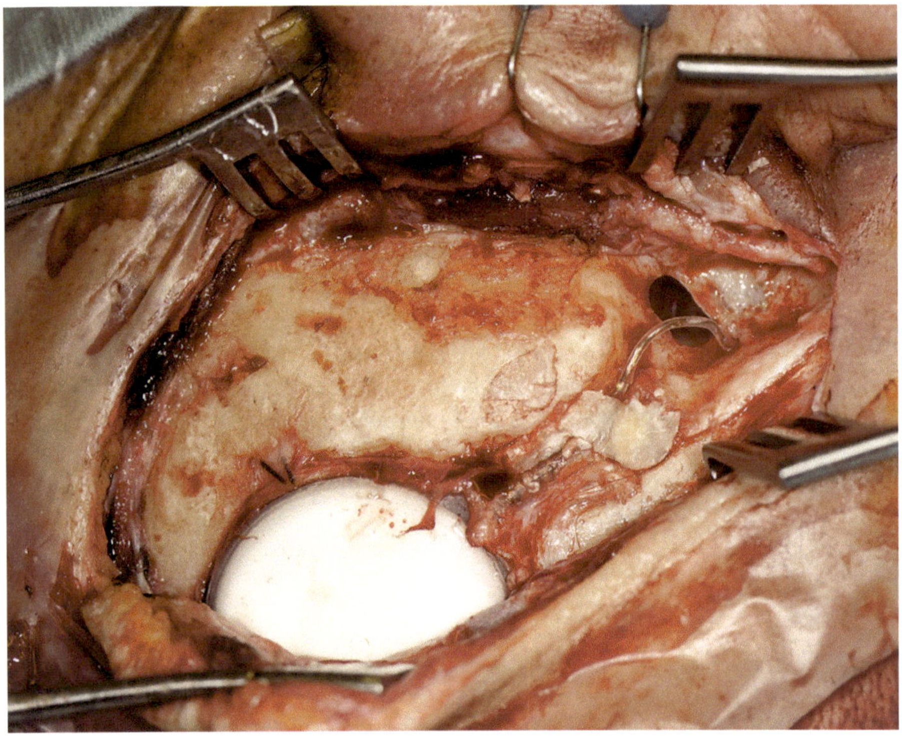

Fig. 7.10.1 A 63-year-old man had been implanted 15 years earlier. During the months before presentation some electrodes had not worked correctly and hearing performance decreased significantly. The patient was then scheduled for explantation and simultaneous re-implantation. At the beginning of the surgery the old implant was identified and exposed.

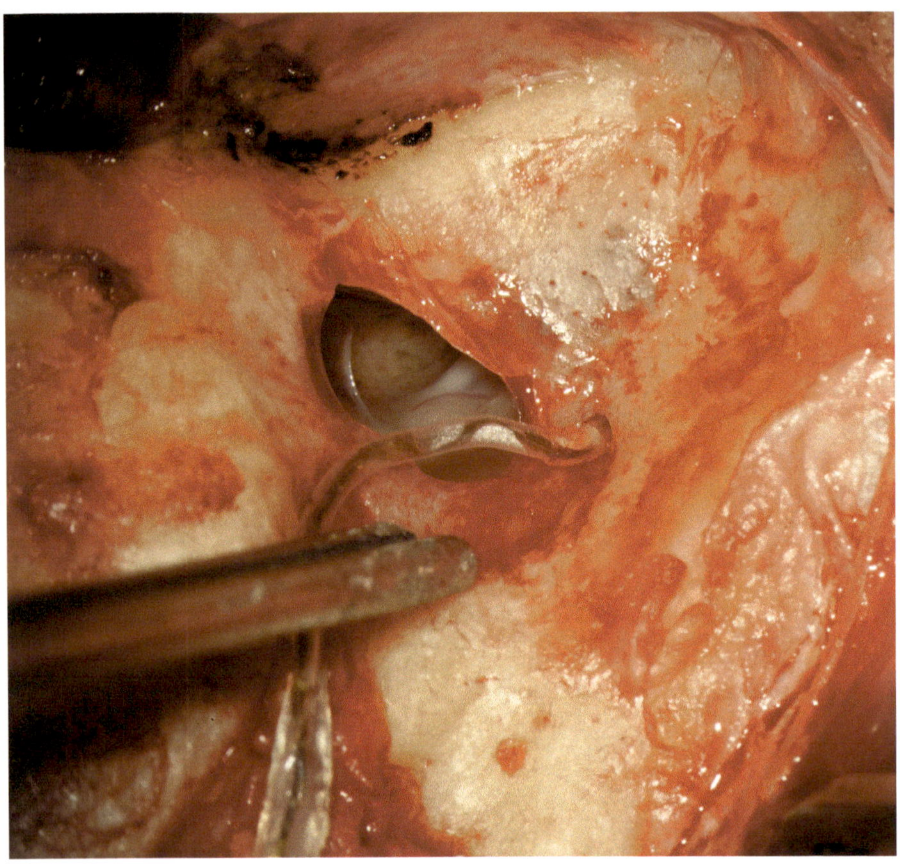

Fig. 7.10.2 At explantation it is often seen that the electrode is trapped within a new formation of cortical bone, as shown here. Stepwise removal of the bone is required to free the electrode.

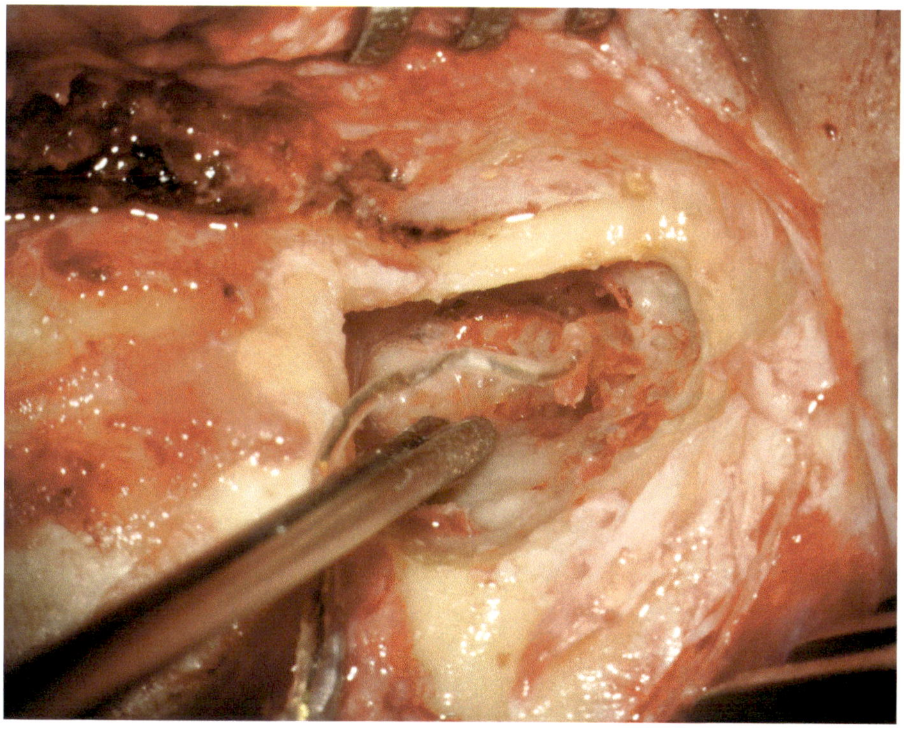

Fig. 7.10.3 In a careful and time-consuming procedure, but without damage to the electrode, the bone is removed and the electrode is ready to be further mobilized.

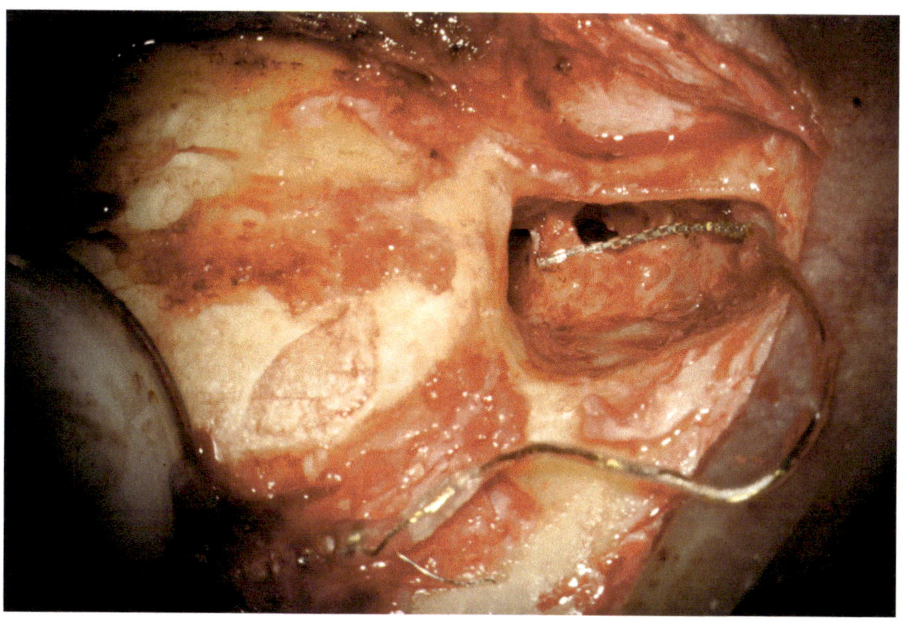

Fig. 7.10.4 Once the posterior tympanotomy is opened and the cochleostomy is seen, the electrode is removed from the cochlea.

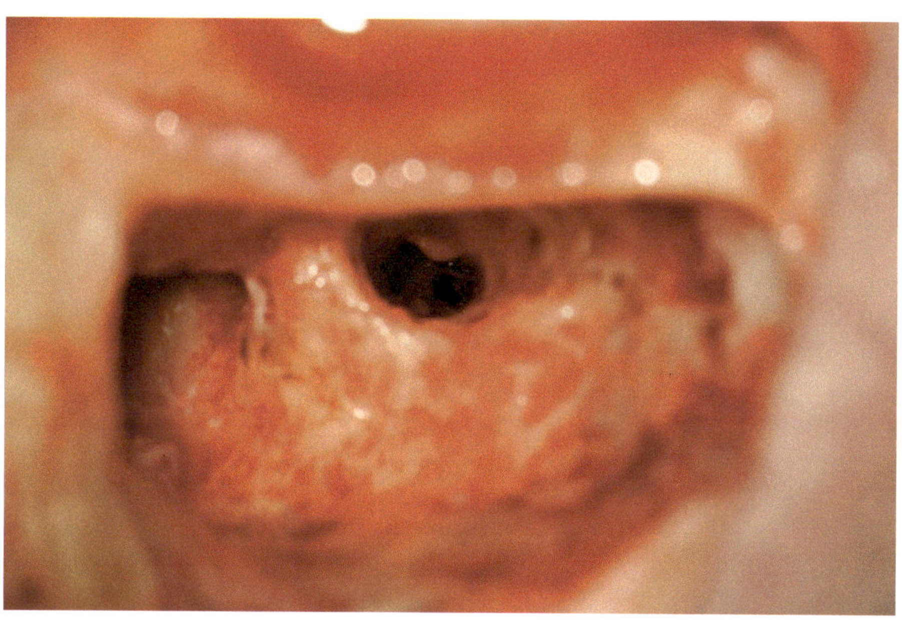

Fig. 7.10.5 The cochleostomy is inspected and fibrous tissue is removed to ensure smooth implantation. If the electrode is the same size as the old one or smaller, no problems should be expected. If there is doubt, a dummy test electrode can be used to make a "test" insertion.

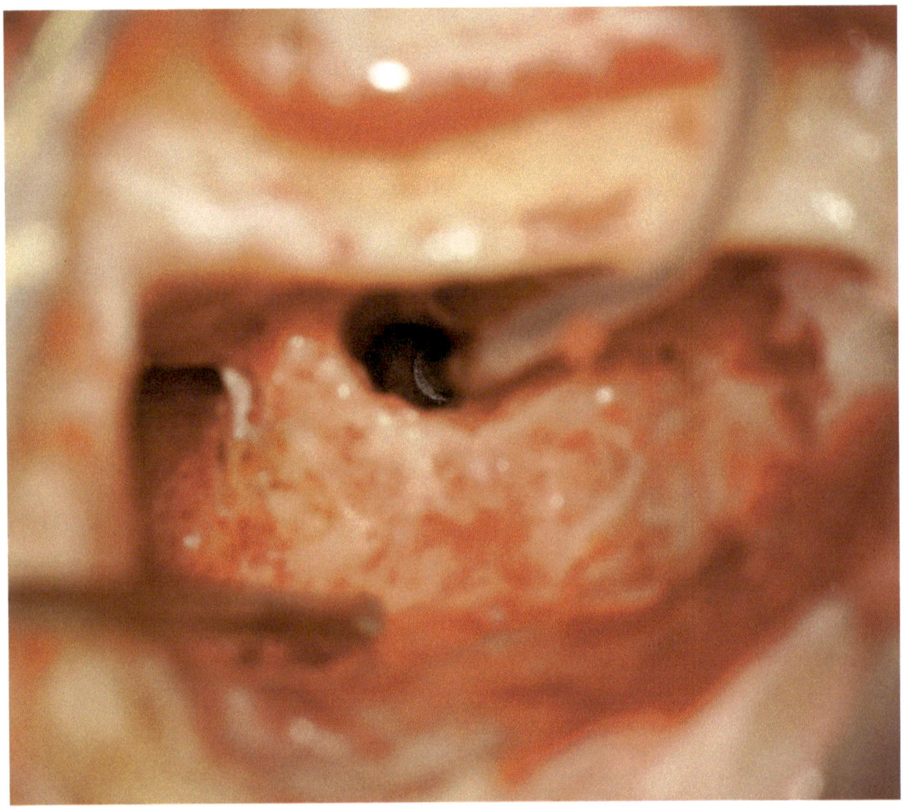

Fig. 7.10.6 The electrode is easily inserted, as shown here.

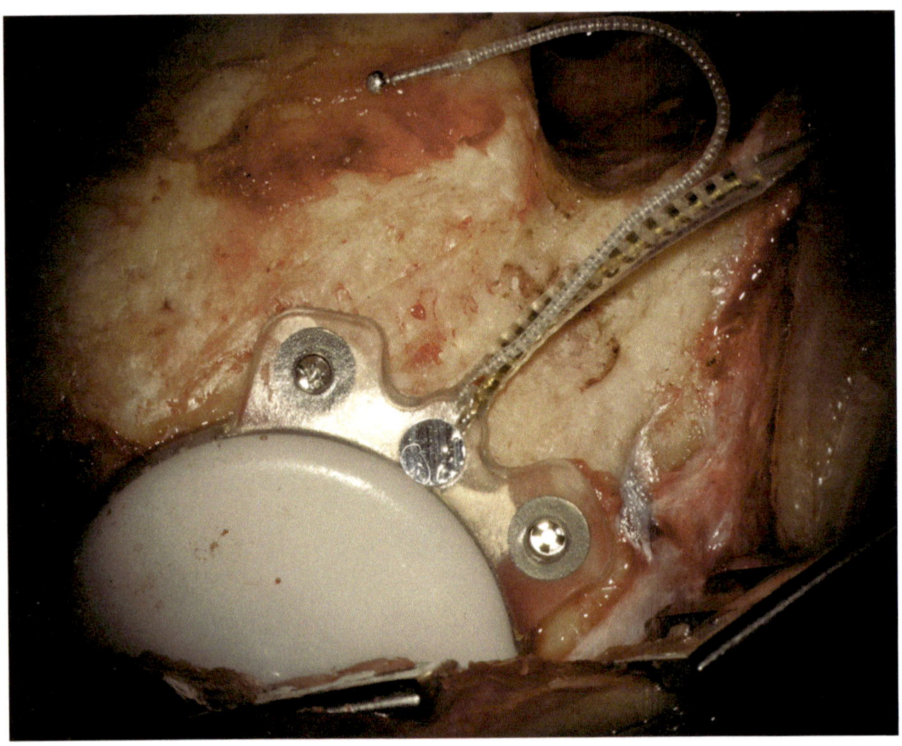

Fig. 7.10.7 The implant is secured on the skull.

Comment

A single procedure explantation and re-implantation is feasible and sometimes necessary in case of device failure. New bone formation can hamper easy explanation.

Pearls and Pitfalls in Cochlear Implantation Complications and Revision Surgery

- Complications in cochlear implantation can be divided into major and minor complications.
- Major complications need special medical attention and often hospital admission, surgery, or even explantation of the implant.
- Major complications occur in 4 to 11% of the cochlear implant surgeries.
- One of the major complications is explantation due to device failure. In children this is often associated with head trauma.
- Device failures can be divided into "hard" and "soft" device failures. Soft failure is the suspicion of a device failure without proof. Hard failure is a proven device failure.
- Other failures can be considered major medical complications as they almost always require re-implantation.
- Antibiotic therapy should be given promptly when an infection, hematoma, or seroma is seen at the implant site.
- To avoid extrusion of the implant the position of the electrode should not be immediately beneath the incision line. The incision lines through the skin and subcutis should be in different planes, preferably crossing or away from the implant and electrodes instead of directly over them.
- In a difficult case, as in postmeningitis ossification of the basal turn, the decision to perform an open approach (in a subtotal petrosectomy procedure) should be easy when misplacement of the electrode is prone.
- Re-implantation is almost always possible according to the literature, but beware in practice that it is not always smooth and easy.
- To avoid (iatrogenic) infection in CI patients, a good history and a bacterial culture of the ear canal can be taken prior to surgery. This will make an adequate preventive antibiotic regime possible.
- In a patient with recurrent otitis and/or sinusitis the best way to avoid infection is to culture prior to surgery, and administer antibiotics for (at least) 1 week with start prior to surgery. Also consider a subtotal petrosectomy with removal of all mucosal lining.
- Removal of a device without damaging the implant is difficult and often takes more time than expected; new bone formation can cover the mastoid cavity and electrodes.
- It is difficult to explant the implant and the electrodes in one piece. Sometimes a clear cut should be made of the electrode at the posterior tympanotomy and sometimes the ground electrode should be cut. New cortical bone formation is often seen around, even over, the electrode.

Reference Video

See Video 7.1.

References

1. Fayad JN, Eisenberg LS, Gillinger M, Winter M, Martinez AS, Luxford WM. Clinical performance of children following revision surgery for a cochlear implant. Otolaryngol Head Neck Surg 2006;134(3):379–384
2. Achiques MT, Morant A, Muñoz N, et al. [Cochlear implant complications and failures]. [Article in Spanish]. Acta Otorrinolaringol Esp 2010;61(6):412–417
3. Masterson L, Kumar S, Kong JH, et al. Cochlear implant failures: lessons learned from a UK centre. J Laryngol Otol 2012;126(1):15–21
4. Hoffman RA, Cohen NL. Complications of cochlear implant surgery. Ann Otol Rhinol Laryngol Suppl 1995;166:420–422
5. Ovesen T, Johansen LV. Post-operative problems and complications in 313 consecutive cochlear implantations. J Laryngol Otol 2009;123(5):492–496
6. Postelmans JTF, Cleffken B, Stokroos RJ. Post-operative complications of cochlear implantation in adults and children: five years' experience in Maastricht. J Laryngol Otol 2007;121(4):318–323
7. Cohen NL, Hoffman RA, Stroschein M. Medical or surgical complications related to the Nucleus multichannel cochlear implant. Ann Otol Rhinol Laryngol Suppl 1988;135:8–13
8. Bhatia K, Gibbin KP, Nikolopoulos TP, O'Donoghue GM. Surgical complications and their management in a series of 300 consecutive pediatric cochlear implantations. Otol Neurotol 2004;25(5):730–739
9. Gosepath J, Lippert K, Keilmann A, Mann WJ. Analysis of fifty-six cochlear implant device failures. ORL J Otorhinolaryngol Relat Spec 2009;71(3):142–147
10. Cohen NL, Hoffman RA. Surgical complications of multichannel cochlear implants in North America. Adv Otorhinolaryngol 1993;48:70–74
11. Beadle EA, McKinley DJ, Nikolopoulos TP, Brough J, O'Donoghue GM, Archbold SM. Long-term functional outcomes and academic-occupational status in implanted children after 10 to 14 years of cochlear implant use. Otol Neurotol 2005;26(6):1152–1160
12. Battmer RD, Linz B, Lenarz T. A review of device failure in more than 23 years of clinical experience of a cochlear implant program with more than 3,400 implantees. Otol Neurotol 2009;30(4):455–463
13. European consensus statement on cochlear implant failures and explantations. Otol Neurotol 2005;26(6):1097–1099
14. Battmer RD, Backous DD, Balkany TJ, et al; International Consensus Group for Cochlear Implant Reliability Reporting. International classification of reliability for implanted cochlear implant receiver stimulators. Otol Neurotol 2010;31(8):1190–1193
15. Rivas A, Marlowe AL, Chinnici JE, Niparko JK, Francis HW. Revision cochlear implantation surgery in adults: indications and results. Otol Neurotol 2008;29(5):639–648
16. Balkany TJ, Hodges AV, Buchman CA, et al. Cochlear implant soft failures consensus development conference statement. Otol Neurotol 2005;26(4):815–818
17. Marlowe AL, Chinnici JE, Rivas A, Niparko JK, Francis HW. Revision cochlear implant surgery in children: the Johns Hopkins experience. Otol Neurotol 2010;31(1):74–82
18. Sparreboom M, van Schoonhoven J, van Zanten BG, et al. The effectiveness of bilateral cochlear implants for severe-to-profound deafness in children: a systematic review. Otol Neurotol 2010;31(7):1062–1071
19. Hoep LS, Merkus P, van Schie A, Rinkel RN, Smit CF. The value of nuclear scans in cochlear implant infections. Eur Arch Otorhinolaryngol 2006;263(10):895–899
20. Antonelli PJ, Lee JC, Burne RA. Bacterial biofilms may contribute to persistent cochlear implant infection. Otol Neurotol 2004;25(6):953–957
21. Merkus P, van Loon MC, Smit CF, Smits C, de Cock AFC, Hensen EF. Decision making in advanced otosclerosis: an evidence-based strategy. Laryngoscope 2011;121(9):1935–1941
22. Toung JS, Zwolan T, Spooner TR, Telian SA. Late failure of cochlear-implantation resulting from advanced cochlear otosclerosis: surgical andprogramming challenges. Otol Neurotol 2004;25(5):723–726
23. Ozmen OA, Falcioni M, Lauda L, Sanna M. Outcomes of facial nerve grafting in 155 cases: predictive value of history and preoperative function. Otol Neurotol 2011;32(8):1341–1346

8 Auditory Brainstem Implantation

8.1 Rationale

Auditory brainstem implantation was originally designed for patients deafened by neurofibromatosis type 2 (NF2) to regain meaningful hearing. However, it can also be indicated in other conditions and has been shown to be useful.[1,2] The auditory brain implant (ABI) device is similar in design and function to a cochlear implant (CI) but its implantation requires a more extended approach gaining access to the brainstem to position the ABI in contact with the cochlear nucleus.[3] Current multichannel ABI technology affords a level of performance in aided speech comprehension but may also just provide a signal function. After programming and training, ~85% of patients experience auditory perception with their ABIs and between 44 and 97% of the ABI-implanted patients do actually use their implants.[4] The results are unpredictable, however, and overall are worse than those with a cochlear implant.[4] Nonetheless, the majority will develop the ability to recognize environmental sounds and the ABI facilitates lip-reading skills.[3]

As well as NF2, several other indications have been reported over the years and seem plausible in cases were no cochlear implant or other means of auditory rehabilitation can be used. Proper diagnostic evaluation needs to be performed before a decision to implant an ABI can be made. Given the current outcomes of auditory brainstem implantation compared with the good and reliable outcomes of cochlear implantation, placement of a CI as the choice for hearing restoration always has to be contemplated first. In many cases a stepwise strategy is appropriate; sometimes a stepwise surgical strategy may have to be completed before a decision about auditory brainstem implantation can be considered.

8.2 Indications

8.2.1 Neurofibromatosis Type 2

NF2 is the most common indication for auditory brainstem implantation,[3,4] but careful counseling is necessary as in some cases of NF2 cochlear implantation might still be possible, depending on the integrity and functionality of the cochlear nerve. Sometimes the decision for ABI or CI has to be taken during surgery.[5–11] See Chapter 16.

8.2.2 Postmeningitis Ossification

In case of bilateral ossified cochleae ABI implantation is only indicated when both cochleae are fully ossified, confirmed by scanning *and* by surgery; a cochlear drill-out procedure is needed to assess whether cochlear implantation is not an option. Since 2003, several papers have discussed this indication for ABI implantation in cases of postmeningitic ossified cochleae.[2,12–14] All point out that a drill-out procedure with an attempt at CI insertion should precede ABI placement.

In *acute meningitis* the hearing should be evaluated early and frequently (see Chapter 12) and MRI should be performed if hearing loss is confirmed. With these precautions, cochlear implantation in the postmeningitic deafened patients can be safeguarded before total obliteration of the cochlea has occurred.[15]

In cases presented *months to years after having had meningitis*, MRI will provide the most reliable information on the patency of the cochlea.[16,17]

When partial or total ossification is present, cochlear implantation surgery should be scheduled and various strategies, such as scala vestibuli insertion,[18,19] partial insertion,[20] basal turn drill-out, or double array insertion,[21] should be considered (see Chapters 11 and 12). If no cochlear lumen can be found during the drill-out procedure, one may convert to translabyrinthine approach for ABI implantation or schedule a separate ABI implantation.

8.2.3 Inner Ear Malformation

In the most common inner ear malformations, such as incomplete partition type 2, common cavity, and other conditions, a cochlear lumen is present.[22] In these cases cochlear implantation is the preferred type of rehabilitation—with the proviso that the cochlear nerve is present—as it has shown to be beneficial in these patients.[23–25] When no cochlear lumen is present or it is insufficient in both ears (i.e., cochlear aplasia, cochlear hypoplasia), a primary indication for an ABI emerges.[1,26] These cases sometimes are associated with a small internal auditory canal and with hypoplasia or aplasia of the cochlear nerve on imaging. Before a final decision to implant (CI or ABI) the existence of a (vestibulo) cochlear nerve should be assessed.[27–29] See Chapter 15.

8.2.4 Cochlear Nerve Aplasia/Cochlear Nerve Deficiency

Vestibulocochlear malformations are often associated with a small internal auditory canal and coupled with hypoplasia or aplasia of the cochlear nerve as seen on imaging.[1] Hypoplasia or even aplasia of the nerve can also be found in solitary cases.[30]

Nevertheless, recent publications point out that the absence of a visible cochlear nerve on imaging does not preclude auditory innervation of the cochlea in some cases.[27–29] Cochlear implantation can be a valuable option for patients with apparent cochlear nerve aplasia as long as they have undergone appropriate audiometric testing.[27,29] Use of electrically evoked ABRs is critical in the evaluation of this group of patients.[27,31,32]

If there is proof of a bilateral absence of the cochlear nerve (on scanning), and possible cochlear nerve fibers (not clear on scanning) cannot be stimulated, or if there is a complete cochlear aplasia or a bilateral Michel deformity, ABI can be the only solution to provide some chance of hearing development.[1] It seems that in the majority of inner ear malformations there is no primary indication for an ABI[33] (see Chapter 15).

8.3 Controversial Indications

8.3.1 Otic Capsule Fracture and Cochlear Nerve Avulsion

Two possible causes of total bilateral deafness after blunt head trauma are mentioned in the literature in relation to ABI: a bilateral posttraumatic fracture of the cochlea/labyrinth or cochlear nerve avulsion. Several patients with posttraumatic deafness, diagnosed as either bilateral fracture or cochlear nerve avulsion, have been implanted with an ABI. These indications are true controversial ABI indications as discussed in literature[33] and in the following two sections.

Otic Capsule Fracture

A fracture of the petrosal bone can be otic capsule–sparing or otic capsule–involving. When the otic capsule is involved in the fracture, total deafness usually occurs. In very rare cases both otic capsules could be fractured, resulting in total bilateral deafness. As soon as the patient is recovering from this huge trauma, occurrence of inflammation and finally ossification of the cochlea should be assessed with CT and especially with MRI to evaluate the patency of the cochlea, as in patients with meningitis. In our opinion, there is an indication for an ABI in cases with complete ossification of both cochleae and after unsuccessful cochlear drill-out attempts (bilateral). In the literature not a single case has been demonstrated with bilateral complete ossification due to head trauma, so this indication for an ABI remains hypothetical. Cochlear implantation is the means of auditory rehabilitation in cases of bilateral otic capsule fractures.[34–37]

Cochlear Nerve Avulsion

The other theoretically valid indication reported for an ABI in deafness due to trauma is bilateral avulsion of the cochlear nerve.[38] This indication has also been mentioned in the consensus paper on the indications of ABI.[26] Surprisingly, in a literature review of all neuroradiologic papers or books concerning this topic there has been reported only a single case presenting a *unilateral* nerve rupture.[39] Cochlear nerve avulsion *in both ears* has never been reported and seems practically impossible without fatal damage to the head and brain. Accordingly, the indication for ABI for this specific entity seems very unlikely (see Chapter 15).

8.3.2 Bilateral or Unilateral Patent Cochlea

Auditory brainstem implantation is not primarily indicated in severe to profoundly deaf patients with an intact nerve and an open cochlea; for these patients cochlear implantation is the first option. Even if the result with a CI is not as good as hoped for or as predicted, the option of refitting/reprogramming the processor, replacing the ipsilateral, or evaluating the contralateral ear for cochlear implantation should be contemplated, before even considering an ABI because a CI in general gives better outcomes in hearing restoration than an ABI[33].

8.3.3 Vestibular Schwannoma in the Only Hearing Ear

In patients with a vestibular schwannoma (VS) in the only hearing ear there seems to be few indications for an ABI. The contralateral deaf ear is almost always compatible for a CI, although the results with a CI will depend on the duration of deafness and more specifically on the development of the auditory pathways serviced by that cochlear nerve. Many options are possible before auditory brainstem implantation enters the picture.[40] The options before surgery of the VS in these cases are: a hearing aid in that ear if surgery can wait, or a cochlear implant in the contralateral ear.[41] The result of cochlear implantation can sometimes be poor, which suggests subsequent auditory brainstem implantation during the tumor removal procedure.[42] However, it does not seem proper to implant an ABI before a contralateral CI has been tried. Two other options should be considered prior to surgery of the tumor: radiotherapy or cochlear implantation on the VS side without tumor removal. Also several options during surgical removal of the VS are possible: the hearing may be preserved during the removal of a small VS[11]; or the cochlear nerve may be preserved and a CI implanted in the same ear[43]; or the tumor may be debulked and a CI inserted. A primary ABI indication seems less favorable in regard to all the above-mentioned options in patients with a VS in the only hearing ear (see Chapters 16 and 17).

8.3.4 Autoimmune Inner Ear Disease

Ossification of the cochlea can occur in autoimmune inner ear diseases similarly to that in postmeningitis cases, but bilateral fully ossified cochleae in these cases have not been reported.[44] See Chapter 11.

8.3.5 Von Hippel–Lindau Disease

In general, Von Hippel-Lindau disease is associated with endolymphatic sac tumors that can destroy the labyrinth and the temporal bone. Bilateral complete destruction of the labyrinth including the cochlea appears to be very exceptional but would represent an ABI indication. However, successful CI placement in similar cases with Von Hippel-Lindau disease have been published.[45]

8.3.6 Auditory Neuropathy

Auditory neuropathy spectrum disease (ANSD) is also mentioned as an ABI indication in the literature.[38] However, this little-known diagnostic entity presents predominantly with a normal cochlea and an intact cochlear nerve. The precise location of the pathology in ANSD is variable, making cochlear implantation an option only for some patients. In patients, mostly children, with ANSD the stepwise rehabilitation should be: hearing aids; cochlear implant; and if the young patient still does not show adequate improvement or when speech and language development has reached a standstill, ABI could then be an option. Thorough and careful analysis and counseling of these patients should be performed as in this variable disease decisions are very individually based. The literature shows average to good results in patients with ANSD and a CI.[46,47]

8.3.7 Otosclerosis

In severe retrofenestral otosclerosis, the temporal bone shows otospongiotic hypodense lesions around the otic capsule and at the same time often intracochlear ossification, most prominently present in the scala tympani.[48] These lesions can hamper the insertion of a cochlear implant and create potential risks, as explained in Chapter 13.[49–51]

Despite these potential complications, cochlear implantation still remains the first choice in hearing rehabilitation in patients with otosclerosis and severe to profound sensorineural hearing loss.[33]

8.4 Indications for ABI/CI: Summary

Auditory brainstem implantation presents a solution for hearing revalidation in a very limited group of patients. The outcomes in hearing with an ABI at present are unpredictable and in general worse than with a CI, which limits the value an ABI. In general, if a patent cochlea and a cochlear nerve are present the first choice for hearing restoring would be cochlear implantation.

ABI is indicated in

- NF2 patients when the cochlear nerve is not preserved and the contralateral ear has no functional hearing.
- NF2 patients when the cochlear nerve is preserved but stimulation via a cochlear implant is not possible.
- Completely ossified cochleae; but a cochlear implantation with drill-out procedure should be attempted first.
- Absence of the cochlear nerve proven on scanning and in audiometric testing.
- Bilateral complete cochlear aplasia (Michel deformity).

CI is first choice of treatment in

- Normal cochlea and cochlear nerve present.
- Posttraumatic deafness.
- Otosclerosis.
- Most of the malformations of the cochlea with some sort of cochlear lumen, in presence of a cochlear nerve.
- Solitary vestibular schwannoma in the only hearing ear (several options of alternative treatment possible).
- Autoimmune inner ear disease, Von Hippel–Lindau disease, auditory neuropathy spectrum disorders (ANSD).

8.5 Surgical Steps of Auditory Brainstem Implantation

8.5.1 Surgical Anatomy

The surgical anatomy of the lateral skull base, brainstem, and cochlear nucleus is addressed in detail in Chapter 2. Since the ABI relies on the electrical stimulation of the cochlear nucleus complex for the perception and recognition of speech, the surgical goal of auditory brainstem implantation is to position the electrode array correctly against the surface of the cochlear nuclei in the lateral recess of the fourth ventricle. Usually, the intraventricular part of the ventral cochlear nucleus and the dorsal cochlear nucleus are both stimulated, although the ventral cochlear nucleus has the best connections with the auditory pathway. The extraventricular ventral cochlear nucleus represents the continuation of the root of the eighth cranial nerve. Access to the lateral recess of the fourth ventricle is gained through the foramen of Luschka (see **Fig. 8.1–Fig. 8.3**).

Landmarks of the Lateral Recess

- Origin of the vestibulocochlear and glossopharyngeal nerve
- The flocculus of the cerebellum
- The choroid plexus exiting the foramen of Luschka (this is the most reliable landmark according to our experience).

It should be emphasized that the anatomy can be distorted in presence of a tumor. The simplest way to identify the foramen of Luschka is to follow the vestibulocochlear nerve proximally. Even when the nerve is transected, its stump can be identified and followed similarly. The cochlear nucleus extends from the floor of the fourth ventricle medially to the entry zone of the vestibulocochlear nerve at the posterolateral surface of the brainstem. The dorsal cochlear nucleus can be seen as a prominence; the auditory tubercle in the anterior wall ("floor") of the lateral recess. The ninth nerve is located just inferiorly to the eighth nerve. The apex of the angle formed by two nerves indicates the inferior margin of the foramen of Luschka.

The choroid plexus projects from the fourth ventricle and exits through the Luschka foramen. Retracting the choroid plexus and flocculus posterior-laterally will give better access to the foramen. This is confirmed by cerebrospinal fluid coming through the foramen when the intracranial pressure is increased by the anesthesiologist on request.

The proposed surgical position of the electrode carrier in relation to the cochlear nucleus and the lateral recess as well as to other cranial nerve nuclei is explained in detail in Chapter 2.

8.5.2 Surgical Approach

The ABI is inserted through an extended translabyrinthine approach (ETLA). The ETLA offers the best angle of approach and direct access to the lateral recess of the fourth ventricle, as previously decribed.[4] A gentle retraction of the flocculus is enough to expose the root of the eighth cranial nerve and choroid plexus. In the retrosigmoidal approach, significantly more retraction of the cerebellum and flocculus is required to visualize these structures because of the angulations. In the translabyrinthine approach, either CPA tumor removal or a cochlear implantation attempt can be performed prior to ABI placement. The retrosigmoid approach for ABI placement will not be described in this book. In some cases the final decision whether to place a CI or an ABI is taken only during surgery. When a CI is attempted first, usually the approach is combined with a subtotal petrosectomy.

8.5.3 Intraoperative Monitoring

Intraoperative monitoring is addressed in detail in Chapter 4. For several reasons, intraoperative monitoring of evoked auditory potentials and monitoring of the trigeminal, facial, and glossopharyngeal nerves are crucial during placement of ABIs. Monitoring of electrical ABR can corroborate accurate electrode placement, whereas monitoring of neighboring cranial nerves may detect inadvertent stimulation of regional structures.

In intraoperative electrical ABR monitoring, the first wave of the ABR observed will be wave III, which represents the cochlear nuclei. Ideally, three waves would be expected: those of the cochlear nuclei (III), the olivary nuclei (IV), and the nuclei of the lateral lemniscus (V). In practice, one to three responses, termed P1–P3, are usually seen. The presence of one or more responses helps corroborate proper electrode placement. No correlations between the number or quality of waveform responses (i.e., P1, P2, and P3) and the efficacy of the ABI have been found, but the number of electrodes functioning is related to the accuracy of array location as well as to hearing outcome.

It should also be noted that electrical ABR monitoring is understood more as an adjunct to anatomical means for localizing the cochlear nuclei. Its role is rather to confirm that the ABI correctly stimulates the cochlear nuclei. Insofar as the surgeon is confident of adequate electrode placement on the basis of reliable anatomical landmarks, even the complete absence of ABR waves does not necessarily predict that the ABI will fail to impart useful hearing.

8.6 Surgical Anatomy in Auditory Brainstem Implantation (Fig. 8.1–Fig. 8.3)

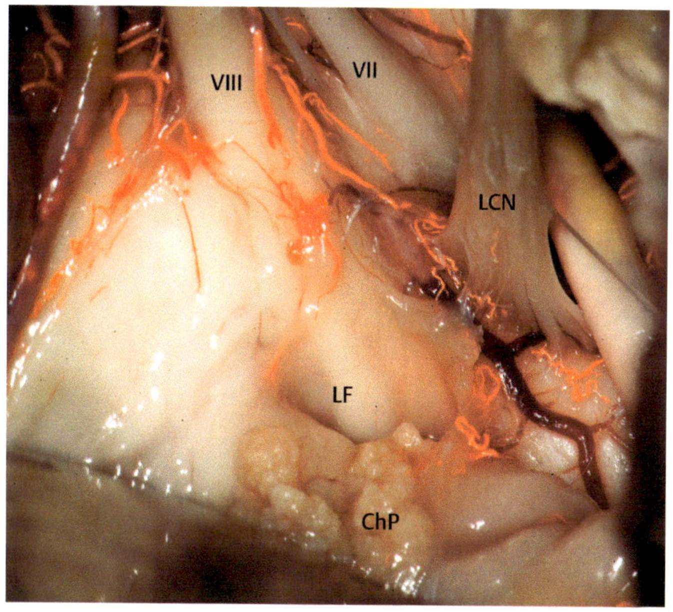

Fig. 8.1 Microscopic view of the foramen of Luschka on an injected specimen. ChP, choroid plexus; VII, facial nerve; VIII, vestibulocochlear nerve; LCN, lower cranial nerves; LF, foramen of Luschka.

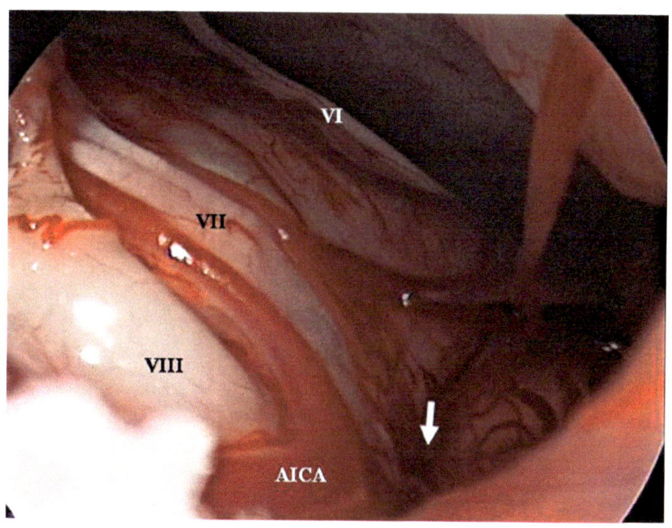

Fig. 8.2 Endoscopic view of the foramen of Luschka (*arrow*). The bulbopontine junction is clearly appreciated. AICA, anterior inferior cerebellar artery; VI, abducens nerve; VII, facial nerve; VIII, vestibulocochlear nerve.

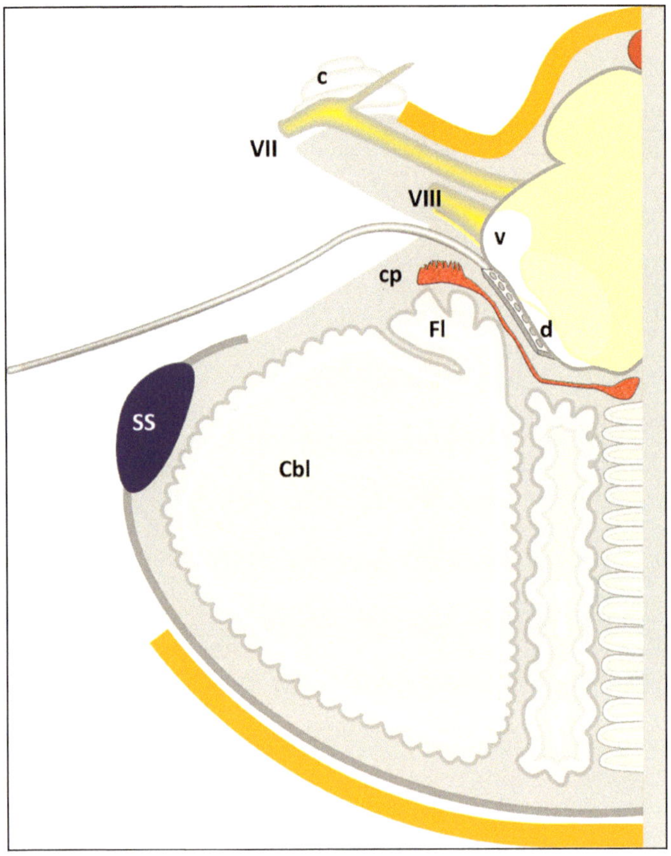

Fig. 8.3 Anatomy of the fourth ventricle and the lateral recess and the location of the cochlear nuclei. This schematic illustration shows an ideal placement of an array of electrodes. The choroid plexus (cp) is shown in red. Cbl, cerebellum; d, dorsal cochlear nucleus; Fl, flocculus; SS, sigmoid sinus; v, ventral cochlear nucleus; VII, facial nerve; VIII, stump of the vestibulocochlear nerve; c, cochlea.

8.7 Surgical Steps in Auditory Brainstem Implantation (Fig. 8.4–Fig. 8.9)

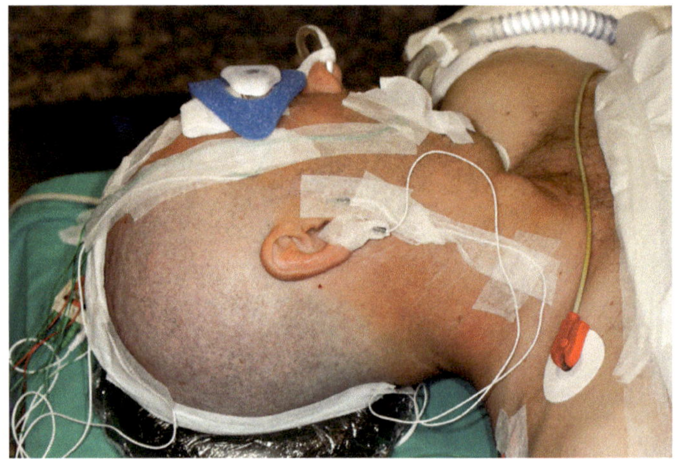

Fig. 8.4 This patient has been prepared for a translabyrinthine ABI placement with monitoring via ABR electrodes and facial nerve electrodes.

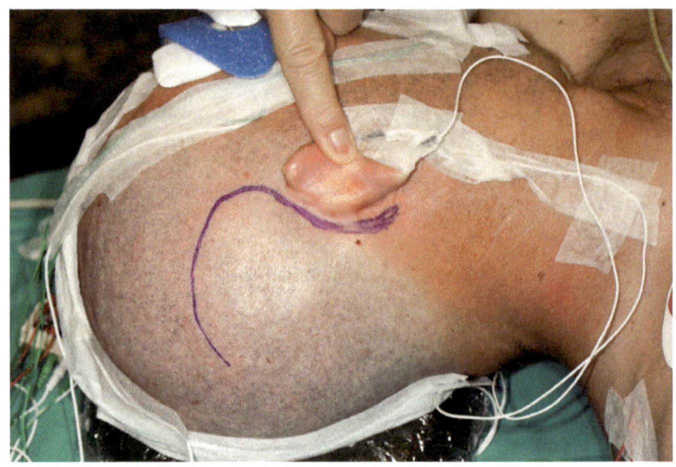

Fig. 8.5 Incision line. S-shaped incision starting just on the mastoid tip and at least 5 cm above the pinna. If previous ear surgery has been performed enlargement of the old incision should be attempted, to avoid skin necrosis due to insufficient blood supply to the skin flap.

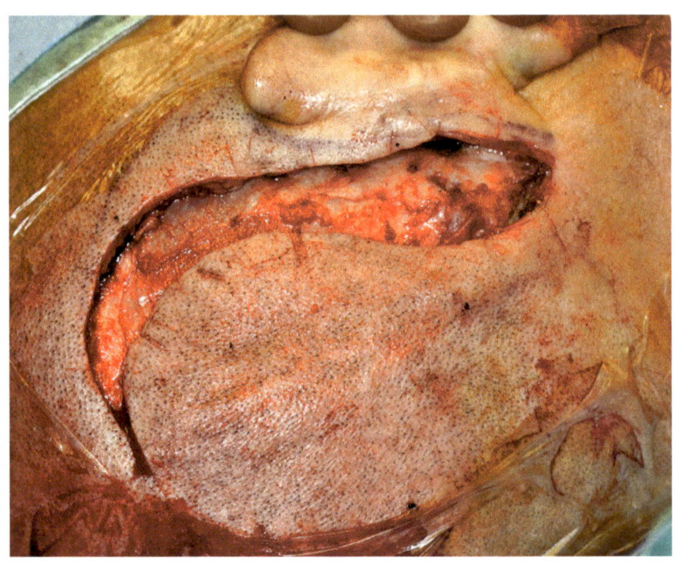

Fig. 8.6 Incision of the skin. First, small skin cuts perpendicular to the incision are made at different locations along the incision line for easier suturing later on. Then the cutaneous and subcutaneous layers are cut, just onto the fascia of the temporal muscle.

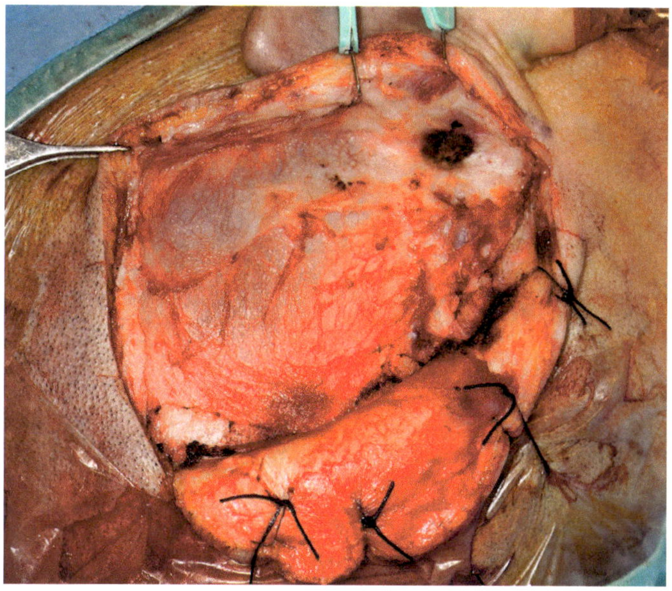

Fig. 8.7 Deflection of the skin flap and development of the cranial-based temporal muscle flap is shown. Before the temporal muscle is deflected, the ear canal is transected.

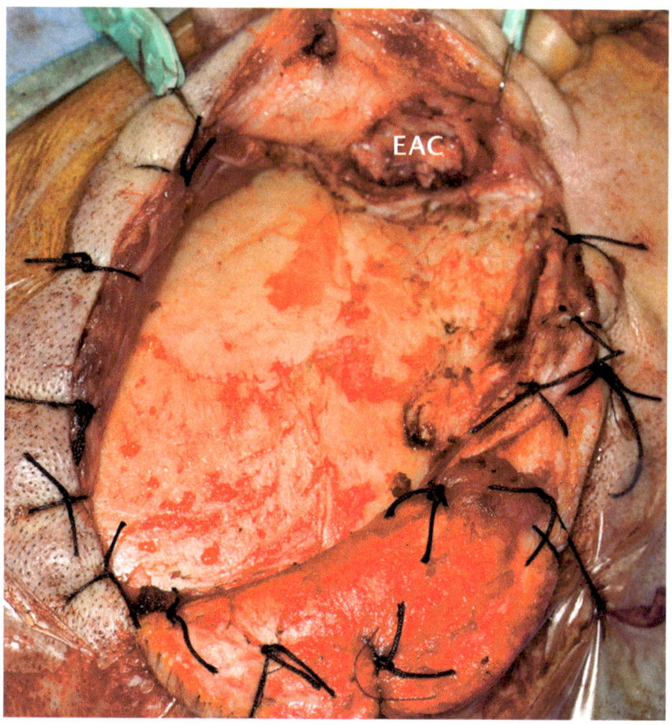

Fig. 8.8 The external auditory canal (EAC) has been cut and the temporal muscle is deflected cranially and secured with firm stitches. The muscle should be preserved as it is needed to cover the complete surgical cavity during closure.

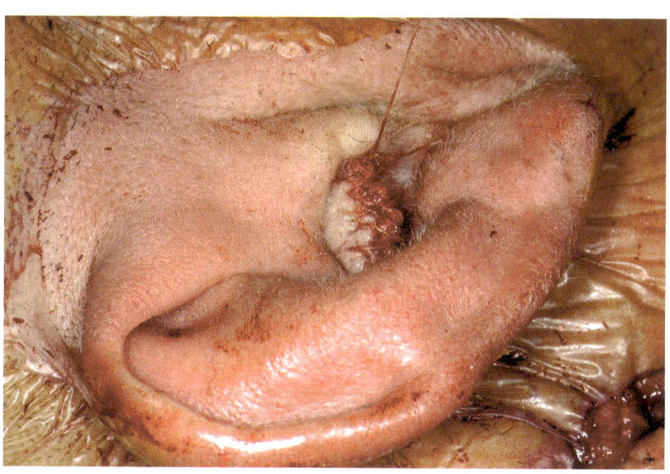

Fig. 8.9 The external auditory canal is closed in several layers in the same fashion as in subtotal petrosectomy approach (see Chapter 10).

8.8 Surgical Steps According to the Indication (Fig. 8.10–Fig. 8.36)

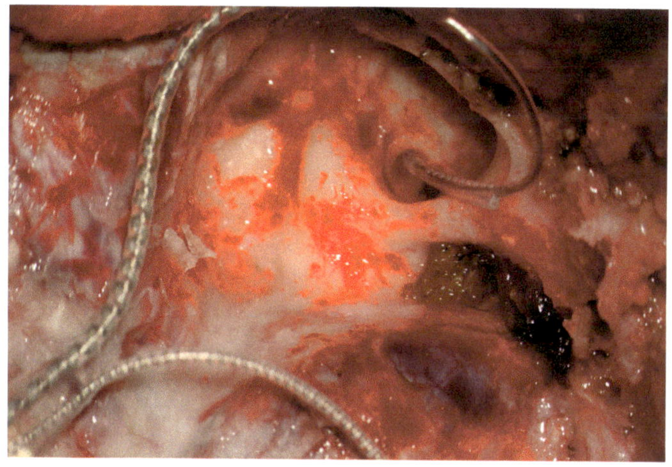

Fig. 8.10 Cochlear implant attempt. In some cases cochlear implantation should be attempted first (cochlear malformation, cochlear nerve deficiency). In case of unsuccessful CI placement (malformation/ossification) or no reaction on EABR, the approach is extended to implant an ABI (see text, Chapter 15 for explanation).

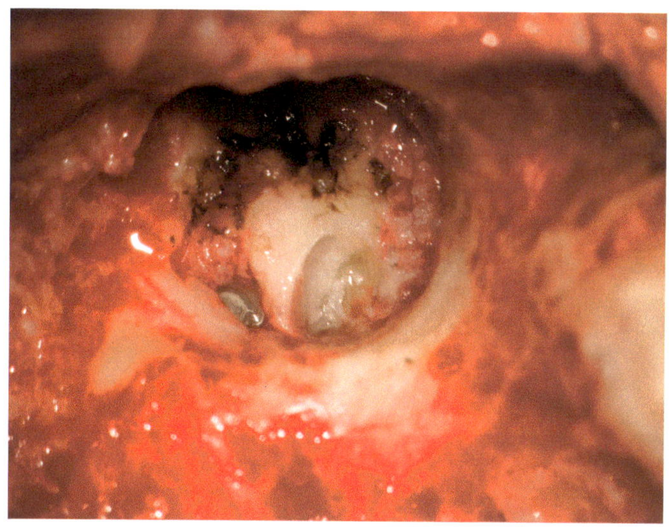

Fig. 8.11 Cochlear drill-out. In some cases there is an attempt at cochlear implantation in an ossified cochlea (see text, Chapters 11 and 12 for explanation).

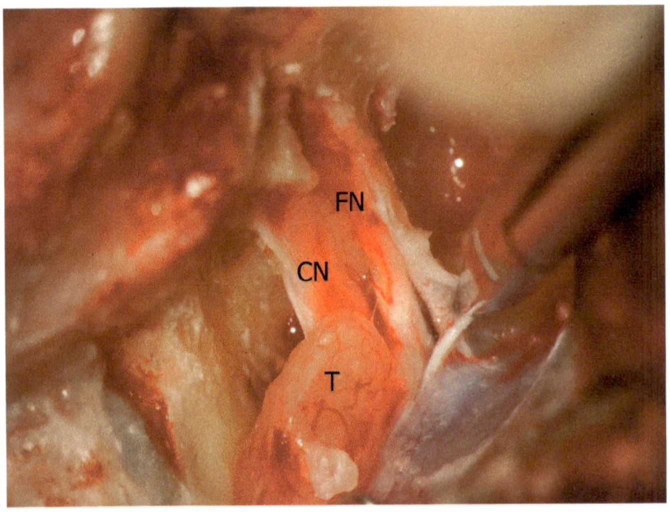

Fig. 8.12 Tumor removal. In some cases it is possible to remove the tumor in a translabyrinthine approach and preserve the cochlear nerve. The functionality of the nerve is essential in making the decision whether to place a CI or an ABI. FN, facial nerve; CN, cochlear nerve; T, tumor.

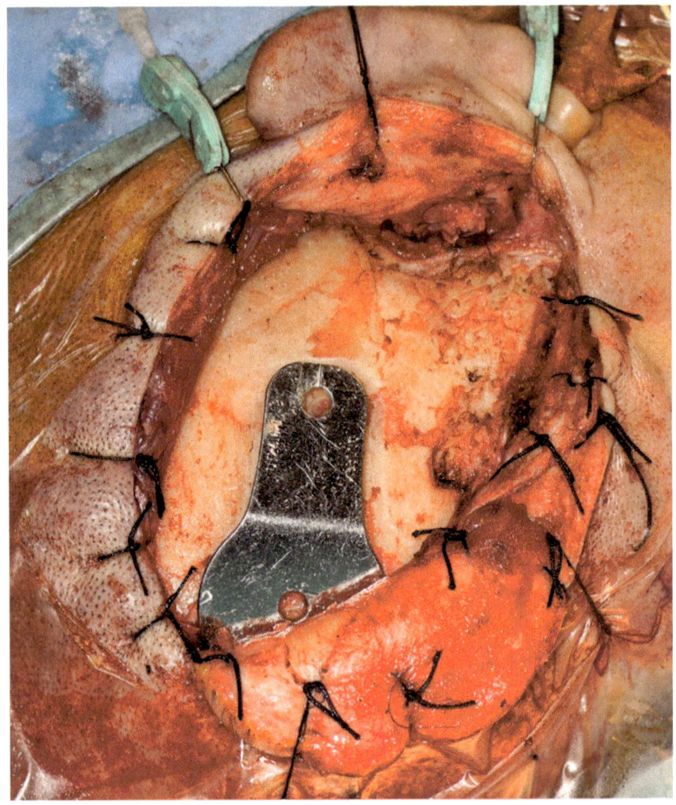

Fig. 8.13 If the decision to place an ABI has been made, the location of the receiver-stimulator well can be drawn on the skull.

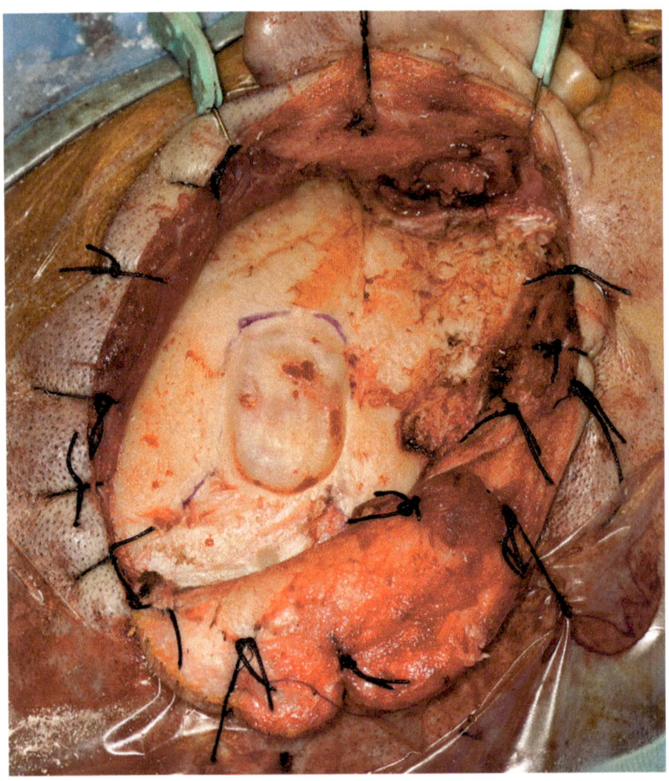

Fig. 8.14 The receiver-stimulator well has been drilled to accommodate the receiver-stimulator and prevent it from turning sideways during placement and closure and afterward. Fixation sutures are applied in a later phase and not shown in this picture.

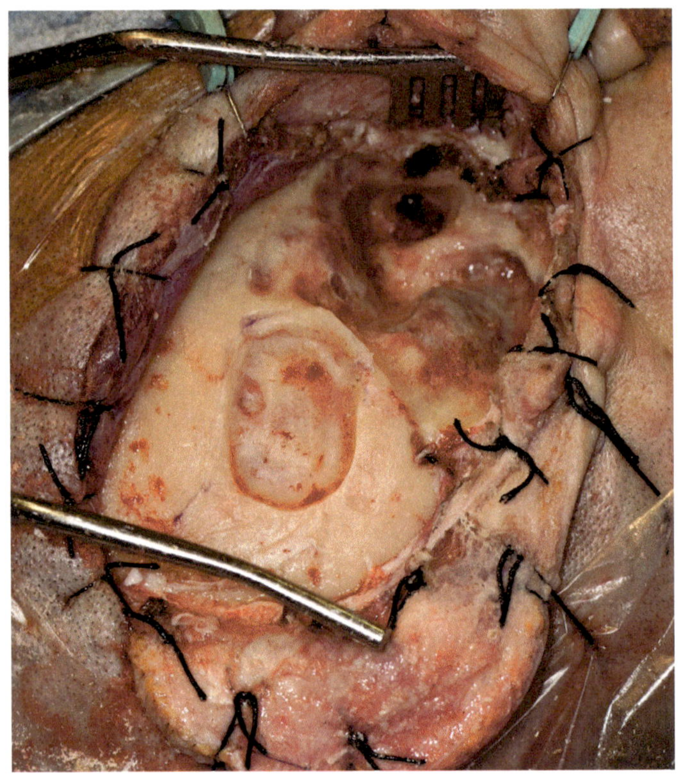

Fig. 8.15 An extended radical mastoidectomy is drilled with exposure of the middle ear, facial nerve, middle cranial fossa, posterior fossa dura, and sigmoid sinus.

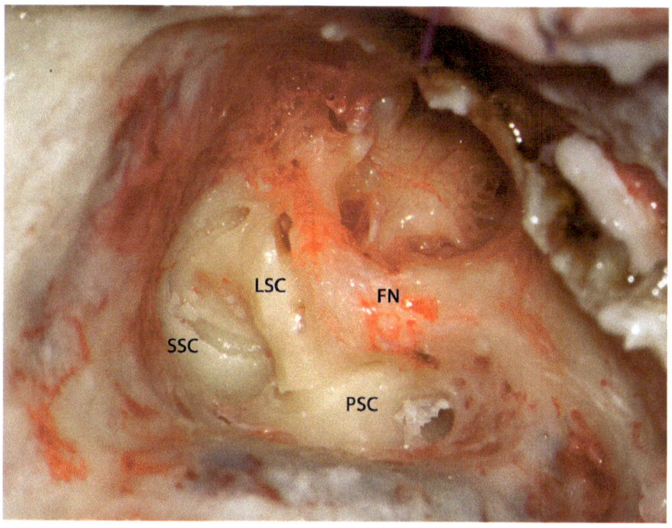

Fig. 8.16 The labyrinthectomy has started with opening of the three canals. LSC, lateral semicircular canal; SSC, superior semicircular canal; PSC, posterior semicircular canal; FN, facial nerve.

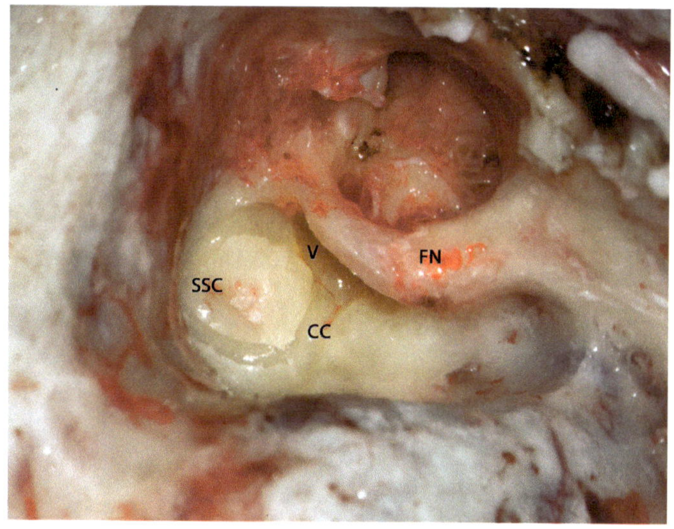

Fig. 8.17 Removal of the posterior and superior semicircular canals allows visualization of the vestibule (V). It will be used as a landmark for internal auditory canal identification. FN, facial nerve; SSC, superior semicircular canal; CC, common crus.

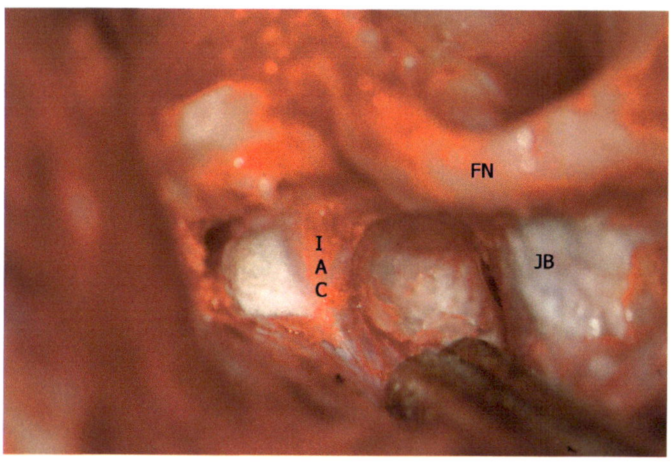

Fig. 8.18 Skeletonizing the internal auditory canal (IAC) can take some time because of the compact bone surrounding the IAC. In this photograph, a large part of the circumference of the IAC is already skeletonized. JB, jugular bulb; FN, facial nerve.

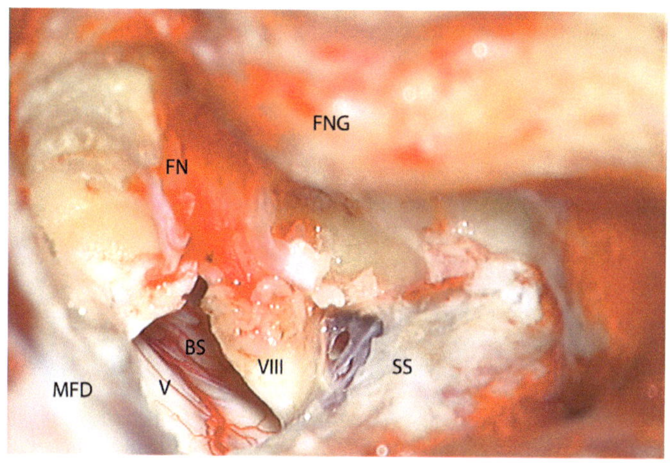

Fig. 8.19 Opening of the CPA (after tumor removal). The anatomical integrity of the cochlear nerve is also preserved. The trigeminal nerve (V) exiting the brainstem (BS) is also observed. FN, facial nerve in the internal auditory canal; FNG, facial nerve genu; MFD, middle fossa dura; SS, sigmoid sinus; VIII, vestibulocochlear nerve.

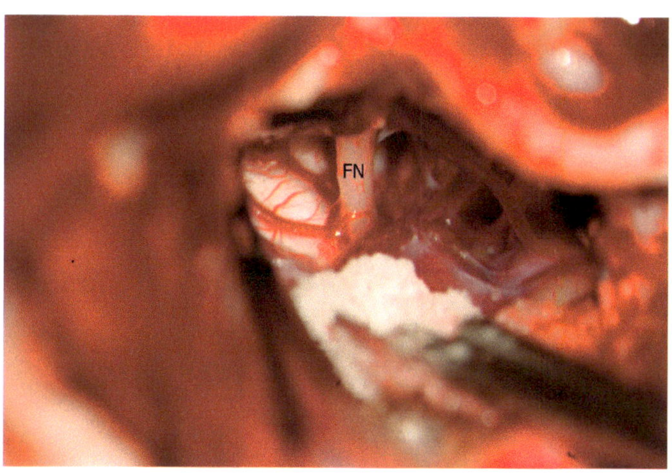

Fig. 8.20 The nerve(s) in the CPA are appreciated after opening of the dura. In this case, with agenesia of the vestibulocochlear nerve, only the facial nerve (FN) can be found.

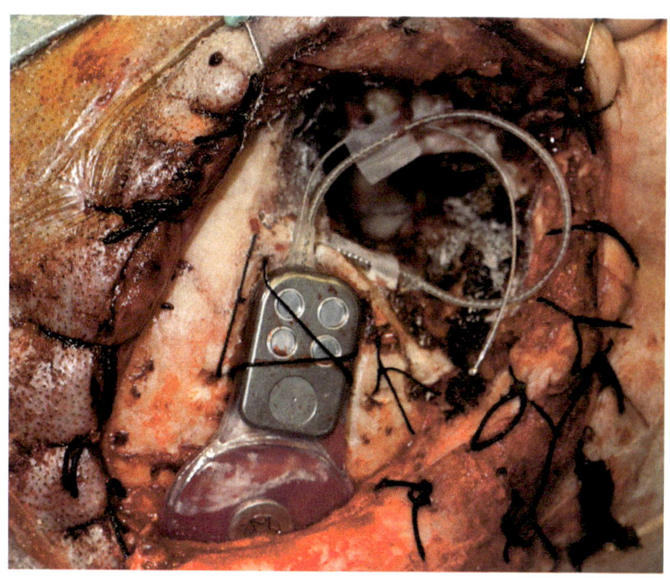

Fig. 8.21 The ABI then is positioned. The holes for the tie-down sutures are created parallel to the well and a nonresorbable suture is applied. While drilling this well the dural opening is covered to avoid bone dust from entering the intradural space. The receiver-stimulator is fixed in its well, the ground electrode is positioned under the muscle, and the ABI array is handled with care before placement.

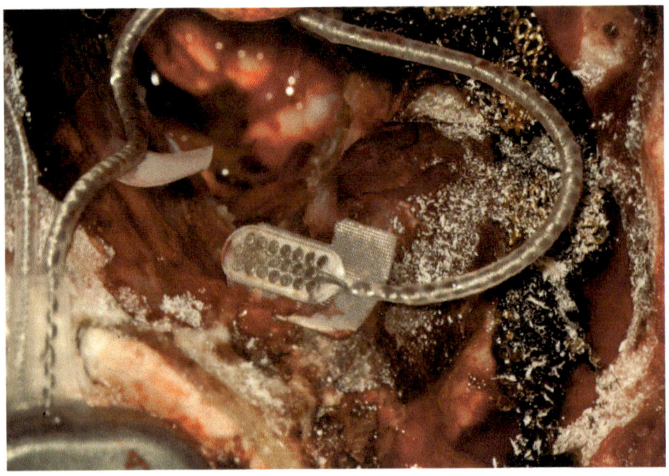

Fig. 8.22 The electrode array has two Dacron mesh strips to handle and fixate the electrode as within the CPA it is not possible to suture or make a groove for fixation.

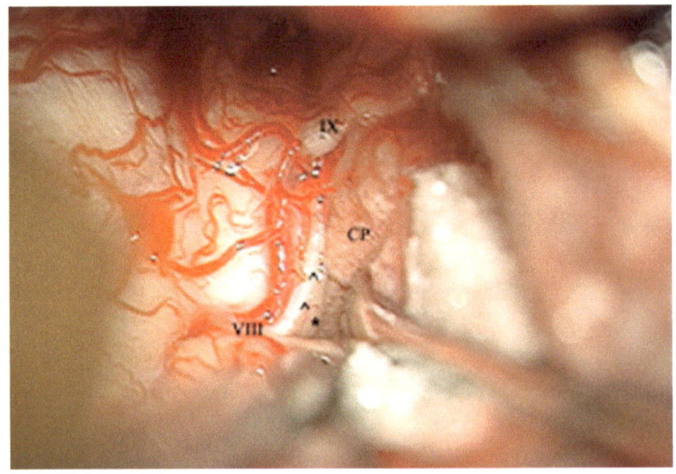

Fig. 8.23 The exact location of the foramen of Luschka is explored. The choroid plexus (CP) is retracted posterior-laterally as it reveals the foramen. Note that the tenia (*arrowheads*) forms a boundary of the lateral recess and the division line between the cochlear nerve (VIII) and the ventral cochlear nucleus. Note also the smooth glistening surface of the ventral cochlear nucleus (✱). IX, glossopharyngeal nerve.

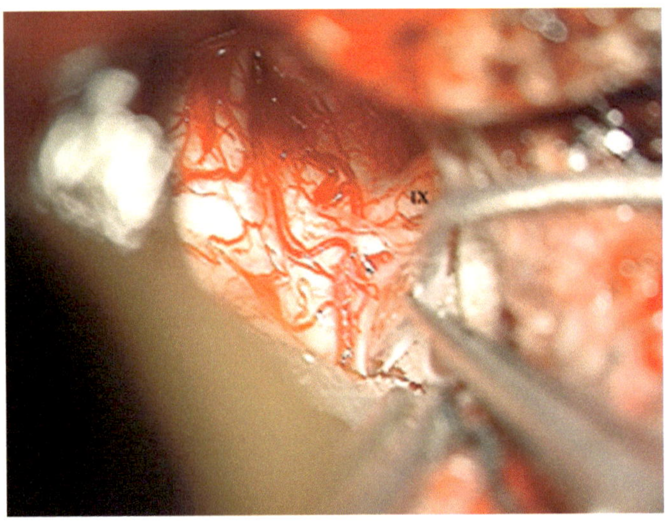

Fig. 8.24 The array of the brainstem implant is held gently using non-toothed forceps. IX, glossopharyngeal nerve.

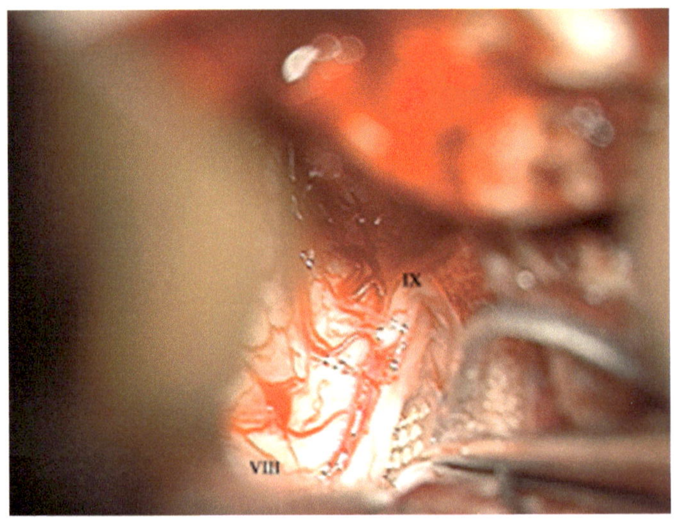

Fig. 8.25 The array is partially inserted. Note that the surface of the electrodes should be directed anterior-superiorly to lie in contact with the uncovered posterior surface of the ventral cochlear nucleus. VIII, vestibulocochlear nerve; IX, glossopharyngeal nerve.

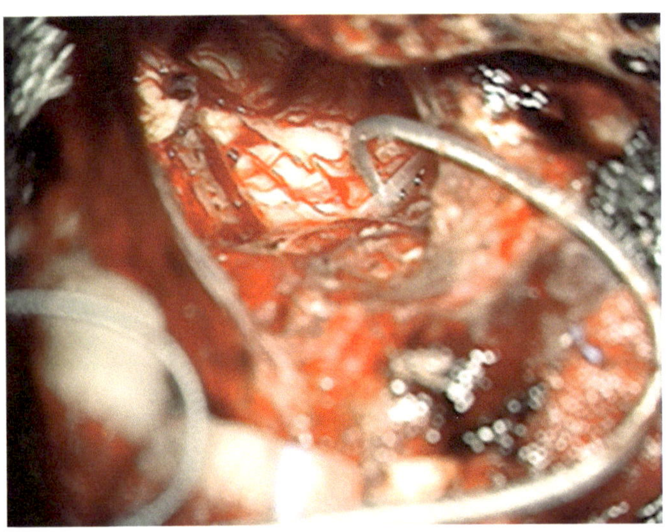

Fig. 8.26 The electrode array is fully inserted.

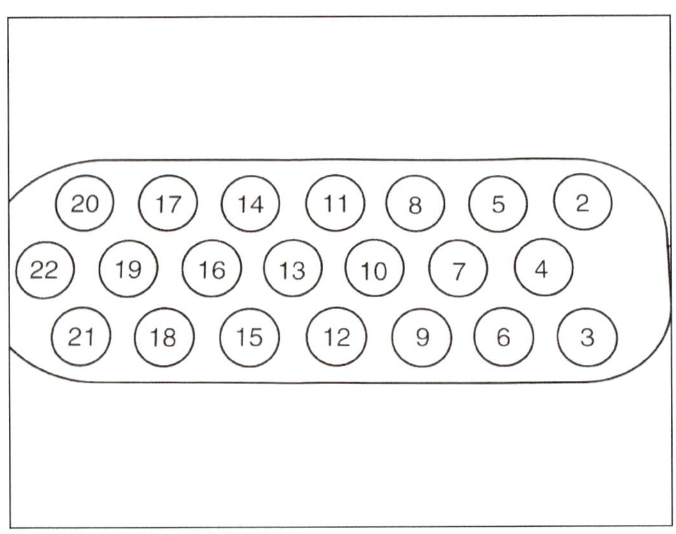

Fig. 8.27 Mapping and intraoperative monitoring: EABR measurement. Electrical auditory brainstem response monitoring is performed to check the position of the array. A worksheet is used by the audiologist during ABR testing to make notes of each electrode.

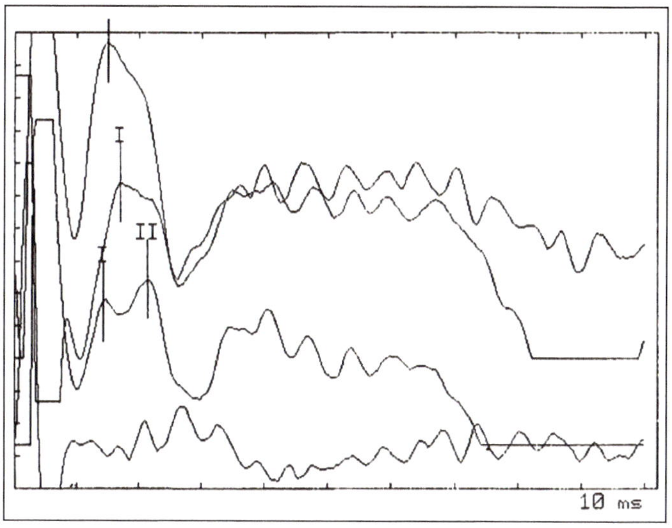

Fig. 8.28 Sample of the intraoperative recording of electrical auditory brainstem response; PI and PII waves are found, indicating hearing stimulation (see Chapter 4 for full explanation).

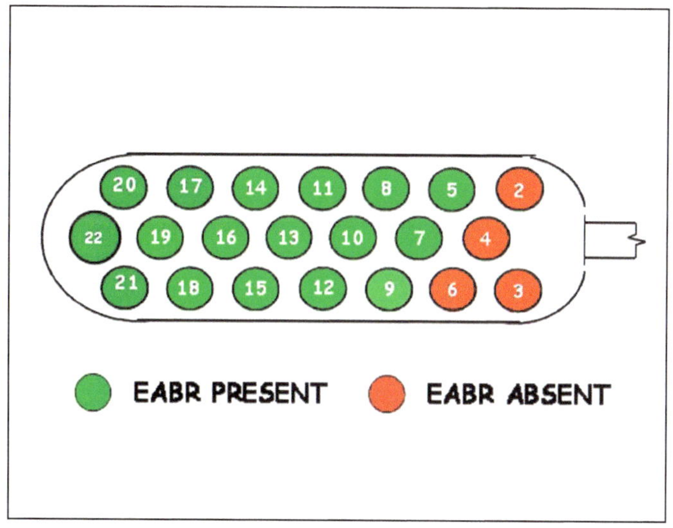

Fig. 8.29 N24 electrode intraoperative mapping indicating that most channels are functioning apart from 2, 3, 4, and 6. In this case, the array may be inserted more medially.

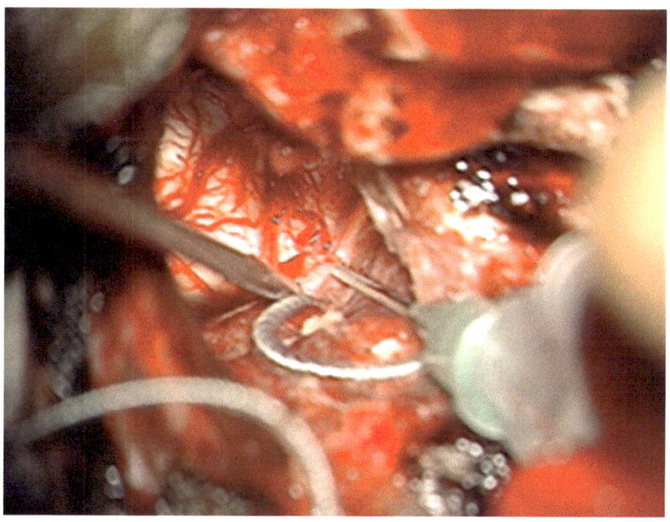

Fig. 8.30 After checking of the correct positioning of the electrode array, fibrin glue and a piece of fascia are used to secure the array in position.

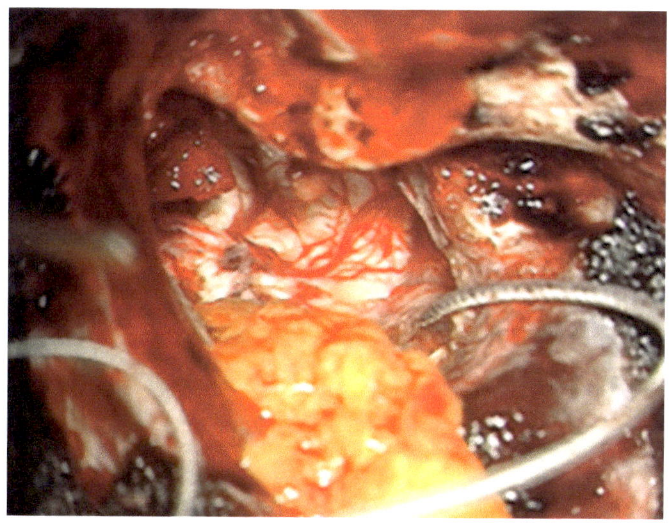

Fig. 8.31 Obliteration of the cavity is started using long strips of abdominal fat.

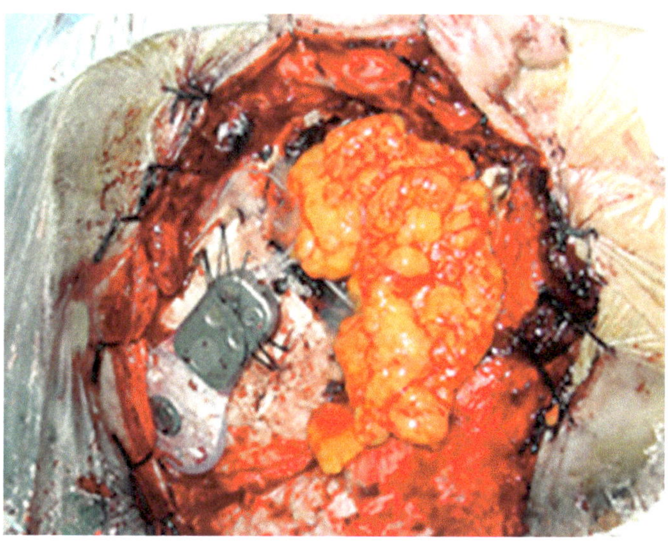

Fig. 8.32 The implant in place with surrounding fat. The wound is now closed in layers in a watertight fashion (not shown here). The temporal muscle covers the receiver-stimulator and is not used to cover the abdominal fat filling the cavity.

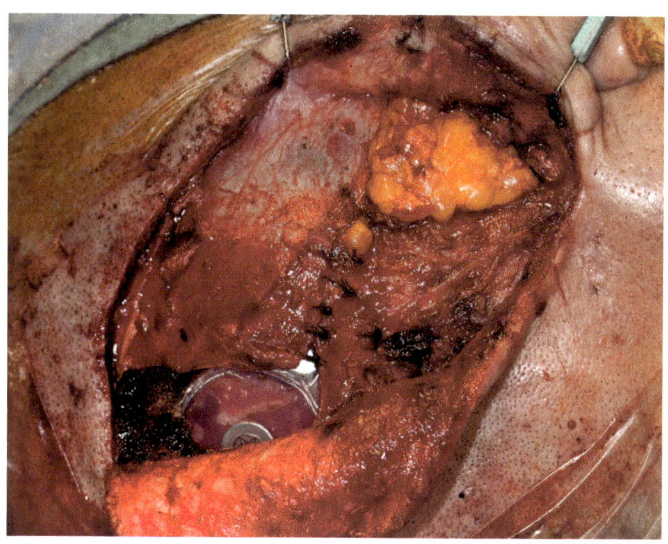

Fig. 8.33 The musculoperiosteal flap is sutured over the fat and the receiver-stimulator.

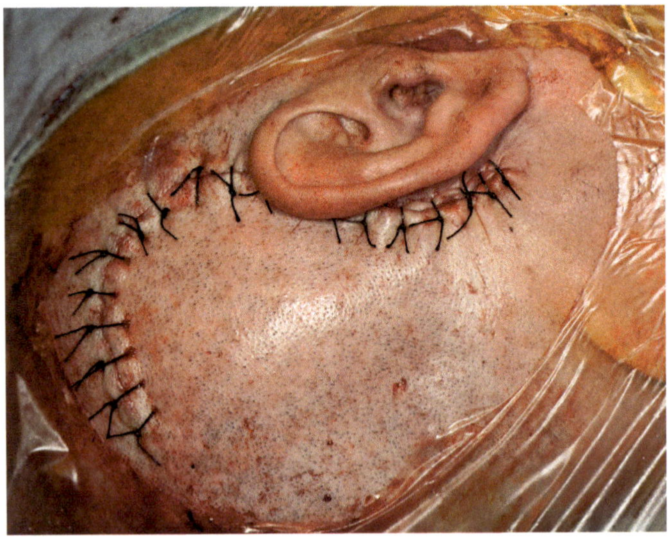

Fig. 8.34 The skin flap is sutured in two layers.

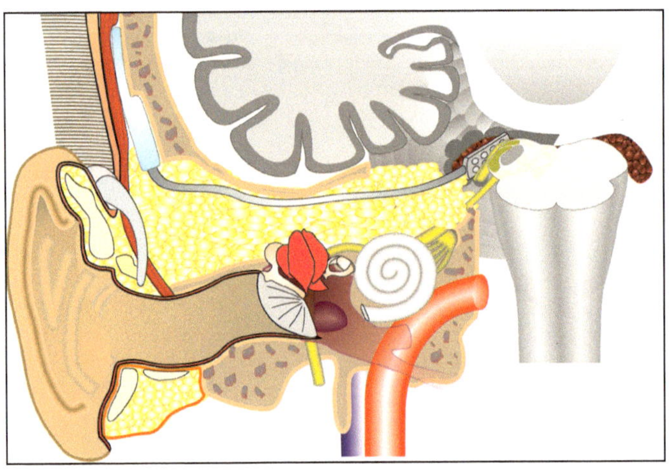

Fig. 8.35 Schematic drawing showing the ABI in place at the end of a standard translabyrinthine approach.

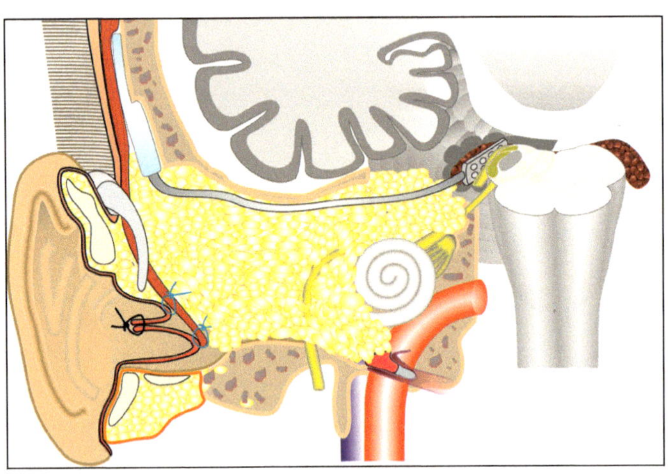

Fig. 8.36 Schematic drawing showing the ABI in place at the end of a standard translabyrinthine approach combined with a subtotal petrosectomy.

8.9 Summary of Auditory Brainstem Implants

- ABIs are designed similar to CIs, but differ from them in that the electrode stimulates the cochlear nuclei directly and bypasses the cochlear nerve.
- ABI is indicated in NF2 patients when the cochlear nerve is not preserved and the contralateral ear has no functional hearing.
- ABI is indicated in NF2 patients when the cochlear nerve is preserved but when stimulation via a cochlear implant has not led to a positive result.
- ABI is indicated in case of completely ossified cochleae; but a drill-out procedure with cochlear implantation (partial or total) should be attempted first.
- ABI is indicated in case of absence of the cochlear nerve proven on scanning and in audiometric testing.
- ABI is indicated in case of bilateral complete cochlear aplasia (Michel deformity).
- ABIs have changed the policy of treatment for patients with NF2 or for patients who had no hearing rehabilitation options in an earlier era, as in complete labyrinth aplasia.
- The side of implantation depends on the patient's hearing abilities, the size of the tumor, other disabilities (such as loss of vision), and surgical risks.
- The best time to implant is at removal of the (first) tumor.
- Appropriate expectations and motivation on the part of the patient are essential. Many ABI patients are initially discouraged by the quality of sound heard through an ABI. They must understand that participation in their auditory rehabilitation program is crucial to continue to improve their proficiency with the device. Such improvement can be expected to continue over many years.
- Almost all patients can expect to obtain some auditory perception and awareness of environmental sounds. Most patients experience a significant improvement in speech comprehension when the implant is used as an adjunct to lip-reading. A minority of patients are able to achieve open-set sound-only speech comprehension.
- During the surgical intervention, intraoperative monitoring of the EABR is essential in making a decision on the concomitant placement of a device. Cochlear implants can be used when the cochlear nerve is preserved, although the outcome can be variable and cannot be predicted in advance.

Pearls and Pitfalls in Auditory Brainstem Implantation Surgery

- The enlarged translabyrinthine approach is best suited for CPA tumor removal and the concomitant placement of an ABI. This enables access to the lateral recess more easily.
- Skin incision for translabyrinthine tumor removal and concomitant ABI is designed as an S-shaped incision, more extended than the regular incision for tumor removal alone or conventional CI placement. Drilling of the bone over the middle cranial fossa dura is limited to leave space for the bed of the implant.
- Landmarks used to identify the foramen of Luschka are the origins of the vestibulocochlear and glossopharyngeal nerves. The flocculus of the cerebellum and the choroid plexus are good indicators as well. CSF leakage can be observed through the foramen of Luschka by increasing the intracranial pressure temporally.
- The array with electrodes must be inserted correctly in the lateral recess, facing the cochlear nucleus complex. Intraoperative electrical ABR monitoring is necessary and a larger number of functioning electrodes may more correctly secure the array and probably give a better hearing result. The position of the array in the lateral recess is adjusted if too few electrodes are functioning.
- Monitoring of other cranial nerves is important to check whether they are stimulated by the electrode array.

Reference Video

See Video 8.1.

References

1. Sennaroglu L, Ziyal I, Atas A, et al. Preliminary results of auditory brainstem implantation in prelingually deaf children with inner ear malformations including severe stenosis of the cochlear aperture and aplasia of the cochlear nerve. Otol Neurotol 2009;30(6):708–715
2. Sanna M, Khrais T, Guida M, Falcioni M. Auditory brainstem implant in a child with severely ossified cochlea. Laryngoscope 2006;116(9):1700–1703
3. Schwartz MS, Otto SR, Brackmann DE, Hitselberger WE, Shannon RV. Use of a multichannel auditory brainstem implant for neurofibromatosis type 2. Stereotact Funct Neurosurg 2003;81(1–4):110–114
4. Sanna M, Di Lella F, Guida M, Merkus P. Auditory brainstem implants in NF2 patients: results and review of the literature. Otol Neurotol 2012;33(2):154–164
5. Arístegui M, Denia A. Simultaneous cochlear implantation and translabyrinthine removal of vestibular schwannoma in an only hearing ear: report of two cases (neurofibromatosis type 2 and unilateral vestibular schwannoma). Otol Neurotol 2005;26(2):205–210
6. Piccirillo E, Hiraumi H, Hamada M, Russo A, De Stefano A, Sanna M. Intraoperative cochlear nerve monitoring in vestibular schwannoma surgery—does it really affect hearing outcome? Audiol Neurootol 2008;13(1):58–64
7. Piccirillo E, Guida M, Flanagan S, Lauda L, Fois P, Sanna M. CNAP to predict functional cochlear nerve preservation in NF-2: cochlear implant or auditory brainstem implant. Skull Base 2008;18(4):281–287
8. Vincenti V, Pasanisi E, Guida M, Di Trapani G, Sanna M. Hearing rehabilitation in neurofibromatosis type 2 patients: cochlear versus auditory brainstem implantation. Audiol Neurootol 2008;13(4):273–280
9. Neff BA, Wiet RM, Lasak JM, et al. Cochlear implantation in the neurofibromatosis type 2 patient: long-term follow-up. Laryngoscope 2007;117(6):1069–1072
10. Lustig LR, Yeagle J, Driscoll CL, Blevins N, Francis H, Niparko JK. Cochlear implantation in patients with neurofibromatosis type 2 and bilateral vestibular schwannoma. Otol Neurotol 2006;27(4):512–518
11. Yamakami I, Yoshinori H, Saeki N, Wada M, Oka N. Hearing preservation and intraoperative auditory brainstem response and cochlear nerve compound action potential monitoring in the removal of small acoustic neurinoma via the retrosigmoid approach. J Neurol Neurosurg Psychiatry 2009;80(2):218–227
12. Grayeli AB, Bouccara D, Kalamarides M, et al. Auditory brainstem implant in bilateral and completely ossified cochleae. Otol Neurotol 2003;24(1):79–82
13. Grayeli AB, Kalamarides M, Bouccara D, Ambert-Dahan E, Sterkers O. Auditory brainstem implant in neurofibromatosis type 2 and non-neurofibromatosis type 2 patients. Otol Neurotol 2008;29(8):1140–1146
14. Sollmann WP, Laszig R, Marangos N. Surgical experiences in 58 cases using the Nucleus 22 multichannel auditory brainstem implant. J Laryngol Otol Suppl 2000;(27):23–26
15. Merkus P, Free RH, Mylanus EAM, et al; 4th Consensus in Auditory Implants Meeting. Dutch Cochlear Implant Group (CI-ON) consensus protocol on postmeningitis hearing evaluation and treatment. Otol Neurotol 2010;31(8):1281–1286
16. Beijen J, Casselman J, Joosten F, et al. Magnetic resonance imaging in patients with meningitis induced hearing loss. Eur Arch Otorhinolaryngol 2009;266(8):1229–1236
17. van Loon MC, Hensen EF, de Foer B, Smit CF, Witte B, Merkus P. Magnetic resonance imaging in the evaluation of patients with sensorineural hearing loss caused by meningitis: implications for cochlear implantation. Otol Neurotol 2013;34(5):845–854
18. Steenerson RL, Gary LB, Wynens MS. Scala vestibuli cochlear implantation for labyrinthine ossification. Am J Otol 1990;11(5):360–363
19. Bacciu S, Bacciu A, Pasanisi E, et al. Nucleus multichannel cochlear implantation in partially ossified cochleas using the Steenerson procedure. Otol Neurotol 2002;23(3):341–345
20. Kemink JL, Zimmerman-Phillips S, Kileny PR, Firszt JB, Novak MA. Auditory performance of children with cochlear ossification and partial implant insertion. Laryngoscope 1992;102(9):1001–1005
21. Lenarz T, Battmer RD, Lesinski A, Parker J. Nucleus double electrode array: a new approach for ossified cochleae. Am J Otol 1997;18(6, Suppl)S39–S41
22. Sennaroglu L, Saatci I. A new classification for cochleovestibular malformations. Laryngoscope 2002;112(12):2230–2241
23. Papsin BC. Cochlear implantation in children with anomalous cochleovestibular anatomy. Laryngoscope 2005;115(1 Pt 2, Suppl 106)1–26
24. Sennaroglu L, Sarac S, Ergin T. Surgical results of cochlear implantation in malformed cochlea. Otol Neurotol 2006;27(5):615–623
25. Mylanus EA, Rotteveel LJ, Leeuw RL. Congenital malformation of the inner ear and pediatric cochlear implantation. Otol Neurotol 2004;25(3):308–317
26. Sennaroglu L, Colletti V, Manrique M, et al. Auditory brainstem implantation in children and non-neurofibromatosis type 2 patients: a consensus statement. Otol Neurotol 2011;32(2):187–191
27. Warren FM III, Wiggins RH III, Pitt C, Harnsberger HR, Shelton C. Apparent cochlear nerve aplasia: to implant or not to implant? Otol Neurotol 2010;31(7):1088–1094
28. Song MH, Kim SC, Kim J, Chang JW, Lee WS, Choi JY. The cochleovestibular nerve identified during auditory brainstem implantation in patients with narrow internal auditory canals: can preoperative evaluation predict cochleovestibular nerve deficiency? Laryngoscope 2011;121(8):1773–1779
29. Buchman CA, Teagle HF, Roush PA, et al. Cochlear implantation in children with labyrinthine anomalies and cochlear nerve deficiency: implications for auditory brainstem implantation. Laryngoscope 2011;121(9):1979–1988
30. Kutz JW Jr, Lee KH, Isaacson B, Booth TN, Sweeney MH, Roland PS. Cochlear implantation in children with cochlear nerve absence or deficiency. Otol Neurotol 2011;32(6):956–961
31. Colletti V, Shannon RV, Carner M, Veronese S, Colletti L. Complications in auditory brainstem implant surgery in adults and children. Otol Neurotol 2010;31(4):558–564

32. Beltrame MA, Bonfioli F, Frau GN. Cochlear implant in inner ear malformation: double posterior labyrinthotomy approach to common cavity. Adv Otorhinolaryngol 2000;57:113–119
33. Merkus P, Di Lella F, Di Trapani G, et al. Indications and contra-indications of auditory brainstem implants. Systematic review and illustrative cases. Eur Arch Otolaryngol 2014;271(1):3–13
34. Camilleri AE, Toner JG, Howarth KL, Hampton S, Ramsden RT. Cochlear implantation following temporal bone fracture. J Laryngol Otol 1999;113(5):454–457
35. Serin GM, Derinsu U, Sari M, et al. Cochlear implantation in patients with bilateral cochlear trauma. Am J Otolaryngol 2010;31(5):350–355
36. Simons JP, Whitaker ME, Hirsch BE. Cochlear implantation in a patient with bilateral temporal bone fractures. Otolaryngol Head Neck Surg 2005;132(5):809–811
37. Medina M, Di Lella F, Di Trapani G, et al. Cochlear implantation versus auditory brainstem implantation in bilateral total deafness after head trauma: personal experience and review of the literature. Otol Neurotol 2014;35(2):260–270
38. Colletti V, Carner M, Miorelli V, Colletti L, Guida M, Fiorino F. Auditory brainstem implant in posttraumatic cochlear nerve avulsion. Audiol Neurootol 2004;9(4):247–255
39. Corrales CE, Monfared A, Jackler RK. Facial and vestibulocochlear nerve avulsion at the fundus of the internal auditory canal in a child without a temporal bone fracture. Otol Neurotol 2010;31(9):1508–1510
40. Di Lella F, Merkus P, Di Trapani G, Taibah A, Guida M, Sanna M. Vestibular schwannoma in the only hearing ear: role of cochlear implants. Ann Otol Rhinol Laryngol 2013;122(2):91–99
41. Thedinger BA, Cueva RA, Glasscock ME III. Treatment of an acoustic neuroma in an only-hearing ear: case reports and considerations for the future. Laryngoscope 1993;103(9):976–980
42. Ramsden R, Khwaja S, Green K, O'Driscoll M, Mawman D. Vestibular schwannoma in the only hearing ear: cochlear implant or auditory brainstem implant? Otol Neurotol 2005;26(2):261–264
43. Aristegui M, Denia A. Simultaneous cochlear implantation and translabyrinthine removal of vestibular schwannoma in an only hearing ear: report of two cases (neurofibromatosis type 2 and unilateral vestibular schwannoma). Otol Neurotol 2005;26:205–210
44. Aftab S, Semaan MT, Murray GS, Megerian CA. Cochlear implantation outcomes in patients with autoimmune and immune-mediated inner ear disease. Otol Neurotol 2010;31(8):1337–1342
45. Jagannathan J, Lonser RR, Stanger RA, et al. Cochlear implantation for hearing loss associated with bilateral endolymphatic sac tumors in von Hippel–Lindau disease. Otol Neurotol 2007;28(7):927–930
46. Breneman AI, Gifford RH, Dejong MD. Cochlear implantation in children with auditory neuropathy spectrum disorder: long-term outcomes. J Am Acad Audiol 2012;23(1):5–17
47. Roush P, Frymark T, Venediktov R, Wang B. Audiologic management of auditory neuropathy spectrum disorder in children: a systematic review of the literature. Am J Audiol 2011;20(2):159–170
48. Rotteveel LJ, Proops DW, Ramsden RT, Saeed SR, van Olphen AF, Mylanus EA. Cochlear implantation in 53 patients with otosclerosis: demographics, computed tomographic scanning, surgery, and complications. Otol Neurotol 2004;25(6):943–952
49. Ramsden R, Bance M, Giles E, Mawman D. Cochlear implantation in otosclerosis: a unique positioning and programming problem. J Laryngol Otol 1997;111(3):262–265
50. Toung JS, Zwolan T, Spooner TR, Telian SA. Late failure of cochlear implantation resulting from advanced cochlear otosclerosis: surgical and programming challenges. Otol Neurotol 2004;25(5):723–726
51. Merkus P, van Loon MC, Smit CF, Smits C, de Cock AFC, Hensen EF. Decision making in advanced otosclerosis: an evidence-based strategy. Laryngoscope 2011;121(9):1935–1941

9 Electroacoustic Stimulation

Cochlear implantation has become the standard treatment for severe to profound hearing loss in adults and children; new implant and electrode designs and speech coding techniques are still being developed for further improvement. At the same time the inclusion criteria for standard cochlear implantation are being extended. From the surgical perspective as well new techniques have been introduced: hearing preservation and the use of combined electric and acoustic stimulation are highly dependent on surgical skills.

9.1 Hearing Preservation and Electroacoustic Stimulation

Several investigators have reported the unintended presence of residual hearing after cochlear implantation surgery, showing that hearing preservation is indeed possible while at the same time opening the cochlea and inserting an electrode. As early as 1993 reports on soft surgery techniques were presented in the search for the most effective surgical principles of hearing preservation.[1] Prevention of blood and bone dust entering the cochlea, as little drilling on the cochlea as possible, very slow and atraumatic insertion of the cochlear electrode in the midportion of the scala tympani, and use of atraumatic, tapered, and flexible implants were some of the measures discussed.

With the introduction of electroacoustic stimulation (EAS) in 1999, hearing preservation became even more important because now this intended residual hearing was in fact being used.[2]

In EAS the low, apical frequencies are preserved and acoustically stimulated, while the high, basal frequencies are electrically stimulated with a cochlear electrode. For this technique a combined electric and acoustic speech processor had to be developed (**Fig. 9.1**) and the length of the cochlear electrode array was shortened in an attempt to preserve the residual hearing in the low frequencies.[3] The audiometric results showed an increase in speech understanding in quiet and in noisy situations in comparison with only cochlear implantation,[4,5] making this a very beneficial option for patients with a ski-slope audiogram, who before this development found themselves caught between hearing aids that gave inadequate amplification and standard cochlear implantation with the attendant risk of losing their residual hearing.[6]

With the special surgical techniques necessary for this approach and the development of a combined electroacoustic speech processor, high success rates can now be achieved.[7,8]

Nevertheless, loss of hearing after EAS still occurs either in the early or in the late phase, without the reasons being completely known. This puts the surgeon's aims in jeopardy, because the success of EAS cannot be predicted preoperatively, while at the same time the decision for the shorter electrode used in EAS has already been made with the intention of not affecting the cochlear apical hair cells. Also, a shorter electrode is not favorable with future progression of the underlying pathology. Current research therefore focuses on hearing preservation using electrodes that are of nearly standard length but thinner and more flexible, to provide better pitch matching and possibilities for use as a "normal" cochlear electrode when residual hearing fades.

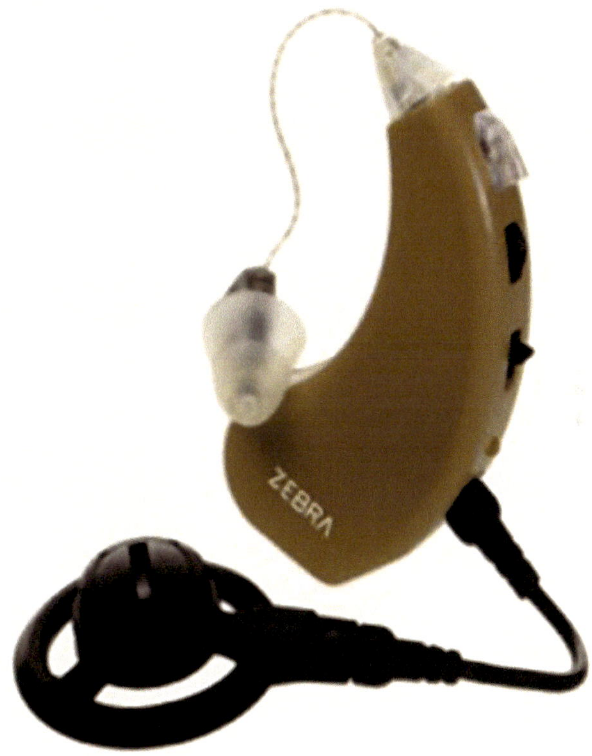

Fig. 9.1 Combined electric and acoustic speech processor/hearing aid combination unit.

These developments in hearing preservation have widened the indications for cochlear implantation but at the same time have increased the interest in preserving the intracochlear structures and the neural tissue in the "normal" cochlear implant population. This is especially of interest for the younger population of cochlear implantees, who might need several implantations during their lifetime and depend on the cochlear implant and the viability of their neural tissues for their hearing restoration in future life. Therefore, the use of the techniques now known and practiced in EAS are worth practicing in all cochlear implant surgery.

9.2 Indication for EAS

Ski-slope audiogram, with preoperative residual hearing in the lower frequencies up to 1 kHz of 60 dB and speech audiometry below 50%.

9.3 Influential Factors in Hearing Preservation

Several factors are considered relevant when attempting to preserve the residual hearing:

- Surgical technique with atraumatic insertion of electrode
- Electrode design to minimize endocochlear trauma
- Perioperative use of medication

9.3.1 Atraumatic Surgical Technique

Round Window Anatomy and Insertion

The round window insertion is used in this type of surgery to achieve adequate positioning of the electrode in the midportion of the scala tympani, without damage to the modiolus or the spiral ganglia.[9,10] As explained in Chapter 2, the round window margin cochleostomy (RWMC) is often used, in which the crista semilunaris and crista fenestrae are removed by drilling for easier introduction (see **Fig. 5.1.14**). The amount of bone removal in this procedure is minimal, ~1 mm.[11] However, a normal round window cochleostomy (RWC) without drilling is even better if anatomy allows. While performing this, care must be taken not to damage the cochlear aqueduct, the basilar membrane, and the osseous spiral lamina, which are all closely related to the bony overhang above the round window.[9] Also the common modiolar vein, which provides drainage of the entire cochlea and is situated closely to the cochlear aqueduct, should be preserved because once it is compromised this will lead to deterioration of cochlear function.

The long axis of the scala tympani is entered from superior-posterior to anterior-inferior (the right angle of insertion), in the middle of the scala tympani, below the basilar membrane and spiral ligament. These techniques will minimize insertion trauma.

Mechanical Trauma Due to Insertion

Fractures of the osseous spiral lamina, disruption of the basilar membrane, tearing of the lateral spiral ligament or of the endothelial layer of the scala tympani, and leakage of traumatized blood vessels can all lead to trauma and subsequently to hearing deterioration in the cochlea.[12] Disruption of the inner ear homeostasis with perilymph and endolymph mixing due to trauma to the separating membranes also leads to toxic effects on the hair cells and loss of the residual hearing. For these reasons, in addition to the RWC or RWMC technique as described, whenever resistance is encountered during introduction of a cochlear electrode, the electrode should not be inserted with force: after pulling it back slightly, a second gentle attempt should be made after rotating the electrode slightly.

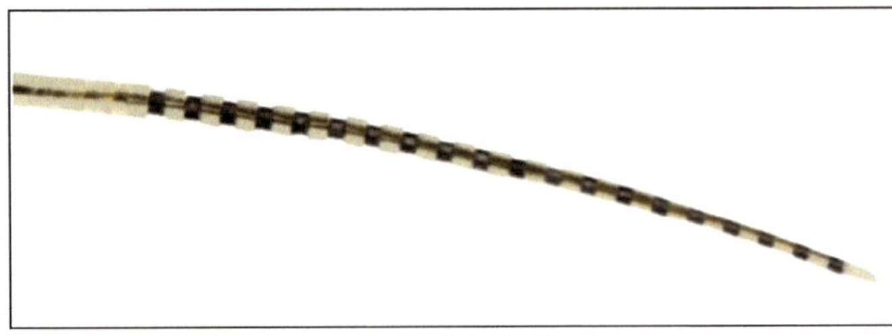

Fig. 9.2 Thinner electrode designed to minimize insertion trauma.

Bone Dust and Blood Entering Cochlea

Once the cochlea has been opened, special care is required to avoid bone dust and blood entering the cochlea. This may be achieved by positioning a small piece of resorbable sponge soaked in physiologic solution as protection for the round window immediately after it is opened. Suction should be absolutely avoided in the round window area after the secondary membrane has been opened.

9.3.2 Atraumatic Electrode Design

Special electrodes have been developed for EAS, starting with the short straight 10-mm electrode of Gantz in 2005.[13] However, current research focuses on electrodes that are of nearly standard length but thinner and more flexible in design (**Fig. 9.2**).

9.3.3 Perioperative Use of Medication

Local (intracochlear) and systemic use of glucocorticosteroids has been reported helpful in hearing preservation during CI surgery.[14,15]

Case 9.1 Cochlear Implantation with Attempt at Hearing Preservation Using Slim Straight Regular Electrode (Fig. 9.1.1–Fig. 9.1.4)

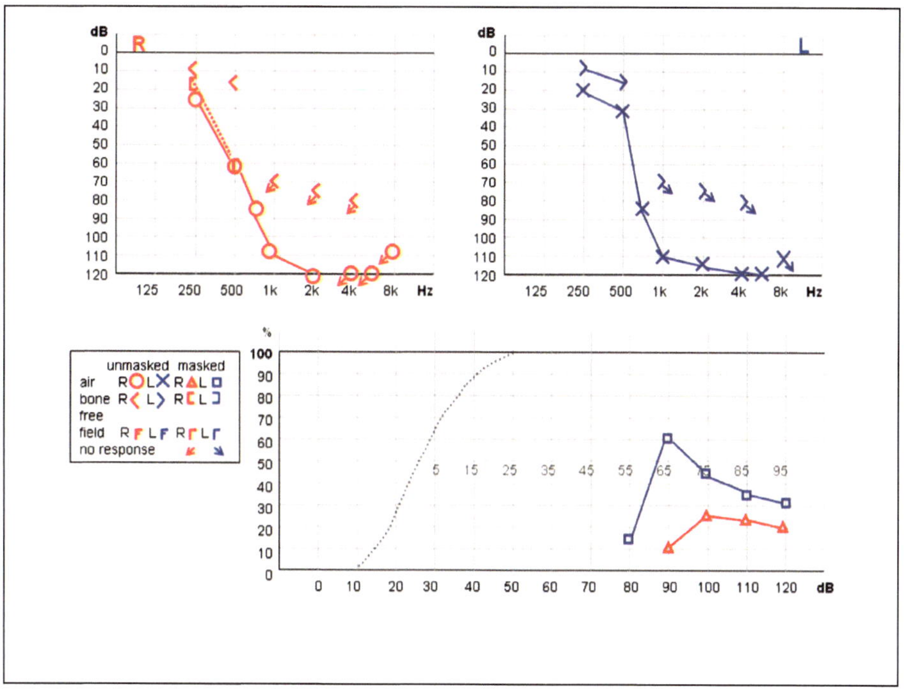

Fig. 9.1.1 Male patient, 45 years old, severe perceptive hearing loss since childhood, progressive in nature. Family history: positive, brother also affected. CT images: normal anatomy, no malformations. Never wore hearing aids because of residual hearing for the low frequencies. Excellent use of voice, although hearing loss is audible in use of speech (Speech Intelligibility Score [SIR]: 4). Since 2008 deterioration in hearing on the right side (see audiogram), also presence of tinnitus. MRI: no CPA tumor. Best ear: left ear (visible in speech audiogram). Decision: because of the presence residual hearing in the left ear, a decision for conventional cochlear implantation in right ear, with slim straight electrode. Objective: hearing preservation with normal-length electrode. Low frequencies safeguarded by left ear.

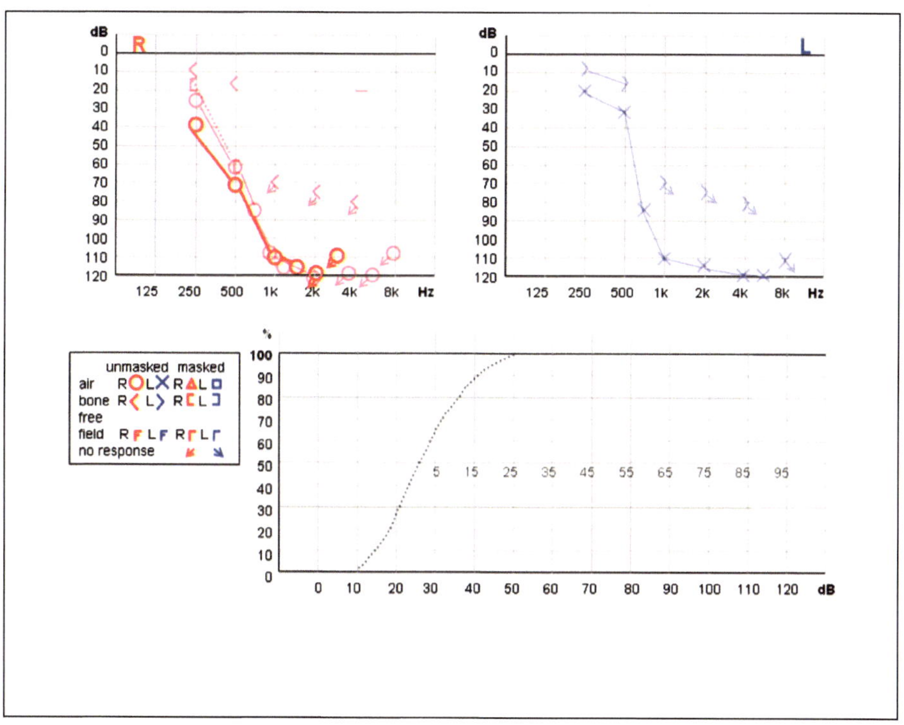

Fig. 9.1.2 Audiometric testing 2 months after cochlear implantation revealed hearing preservation on the right ear; not more than maximum 15 dB decrease in threshold was measured. Soft surgery techniques were employed. Additionally, dexamethasone 5 mg 4× daily was administered intravenously during the first 2 days starting 1 hour before the opening of the cochlea, after which 2 mg 4× daily orally was given for 2 days. The objective of this medication was to suppress the intracochlear immune response to the insertion of the electrode.

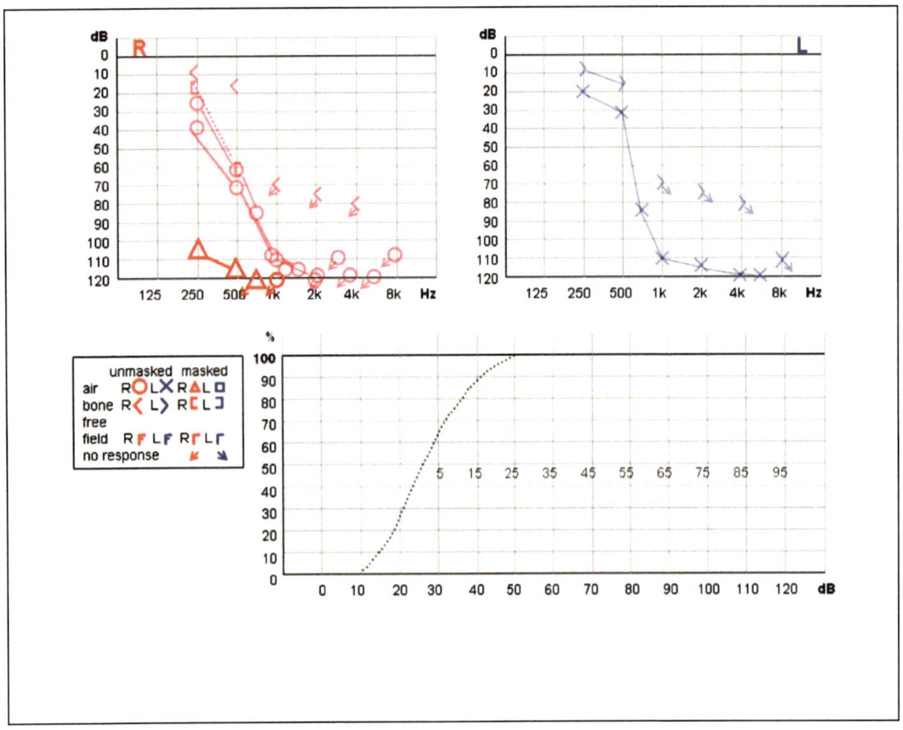

Fig. 9.1.3 Unfortunately, 6 months postoperatively the hearing threshold for the low frequencies deteriorated severely, resulting in a total loss of residual hearing on the right ear. With the cochlear implant, speech perception levels of 70 dB were measured.

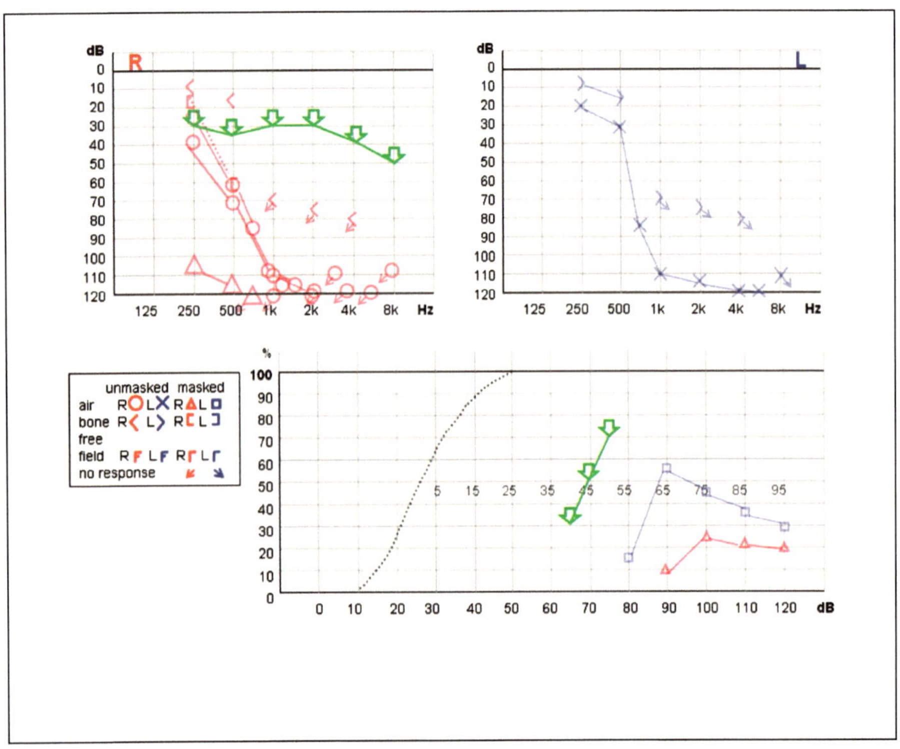

Fig. 9.1.4 Threshold levels for pure tone audiometry using the cochlear implant are visible in this audiogram: around 25 dB, while speech perception thresholds are measured at 70 dB.

Case 9.2 Cochlear Implantation with Attempt at Hearing Preservation Using Hybrid Electrode (Fig. 9.2.1–Fig. 9.2.4)

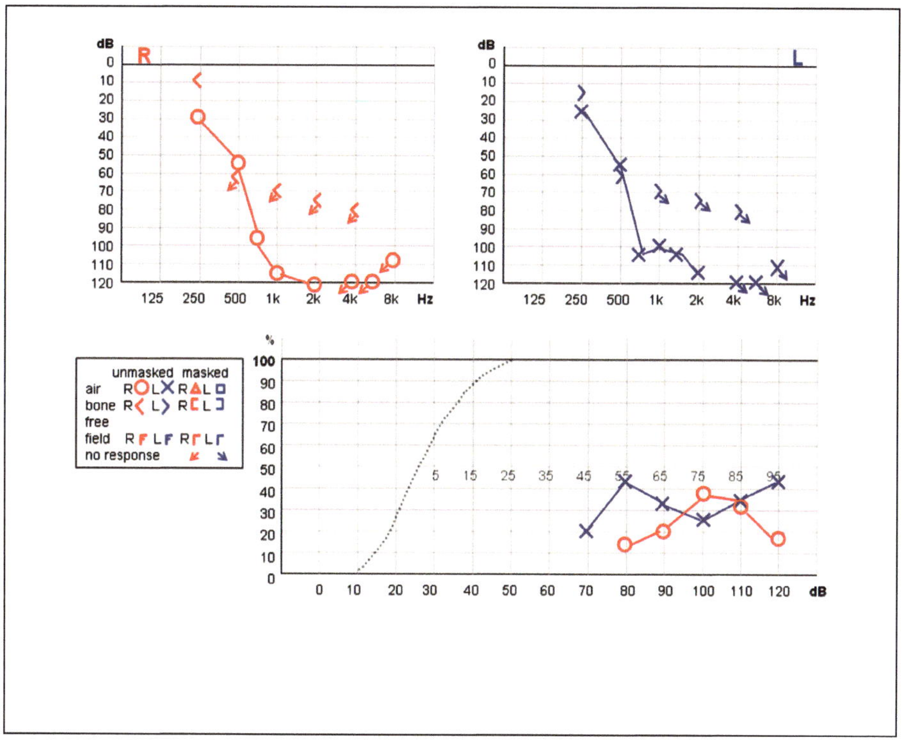

Fig. 9.2.1 Female patient, 68 years old, severe perceptive hearing loss since age 55 years, progressive in nature. Family history: positive, brothers also affected. CT images: normal anatomy, no malformations. Wears hearing aids on the left ear since 2007, this is best hearing ear. Excellent use of voice (Speech Intelligibility Score [SIR]: 5). Best hearing ear: left ear (subjective). Decision: because of presence residual hearing in both ears, a decision for hybrid cochlear implantation in right ear. Objective: hearing preservation at lower frequencies.

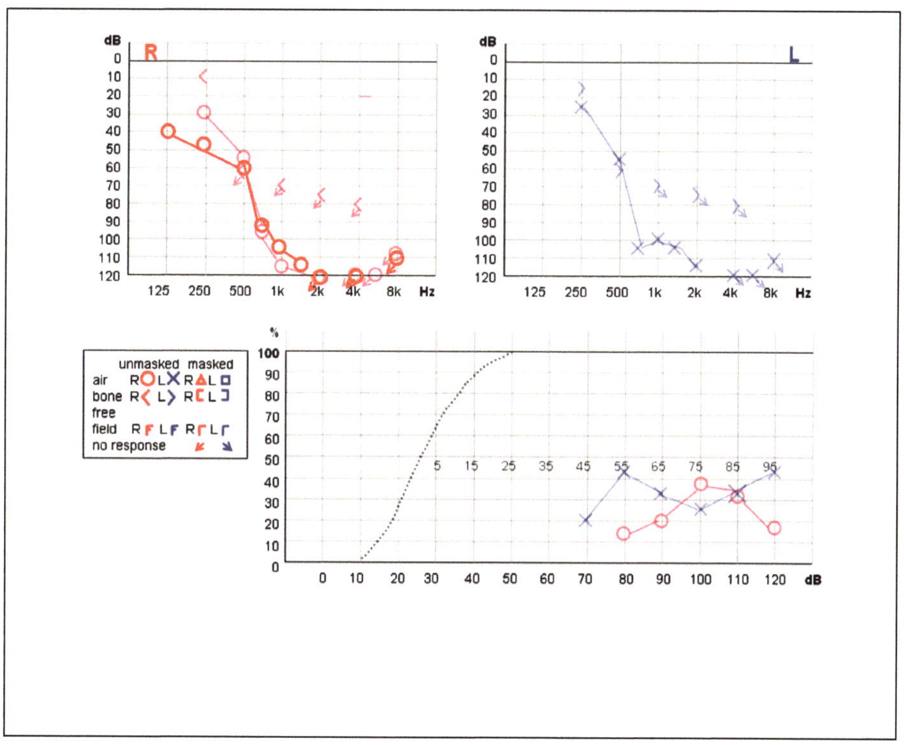

Fig. 9.2.2 Four months postoperatively the hearing thresholds for the lower frequencies are spared: maximum loss 15 dB (at 250 Hz). During surgery dexamethasone 10 mg 4× daily was started, 1 hour before the opening of the cochlea; this was given for 48 hours. The cochlea was opened via the round window, using a slit opening. Care was taken to introduce the hybrid electrode with a slow and constant movement.

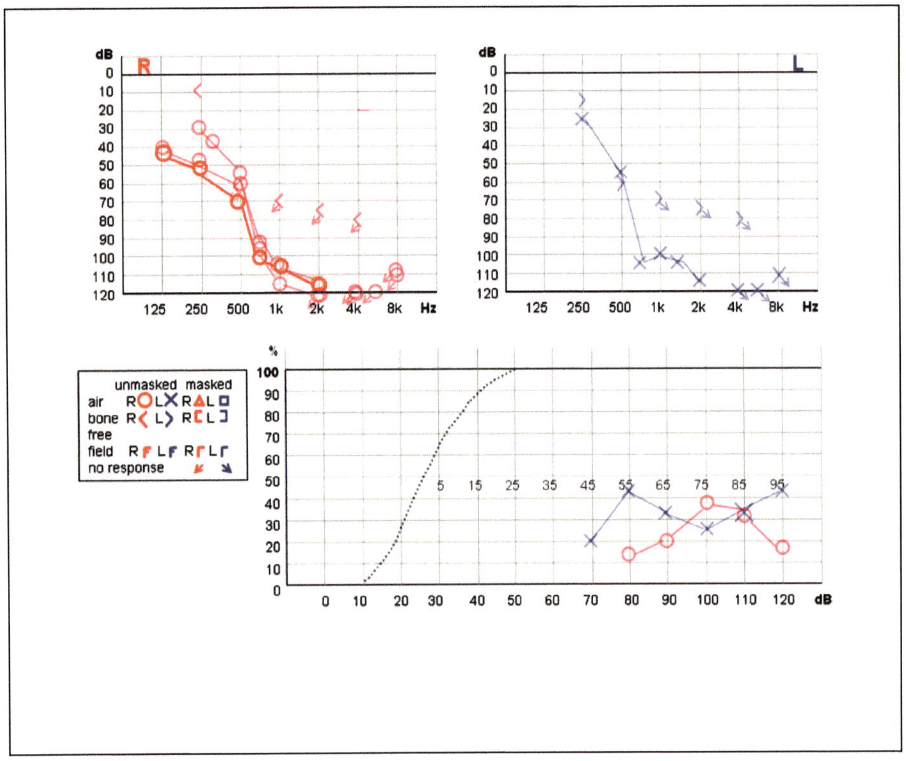

Fig. 9.2.3 At 27 months after cochlear implantation the hearing thresholds for the lower frequencies are still preserved.

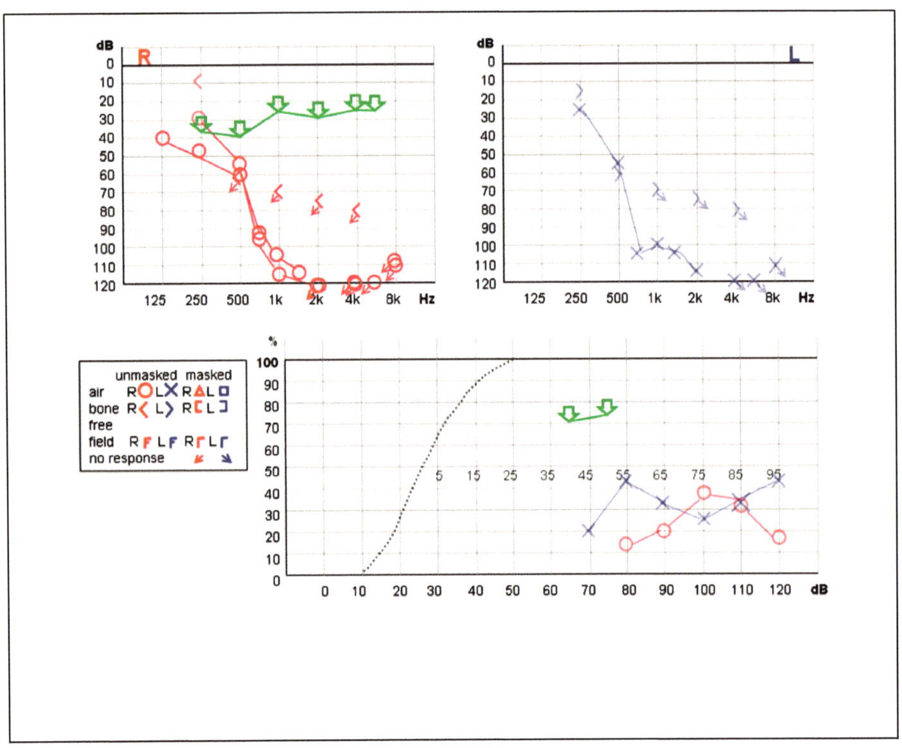

Fig. 9.2.4 Threshold levels for pure tone audiometry using the cochlear implant are visible in this audiogram as around 30 dB, while speech perception thresholds are measured at 75 dB.

References

1. Lehnhardt E. [Intracochlear placement of cochlear implant electrodes in soft surgery technique]. [Article in German]. HNO 1993;41(7):356–359
2. von Ilberg C, Kiefer J, Tillein J, et al. Electric-acoustic stimulation of the auditory system. New technology for severe hearing loss. ORL J Otorhinolaryngol Relat Spec 1999;61(6):334–340
3. Adunka O, Kiefer J, Unkelbach MH, Lehnert T, Gstoettner W. Development and evaluation of an improved cochlear implant electrode design for electric acoustic stimulation. Laryngoscope 2004;114(7):1237–1241
4. Kiefer J, Pok M, Adunka O, et al. Combined electric and acoustic stimulation of the auditory system: results of a clinical study. Audiol Neurootol 2005;10(3):134–144
5. Gantz BJ, Turner C. Combining acoustic and electrical speech processing: Iowa/Nucleus hybrid implant. Acta Otolaryngol 2004;124(4):344–347
6. James CJ, Fraysse B, Deguine O, et al. Combined electroacoustic stimulation in conventional candidates for cochlear implantation. Audiol Neurootol 2006;11(Suppl 1):57–62
7. Mahmoud AF, Massa ST, Douberly SL, Montes ML, Ruckenstein MJ. Safety, efficacy, and hearing preservation using an integrated electro-acoustic stimulation hearing system. Otol Neurotol 2014;35(8):1421–1425
8. Gifford RH, Dorman MF, Skarzynski H, et al. Cochlear implantation with hearing preservation yields significant benefit for speech recognition in complex listening environments. Ear Hear 2013;34(4):413–425
9. Roland PS, Wright CG, Isaacson B. Cochlear implant electrode insertion: the round window revisited. Laryngoscope 2007;117(8):1397–1402
10. Briggs RJ, Tykocinski M, Stidham K, Roberson JB. Cochleostomy site: implications for electrode placement and hearing preservation. Acta Otolaryngol 2005;125(8):870–876
11. Takahashi H, Sando I. Computer-aided 3-D temporal bone anatomy for cochlear implant surgery. Laryngoscope 1990;100(4):417–421
12. Roland PS, Wright CG. Surgical aspects of cochlear implantation: mechanisms of insertional trauma. Adv Otorhinolaryngol 2006;64:11–30
13. Gantz BJ, Turner C, Gfeller KE, Lowder MW. Preservation of hearing in cochlear implant surgery: advantages of combined electrical and acoustical speech processing. Laryngoscope 2005;115(5):796–802
14. O'Leary SJ, Monksfield P, Kel G, et al. Relations between cochlear histopathology and hearing loss in experimental cochlear implantation. Hear Res 2013;298:27–35
15. van de Water TR, Dinh CT, Vivero R, Hoosien G, Eshraghi AA, Balkany TJ. Mechanisms of hearing loss from trauma and inflammation: otoprotective therapies from the laboratory to the clinic. Acta Otolaryngol 2010;130(3):308–311

Further Readings

Adunka OF, Pillsbury HC, Buchman CA. Minimizing intracochlear trauma during cochlear implantation. Adv Otorhinolaryngol 2010;67:96–107. doi: 10.1159/000262601. Epub 2009

Briggs RJ, Tykocinski M, Stidham K, Roberson JB. Cochleostomy site: implications for electrode placement and hearing preservation. Acta Otolaryngol 2005 Aug;125(8):870–876

Havenith S, Lammers MJ, Tange RA, et al. Hearing preservation surgery: cochleostomy or round window approach? A systematic review. Otol Neurotol 2013 Jun;34(4):667–674. doi: 10.1097/MAO.0b013e318288643e

Santa Maria PL, Gluth MB, Yuan Y, Atlas MD, Blevins NH. Hearing preservation surgery for cochlear implantation: a meta-analysis. Otol Neurotol 2014 Dec;35(10):e256–e269. doi: 10.1097/MAO.0000000000000561

Seyyedi M, Nadol JB Jr. Intracochlear inflammatory response to cochlear implant electrodes in humans. Otol Neurotol 2014 Oct;35(9):1545–1551. doi: 10.1097/MAO.0000000000000540

10 Subtotal Petrosectomy in Cochlear Implantation

In some specific situations in cochlear implant (CI) surgery, a different surgical technique is necessitated. The objective of subtotal petrosectomy (SP) with closure of the external auditory canal and eustachian tube, in combination with obliteration of the cavity with abdominal fat, is to isolate the cavity from the external environment.[1,2] An additional reason for using this technique is to obtain easier access to and better visibility of the middle ear and cochlea.[3] The decision to perform SP is not taken lightly when normal hearing is still present, but in a cochlear implant candidate this consideration is of importance only if residual hearing is present and electroacoustic stimulation is intended. Subtotal petrosectomy is easy to combine with cochlear implantation in the same procedure and should be among the surgical options in cochlear implant surgery.

In general the **objectives of subtotal petrosectomy** are

- To deal with chronic infections of middle ear or cavity
- To minimize cerebrospinal fluid (CSF) leakage and/or the risk of meningitis
- To reduce the risk of extrusion of the array
- To provide better access and visibility

Indications for a subtotal petrosectomy combined with cochlear implantation

- Chronic otitis media/cholesteatoma/osteoradionecrosis of the temporal bone
- Presence of a radical cavity/canal wall down technique
- Cochlear ossification/obliteration
- Inner ear malformations
- Fracture of temporal bone with involvement of the otic capsule
- Sometimes in revision surgery
- Unfavorable anatomical conditions
- Skull base lesions, with preservation of the cochlear nerve and cochlea

In certain skull base cases with preservation of the cochlear nerve and cochlea, the last indication mentioned above, cochlear implantation is a possibility for hearing revalidation. The approaches are a combination of the technique of subtotal petrosectomy with obliteration of the cavity in combination with the skull base procedure. These are discussed in Chapters 16 and 17.

For all the indications mentioned, the patient follows the same route with the same inclusion criteria for cochlear implantation as used in patients without the need for SP; this includes extensive audiometric testing and evaluation by a multidisciplinary team, which finalizes the decision to implant or not to implant.

10.1 Indications

10.1.1 Chronic Otitis Media/Cholesteatoma/ Osteoradionecrosis of the Temporal Bone

The most important risks of cochlear implantation in patients with chronic otitis media are represented by returning infection leading either to labyrinthitis or meningitis or to extrusion of the implant. The latter can be either extrusion of the electrode array out of the cochlea or through the tympanic membrane, or breakdown of the retroauricular skin covering the receiver-stimulator.[4–6]

The fact that the cochlear implant might be introduced through a contaminated field during a single-stage procedure has to be considered. In chronic suppurative otitis media, tympanoplasty or tympanomastoidectomy in the same procedure or in a staged procedure is the alternative option, but still with the risk of recurrence of disease.[4–9]

In case of recurrence of disease, revision surgery in the presence of a CI is always a challenge accompanied by a serious risk of accidently sacrificing the CI during the procedure. It is difficult, if not impossible, to spare the CI during the revision procedure while at the same time performing radical surgery with removal of all pathology. On the other hand, a staged procedure means postponing the cochlear implantation, which is not always favorable.

In patients with cholesteatoma of course this has to be removed meticulously, but they can be operated in a single-stage procedure when the surgeon is convinced of total removal of all disease and matrix. In case of doubt about total removal, a staged procedure, that is, second-look surgery in combination with cochlear implantation after 6–12 months, is recommended. However, in cholesteatoma surgery there is never an absolute guarantee of total removal of disease; residual or recurrent cholesteatoma might return after 12 months or even longer.

In both types of pathology (chronic otitis media with/without cholesteatoma) subtotal petrosectomy gives more certainty of removal of all disease.[2,10,11] However, radiologic follow-up remains necessary due to the risk of residual cholesteatoma in the obliterated cavity.

In addition, the packing of the eustachian tube during SP avoids any connection with the nasopharynx, excluding infections from contact with the middle ear and cochlear implant. An atelectatic middle ear is common in chronic otitis media and may lead to the development of cholesteatoma, one should therefore consider performing an SP in these cases.[7] One might also consider SP in patients with a cleft palate or other reasons for impaired eustachian tube function.[5]

In case of osteoradionecrosis the blood supply to the temporal bone is compromised, with bone necrosis as a result. This pathology can be treated with local débridement, local antibiotics, and hyperbaric oxygen; sometimes surgical removal of bone sequesters is necessary. Cochlear function often decreases over time due to the irradiation of tonsillar, nasopharyngeal, or parotid tumors[12]; this can result in bilateral hearing loss with or without bilateral osteoradionecrosis. Management of these cases can be challenging, but an ear without any infection and rehabilitated with a cochlear implant is not an impossible end result.[13] Although some suggest obliteration with a muscular flap instead of fat,[13] SP in combination with a cochlear implant seems a reasonable solution in these rare cases.

10.1.2 Presence of a Radical Cavity/Canal Wall Down Technique

Early attempts to insert the CI in a radical cavity/canal wall down procedure resulted in a high rate of complications, mainly extrusion of the array through the very thin epithelial lining of the cavity.[1,4,9,14] Also, cavities are in direct contact with the external environment and can easily and repeatedly become infected. These patients usually need cleaning of the cavity once or twice a year, and this outpatient procedure can lead to damage of the epithelial lining with potential risk to the implant. Infections of the cavity involve a higher risk of developing labyrinthitis and meningitis and of implant extrusion. Although there are different techniques for covering the array (using muscle or cartilage) and also a technique with closure of the external ear canal and eustachian tube without abdominal fat obliteration,[15] we feel that SP with abdominal fat is the safest and most permanent solution in these cases. Knowledge of this technique and consensus for adopting it in previous canal wall down procedures are growing.

More information on cochlear implantation in chronic otitis media or a previous radical cavity can be found in Chapter 14.

10.1.3 Cochlear Ossification/Obliteration

A partially or totally obliterated cochlea can be present as a result of[16–20]

- Bacterial meningitis
- Autoimmune inner ear disease
- Fracture of the labyrinth/intracochlear hemorrhage/persistent perilymphatic fistula
- Chronic middle ear or cavity infection
- Loss of labyrinthine blood supply (e.g., after translabyrinthine surgery)
- Otosclerosis

In the presence of such pathology, a drill-out procedure of the cochlea would be the first step in hearing revalidation, because it is expected that cochlear implantation will give better outcome than hearing restoration with a possible auditory brainstem implant (ABI).

Theoretically, the drill-out procedures may be performed through a posterior tympanotomy approach. However, this may result in a challenging and risky situation, because the narrow approach does not permit control of all landmarks and makes it difficult to perform surgical maneuvers. A dangerous possible complication of a drill-out procedure is damage to the carotid artery, situated in close relationship to the most anterior part of the basal and middle turns.[21–24] The canal wall down technique in SP offers an unobstructed view of all middle ear anatomy and, if required, offers the possibility to identify additional structures such as the carotid artery and jugular bulb, making damage less likely. The more open approach offers the opportunity to perform safer maneuvers with better access. Unfortunately, not all attempted drill-out procedures lead to successful implantation as the cochlear lumen cannot always be found. It is therefore advisable to undertake these difficult CI cases in a center where conversion to ABI surgery can be done during the same procedure once the drill-out procedure has failed.[25] More information on drill-out procedures can be found in Chapter 11.

10.1.4 Inner Ear Malformations

There are three reasons to perform cochlear implantation using the SP technique in inner ear malformations.

First, there is the need to identify the available landmarks; aberrations of middle ear structures such as the round window niche and facial nerve can be present. Second, the possibility of an intraoperative CSF leak/gusher is higher in inner ear malformations.[26–31] In the literature, up to 45% of the CI cases with various kinds of malformations resulted in a CSF leakage during surgery.[32] The CSF leak/gusher is best controlled by obliteration of the eustachian tube orifice with removal of all peritubal cells, closure of the external ear canal, and obliteration of the cavity. Third, in inner ear malformations the risk of developing meningitis during the patient's lifetime is higher than in the normal population, even without CI surgery.[28] In some inner ear malformations (especially in incomplete partition types I and type III), a cystic structure filled with perilymph/CSF may be present at the oval window niche, with the bony footplate being incomplete.[28,32,33] SP is recommended to reduce the lifelong risk of meningitis in these cases, especially for the more severe malformations.

With common cavity malformations the introduction of a straight electrode is easiest done via a transmastoid translabyrinthotomy technique; however, in this type of malformation we also advise combination with subtotal petrosectomy because of the risk of postoperative gusher and higher risk of meningitis during the patient's lifetime.[34]

More information on the approach for each type of malformation can be found in Chapter 15.

10.1.5 Fracture of the Temporal Bone with Otic Capsule Involvement

In severe trauma leading to a fracture of the otic capsule with loss of sensorineural hearing, a cochlear implantation is a possible solution for hearing revalidation when the cochlear nerve is still intact and the cochlear lumen is patent.[35–39] As fractures of the otic capsule heal not with formation of new bone but only by fibrous bonding, a lifelong risk of developing meningitis is present even without cochlear implantation. This risk remains high with a standard CI approach.[40] In these cases SP in combination with cochlear implantation is mandatory. Additionally, this procedure will also give better access and overview of the fractured temporal bone. As fractures of the otic capsule can lead to ossification of the cochlea, urgent evaluation for cochlear implantation, including urgent imaging, is necessary in case of bilateral fractures (see Chapter 11). More information on fractures can be found in Chapter 17.

10.1.6 Revision Cases

Some revision cases in which the previous surgeon was (repeatedly) unable to correctly insert the array might be better treated by means of SP, which allows an unobstructed view of all the middle ear landmarks as well as opportunities for better drill-out.

10.1.7 Unfavorable Anatomical Conditions for Posterior Tympanotomy

In cases with a very anteriorly positioned sigmoid sinus or other anatomical limitations, a posterior tympanotomy will not be easy to perform; changing to a canal wall down approach will give much easier access in these cases. In the presence of a meningocele or preexistent CSF leakage, SP + CI would also be the preferred treatment.[3,41]

10.2 Contraindications

The absolute contraindication for subtotal petrosectomy is the presence of residual hearing to be spared and utilized by means of electroacoustic stimulation.[42] For this technique the speech processor is augmented with an intrameatal (acoustic) hearing aid (see **Fig. 9.1**). An open external auditory canal is mandatory for the acoustic part of this stimulation; this is no longer available after SP surgery.

Relative contraindications can arise in the presence of active purulent infection of middle ear or cavity. Especially in infections with multidrug-resistant microorganisms or tuberculosis, this is of importance. The procedure can be staged when the risks of developing meningitis or failure to control the infection is considered too high. In these cases separate SP with total eradication of the infection under antibiotic coverage has to be performed. After 3 to 6 months, when there is no sign of infection, the obliterated cavity can be reopened and the cochlear implantation can be pursued. In case of bone involvement (osteomyelitis), nuclear scanning can be used to follow up on the infection.[43] The use of fat instead of muscle to obliterate the cavity makes landmark identification easier during second-stage surgery, due to the fact that there are fewer adhesions.

The same principle applies to cholesteatoma cases when the surgeon is not sure of total removal of the disease.

10.3 Surgical Procedure

The surgery requires proper positioning, more extensive hair shaving than in normal cochlear implantation, and facial nerve monitoring. The use of antibiotics, the required instruments, monitoring, and other perioperative management is discussed in Chapter 4.

Surgical steps in subtotal petrosectomy with cochlear implantation include:

- Skin incision
- Anterior pedicled flap
- Blind-sac closure of the external meatus
- Removal of the skin of the lateral portion of the external ear canal
- Canal wall down mastoidectomy
- Removal of the skin of the medial portion of the external ear canal with annulus, malleus, and incus
- Exposure and closure of the eustachian tube
- Drill-out of the receiver well
- Harvesting of abdominal fat
- Exposure of the round window
- Insertion of the cochlear electrode
- Electrophysiologic testing
- Fixation of the implant
- Obliteration of the cavity with fat
- Closure

10.3.1 Skin Incision

A wide retroauricular incision along the hairline gives best access; the pinna and subcutaneous tissue should be reflected anteriorly for the work on the blind-sac closure.

10.3.2 Anterior Pedicled Flap

A broad, anteriorly pedicled periosteal or subcutaneous flap is created, following the classic subtotal petrosectomy approach.[44] It is left attached anteriorly and is used for closure of the second layer of the external auditory canal. Cartilage of the tragus can additionally be used as an extra layer. A superiorly or inferiorly pedicled flap can also be used, depending on amount of tissue and the preference of the surgeon.

10.3.3 Blind-sac Closure of the External Meatus

The skin and cartilage of the external auditory canal are transected in the plane beneath the pedicled flap. Anteriorly a clamp can be passed underneath the subcutaneous tissue anterior to the tragal cartilage for protection of the vascular capsule of the parotid gland and branches of the facial nerve. More lateral transection of the skin and cartilage of the external ear canal pose less risk to the parotid capsule and facial nerve branches. The skin of the lateral part of the external canal is elevated from the cartilage for a length of 1 cm and is subsequently everted. Use of a microscope or ocular loupes will make this easier. The skin edges, now on the outside, are sutured with resorbable 4–0 sutures. The second layer consisting of subcutaneous tissue or tragal cartilage is now folded back and sutured to the anterior rim of the remaining cartilage.

10.3.4 Removal of the Skin of the Lateral Portion of the External Ear Canal

The skin of the external ear canal is elevated up to the level of the annulus. The lateral part of the skin is removed. The more medial part is removed in a later stage together with the tympanic membrane, annulus, and ossicles.

10.3.5 Canal Wall Down Mastoidectomy

After mobilizing the subcutaneous tissue and temporal muscle, now the canal wall down mastoidectomy can be drilled, removing as many pneumatized cells as possible. Some surgeons also remove the mastoid tip.

10.3.6 Removal of the Skin of the Medial Portion of the External Ear Canal with Annulus, Malleus, and Incus

The medial remnant of the skin of the external ear canal with the annulus is now elevated. The incudostapedial joint is separated. Skin, annulus, and tympanic membrane with malleus and incus can now be removed en bloc to reduce the risk of leaving some skin behind.

10.3.7 Exposure and Closure of Eustachian Tube

Bone around the eustachian tube orifice can be removed. Peritubal cells should also be eradicated because they can form the route for CSF to the nasopharynx bypassing the closed eustachian tube. The mucosal lining of the eustachian tube entrance is mobilized and folded back into the eustachian tube. The mucosa can be cauterized with bipolar coagulation, after which the orifice is filled with muscle, cartilage, and bone wax to close it off from the tympanic cavity. A layer of fascia can be used as a second layer. Additionally, all mucosa is removed from the tympanic cavity; this might give better adhesion of the fat to the bone and also prevents mucosal cysts.

10.3.8 Drill-out of the Receiver Well

Depending on the type of implant a receiver well is drilled or just a pocket underneath the temporal muscle is created.

10.3.9 Harvesting of Abdominal Fat

Abdominal fat is harvested just below and medial to the level of the spina iliaca anterior using a horizontal incision of ~2 cm. Preferably the fat is harvested on the left side to avoid confusion with an appendectomy incision in future. Hemostasis is important, as many small vessels run in the fat, and is performed using bipolar coagulation or sutures. The abdominal wound is closed in two layers.

10.3.10 Exposure of the Round Window

Similarly to normal cochlear implantation, the round window niche is widened by removing the superior and anterior inferior overhangs by drilling.

10.3.11 Insertion of the Cochlear Electrode

Either the round window is inserted comparably to standard cochlear implantation, or drill-out of the cochlea is undertaken, depending on the pathology. The techniques of drill-out surgery can be found in Chapter 11.

10.3.12 Electrophysiologic Testing

Impedances, stapedial reflexes, and neural response telemetry (NRT) are measured. More information on eletrophysiologic testing can be found in Chapter 4.

10.3.13 Fixation of the Implant

The electrode array is fixated with a small piece of fascia in the round window niche. The receiver stimulator is fixated with a nonresorbable suture, through two drilled bony canals, or by screws depending on the type of implant. The temporal muscle covers and protects the receiver-stimulator and remains at its anatomical location.

10.3.14 Obliteration of Cavity with Fat

The cavity is then filled with the abdominal fat, which is cut in small pieces. Fibrin glue can be used.

10.3.15 Closure

The wound is closed in two or three layers using non-resorbable sutures. The periost flaps and superiorly the temporal muscle, which remains in its anatomical position to cover and protect the receiver stimulator, cover the fat. A head bandage is carried for at least 48 hours.

Case 10.1 Surgical Steps

Subtotal Petrosectomy with Cochlear Implantation (Fig. 10.1.1–Fig. 10.1.38)

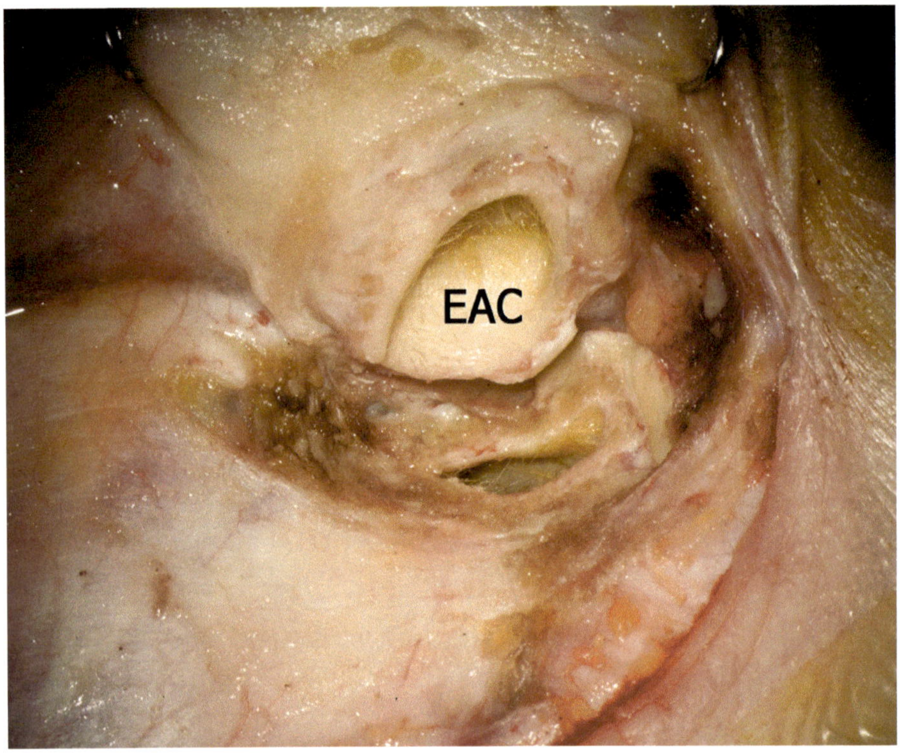

Fig. 10.1.1 After the wide retroauricular incision that extends superior and inferior more anteriorly for better access and possibly to reflect the pinna, the skin and cartilage of the external ear canal (EAC) are transected. Transection should not be performed too medially as the skin is thinner here, making dissection of the lateral part more difficult.

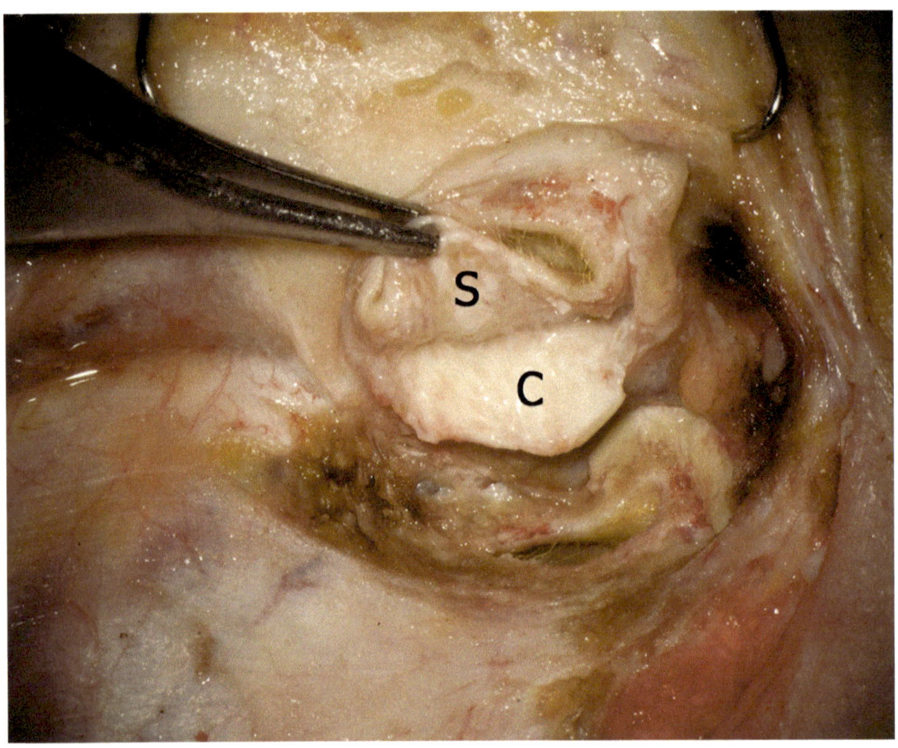

Fig. 10.1.2 The skin (S) of the lateral part of the external meatus is then circumferentially elevated for ~1 cm. Note the tragal cartilage (C) anteriorly. This can be used for the second layer closure of the blind-sac closure. For elevation of the skin the microscope or loop glasses can be used for better visualization.

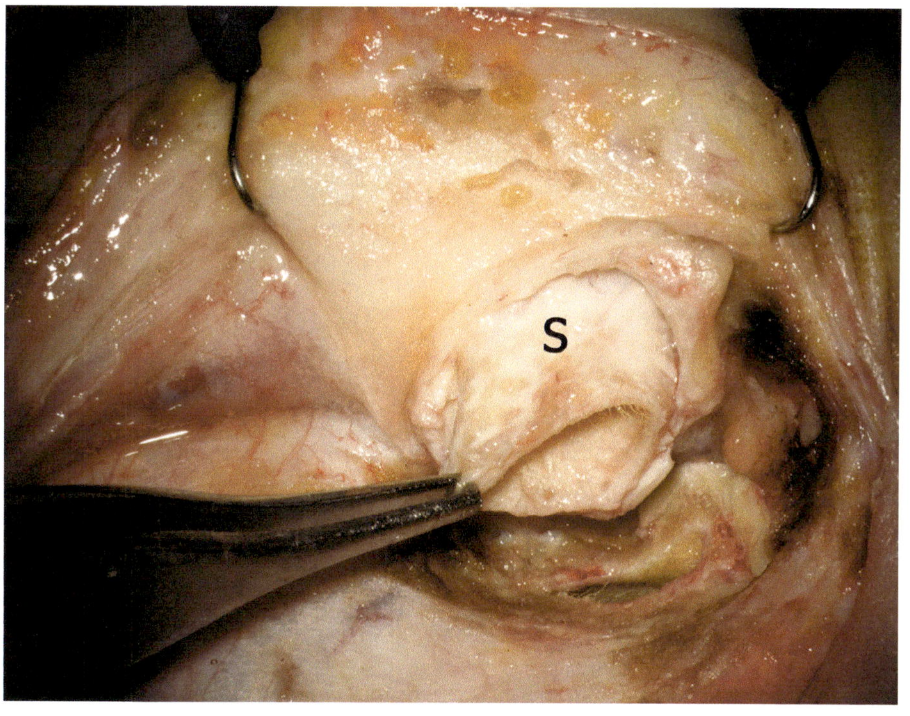

Fig. 10.1.3 The skin (S) is loosened circumferentially and can now be everted. For this maneuver also sutures can be used.

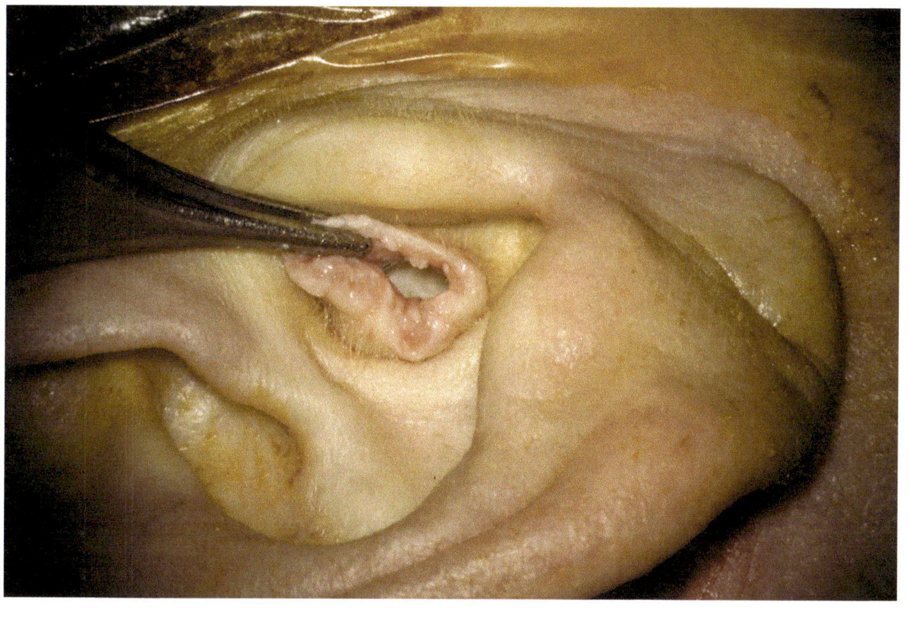

Fig. 10.1.4 The skin of the external ear canal is everted.

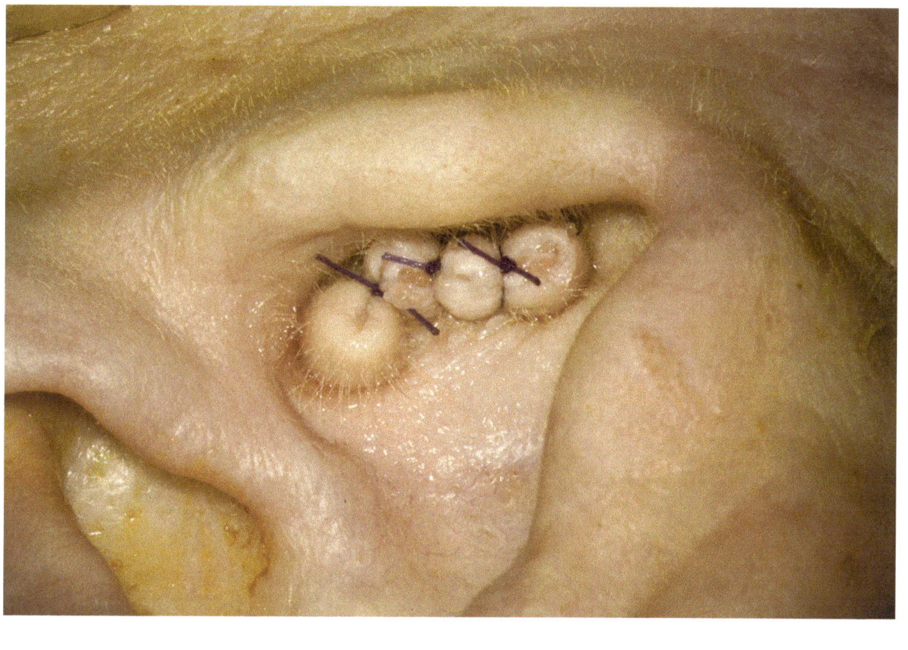

Fig. 10.1.5 The external ear canal is closed off using nonabsorbable sutures 4–0. The everted tissue will shrink after some time and not be as visible as on this picture.

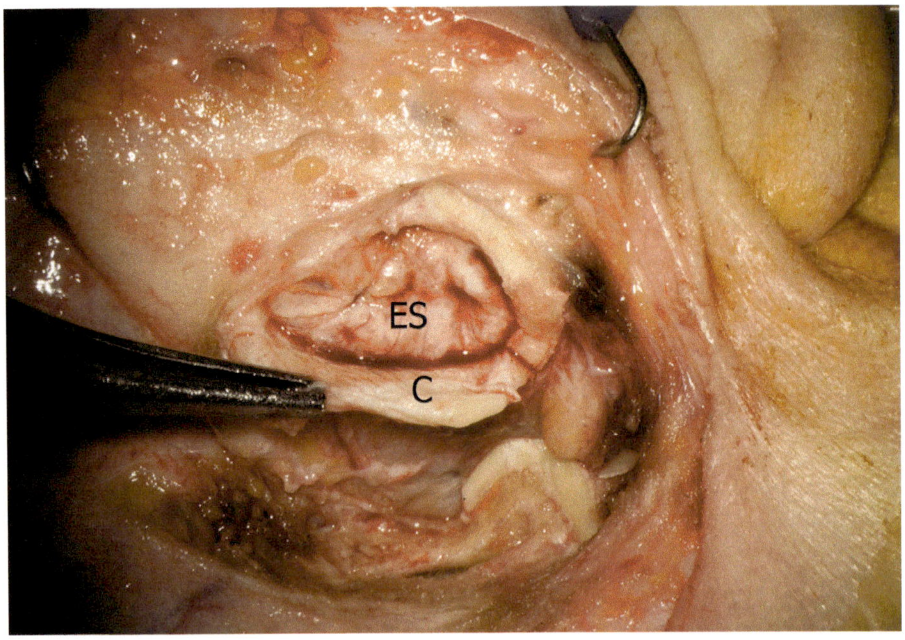

Fig. 10.1.6 Tragal cartilage (C) is used for the second layer of the blind-sac closure. It is attached to either the posterior rim of cartilage of the pinna, respectively, to the anterior remnant of cartilage. ES, internal surface of the everted skin.

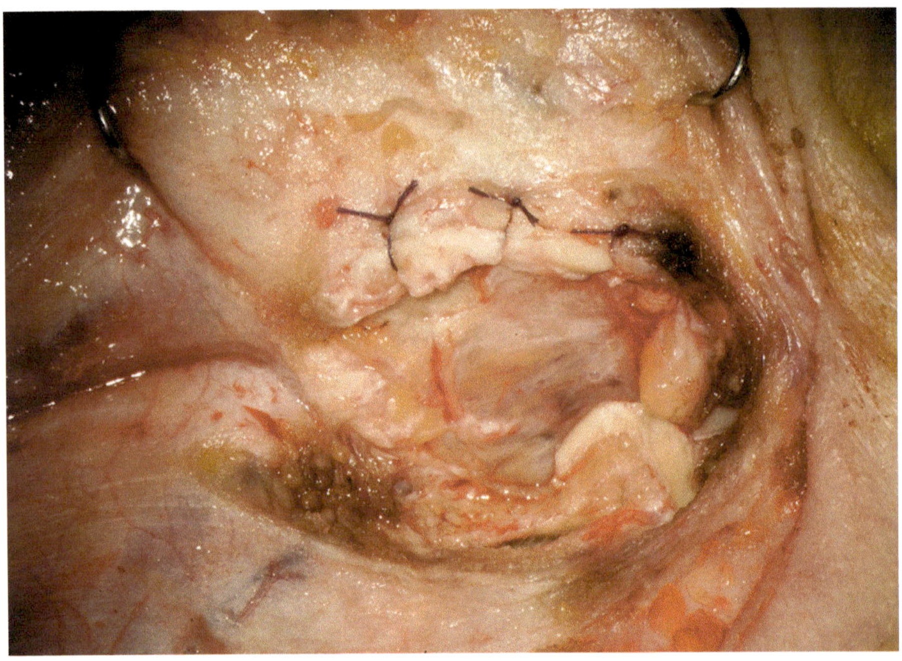

Fig. 10.1.7 The second layer is fixated with sutures.

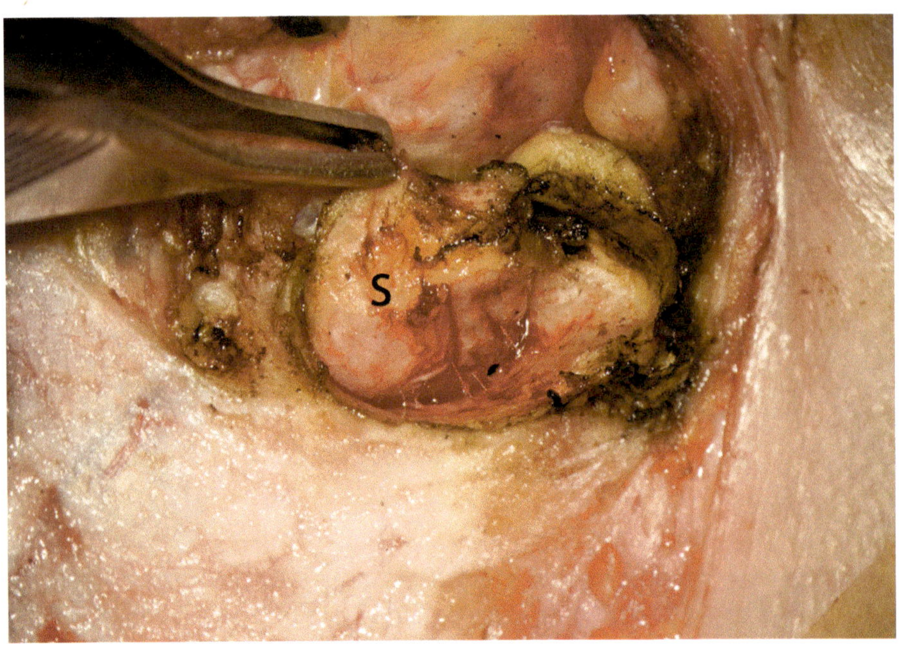

Fig. 10.1.8 After blind-sac closure, the skin of the medial portion of the external canal is elevated. This can be done using a cottonoid. It is important that all skin is removed, because of the risk of inclusion cholesteatoma when skin remnants are left behind.

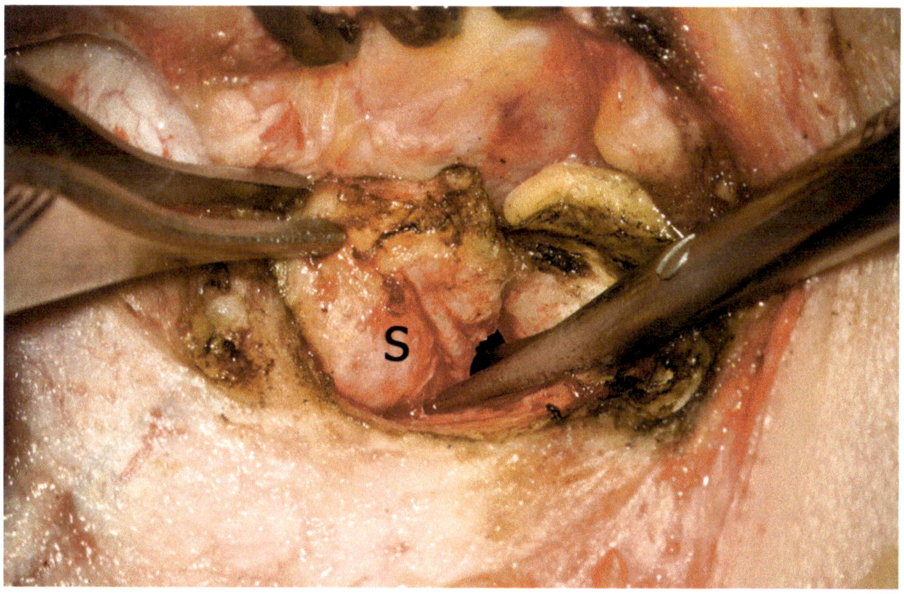

Fig. 10.1.9 The mobilized skin (S) is removed.

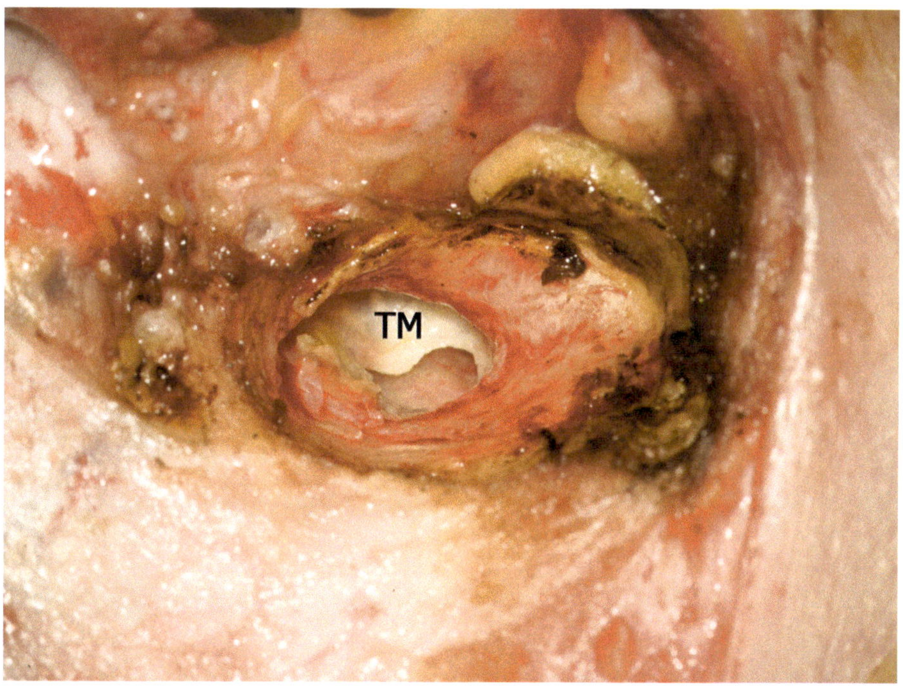

Fig. 10.1.10 All skin is now removed, the tympanic cavity is visible through a tympanic membrane (TM) perforation.

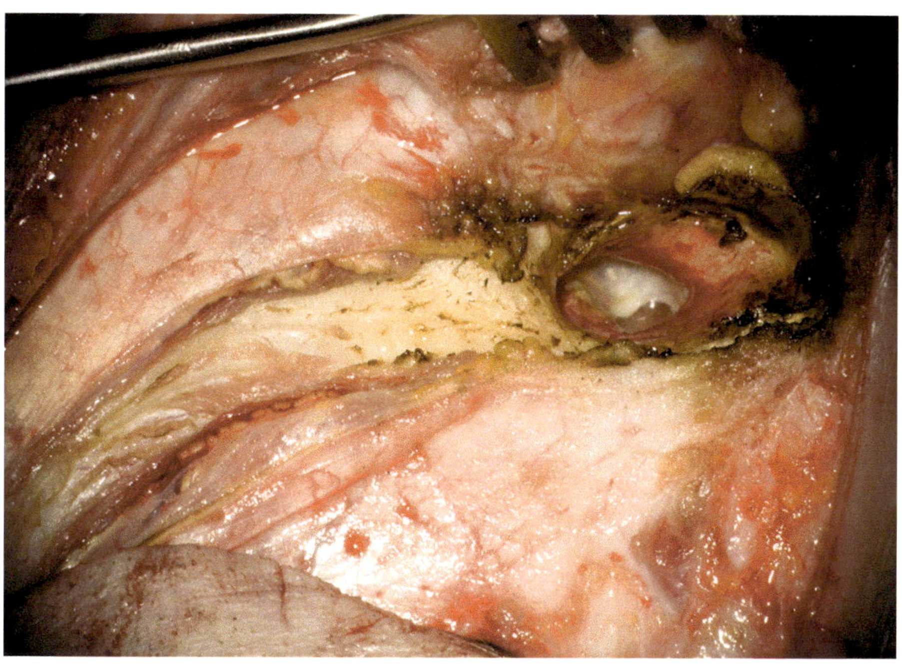

Fig. 10.1.11 The subcutaneous tissue and temporal muscle are cut.

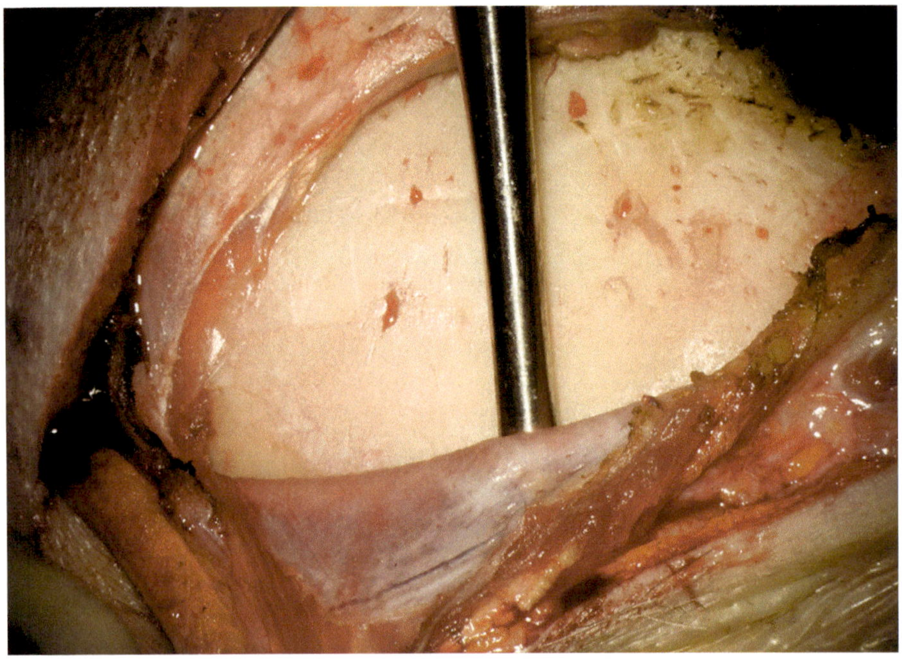

Fig. 10.1.12 A pocket is created underneath the temporal muscle for placement of the receiver-stimulator.

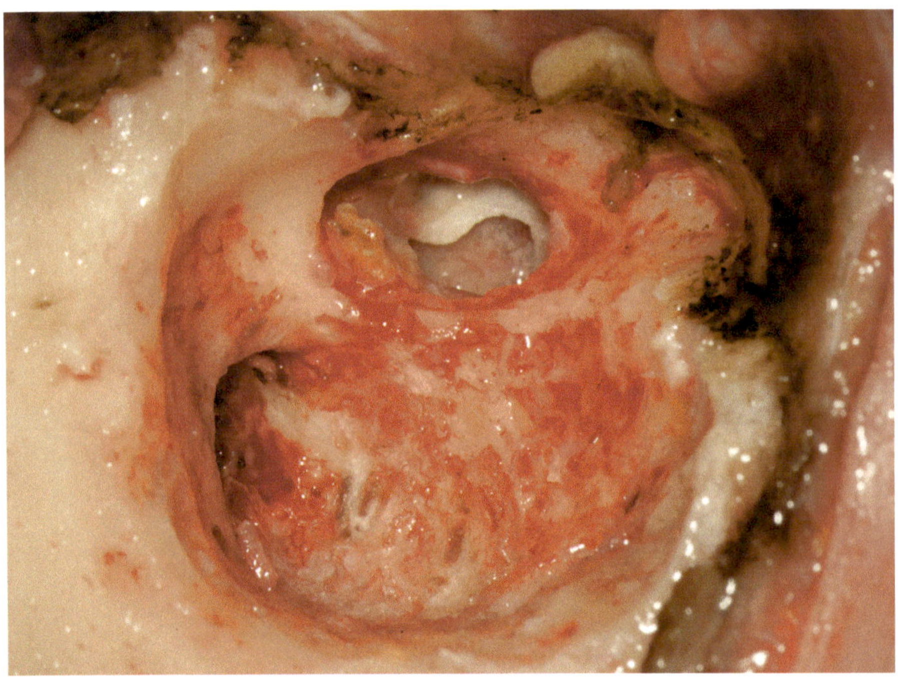

Fig. 10.1.13 Canal wall down mastoidectomy is performed, but incompletely. The tympanic membrane and ossicles are still present. Superiorly there is still some skin present attached to the pars flaccida of the tympanic membrane.

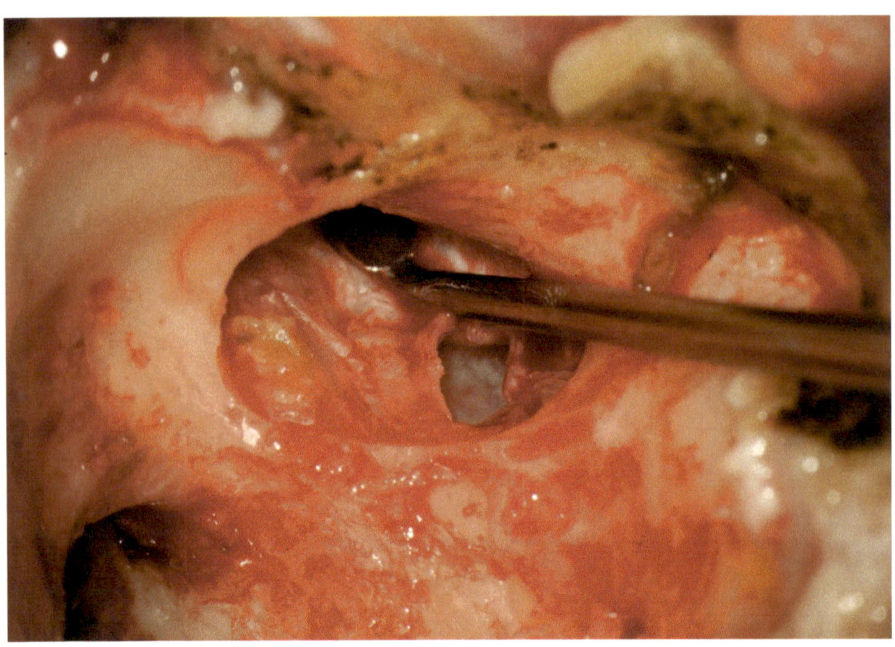

Fig. 10.1.14 The tympanic membrane with the annulus, malleus, and incus are now mobilized including the superior remnant of skin of the external ear canal.

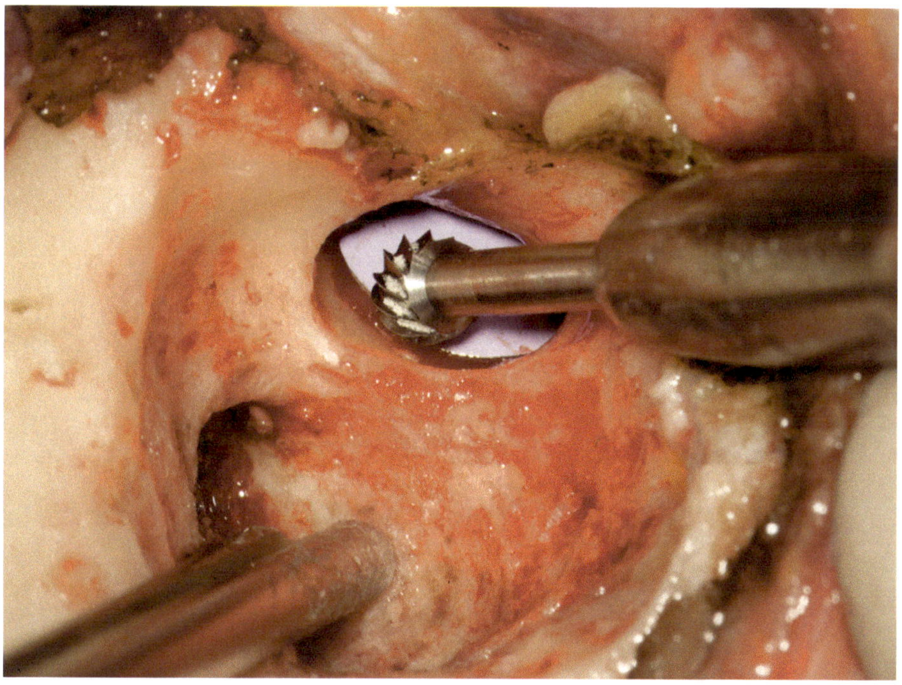

Fig. 10.1.15 During drilling of the canaloplasty the middle ear is protected from bone dust and the annulus from damage by drilling by using a circular piece of aluminum made from the package of suture material. The canaloplasty is done for better visualization of the annulus, to be able to remove all skin together with the annulus in one piece.

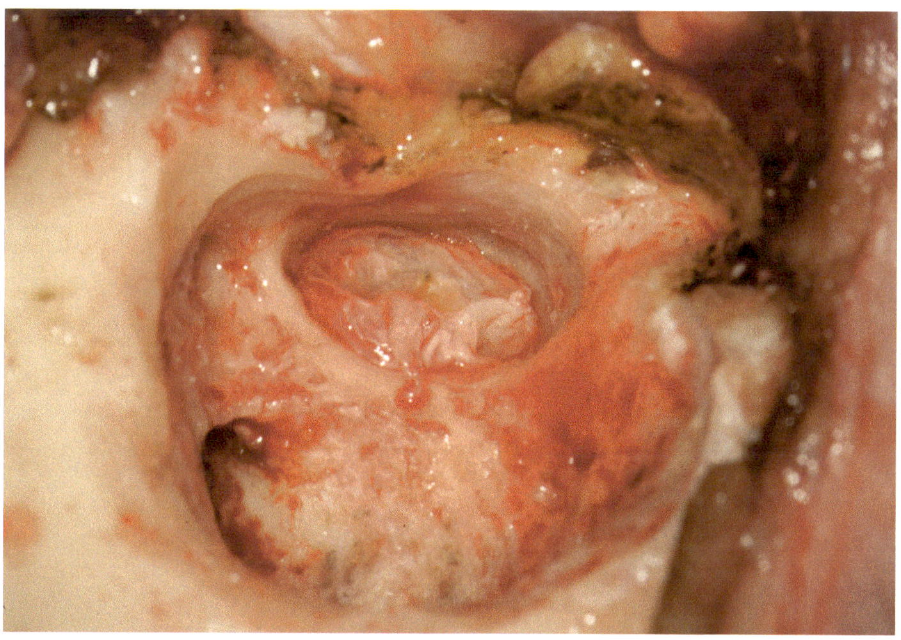

Fig. 10.1.16 After canaloplasty the complete annulus can be visualized.

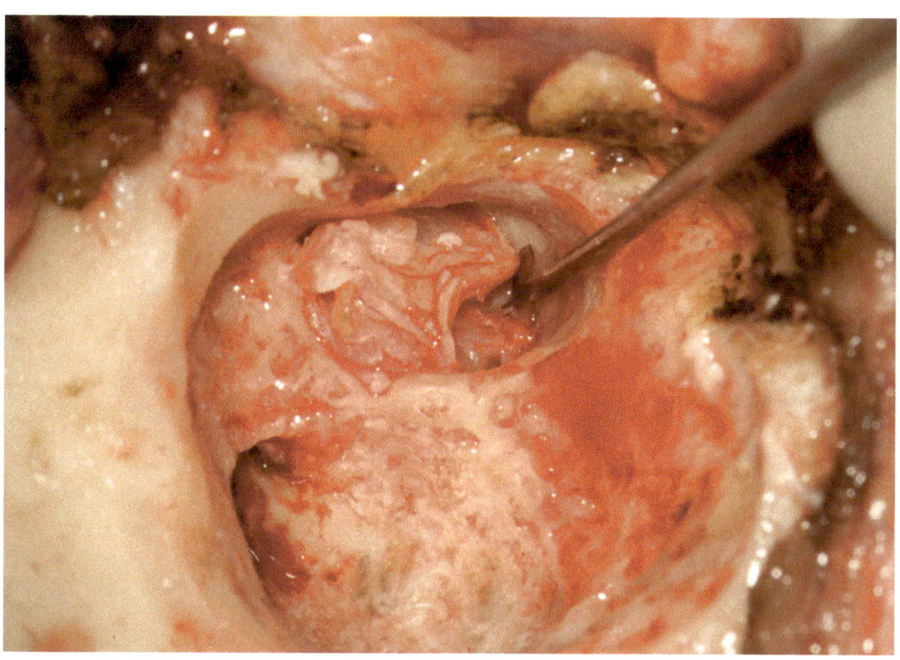

Fig. 10.1.17 The tympanic membrane, the remnant of medial skin of the external ear canal, and the annulus, malleus, and incus are now prepared for removal.

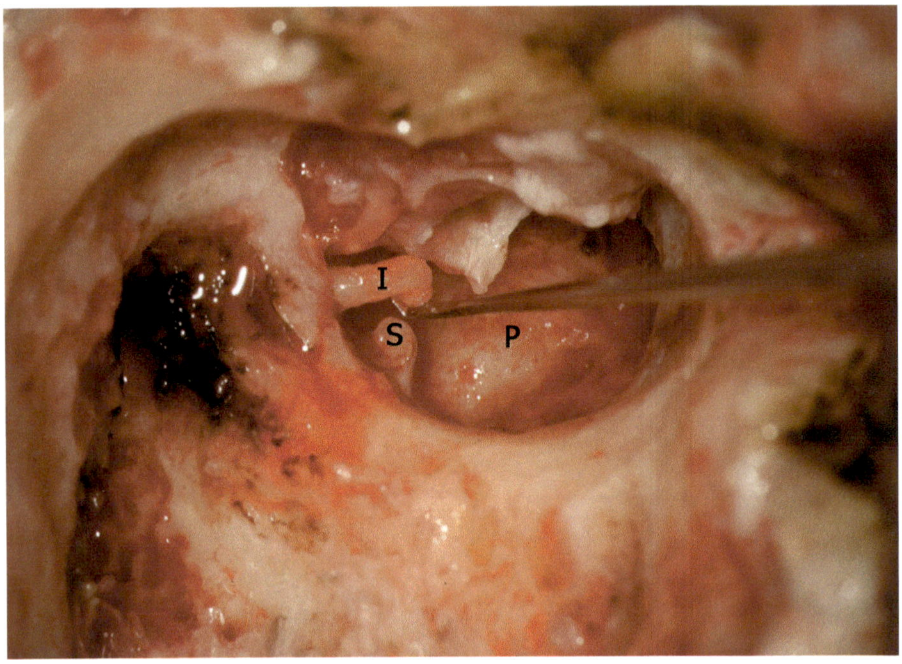

Fig. 10.1.18 The long process of the incus (I) with lenticular process is detached from the stapes (S). P, promontory.

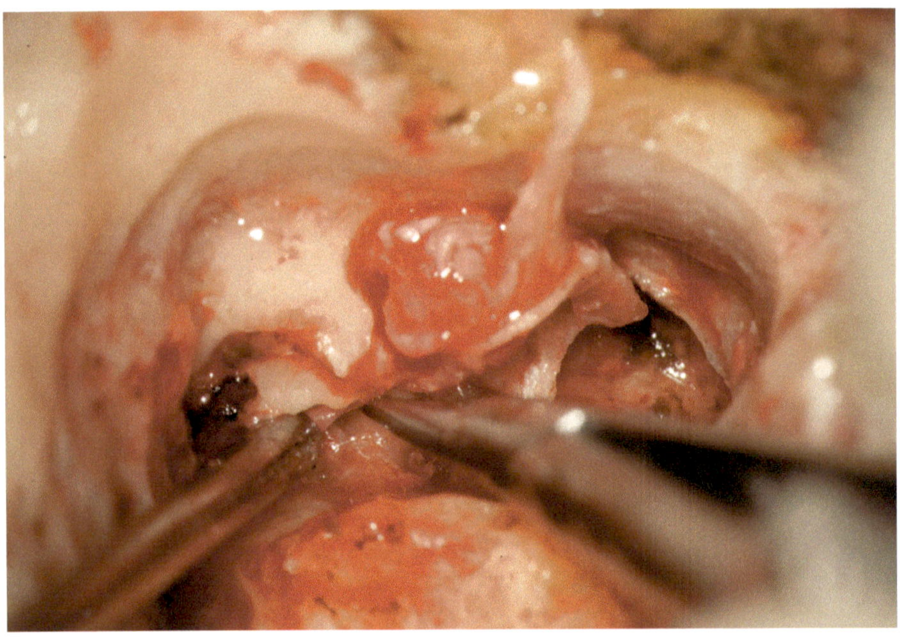

Fig. 10.1.19 The tendon of the tensor tympani muscle is cut.

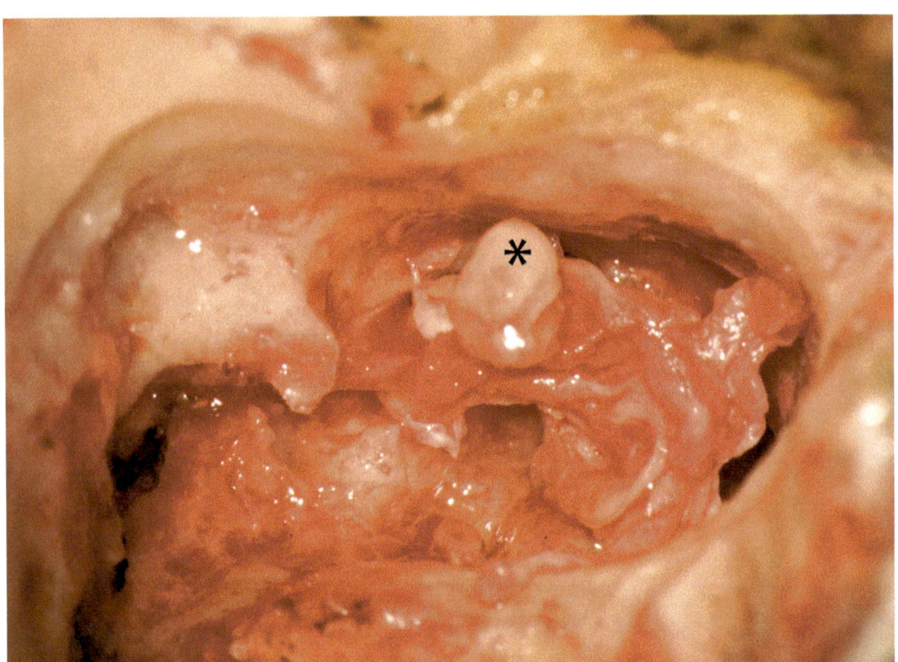

Fig. 10.1.20 Tympanic membrane with annulus, incus, and malleus can now be removed en bloc. Note the head of the malleus (*) centrally in the figure. The anterior buttress needs still to be removed.

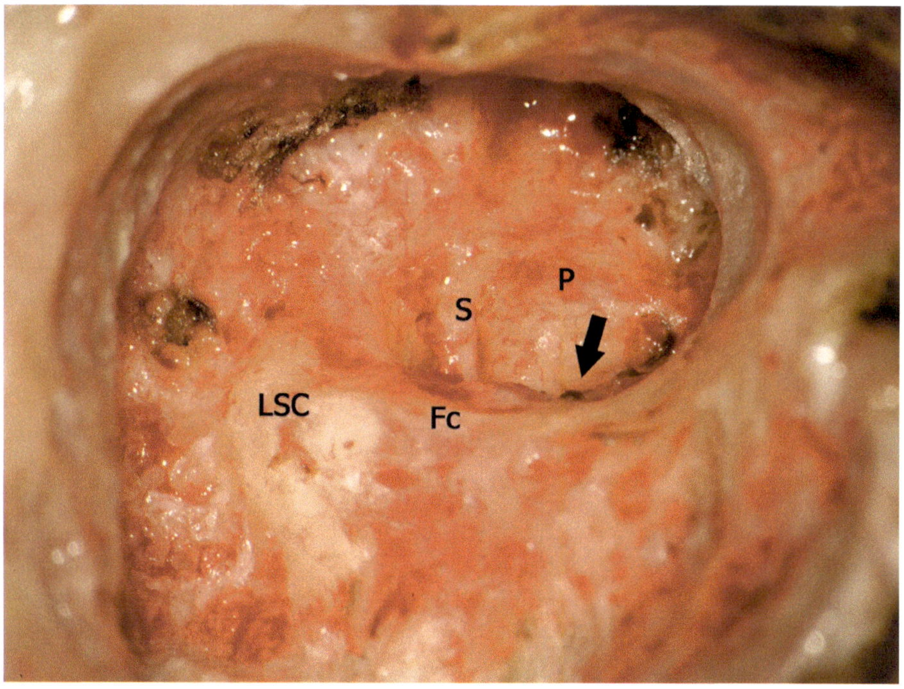

Fig. 10.1.21 After removal. The round window niche is slightly visible (*arrow*), the stapes (S) can be well appreciated. The anterior buttress is removed. P, promontory; LSC, lateral semicircular canal; Fc, fallopian canal.

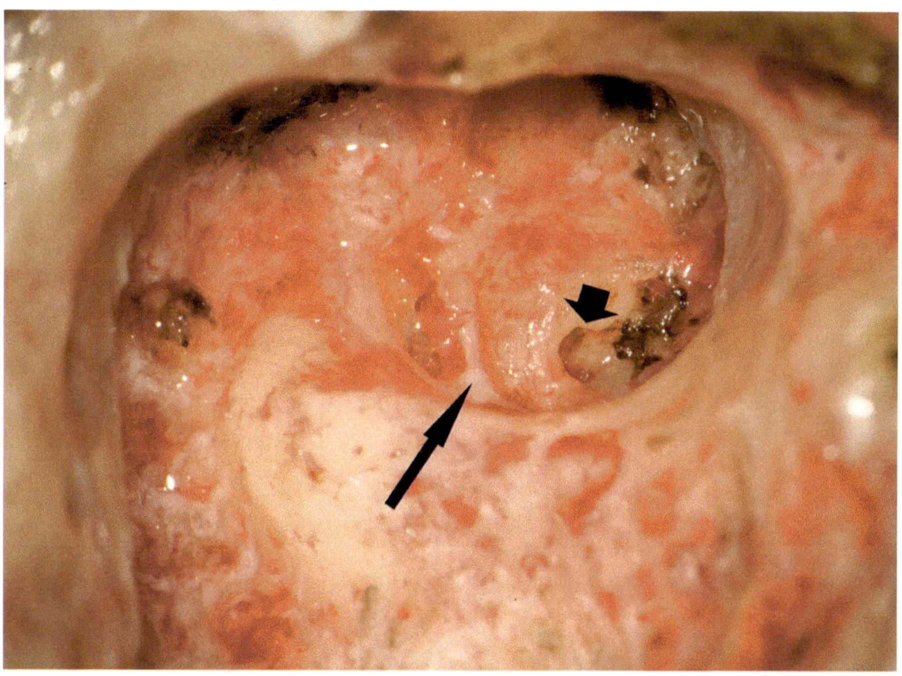

Fig. 10.1.22 After lowering of the facial ridge the eminentia pyramidalis (*long arrow*), stapes, and round window niche (*short arrow*) can easily be seen.

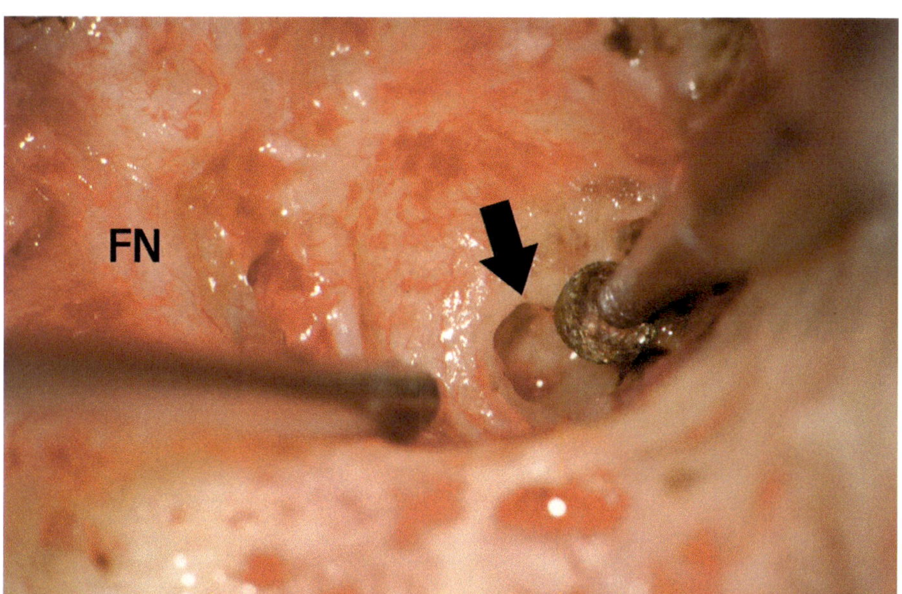

Fig. 10.1.23 Round window niche (*arrow*) in detail: note the superior overhang and the anterior inferior lip. These structures can now be removed without opening the round window. A small diamond drill is used. FN, tympanic portion of the facial nerve.

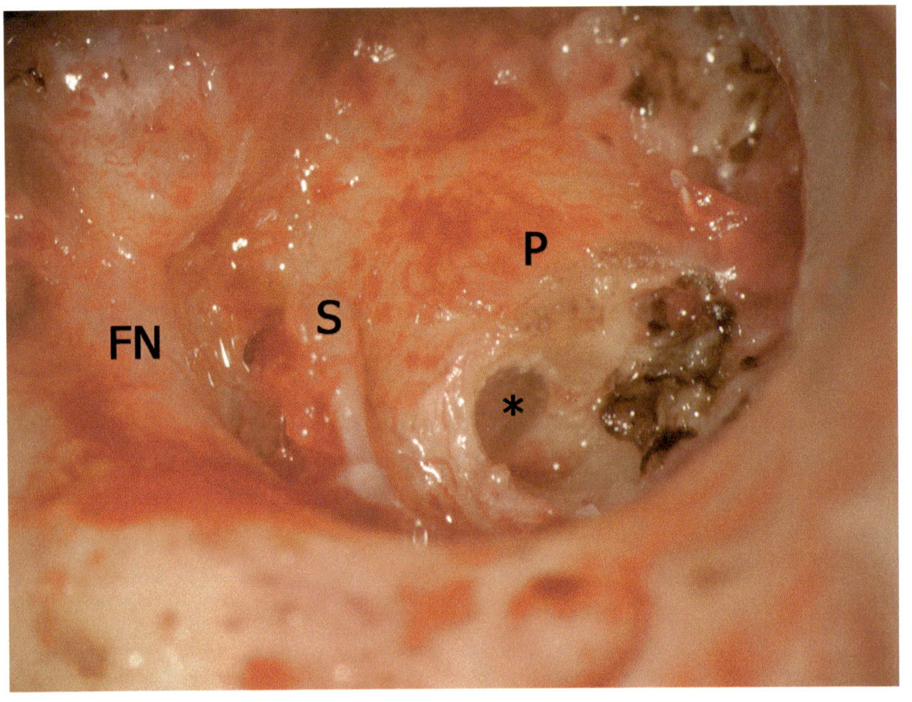

Fig. 10.1.24 After removal of both superior overhang and anterior inferior lip the whole round window membrane is visible (✱). S, stapes; FN, tympanic portion of the facial nerve; P, promontory.

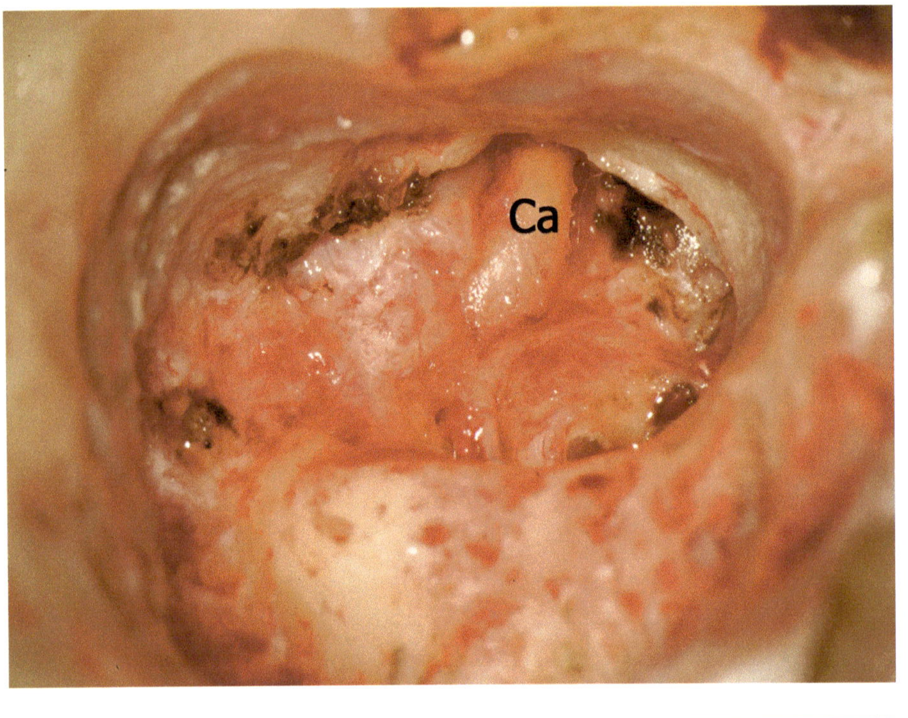

Fig. 10.1.25 The eustachian tube is closed off with cartilage (Ca).

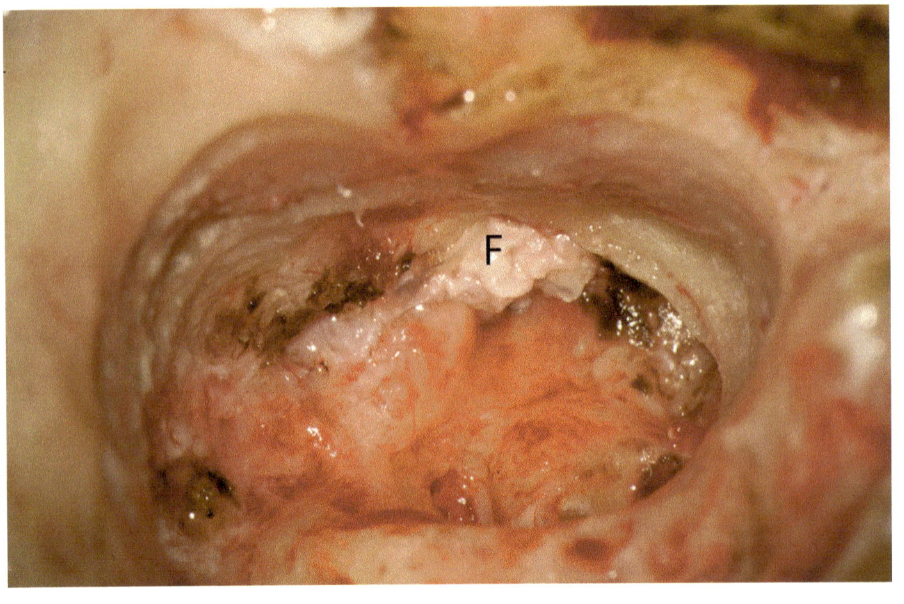

Fig. 10.1.26 The eustachian tube is additionally closed off with fascia (F).

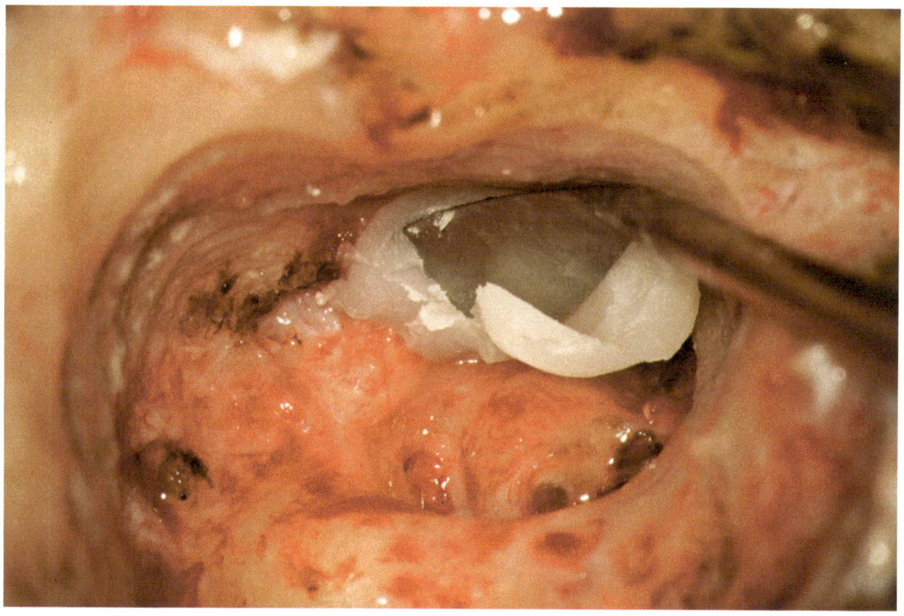

Fig. 10.1.27 Finally bone wax is applied to seal the eustachian tube.

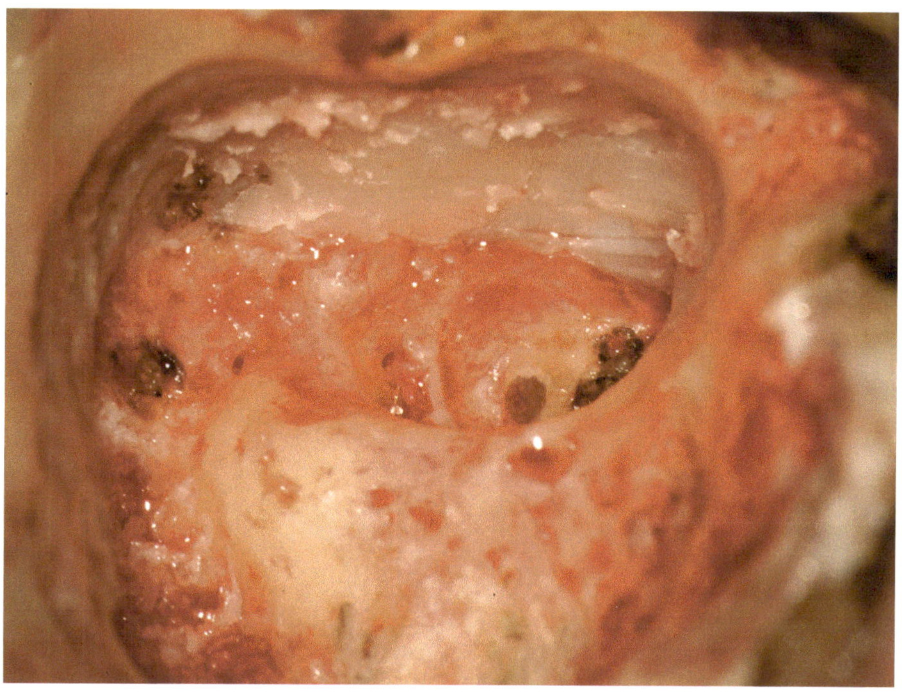

Fig. 10.1.28 The eustachian tube is now sealed off.

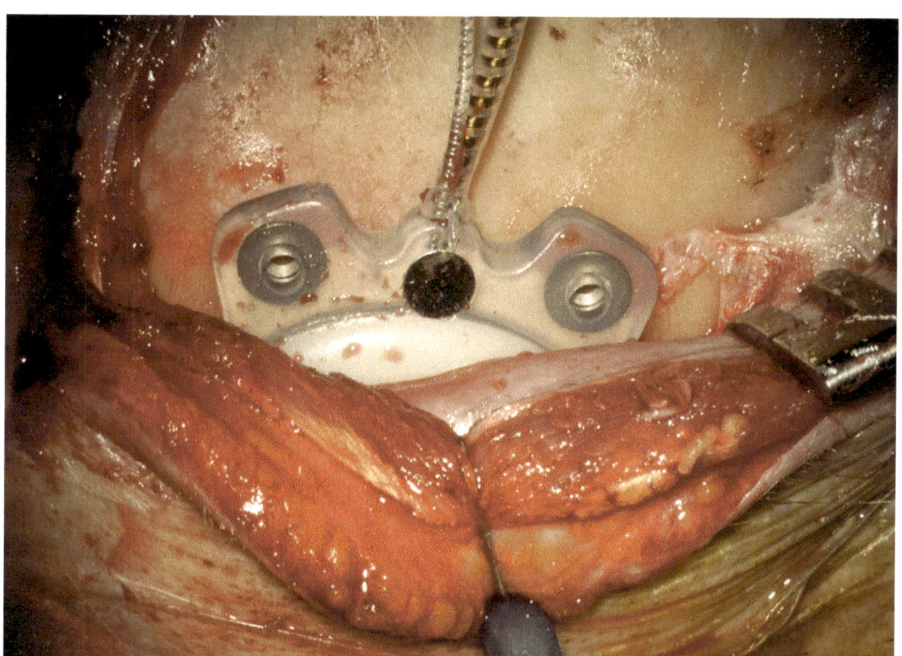

Fig. 10.1.29 The implant is introduced underneath the musculocutaneous flap.

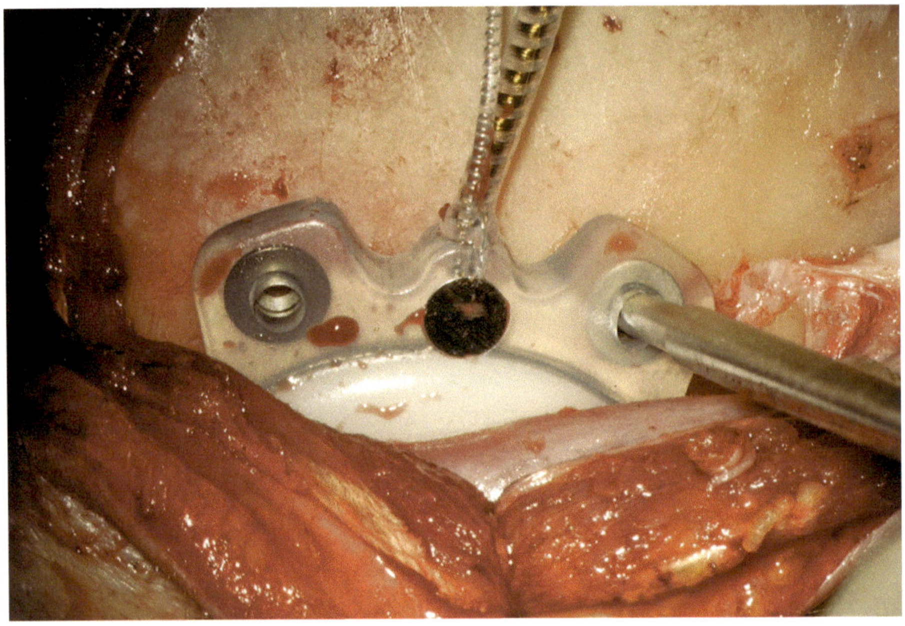

Fig. 10.1.30 The implant is fixated with a screw.

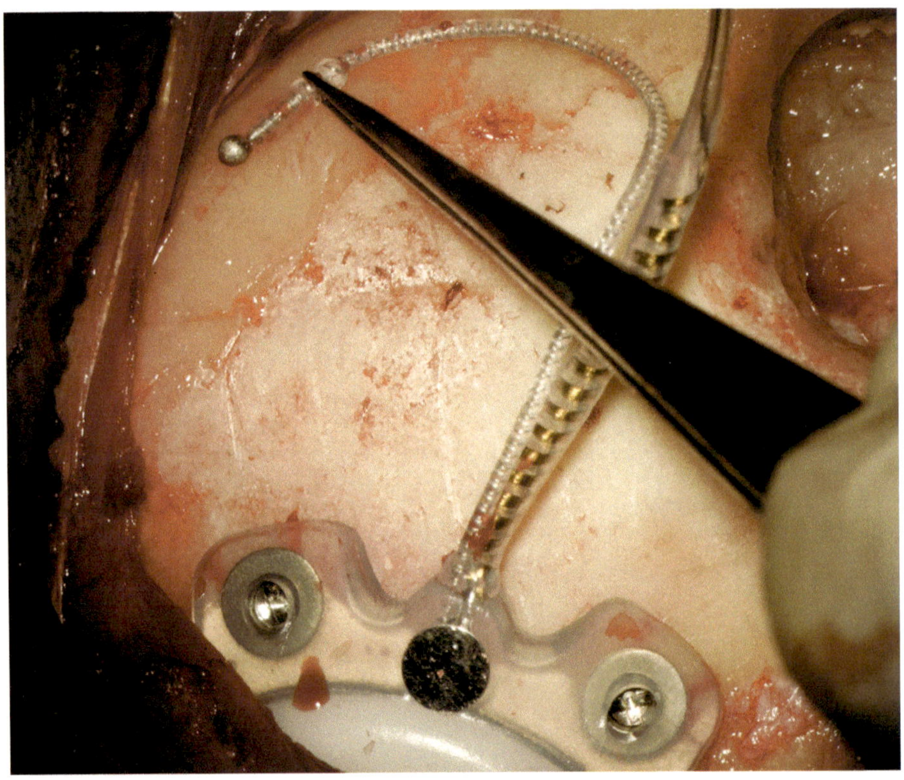

Fig. 10.1.31 The reference electrode is positioned underneath the anterior part of the temporalis muscle.

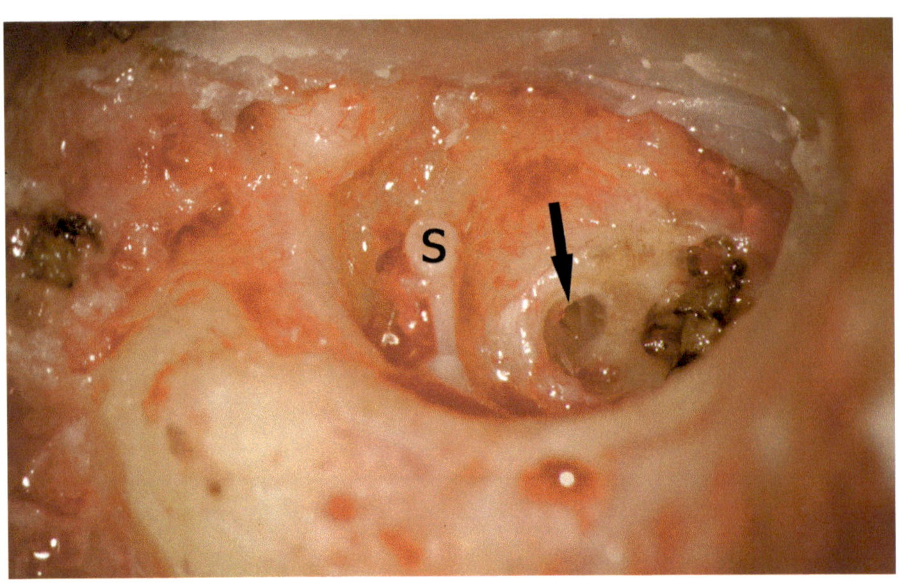

Fig. 10.1.32 The insertion can be done through the round window in this case; a small incision (*arrow*) in the round window membrane is made with a hooked instrument. S, stapes.

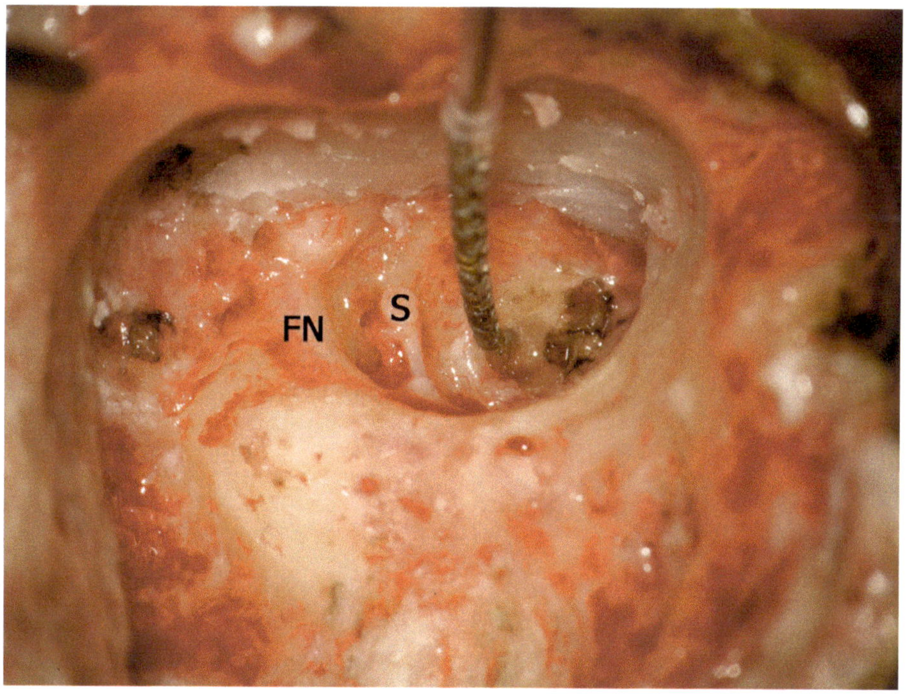

Fig. 10.1.33 The electrode array is inserted in a fluid movement without force. The angle of approach is from superior-posterior to anterior-inferior. S, stapes; FN, tympanic portion of the facial nerve.

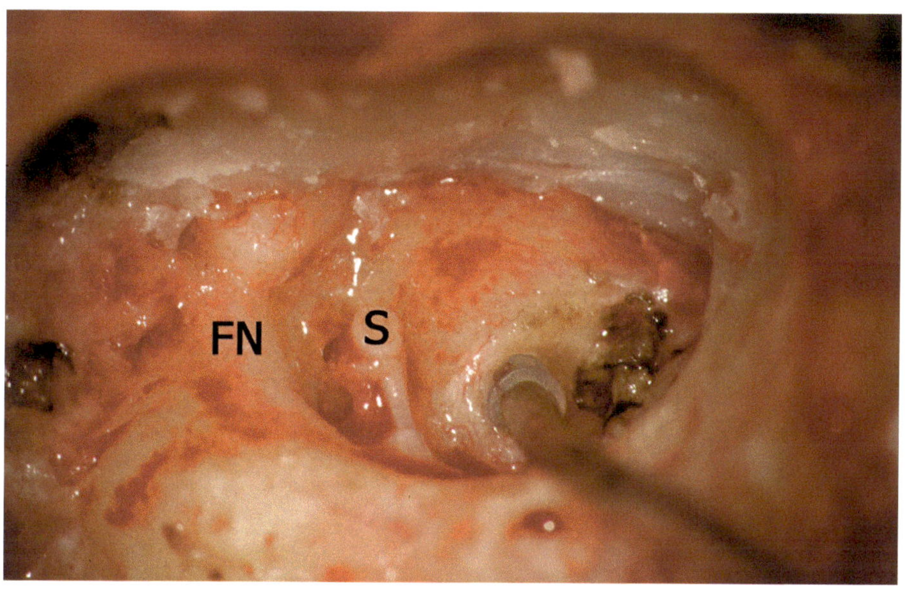

Fig. 10.1.34 A complete insertion is achieved. S, stapes; FN, tympanic portion of the facial nerve.

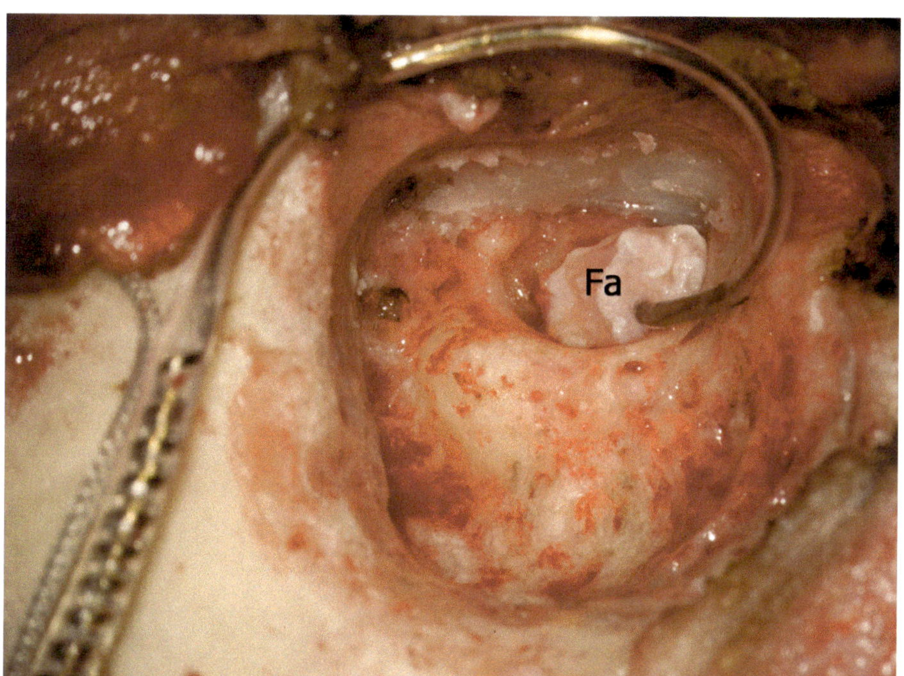

Fig. 10.1.35 The array is fixated with fascia (Fa) in the round window cochleostomy.

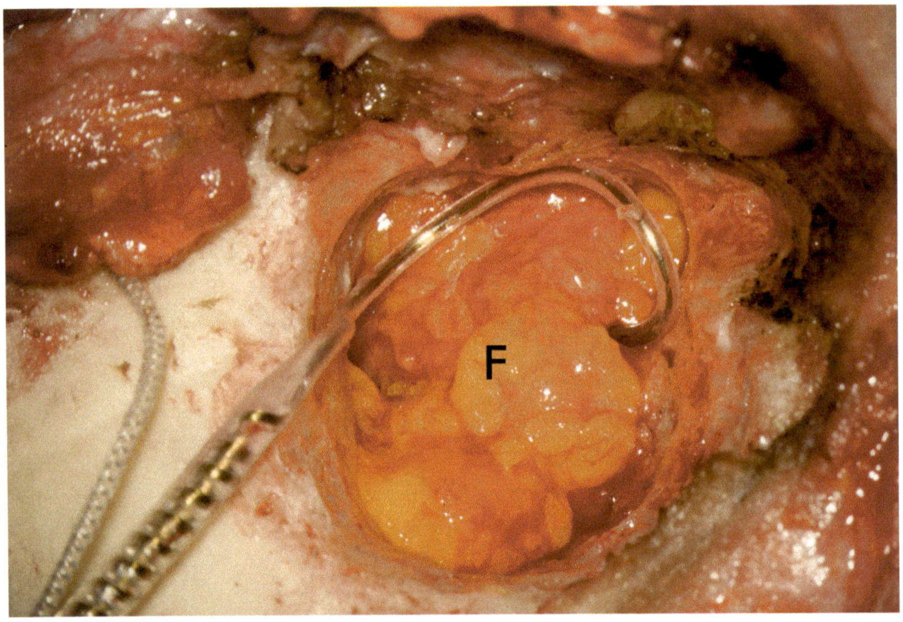

Fig. 10.1.36 The cavity is filled with abdominal fat (F) marinated in an antibiotic solution (yellow color).

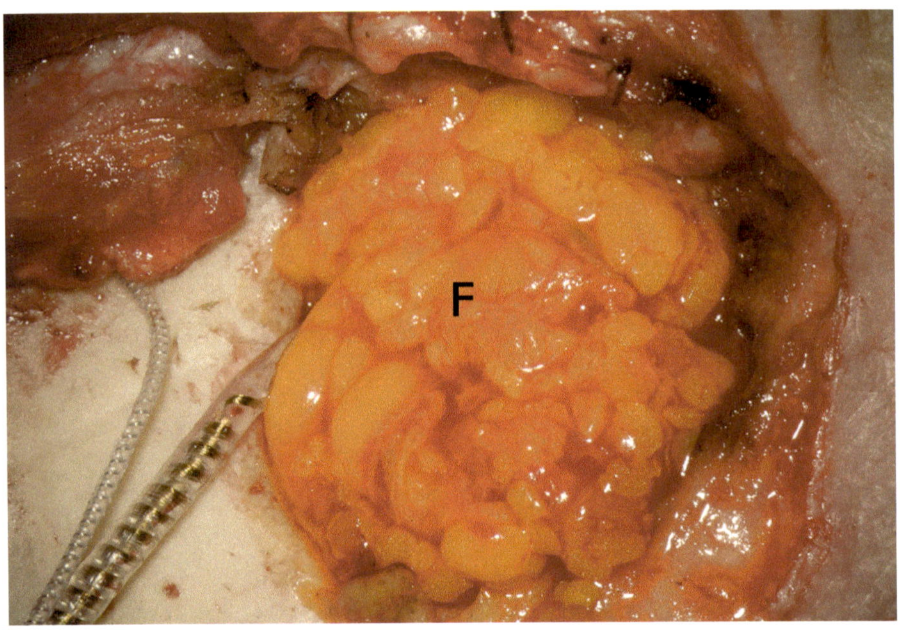

Fig. 10.1.37 Some overfilling with fat (F) is necessary in anticipation of fat resorption.

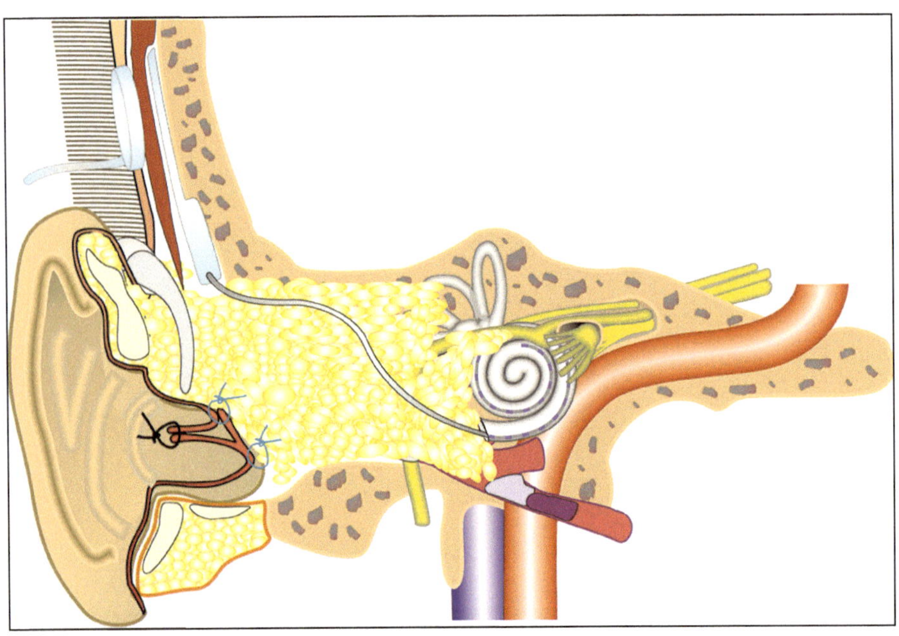

Fig. 10.1.38 Schematic drawing showing final appearance of the cochlear implant in place after a subtotal petrosectomy procedure.

10.4 Risks and Complications of Subtotal Petrosectomy

The risks specifically ascribed to the subtotal petrosectomy approach are infection of the abdominal fat, breakdown of the blind sac closure, and entrapment of cholesteatoma in the closed cavity ("entrapped cholesteatoma"). Additional risks are related to the abdominal wound for harvesting of the fat: infection or subcutaneous hematoma can arise. General risks and complications of cochlear implantation are discussed in Chapter 7.

Infected fat in an existing SP is difficult to treat adequately with antibiotic therapy and might necessitate revision surgery. During surgery the fat needs to be harvested shortly before use in the cavity and, to minimize the risk of infection as much as possible, can be kept in rifampicin solution (Rifocin 250 mg/3 ml) for about 30 minutes, protected from airborne infection, before use in the cavity.

A retroauricular retraction may develop due to **fat resorption** in the cavity. Overfilling of the cavity with abdominal fat might partially reduce the incidence of retraction.

The **blind-sac closure** of the external auditory canal in subtotal petrosectomy is considered the most vulnerable part of the skin suturing. Breakdown of the blind-sac closure can allow open access to the cavity, with risk of infection of cavity and fat. Ingrowth or entrapment of skin, leading to cholesteatoma, also poses a risk. Accordingly, this closure needs to be performed with utmost care and always in two layers.

The risk of **entrapped cholesteatoma** in the obliterated cavity should always be considered; however, a meticulous surgical technique may reduce this risk to almost zero.[45,46] Removal of all skin using cottonoid dissection and smoothing the remaining bony walls subsequently by drilling will lower this risk considerably. In situations considered at high risk for a residual lesion, a staged procedure may be carried out. Besides these precautions, all patients need prolonged postoperative follow-up and routine CT scanning.

10.5 Postoperative Imaging

Follow-up with imaging is required after subtotal petrosectomy because of the risk of entrapped cholesteatoma. The routine use of MRI for follow-up of SP cavities is impeded in the presence of a cochlear implant, although MRI up to 1.5 T can be used safely after application of a head bandage to fixate the implant.[47,48] However, the visibility of a possible cholesteatoma on MRI will be poor because of the presence of artifacts. Removal of the magnet requires only two small procedures (removal and replacement) performed under local anesthesia, but will hardly give better detection because artifacts from the cochlear implant will still be present. Moreover, both procedures may lead to infection of the surgical site and weakening of the pocket carrying the magnet, giving more risk for displacement.[48]

Although not the gold standard for detection of residual cholesteatoma, CT imaging of the patient at 1, 3, 5, and 10 years postoperatively is a good option for follow-up. The capacity of CT in this situation is improved by the presence of the abdominal fat, which creates an ideal interface for differentiation (**Figs. 10.1 and 10.2**). Repeated CT examinations might reveal growth of the lesion and thus increase suspicion of cholesteatoma.

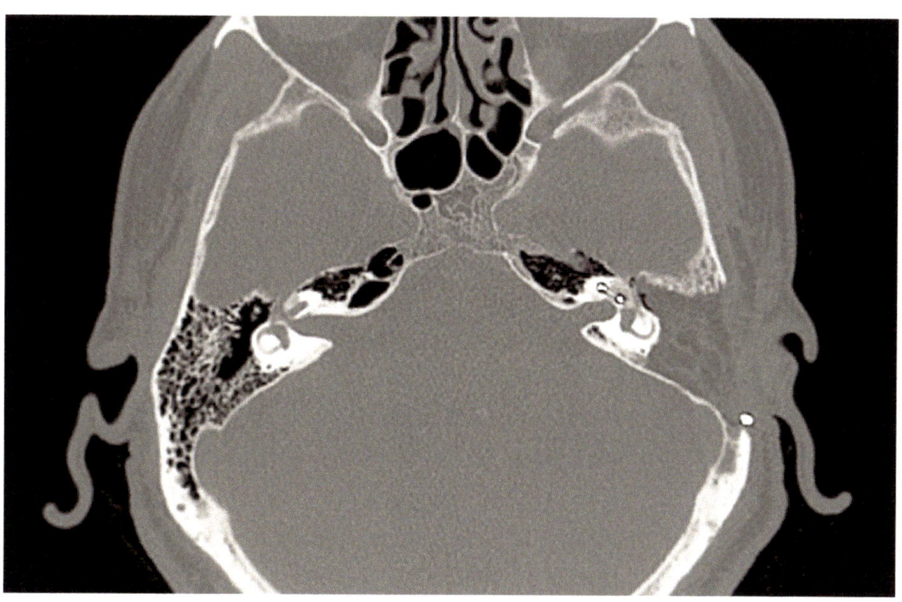

Fig. 10.1 Postoperative CT image of subtotal petrosectomy with fat obliteration. A homogeneously filled cavity is present on the left side.

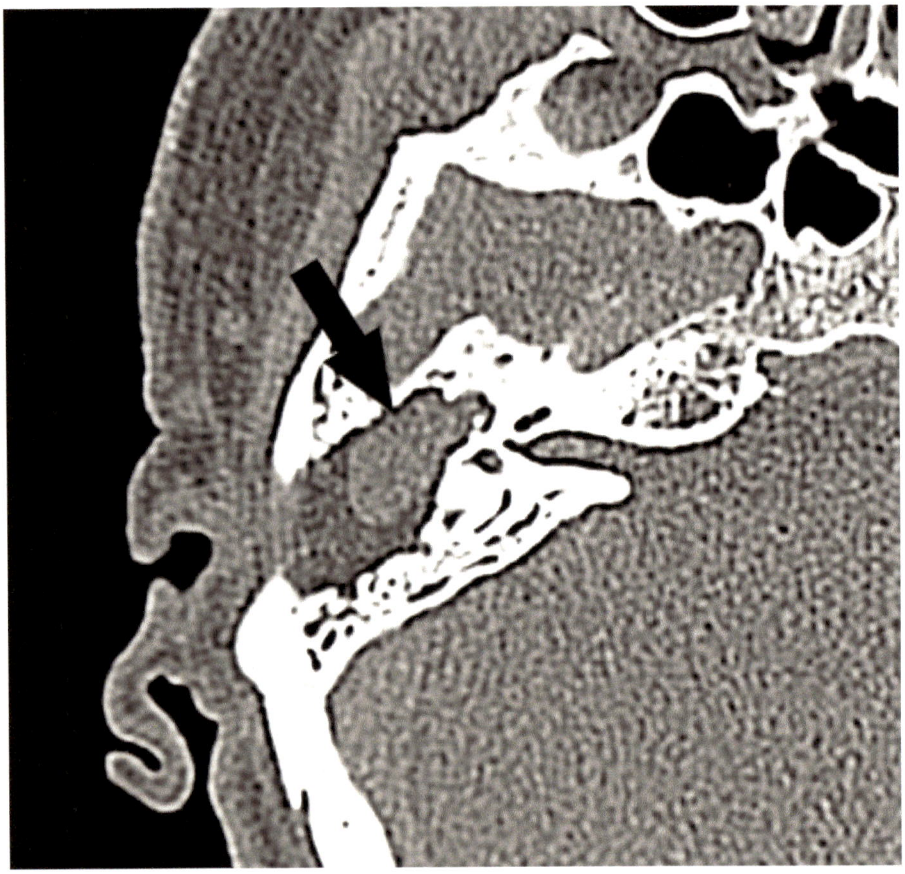

Fig. 10.2 Postoperative transverse axial CT follow-up image of subtotal petrosectomy cavity (without cochlear implant present) with entrapped cholesteatoma (*arrow*) in the right ear. Note the difference in intensity between the fat and the cholesteatoma.

Pearls and Pitfalls in Subtotal Petrosectomy Surgery Combined with Cochlear Implantation

- The blind-sac closure of the external auditory canal is easier to perform when the transection of the skin and cartilage is done more laterally. The skin is thicker at this site, making dissection easier.
- Suturing of the blind-sac closure is done with resorbable sutures because the removal of any nonresorbable sutures might open up the wound edges anew, giving the risk of skin ingrowth or infection of the cavity.
- For better visualization during elevation of the skin, the microscope can be used.
- Removal of all skin from the external ear canal leaving no remnant in the cavity is important because of the risk of development of cholesteatoma in the occluded cavity. The use of a cottonoid to elevate and remove the skin followed by drilling of the remaining ear canal wall minimizes the chance of leaving any remnants of skin.
- The stapes is left in the cavity, although some surgeons prefer to remove the superstructure. The rationale for removal is that in theory the stapes could tilt and create a perilymphatic fistula or additional damage to the labyrinth. This can be prevented by carefully positioning small pieces of fat around the stapes. Also the possibility of observing stapedial reflexes after cochlear implantation then remains. A good reason for removal of the superstructure is possible epidermization on it.
- Tight closure of the eustachian tube is difficult because this is a dynamic structure; closure in several layers will give the best results to occlude the cavity from the nasopharynx.
- Subtotal petrosectomy gives opportunity for more aggressive removal of disease because the cavity will be closed off from the environment. For example, in removal of cholesteatoma or inflammatory tissue, more bone can be removed or a bare dura can be left behind.
- In SP + CI care must be taken that blood and bone dust do not enter the cochlea, and suction on the perilymphatic spaces must be avoided for protection of the intracochlear structures. Hearing preservation will not be relevant because of the blind-sac closure of the ear canal, but preservation of the intracochlear structures remains desirable.
- Subtotal petrosectomy provides better access and more comfortable surgery in drill-out procedures with better control of the landmarks.
- When the basal turn or middle turn are opened in drill-out procedures there is a higher chance of meningitis developing, and also of extrusion of the array from the grooves in the cochlea. In these cases the array has to be carefully fixated with fascia, muscle, and fibrin glue, preferably in several layers, and an extra tight filling with fat over the cochlea is advisable. This can also be done in fractures of the otic capsule. In malformations, extra care must be taken in sealing off the cochleostomy site to prevent a possible gusher, but at the same time the sites of the (presumably) round and oval windows can be carefully sealed off, given the opportunity of doing so during this procedure.
- A wider skin incision, more drilling, and a fat filled cavity sometimes result in a lower position of the pinna (0.5–1 cm). This can be of esthetic value to the patient and needs to be included in counseling preoperatively.
- In subtotal petrosectomy it is advisable to fixate the receiver-stimulator because of the wider incision.
- The harvesting of fat needs to be done shortly before use, to minimize the risk of airborne bacterial contamination as much as possible.
- After SP with cochlear implantation, extra care in hemostasis and a tight head bandage for at least 48 hours are advisable.
- Subtotal petrosectomy gives better control and visibility of the landmarks, gives better access, and reduces the risks of postoperative infection by isolating the cavity from the external environment.

Reference Video

See Video 10.1.

References

1. Issing PR, Schönermark MP, Winkelmann S, Kempf HG, Ernst A. Cochlear implantation in patients with chronic otitis: indications for subtotal petrosectomy and obliteration of the middle ear. Skull Base Surg 1998;8(3):127–131
2. Bendet E, Cerenko D, Linder TE, Fisch U. Cochlear implantation after subtotal petrosectomies. Eur Arch Otorhinolaryngol 1998;255(4):169–174
3. Free RH, Falcioni M, Di Trapani G, Giannuzzi AL, Russo A, Sanna M. The role of subtotal petrosectomy in cochlear implant surgery—a report of 32 cases and review on indications. Otol Neurotol 2013;34(6):1033–1040
4. Leung R, Briggs RJS. Indications for and outcomes of mastoid obliteration in cochlear implantation. Otol Neurotol 2007;28(3):330–334
5. Roehm PC, Gantz BJ. Cochlear implant explantation as a sequela of severe chronic otitis media: case report and review of the literature. Otol Neurotol 2006;27(3):332–336
6. Incesulu A, Kocaturk S, Vural M. Cochlear implantation in chronic otitis media. J Laryngol Otol 2004;118(1):3–7
7. Xenellis J, Nikolopoulos TP, Marangoudakis P, Vlastarakos PV, Tsangaroulakis A, Ferekidis E. Cochlear implantation in atelectasis and chronic otitis media: long-term follow-up. Otol Neurotol 2008;29(4):499–501
8. Hellingman CA, Dunnebier EA. Cochlear implantation in patients with acute or chronic middle ear infectious disease: a review of the literature. Eur Arch Otorhinolaryngol 2009;266(2):171–176
9. Postelmans JTF, Stokroos RJ, Linmans JJ, Kremer B. Cochlear implantation in patients with chronic otitis media: 7 years' experience in Maastricht. Eur Arch Otorhinolaryngol 2009;266(8):1159–1165
10. Sanna M, Dispenza F, Flanagan S, De Stefano A, Falcioni M. Management of chronic otitis by middle ear obliteration with blind sac closure of the external auditory canal. Otol Neurotol 2008;29(1):19–22
11. Sanna M, Pandya Y, Mancini F, Sequino G, Piccirillo E. Petrous bone cholesteatoma: classification, management and review of the literature. Audiol Neurootol 2011;16(2):124–136
12. van der Putten L, de Bree R, Plukker JT, et al. Permanent unilateral hearing loss after radiotherapy for parotid gland tumors. Head Neck 2006;28(10):902–908
13. Adunka OF, Buchman CA. Cochlear implantation in the irradiated temporal bone. J Laryngol Otol 2007;121(1):83–86
14. Pasanisi E, Vincenti V, Bacciu A, et al. Multichannel cochlear implantation in radical mastoidectomy cavities. Otolaryngol Head Neck Surg 2002;127(5):432–436
15. El-Kashlan HK, Arts HA, Telian SA. External auditory canal closure in cochlear implant surgery. Otol Neurotol 2003;24(3):404–408
16. Durisin M, Bartling S, Arnoldner C, et al. Cochlear osteoneogenesis after meningitis in cochlear implant patients: a retrospective analysis. Otol Neurotol 2010;31(7):1072–1078
17. Wang JR, Yuen HW, Shipp DB, et al. Cochlear implantation in patients with autoimmune inner ear disease including cogan syndrome: a comparison with age- and sex-matched controls. Laryngoscope 2010;120(12):2478–2483
18. Aftab S, Semaan MT, Murray GS, Megerian CA. Cochlear implantation outcomes in patients with autoimmune and immune-mediated inner ear disease. Otol Neurotol 2010;31(8):1337–1342
19. Merkus P, Free RH, Mylanus EA, et al; 4th Consensus in Auditory Implants Meeting. Dutch Cochlear Implant Group (CI-ON) consensus protocol on postmeningitis hearing evaluation and treatment. Otol Neurotol 2010;31(8):1281–1286
20. Rotteveel LJ, Proops DW, Ramsden RT, Saeed SR, van Olphen AF, Mylanus EA. Cochlear implantation in 53 patients with otosclerosis: demographics, computed tomographic scanning, surgery, and complications. Otol Neurotol 2004;25(6):943–952
21. Lin K, Marrinan MS, Waltzman SB, Roland JT Jr. Multichannel cochlear implantation in the scala vestibuli. Otol Neurotol 2006;27(5):634–638
22. Isaacson B, Roland PS, Wright CG. Anatomy of the middle-turn cochleostomy. Laryngoscope 2008;118(12):2200–2204
23. Roland JT Jr, Coelho DH, Pantelides H, Waltzman SB. Partial and double-array implantation of the ossified cochlea. Otol Neurotol 2008;29(8):1068–1075
24. Balkany T, Bird PA, Hodges AV, Luntz M, Telischi FF, Buchman C. Surgical technique for implantation of the totally ossified cochlea. Laryngoscope 1998;108(7):988–992
25. Sanna M, Khrais T, Guida M, Falcioni M. Auditory brainstem implant in a child with severely ossified cochlea. Laryngoscope 2006;116(9):1700–1703
26. Papsin BC. Cochlear implantation in children with anomalous cochleovestibular anatomy. Laryngoscope 2005;115(1 Pt 2, Suppl 106)1–26
27. Arndt S, Beck R, Schild C, Grauvogel TD, Laszig R, Aschendorff A. Management of cochlear implantation in patients with malformations. Clin Otolaryngol 2010;35(3):220–227
28. Kaddour HS. Recurrent meningitis due to a congenital fistula of the stapedial footplate. J Laryngol Otol 1993;107(10):931–932
29. Graham JM, Phelps PD, Michaels L. Congenital malformations of the ear and cochlear implantation in children: review and temporal bone report of common cavity. J Laryngol Otol Suppl 2000;25:1–14
30. Valencia DM, Rimell FL, Friedman BJ, Oblander MR, Helmbrecht J. Cochlear implantation in infants less than 12 months of age. Int J Pediatr Otorhinolaryngol 2008;72(6):767–773
31. Beltrame MA, Bonfioli F, Frau GN. Cochlear implant in inner ear malformation: double posterior labyrinthotomy approach to common cavity. Adv Otorhinolaryngol 2000;57:113–119
32. Sennaroglu L. Cochlear implantation in inner ear malformations—a review article. Cochlear Implants Int 2010;11(1):4–41
33. Ehmer DR Jr, Booth T, Kutz JW Jr, Roland PS. Radiographic diagnosis of trans-stapedial cerebrospinal fluid fistula. Otolaryngol Head Neck Surg 2010;142(5):694–698
34. McElveen JT Jr, Carrasco VN, Miyamoto RT, Linthicum FH Jr. Cochlear implantation in common cavity malformations using a transmastoid labyrinthotomy approach. Laryngoscope 1997;107(8):1032–1036
35. Camilleri AE, Toner JG, Howarth KL, Hampton S, Ramsden RT. Cochlear implantation following temporal bone fracture. J Laryngol Otol 1999;113(5):454–457
36. Serin GM, Derinsu U, Sari M, et al. Cochlear implantation in patients with bilateral cochlear trauma. Am J Otolaryngol 2010;31(5):350–355
37. Simons JP, Whitaker ME, Hirsch BE. Cochlear implantation in a patient with bilateral temporal bone fractures. Otolaryngol Head Neck Surg 2005;132(5):809–811
38. Greenberg SL, Shipp D, Lin VY, Chen JM, Nedzelski JM. Cochlear implantation in patients with bilateral severe sensorineural hearing loss after major blunt head trauma. Otol Neurotol 2011;32(1):48–54
39. Colletti V, Carner M, Miorelli V, Colletti L, Guida M, Fiorino F. Auditory brainstem implant in posttraumatic cochlear nerve avulsion. Audiol Neurootol 2004;9(4):247–255
40. Sudhoff H, Linthicum FH Jr. Temporal bone fracture and latent meningitis: temporal bone histopathology study of the month. Otol Neurotol 2003;24(3):521–522
41. Feenstra L, Sanna M, Zini C, Gamoletti R, Delogu P. Surgical treatment of brain herniation into the middle ear and mastoid. Am J Otol 1985;6(4):311–315
42. von Ilberg CA, Baumann U, Kiefer J, Tillein J, Adunka OF. Electric-acoustic stimulation of the auditory system: a review of the first decade. Audiol Neurootol 2011;16(Suppl 2):1–30
43. Hoep LS, Merkus P, van Schie A, Rinkel RN, Smit CF. The value of nuclear scans in cochlear implant infections. Eur Arch Otorhinolaryngol 2006;263(10):895–899
44. Fisch U, Mattox D. Microsurgery of the Skull Base. Stuttgart: Thieme; 1988
45. Vercruysse JP, De Foer B, Somers T, Casselman JW, Offeciers E. Mastoid and epitympanic bony obliteration in pediatric cholesteatoma. Otol Neurotol 2008 Oct;29(7):953–960. doi: 10.1097/MAO.0b013e318184f4d6

46. De Foer B, Vercruysse JP, Pouillon M, Somers T, Casselman JW, Offeciers E. Value of high-resolution computed tomography and magnetic resonance imaging in the detection of residual cholesteatomas in primary bony obliterated mastoids. Am J Otolaryngol 2007;28(4):230–234
47. Wackym PA, Michel MA, Prost RW, Banks KL, Runge-Samuelson CL, Firszt JB. Effect of magnetic resonance imaging on internal magnet strength in Med-El Combi 40+ cochlear implants. Laryngoscope 2004;114(8):1355–1361
48. Crane BT, Gottschalk B, Kraut M, Aygun N, Niparko JK. Magnetic resonance imaging at 1.5 T after cochlear implantation. Otol Neurotol 2010;31(8):1215–1220

Further Reading

Antonelli PJ, Lee JC, Burne RA. Bacterial biofilms may contribute to persistent cochlear implant infection. Otol Neurotol 2004;25(6):953–957

Cristobal R, Edmiston CE Jr, Runge-Samuelson CL, Owen HA, Firszt JB, Wackym PA. Fungal biofilm formation on cochlear implant hardware after antibiotic-induced fungal overgrowth within the middle ear. Pediatr Infect Dis J 2004;23(8):774–778

Gray RF, Irving RM. Cochlear implants in chronic suppurative otitis media. Am J Otol 1995;16(5):682–686

Husseini ST, Guida M, Negri M, Falcioni M. Bilateral cochlear implantation in a patient with petrous bone cholesteatoma in the only hearing ear: case report. J Laryngol Otol 2011;125(12):1272–1274

Pawlowski KS, Wawro D, Roland PS. Bacterial biofilm formation on a human cochlear implant. Otol Neurotol 2005;26(5):972–975

11 Cochlear Implantation in Cochlear Ossification

Cochlear fibrosis and subsequently a partially or totally ossified cochlea may have several different causes. Apart from bacterial meningitis and otosclerosis, which are discussed in Chapters 12 and 13, a wide variety of other pathology can result in labyrinthitis ossificans (LO). LO is a pathologic process of intracochlear new bone formation in response to or as a result of inflammation. This can be tympanogenic, meningogenic, or hematogenic in origin,[1] and can be caused by an infection, a systemic (autoimmune) or local (otosclerosis) disease, a destructive process or trauma, or can be caused by a lack of vascular supply.[2]

The most common conditions leading to labyrinthitis ossificans are[3–7]

- Bacterial meningitis
- Autoimmune inner ear disease
- Fracture of the labyrinth/intracochlear hemorrhage/persistent perilymphatic fistula
- Chronic middle ear or cavity infection
- Loss of labyrinthine blood supply (e.g., after translabyrinthine surgery)
- Otosclerosis

Sporadic cases of LO presenting in patients with Usher syndrome,[8] with sickle cell disease,[9] with leukemia,[10] after rubella vaccination,[11] in Paget disease, in fibrous dysplasia, and after radiation therapy[12] have been published, showing that this process seems to be a universal reaction of the cochlea.

The presence of such pathology is challenging for CI surgeons because its management and follow-up need specific radiologic knowledge and sometimes quick handling; new drilling techniques need to be mastered and different surgical steps during a drill-out procedure of the cochlea might be needed.

There are two important issues in the assessment of patients with a higher risk of cochlear ossification:

- Evaluation of the *presence* and the *phase* of the intracochlear inflammation in the acute situation. This can only be evaluated by contrast-enhanced MRI.
- Evaluation of the *extent* of the intracochlear obliteration (fibrosis and/or ossification). This can be necessary in the acute phase, but also years after the primary disease resulting in LO. This can be evaluated best by the combination of MRI and CT.

The presence and phase of the intracochlear inflammation in relation to the onset of hearing loss and primary disease will influence the *speed* and *method* of management. It might necessitate urgent CI surgery, while the extent of the intracochlear disease will dictate the *surgical technique*, the *surgical approach*, and the *type of auditory implant* used.

The outcome of cochlear implantation in this group is difficult to predict because the number of cases with this type of pathology per center is small and also because the original diseases leading to the ossification can induce central hearing loss or affect the peripheral neural tissues.[11,13–16]

The process of inflammation and ossification itself can also negatively affect the neural tissue in the cochlea, with damage to the remaining spiral ganglion cells or additional decrease in their number.[16] Even the conditions for the spread of electrical current in the cochlea can be influenced by the LO process.[11] As a rule, more extensive ossification is related to worse results in hearing outcome, sometimes because only partial insertion of the electrode array is possible.[15] This has to be discussed with the patient or parents; support of lip-reading skills (level II, see Chapter 5) should be included in counseling as the most likely outcome of the procedure, although sometimes only signal function (level I) can be achieved.

11.1 Fibrosis and Ossification Process

The process of intracochlear fibrosis and ossification seems to be a general reaction to stimuli of various origins.[17–19] The time course can be variable. Otosclerosis can be considered as a separate, distinct entity because it presents not only with otosclerotic lesions in the cochlea (intracochlear ossification) but also with otospongiotic lesions around the cochlea. These are not found in LO.

A certain chronological pattern in the progression of the LO process can be distinguished. Studies have been done in animals and humans on the pattern of ossification in relation to location and extent over time,[2,18,20] showing that the area of the round window, close to the cochlear aqueduct, followed by the scala tympani of the basal turn are usually affected first and most severely. A relatively small proportion of cases do not follow this pattern and present with isolated patches of ossification only in the middle or apical turn of the cochlea.[21] Total ossification of the cochlea is only rarely encountered.[21]

Different phases in the development of intracochlear fibrosis and ossification are described in the histopathologic literature.[2,18,20,22]

Four phases of cochlear fibrosis and ossification can be distinguished:

1. *Acute phase:* Inflammation of the intracochlear tissues: acute labyrinthitis: a purulent effusion fills the perilymphatic spaces, fibrin deposits, and granulation tissue are formed.
2. *Middle phase:* Start of fibrosis. Fibroblastic proliferation with collagen deposition followed by fibrosis. Angiogenesis is also present.
3. *Late phase:* Advanced fibrosis, start of ossification. Next to fibrosis new bone is formed, which usually starts in the scala tympani of the basal turn with deposition of osteoid. This is

followed by neo-ossification/osteoid mineralization, and bone remodeling, which is the resorption of disorganized bone and replacement with new bone. This can last up to 6 to 12 months.[18]
4. *Final phase* or *end stage* of ossification: the process of inflammation and the bone remodeling phase have ceased.

Animal and human studies have shown that the first signs of fibrosis and ossification can be present within 3 days after infection.[20,23] The cochlea can be totally ossified in humans within 3 weeks up to 2 months; therefore, diagnostic and therapeutic interventions need to be performed urgently.[6,18,24] The chances for good access to the cochlea are best when intracochlear fibrosis is not yet visible on MRI, leading to unforced electrode insertion and better hearing outcome during this (short) window of opportunity.[18]

Among the factors influencing the presence, pace, and extent of the LO process are the immunologic status of the patient, the type of primary pathology or the microorganism causing the primary disease, and also individual immunotypical patient factors in relation to the specific primary pathology or microorganism. These factors explain the large interindividual differences. It is important to remember that not every patient with these pathologies develops a sensorineural hearing loss, and that not all of the hearing losses found in these patients are combined with intracochlear obliteration.

Two types of bone have been described in cochlear ossification: (1) *metaplastic bone*, highly cellular without osteoblasts or lamellar structure of bone, thought to be formed as a result of interference with the cochlear blood supply; and (2) *osteoplastic bone*, with low cellularity, presence of osteoblasts, and lamellar structure, and connected to the endosteal layer. The osteoplastic bone formation seems to be the result of damage to the endosteum, either surgical or through disease.[1] According to these etiologic concepts, both types of bone can be present in labyrinthitis ossificans.

11.2 Management Work-up

In cases with a risk of intracochlear obliteration, several steps in the diagnostic work-up are necessary. Generally two different work-ups apply. (1) A fast diagnostic work-up in cases with rapid loss of hearing (several days or less to 3 weeks) combined with a high risk of ossification: this can be the case in bacterial meningitis, autoimmune inner ear diseases, fractures, and hemorrhage. MRI and audiometric evaluation need to be performed urgently. (2) The extended diagnostic work-up will apply to all other cases with the pathology mentioned earlier and comprises additional T2-weighted (T2W) MRI.

A management plan and surgical strategy can be developed based on the information gathered during the work-up.

11.2.1 Fast Diagnostic Work-up

- Especially in bacterial meningitis, autoimmune inner ear diseases, fractures, and hemorrhage, the LO process can develop rapidly. Therefore, hearing evaluation has to be performed in all patients soon after diagnosis (within days to a maximum of 1.5 weeks or as soon as possible if these deadlines are missed) followed by urgent MRI evaluation in patients with severe or even moderate (>30 dB and progressive) hearing loss. These steps, the short time frame, and the follow-up are explained and discussed in Chapter 12. If the primary pathology developed more than a year previously, the work-up is similar to that for other pathology listed below in the extended diagnostic work-up.
- Autoimmune inner ear diseases can develop as quickly as bacterial meningitis but are the only conditions that are reversible by treatment with corticosteroids. Urgent consultation with an immunologist or pediatrician is necessary for starting this treatment within 2 to 3 weeks.
- In cases with head trauma, labyrinth fractures, hemorrhage, and bacterial cochleitis, the hearing deterioration can be very variable, ranging from immediate complete deafness to some hearing loss that remains stable or deteriorates slowly. It seems that the more severe the trauma/fracture/infection or hemorrhage the more likely the development of hearing loss and ossification, but the literature is only suggestive and not conclusive on this. No good guideline for hearing follow-up can be given, but it must be clear that hearing follow-up cannot be abandoned.[25] We therefore advise audiometric follow-up at 1, 2, 3, 6, and 12 months in these cases.

11.2.2 Extended Diagnostic Work-up

In all the other pathologies, acute and complete bilateral cochlear obliteration is much less likely; the primary pathology is a longer ongoing process. An extended diagnostic work-up, but in a less urgent time frame, is required in the following cases:

- Persistent perilymphatic fistula
- Chronic middle ear or cavity infection
- Loss of labyrinthine blood supply
- Otosclerosis

The extended diagnostic work-up includes additional MRI scanning, most importantly T2W (heavily weighted) MRI. This will provide a blueprint of the scala tympani and scala vestibuli of the basal turn next to the middle and apical turns, and will show the presence or absence of intracochlear fluids. CT scanning can provide additional information about the cochlear ossification of the obliterated part of the cochlear lumen, although its sensitivity is low, especially for metaplastic bone.

In autoimmune inner ear disease the location of fibrosis and ossification can be more diffuse, whereas in otosclerosis it is predominantly in the scala tympani of the basal turn (see Chapter 13). In fractures or hemorrhage it also depends on the location of the lesion.

11.3 Audiometric Evaluation

Audiometric evaluation is as important in this group of patients as in "normal" CI candidates, but in the LO group audiometric testing can also reveal a still limited but progressive hearing loss while LO is developing. This means that moderate loss (>30 dB and progressive) requires MRI evaluation to identify the presence and phase of intracochlear inflammation.

Audiometric evaluation can also be used as a screening tool to keep track of possible development of intracochlear disease (post meningitis, autoimmune conditions, fracture, hemorrhage). Both aspects are more important during the fast diagnostic work-up. After the first assessment of sensorineural hearing loss (30 dB and progressive) leading to imaging, the hearing can deteriorate further and late fibrosis/ossification (up to 6–12 months) is also reported.[26] Therefore, all cases with sensorineural hearing loss related to the diseases mentioned (especially the more acute ones), with and without presence of LO as found on MRI, need audiometric follow-up at 1, 2, 3, 6, and 12 months after the primary disease to check for late LO development when urgent cochlear implantation has not already been carried out. Of course, additional audiometric testing can be useful when there is doubt about the course of the hearing loss. If the sensorineural hearing deteriorates during the follow-up, MRI needs to be repeated to document possible progression of intracochlear pathology.

More information on audiometric evaluation and management in the acute phase (of bacterial meningitis) can be found in Chapter 12.

11.4 CT and MRI

The four phases of intracochlear fibrosis and ossification as seen histopathologically can also be detected on imaging (see also Chapter 12):

1. *Acute phase.* Inflammation causing labyrinthitis is visible on T1W MRI by contrast enhancement of the cochlea and labyrinth; on T2W imaging there is no sign of loss of intracochlear/intralabyrinthine fluid. On T1W imaging without contrast, the cochlea and labyrinth can be more hyperintense than in the normal situation.
2. *Middle phase.* Start of fibrosis, with contrast enhancement on T1W MRI of the cochlea and labyrinth (caused by inflammation and angiogenesis) and also loss of fluid in the cochlea/labyrinth on T2W MRI (caused by fibrosis). On T1W images without contrast, the cochlea and labyrinth may be more hyperintense.
3. *Late phase.* Advanced fibrosis and start of ossification with no sign or few signs of enhancement remaining on T1W MRI with contrast. Mild hyperintensity of the cochlear turns may be present; on T2W MRI clear loss of intracochlear/intralabyrinthine fluid. Differentiation between fibrosis or ossification as the cause of the loss of fluid might be possible by combining the information found on MRI imaging with that found on CT imaging.
4. *Final phase* or *end stage of ossification.* No signs of active inflammation remain: no enhancement on T1W imaging with contrast. Loss of fluid on T2W imaging. The ossification can usually be visualized with CT (but beware of low sensitivity) and can be graded (for classification see later). This final stage of ossification is reached after 6 to 12 months of the start of the primary pathology or may not be attained in case of a chronic ongoing infection (e.g., chronic infection in radical cavity).

11.4.1 Fibrosis and Ossification on Imaging

Magnetic resonance (T2W) imaging is superior to CT scanning for detection of the loss of intralabyrinthine fluid.[12,14,23,27] However, ossification in the third and fourth histopathological phases might be visible on CT, whereas this cannot be differentiated from fibrosis on MRI.

The literature reports that metaplastic bone is more difficult to detect on CT than osteoplastic bone, due to its low mineralization.[12] For this reason, cochlear ossification can be found incidentally, demonstrating that CT does not identify all ossification cases; its sensitivity is found to be low.[3,28] The time interval between imaging and the surgical procedure might be a contributing factor when the remodeling of bone is still ongoing. Limitations of imaging techniques might also be factors.

Fibrous tissue that is present during or after LO without further transformation into ossification cannot be seen on CT, but the combination of loss of fluid on T2W MRI and absence of ossification on CT suggests (noncalcified) fibrosis or undetected ossification. CT and MRI therefore are complementary modalities for the evaluation of this kind of pathology.[3,12]

The intracochlear neo-osteogenesis as well as the fibrotic tissue can usually also be clearly recognized during surgery. Information on the patency of the scala vestibuli is provided by T2W MRI.

Best imaging modalities according to histopathological phase of labyrinthitis ossificans

- Presence of acute labyrinthitis:
  - MRI T1W with gadolinium enhancement
- Presence of fibrosis or ossification:
  - MRI T2W: loss of intralabyrinthine fluid
- Presence of intracochlear ossification:
  - CT scanning: limited sensitivity (62–95%)

Besides the cochlea, the lateral semicircular canal (LSCC) can provide information on patency; it can show signs of ossification before the cochlea does and therefore can serve as a screening tool, especially on CT imaging.[14,26,29,30] If calcification is visible on CT (LSCC or intracochlear), MRI should determine unambiguously the patency or non-patency of the cochlea.

11.5 Surgical Planning

MRI and CT images help in the decision-making process and show the patency of the cochlear lumen and thus the extent of the LO. A surgical plan can now be made with the proper imaging and with the assistance of the following classification and guideline.

11.5.1 Classification of Ossification and Surgical Strategy

Labyrinthitis ossificans seems to be a universal process in reaction to a specific inflammatory stimulus; however, in different patients and even in different cochlea, differences in the location and extent of the ossification can be found. The following classification is a guide to the appropriate surgical strategy with best hearing outcomes and possibly smallest damage to the intracochlear structures (see **Table 11.1** and **Fig. 11.1–Fig. 11.6**).

Table 11.1 Classification of the grade of ossification with suggested surgical strategy and suggested surgical approach

	Location of ossification on CT and MRI	Surgical procedure + approach	Expected level of postoperative hearing
Grade 0	No fibrosis or ossification visible on CT or MRI	Normal cochlear implantation	
Grade I	Ossification only at round window (IA) or up to half of the scala tympani in the basal turn (IB)	Drill-out round window niche and part of scala tympani of basal turn via PT or extended PT approach	Comparable with standard cochlear implantation
Grade II	Ossification in more than half of the scala tympani in basal turn; scala vestibuli basal turn at least partially accessible	Scala vestibuli insertion via PT or extended PT approach	Better results in scala vestibuli insertion (than basal turn drill-out), less damage due to drilling,[a] but more risks of vertigo and loss of residual hearing
Grade III	Ossification of the basal turn (scala tympani and vestibuli); either with ascending basal turn accessible (IIIA) or not accessible (IIIB). Middle and apical turn open	1. Drill-out of basal turn, normal electrode insertion using SP if the ascending portion of the basal turn is accessible or 2. Drill-out of basal turn with middle turn cochleostomy and double array electrode via SP[b]	Worse results than standard CI due to drilling and neural tissue affected by inflammation and ossification process
Grade IV	Total ossification of the cochlea	1. Drill-out of basal turn with middle turn cochleostomy drill-out and double or triple array electrode via SP[b] or 2. If no cochlear lumen is identified, ABI (possibly in the same procedure via translabyrinthine approach)	Worse results than standard CI due to drilling and neural tissue affected by inflammation and ossification process In general ABI presents worse results than a cochlear implant in a drilled out cochlea[c]

Abbreviations: ABI, auditory brainstem implant; PT, posterior tympanotomy; SP, subtotal petrosectomy. Note: The scala tympani of the middle turn can only be reached through the scala vestibuli of the middle turn or by removal of the scala vestibuli of the basal turn first. Also, the medial part of the basal turn cannot be reached without removal of part of the middle turn (see anatomical illustrations in Chapter 2, **Figs. 2.16 and 2.17**).

[a] Scala vestibuli insertion will result in less drilling than ¾ to total scala tympani drill-out, but in scala vestibuli insertion the risk of damage to the basilar membrane and Reissner membrane is higher.13,16 When a complete basal turn drill-out is performed, anatomically in the anterior segment of the basal turn the scala vestibuli might also be opened.

[b] Using the subtotal petrosectomy approach in basal turn drill out with or without middle turn drill out, not only allows better access and visibility, but also will lower the changes for meningitis or cochlear electrode extrusion (out of the drilled out cochlea), because the implant can be better fixated into the cochlea and in the cavity due to the obliteration with abdominal fat. These are two further reasons for the subtotal petrosectomy approach.

[c] Results with an ABI are in general much worse than with normal cochlear implantation, leading at best to support of lip-reading skills but very often only to signal function. Also, the results of ABI remain worse than those from a cochlear drill-out procedure with cochlear implantation.

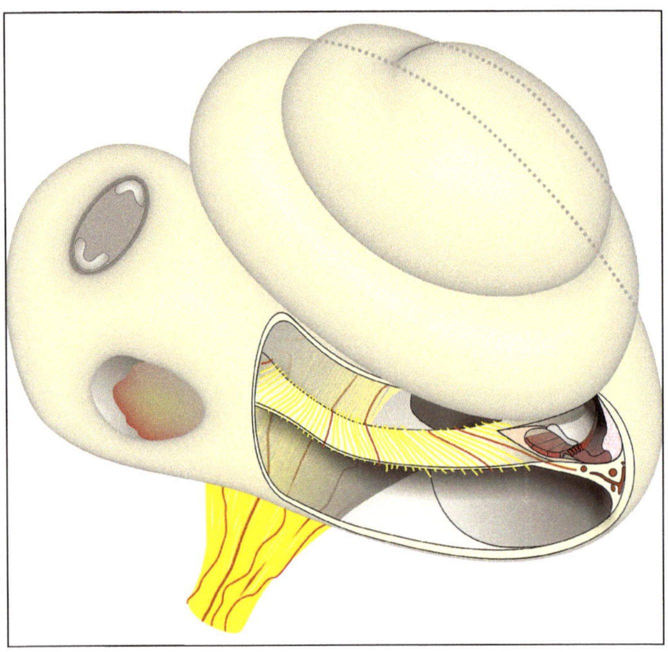

Fig. 11.1 Schematic presentation of Grade I (IA) ossification: only the area of the round window is affected.

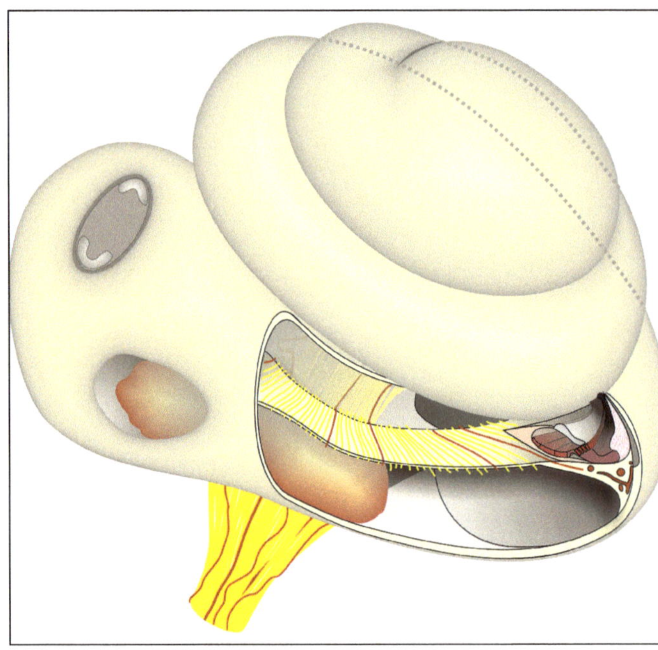

Fig. 11.2 Grade I (IB) ossification: up to half of the scala tympani of the basal turn is affected.

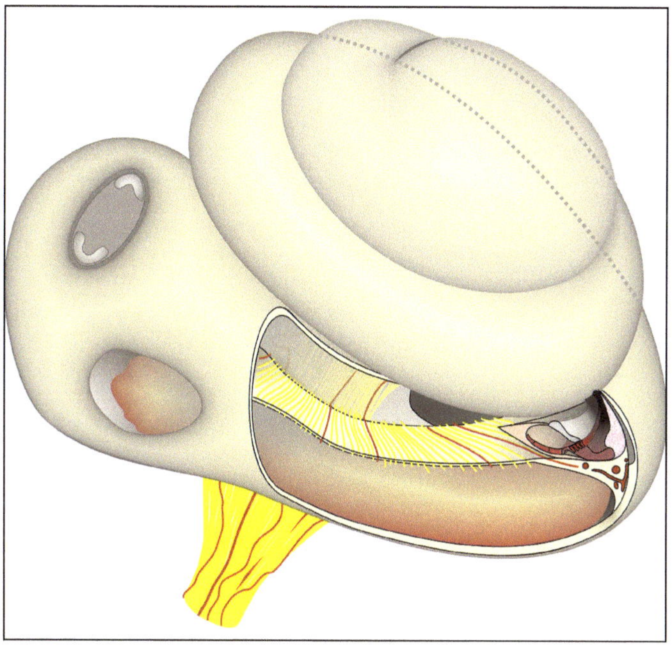

Fig. 11.3 Grade II: more than half up to whole of the scala tympani of the basal turn is affected.

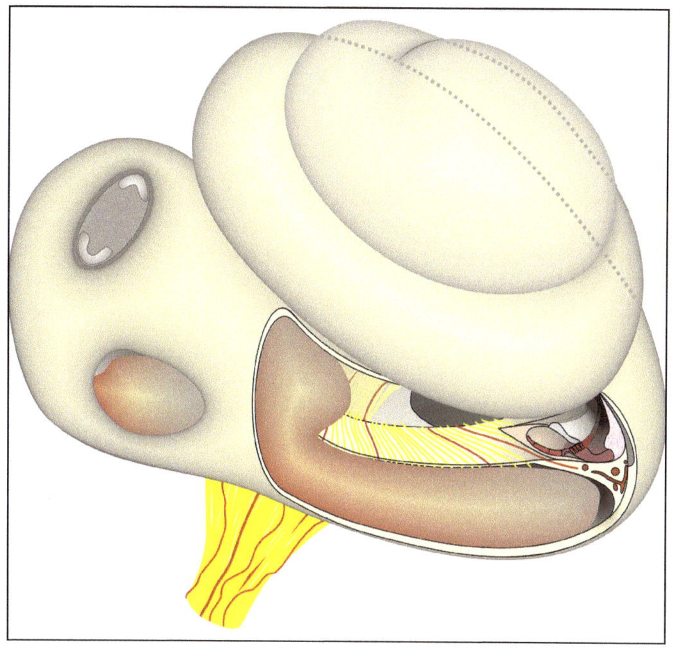

Fig. 11.4 Grade II: the scala tympani of the basal turn is completely ossified; the scala vestibuli is less than half ossified, also grade II.

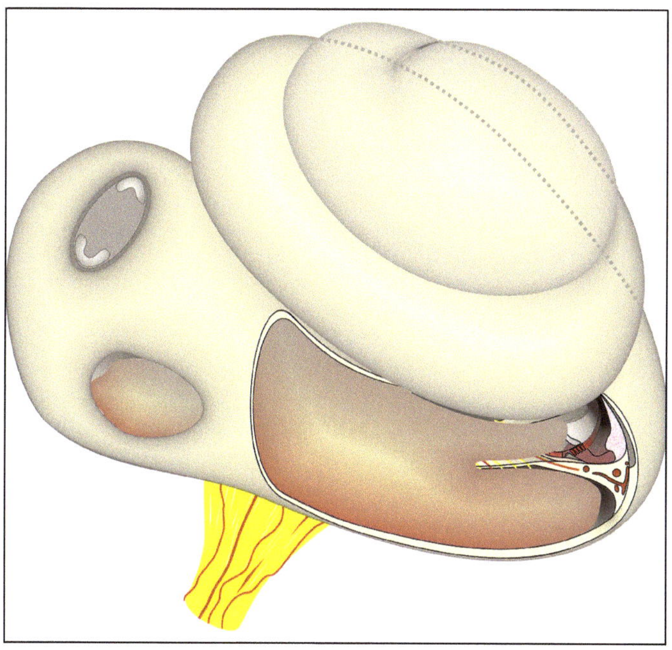

Fig. 11.5 Grade III: both the scala tympani and scala vestibuli of the basal turn are ossified, while the middle and apical turns are patent. This can occur with the ascending part of the basal turn being accessible (IIIA) or inaccessible (IIIB).

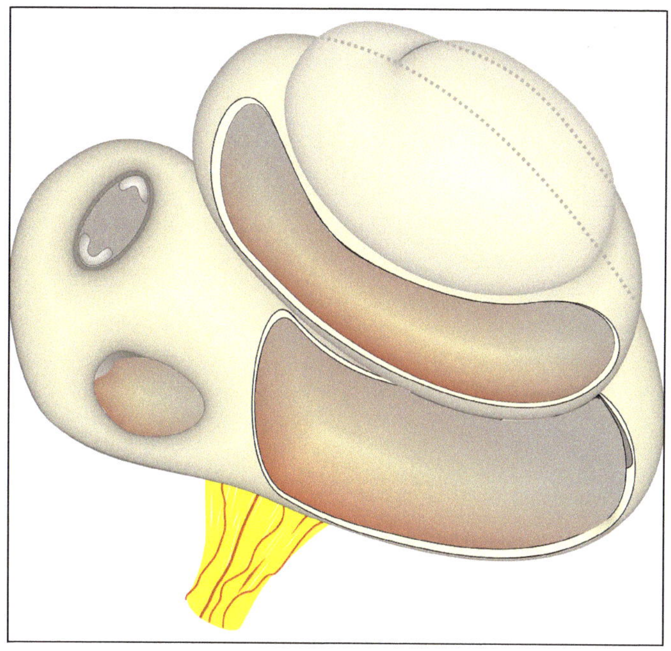

Fig. 11.6 Grade IV: totally ossified cochlea.

Grade I

Usually the first location of ossification is the area of the round window, close to the entrance of the cochlear aqueduct, grade IA. The ossification will then spread to the first third to half of the scala tympani in the basal turn (grade IB). Both classify as grade I.

Grade II

The second grade represents ossification of the basal turn involving more than half to the whole of the scala tympani (grade II), while the scala vestibuli of the basal turn remains at least partially accessible. Grade II also represents a total ossification of the scala tympani of the basal turn, while the scala vestibuli is ossified for less than half of the basal turn. The ascending part of the basal turn, the middle turn, and the apical turn are patent.

Grade III

Grade III represents the situation in which both the scala tympani and the scala vestibuli of the basal turn are totally ossified.

Grade IV

Finally grade IV represents total ossification of the cochlea.

11.5.2 Autoimmune Inner Ear Disease

The group of autoimmune inner ear diseases (AIED; primary or secondary/systemic) is the only pathology with intracochlear inflammation that has been proven to be reversible when treated promptly (within 14–30 days), and therefore demands a different approach regarding cochlear implantation and follow-up.[4,5,12,31]

This condition presents with a sudden onset of hearing loss bilaterally in days to weeks. It differs from ISSHL (idiopathic sudden sensorineural hearing loss), which presents unilaterally and within 24 to 48 hours. A history of weight loss, uveitis, keratitis, joint disease, bowel complaints, or skin rashes points in the direction of systemic disease.

These patients need to be seen urgently by an immunologist/pediatric immunologist; treatment with immunosuppressive medication has to be started quickly and will prove to be a diagnostic tool, but only after further diagnostic evaluation by nasendoscopy (with biopsy), a consultation by internal medicine, and blood tests (e.g., ESR, ANA, ANCA, RF) have been performed.[32,33]

Follow-up on the hearing thresholds and presence of labyrinthine enhancement with repeated T1W MRI with gadolinium enhancement will demonstrate the effect of the medical treatment.[31] Some of these patients will not react to the medication, others might need stronger immunosuppressive (methotrexate, azathioprine) or even cytostatic medication (cyclophosphamide) with negative side effects or unwanted side effects (loss of fertility, loss of hair, induction of bladder cancer), making cochlear implantation sometimes the preferable option compared with the continuation of this kind of medication.[33] This group of patients can present with acute loss of vestibular function in addition to the hearing loss.

- **Primary autoimmune inner ear disease (AIED)** is characterized by bilateral perceptive sensorineural hearing loss that presents in days to weeks, without an underlying systemic disease present. Patients can react well on immune suppressive medication ("prednisolone-responsive disease").
- **Secondary autoimmune inner ear disease** can be due to Wegener disease, Cogan disease, rheumatoid arthritis, systemic lupus erythematosus, Sjögren syndrome, polyarthritis nodosa, relapsing polychondritis, sarcoidosis, inflammatory bowel diseases (colitis ulcerosa, Crohn disease), Hashimoto disease, Churg–Strauss syndrome, or Behçet syndrome.

11.6 Indication for Bilateral Implantation

Labyrinthitis ossificans poses the risk of losing the best and possibly only chance of insertion of a cochlear electrode, usually affects both cochleae, and can in the long term lead to loss of intracochlear neural structures that might be stimulated in future. For these reasons, proper audiologic follow-up and imaging are required, and if bilateral obliteration is expected then bilateral implantation is advised.[3]

Autoimmune inner ear disease is the only entity in which the pathology may be reversible by prompt treatment with corticosteroids or other immunosuppressant medication; for this reason a different delivery of treatment is necessary (as explained above).

11.7 Creating Awareness

ENT surgeons are usually not the first medical specialists to treat patients with bacterial meningitis or autoimmune diseases affecting the inner ear. It is wise to create awareness, especially in pediatricians, immunologists, neurologists, and intensive care doctors working in your hospital or area who first see the patients prone to rapid loss of hearing and at risk of a prompt obliteration of the cochlea. Also the audiologists and audiologic centers should be informed. These colleagues should be familiar with the need for urgent management and consultation regarding the hearing loss and possibilities for hearing restoration.[6]

11.8 Surgical Steps in Ossification

Different surgical steps during the same procedure might be necessary, although based on CT and MRI imaging a preliminary strategy following the classification can be planned. The order of these approaches is arranged in such a way as to harm the cochlea and its neural structures as little as possible with likely the best results in hearing. However, not many results in literature on the hearing outcome comparing the different approaches are available yet.

Overview of suggested surgical approaches in obliterated cochlea

- Partial drill-out of the basal turn
  - Round window and beginning of basal turn
  - Half of the scala tympani of the basal turn
- Scala vestibuli insertion
- Complete drill-out of the basal turn
- Complete drill-out of the basal turn with middle turn cochleostomy with double array insertion
  - Anterograde insertion
  - Retrograde insertion
- Complete drill-out of the basal turn with middle turn drill-out with incomplete double array insertion
  - Anterograde insertion
  - Retrograde insertion
- No lumen found: Indication for ABI

These drill-out procedures can be performed via a posterior tympanotomy approach (PT) or via *an extended PT approach*—a PT approach with removal of the buttress and the incus for better access to the round window niche and more ease in maneuvering. In addition, a canal wall down approach can be performed using subtotal petrosectomy (SP) with obliteration of the cavity (see Chapter 10).

Which approach should be chosen depends on the individual anatomy of the temporal bone, the extent of the ossification, and the surgeon's preference and experience. In case of fractures of the otic capsule we have a strong preference always to undertake the SP + CI approach, because there is a higher risk of meningitis in this type of pathology due to the fibrotic-only repair of the fractures.[34]

In more extensive drill-out procedures the SP approach will give better access and an unobstructed view of all middle ear anatomy, with the possibility of identifying additional structures such as the carotid artery and the jugular bulb.[35] At the same time, the higher risk of developing meningitis and the higher risk of extrusion of the array out of the drilled out cochlea will make SP with obliteration of the cavity the better option. Conversion during surgery to the SP approach is a little more difficult and the choice of SP approach is best made before the procedure.

11.8.1 Partial Drill-out of the Basal Turn

For the partial drill-out procedures necessary in a grade I ossification, the basal turn is opened by drilling at the location of the round window, which can usually be visualized but which is ossified. Instead of dark gray it will then have a white color, resembling the color of a pseudomembrane. Additional landmarks are the round window niche, stapes, tympanic segment of the facial nerve, cochleariform process, and promontory (see Case 11.1).

The osteoneogenesis will be visible as a white, crystalline structure during the drill-out procedure; this bone has to be removed. The true bone of the cochlea is more yellow in appearance. The drilling should be performed anterior-inferiorly in the direction of the basal turn to avoid damage to the basilar membrane, scala vestibuli, or modiolus.

Round Window and Beginning of Basal Turn Drill-out

For ossification grade IA a standard cochlear implantation technique employing the posterior tympanotomy approach can be used. The osteoneogenesis can simply be removed by drilling: the amount of drilling is limited. Additional fibrous intracochlear tissue can be removed using a small hooked instrument, taking care not to damage the basilar membrane. The procedure continues using the normal steps of surgery.

Half Basal Turn Drill-out

For the drill-out in grade IB more space for maneuvering is required and it might be necessary to remove the incus and the buttress (extended PT). The drilling in grade IB is more extensive and might damage the inner ear because of the noise and vibrations[36]; however, the scala tympani can still be opened up and the lumen can be found. It is important to drill from inferiorly to avoid damage to the scala vestibuli or modiolus.

11.8.2 Scala Vestibuli Insertion

When opening the scala tympani of the basal turn is not possible and T2W MRI shows that the scala vestibuli is still accessible or partly accessible (grade II), extending the drilling at the round window niche more superiorly will give access to the scala vestibuli.[37] The anatomical relations are visible in the figures of Case 11.3. A dummy electrode or depth gauge, manufactured by the company, can be used to measure the depth and patency of the opened scala vestibuli. The scala vestibuli is slightly smaller in diameter in the basal turn than the scala tympani, but larger in the middle and apical turns; therefore, a normal or slightly more slender, but not tapered, electrode is best used.

Comparisons of scala vestibuli insertion with normal scala tympani insertion appear to find equal outcomes,[28,37] without a difference in trauma to intracochlear neural structures or in insertion depth of the electrode.[13] At the time of writing, no comparative studies between basal turn drill-out procedures and scala vestibuli insertions are available.

A partial basal turn drill-out (for grade I ossification) might at the start unintentionally give access to the scala vestibuli as this is oriented more superiorly in the anterior part of the cochlea. Once the lumen is found, the opening can be extended inferiorly to find the lumen in the scala tympani and perform insertion in the scala tympani (see Case 11.3). The scala tympani insertion will enable preservation of the Reissner membrane, will position the cochlear electrode closer to the spiral ganglion cells, and will produce fewer complaints of vertigo, making this the preferred alternative to scala vestibuli insertion.

In a complete basal turn drill-out, however, more damage from the noise and vibration and injury due to damage of the inner ear osseous and neural structures can be expected than is experienced with scala vestibuli insertion.[13,36,37] For these reasons we prefer scala vestibuli insertion in grade II ossification.

11.8.3 Complete Basal Turn Drill-out

For grade III ossification a complete (lateral) basal turn drill-out needs to be performed, as first described by Cohen and Waltzman in 1993. Starting from the ossified round window, the white osteoneogenesis is drilled out until the lumen is reached at the start of the ascending part of the basal turn; this measures around 10 mm.[38,39] For this approach, drilling (using a 1-mm drill or smaller) from inferiorly is advised, thus preserving the modiolus. Care must be taken not to damage the carotid artery, which can be seen as a blue/reddish structure anterior to the basal turn. Fibrous tissue can be removed from the lumen using a small hooked instrument. For better access and safety, a canal wall down procedure using subtotal petrosectomy approach can be carried out.

Gantz et al[40] described a total cochlear drill-out combined with SP, in which a channel around the modiolus is created, but we prefer the lateral basal turn drill-out of Balkany et al.[39] This approach presents less trauma to the cochlea, with smaller risk of damaging the modiolus or facial nerve. The electrode can usually be inserted fully when the ascending part of the basal turn is accessible. The proximal part of the array positioned in the drilled out well needs to be packed with fascia and fibrin glue for fixation. The outcome of implantation using the lateral basal turn drill-out is usually comparable to or worse than that of normal implantation due to insertion and/or the use of fewer electrodes, loss of neural tissue due to the inflammation/ossification or to surgery, and the possibly extended time between ossification and implantation.[39] Because of discomfort, facial nerve stimulation, or pain, some (proximal) electrodes might need to be switched off, leaving fewer functional electrodes.

For grade IIIB in which the ascending part of the basal turn is not accessible, preparations need to be made for a double array insertion. Without double-array technique only 9 or 10 electrodes can be placed in the drilled-out basal turn groove[38,41]; this represents about the minimum number of electrodes for speech perception. In combination with a middle turn cochleostomy, on average 17 electrodes (range 13–21) can be inserted using a double array implant.

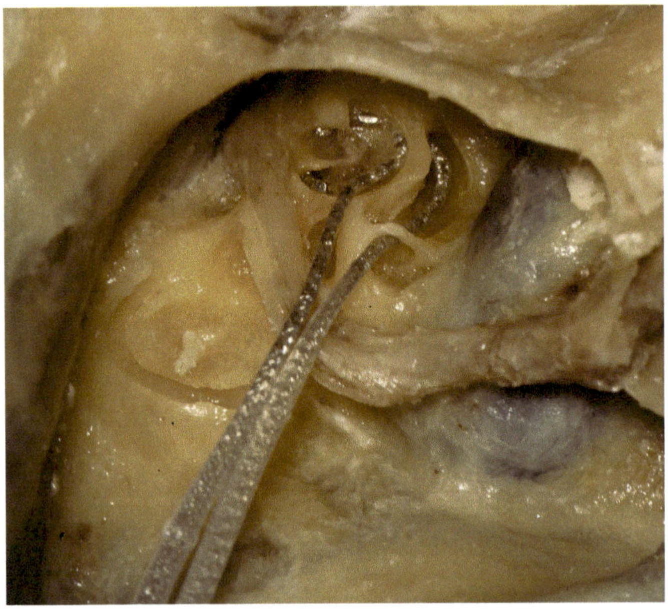

Fig. 11.7 An example of a double array insertion; both arrays are inserted anterogradely.

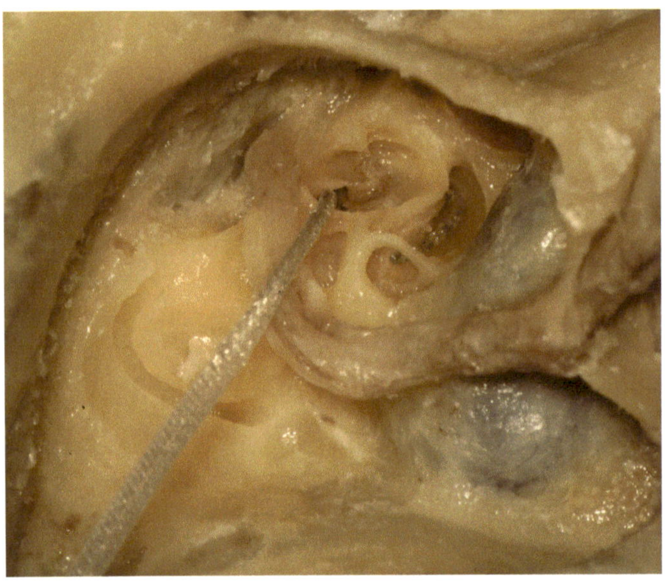

Fig. 11.8 An example of a retrograde electrode introduced via middle turn cochleostomy.

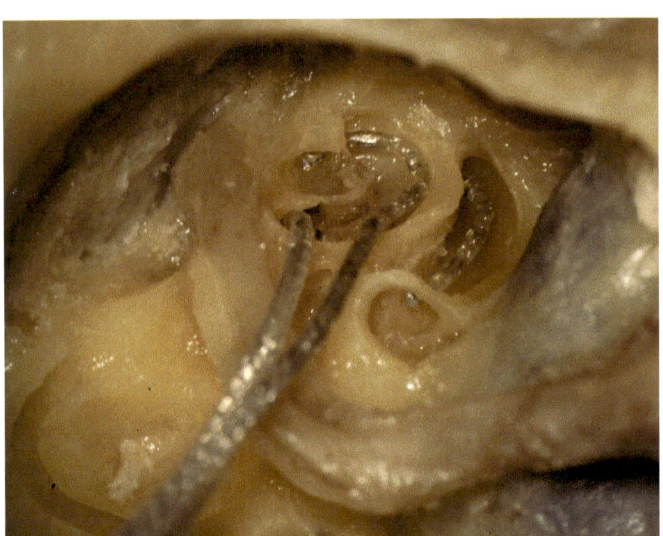

Fig. 11.9 An example of the combination of a retrograde basal turn electrode and anterograde middle turn insertion.

11.8.4 Middle Turn Cochleostomy with Double Array Insertion

When opening of the basal turn does not reveal a lumen at the anterior medial side, showing the ascending part of the basal turn to be ossified, and if also scala vestibuli insertion (as the first choice option) is not a possibility, a double array/split array implant (from Cochlear or MED-EL) will be the next step in the surgical management.

These types of implants have two shorter electrode arrays with around 10 electrodes each. The basal electrode array is positioned with as many electrodes as possible in the lateral drilled out basal turn. The second electrode array will be introduced in the scala vestibuli of the middle turn of the cochlea through a middle turn cochleostomy drilled 2 to 3 mm anterior from the oval window below the cochleariform process with a 1-mm diamond drill.[11] For better access to this middle turn cochleostomy an SP or extended PT is advised. Opening the middle turn cochleostomy would risk opening the scala vestibuli of the basal turn, which is situated more inferiorly and posteriorly than the middle turn (see **Fig. 11.7–Fig. 11.10**).

The surgical steps of the procedure are first to execute the basal turn drill-out, ascertaining the ascending part to be ossified, and then to create the middle turn cochleostomy. Subsequently, first implantation of the basal turn electrode with fixation should be done, followed by middle turn insertion. Both arrays need to be fixated using pieces of muscle or fascia with fibrin glue around both cochleostomies to create a firm seal.

Because more electrodes can now be introduced in a (partially) ossified cochlea (8–11 in the basal turn, 4–10 in the middle turn), significantly better auditory results and speech understanding are achieved. There is a gap in pitch scale between the basal and apical array because of the unstimulated area of the ascending part of the basal turn. In time, though, this gap is corrected for by brain plasticity. Also the basal array contributes more to the outcome in terms of speech perception than does the apical array.[42]

The electrode array in the middle turn can be inserted either anterogradely[11,42] or retrogradely,[43] depending on the exact position of the opening of the middle turn and the presence of ossification or fibrosis. The retrograde approach will require reprogramming of the order of electrodes by the audiologist, but there will be no gap in pitch scale.

Opening the middle turn cochleostomy can give access to the scala vestibuli or to the scala tympani. Isaacson et al[44] showed that in this technique the scala vestibuli of the middle turn is usually opened and that the scala media and Reissner membrane are nearly always severely damaged. Fractures of the modiolus or osseous spiral lamina were not found. For these reasons the double array technique leaves no room for residual hearing, and very precise insertion in the middle turn is difficult; a false route to the apical turn or scala vestibuli of the basal turn has been described using this technique. Lenarz showed that 8 to 10 electrodes can be introduced via the middle turn cochleostomy into the middle and apical turn.[41]

An additional reason to use this technique (as opposed to basal turn drill-out with partial insertion) is that the neural tissue of the ossified parts of the cochlea will deteriorate, whereas the neural tissue of the nonossified middle turn will still be functional and of better quality, giving better outcome in hearing.

Longer duration of deafness will, however, lead to worse results in outcome, for the nonossified areas as well.

As a rule of thumb, for best hearing a minimum of 8 to 10 electrodes need to be introduced in the cochlea, either in the basal turn or combined in the basal and medial turns of the cochlea. Insertion of more electrodes gives a better outcome.[42]

11.8.5 Middle Turn Drill-out with Double Array Insertion

When the middle turn is also ossified, a total circular cochlear drill-out of basal and middle turns is possible.[40] One of the risks of this procedure is damage to the modiolus.

We prefer a middle turn drill-out procedure to keep this risk as low as possible, while still being able to introduce around 14 or 15 electrodes. For this procedure the middle turn cochleostomy is extended posteriorly and anteriorly, parallel to the groove already drilled out for the basal turn. A bone bed of 6 to 7 mm can thus be created in which the second array of the double array can be placed and fixated, while the first array is harbored in the groove of the basal turn.[11]

Risks of the middle turn drill-out are damage to the modiolus, damage to the horizontal and possibly labyrinthine parts of the facial nerve, and damage to the carotid artery. Intraoperative CSF leakage from the middle turn cochleostomy has also been described, which can be solved by packing pieces of muscle with fibrin glue around the array.[11] Some electrodes might have to be deactivated because of pain sensations or facial nerve stimulation.

This procedure can best be performed using the SP approach.

11.8.6 No Lumen Found: Indication for ABI

Unfortunately, not all attempted drill-out procedures lead to successful implantation. Some cases have to be converted to auditory brainstem implantation because no cochlear lumen can be detected. It is therefore advisable to perform these difficult CI cases in a center where conversion to an ABI can be made during the same surgical procedure.

As cochlear implantation in ossification cases usually gives better hearing rehabilitation than an ABI, an attempted drill-out procedure followed by cochlear implantation always has to be the first choice for hearing restoration. More information on auditory brainstem implantation can be found in Chapter 8.

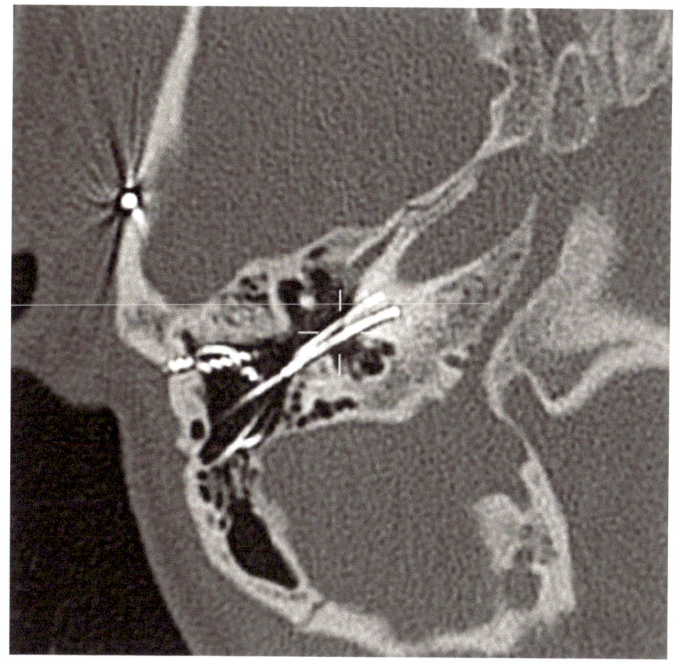

Fig. 11.10 Postoperative CT image of a patient in whom a double array implant was inserted.

11.9 Types of Electrodes

For this type of surgery an electrode with a stylet allows the possibility to exercise some force during insertion (in presence of fibrous tissue). A normal to slightly smaller diameter electrode array is best used for scala vestibuli insertion (the diameter of the scala vestibuli and media together is more or less equal to that of the scala tympani).[45,46] The double array/Gemini electrode will serve during a double cochleostomy approach[11] (see **Fig. 11.7–Fig. 11.10**). Also an implant with three electrodes has been reported.[47]

11.9.1 Dummy Electrode

Dummy electrodes can be used to keep the lumen of the cochlea patent for future implantation, when cochlear implantation is not immediately possible: for example, in countries where reimbursement or guarantee of cochlear implantation needs time to be organized.[48] A dummy electrode (a sterile nonfunctional electrode) can be provided on request by the companies supplying the CIs: the diameter needs to be the same size as the electrode of the planned cochlear implant. During the replacement the fibrous sheath surrounding the dummy electrode is easily recognized and the functional electrode array can be inserted using this sheath to give proper access (see also Chapter 14).

Case 11.1 Round Window Drill-out

Cochlear Implantation with Obliterated Round Window (Grade IA) in Open Cavity Left Ear (Fig. 11.1.1–Fig. 11.1.10)

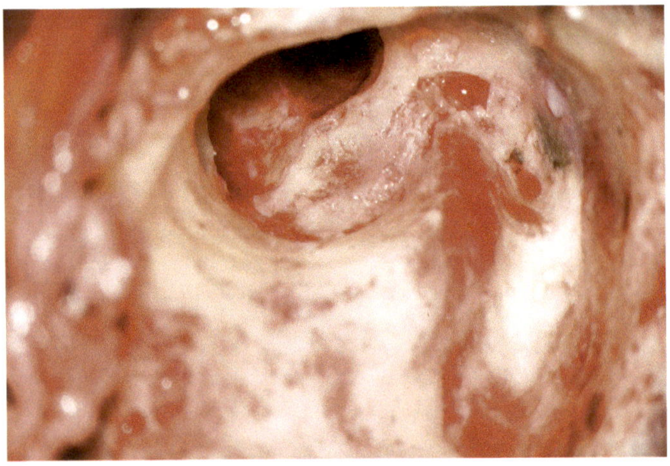

Fig. 11.1.1 The patient had previously undergone left middle ear surgery with canal wall down technique. The skin covering the cavity and the tympanic membrane is completely removed, and the cavity is smoothed by drilling. The round window and the oval window are both ossified.

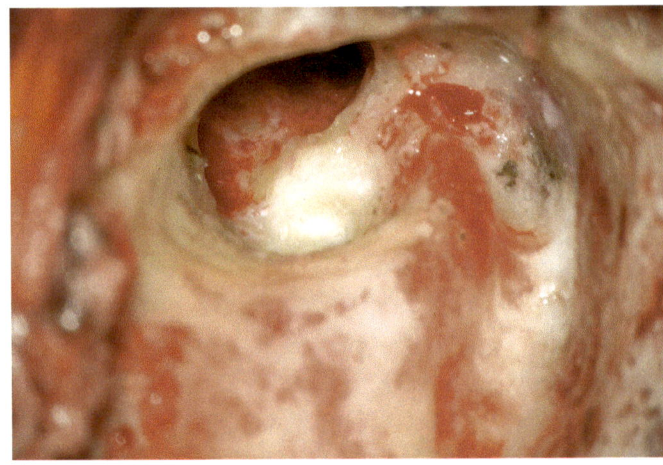

Fig. 11.1.2 The area of the round window and the basal turn of the cochlea are drilled out gradually. The facial nerve, the oval niche, and the cochleariform process are used as landmarks. To avoid opening the scala vestibuli or middle turn of the cochlea, the drilling is started inferiorly.

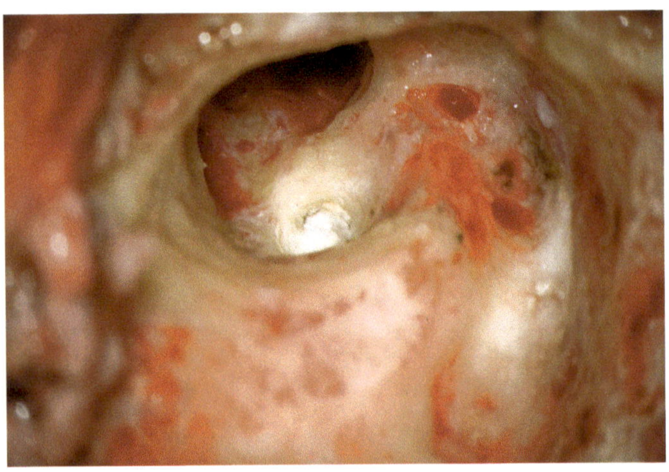

Fig. 11.1.3 The round window is ossified; the osteoneogenesis in the scala tympani of the basal turn is removed by drilling. Note that the ossification is whiter in color than the original bone of the otic capsule, which is yellow. Also the structure of the osteoneogenesis is more crystalline, more brittle.

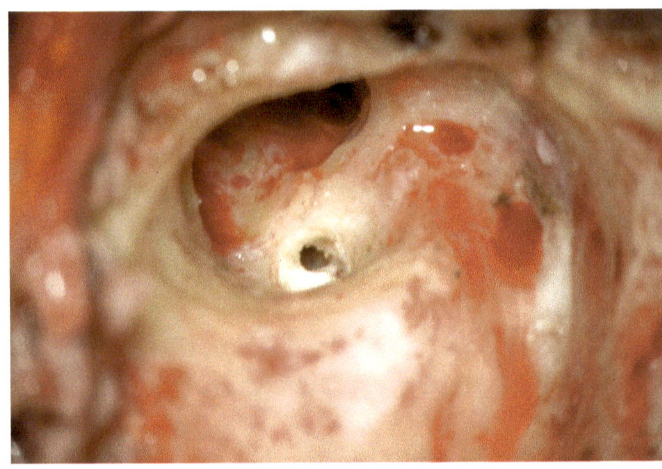

Fig. 11.1.4 After more drilling, the scala tympani of the basal turn is found and is accessible for electrode insertion.

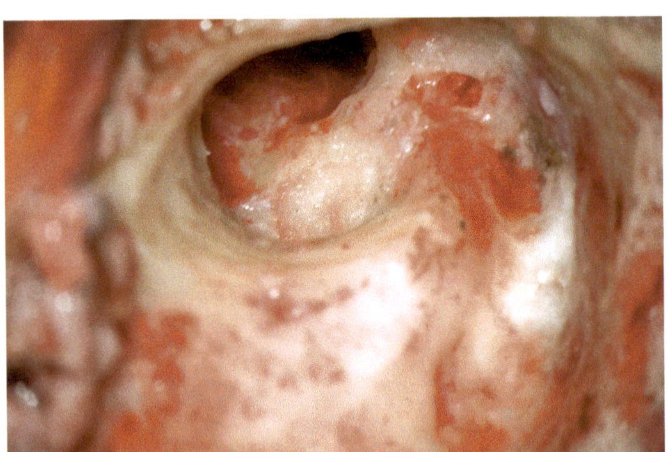

Fig. 11.1.5 Before the receiver well is drilled, the opening to the cochlea is covered with Gelfoam soaked in saline solution to prevent bone dust and blood from entering the cochlea. Alternatively, the receiver well can be drilled before the cochlea is opened or hyaluronic acid solution can be used at the entrance of the cochlea. This viscous solution will also keep the blood and bone dust out of the cochleostomy.

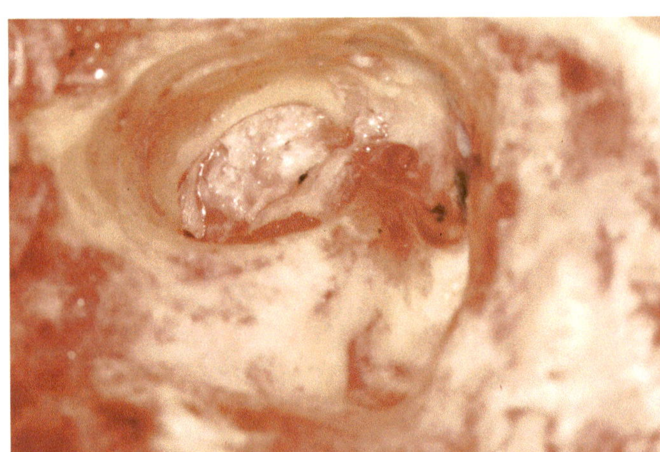

Fig. 11.1.6 The orifice of the eustachian tube is obliterated with muscle, cartilage, or bone wax and covered with a layer of periosteum or fascia. This is done before the insertion of the cochlear electrode.

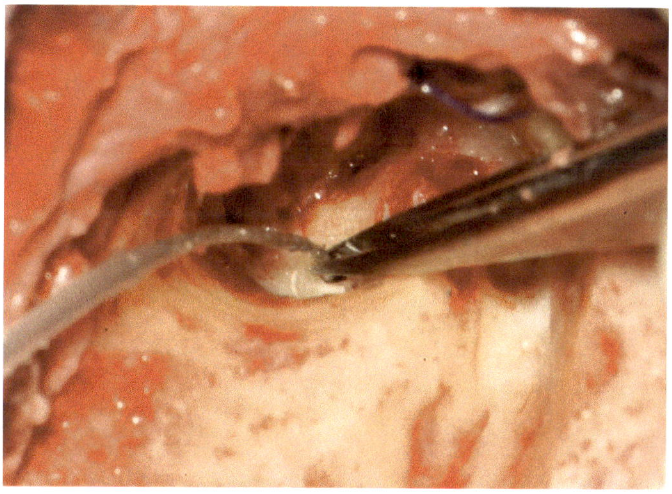

Fig. 11.1.7 The insertion of the cochlear electrode array. A watchmaker's forceps is used. The array should be inserted with a slow, gentle movement. Possible fibrotic tissue can be encountered in this group of patients.

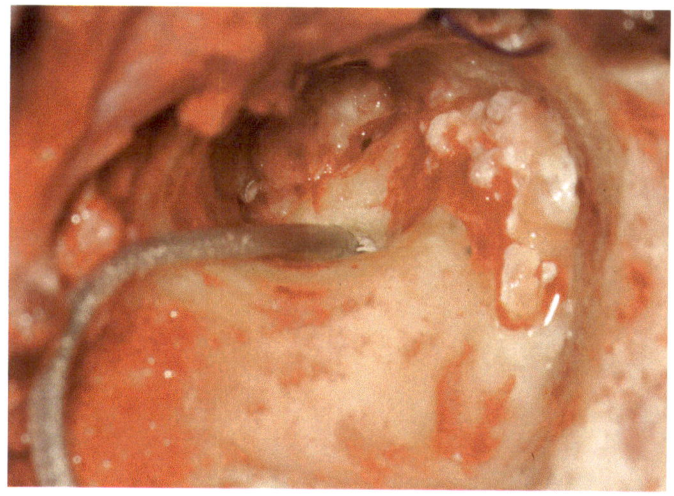

Fig. 11.1.8 Full insertion has been achieved.

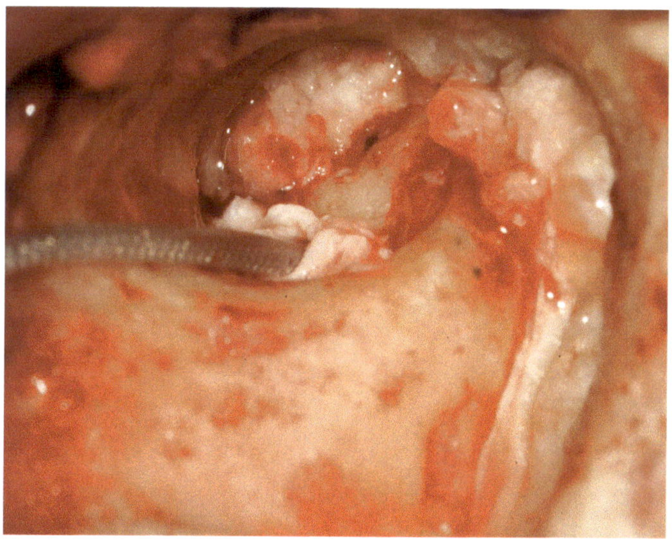

Fig. 11.1.9 Small pieces of fascia and fibrin glue are used to fixate the electrode array at the cochleostomy.

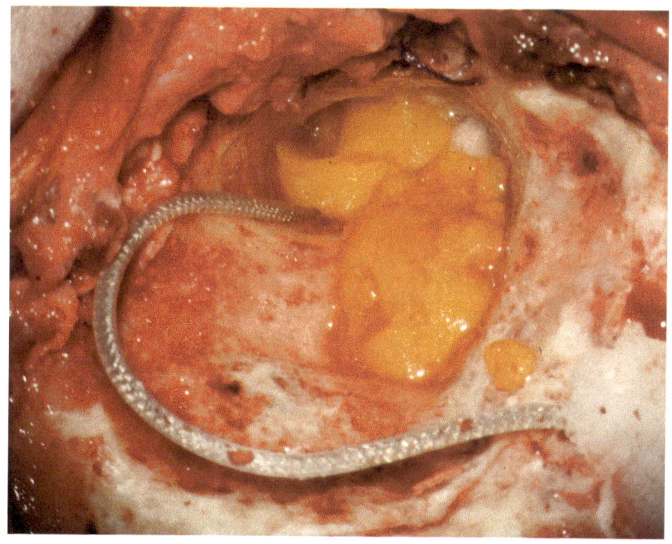

Fig. 11.1.10 Finally the cavity is obliterated with abdominal fat.

Case 11.2 Basal Turn Drill-out

Cochlear Implantation in Ossified Basal Turn (Grade IIB) in a Case of Bony Dysplasia Right Ear; Canal Wall Down Procedure (Fig. 11.2.1–Fig. 11.2.8)

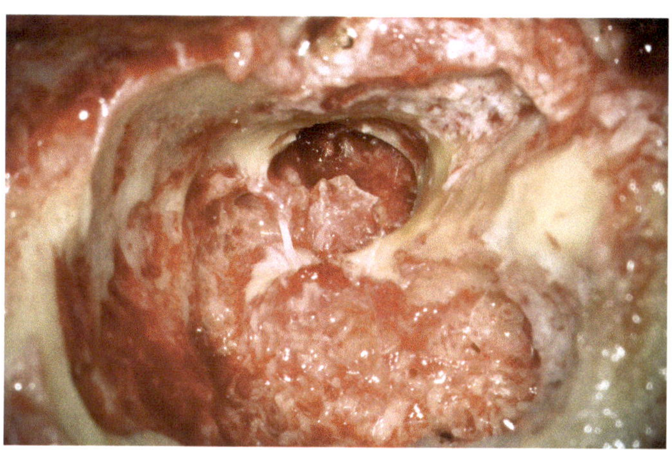

Fig. 11.2.1 After blind-sac closure of the external auditory canal, the meatal skin and tympanic membrane are completely removed, and a canal wall down mastoidectomy is performed. The promontory is covered with a tympanosclerotic plaque.

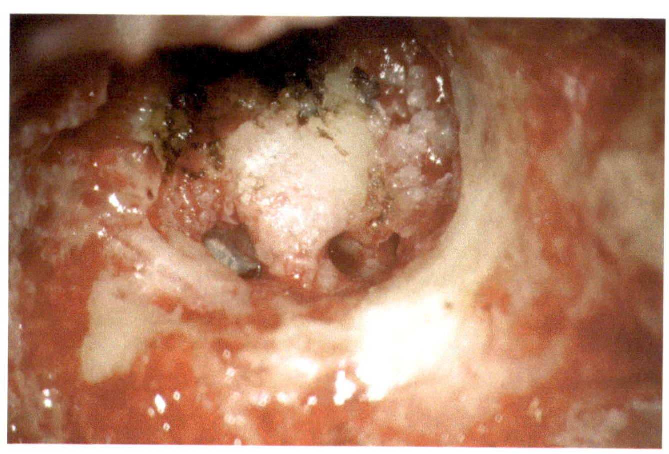

Fig. 11.2.2 Removal of the tympanosclerotic plaque has revealed the footplate of the stapes and the round window niche.

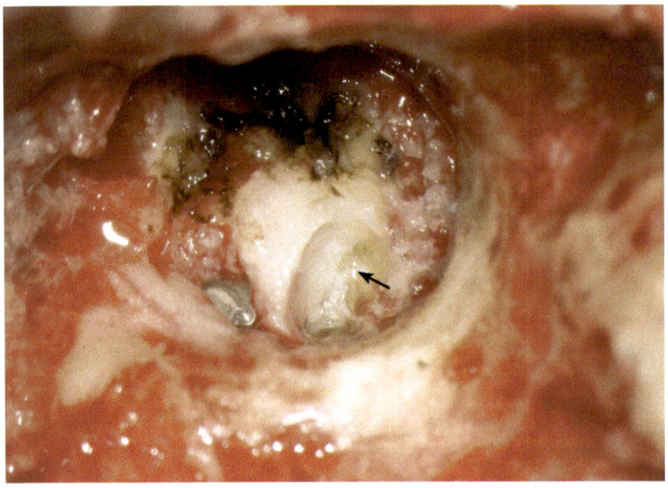

Fig. 11.2.3 Since the round window membrane is totally ossified, drilling over the posterior-inferior aspect of the promontory to open the basal turn is performed. The drilling proceeds anteriorly, following the ossified cochlea. Note the different color and aspect of the ossified basal turn in comparison to the original otic capsule *(arrow)*.

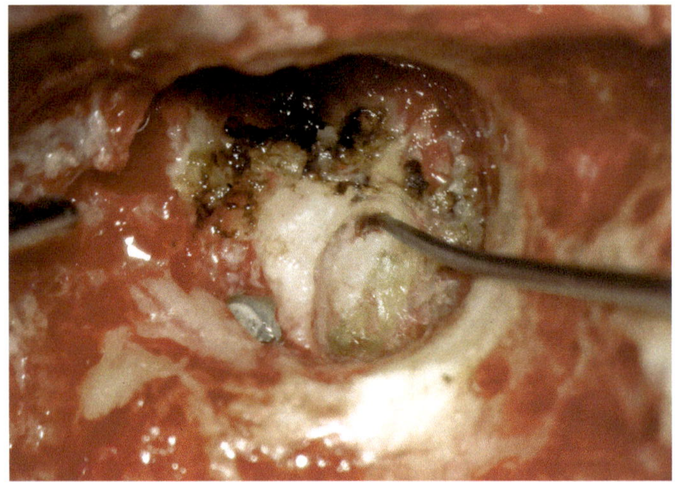

Fig. 11.2.4 A small lumen is found at the anterior end of the basal turn after drill-out. Anatomically this should be the scala tympani of the basal turn.

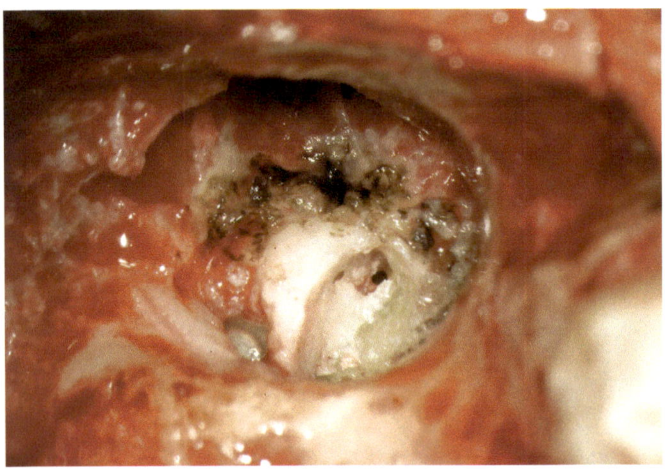

Fig. 11.2.5 Obliterating tissue is still present all around the identified lumen.

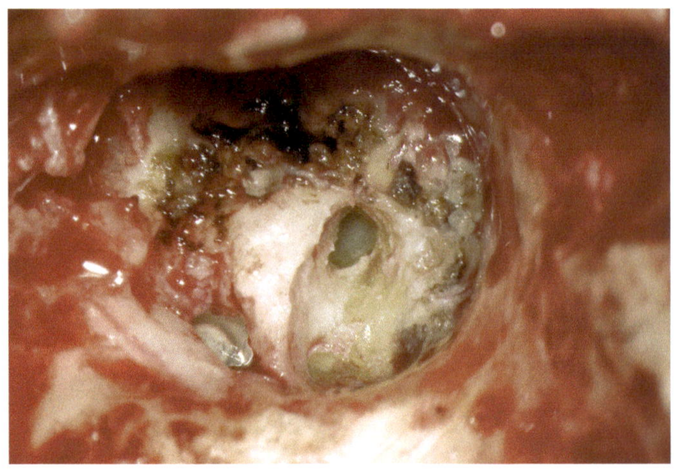

Fig. 11.2.6 The opening is enlarged with a small diamond bur in the inferior direction to further open up the scala tympani. Care is taken not to damage the modiolus located superiorly.

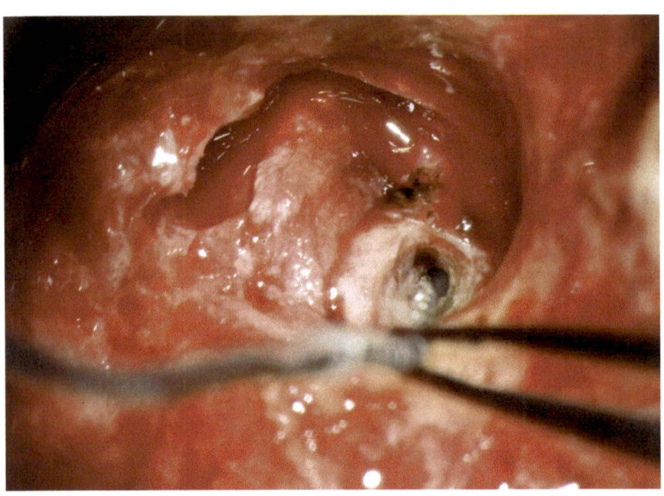

Fig. 11.2.7 The eustachian tube is obliterated with small pieces of muscle, cartilage, or bone wax. The electrode array is completely inserted into the scala tympani.

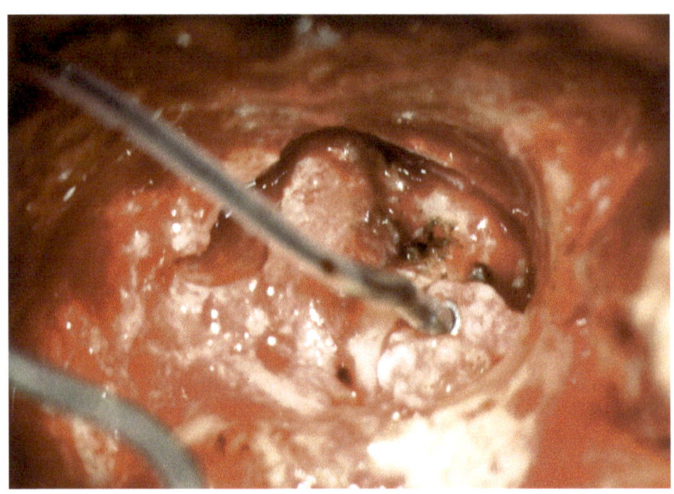

Fig. 11.2.8 The electrode is inserted in the scala tympani and stabilized with fascia and muscle. Because of the larger opening of the cochlea, there is a higher risk of developing meningitis. The risk of extrusion of the implant is also higher. After the cavity has been filled with abdominal fat, the retroauricular incision is closed in three layers.

Case 11.3 Scala Tympani Insertion with Vision of Scala Vestibuli (Left Ear) (Fig. 11.3.1–Fig. 11.3.10)

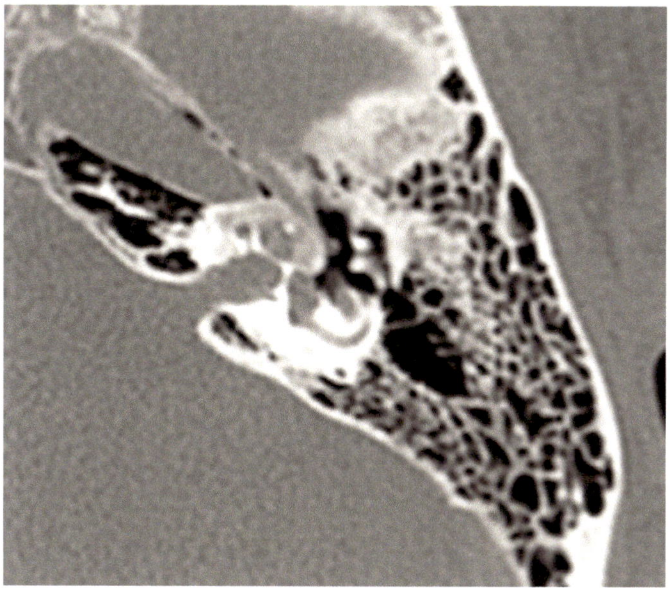

Fig. 11.3.1 A 60-year-old man with bilateral progressive hearing loss due to otosclerosis showed retrofenestral otosclerosis with total otic capsule involvement on CT imaging.

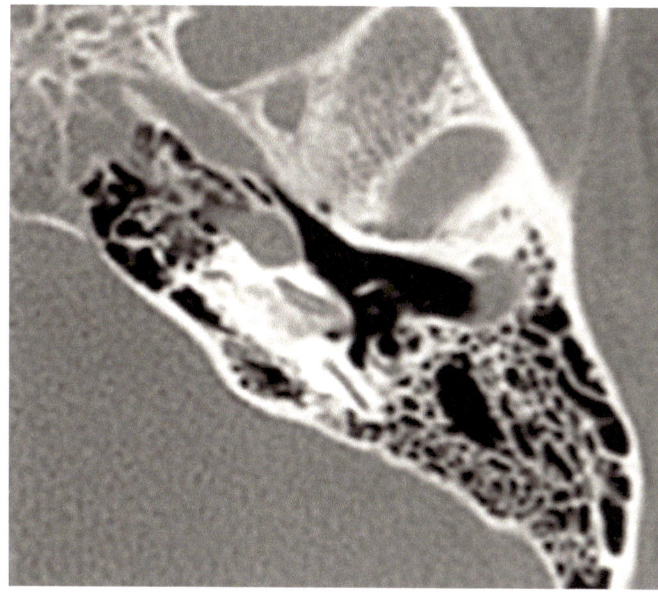

Fig. 11.3.2 The basal turn is especially affected around the round window but a double ring is not seen. The basal turn seems mostly noncalcified but the round window area is "blurry." A clear notion of what to expect during surgery cannot be derived from this picture.

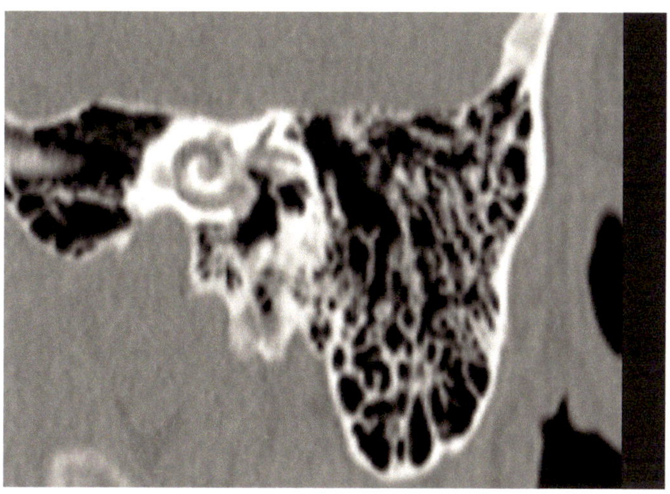

Fig. 11.3.3 On coronal imaging the otosclerotic lesions are concentrated at the center axis of the labyrinth and involve the round as well as the oval window.

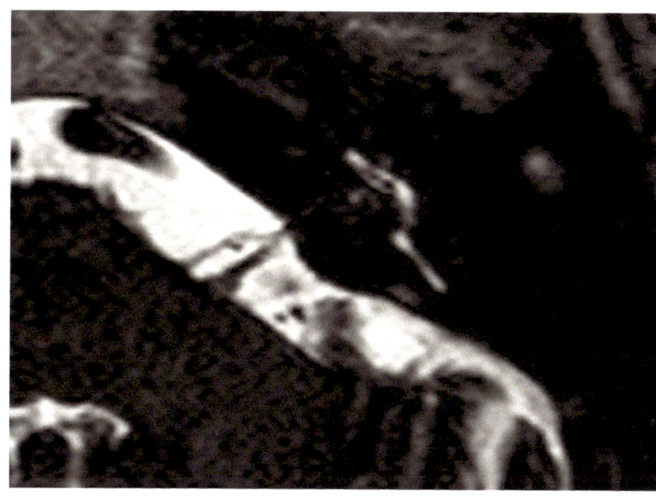

Fig. 11.3.4 In spite of the clear abnormalities on CT images, inner ear fluids are preserved, as shown here on MRI.

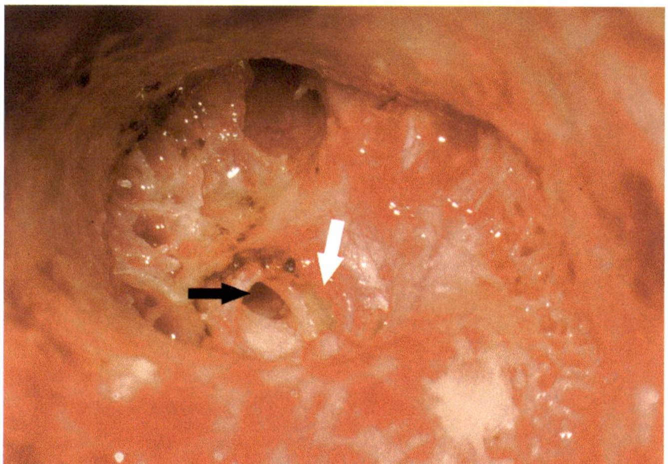

Fig. 11.3.5 After partial drilling of the basal turn, both the scala tympani (*black arrow*) and scala vestibuli (*white arrow*) are clearly visible and accessible in this patient. Note also the basilar membrane and osseous spiral ligament separating both scalae.

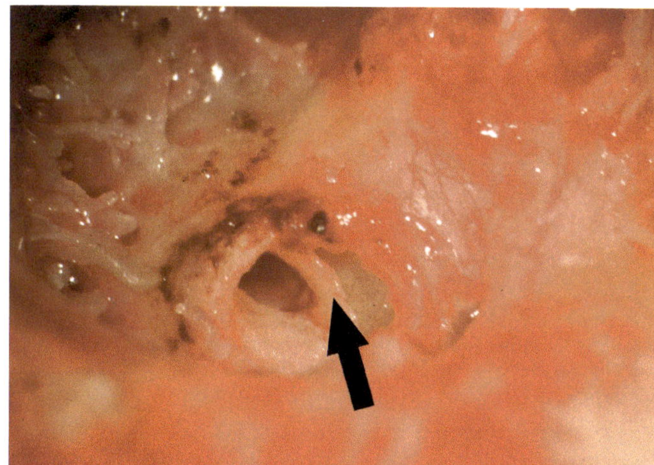

Fig. 11.3.6 A view in greater detail: note the basilar membrane and osseous spiral lamina (*black arrow*) separating both scalae. Remnants of the osteoneogenesis are still visible in the inferior part of the scala tympani.

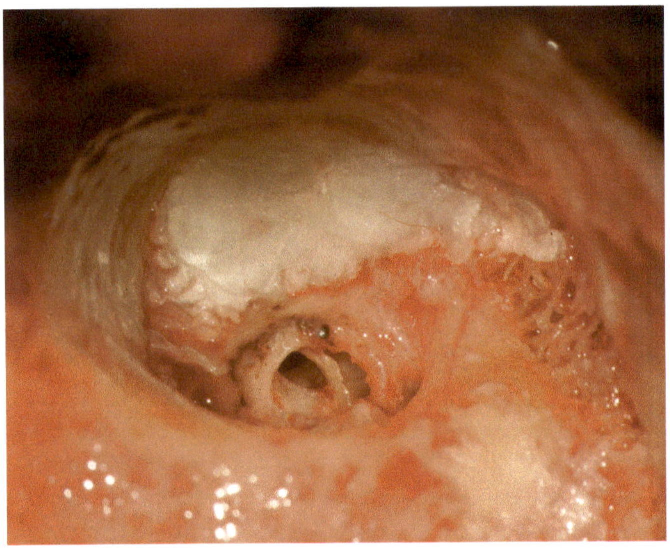

Fig. 11.3.7 The eustachian tube is closed off using bone wax.

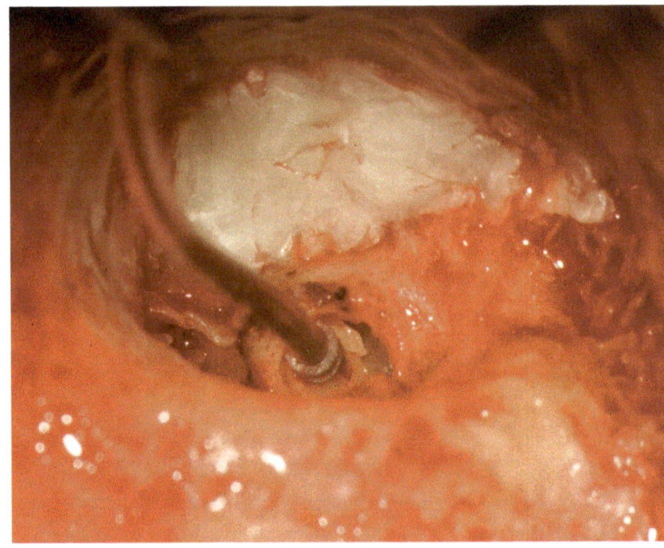

Fig. 11.3.8 The electrode array is inserted in the scala tympani, which is preferable because it is wider in diameter and closer to the spiral ganglion cells, and there is less risk of damage to the basilar membrane and Reissner membrane than with a scala vestibuli insertion.

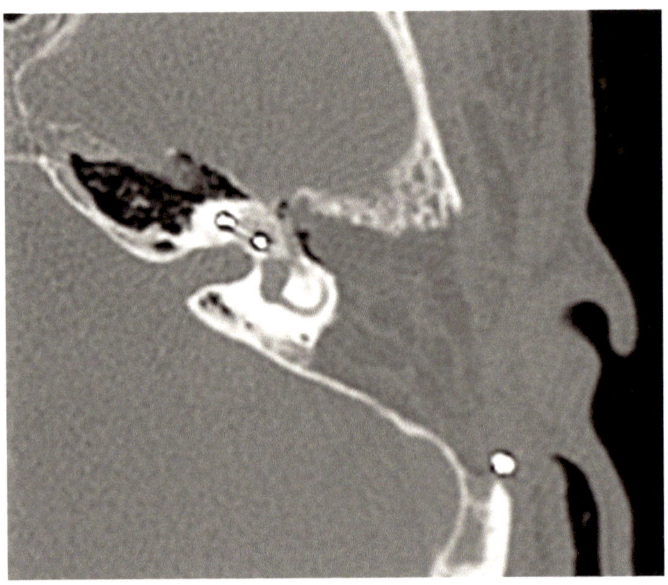

Fig. 11.3.9 Postoperative CT imaging confirms the correct positioning of the electrode array. The cavity of the subtotal petrosectomy is filled with abdominal fat.

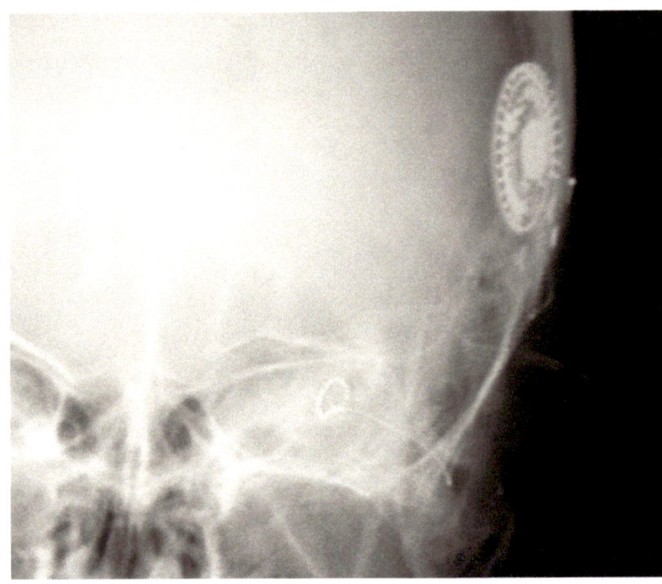

Fig. 11.3.10 Postoperative anterior-posterior radiograph shows a good position of the electrode.

11.10 Risks in Surgery for Ossified Cochlea

- Trauma of the modiolus, spiral ganglion cells, and osseous spiral lamina during the drill-out procedure. Damage to the basilar membrane, osseous spiral lamina, and Reissner membrane is very likely in the total drill-out procedures and can hardly be prevented. However, the function of these structures is usually already lost because of the extensive ossification.
- Trauma of the carotid artery: a dangerous complication of a drill-out procedure is damage to the carotid artery, situated in close relation to the most anterior part of the basal turn.[15,44,49,50] When a drill-out needs to be extended far anteriorly, identification of the carotid is advisable.
- A possible false route of the electrode array.
- Vertigo in scala vestibuli insertion.[13]
- In scala vestibuli insertion damage to the Reissner membrane, the organ of Corti, and the basilar membrane is more common.[13]
- Due to the larger distance from the intracochlear neural tissues higher electrical stimulation levels are needed in scala vestibuli insertion.[16]
- Damage to the facial nerve, due to more extensive drilling with fewer available landmarks.
- Higher risk of developing meningitis because of a larger opening to the cochlea in the more extended drill-out procedures of the middle turn and basal turns.
- Higher risk of extrusion of the electrode array in the more extended drill-out procedures of the middle turn and basal turns when the array is simply accommodated in a groove.

Pearls and Pitfalls in Cochlear Ossification Surgery

- Drill-out surgery is challenging and exciting surgery!
- The rule of thumb is to introduce at least 8 to 10 electrodes into the cochlea; introduction of more electrodes is generally better.[41,51]
- For extensive drill-out procedures an SP approach will give better access and visualization (Chapter 10).

Reference Video

See Video 11.1.

References

1. Kotzias SA, Linthicum FH Jr. Labyrinthine ossification: differences between two types of ectopic bone. Am J Otol 1985;6(6):490–494
2. Xu HX, Joglekar SS, Paparella MM. Labyrinthitis ossificans. Otol Neurotol 2009;30(4):579–580
3. Durisin M, Bartling S, Arnoldner C, et al. Cochlear osteoneogenesis after meningitis in cochlear implant patients: a retrospective analysis. Otol Neurotol 2010;31(7):1072–1078
4. Wang JR, Yuen HW, Shipp DB, et al. Cochlear implantation in patients with autoimmune inner ear disease including cogan syndrome: a comparison with age- and sex-matched controls. Laryngoscope 2010;120(12):2478–2483
5. Aftab S, Semaan MT, Murray GS, Megerian CA. Cochlear implantation outcomes in patients with autoimmune and immune-mediated inner ear disease. Otol Neurotol 2010;31(8):1337–1342
6. Merkus P, Free RH, Mylanus EA, et al; 4th Consensus in Auditory Implants Meeting. Dutch Cochlear Implant Group (CI-ON) consensus protocol on postmeningitis hearing evaluation and treatment. Otol Neurotol 2010;31(8):1281–1286
7. Rotteveel LJ, Proops DW, Ramsden RT, Saeed SR, van Olphen AF, Mylanus EA. Cochlear implantation in 53 patients with otosclerosis: demographics, computed tomographic scanning, surgery, and complications. Otol Neurotol 2004;25(6):943–952
8. Ruiz AP, Garcia Gomez JM. Labyrinthitis ossificans in a cochlear implant patient with Usher syndrome. Otol Neurotol 2013;34(3):e10–e11
9. Liu BP, Saito N, Wang JJ, Mian AZ, Sakai O. Labyrinthitis ossificans in a child with sickle cell disease: CT and MRI findings. Pediatr Radiol 2009;39(9):999–1001
10. Sando I, Egami T. Inner ear hemorrhage and endolymphatic hydrops in a leukemic patient with sudden hearing loss. Ann Otol Rhinol Laryngol 1977;86(4 Pt 1):518–524
11. Lenarz T, Lesinski-Schiedat A, Weber BP, et al. The nucleus double array cochlear implant: a new concept for the obliterated cochlea. Otol Neurotol 2001;22(1):24–32
12. Hegarty JL, Patel S, Fischbein N, Jackler RK, Lalwani AK. The value of enhanced magnetic resonance imaging in the evaluation of endocochlear disease. Laryngoscope 2002;112(1):8–17
13. Adunka O, Kiefer J, Unkelbach MH, Radeloff A, Gstoettner W. Evaluating cochlear implant trauma to the scala vestibuli. Clin Otolaryngol 2005;30(2):121–127
14. Isaacson B, Booth T, Kutz JW Jr, Lee KH, Roland PS. Labyrinthitis ossificans: how accurate is MRI in predicting cochlear obstruction? Otolaryngol Head Neck Surg 2009;140(5):692–696
15. Roland JT Jr, Coelho DH, Pantelides H, Waltzman SB. Partial and double-array implantation of the ossified cochlea. Otol Neurotol 2008;29(8):1068–1075
16. Steenerson RL, Gary LB. Multichannel cochlear implantation in children with cochlear ossification. Am J Otol 1999;20(4):442–444
17. Harris JP, Heydt J, Keithley EM, Chen MC. Immunopathology of the inner ear: an update. Ann N Y Acad Sci 1997;830(830):166–178
18. Nabili V, Brodie HA, Neverov NI, Tinling SP. Chronology of labyrinthitis ossificans induced by Streptococcus pneumoniae meningitis. Laryngoscope 1999;109(6):931–935
19. Tinling SP, Nabili V, Brodie HA. Fine structure histopathology of labyrinthitis ossificans in the gerbil model. Ann Otol Rhinol Laryngol 2005;114(2):161–166
20. Tinling SP, Colton J, Brodie HA. Location and timing of initial osteoid deposition in postmeningitic labyrinthitis ossificans determined by multiple fluorescent labels. Laryngoscope 2004;114(4):675–680
21. Green JD Jr, Marion MS, Hinojosa R. Labyrinthitis ossificans: histopathologic consideration for cochlear implantation. Otolaryngol Head Neck Surg 1991;104(3):320–326
22. Brodie HA, Thompson TC, Vassilian L, Lee BN. Induction of labyrinthitis ossificans after pneumococcal meningitis: an animal model. Otolaryngol Head Neck Surg 1998;118(1):15–21
23. van Loon MC, Hensen EF, de Foer B, Smit CF, Witte B, Merkus P. Magnetic resonance imaging in the evaluation of patients with sensorineural hearing loss caused by meningitis: implications for cochlear implantation. Otol Neurotol 2013;34(5):845–854
24. Aschendorff A, Klenzner T, Laszig R. Deafness after bacterial meningitis: an emergency for early imaging and cochlear implant surgery. Otolaryngol Head Neck Surg 2005;133(6):995–996
25. Bergemalm PO. Progressive hearing loss after closed head injury: a predictable outcome? Acta Otolaryngol 2003;123(7):836–845
26. Beijen J, Casselman J, Joosten F, et al. Magnetic resonance imaging in patients with meningitis induced hearing loss. Eur Arch Otorhinolaryngol 2009;266(8):1229–1236
27. Beijen J, Casselman J, Joosten F, et al. Magnetic resonance imaging in patients with meningitis induced hearing loss. Eur Arch Otorhinolaryngol 2009:266:1229–1236
28. Bacciu S, Bacciu A, Pasanisi E, et al. Nucleus multichannel cochlear implantation in partially ossified cochleas using the Steenerson procedure. Otol Neurotol 2002;23(3):341–345
29. Chan CC, Saunders DE, Chong WK, Hartley BE, Raglan E, Rajput K. Advancement in post-meningitic lateral semicircular canal labyrinthitis ossificans. J Laryngol Otol 2007;121(2):105–109
30. Muren C, Bredberg G. Postmeningitic labyrinthine ossification primarily affecting the semicircular canals. Eur Radiol 1997;7(2):208–213
31. Malik MU, Pandian V, Masood H, et al. Spectrum of immune-mediated inner ear disease and cochlear implant results. Laryngoscope 2012;122(11):2557–2562
32. Bovo R, Ciorba A, Martini A. The diagnosis of autoimmune inner ear disease: evidence and critical pitfalls. Eur Arch Otorhinolaryngol 2009;266(1):37–40
33. Ruckenstein MJ. Autoimmune inner ear disease. Curr Opin Otolaryngol Head Neck Surg 2004;12(5):426–430
34. Sudhoff H, Linthicum FH Jr. Temporal bone fracture and latent meningitis: temporal bone histopathology study of the month. Otol Neurotol 2003;24(3):521–522
35. Free RH, Falcioni M, di Trapani G, Gianucci AL, Russo A, Sanna M. The role of subtotal petrosectomy in cochlear implant surgery--a report of 32 cases and review on indications.. Otol Neurotol 2013;34:1033–1040
36. Pau HW, Just T, Bornitz M, Lasurashvilli N, Zahnert T. Noise exposure of the inner ear during drilling a cochleostomy for cochlear implantation. Laryngoscope 2007;117(3):535–540
37. Steenerson RL, Gary LB, Wynens MS. Scala vestibuli cochlear implantation for labyrinthine ossification. Am J Otol 1990;11(5):360–363
38. Cohen NL, Waltzman SB. Partial insertion of the nucleus multichannel cochlear implant: technique and results. Am J Otol 1993;14(4):357–361
39. Balkany T, Gantz BJ, Steenerson RL, Cohen NL. Systematic approach to electrode insertion in the ossified cochlea. Otolaryngol Head Neck Surg 1996;114(1):4–11
40. Gantz BJ, McCabe BF, Tyler RS. Use of multichannel cochlear implants in obstructed and obliterated cochleas. Otolaryngol Head Neck Surg 1988;98(1):72–81
41. Lenarz T, Battmer RD, Lesinski A, Parker J. Nucleus double electrode array: a new approach for ossified cochleae. Am J Otol 1997; **18**(6, Suppl)S39–S41
42. Lenarz T, Büchner A, Tasche C, et al. The results in patients implanted with the nucleus double array cochlear implant: pitch discrimination and auditory performance. Ear Hear 2002;23(1, Suppl)90S–101S

43. Bredberg G, Lindström B, Baumgartner WD, et al. Open-set speech perception in adult cochlear implant users with ossified cochleae. Cochlear Implants Int 2003;4(2):55–72
44. Isaacson B, Roland PS, Wright CG. Anatomy of the middle-turn cochleostomy. Laryngoscope 2008;118(12):2200–2204
45. Gulya AJ, Steenerson RL. The scala vestibuli for cochlear implantation. An anatomic study. Arch Otolaryngol Head Neck Surg 1996;122(2):130–132
46. Zrunek M, Lischka M. Dimensions of the scala vestibuli and sectional areas of both scales. Arch Otorhinolaryngol 1981;233(1):99–104
47. Richardson HC, Beliaeff M, Clarke G, Hawthorne M. A three-array cochlear implant: a new approach for the ossified cochlea. J Laryngol Otol 1999;113(9):811–814
48. Kirtane MV, More YI, Mankekar G. Cochlear stenting: how I do it. Eur Arch Otorhinolaryngol 2010;267(6):985–987
49. Lin K, Marrinan MS, Waltzman SB, Roland JT Jr. Multichannel cochlear implantation in the scala vestibuli. Otol Neurotol 2006;27(5):634–638
50. Balkany T, Bird PA, Hodges AV, Luntz M, Telischi FF, Buchman C. Surgical technique for implantation of the totally ossified cochlea. Laryngoscope 1998;108(7):988–992
51. Hartrampf R, Dahm MC, Battmer RD, et al. Insertion depth of the Nucleus electrode array and relative performance. Ann Otol Rhinol Laryngol Suppl 1995;166:277–280

Further Reading

Belal A Jr. The effects of vascular occlusion on the human inner ear. J Laryngol Otol 1979;93(10):955–968

Hinojosa R, Green JD Jr, Marion MS. Ganglion cell populations in labyrinthitis ossificans. Am J Otol 1991;12(Suppl):3–7, discussion 18–21

Kerr J, Backous DD. Cochlear implantation in the partially ossified cochlea. Oper Tech Otolaryngol 2005;16:113–116

Kesser BW, Hashisaki GT, Spindel JH, Ruth RA, Scheld WM. Time course of hearing loss in an animal model of pneumococcal meningitis. Otolaryngol Head Neck Surg 1999;120(5):628–637

Pasanisi E, Bacciu A, Vincenti V, et al. [Multi-channel cochlear implant in cochlear ossification]. Acta Otorhinolaryngol Ital 2002;22(3):127–134

Smullen JL, Balkany TJ. Implantation of the ossified cochlea. Oper Techn Otolaryngol 2005;16:117–220

deSouza C, Paparella MM, Schachern P, Yoon TH. Pathology of labyrinthine ossification. J Laryngol Otol 1991;105(8):621–624

12 Meningitis and Implantation

12.1 Introduction

Worldwide, vaccination against *Haemophilus influenzae, Neisseria meningitidis*, and *Streptococcus pneumoniae* has led to an absolute decline in numbers of patients suffering from bacterial meningitis. *S. pneumoniae* is nowadays the leading causative pathogen, accountable for ~68% of the bacterial meningitis infections in developed countries. In patients surviving bacterial meningitis, it is important to assess hearing in an early postmeningitic phase to identify patients who would benefit from cochlear implantation. Some of these patients are at risk for development of cochlear obliteration and delayed detection could lead to complicated cochlear implantation[1,2] or diminished cochlear implant (CI) performance, or even preclude cochlear implantation at all[3–5] (see also Chapter 11). Various audiologic tests and radiologic modalities are available to guide clinical decision making. A stepwise approach for the audiologic and radiologic evaluation and treatment of hearing loss in postmeningitis patients will be discussed. Furthermore, in cases with full obliteration the placement of an auditory brainstem implant (ABI) could be of benefit.

12.2 Hearing Loss after Bacterial Meningitis

Bacterial meningitis is the most common etiology for acquired hearing loss in children.[6,7] Sensorineural hearing loss (SNHL) as a complication will occur in ~5 to 36% of bacterial meningitis patients. Severe to profound bilateral SNHL will occur in 3 to 9%, predominantly among pneumococcal meningitis survivors.[8–11] Unfortunately, SNHL is not always noticeable or detected in the acute phase, leaving SNHL sometimes undetected for a long period, thereby postponing adequate follow-up and delaying treatment.[6,11,12]

12.3 Audiologic Follow-up after Meningitis

A protocol for the follow-up of survivors of bacterial meningitis is important. Delayed audiologic assessment and/or delayed referral for cochlear implantation might lead to a worse hearing outcome.

Especially in young children, hearing loss may be discovered *only* by formal assessment, and be delayed or missed without assessing the hearing, despite the fact that at this age it may critically affect the development of speech.[13] A good evaluation of hearing, appropriate imaging as soon as possible, and CI counseling are crucial to obtaining the best rehabilitation options. A postmeningitis hearing evaluation protocol, such as proposed by Merkus et al,[14] can lead to an accurate and swift assessment of all children (and adults) so that the severely hearing impaired can be implanted soon after their meningitis. The two key audiologic items of this protocol are: (1) hearing assessment before discharge or as soon as the patient is capable; (2) direct referral to an audiologic center/CI center if there is a hearing loss (>30 dB, in at least one ear).

The first months are the most important in the follow-up of patients without hearing loss or with only mild hearing loss to confirm the stability of the hearing. When a (delayed) progression is noted, referral and further investigation are needed. In very young children (less than 12 months) it is preferable to have a specialized team to assess the hearing.

Sensorineural hearing loss of 30 dB or more should lead to MRI scanning and follow-up. The hearing can deteriorate further and also late fibrosis/ossification (up to 6–12 months) is reported.[15] Therefore, all cases with sensorineural hearing loss after meningitis, with or without the presence of labyrinthitis ossificans, need audiometric follow-up at 1, 2, 6, and 12 months after the first hearing test. Additional audiometric testing can be useful when there is doubt about the course of the hearing loss. When sensorineural hearing deteriorates during the follow-up, MRI needs to be repeated to identify possible progression of intracochlear pathology such as labyrinthitis ossificans. Hearing deterioration to audiometric thresholds between 30 and 70 dB needs follow-up with audiometric testing and MRI scanning for evaluation.[14]

12.4 Postmeningitis Hearing Evaluation and Treatment Flowchart

(See **Figs. 12.1** and **12.2**.)

Hearing assessment should be done as soon as possible (preferably before discharge from the hospital) in *all* survivors of meningitis, children as well as adults, irrespective of the suspicion of hearing loss before the first audiologic tests. A protocolized follow-up scheme of formal hearing tests should be adopted in the following months, as the hearing loss can be progressive up to at least 6 months after the meningitis, with a check that the hearing is stable at 12 months. We have not seen any cases with postmeningitis hearing deterioration and development of cochlear fibrosis after 12 months of follow-up.

If SNHL is present, immediate referral to a CI center is advocated for audiologic assessment and imaging of the cochlea; see part 2 of the flowchart (**Fig. 12.2**).

With the introduction of the protocol, a crucial step is taken toward better awareness among pediatricians and neurologists/intensivists of the risk of SNHL after meningitis and the need for a swift evaluation. They are the "gatekeepers" of this protocol, as they see these patients at admission and during the clinical phase of the meningitis treatment. A close collaboration with pediatricians and neurologists/intensivists in the region is therefore of utmost importance for every CI team.

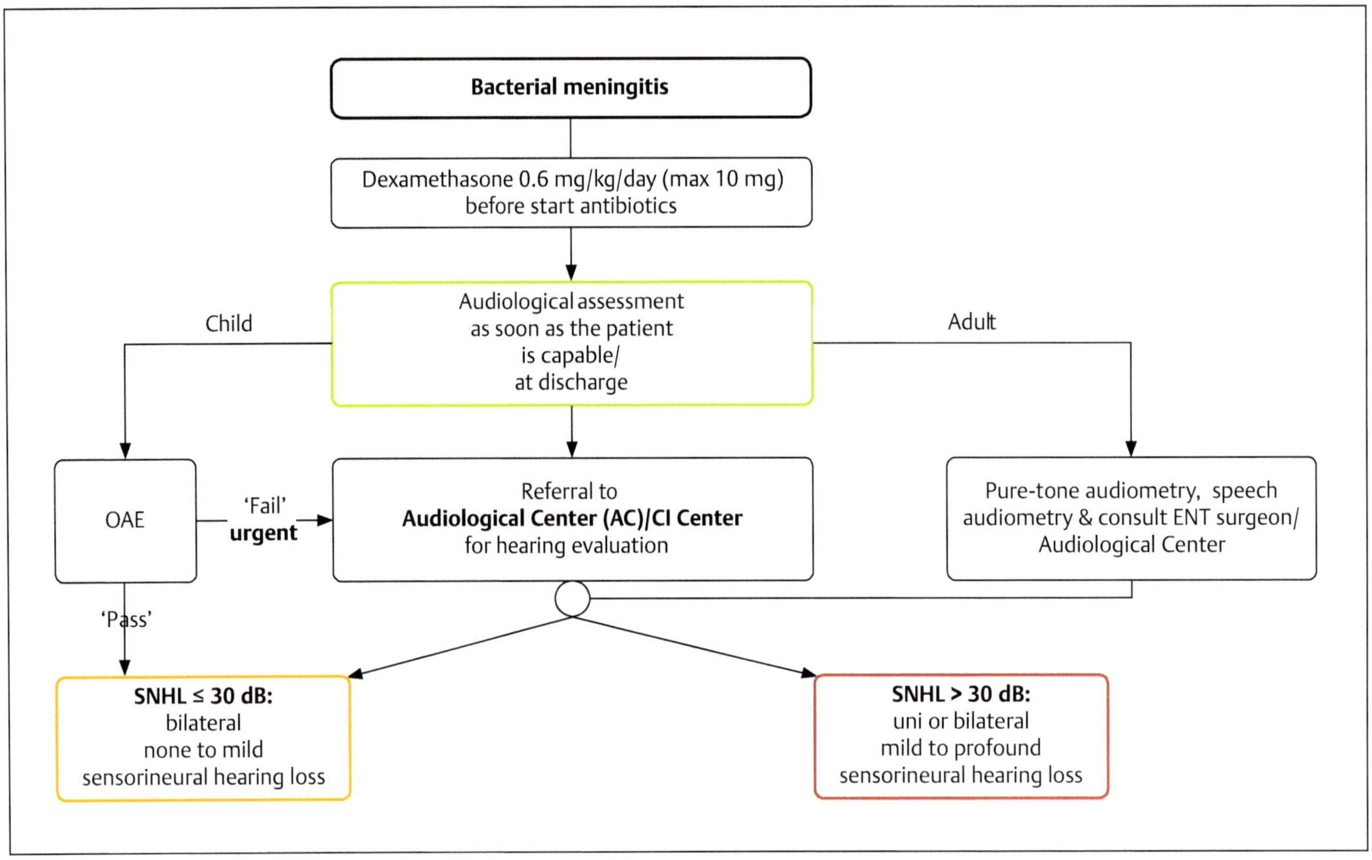

Fig. 12.1 Postmeningitis hearing evaluation and treatment flowchart part 1. ABR in children. "Urgent" is within 2 weeks ENT, ear, nose, throat; OAE, otoacoustic emission; SNHL, sensorineural hearing loss.. (This flowchart is adapted from Merkus et al 2010,[11] for explanation see text.)

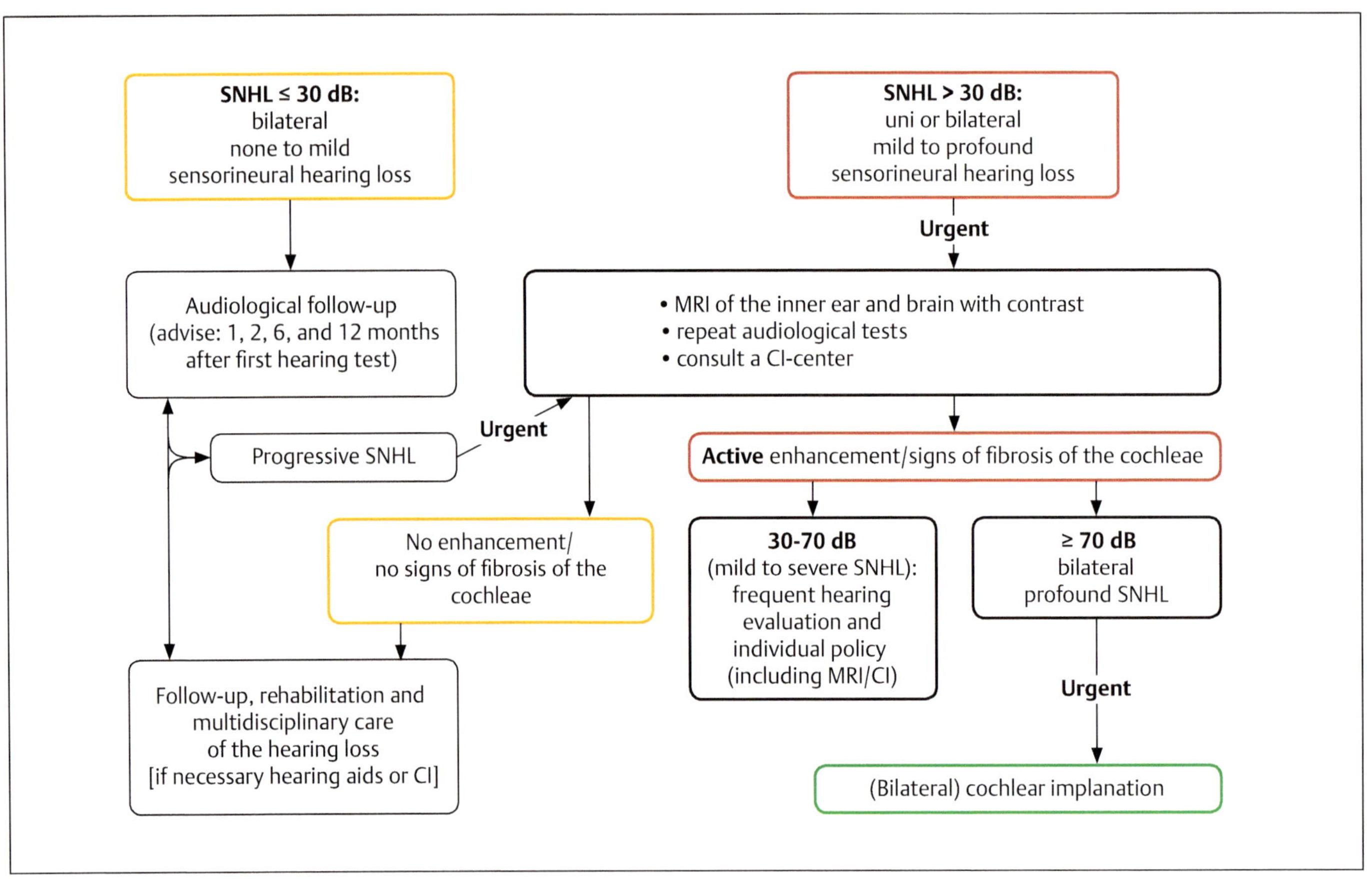

Fig. 12.2 Postmeningitis hearing evaluation and treatment flowchart part 2. "Urgent" is within 2 weeks CI, cochlear implant; MRI, magnetic resonance imaging; SNHL, sensorineural hearing loss. (This flowchart is adapted from Merkus et al 2010,[11] for explanation see text.)

12.4.1 First Hearing Evaluation

Bacterial meningitis is found more frequently in children before the age of 2 years. In this group especially, objective hearing evaluation using otoacoustic emissions (OAE)[16] and auditory brainstem response (ABR) is necessary. *In case of a passed OAE* follow-up should be frequent, since hearing deterioration is possible and if it occurs it is most likely soon after the meningitis. Follow-up should be done in an audiologic center, but if this is not feasible, at least OAE should be done followed by a quick referral in case of progression. *In case of a failed OAE* the referral should be immediate and objective measurements should be done within 2 weeks.

This consensus protocol was intended to provide easily accessible and usable guidance for all the professionals involved in every hospital. Moreover, due to the vaccination programs for *H. influenzae* and *S. pneumoniae*, the number of meningitis cases is decreasing, making the routine of hearing follow-up in every meningitis case less frequent and correspondingly more vulnerable to being overlooked.

12.4.2 Dexamethasone

Administration of dexamethasone prior to antibiotic treatment in meningitis in adults and children will reduce the neurologic complications and the risk of hearing loss.[17–21]

We therefore advocate in children dexamethasone 0.6 mg/kg/day in 4 doses for 4 days starting prior to the first antibiotic infusion, and in adults 10 mg every 6 hours for 4 days (40 mg/day), especially if a pneumococcal infection is present.

As the lysis of bacteria in the cochlea is supposedly one of the triggers leading to the intracochlear immune response, it seems important to start with the dexamethasone therapy at least 10 to 30 minutes prior to the first antibiotic administration.[18,20]

12.4.3 Obliteration

An unresolved question is how quickly the obliteration of the cochlea can become manifest. According to animal experiments, case reports, and the experience in our group it seems to be a matter of weeks.[1,2,22] It is recommended that if the OAE test at discharge is failed, a decision whether cochlear implantation is needed should be made within 2 to 3 weeks.

A cascade of actions needs to be completed to enable such a decision to be made. First of all prompt referral to a cochlear implant center is essential. Referral to a cochlear implant center is especially important in these cases as counseling, diagnosis, and expertise are needed in a timely manner within a multidisciplinary approach. This is particularly so because the hearing loss does not appear to be an emergency case to the parents or even the doctors around them in a sometimes otherwise healthy child or adult.

12.4.4 Hearing Loss of 30 dB or More

The cochlear implant center will evaluate all patients with a sensorineural hearing loss of 30 dB or more and screen postmeningitic patients with < 30 dB loss or still normal hearing. In our experience this is a safe and valuable cut-off point for deciding between non-affected ears and affected ears. Thus, children or adults with a > 30 dB hearing loss should be considered "at risk" for developing irreversible SNHL; moreover, children are prone to develop a problem in speech and language development. See flowchart part 2 (**Fig. 12.2**). Although 30 dB hearing loss alone is not enough for cochlear implantation, signs of fibrosis on MRI and a 30 to 70 dB hearing loss should be very closely monitored via frequent hearing tests and MR imaging. In case of progression of hearing loss or fibrosis on the MRI scan, cochlear implantation is inevitable. More than 70 dB hearing loss and signs of labyrinthitis or fibrosis on the MRI (see next section) are reason to perform an urgent cochlear implantation. Below 30 dB loss a "follow-up policy" is adequate: in this "at risk" group, repeated hearing assessment and, when indicated, MRI are the keystones in the follow-up. When considering placement of a CI, it is wise also to scan the complete brain as the CI magnet will hamper visualization of the brain post implantation (see Chapter 3).

12.4.5 Radiologic Phases of Inflammation, Fibrosis, and Ossification[14,23,24]

(See **Fig. 12.3**.)

Different Phases of Postmeningitic Cochlear Inflammation as Seen on MRI and HRCT

Normal

- No cochlear enhancement on gadolinium-enhanced T1W MRI (GdMRI)
- No loss of fluid on heavily T2-weighted MRI (T2W MRI)
- No calcification on high-resolution CT (HRCT)

Acute phase

- Cochlear enhancement on GdMRI (*yellow arrow*)
- No loss of fluid on T2W MRI

Intermediate phase

- Cochlear enhancement on GdMRI
- Loss of fluid on T2W MRI (*red arrow*)

Final phase

- *No* cochlear enhancement is present, fairly significant loss of fluid is seen on T2W MRI.

To distinguish whether cochlear obliteration is caused by either fibrosis or ossification, the combination of T2W MRI and HRCT (*blue arrow*) is needed.

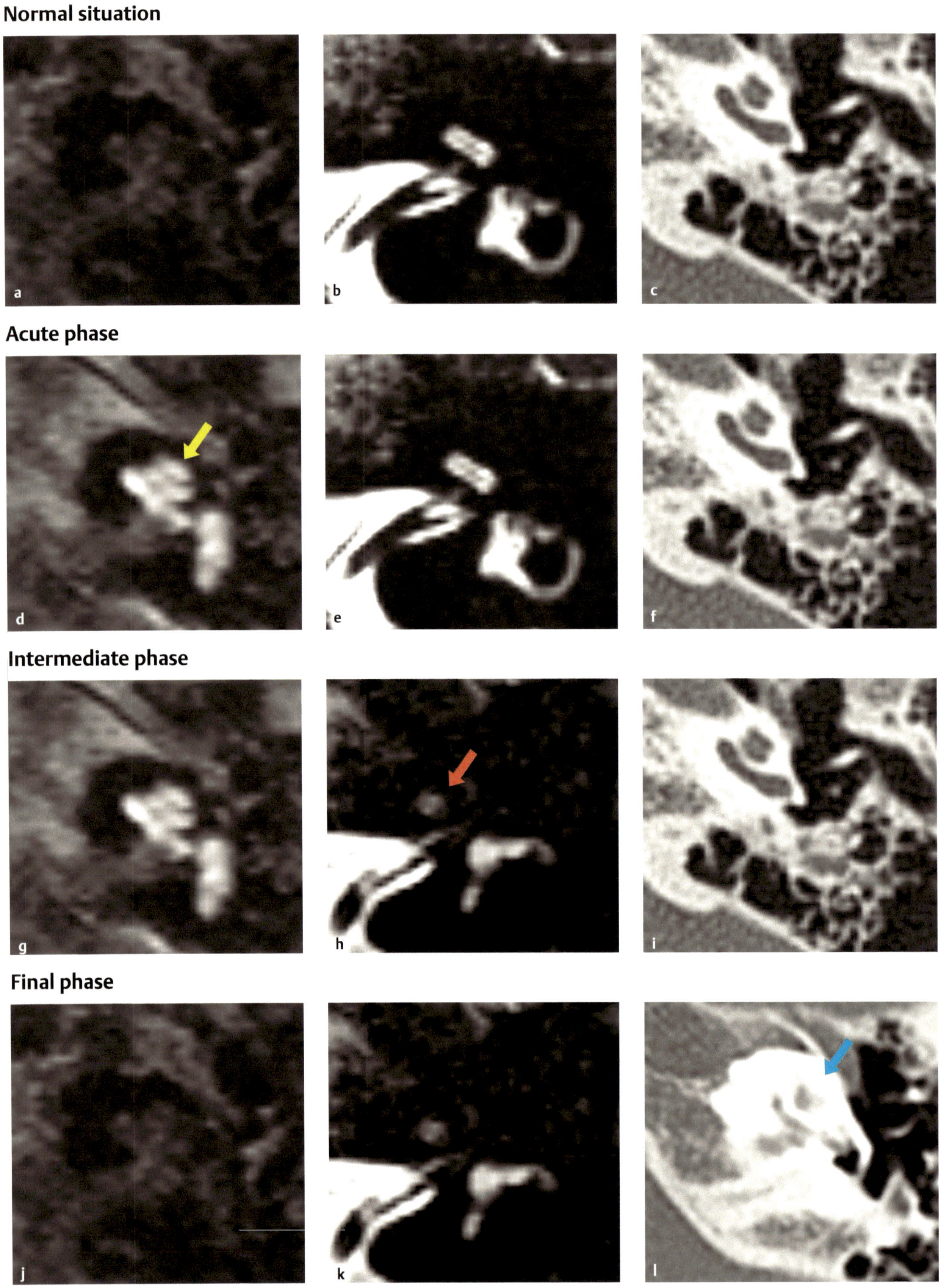

Fig. 12.3a–l Radiologic phases of inflammation, fibrosis, and ossification. First column GdMR images, second column T2W MR images, and third column HRCT images. (Adapted from references [14, 23, 24] with permission of *Otology & Neurotology*.)

12.5 Early Postmeningitis Radiology and Decision Making

Relatively recently it has been recognized that there is a strong correlation between the development of hearing loss and enhancement on T1W images.[23] One can expect deterioration of the hearing in a postmeningitis child with enhancement on the T1W image. The quality of the image and the slice thickness is important if there is any doubt about candidacy for a CI. The imaging will indicate location of the most inflamed area within the cochlea and accordingly the outcome of hearing loss. See **Figs. 12.4 and 12.5**, illustrating cases in which the decision *not* to implant was based on the MR image in combination with the hearing result.

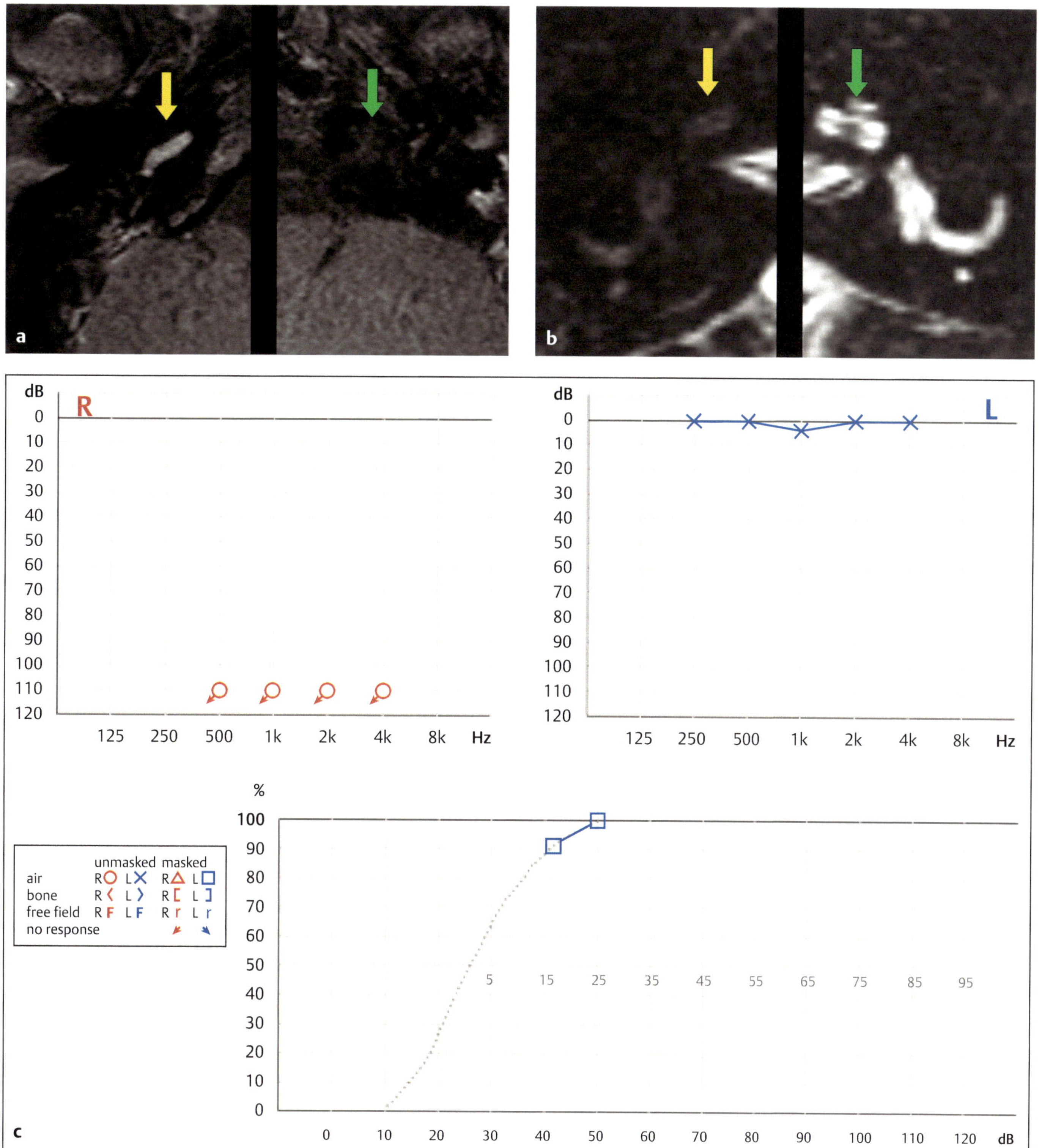

Fig. 12.4a–c Unilateral hearing loss and enhancement.

a In this case of an 11-month-old infant, hearing evaluation was performed 2 weeks after start of the meningitis. The ABR showed a deafened right ear and a normal functioning left ear. On contrast-enhanced T1W MR images, the right deaf ear (*yellow arrow*) showed an enhancement, whereas no enhancement was present in the left ear (*green arrow*).

b The heavily weighted T2W MR images showed a decrease in fluid filling of the cochlea on the inflamed right side (*yellow arrow*). On the other side a normal fluid distribution was seen within the complete labyrinth. (The left side lateral canal was completely fluid filled, adjacent image not shown here.) The decision for unilateral cochlear implantation or no implantation is debatable in this case.

c The hearing of the unaffected left ear was followed during the next 12 months by audiometric testing at 1, 2, 6, and 12 months and remained stable over years.

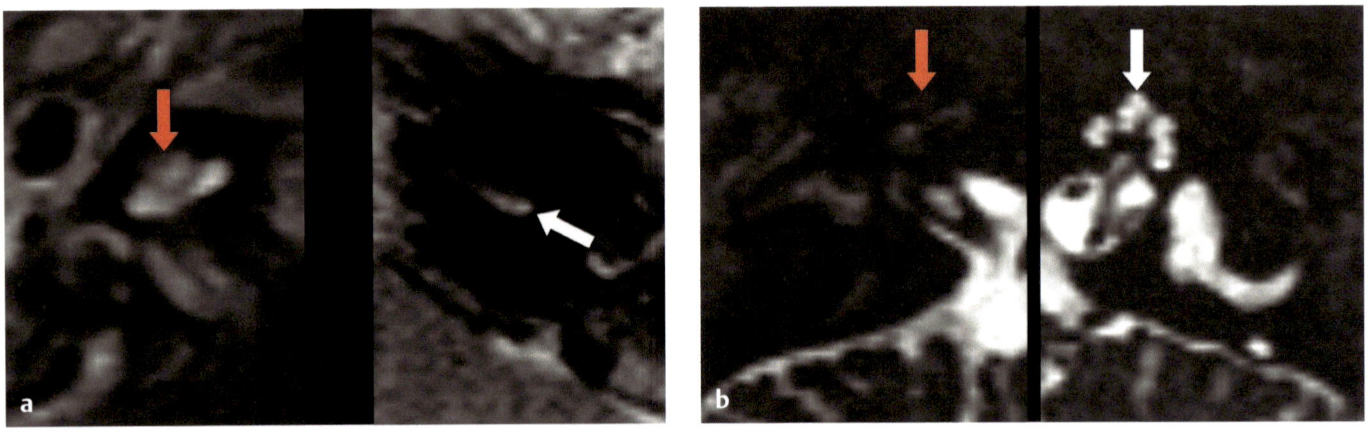

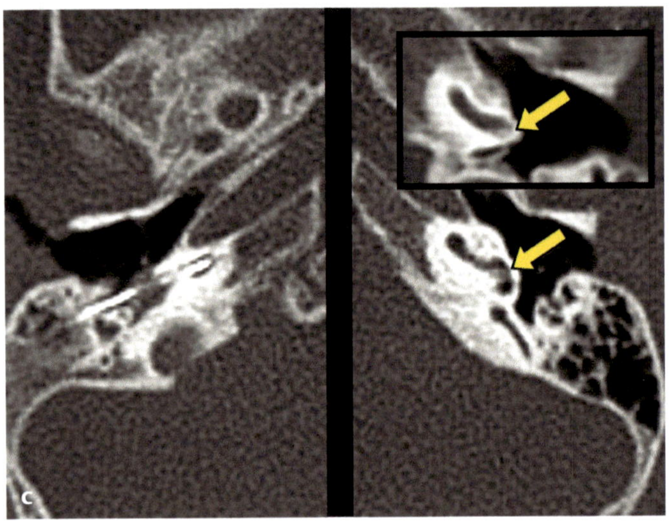

Fig. 12.5a–d Asymmetric hearing loss; a tailored approach.

a In this case we encountered slight enhancement on contrast-enhanced T1W MR imaging, only in the left basal turn (scala tympani, *white arrow*), as shown here. The other ear (*red arrow*) had become deaf directly post meningitis and the cochlea showed contrast-enhancement. Hearing on the left remained stable during three sequential ABRs (3000 Hz) over 3 weeks, showing a stable high-frequency hearing loss of 60 dB.

b The T2W MR image showed a normal fluid-filled cochlea on the left side, and hypointense "fluid loss" on the right side. Because of the unenhanced lower frequency area at the middle and apical turn on the left side and the stable results of the ABRs we scheduled this child for a CI in the deafened right ear and a hearing aid rehabilitation for the high-frequency hearing loss in the left ear.

c The left side had some enhancement at the region of the round window in the week directly post meningitis. CT investigation was done one year and several years later. A closer view of the round window region (*yellow arrows*) showed calcification of the round window area. It appears that MRI enhancement in the acute phase and obliteration/ossification in the end stage are closely related.

d The hearing remained stable over several years and the hearing aid in the left ear is used daily. Notable is the mixed-type hearing loss, which suggests that the calcified round window (*yellow arrow* in [**c**]) is causing a conductive low-frequency component in addition to the postmeningitis SNHL.

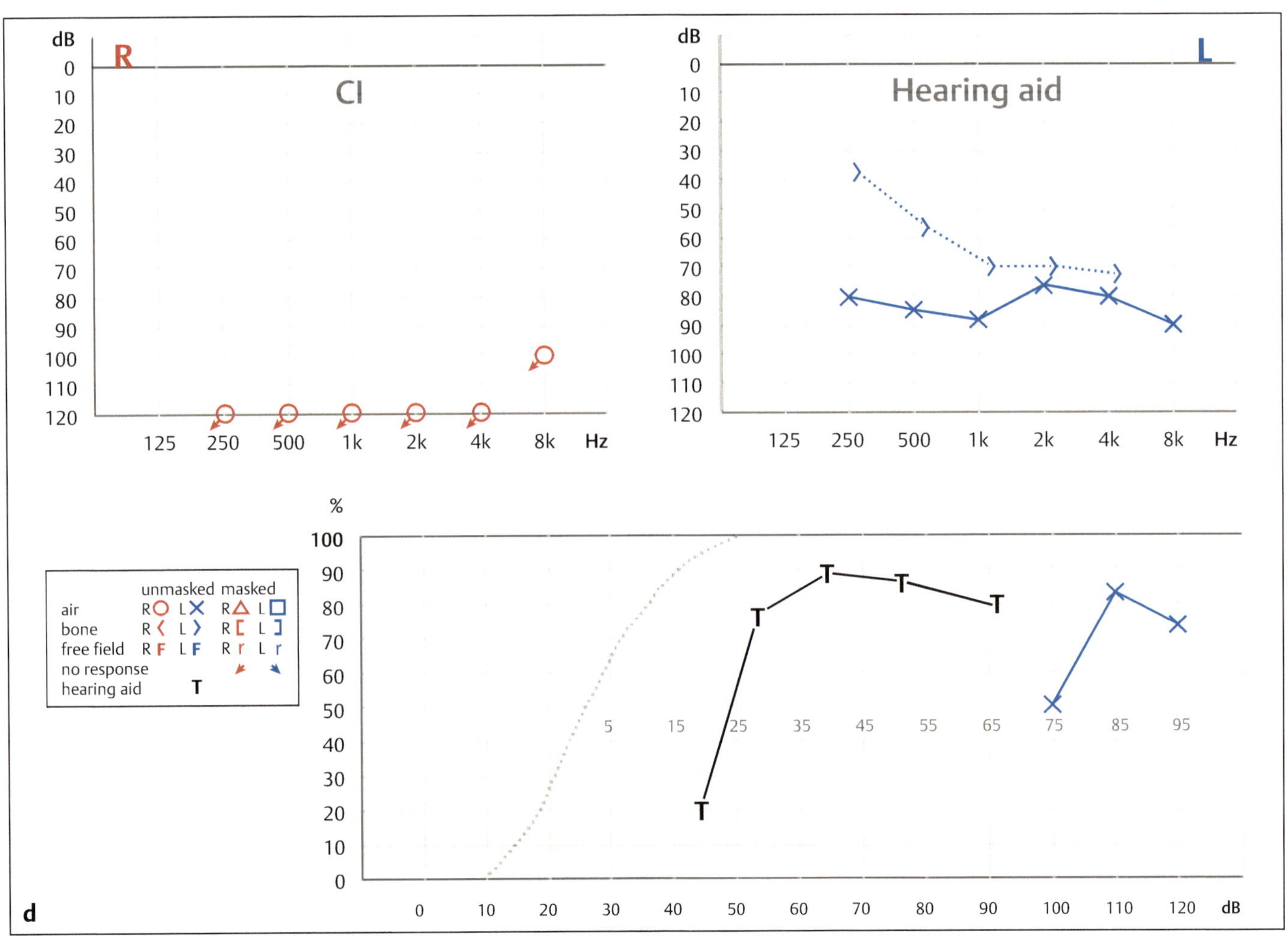

12.5.1 Unilateral Hearing Loss and Radiology

Abnormalities on postmeningitis T2W images will appear later than on the contrast-enhanced T1W images. T1W images will show the inflammation in the acute phase and T2W images will show loss of fluid, which is due to obliteration with either fibrosis or calcified (fibrous) tissue. Patients should be considered as CI candidates as soon as there is any loss of fluid in the weeks following onset of meningitis. Only when there is a single side affected (unilateral hearing loss and MRI abnormalities) and stable normal hearing remaining on the contralateral side, can unilateral implantation or *no* implantation be considered. The hearing of the normal hearing side must be monitored closely in the following months. If only one cochlea is enhanced it is very likely that the normal hearing of the unenhanced cochlea will be preserved.[23]

12.5.2 Bilateral 0–30 dB Loss and Radiology

A good hearing follow-up is needed in this patient group, as explained in earlier sections. There is no routine need for MRI, but if there is deterioration of the hearing then referral to a CI team and urgent MRI are necessary.

12.5.3 Bilateral 30–70 dB Loss and Radiology

This is the most difficult group when it comes to decision making. The hearing is too good for placement of a CI, but is definitely deteriorated. Further deterioration might become apparent in time. With the help of audiometric follow-up and T1W MRI, certain assumptions can be made that help in the decision process. Reimbursement policies may also influence decisions in this group as well as differences in hearing thresholds between the ears. It is wise is to follow up closely with appropriate hearing evaluation (ABR in young children) and when in doubt perform a second MRI. If obliteration, as seen on T2W MRI, sets in there is no time to waste.

12.5.4 Bilateral > 70 dB Loss and Radiology

This is the group often referred to in discussion of simultaneous bilateral cochlear implantation.[25] Fortunately, it seems to involve a minority of patients with postmeningitis hearing loss, but it is the most demanding one. These are the patients in whom there is no time to lose and in whom rapid bilateral cochlear implantation should be performed. MRI can inform the surgeons whether the stage is still *acute* or in case of obliteration is already *intermediate* or even *final*. In the acute phase, cochlear implantation should not present a problem. In the intermediate phase, it depends strongly on the amount of obliteration and the time between the scan and the operation. In the final phase, no enhancement can any longer be seen. In addition, obliteration will be seen on T2W MRI in this phase, but it is unknown whether (a part of) the obliterated intracochlear area is calcified. Combination imaging with HRCT is needed. One must remember that obliteration can be both fibrosis and/or calcification[23] and that these imaging modalities are complementary. The calcification process is thought to start within weeks, but as yet it is unknown when this period ends.

12.6 Difficulties in the Assessment Phase

Bacterial meningitis can occur at all ages, but young children and even infants are more prone due to their immunologic status. This age group needs extra expertise in the assessment and rehabilitation phase. Difficulties in the audiologic and radiologic assessment are discussed here, along with sequelae and the counseling of the parents.

12.6.1 Audiologic Assessment in Infants

The method of hearing evaluation in young CI candidates depends on the developmental age and cooperation of the child.[26] Especially in the age group from birth to approximately 5 or 6 months, behavioral measurements cannot be used to obtain reliable thresholds; objective methods are needed in this age group. Measurement of auditory brainstem responses (ABR) is well-established for predicting the hearing threshold around 3 kHz. In some cases, more frequency-specific information is needed. For instance, children with moderate to severe hearing losses in the lower and middle frequencies and hearing losses larger than 100 dB in the higher frequencies may show an absent click ABR.[27] These children could benefit greatly from hearing aids and are not cochlear implant candidates per se.[28] Other objective measurements such as auditory steady-state responses (ASSR), tone burst ABR, and electrocochleography (ECochG) may provide better frequency-specific information. A hearing aid trial is considered standard procedure in most cochlear implant centers, though the necessity of a hearing aid trial prior to cochlear implantation has been questioned recently because it may delay cochlear implantation in some children. We consider it an important part of the diagnostic protocol in most infants, especially because it enables behavioral assessment at this stage. Furthermore, amplification prior to cochlear implantation is important because it could improve the outcomes of the procedure, as it activates the auditory pathway. Also the wearing of hearing aids facilitates the use of the behind-the-ear CI processor.

The preoperative evaluation of young children with hearing loss after meningitis differs from that of other hearing-impaired children in many respects. The interval between establishing hearing loss and implantation of the cochlear implant can be as short as one week. In this short period the parents need to be informed about hearing loss and about the possibility of cochlear implantation, and counseled in the decision making. It is a difficult period in which to expect parents to take well thought-out decisions since they are naturally in a stressful situation as their child has just recovered from a life-threatening disease. It is important that parents fully realize the fact that the child has a permanent and profound damage of the inner ears and is suffering from subsequent hearing loss. In this process, behavioral observation audiometry may be helpful. A hearing aid trial is omitted for reasons of urgency when bilateral severe to profound hearing loss is confirmed in combination with signs of fibrosis on MRI. The interval between establishing hearing loss and implantation is often too short for parents to absorb and appreciate all the consequences of the hearing loss, cochlear implantation, and possible long-term effects of meningitis. However, the time between implantation and first fitting of the implant can be used for this purpose, including the process of setting realistic expectations of the cochlear implant. The expectations may be lower for these children than for other children with cochlear implants because of long-term effects of meningitis that cannot be fully predicted at the time of implantation.

Especially in the postmeningitis population it is of importance that the diagnostic process is embedded in a multidisciplinary approach, which comprises surgical, audiologic, communicative, and psychosocial disciplines.

12.6.2 Imaging in Infants

The preferred imaging modality in postmeningitis patients is MRI. The preferred scanning sequences are T1W, gadolinium-enhanced T1W, T2W, heavily weighted T2 (CISS/Fiesta C), and general brain scan sequence. All these sequences together will take at least 45 minutes to perform. The small slice thickness and the duration will make the scan vulnerable to movement and therefore unsuitable for young children without general anesthesia. Up to an age of at least 5 years general anesthesia is required in order to obtain the necessary images as soon as possible. A positive side effect is that in some hospitals this general anesthesia can also be used in performing an ABR.

12.6.3 Other Sequelae of Meningitis

The cochlear implant team is focused on the rehabilitation of hearing but should not forget that meningitis can be devastating in many ways. First of all, parents and patients are relieved the child is still alive and hearing is sometimes not the key issue in their lives. Numerous sequelae can follow meningitis. Fortunately, many problems improve over time.

Sequelae after meningitis

- Paresis/weakness of one or more limbs
- Cognitive impairment, which will interfere with the assessment of learning ability and rehabilitation
- Memory loss/lack of concentration, which will interfere with rehabilitation
- Loss of balance/dizziness
- Clumsiness
- Residual headaches
- Epilepsy/seizures
- Loss of sight

12.6.4 Counseling Parents

Bacterial meningitis is potentially lethal and parents naturally relieved that their son or daughter has survived this devastating disease. They are sometimes taken aback that there is then a new emerging dilemma apparent: the hearing loss or even deafness of their child. The cochlear implant team has to make a special effort to give the parents time to adjust to the new situation while still emphasizing the importance of a swift diagnostic follow-up. Some parents feel it a real burden to have to decide whether a cochlear implant will be the best for their child's future. Parents want their child to hear very well after the surgery and rehabilitation. This is not a realistic prospect, as only in some of the children will the hearing be perfect with the use of a CI (categories of auditory performance [CAP] = 5–6; speech intelligibility rating [SIR] = 5), whereas others will perform poorly after meningitis (CAP = 3; SIR = 0).[29]

The variability of outcomes is due to sequelae other than hearing loss, which are not always visible at a young age, and arise from the unknown extent of neural damage. It is still uncertain whether a complete electrode insertion is possible. These uncertainties should be discussed and any predictions about the final result should be tempered accordingly. Luckily, recent research has shown that in case of no loss of fluid on T2W MRI the likelihood of an unsuccessful insertion is nil,[23] so it is possible to offer some hopeful statements about success. Anesthesiologic concerns are stated in Chapter 6, Section 6.6.[30,31,32]

12.7 Decision Making

When a patient is assessed for cochlear implantation and the (possible) cause of deafness is meningitis, this patient should be assessed and counseled with care. The meningitis could have been years ago and the history is not always very clear, especially with adult patients who experienced their hearing loss and had the meningitis at a young age. The status of cochlear ossification should be clear before any prognosis of the result of cochlear implantation can be discussed with the patient.

12.7.1 Hearing and MRI Assessment

After a couple of months the sequelae of meningitis are mostly well-known and at a final stage. Depending on the age of the patient, sometimes the hearing loss and the cognitive disabilities are the last to be discovered. If a CI is not considered in the direct postmeningitis phase, it is usually several years before the question arises again. In these patients the urgency to perform an implantation before the cochlea is obliterated no longer applies. They should be assessed like any other CI implant candidate, except for an additional MRI scan. Counseling should be done with care, considering the expectations and surgical results. In the diagnostic work-up the assessment of the cochlear patency via MRI is essential. If obliteration is seen it is correlated with less favorable outcomes.[23]

12.7.2 Ossification

In case of fibrosis or ossification in (a part of) the cochlea, certain surgical options are available. A partial basal turn drill-out, a scala vestibuli insertion, a complete basal turn drill-out in a canal wall down procedure, and a double array placement are options. A guideline and the surgical techniques are described in Chapter 11. When there is no possibility for cochlear implantation within the obliterated cochlea, an ABI should be considered.

12.7.3 ABI in Postmeningitis Cases

The literature is not clear about the primary advice in case of a fully obliterated cochlea. Should placement of a CI be attempted, followed by ABI placement if the CI placement is unsuccessful? Or should a direct decision for an ABI be made? Or should sign language alone be advised? The best chances of regaining some hearing are with a CI, but in individual cases an ABI can be successful. Substantial case series to support any of the strategies are lacking. In our opinion an attempt to find an opening within the cochlea in a canal wall down procedure is the best way to confirm the possibility of CI insertion. If this is unsuccessful, an ABI and/or use of sign language are both still possible.

Case 12.1 Bilateral CI in a Young Patient with Active Postmeningitis Enhancement of the Cochlea (Fig. 12.1.1–Fig. 12.1.7)

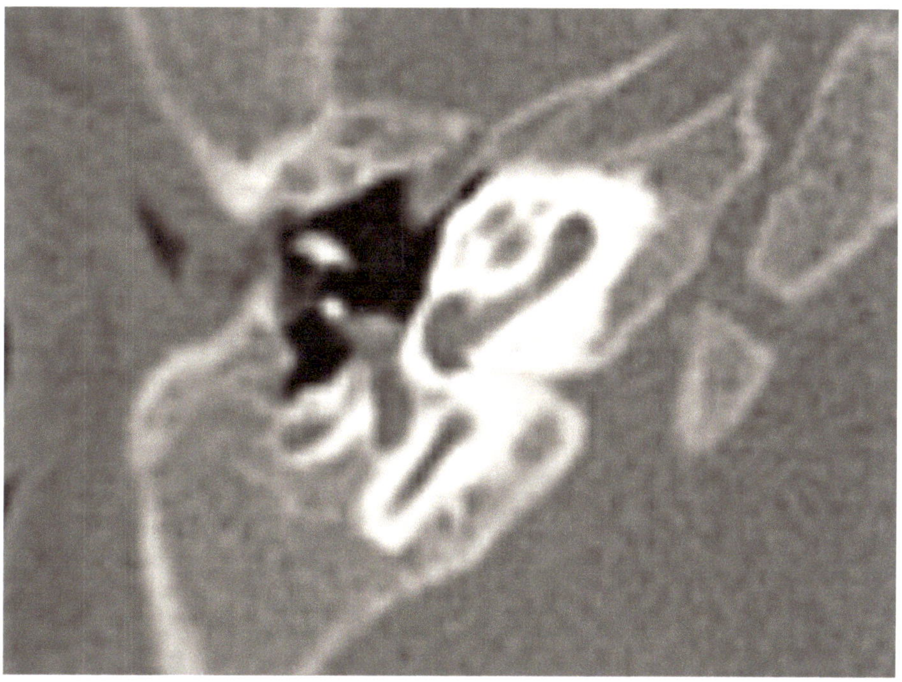

Fig. 12.1.1 An infant girl of 3 months had pneumococcal meningitis and received dexamethasone and 14 days of antibiotics in the intensive care unit. She recovered well but did not move her left leg adequately. There were some doubts about her hearing. At ABR testing she was shown to be deaf. Imaging followed swiftly and the CT scan showed no abnormalities, as shown here.

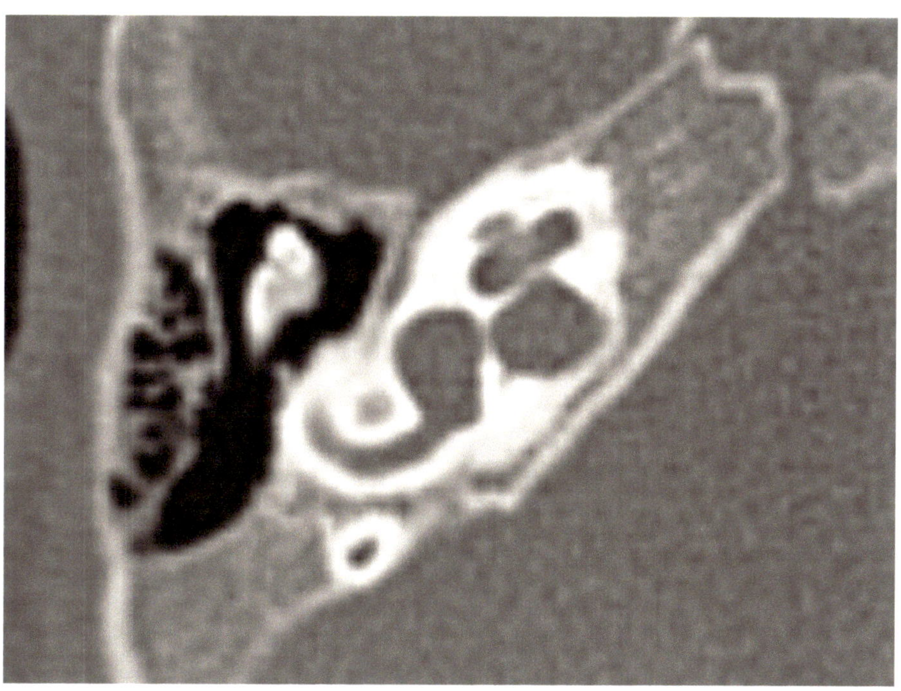

Fig. 12.1.2 The other parts of the labyrinth did not shown any signs of loss of patency. The mastoid of a 3-month-old child is still small with only one "cell" present; the antrum. The ossicular chain and cochlea have reached their normal size. The mastoid bone is mostly noncalcified and probably still full of bone marrow.

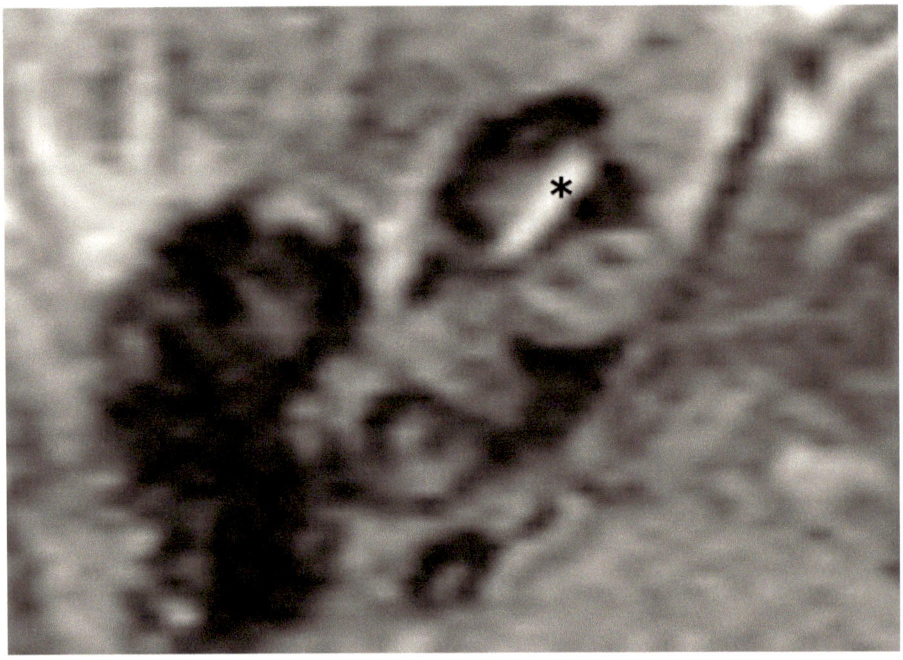

Fig. 12.1.3 MRI scanning was done 13 days after the start of the meningitis; the contrast-enhanced T1W images showed an enhancement of the basal turn of the cochlea (✱). The enhancement is seen as a white line at the position of the basal turn (most likely the scala tympani in congruence with the T2W images). The lateral semicircular canal was not enhanced and is vaguely visible in this image.

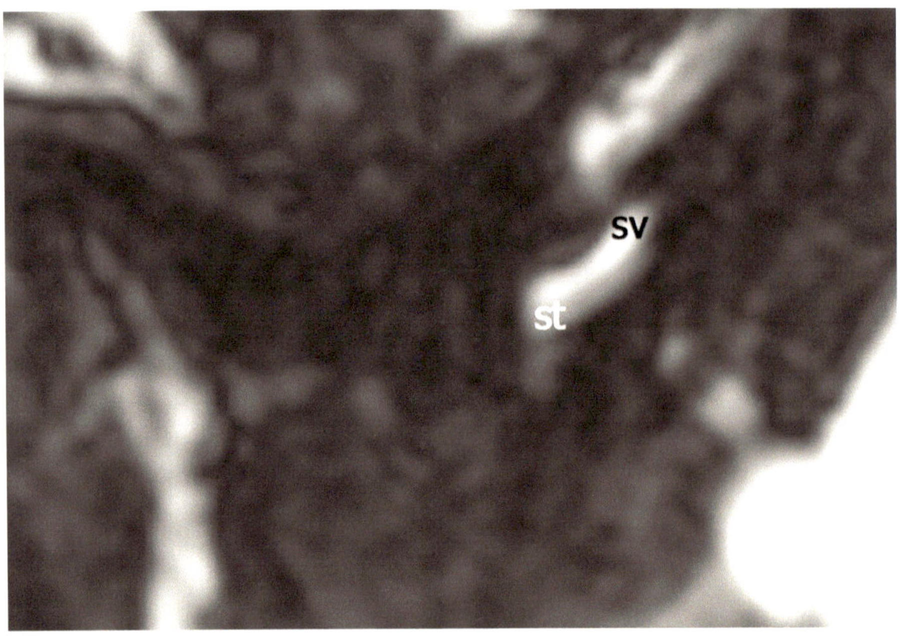

Fig. 12.1.4 On the heavily weighted T2W MRI images the cochlea is visible because of the fluid-filled space. A clear difference between the scala tympani and scala vestibuli is seen: a more gray (isointense) line representing the scala tympani (st) and more white (hyperintense) scala vestibuli (sv). The increased number of cells within the perilymph of the scala tympani has made the perilymph aspect more "gray"/isointense or even hypointense.

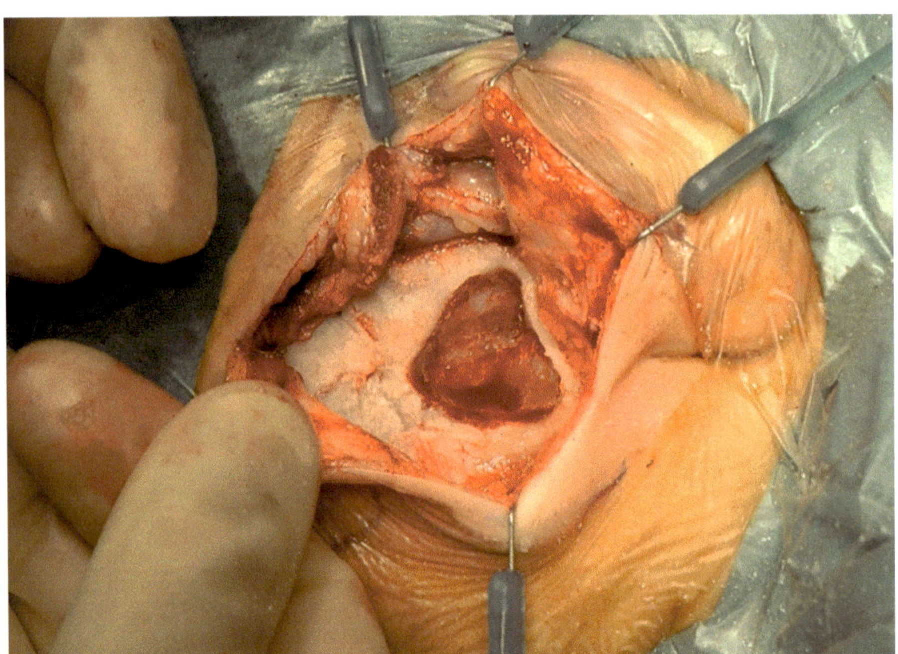

Fig. 12.1.5 Bilateral cochlear implant surgery was performed 34 days after onset of the meningitis, when the girl was just 4 months old. The mastoid was opened, as here, revealing a single cavity, a lot of oozing bone marrow, and a normal sized middle ear.

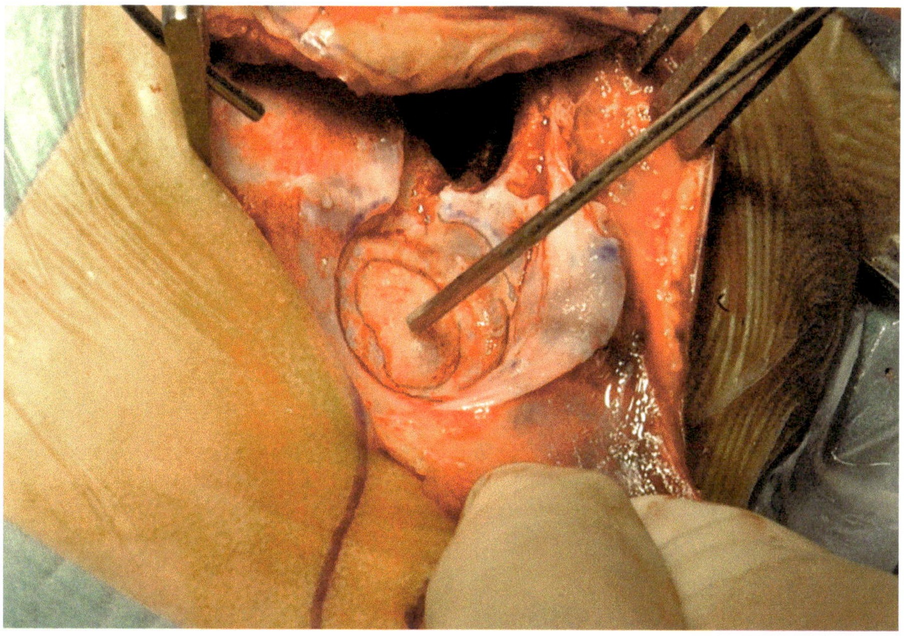

Fig. 12.1.6 With a very shallow cortical bone a bony island was created for the well of the receiver-stimulator. The implantation was without problems, with full bilateral insertion. Noteworthy was the debris found immediately behind the round window, which appeared as a "whitish plug." The perilymph behind it was not clear but rather milk-like.

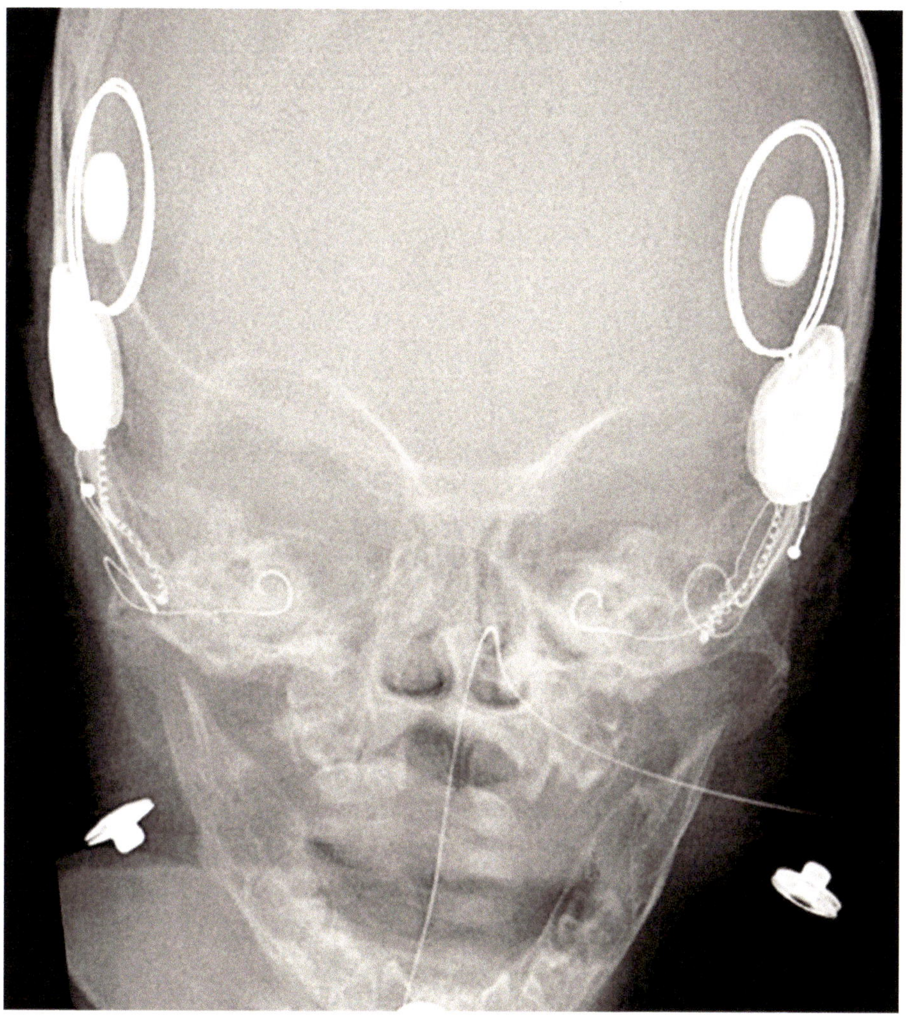

Fig. 12.1.7 Postoperative radiograph shows the infant with good positioning of both electrodes. A gastric nasal tube is also visible. The girl developed well but had a hemiparesis of the left leg, which slowly improved over time. Her audiologic performance developed: one year postoperatively she had a CAP score of 4 (discrimination of speech sounds without lip reading).

Comment 1

In all postmeningitis cases the hearing should be assessed as soon as the patient is capable, at least before discharge.

Comment 2

There is no age limit for cochlear implantation.

Case 12.2 Bilateral CI in a Case with Active Postmeningitis Enhancement of the Cochlea with Intracochlear Fibrosis (Fig. 12.2.1–Fig. 12.2.10)

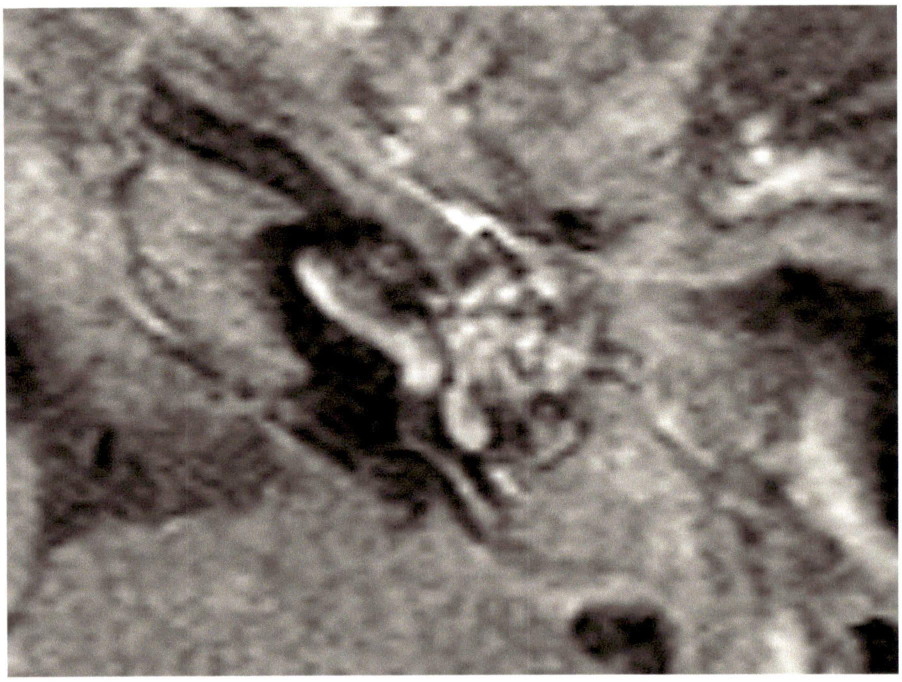

Fig. 12.2.1 In a 7-month-old boy with meningitis it became clear that his hearing was lost as soon as his situation became less critical. ABR confirmed deafness, and MR images were acquired during general anesthesia. Here we see the basal turn (scala tympani) of the left cochlea enhancing with contrast (T1W MRI).

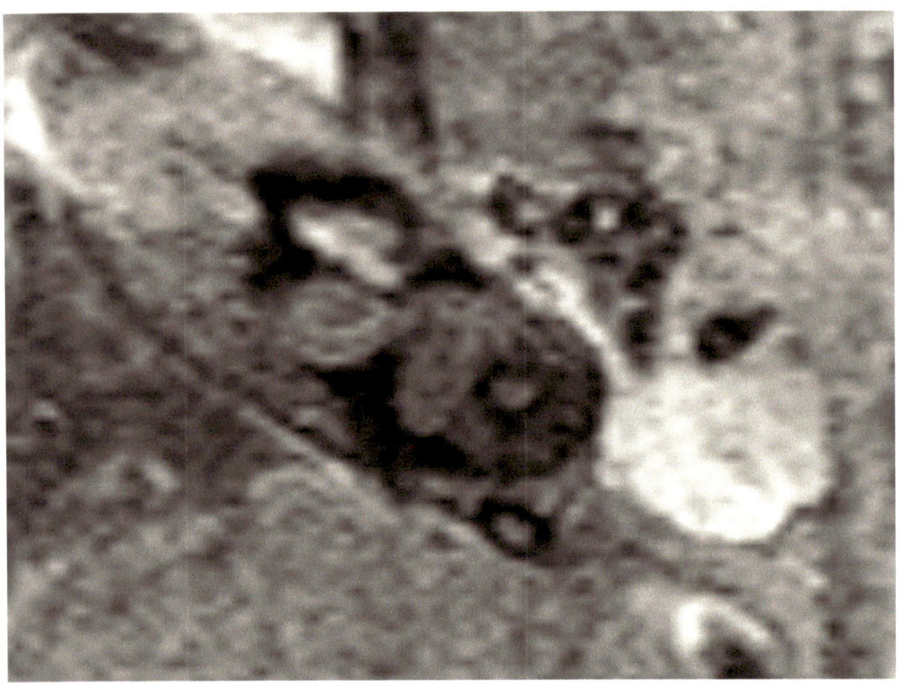

Fig. 12.2.2 The rest of the cochlea was also enhanced and the lateral canal did not enhance. The mastoid and middle ear also showed some (enhancing) fluid.

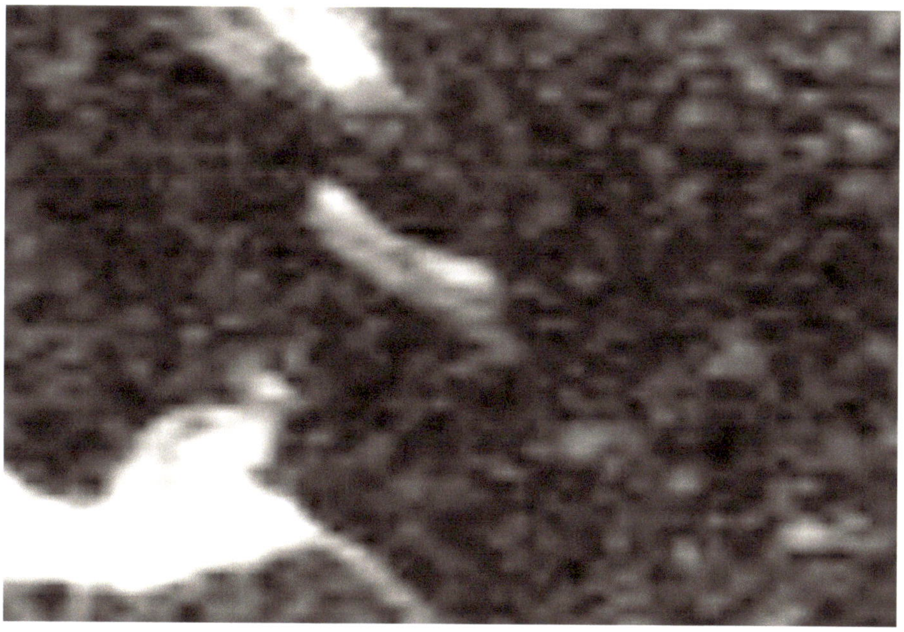

Fig. 12.2.3 On CISS (heavily T2-weighted) images the basal turn appeared partly hypointense. The scala tympani has a less bright appearance than the scala vestibuli, which is suggestive of the start of fibrosis within the scala tympani.

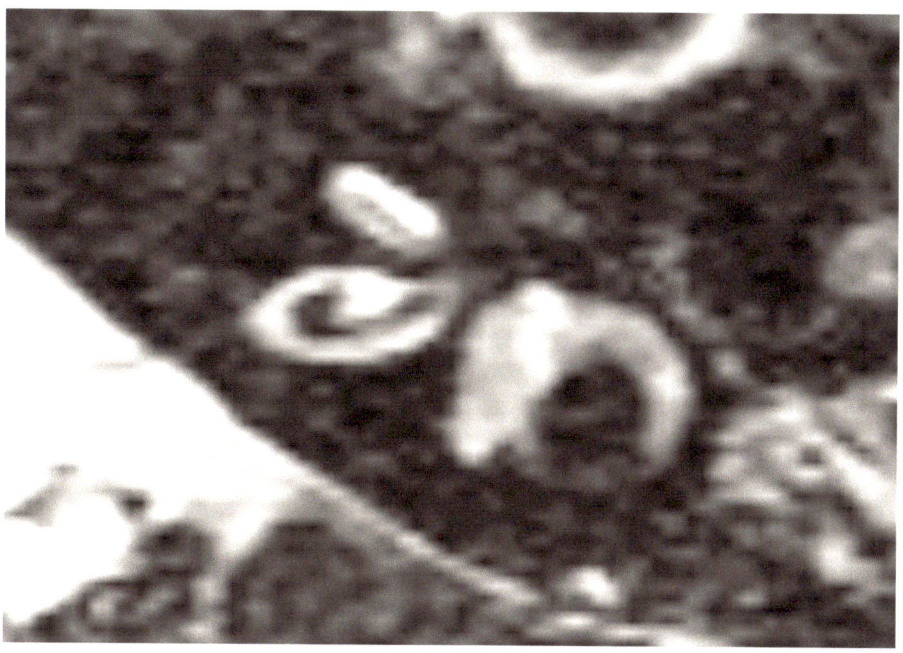

Fig. 12.2.4 The same effect is seen within the middle turn. The scala tympani is isointense and the scala vestibuli is hyperintense.

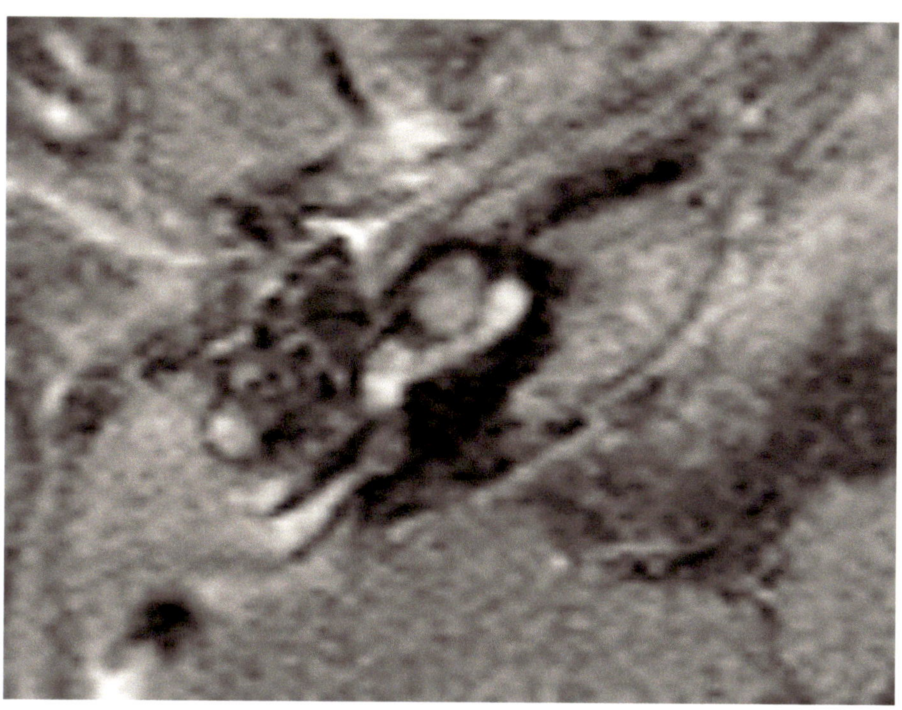

Fig. 12.2.5 On the right side a similar aspect of the enhancement is seen again. A contrast-enhanced T1W MR image shows an inflamed enhancing basal turn.

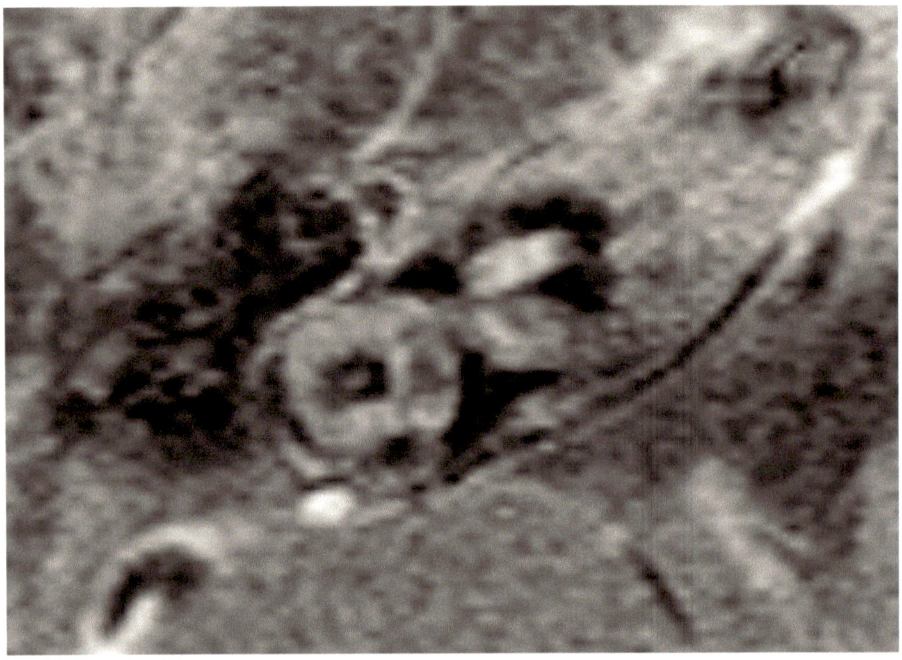

Fig. 12.2.6 The rest of the cochlea is also enhancing, whereas the labyrinth is somewhat more visible, but not clearly enhancing.

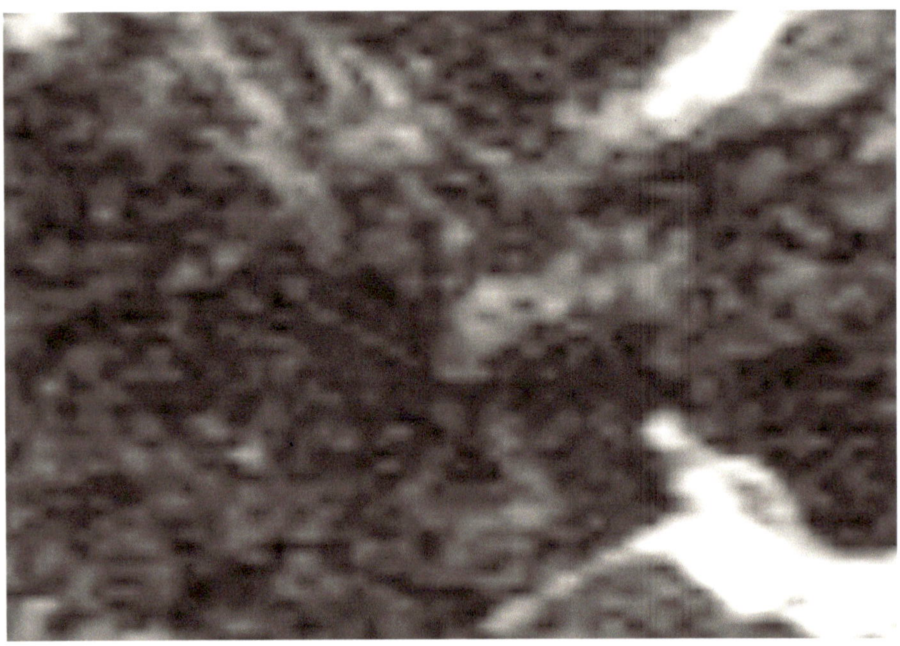

Fig. 12.2.7 The appearance of this CISS image on the right side is different from that of the left ear. There is almost no visible contour of the cochlea; the shape is vaguely discernible. It seems that the perilymph has been replaced by inflammatory cells or fibrosis. CT to rule out ossification was done without general anesthesia, but was not usable because there were too many movement artifacts.

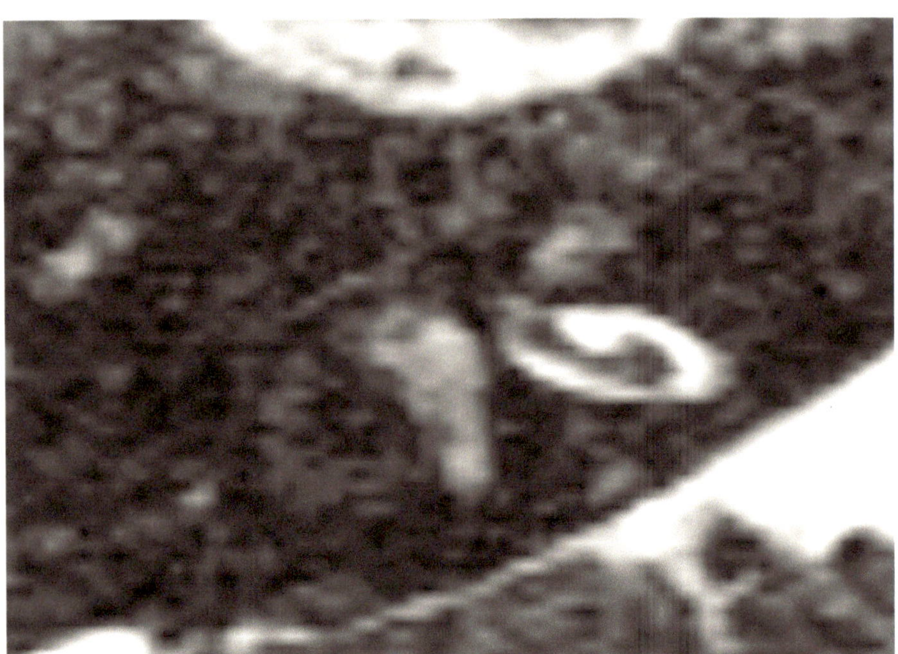

Fig. 12.2.8 Some fluid could still be seen in the vestibule, as shown here. It was decided to undertake a bilateral CI placement, which was performed 8 days after the MRI, 15 days after the first post-meningitis hearing test.

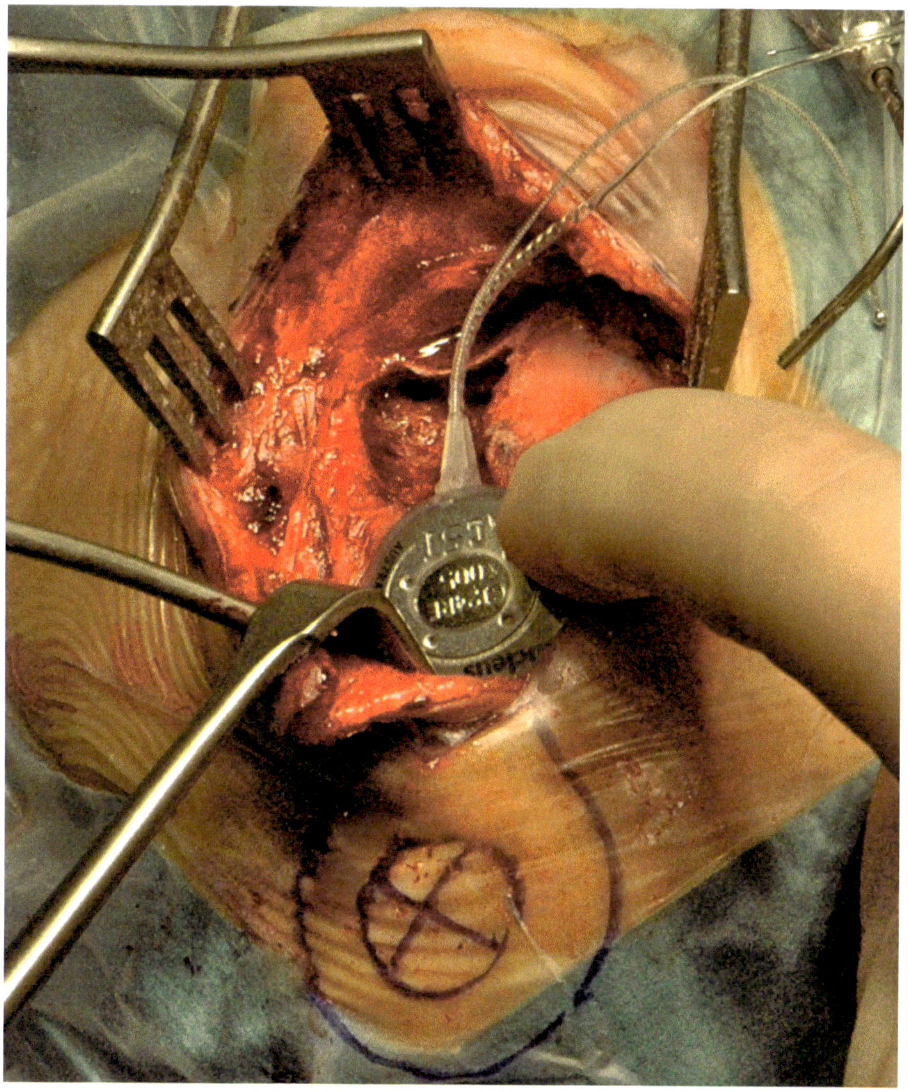

Fig. 12.2.9 The surgery was started at the ear with the best potential for electrode insertion. The insertion on the left side proceeded perfectly. On the right side, at the opening of the cochlea there was some white debris but still a good lumen for the dummy electrode. Insertion was carried out in an advanced-off stylet procedure and despite some resistance a full insertion was possible.

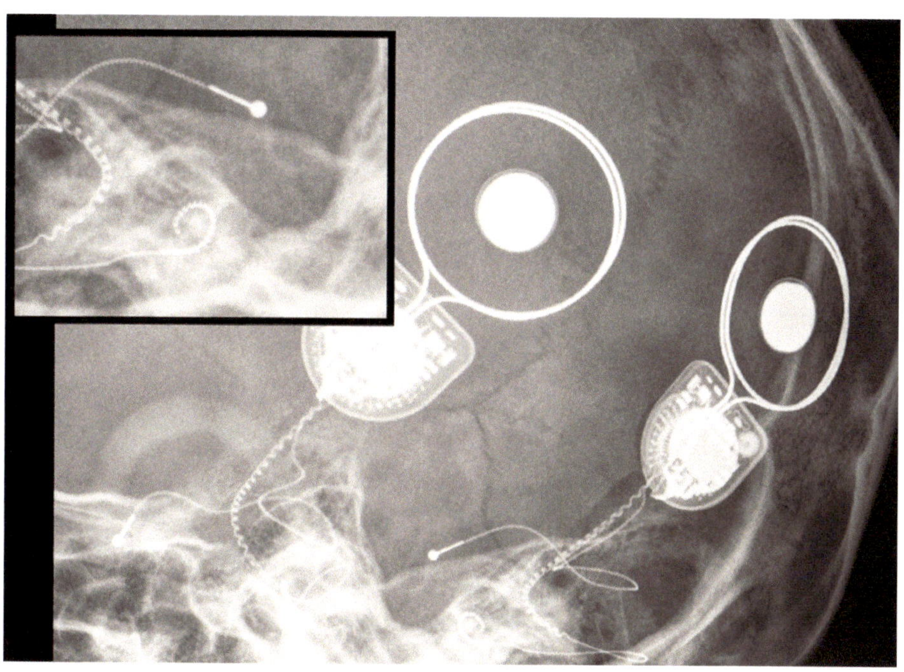

Fig. 12.2.10 Complete insertion is shown here with the postoperative radiographs. The boy developed well, despite other postmeningitis sequelae such as attention deficit and hemiparesis of the tongue. His performance now is CAP 5 (understanding common phrases without lip reading) and SIR 5 (connected speech is intelligible to all listeners). The child is understood easily in everyday contexts.

Comment

Despite the cochlear fluid having almost vanished on the T2W MRI image, it was possible to achieve a full insertion. Nevertheless, hypointensity of the cochlear fluid on T2W images is associated with an increased risk of partial insertion.[23]

Case 12.3 Scala Vestibuli Insertion in a Young Boy (Fig. 12.3.1–Fig. 12.3.6)

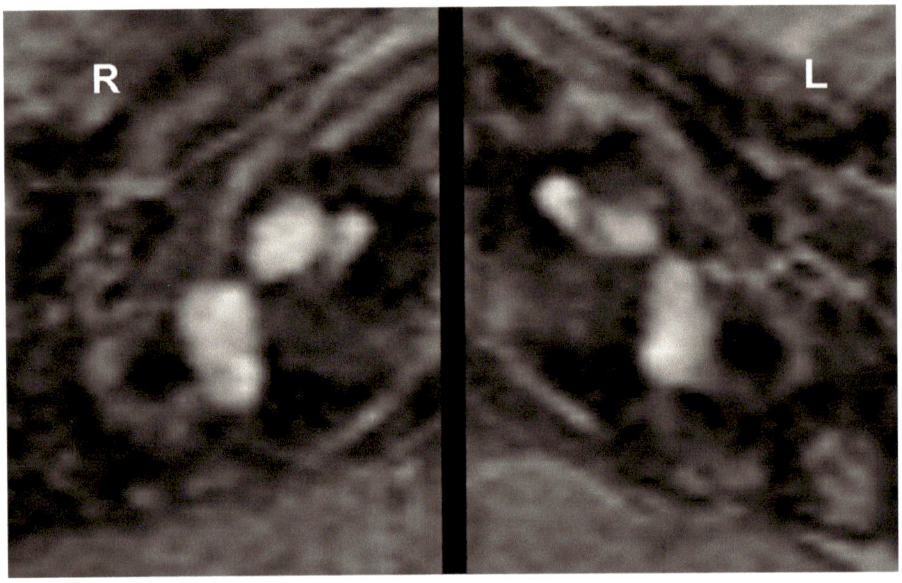

Fig. 12.3.1 This 2-year-old boy had hearing deterioration during the first days of his bacterial meningitis caused by *S. pneumoniae*. A week later, ABR confirmed that no thresholds were measurable. Due to delay by the patient's parents and the doctor, MR imaging took 4 weeks to plan. Contrast-enhanced T1W MRI images showed bilateral enhancement of the middle turn and vestibule.

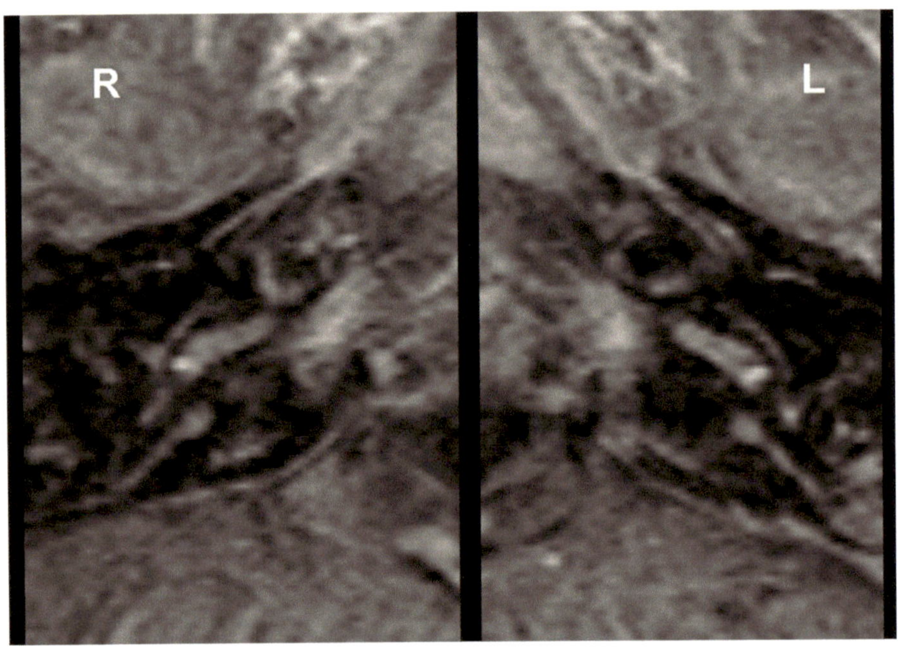

Fig. 12.3.2 The basal turn appeared less enhancing. Was this a good sign? Was there less inflammation in the basal turn, or inflammation that had already turned into fibrosis?

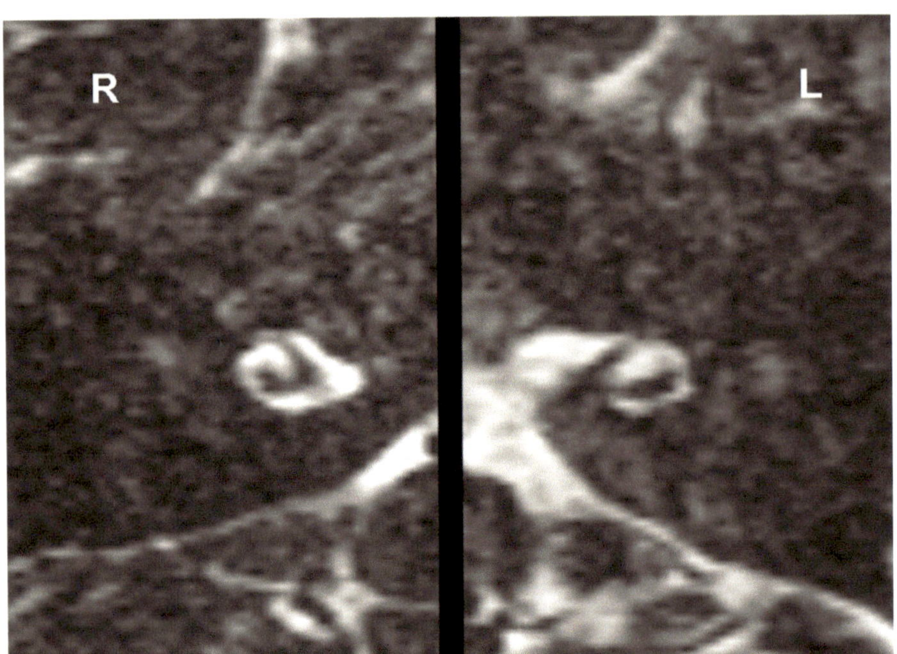

Fig. 12.3.3 The heavily weighted T2W images showed a "black cochlea," suggestive of intracochlear fibrosis. Cochlear implantation was planned immediately, but the parents still had to be persuaded that it was an emergency.

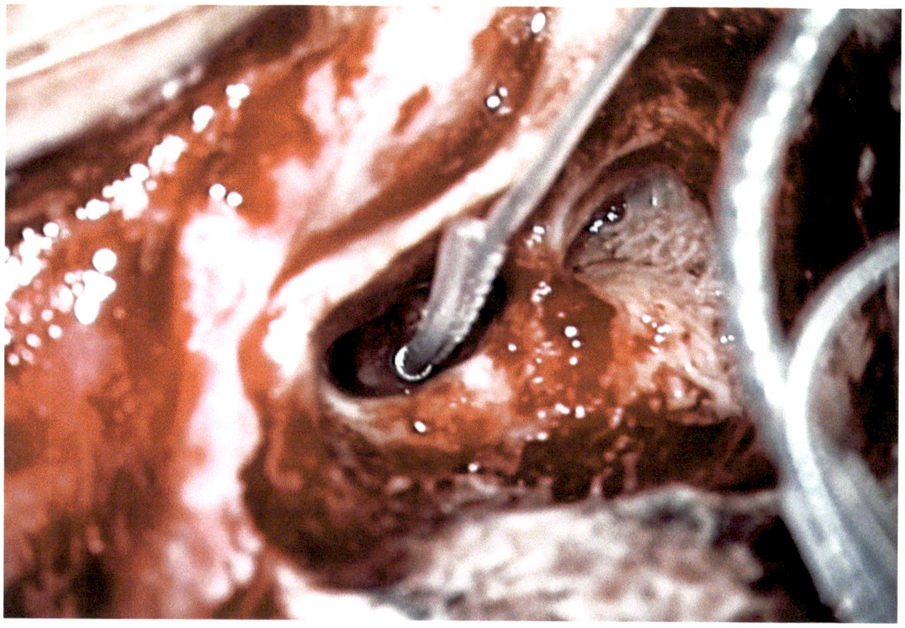

Fig. 12.3.4 During surgery the scala tympani was full of fibrosis/granulation tissue. The cochleostomy was extended further anteriorly toward the scala vestibuli. The intrascalar fibrous tissue seemed less prominent at the scala vestibuli and an attempt was made to insert.

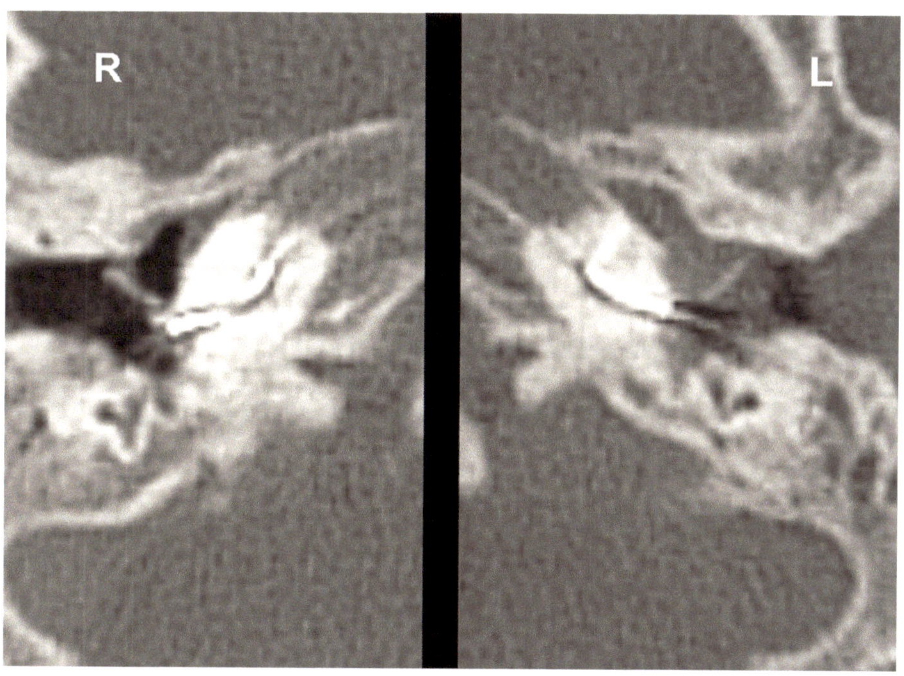

Fig. 12.3.5 On the postoperative CT scan the electrode in the scala vestibuli can be seen at the basal turn.

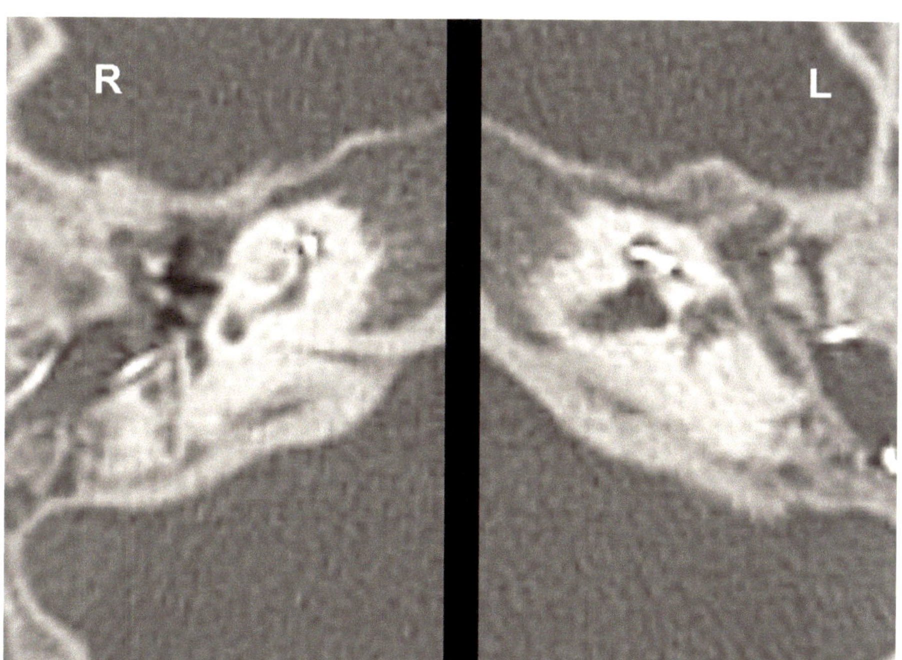

Fig. 12.3.6 At the middle turn the electrode encountered too much resistance and 4 out of 21 electrodes could not be inserted on the left side. Five electrodes remained outside the cochlea on the right side. The result was bilateral incomplete insertion due to fibrosis, 2 months after the start of the meningitis.

Comment

In acute postmeningitis cases the obliteration can occur within weeks and no time should be lost before hearing testing, imaging, and good counseling.

Case 12.4 Double Array Insertion Due to Post Meningitis Fibrosis and Ossification (Fig. 12.4.1–Fig. 12.4.9)

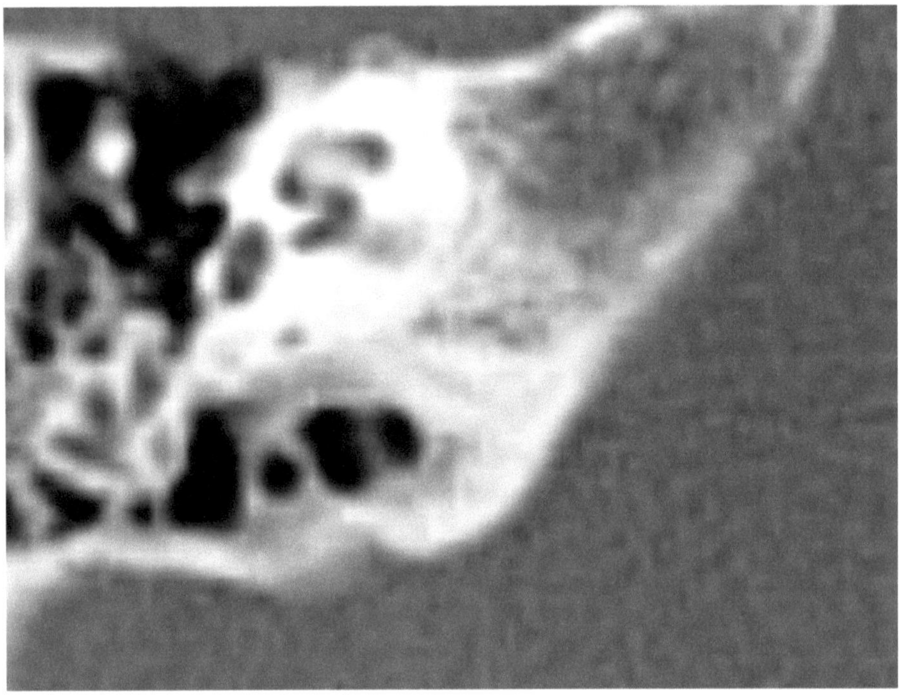

Fig. 12.4.1 A 79-year-old woman was admitted with *S. pneumoniae* meningitis. After almost 2 months in the intensive and medium care unit she emerged from her coma. Ataxia, memory loss, and imprinting problems remained. Because of her poor physical condition it took some time before her hearing was properly tested and imaging was performed.

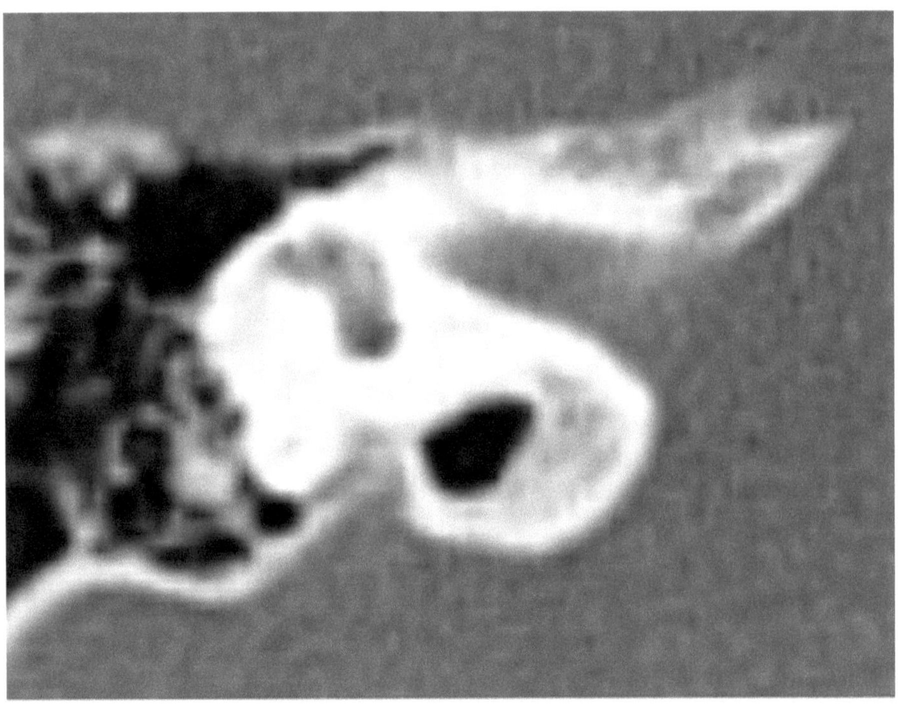

Fig. 12.4.2 The previous image and this image show the partial ossification of the right-side labyrinth and cochlea. The patient was bilaterally deaf, with some functioning but poor hearing on the left side (thresholds above 100 dB).

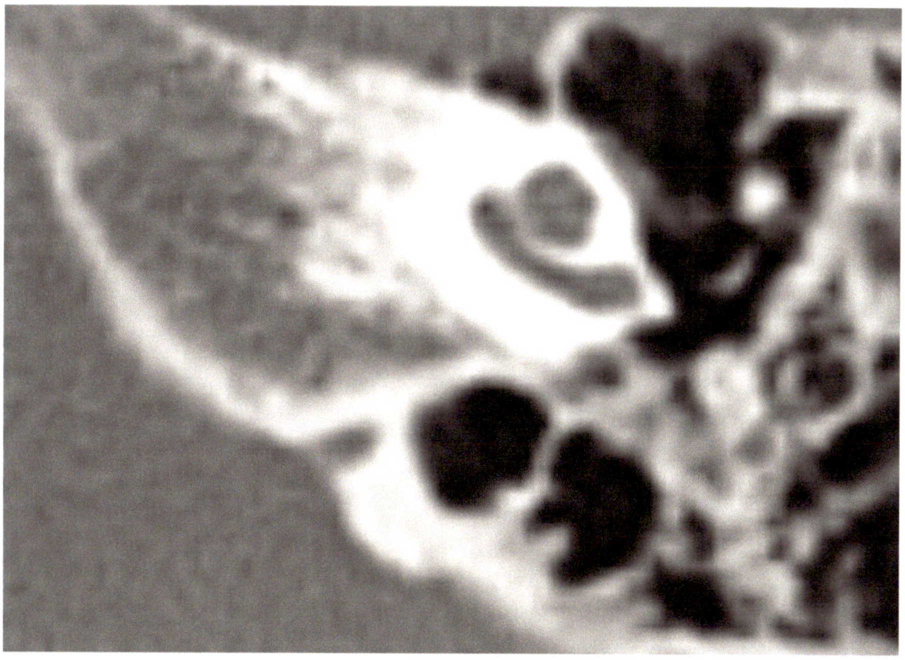

Fig. 12.4.3 The CT scan revealed a nonossified cochlea on the left side, which gave us hope for a successful CI insertion. The memory loss and imprinting problems gave us concern about the ability to learn.

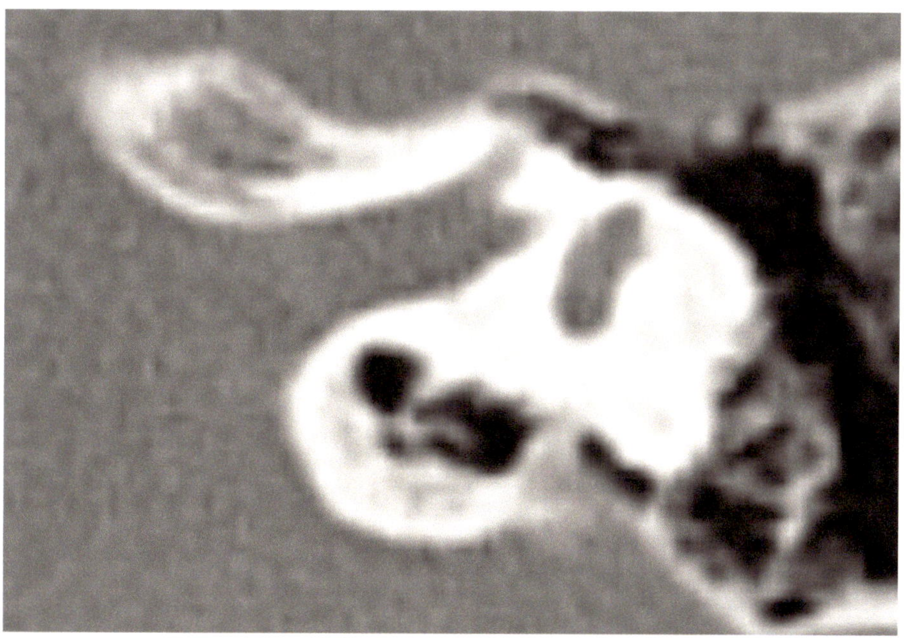

Fig. 12.4.4 The left lateral canal was ossified for a great part, in contrast to the cochlea on the same side, as shown here. MRI was definitely necessary to assess the patency of the cochlea.

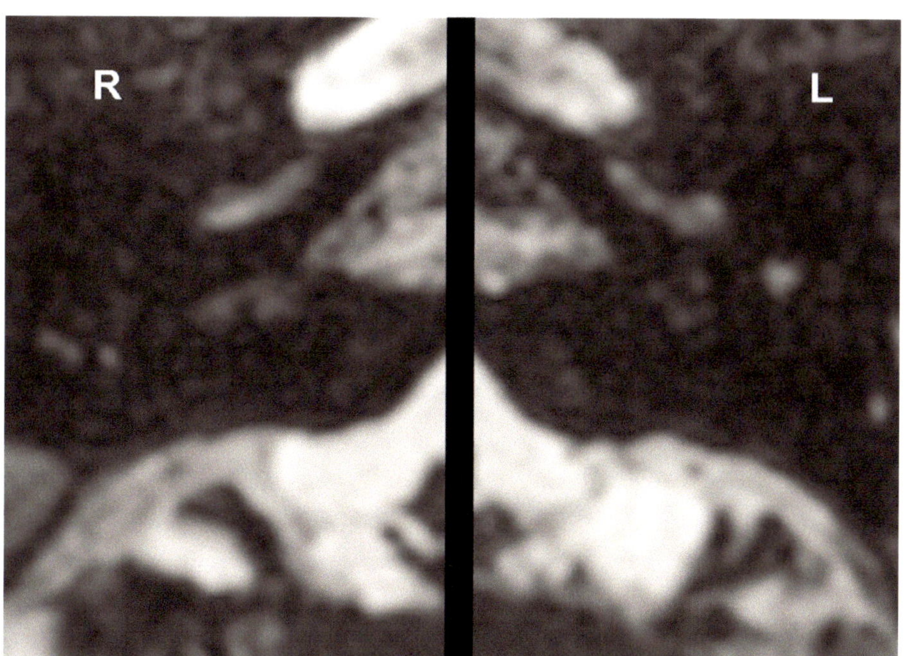

Fig. 12.4.5 MRI showed a somewhat similar pattern on both sides. The cochlea was hardly visible and a great deal of fibrosis was expected during implantation. These MR images and the time between the meningitis and the cochlear implantation, which was several months, gave us concerns about the accessibility of the cochlea.

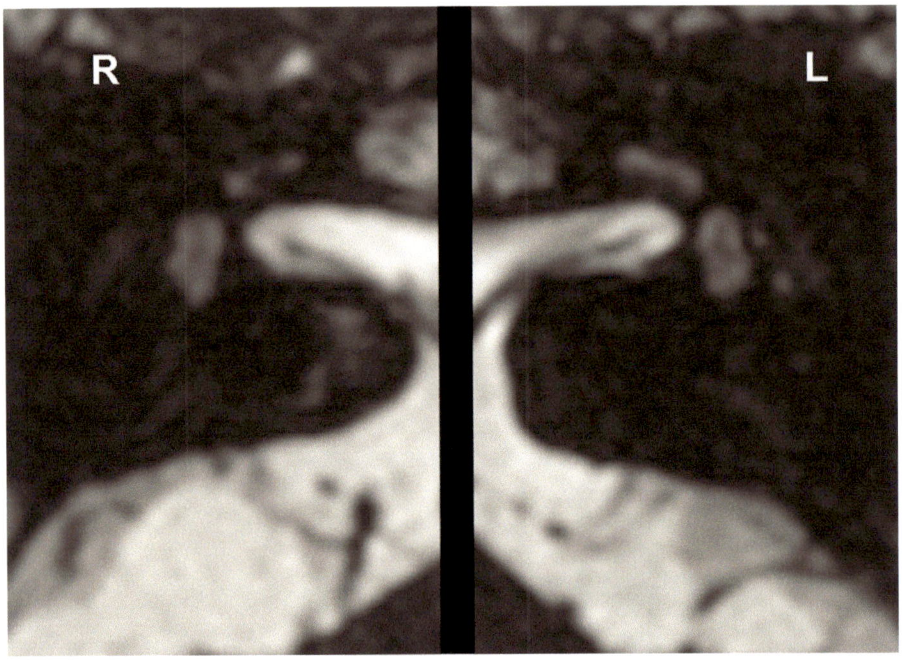

Fig. 12.4.6 Some fluid could still be seen in the vestibule and cochlea, as shown in these images, so an attempt was made to insert on both sides.

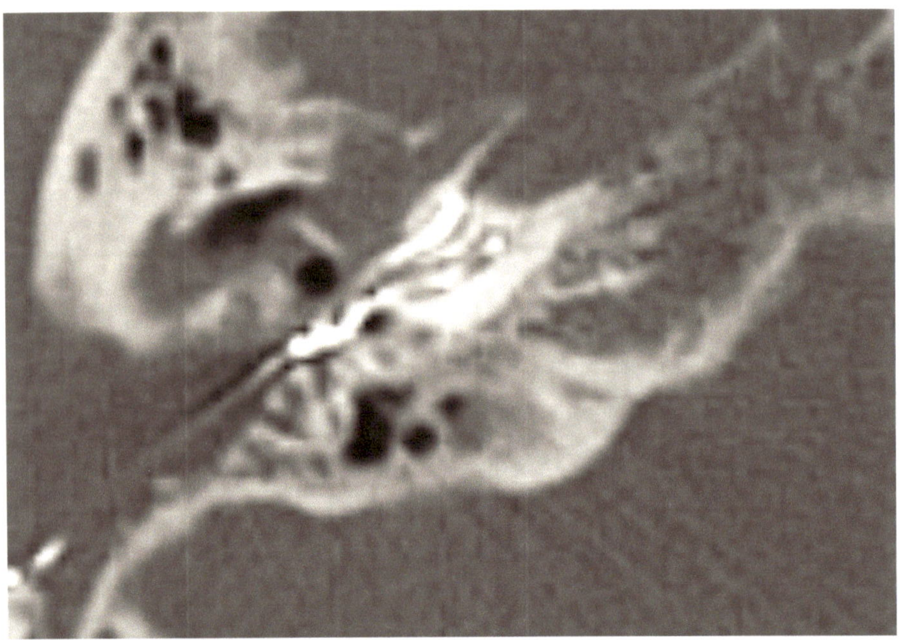

Fig. 12.4.7 During surgery the depth gauge (electrode dummy) was used to measure the possible depth of insertion. The basal turn was well accessible but at the first turn there was no way to push the electrode dummy further in. It was decided to use a double array in this case. The incus was removed and at the side of the cochleariform process the cochlea was opened with a second cochleostomy. CT of the right cochlea: postoperative parallel position of both electrode arrays.

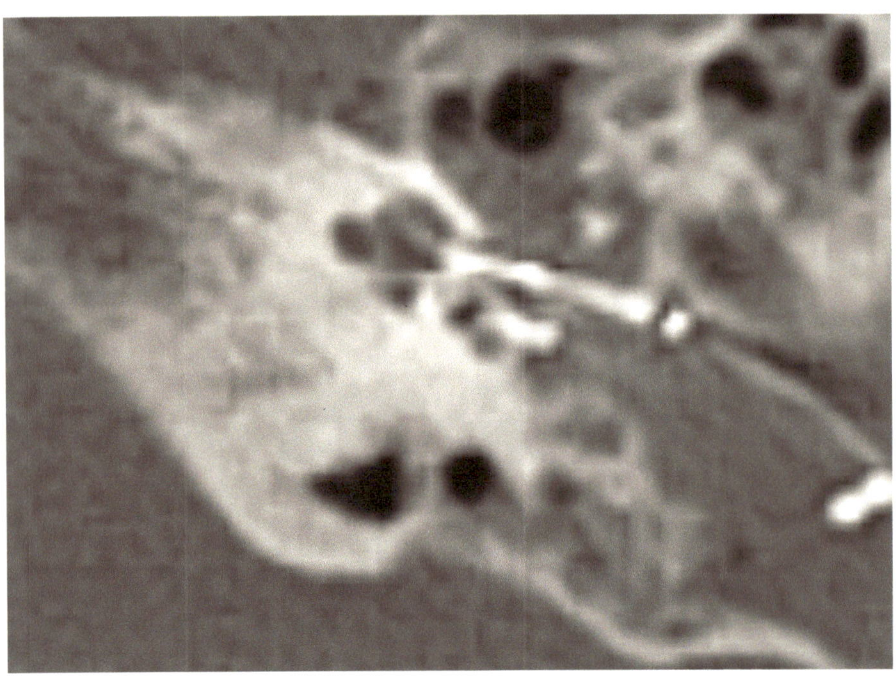

Fig. 12.4.8 On the left side also, despite the encouraging preoperative CT scan, the electrode array could not be inserted completely. Shown here is an image in which the alignment of the electrodes when entering the cochlea is well seen. This inability to completely insert the electrode in the cochlea, even though the preoperative CT shows a patent cochlea, demonstrates the superiority of MRI as means to assess cochlear accessibility.

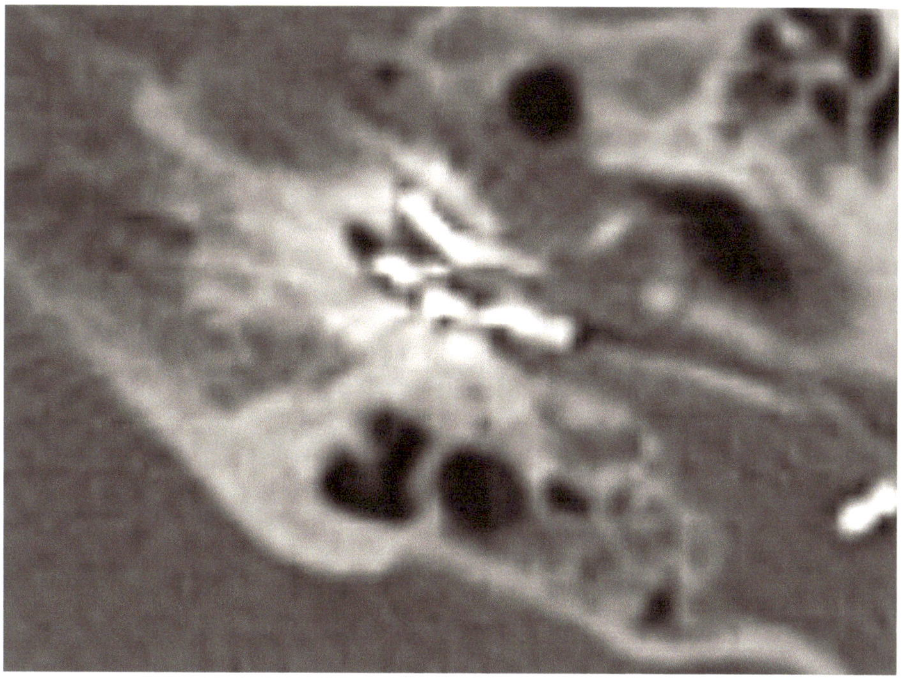

Fig. 12.4.9 In both cochleae we achieved a complete insertion of all four electrodes of the double array. The patient achieved some hearing improvement but it never reached speech understanding. Sound identification was the best outcome attainable.

Comment

Normal patency on a preoperative CT scan in a postmeningitis case does not ensure true cochlear patency. MRI is superior in the assessment of cochlear accessibility.

Case 12.5 Drill-out after CI Insertion Attempts (Fig. 12.5.1–Fig. 12.5.11)

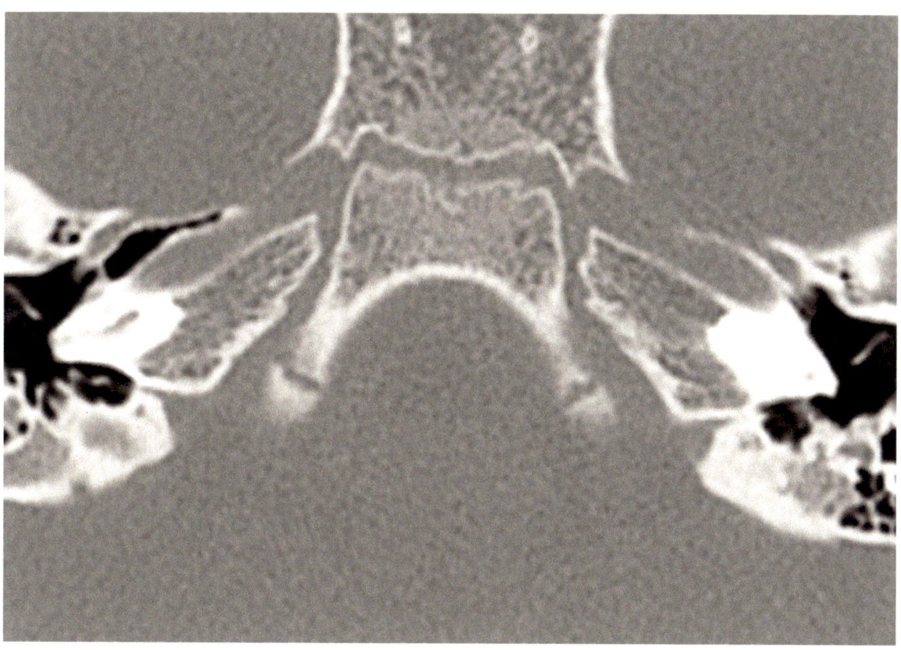

Fig. 12.5.1 This patient had been operated on three times in the referring hospital in an attempt to insert a CI. Because of the failure of this procedure the patient was referred to us to place an ABI. On CT we saw a complete obliteration of the left cochlea. The right cochlea showed a noncalcified portion in the anterior part of probably the scala vestibuli basal turn.

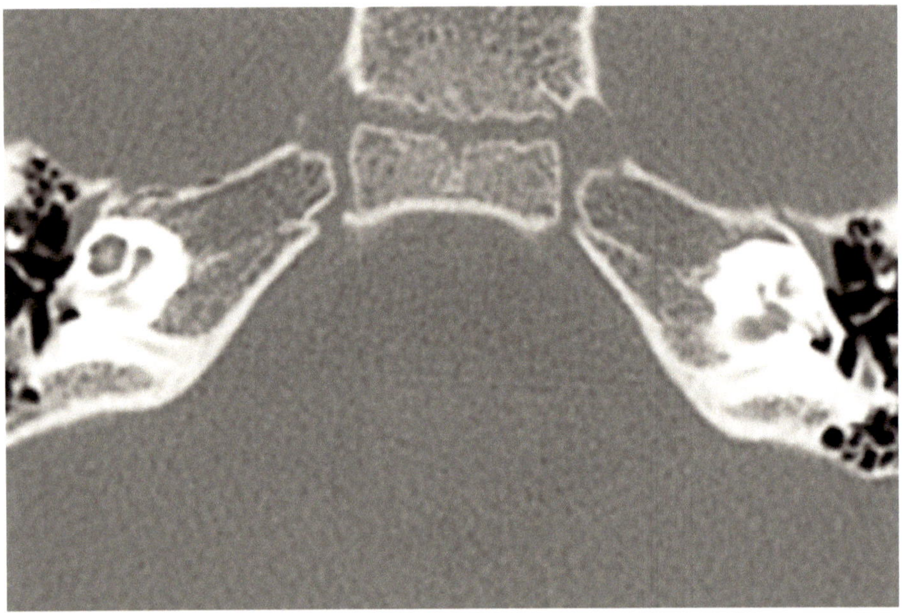

Fig. 12.5.2 The more superior part of the right cochlea showed a noncalcified middle and apical cochlea (this image and next). The left side is much worse. Diffuse calcification in the basal turn and more apically.

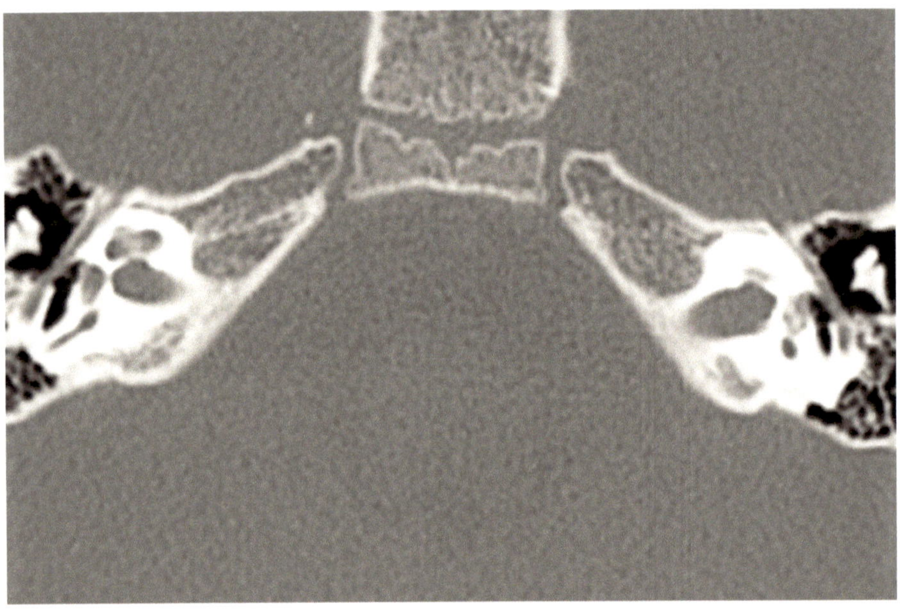

Fig. 12.5.3 The middle turn of the right cochlea is not calcified. MR imaging is still needed, though, to make sure that the lumen is noncalcified but also not obliterated. Obliteration is best seen on MRI.

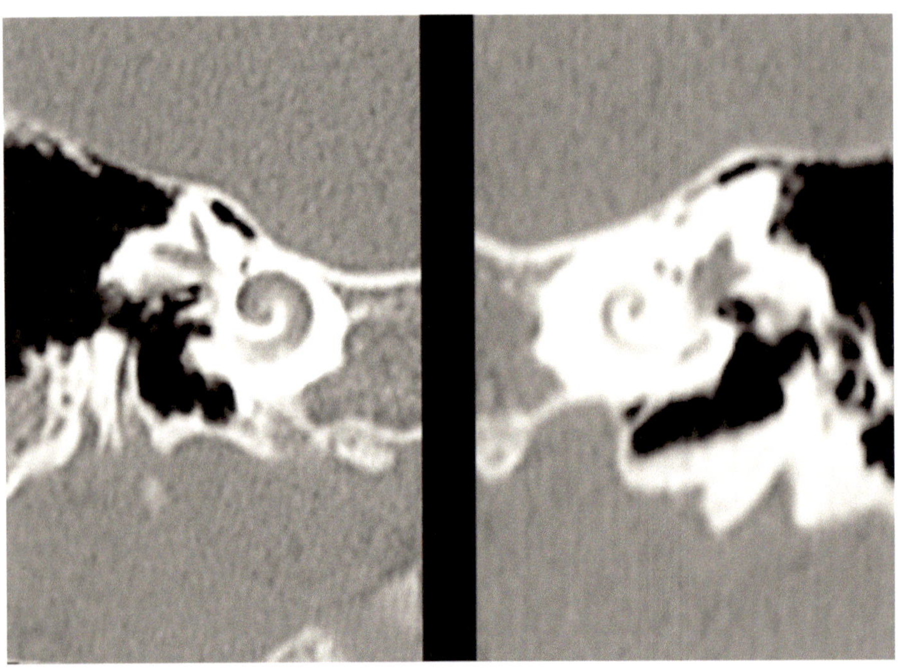

Fig. 12.5.4 Left and right cochleae in a coronal CT image with the axis of imaging in the basal turn plane. The left cochlea is almost completely calcified, whereas only the proximal part of the cochlea is calcified at the right side. The CT scan encouraged us to explore the possibility of a drill-out of the basal turn on the right side.

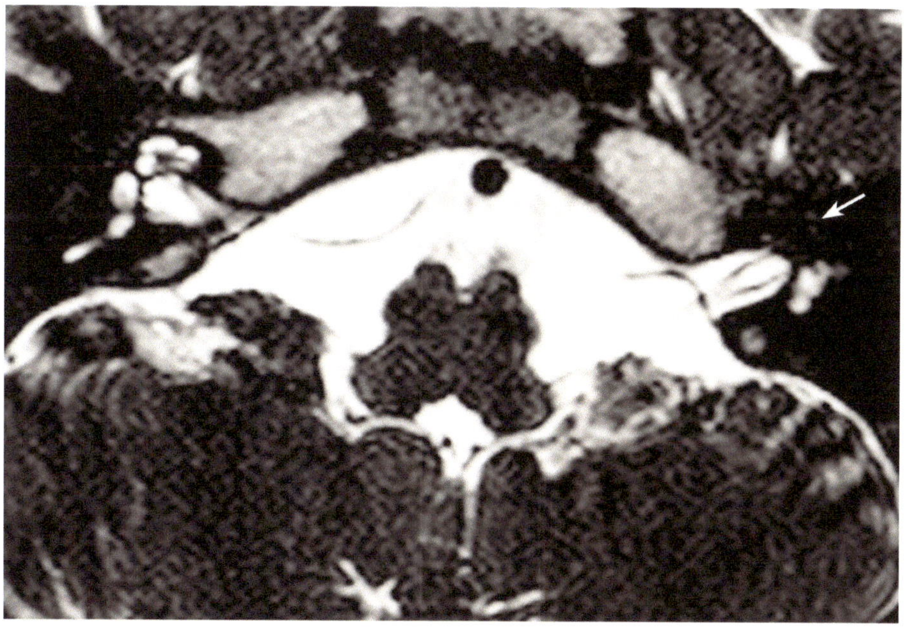

Fig. 12.5.5 MR image with total loss of fluid in the left cochlea (*arrow*) and a still partly open cochlea on the right side.

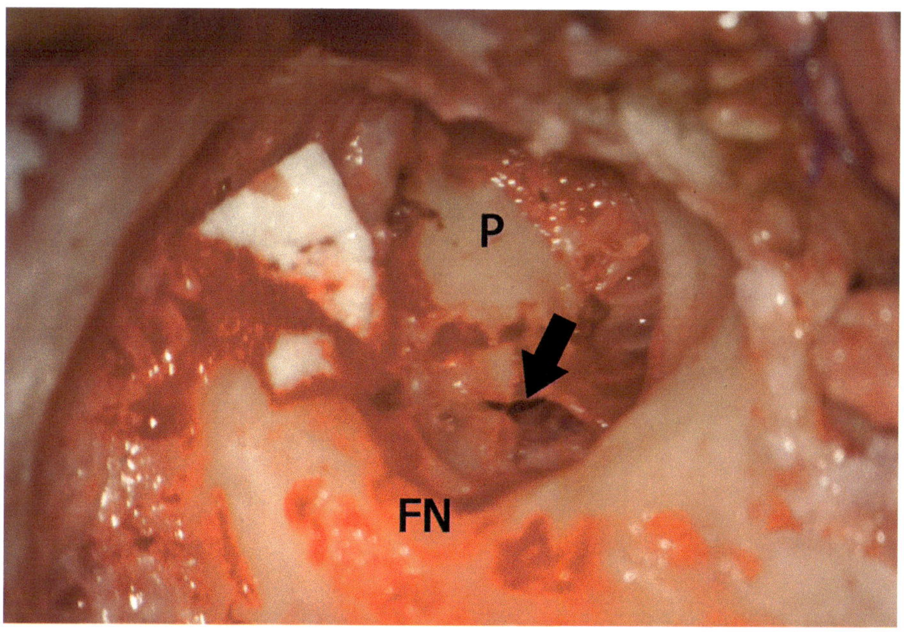

Fig. 12.5.6 The cochlear implant was attempted in a canal wall down procedure to give better exposure of the round window niche (*arrow*) and lessen risk in this drill-out procedure. FN, facial nerve; P, promontory.

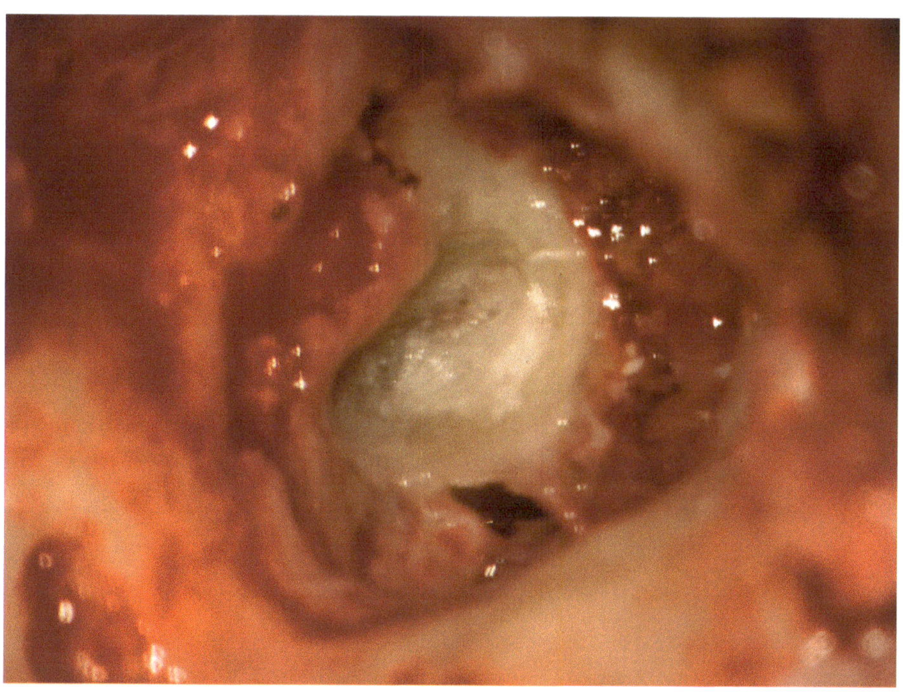

Fig. 12.5.7 The promontory was drilled to open the basal turn. No lumen was found.

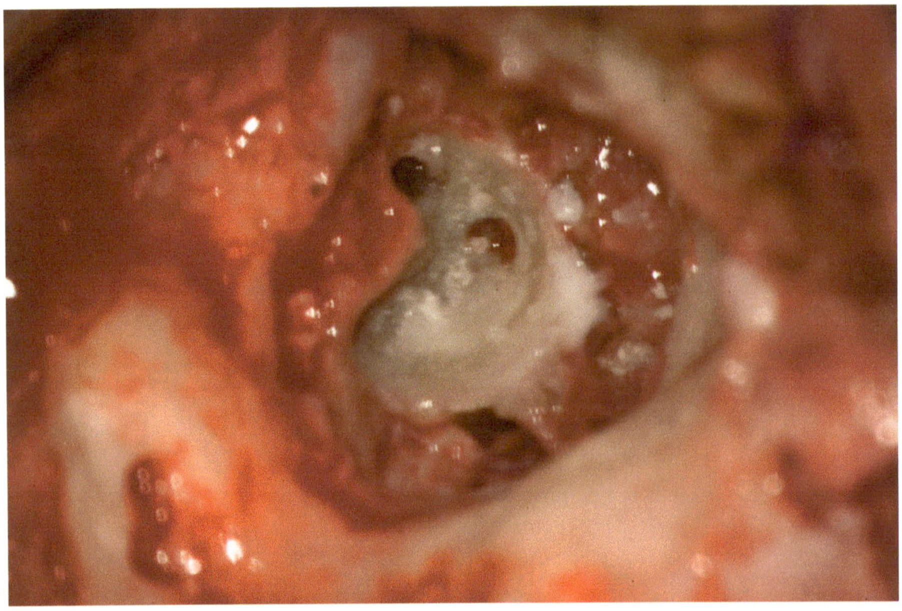

Fig. 12.5.8 As drilling proceeded more anteriorly, a small opening became visible.

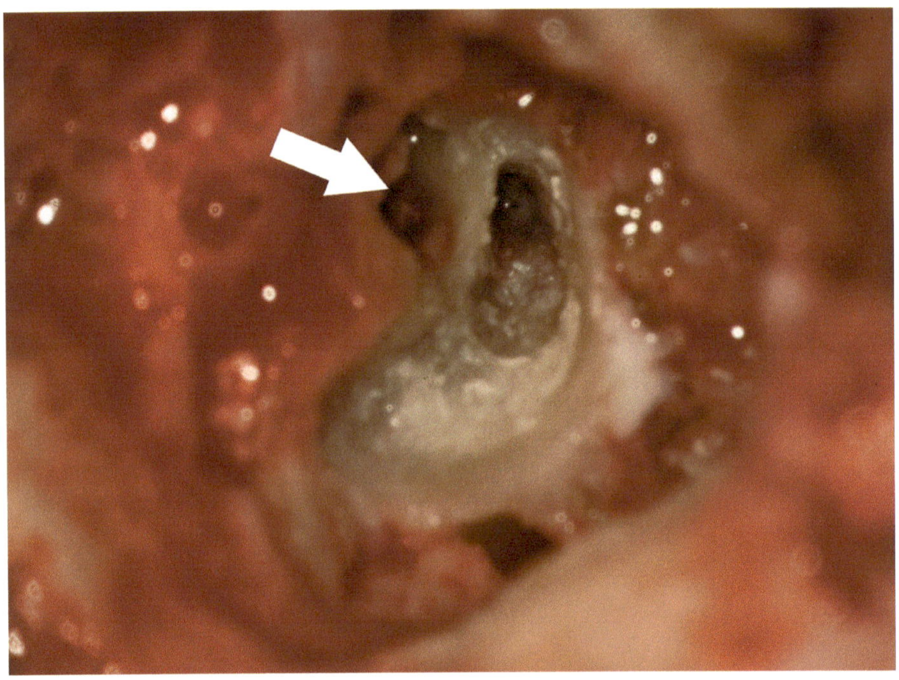

Fig. 12.5.9 The opening in the cochlea was slowly widened with a hook and small bur. The lumen found appeared to be a good opening of one of the scalae. The second turn was also opened during drilling (*arrow*).

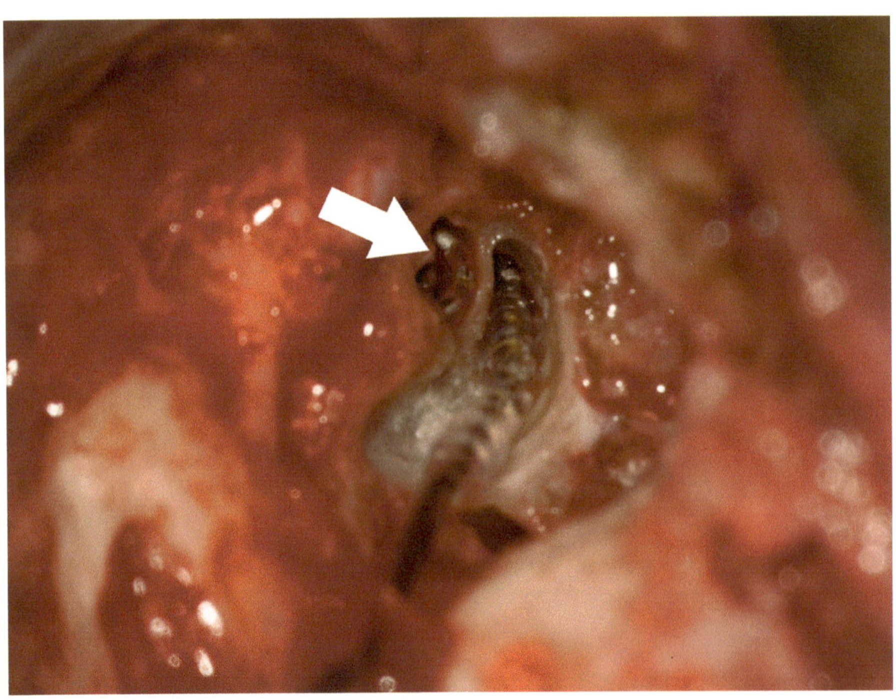

Fig. 12.5.10 The electrode array is inserted from the cochleostomy. The array in the second turn is also seen (*arrow*).

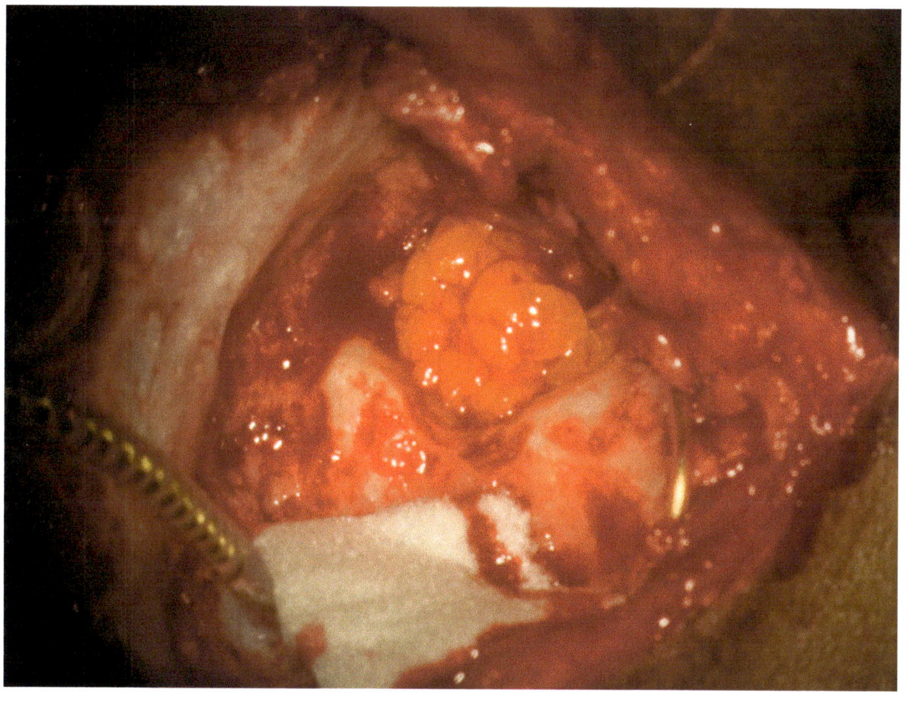

Fig. 12.5.11 At closure, the cochleostomy was securely packed with periosteal pieces and the complete cavity was closed off with abdominal fat.

Comment

MRI and CT will provide adequate information on the patency of the cochlear lumen. If a part of the basal turn is obliterated, experienced surgeons should attempt to perform a drill-out of the basal turn in a canal wall down approach.

Case 12.6 ABI after Cochlear Drill-out Attempt (Fig. 12.6.1–Fig. 12.6.12)

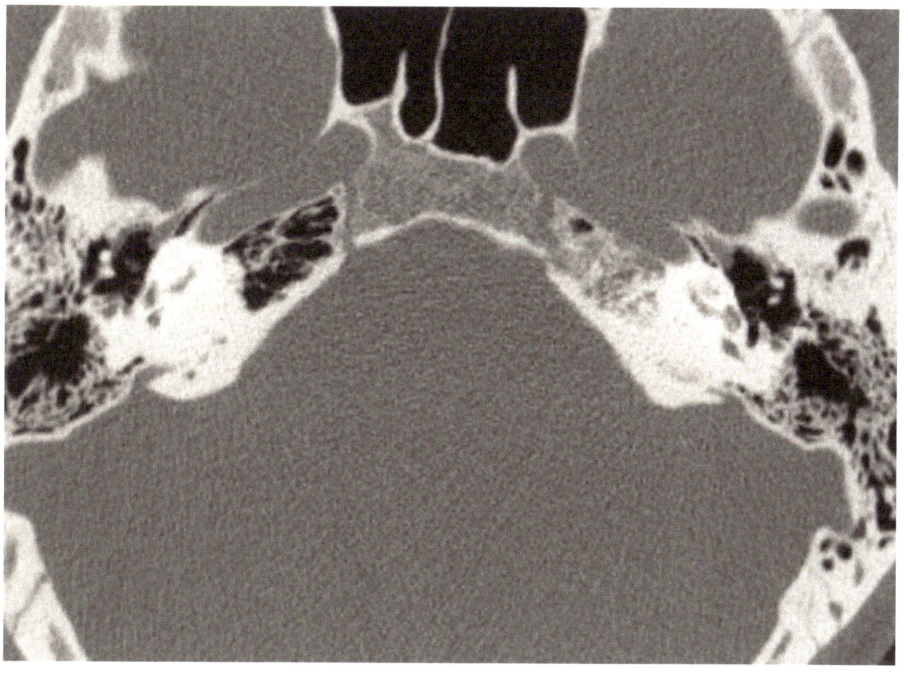

Fig. 12.6.1 In this postmeningitis case, both cochleae were obliterated. The patient had become deaf as a result of bacterial meningitis. Referral to our center took several months. On CT scan we saw a bilateral ossified cochlea with almost complete obliteration. This case was previously presented as a case report by Sanna et al in 2006.[33]

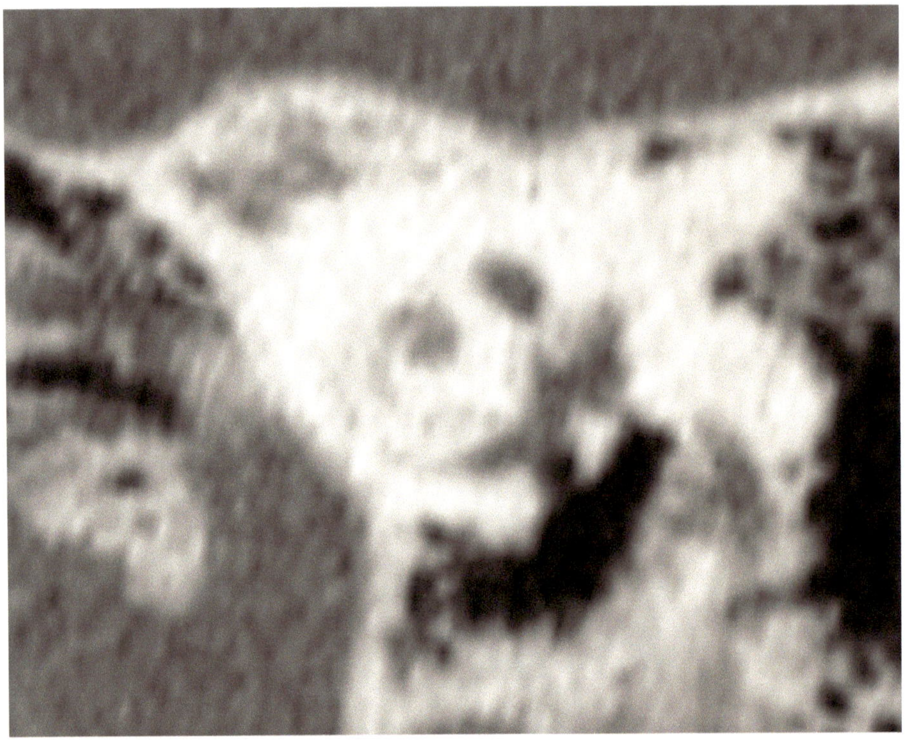

Fig. 12.6.2 Coronal imaging of both sides (here the left cochlea is shown) confirms the complete ossification of the cochlea.

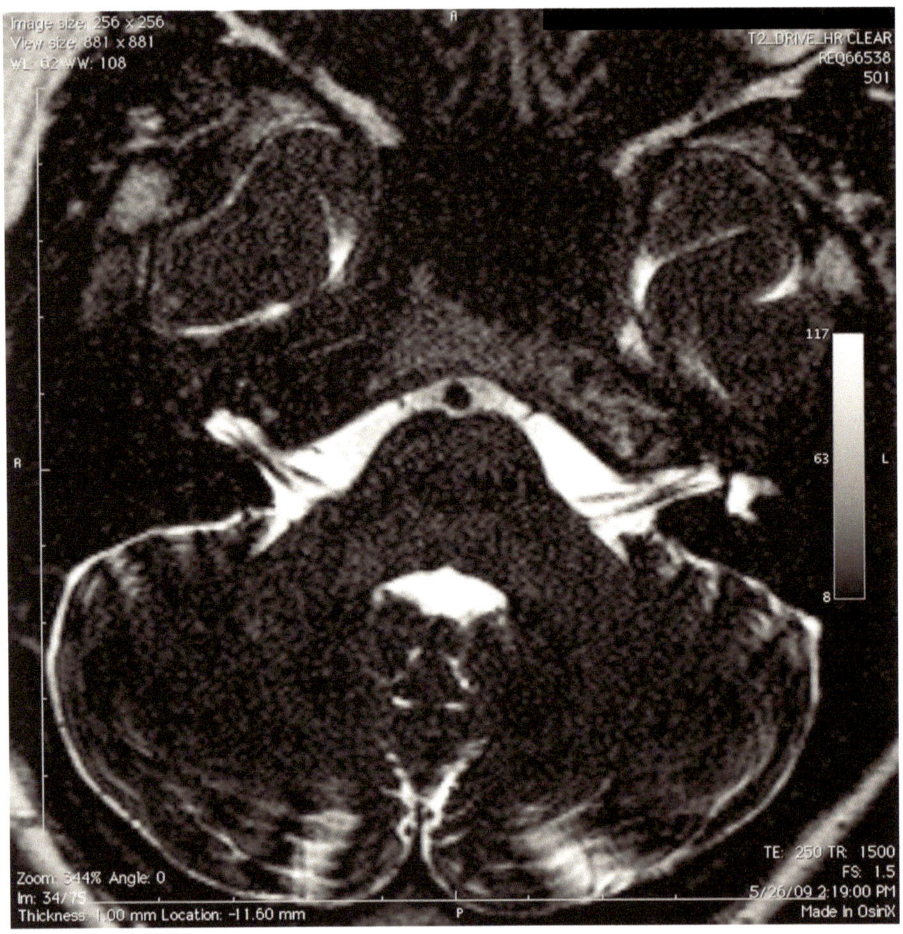

Fig. 12.6.3 The CISS MRI sequence shows two "black cochleae," with no intracochlear fluid visible. Complete obliteration of both cochleae.

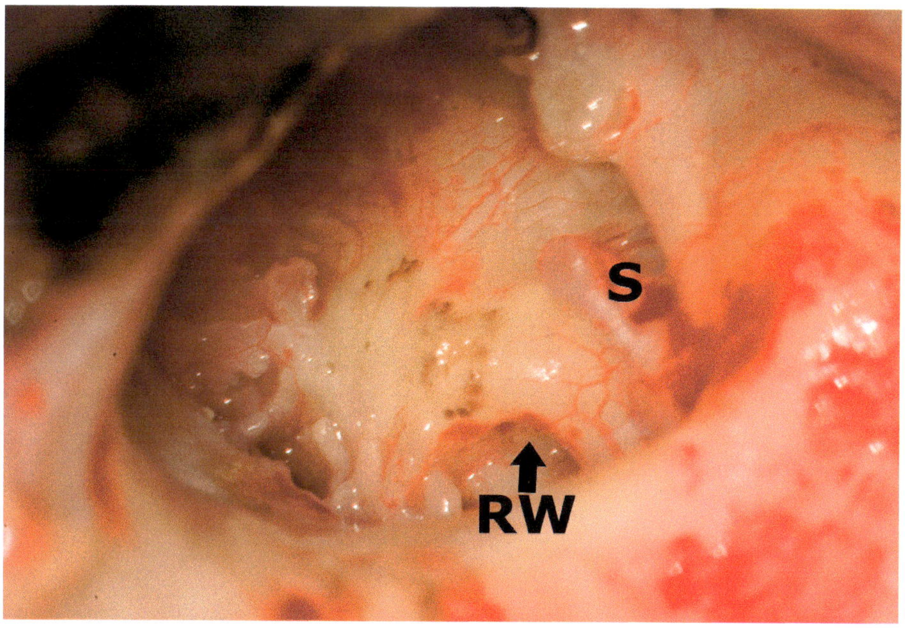

Fig. 12.6.4 The surgery was planned in a subtotal petrosectomy approach to the cochlea, to enable conversion in the same surgery to a translabyrinthine approach to the brainstem. In this intraoperative image of the left ear, the round window (RW) niche and the stapes (S) are seen.

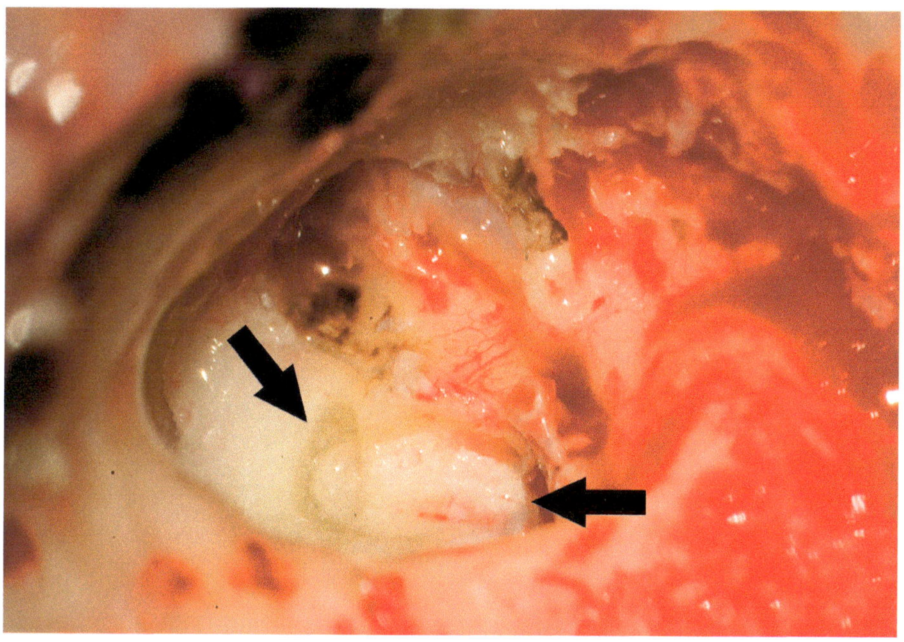

Fig. 12.6.5 The area where the basal turn lumen used to be is marked in this image (between the *arrows*). The drill-out procedure did not reveal any lumen of the cochlea. It was decided to proceed with the translabyrinthine approach for ABI placement.

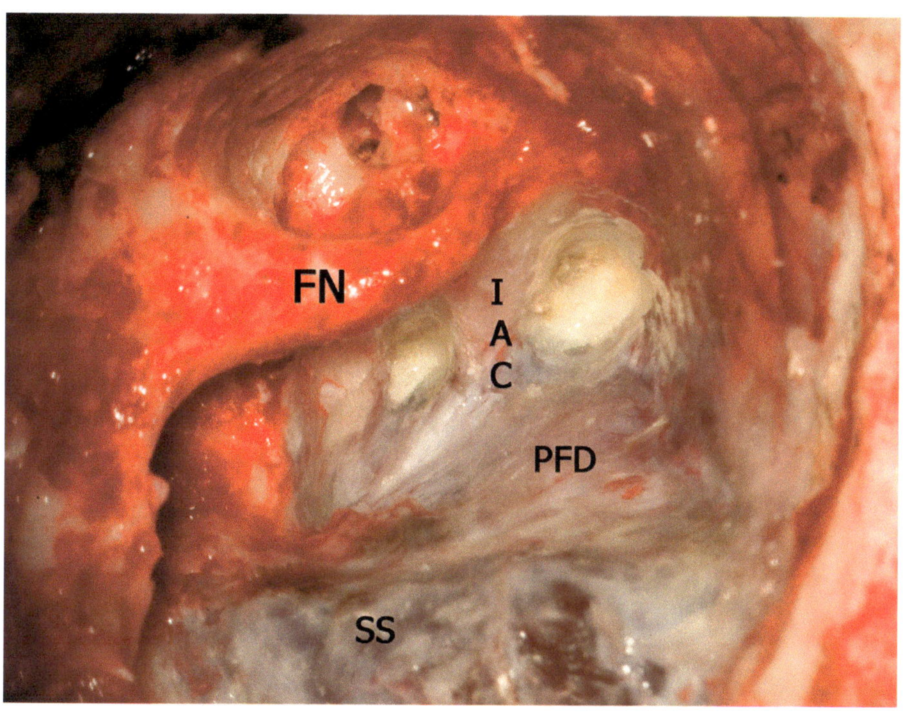

Fig. 12.6.6 The labyrinthectomy was performed using a wide approach with skeletonization of the posterior fossa dura (PFD), the sigmoid sinus (SS), the facial nerve (FN), and the internal acoustic canal (IAC). All mastoid cells are either removed or filled with bone wax to avoid CSF leakage. The eustachian tube will also be closed.

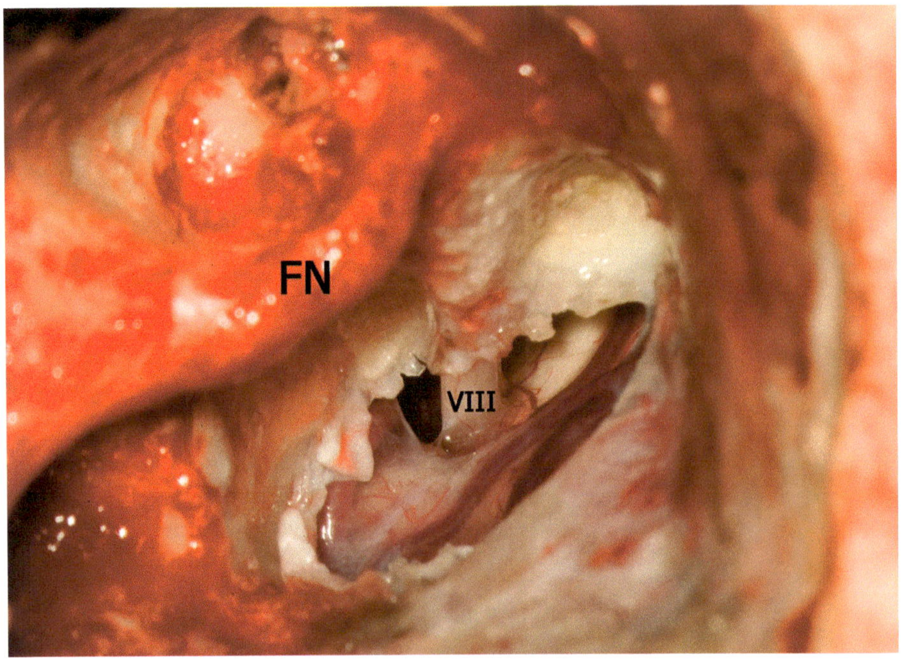

Fig. 12.6.7 The dura was opened toward the brainstem, leaving the fundus of the IAC covered with some bone. If access is inadequate, this bone can still be removed but its presence ensures protection of the facial and cochlear nerves. FN, facial nerve; VIII, vestibulocochlear nerve.

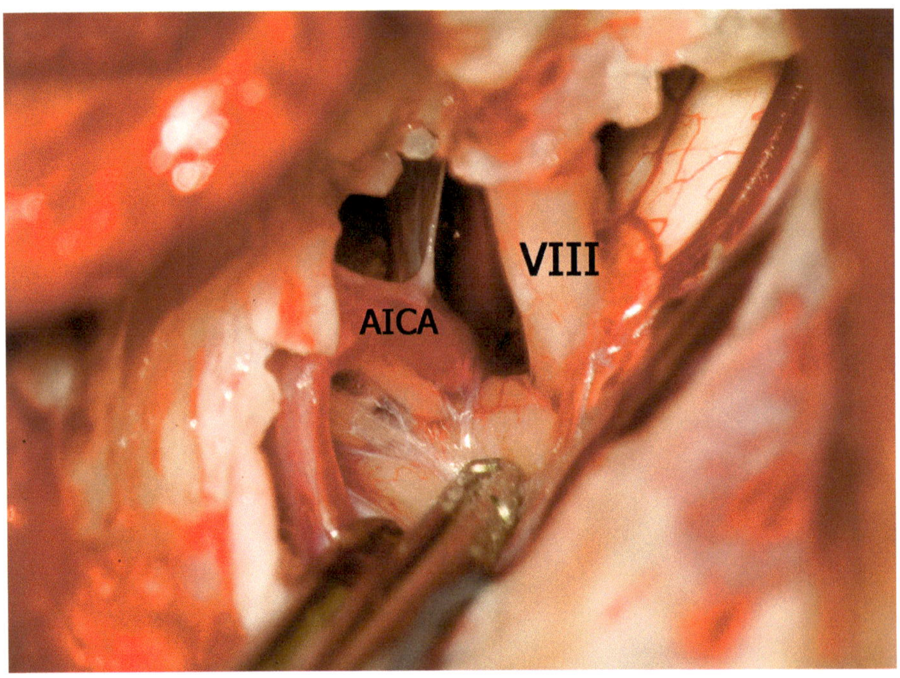

Fig. 12.6.8 At close-up view: with gentle pressure the foramen of Luschka is identified. Also the anterior inferior cerebellar artery (AICA) is well visible just inferior of the suction tube. VIII, vestibulocochlear nerve.

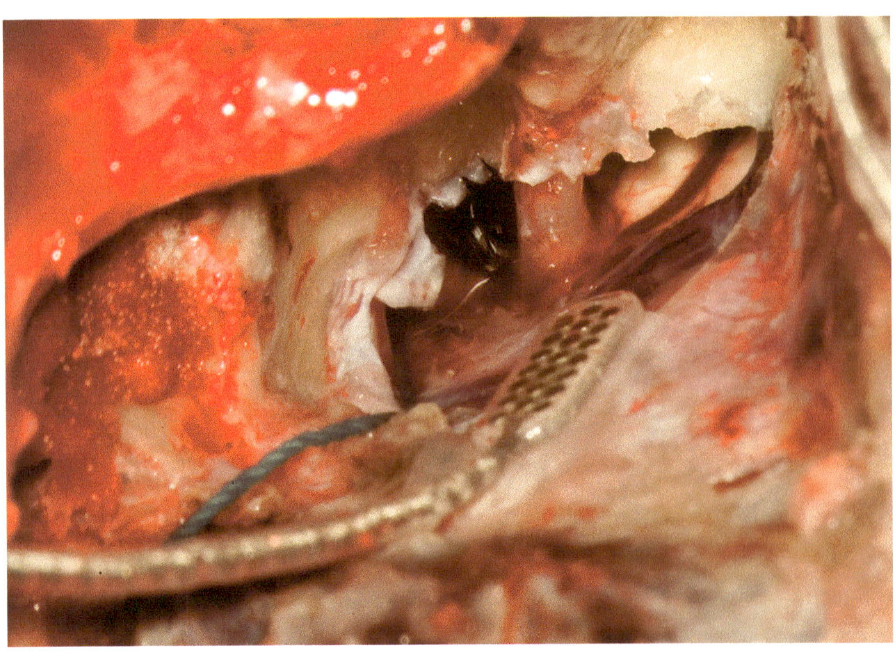

Fig. 12.6.9 The ABI is inserted in the cerebellopontine angle just before placement into the recess of the fourth ventricle.

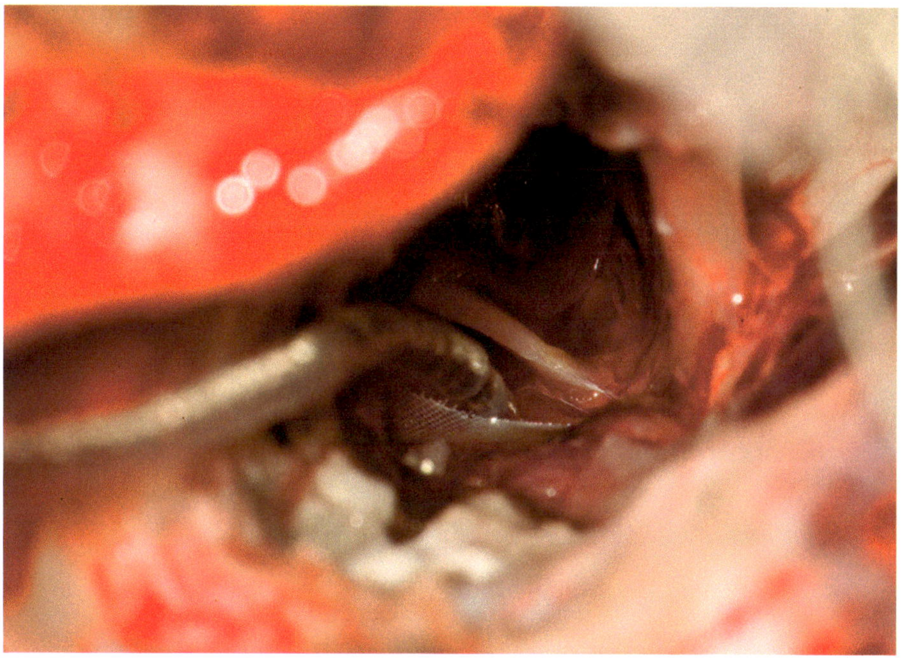

Fig. 12.6.10 The ABI electrode array is gently positioned.

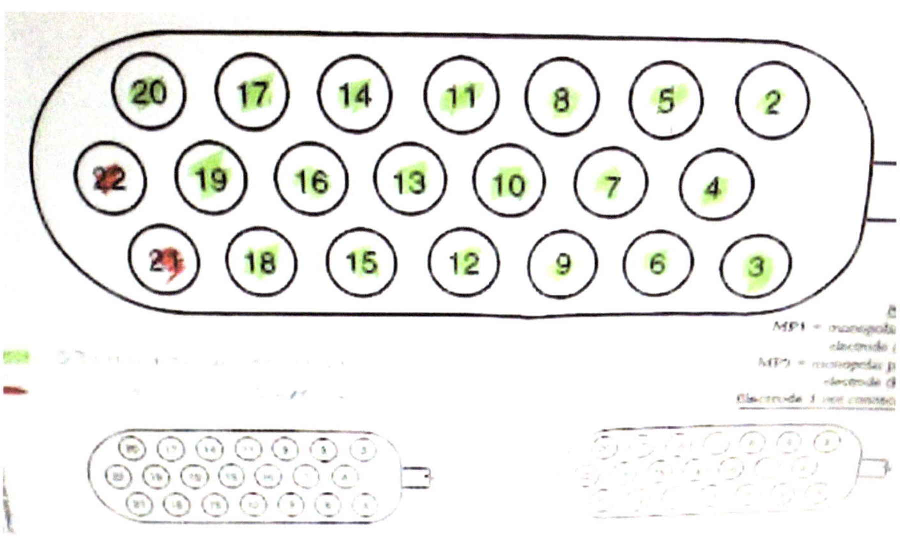

Fig. 12.6.11 Intraoperative EABR measurements are done to optimize and check proper positioning. Lack of auditory stimulation of two electrodes is seen in this patient. A good result with 19 electrodes stimulating the auditory cortex.

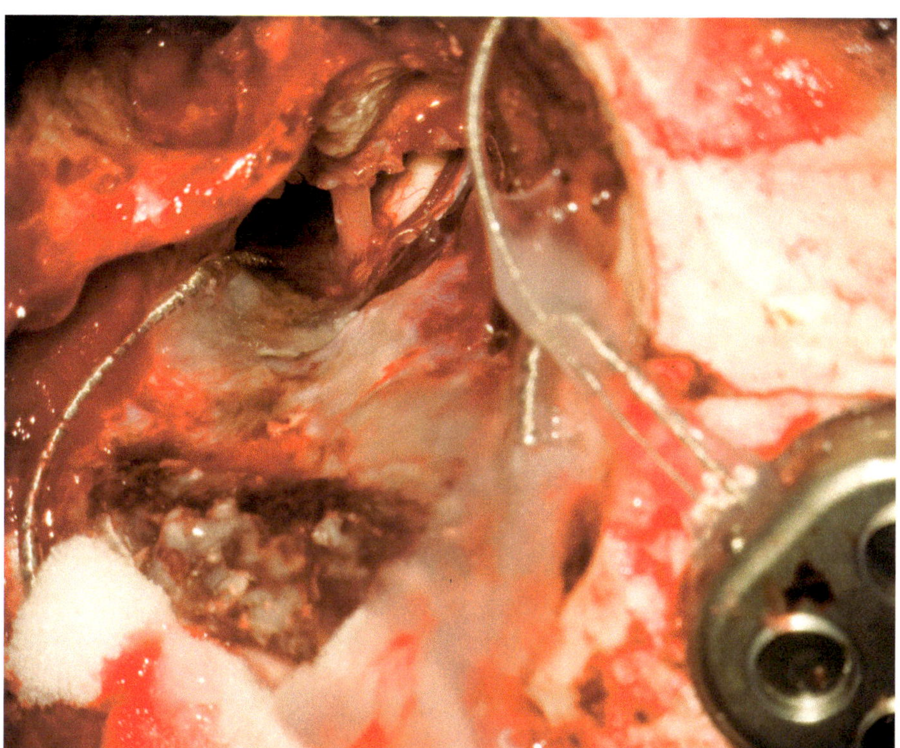

Fig. 12.6.12 Once the ABI electrode array is well positioned, the lead can be glued and reinforced with Gelfoam. Long strips of fat are then used to ensure a corklike closure of the CPA, without any sutures of the dura. This patient had a very good result from her ABI and is able to talk on the telephone with known speakers or relatives.

Comment

A drill-out CI implantation attempt and ABI placement in postmeningitis cases can be done in a single procedure. The subtotal petrosectomy is extended into a translabyrinthine approach.

References

1. Tinling SP, Colton J, Brodie HA. Location and timing of initial osteoid deposition in postmeningitic labyrinthitis ossificans determined by multiple fluorescent labels. Laryngoscope 2004;114(4):675–680
2. Aschendorff A, Klenzner T, Laszig R. Deafness after bacterial meningitis: an emergency for early imaging and cochlear implant surgery. Otolaryngol Head Neck Surg 2005;133(6):995–996
3. Rotteveel LJC, Snik AFM, Vermeulen AM, Mylanus EAM. Three-year follow-up of children with postmeningitic deafness and partial cochlear implant insertion. Clin Otolaryngol 2005;30(3):242–248
4. Rauch SD, Herrmann BS, Davis LA, Nadol JB Jr. Nucleus 22 cochlear implantation results in postmeningitic deafness. Laryngoscope 1997;107(12 Pt 1):1606–1609
5. El-Kashlan HK, Ashbaugh C, Zwolan T, Telian SA. Cochlear implantation in prelingually deaf children with ossified cochleae. Otol Neurotol 2003;24(4):596–600
6. Fortnum H, Davis A. Hearing impairment in children after bacterial meningitis: incidence and resource implications. Br J Audiol 1993;27(1):43–52
7. Durisin M, Arnoldner C, Stöver T, Lenarz T, Lesinski-Schiedat A. Audiological performance in cochlear implanted patients deafened by meningitis depending on duration of deafness. Eur Arch Otorhinolaryngol 2008;265(4):381–388
8. Dodge PR, Davis H, Feigin RD, et al. Prospective evaluation of hearing impairment as a sequela of acute bacterial meningitis. N Engl J Med 1984;311(14):869–874
9. Nadol JB Jr, Hsu WC. Histopathologic correlation of spiral ganglion cell count and new bone formation in the cochlea following meningogenic labyrinthitis and deafness. Ann Otol Rhinol Laryngol 1991;100(9 Pt 1):712–716
10. Wellman MB, Sommer DD, McKenna J. Sensorineural hearing loss in postmeningitic children. Otol Neurotol 2003;24(6):907–912
11. Koomen I, Grobbee DE, Roord JJ, Donders R, Jennekens-Schinkel A, van Furth AM. Hearing loss at school age in survivors of bacterial meningitis: assessment, incidence, and prediction. Pediatrics 2003;112(5):1049–1053
12. Riordan A, Thomson A, Hodgson J, Hart A. Children who are seen but not referred: hearing assessment after bacterial meningitis. Br J Audiol 1993;27(6):375–377
13. Davis JM, Elfenbein J, Schum R, Bentler RA. Effects of mild and moderate hearing impairments on language, educational, and psychosocial behavior of children. J Speech Hear Disord 1986;51(1):53–62
14. Merkus P, Free RH, Mylanus EAM, et al; 4th Consensus in Auditory Implants Meeting. Dutch Cochlear Implant Group (CI-ON) consensus protocol on postmeningitis hearing evaluation and treatment. Otol Neurotol 2010;31(8):1281–1286
15. Beijen J, Casselman J, Joosten F, et al. Magnetic resonance imaging in patients with meningitis induced hearing loss. Eur Arch Otorhinolaryngol 2009;266(8):1229–1236
16. Richardson MP, Williamson TJ, Reid A, Tarlow MJ, Rudd PT. Otoacoustic Emissions as a Screening Test for Hearing Impairment in Children Recovering From Acute Bacterial Meningitis. Pediatrics 1998;102:1364–1368
17. Gans de J, Beek van de D. European Dexamethasone in Adulthood Bacterial Meningitis Study Investigators. Dexamethasone in adults with bacterial meningitis. N Engl J Med 2002;347(20):1549–1556
18. van de Beek D, de Gans J, McIntyre P, Prasad K. Corticosteroids for acute bacterial meningitis. Cochrane Database Syst Rev 2007;(1):CD004405
19. Odio CM, Faingezicht I, Paris M, et al. The beneficial effects of early dexamethasone administration m infants and children with bacterial meningitis. N Engl J Med 1991;324:1525–1531
20. Schaad UB, Lips U, Gnehm HE, Blumberg A, Heinzer I, Wedgwood J. Dexamethasone therapy for bacterial meningitis in children. Swiss Meningitis Study Group. Lancet 1993;342(8869):457–461
21. McIntyre PB, Berkey CS, King SM, et al. Dexamethasone as adjunctive therapy in bacterial meningitis. A meta-analysis of randomized clinical trials since 1988. JAMA 1997;278:925–931
22. Nabili V, Brodie HA, Neverov NI, Tinling SP. Chronology of labyrinthitis ossificans induced by Streptococcus pneumoniae meningitis. Laryngoscope 1999;109(6):931–935
23. van Loon MC, Hensen EF, de Foer B, Smit CF, Witte B, Merkus P. Magnetic resonance imaging in the evaluation of patients with sensorineural hearing loss caused by meningitis: implications for cochlear implantation. Otol Neurotol 2013;34(5):845–854
24. Merkus P, van Loon MC, Hensen EF. Cochlear implantation in young post-meningitis patients: decision making based on hearing evaluation and imaging. Audiol Neurootol 2013;18(Suppl 1):19–23
25. Offeciers E, Morera C, Müller J, Huarte A, Shallop J, Cavallé L. International consensus on bilateral cochlear implants and bimodal stimulation. Acta Otolaryngol 2005;125(9):918–919
26. Cosetti M, Roland JT Jr. Cochlear implantation in the very young child: issues unique to the under-1 population. Trends Amplif 2010;14(1):46–57
27. Marttila TI, Karikoski JO. Comparison between audiometric and ABR thresholds in children. Contradictory findings. Eur Arch Otorhinolaryngol 2006;263(5):399–403
28. Leigh J, Dettman S, Dowell R, Sarant J. Evidence-based approach for making cochlear implant recommendations for infants with residual hearing. Ear Hear 2011;32(3):313–322
29. Roukema BY, Van Loon MC, Smits C, et al. Cochlear implantation after bacterial meningitis in infants younger than 9 months. Int J Otolaryngol 2011;2011:845879
30. Battersby EF. Paediatric anaesthesia. In Adams DA, Cinnamond MJ, eds. Scott-Brown's Otolaryngology. Oxford: Butterworth-Heinemann; 1997:6–24
31. Cross KW, Hey EN, Kennaird DL, Lewis SR, Urich H. Lack of temperature control in infants with abnormalities of central nervous system. Arch Dis Child 1971;46(248):437–443
32. Hannallah RS. Who benefits when parents are present during anaesthesia induction in their children? Can J Anaesth 1994;41(4):271–275
33. Sanna M, Khrais T, Guida M, Falcioni M. Auditory brainstem implant in a child with severely ossified cochlea. Laryngoscope 2006;116(9):1700–1703

Further Reading

Kopelovich JC, Germiller JA, Laury AM, Shah SS, Pollock AN. Early prediction of postmeningitic hearing loss in children using magnetic resonance imaging. Arch Otolaryngol Head Neck Surg 2011;137(5):441–447

Yoon PJ. Pediatric cochlear implantation. Curr Opin Pediatr 2011;23(3):346–350

13 Auditory Implantation in Otosclerosis Patients

13.1 Otosclerosis

Otosclerosis is a process of bone resorption of the petrous bone (otospongiosis) followed by replacement with thick, irregular, sclerotic bone (otosclerosis) often leading to hearing loss. The most commonly affected location is around the oval window, which can result in conductive hearing loss due to stapes footplate fixation (fenestral otosclerosis). In ~10% of patients, otosclerotic foci will also affect the otic capsule (retrofenestral otosclerosis), resulting in cochlear otosclerosis accompanied by sensorineural hearing loss.[1] Next to the radiologic diagnosis, there exists a functional diagnosis for otosclerosis with severe mixed hearing loss called far advanced otosclerosis (FAO). FAO was first described by House and Sheehy[2] as an air conduction threshold of at least 85 dB and an unmeasurable bone conduction threshold (due to the limitations of audiometers at that time). Nowadays, in the era of cochlear implantation, it is more likely that speech discrimination scores will be used instead of pure tone thresholds. Hence, the term FAO is no longer applicable and in this chapter we use the term *advanced otosclerosis* when referring to patients with sensorineural hearing loss and diminished (<100%) speech discrimination scores. Advanced otosclerosis is a purely audiologically based term in contrast to fenestral and retrofenestral otosclerosis (explained below).

13.2 CT Classification in Otosclerosis

High-resolution computed tomography (HRCT) scanning can reveal subtle bone formations and demineralization of the cochlea. It is therefore considered to be the imaging technique of choice for the diagnosis of otosclerosis. HRCT may predict additional difficulties during surgery, as it can detect subtle otosclerotic foci in and around the cochlea. For instance, the necessity for extra drilling to achieve successful electrode insertion is related to the extent of fenestral involvement and/or narrowing of the basal turn,[3–5] both visible on HRCT.

In radiologic terms, otosclerosis can be divided into *fenestral otosclerosis* (demineralization of the bone adjacent to the oval window) and *retrofenestral otosclerosis* (demineralization of the bone around the cochlea).

Different grading systems (Rotteveel[1] and Symons and Fanning[5]) are available for the classification of otosclerosis (**Fig. 13.1**). In general, they are based on the location of the otosclerotic lesions: purely fenestral (grade 1), patchy retrofenestral (grade 2), and diffuse confluent retrofenestral involvement (grade 3).[1,5–7]

Difficulties in electrode insertion tend to be associated with cochlear involvement on CT (grades 2 and 3), even though no statistical significance was found.[1,6] The severity of otosclerosis on CT is also associated with the risk of postoperative facial nerve stimulation: patients with a higher CT classification are significantly more likely to develop facial nerve stimulation.[1,5,6]

13.3 Decision Making in Otosclerosis

Unfortunately, there are no standard guidelines regarding the rehabilitation of advanced otosclerosis. In advanced otosclerosis three treatment options can be proposed to the patient: (1) no intervention and continuation of the use of hearing aids; (2) stapedotomy and hearing aid use; or (3) the placement of a cochlear implant (CI). In some patients with advanced otosclerosis the decision can be difficult because of two factors: first, with mixed hearing loss it is hard to predict the success rate of stapedotomy, especially if compared with cochlear implantation as an alternative intervention. Second, extensive imminent otosclerotic foci around the otic capsule can lead to surgical complications during implantation.[1,8,9]

As well as the role of the success rate in the decision, each intervention has specific advantages and disadvantages. Stapedotomy is a relatively simple, safe, and low-cost procedure that can accomplish very good results. However, the results of stapedotomy in severe mixed hearing loss are unpredictable and variable because stapedotomy is not applicable for treatment of the sensorineural component of hearing loss.[10,11] The Weber test can be of help in deciding the best side for stapedotomy, as it will indicate the ear with the better bone conduction and the more severe air–bone gap. One has to be aware that in case of a calcified round window the success of the stapedotomy might be disappointing. Moreover, a feared complication of stapedotomy is an increase of sensorineural hearing loss, which in advanced otosclerosis could result in a functionally deaf ear. Cochlear implantation has yielded excellent results and seems to be a good treatment for patients with advanced otosclerosis, provided that the electrode can be inserted.[3,12,13] On the debit side, it is an expensive and more complex procedure that requires experienced surgeons especially because otospongiosis and otosclerosis can cause difficulties during implantation. Furthermore, programming of the CI can be challenging since the progression of otosclerosis can cause postoperative impairment in performance of the CI.[14]

A treatment algorithm is presented in **Fig. 13.2.** Patients are divided into three main groups using standard speech audiometry, as explained below.

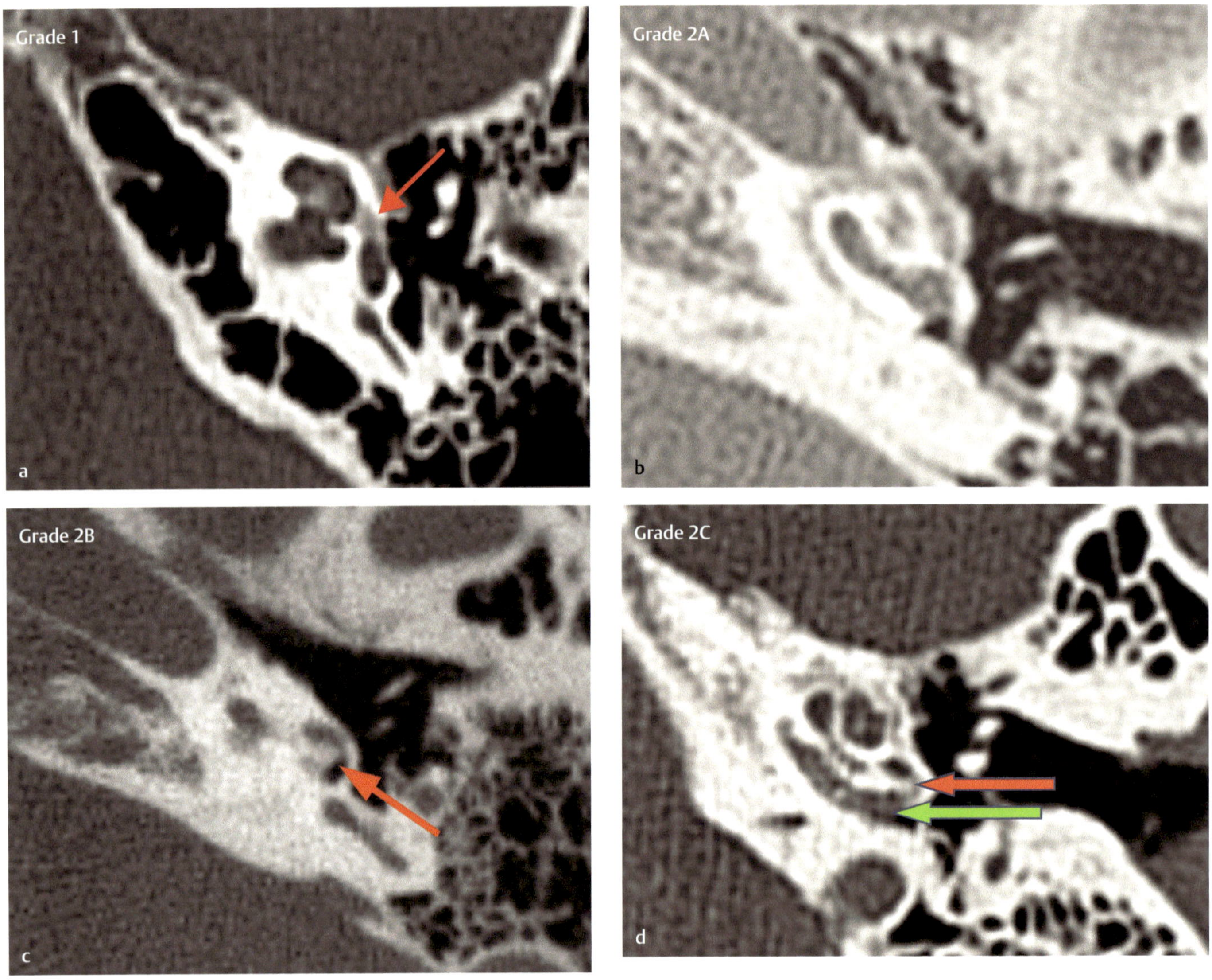

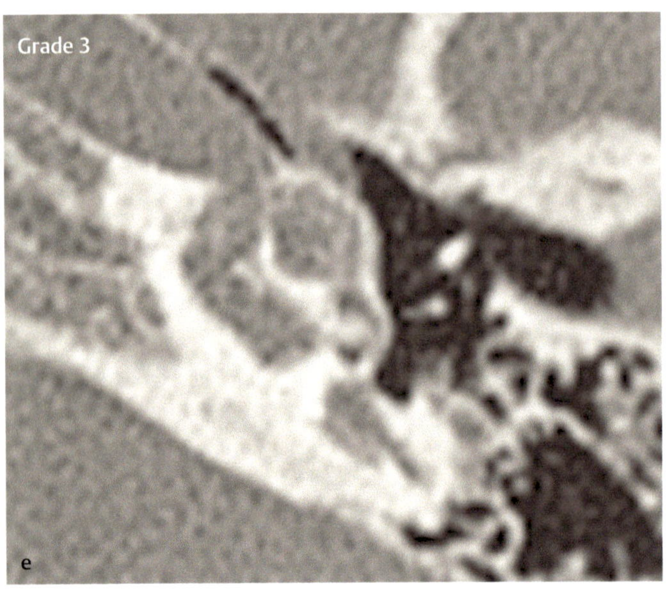

Fig. 13.1a–d Grading of otosclerosis on computed tomography images (according to Rotteveel et al[1]). Axial CT scan of the petrous bone in patients with otosclerosis.

- **a** Grade 1: Fenestral involvement, otospongiotic lesion on the anterior border of the vestibulum (fissura ante fenestram) (*red arrow*).
- **b** Grade 2A: Retrofenestral otosclerosis: the double ring effect. Also described as "halo sign" or the "ring of Valvasori."
- **c** Grade 2B: The basal turn is calcified within the scala tympani (*red arrow*), which makes it grade 2B.
- **d** Grade 2C: The ossification of the basal turn is visible (*green arrow*), but also the double ring around the cochlea (*red arrow*). This situation has an increased risk of a false route of insertion. The narrow and mostly white round window membrane, next to a new (but false) lumen in the same direction as the basal turn. See Case 13.6 at the end of this chapter.
- **e** Grade 3: Diffuse confluent cochlear involvement with an unrecognizable cochlea.

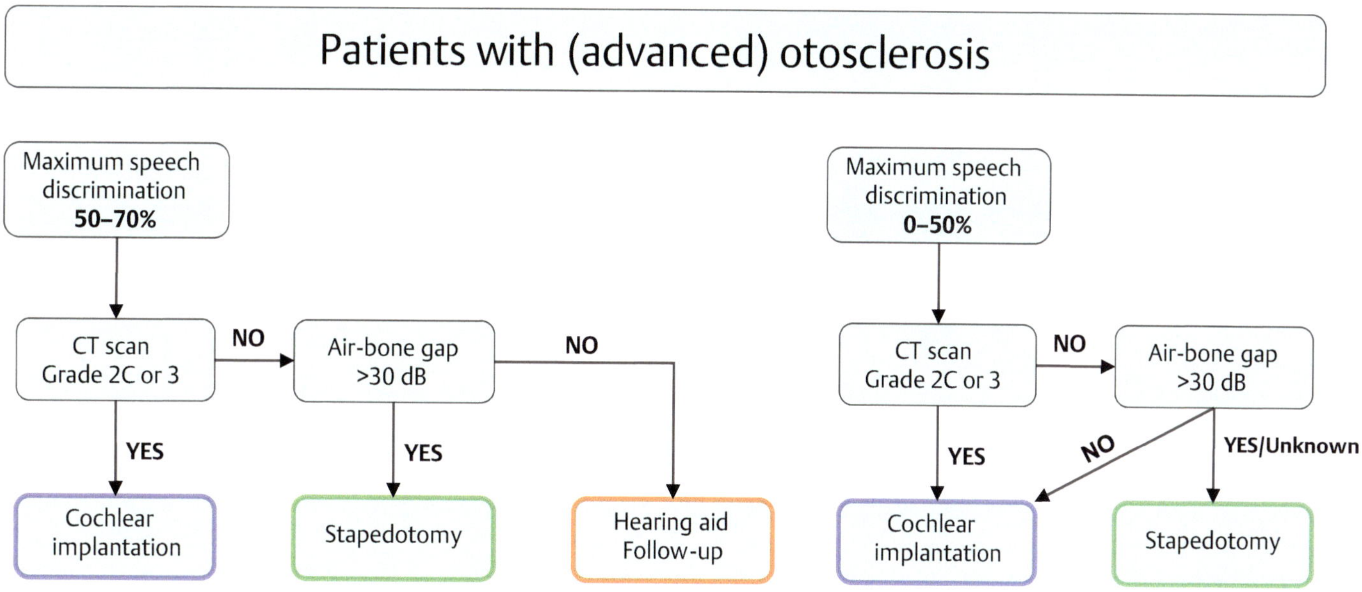

Fig. 13.2 Treatment algorithm in otosclerosis patients with less than 70% speech discrimination. (Adapted from Merkus et al 2011[15] with permission of *Laryngoscope*.) New evidence has shown benefit of stapedotomy also if the air-bone gap is unknown.[16]

13.4 Treatment Algorithm

The presented algorithm[15,16] divides patients into two main groups based on maximum speech discrimination scores: 0–50% and 50–70% (**Fig. 13.2**). Based on the radiologic findings and the extent of the air–bone gap (ABG), patients will be treated with a CI, with a stapedotomy, or with a hearing aid and follow-up.

Patients with speech discrimination between 0 and 50% (open-set monosyllables[16,17]) may be treated with either cochlear implantation or stapedotomy. In case of severe retrofenestral otosclerosis on HRCT (grade 2C or 3), CI is the better option because of the very good results for hearing and the likely progression of cochlear pathology that could make CI very difficult if postponed. If the CT scan shows less cochlear involvement (radiologic grade 1, 2A, or 2B), ABG will guide the surgeon to either stapedotomy or cochlear implantation. If the ABG is 30 dB or more, a stapedotomy seems to be a cost-effective option with good chances of improvement of hearing.

If hearing remains insufficient or decreases with time after stapedotomy, patients can still be treated with CI. If the ABG is 30 dB or less, patients should be treated with CI rather than stapedotomy because in this patient group stapedotomy yields insufficient improvement of hearing.

Patients with a speech discrimination of 50 to 70% can be candidates for stapedotomy, rehabilitation with hearing aids, or in some cases even CI placement. Patients with limited cochlear involvement on HRCT (grade 1, 2A, or 2B) and an ABG of 30 dB or more should be treated with stapedotomy. When the ABG is 30 dB or less and HRCT shows limited cochlear involvement, patients will generally benefit from hearing aids and follow-up. If, on the other hand, HRCT shows extensive retrofenestral otosclerosis (grade 2C or 3), CI seems a viable option in this patient group. To date, SD scores of 50 to 70% are not universally accepted as an indication for CI and in some countries reimbursement may be a problem. However, extensive cochlear involvement on HRCT with impending cochlear obliteration may constitute an indication for CI because speech perception as well as the chances of successful cochlear implantation will diminish further with time. There seems to be a window of opportunity for successful implantation, and CI should be considered as a treatment option in this category of patients.[1,6,15]

13.5 Surgical Difficulties and Management in Cochlear Implantation in Advanced Otosclerosis

Many authors have described surgical difficulties during cochlear implantation in otosclerosis patients such as fenestral and basal turn ossification, the necessity for extra drilling, partial electrode insertion, and scala vestibuli insertion (**Table 13.1**). **Table 13.2** shows the incidence of these difficulties and the occurrence of postoperative facial nerve stimulation as reported in the literature.

Fenestral ossification frequently requires extra drilling to identify the lumen of the scala tympani to achieve successful electrode insertion in this scala.[1,3,4,10,12,15]

Basal turn ossification caused by osteoneogenesis is a serious pathology as almost all patients (80–100%) with a partial electrode insertion or misplacement during surgery have basal turn

Table 13.1 Surgical difficulties encountered during or after cochlear implantation of advanced otosclerosis patients

Surgical difficulties	Sclerotic obliteration of the round window
	Scala tympani obliteration, or both scalae
	"Double ring" creating a false lumen
	Previous chain reconstruction, missing stapes as landmark
	Partial insertion
In severe otospongiosis (CT grade 3)	CSF gusher/ CSF leakage
	Progression of the electrode into a false route (internal auditory canal, carotid canal, etc.)
Postoperative difficulties	Partial insertion, shifting programming
	Facial nerve stimulation, fewer electrodes usable for stimulation
	CSF leakage

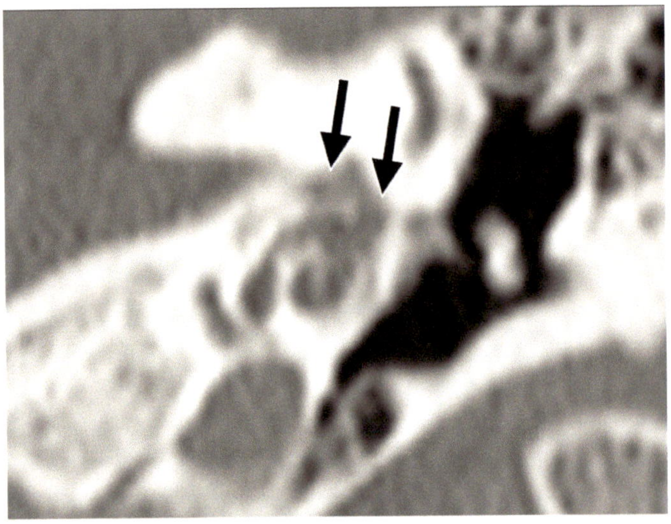

Fig. 13.3 Facial nerve stimulation in severe retrofenestral otospongiotic lesions. Coronal scan of a patient prior to implantation. The otospongiotic bone lesions are seen all around the cochlea and are confluent with the bony facial nerve canal between the internal auditory canal and the geniculate ganglion (*black arrows*). When a cochlear implant is in position within this cochlea, the electrical current in the cranial part of the electrode will stimulate the spiral ganglia of the cochlear nerve as well as the facial nerve. The CI should then be reprogrammed and the middle electrodes should be turned off.

ossification.[1,13,15] Obliteration of the scala tympani requires *scala vestibuli electrode insertion* in 2 to 25% of the cases.[1,10,15,18] This method of insertion is described in Chapter 11.

Some authors suggest that advanced otosclerosis could also be an indication for an auditory brainstem implant (ABI), but in our opinion this is not, as in all otosclerosis cases a CI can be implanted.[19] This could be difficult, as explained above, and one should sometimes plan a subtotal petrosectomy for better access and visibility, but cochlear implantation is usually feasible (for auditory brainstem implantation indications see Chapter 8; for subtotal petrosectomy see Chapter 10).

In severe otospongiosis a cerebrospinal fluid (CSF) gusher can occur due to the otospongiotic bone and connection to the internal auditory canal (see the cases presented in this chapter). Three important steps are suggested to overcome difficulties in case of a cerebrospinal fluid (CSF) gusher:

Table 13.2 Percentage of reported surgical difficulties or complications encountered during or after cochlear implantation of advanced otosclerosis patients

Surgical difficulty/complication in literature	Range	Average
Round window ossification	0–89%	38%
Basal turn ossification	3–60%	31%
Extra drilling	0–60%	28%
Facial nerve stimulation	0–75%	25%
Scala vestibuli insertion	2–25%	5%
Partial insertion	0–19%	5%

Source: Adapted from Merkus et al[15] in a review of 13 studies.

1. Perform a subtotal petrosectomy. This will give you access, orientation, and most importantly a secure closure after surgery with minimal risks of meningitis.
2. Make a large enough cochleostomy that can firmly be packed with periosteum or fascia around the cochlear electrode.
3. Make sure the electrode is directed in the correct angle (superior-posterior to anterior-inferior). A false route is easily adopted. A perioperative CT scan can be an option.

Postoperatively, an electrical shunt between the implant and the facial nerve can cause *facial nerve stimulation (FNS)*. FNS is a worrying complication of cochlear implantation occurring on average in 25% of patients with otosclerosis.[15] The incidence of FNS was significantly higher in patients with otosclerosis compared with control patients in whom FNS was a rarely reported complication.[5,8,12,13,20–22] This high occurrence of FNS can be explained by an increased conductivity of the otospongiotic bone, making it easier to stimulate the facial nerve.[23] The management of facial nerve stimulation consists of a reduction in the stimulus levels of the cranially located electrodes, the total deactivation of the causative electrodes, or even reimplantation.[1,13,20,22] Because the perigeniculate area is the facial nerve segment most frequently involved, the use of a precurved electrode will place the electrode endings farther away from the facial nerve and would therefore seem a more appropriate choice of electrode in otosclerosis patients. (See **Fig. 13.3**.)

Case 13.1 Stapedotomy in a Cochlear Implant Candidate with Otosclerosis (Fig. 13.1.1–Fig. 13.1.4)

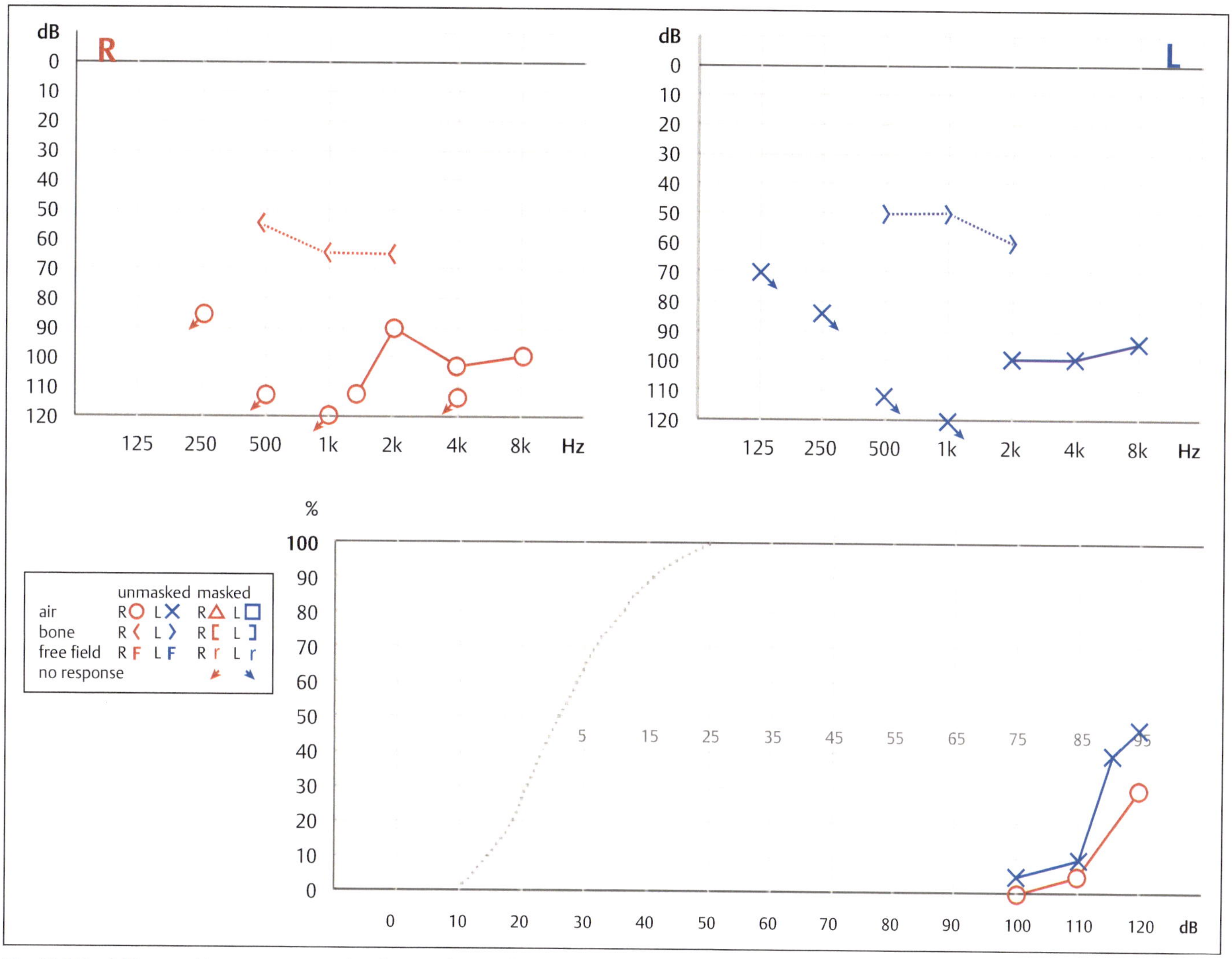

Fig. 13.1.1 A 51-year-old woman presented with severe hearing loss, as shown on this audiogram. She was unaware that she probably had otosclerosis: she had been wearing hearing aids for years and had not had ear surgery in the past.

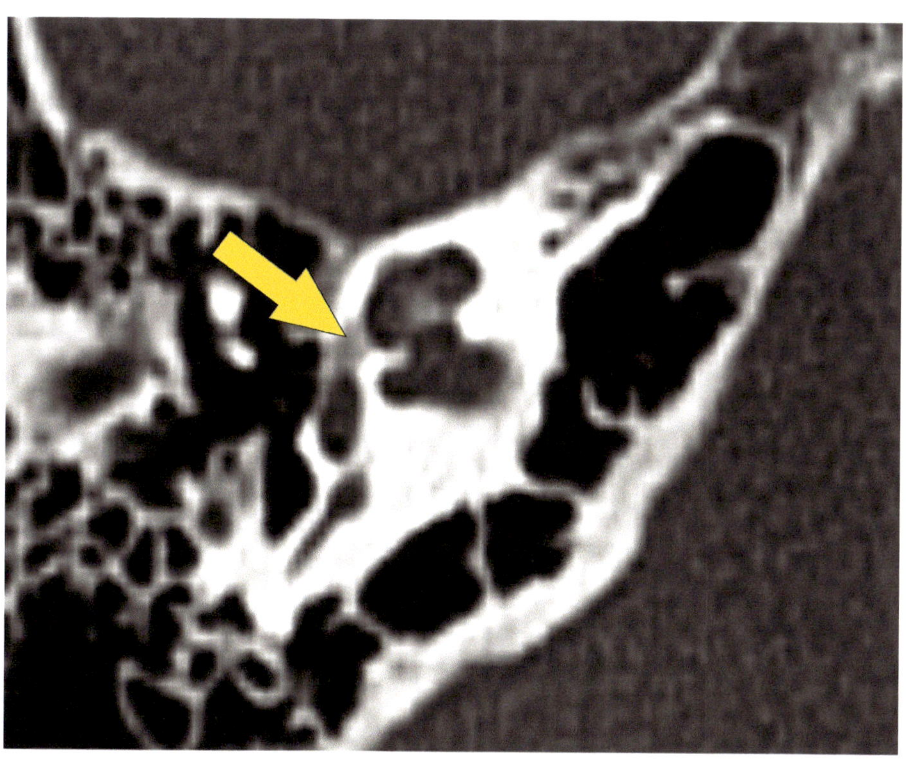

Fig. 13.1.2 On CT the extent of otosclerotic decalcification was entirely anterior of the oval window (grade 1: fenestral, *yellow arrow*). This case shows that the severity of the hearing loss is not directly related to the severity of the fenestral/retrofenestral decalcification.

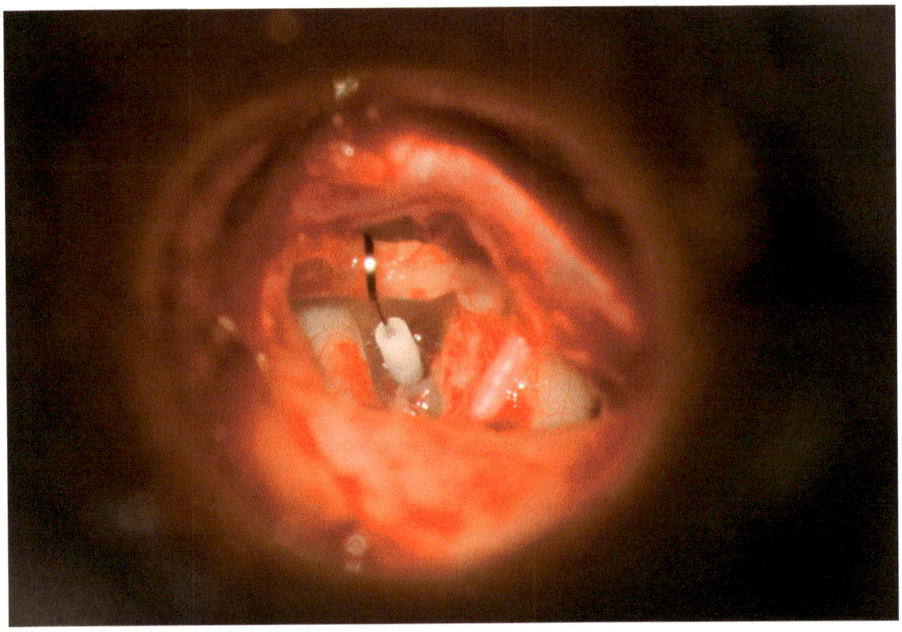

Fig. 13.1.3 An uncomplicated stapedotomy was performed at the right ear.

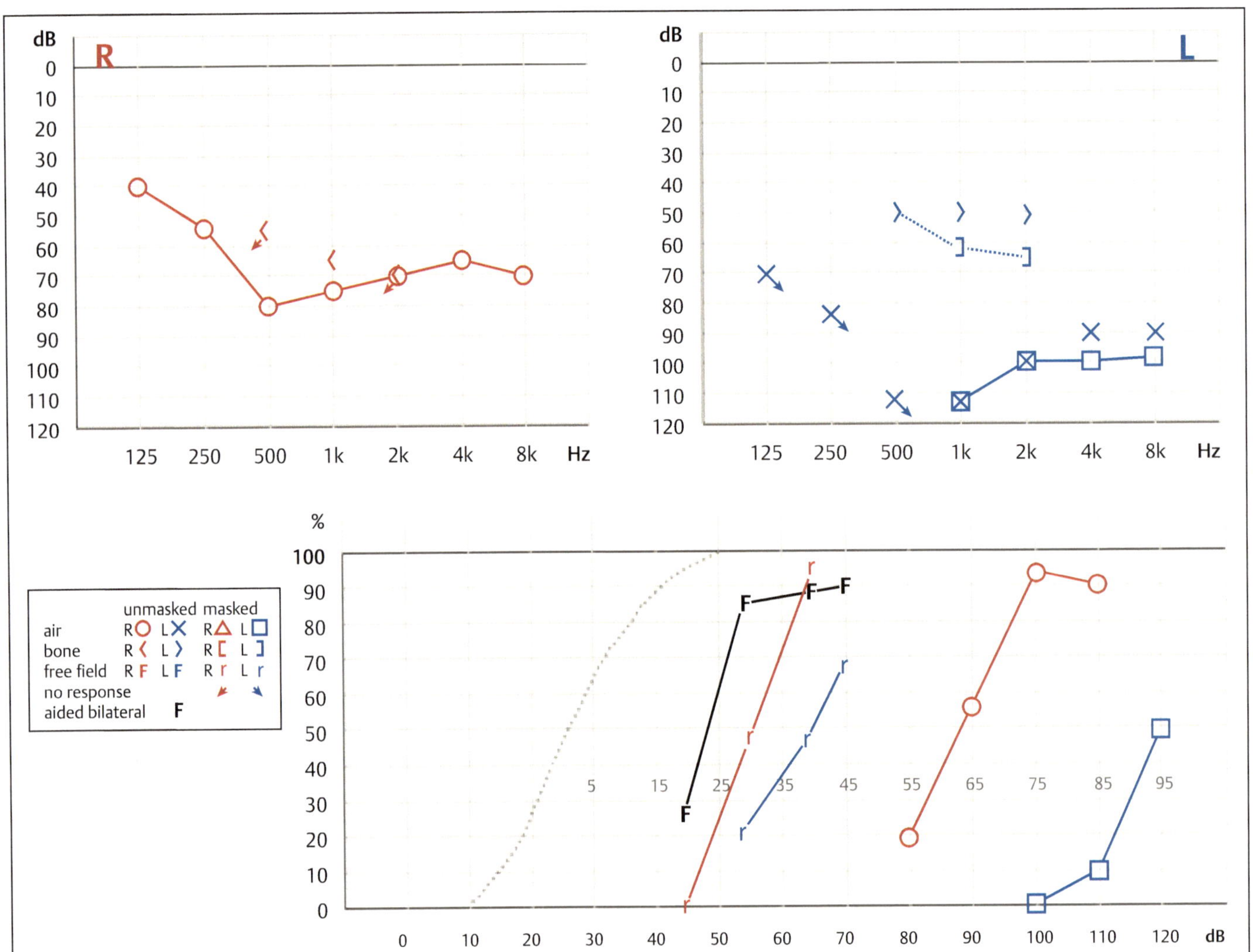

Fig. 13.1.4 Three months postoperatively, the air–bone gap on the right side showed significant improvement as did the speech performance also. She is still wearing bilateral hearing aids, but with less fatigue. This patient is no longer a CI candidate. She is now considering a stapedotomy on her left ear.

Comment

A stapedotomy should be considered in otosclerosis CI candidates with an air–bone gap and without severe otospongiotic bone remodeling.[16]

Case 13.2 Retrofenestral Otosclerosis with Round Window Ossification (Right Ear)
(Fig. 13.2.1–Fig. 13.2.9)

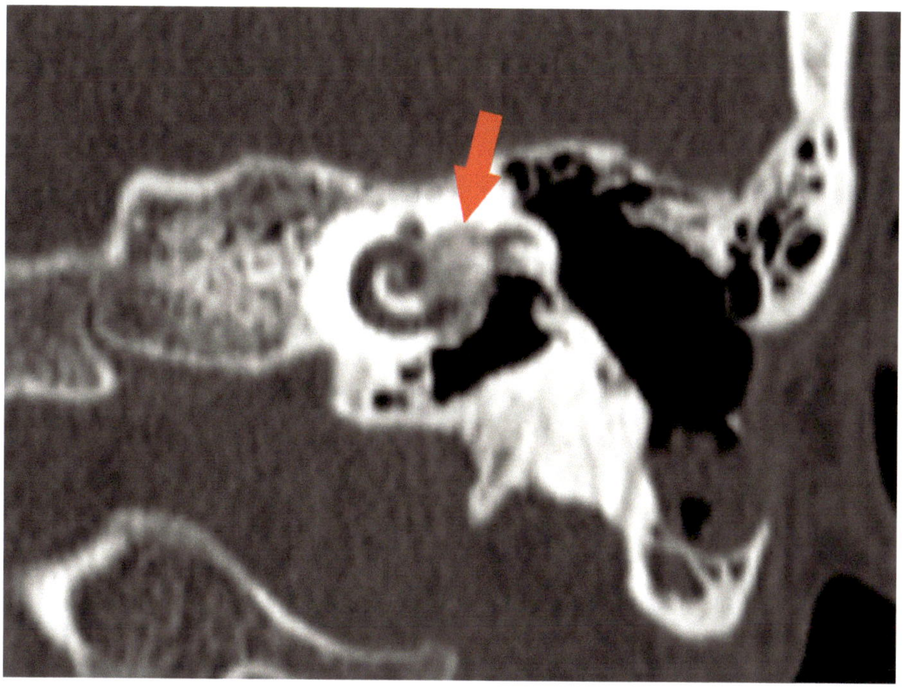

Fig. 13.2.1 A 73-year-old woman with a left-sided canal wall down procedure due to a cholesteatoma. On this left side retrofenestral otosclerosis is seen (*arrow*). She was profoundly deaf in this left ear.

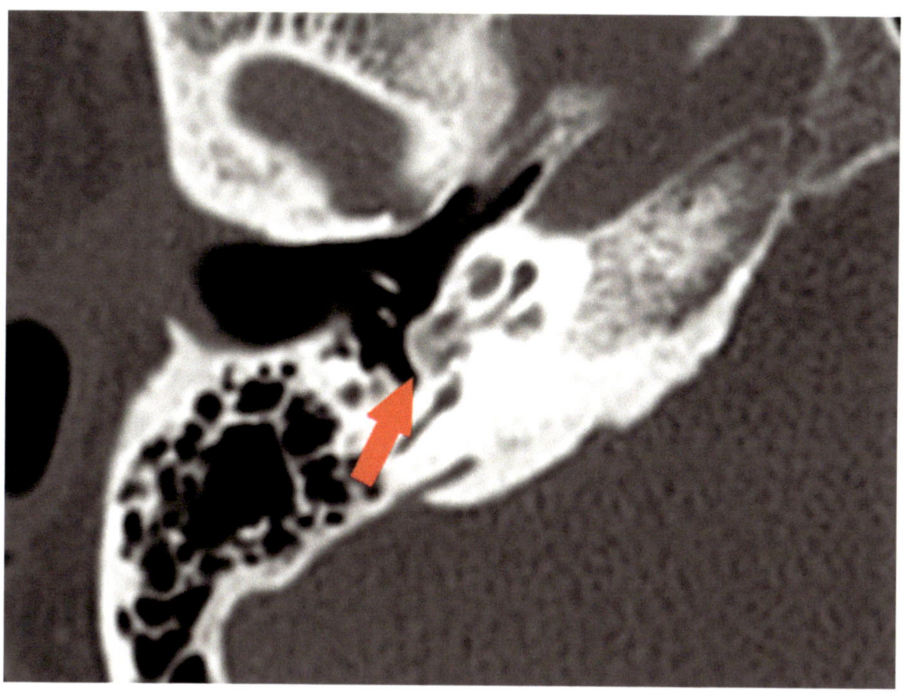

Fig. 13.2.2 On the right ear a more modest retrofenestral otosclerotic lesion is seen (*arrow*). The majority of the otospongiotic bone is present around the round window. A stapedotomy was performed some years previously on this side. Her hearing had deteriorated to the level that her hearing aids were no longer useful.

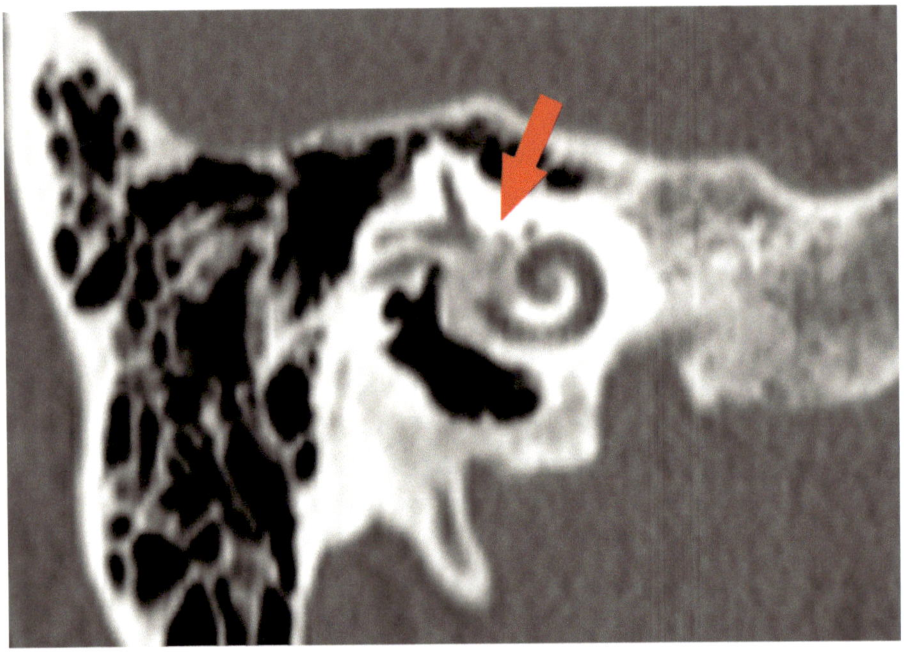

Fig. 13.2.3 The coronal CT scan of the right cochlea shows a decalcification of the complete central part of the labyrinth (*arrow*). The round window area of the basal turn is affected, whereas the rest of the basal turn is not.

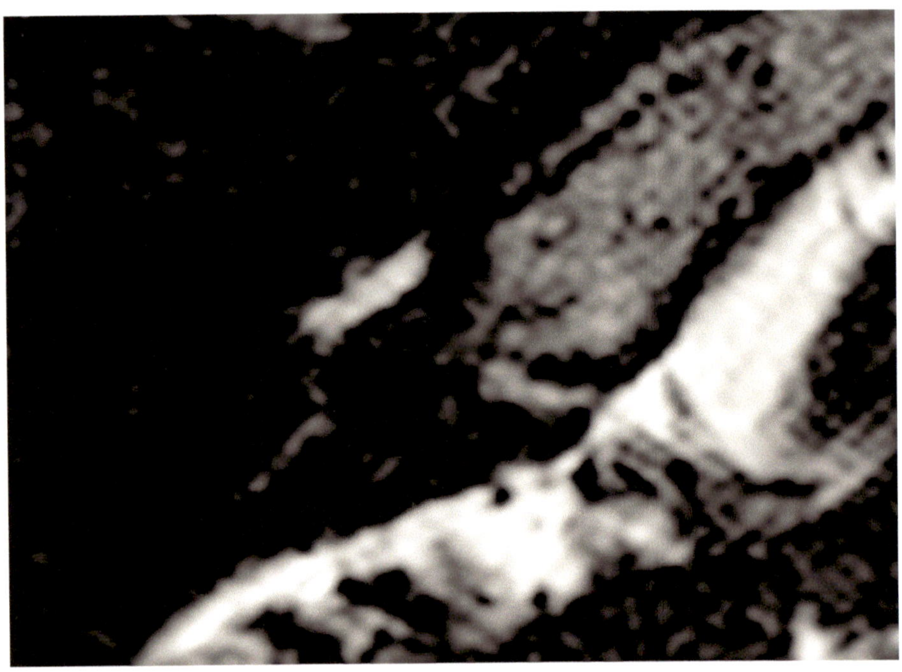

Fig. 13.2.4 On MRI the cochlea on the right showed an open scala tympani. The patient was assigned for cochlear implantation through a posterior tympanotomy and we aimed for a regular scala tympani insertion.

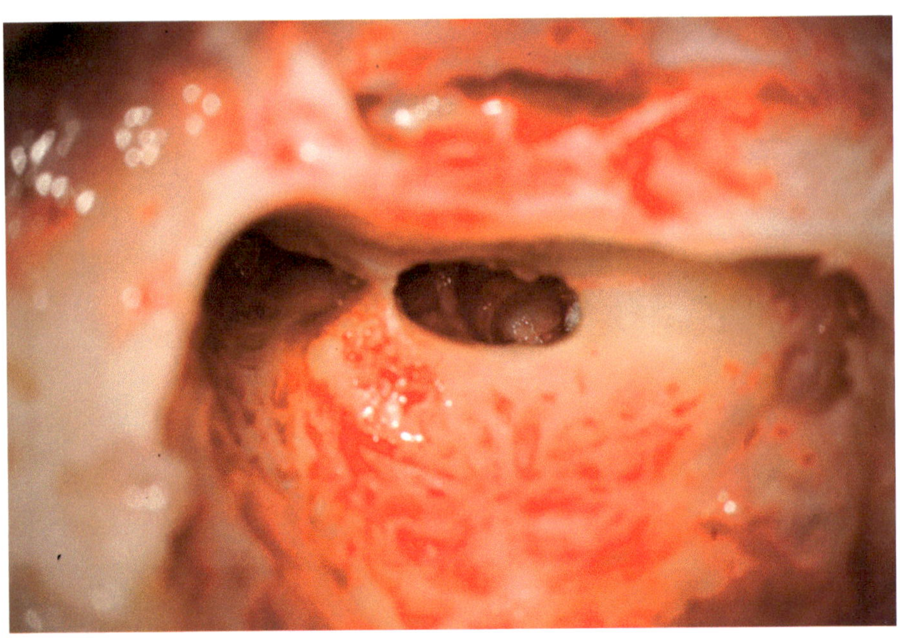

Fig. 13.2.5 During surgery of her right ear a fully calcified round window was seen through the posterior tympanotomy.

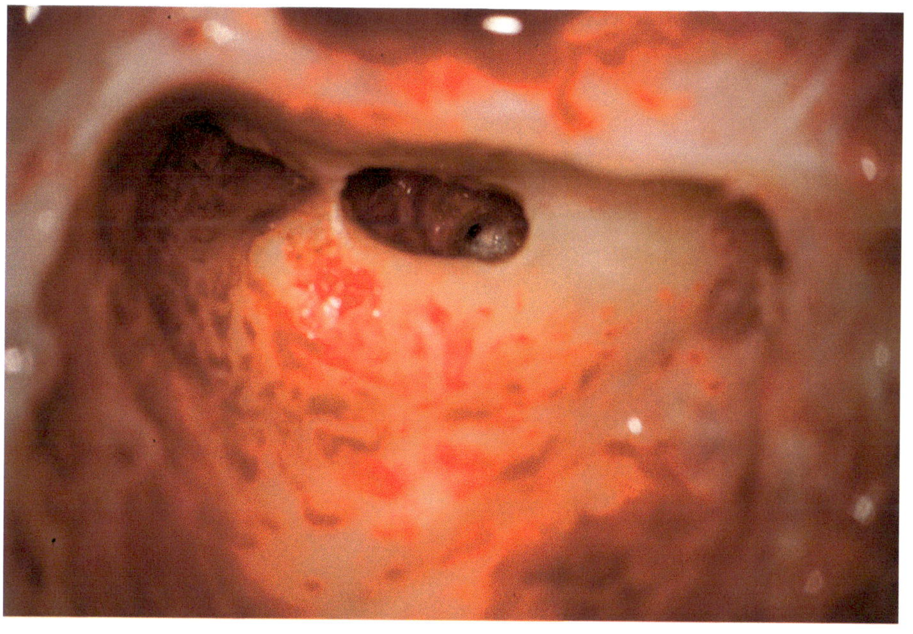

Fig. 13.2.6 An opening was made into the scala tympani with a small bur. The opening was enlarged with small hooks. Hyaluronic acid can be used to avoid bone dust entering the cochlea (not shown here).

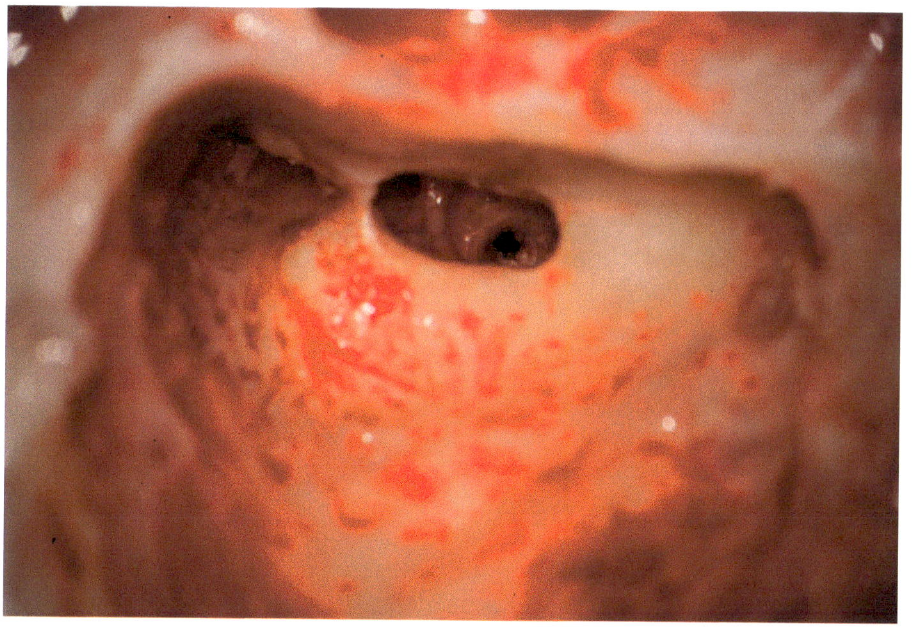

Fig. 13.2.7 As soon as the opening seemed sufficient for an easy insertion of the electrode, the implant was prepared for implantation.

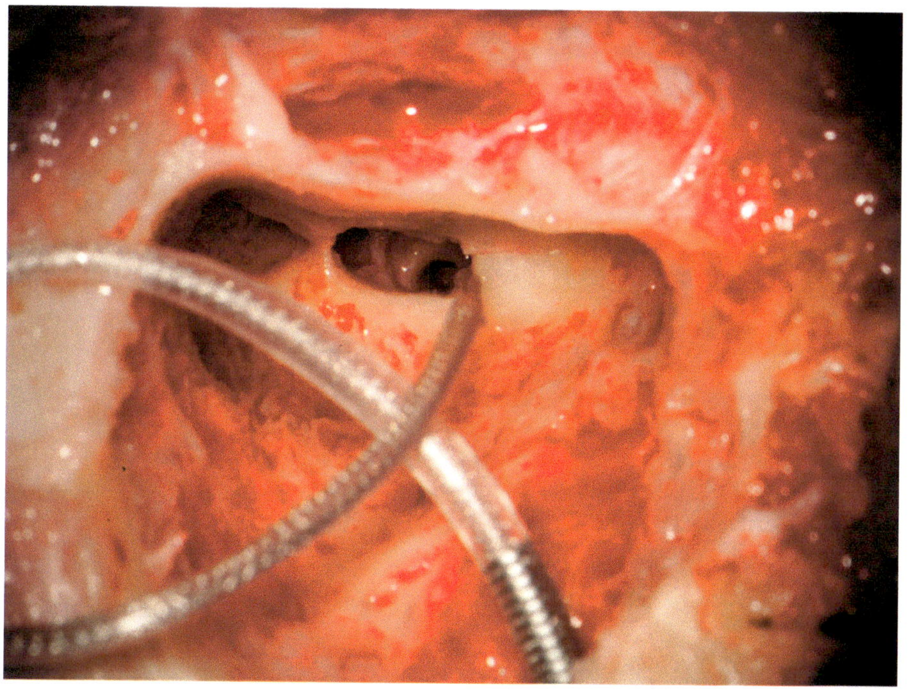

Fig. 13.2.8 The electrode is gently introduced into the scala tympani.

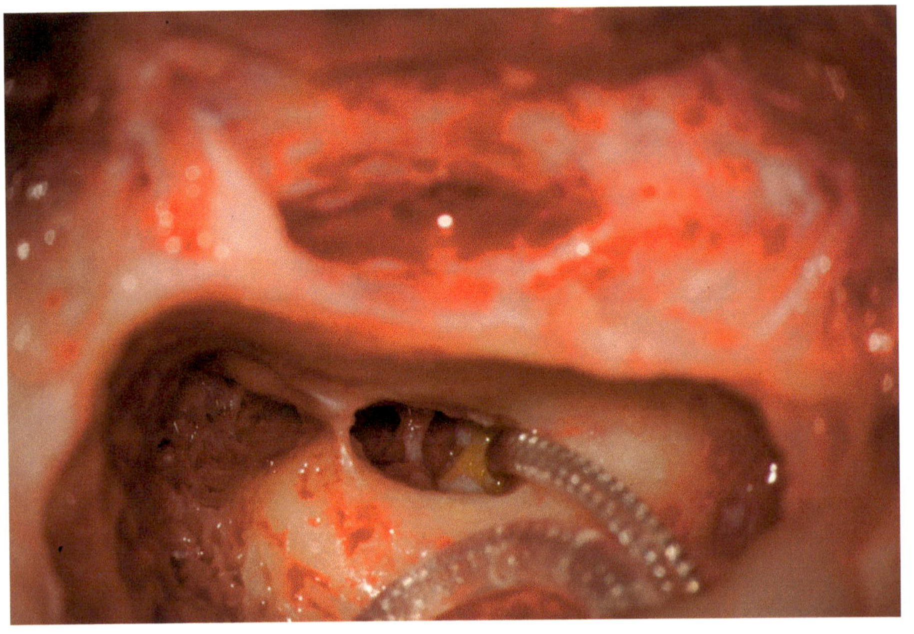

Fig. 13.2.9 The round window opening is then sealed with pieces of soft tissue. This patient is still in her first year of rehabilitation and has increasing speech performance scores.

Comment

Insertion with (only) round window thickening is well possible through a standard posterior tympanotomy.

Case 13.3 Round Window and Oval Window Ossification: Subtotal Petrosectomy and CI

(Fig. 13.3.1–Fig. 13.3.5)

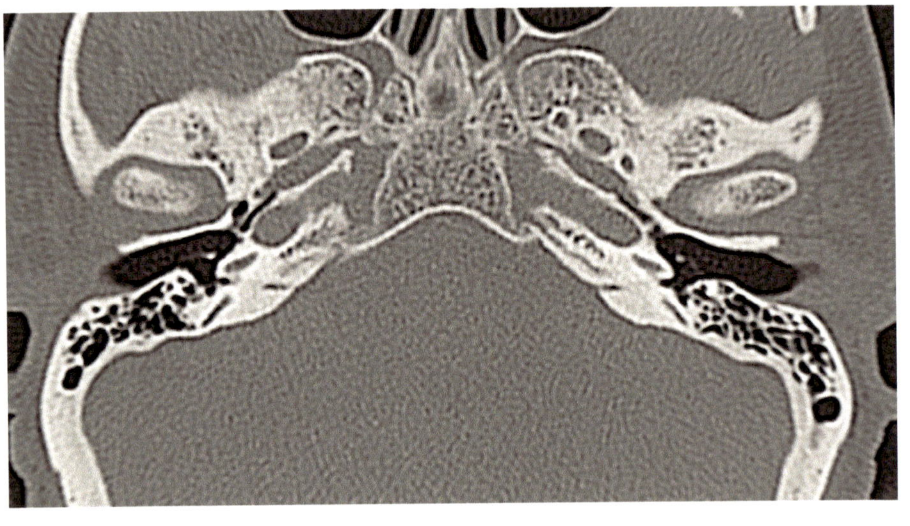

Fig. 13.3.1 A 61-year-old woman with bilateral otosclerosis. A mild ossification of the round window may be appreciated bilaterally. Because of the difficult anatomy encountered during the previous attempt at revision stapedectomy, left, a subtotal petrosectomy was selected.

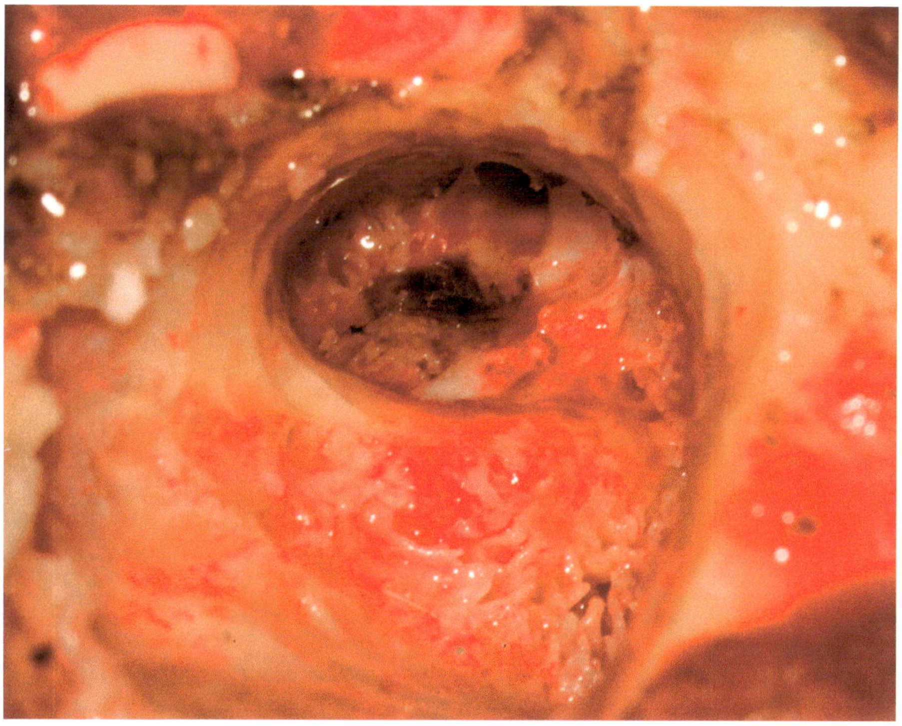

Fig. 13.3.2 In the subtotal petrosectomy approach the middle ear anatomy can be fully seen. There was a lot of thickened mucosa and the round window could not easily be located.

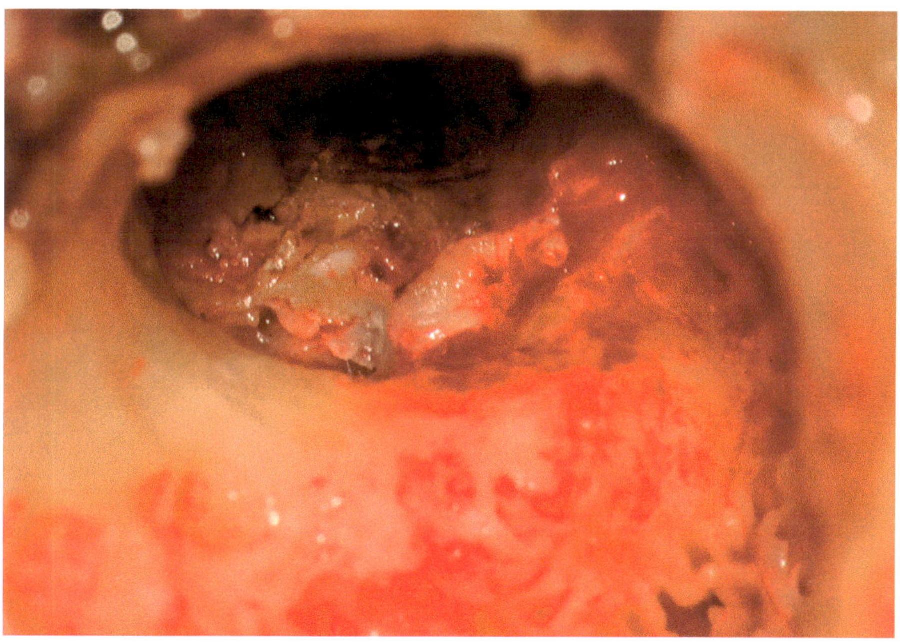

Fig. 13.3.3 Anatomical landmarks were difficult, as already known from the previous surgery. The perichondrium that had been used to seal the oval window during the stapedectomy attempt hindered the anatomical interpretation. After removal of the mucosal layer at the location of the round window, a window was vaguely seen. The calcification of the window obscured a clear view at the window.

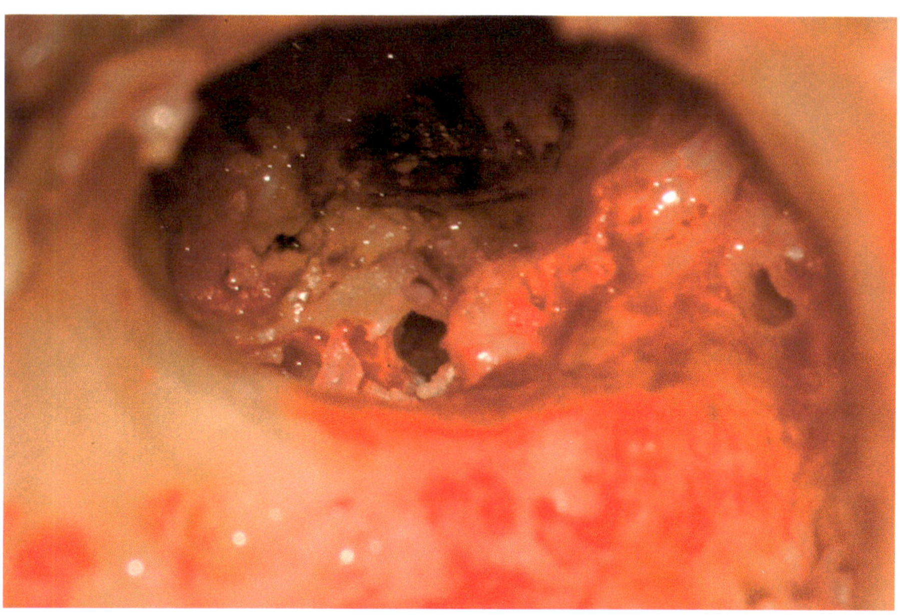

Fig. 13.3.4 The scala tympani was opened with slow drilling at the round window.

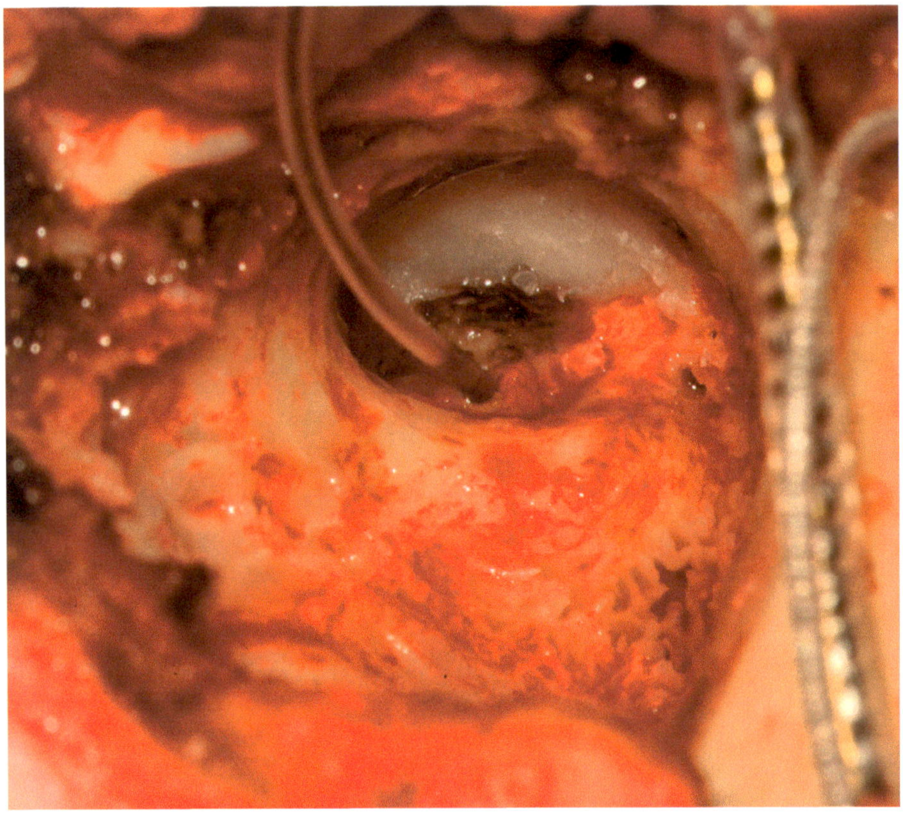

Fig. 13.3.5 The eustachian tube was closed with bone wax (white wax anterior to the electrode). And the electrode was introduced into the cochlea. All electrodes evoked a spiral ganglion and nerve reaction in the neural measurements.

Comment

Subtotal petrosectomy can provide a more complete overview of the round window area and secure scala tympani insertion.

Case 13.4 Cochlear Implantation in a Patient with an Otosclerotic Scala Tympani Ossification at the Basal Turn (Fig. 13.4.1–Fig. 13.4.6)

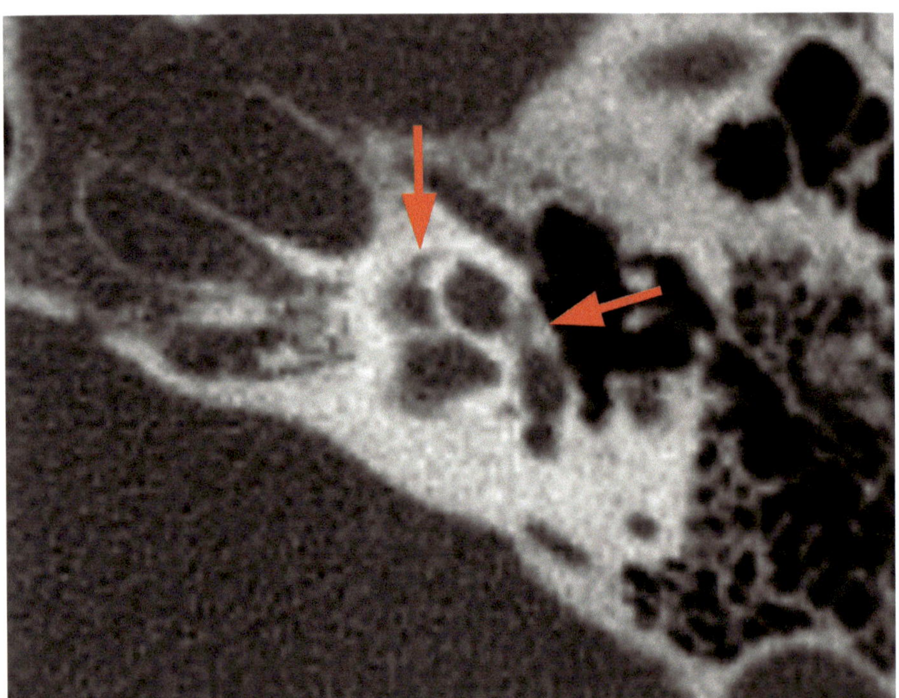

Fig. 13.4.1 A 38-year-old man had undergone a right-side stapedotomy 7 years before with temporary improvement, but was now facing profound (progressive) hearing loss in both ears with minimal benefit from hearing aids. The CT images on both sides show the same pathology. A retrofenestral otosclerosis with otospongiotic lesions around the cochlea (see *red arrows*). The cochlea is still recognizable.

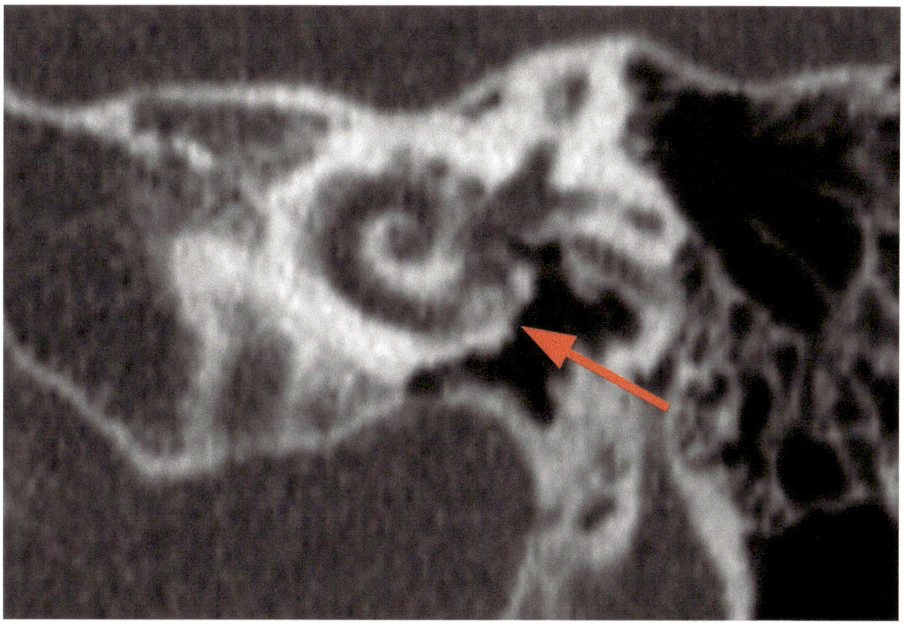

Fig. 13.4.2 In a coronal plane the calcification of the round window area is well visible (*red arrow*). Also, the decalcified spots around the otic capsule can be appreciated on this image.

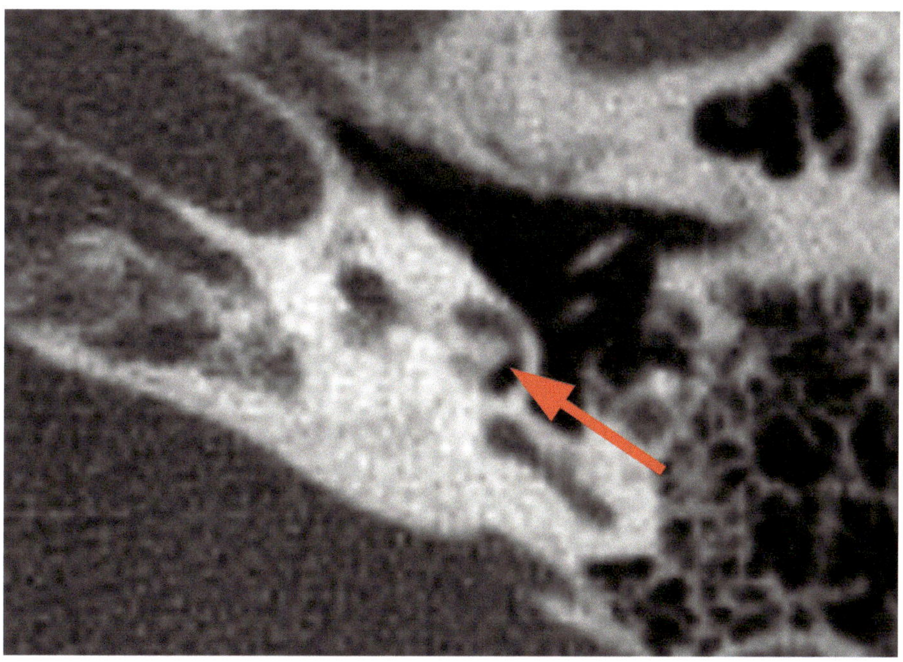

Fig. 13.4.3 The basal turn is calcified within the scala tympani. On CT there appears to be a calcified lesion from the round window up to half way along the basal turn *(red arrow)*. The scala vestibuli appears open, but MRI was performed for confirmation.

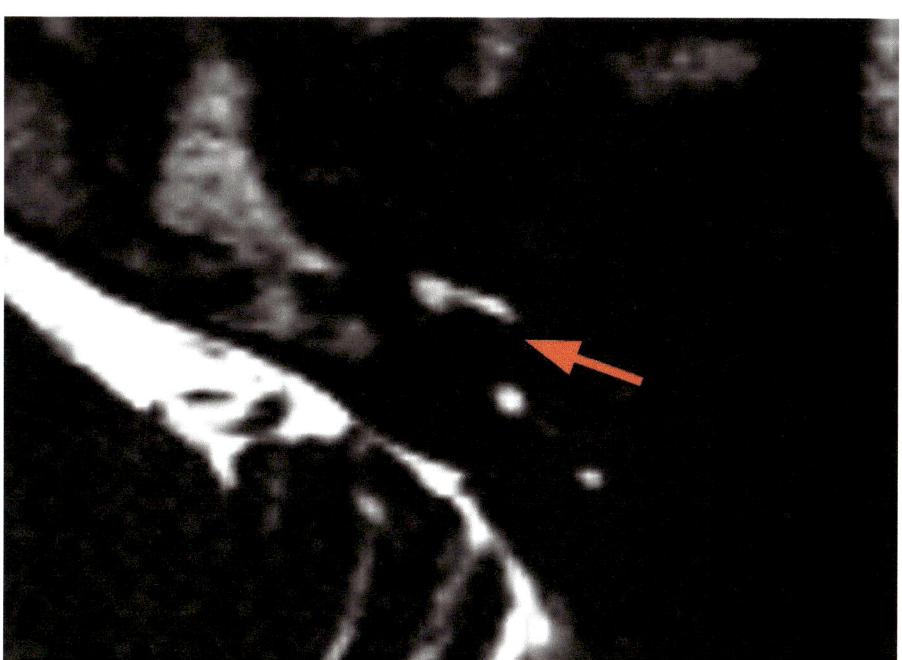

Fig. 13.4.4 On MRI the area of the obliteration (calcification/ossification on CT) of the basal turn can be well distinguished *(red arrow)*. The scala vestibuli is still patent and unaffected by the calcification due to the otosclerosis.

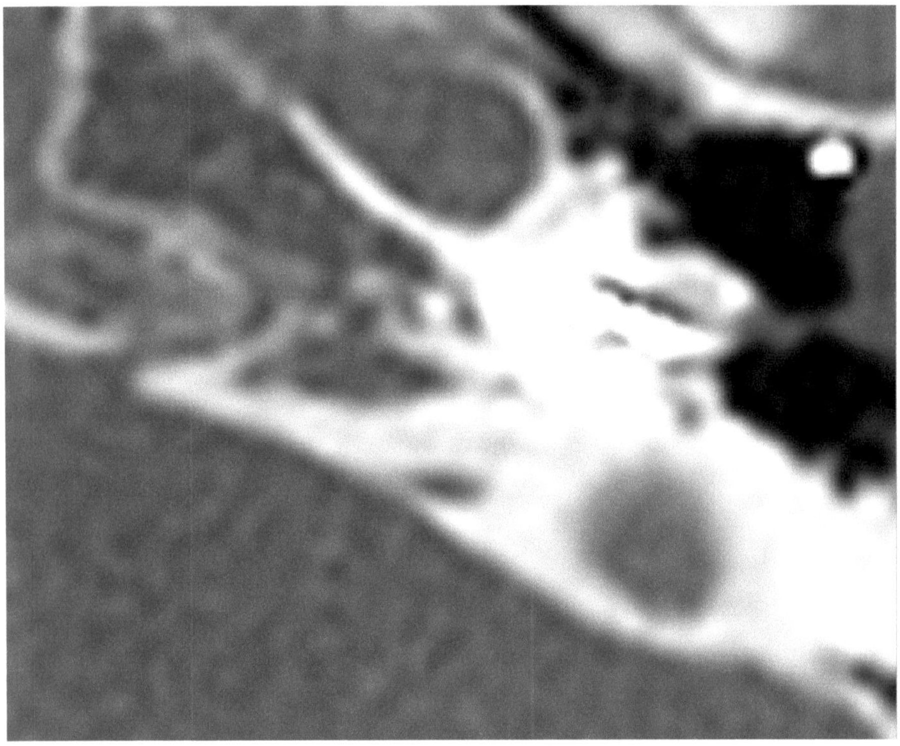

Fig. 13.4.5 The CI is placed after a drill-out procedure through a scala tympani insertion (see Chapter 11 on cochlear ossification).

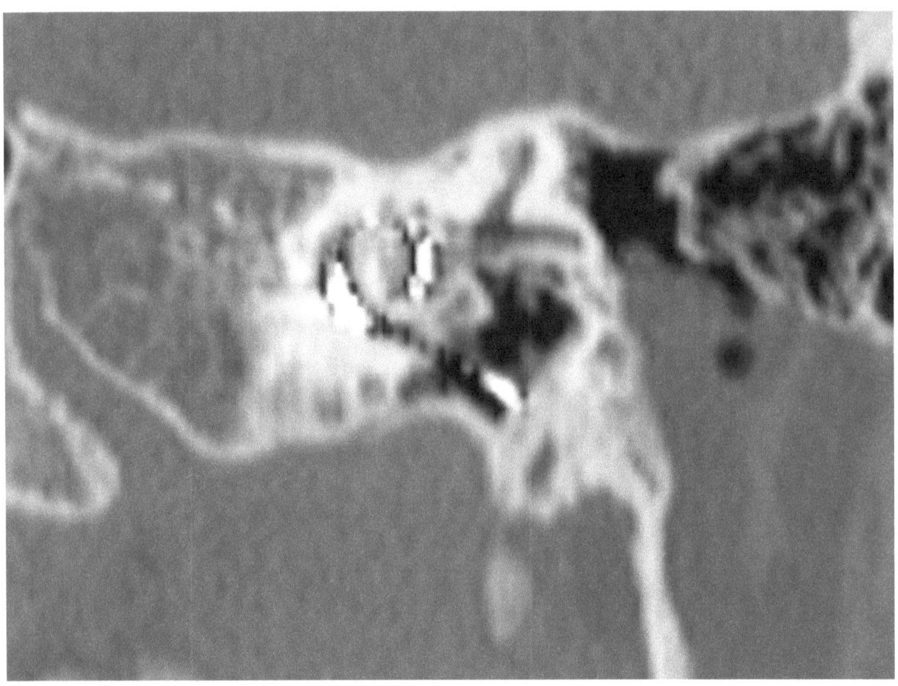

Fig. 13.4.6 The electrode was fully inserted without any resistance. There was no facial nerve stimulation and all electrodes could be activated. The open-set speech performance increased to 90% within 6 months.

Comment

With half of the basal turn obliterated in otosclerosis, it is easier to perform a scala vestibuli insertion, although a scala tympani insertion after drill-out is possible.

Case 13.5 Cochlear Implantation with Subtotal Petrosectomy in a Patient with Basal Turn Ossification (Fig. 13.5.1–Fig. 13.5.14)

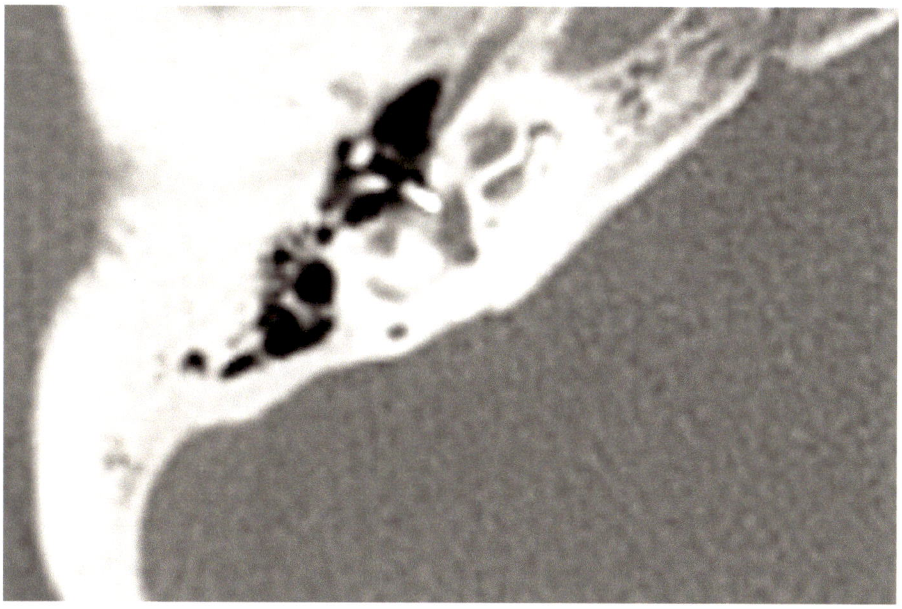

Fig. 13.5.1 A 71-year-old man with a positive family history of otosclerosis and bilateral stapedotomy 30 years earlier. Revision surgery did not improve the hearing. Axial right ear CT scan image in which the stapes prosthesis is clearly visible. Ossification of the basal turn can also be seen.

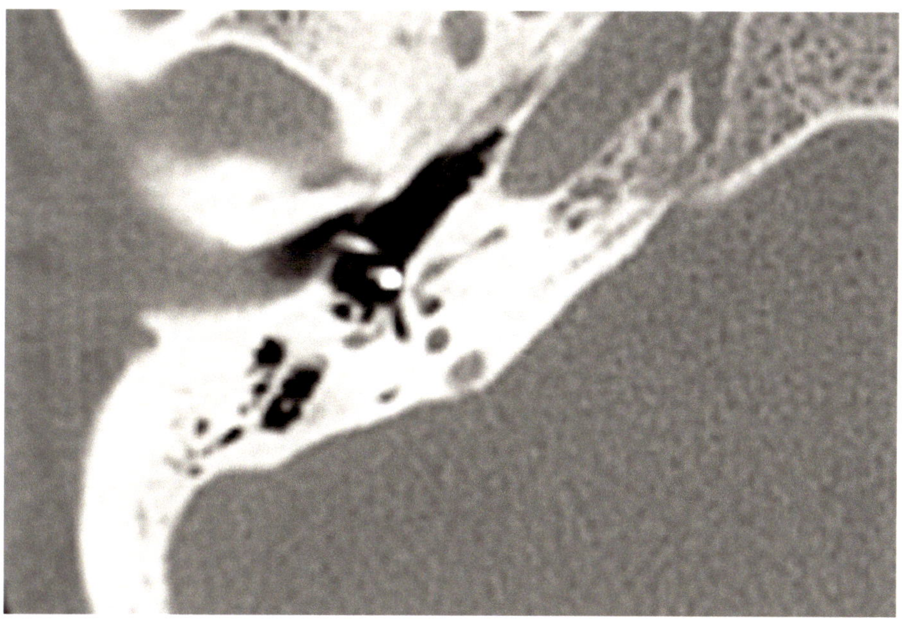

Fig. 13.5.2 Ossification of the scala tympani of the complete basal turn of the cochlea of the right ear appears to be present, while the scala vestibuli seems open. MRI was performed to confirm the patency of the scala vestibuli.

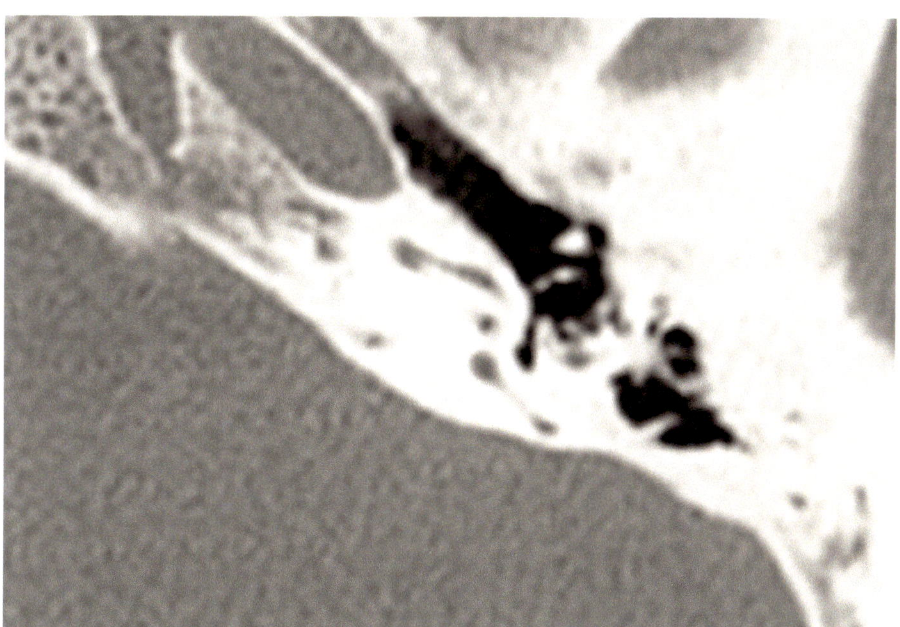

Fig. 13.5.3 Less ossification is seen in the left ear. Two-thirds of the scala tympani in the basal turn is ossified. The scala vestibuli appears patent but MRI is needed to confirm this.

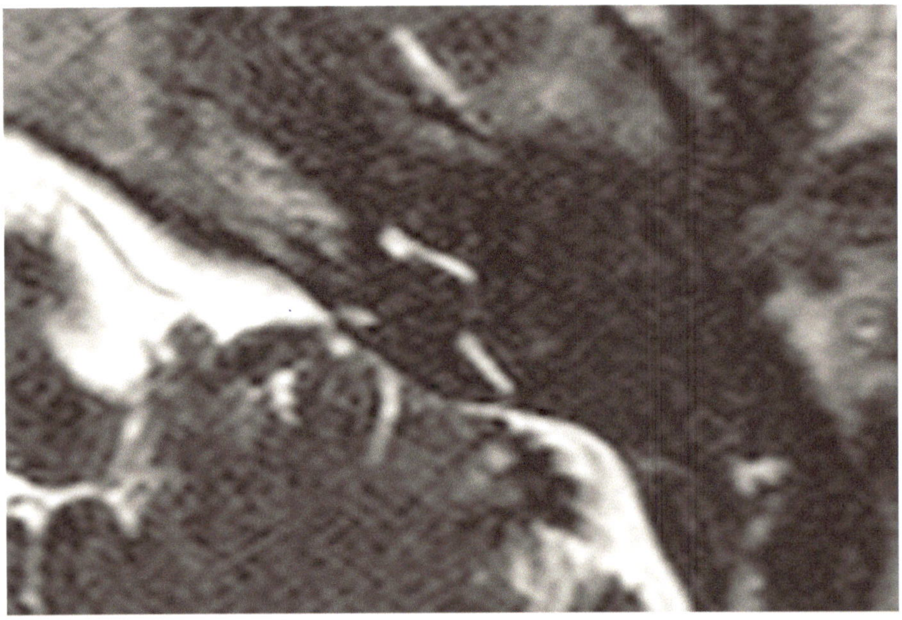

Fig. 13.5.4 On MRI the patency of the scala vestibuli is confirmed and the obliteration of the scala tympani corresponds with the ossified part seen on CT scan.

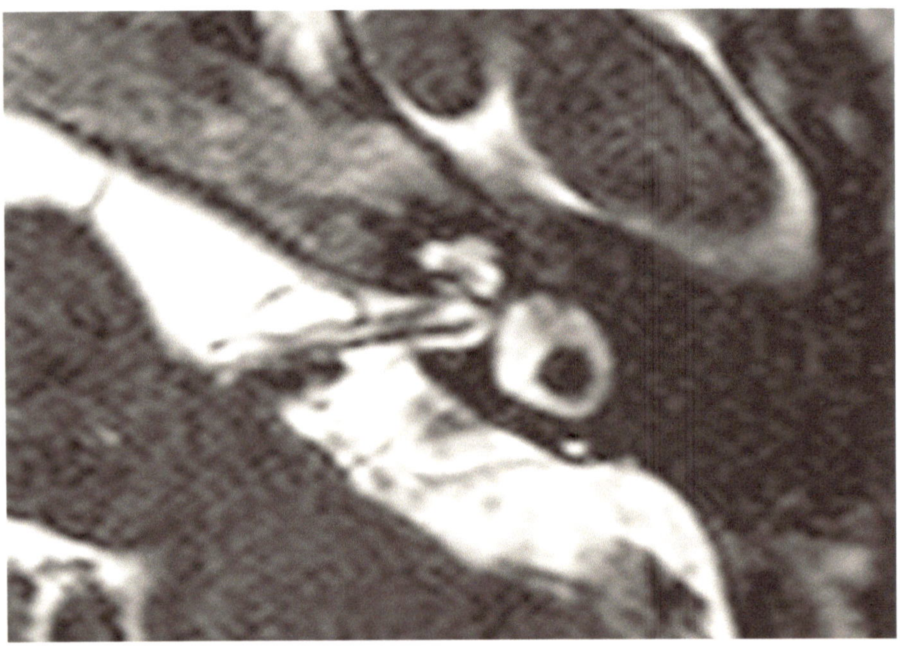

Fig. 13.5.5 The middle turn of the cochlea seems fully patent, as the MRI shows no loss of fluid.

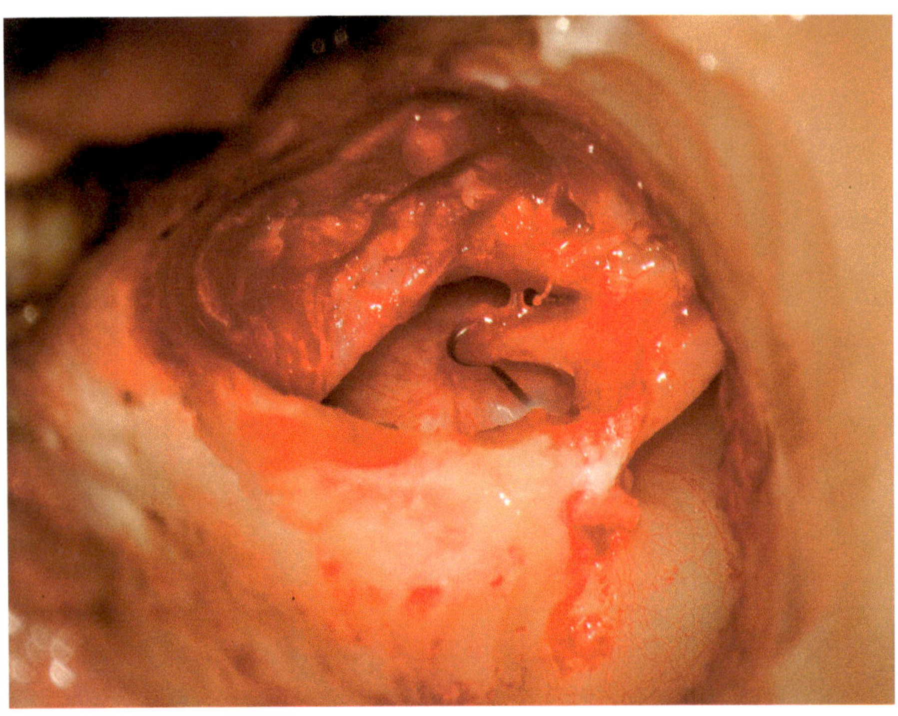

Fig. 13.5.6 The decision was made to implant the left ear because of less ossification there. A subtotal petrosectomy was chosen to provide better access and overview when performing a drill-out procedure.

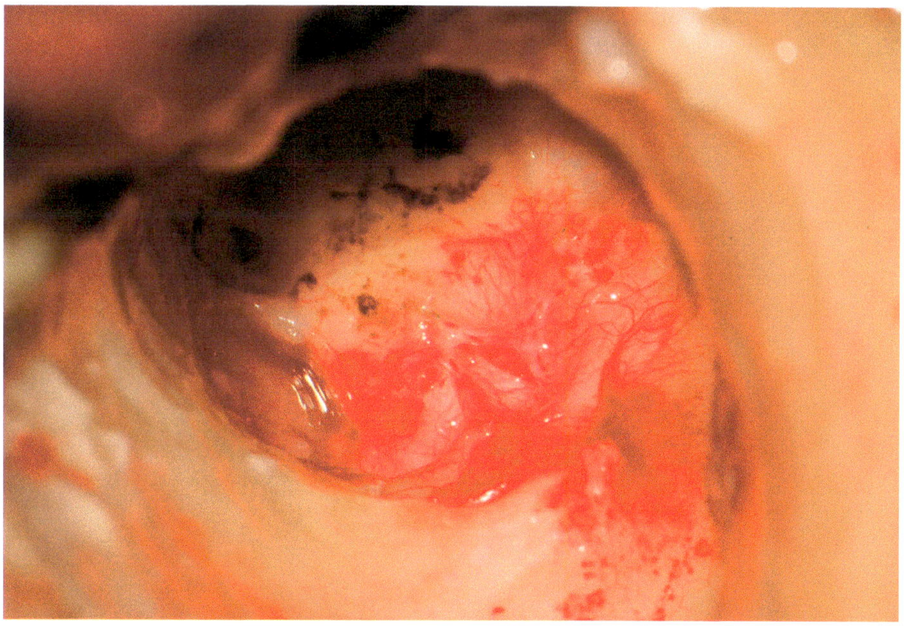

Fig. 13.5.7 After removing the canal wall, the eardrum, and the remaining ossicles, the round window area is focused on. The soft tissue is removed and, with the oval window and round window as landmarks, the drill-out procedure is started.

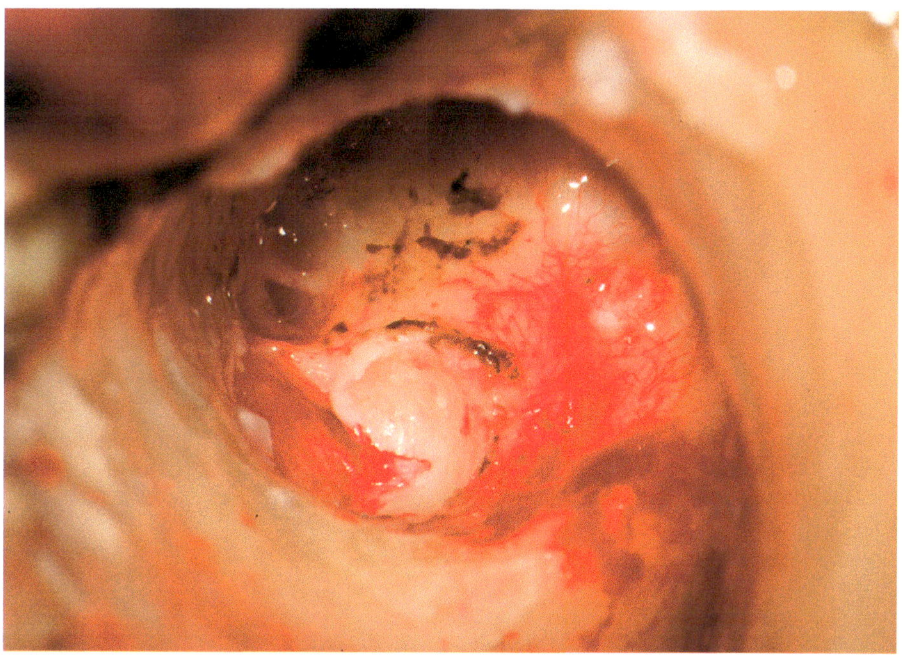

Fig. 13.5.8 As expected, no lumen is visible in the scala tympani area.

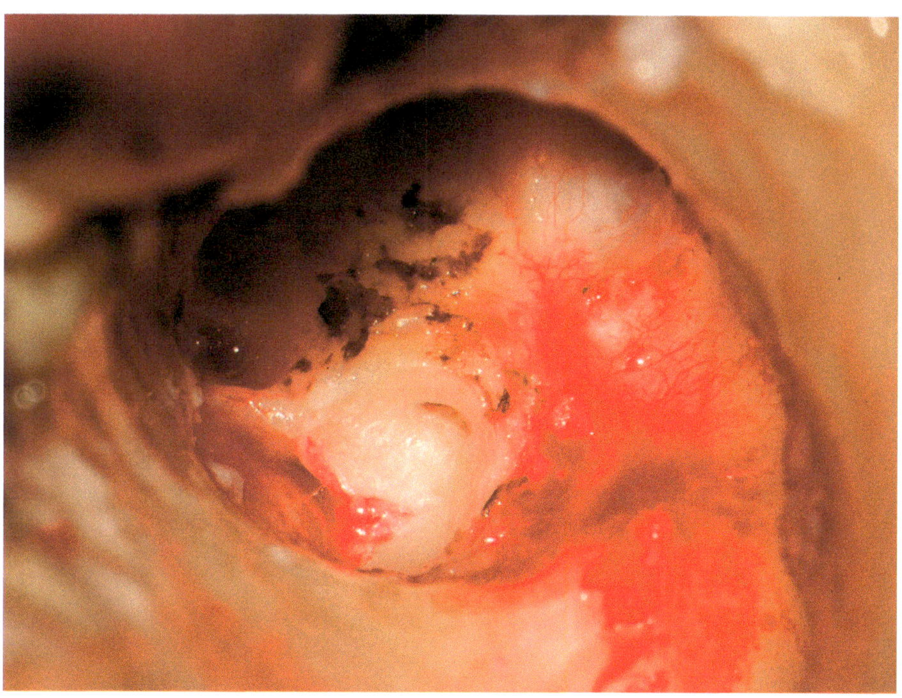

Fig. 13.5.9 With drilling more anteriorly and superiorly, the scala vestibuli appears.

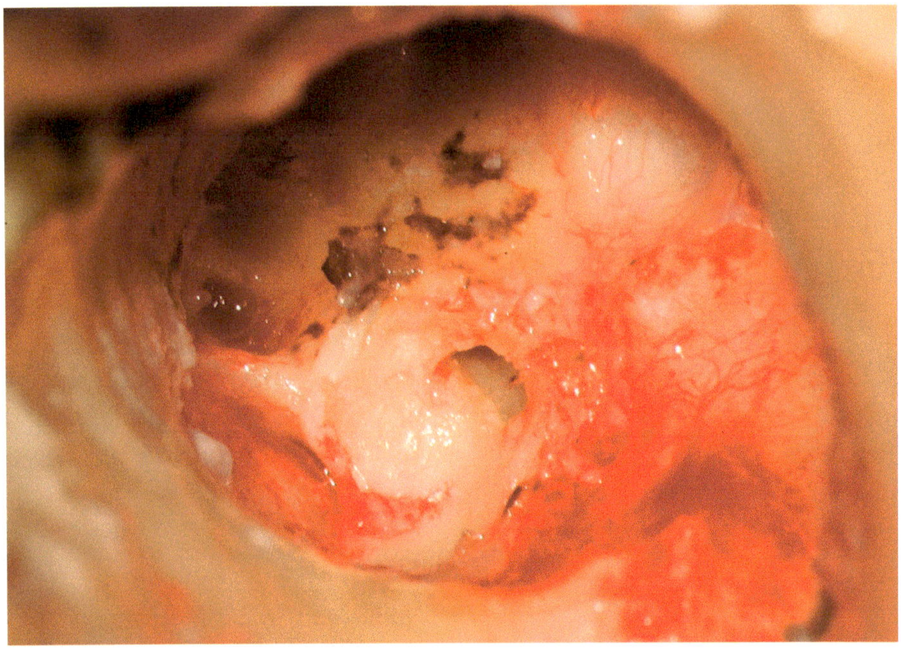

Fig. 13.5.10 The scala vestibuli opening is enlarged.

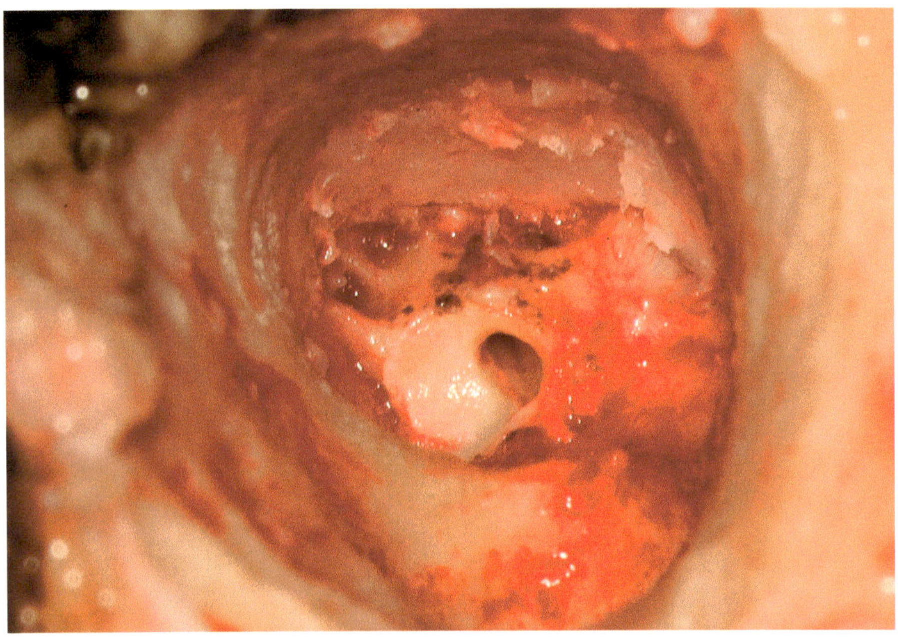

Fig. 13.5.11 When a sufficient opening has been created, the eustachian tube is closed. The ear canal is already closed and abdominal fat is harvested (not shown here). The implant is prepared for placement.

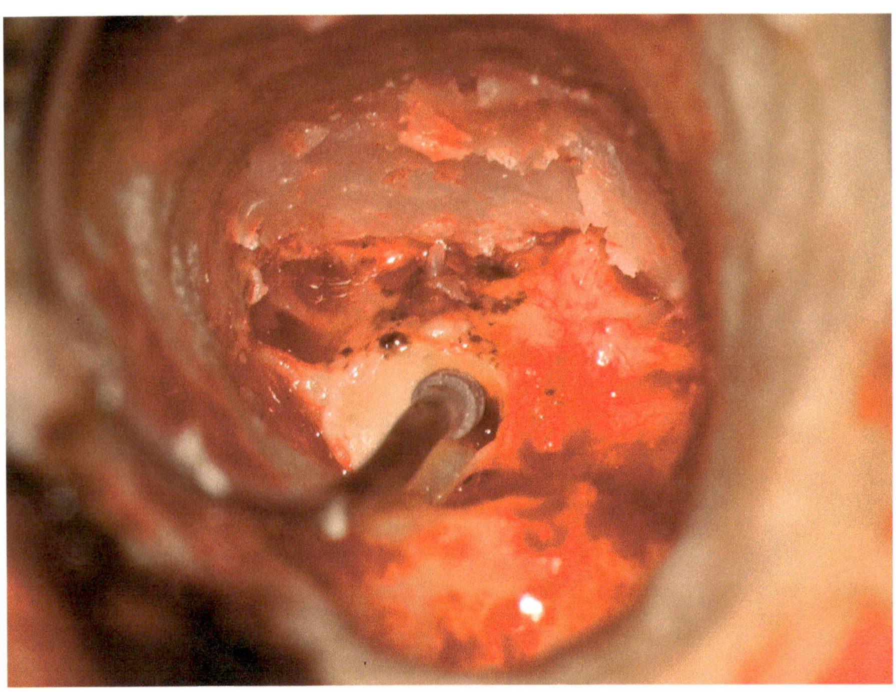

Fig. 13.5.12 A full implantation through this scala vestibuli approach is achieved. Neural response measurements confirmed a functional implant and a correct placement.

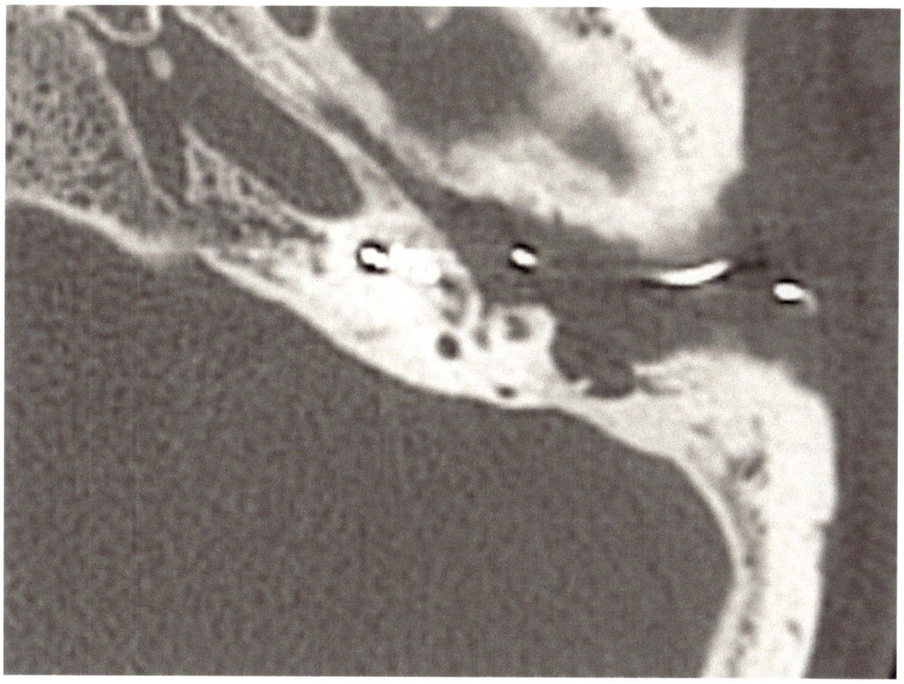

Fig. 13.5.13 Postoperative CT scan shows the more anterior position within the basal turn according to the scala vestibuli position.

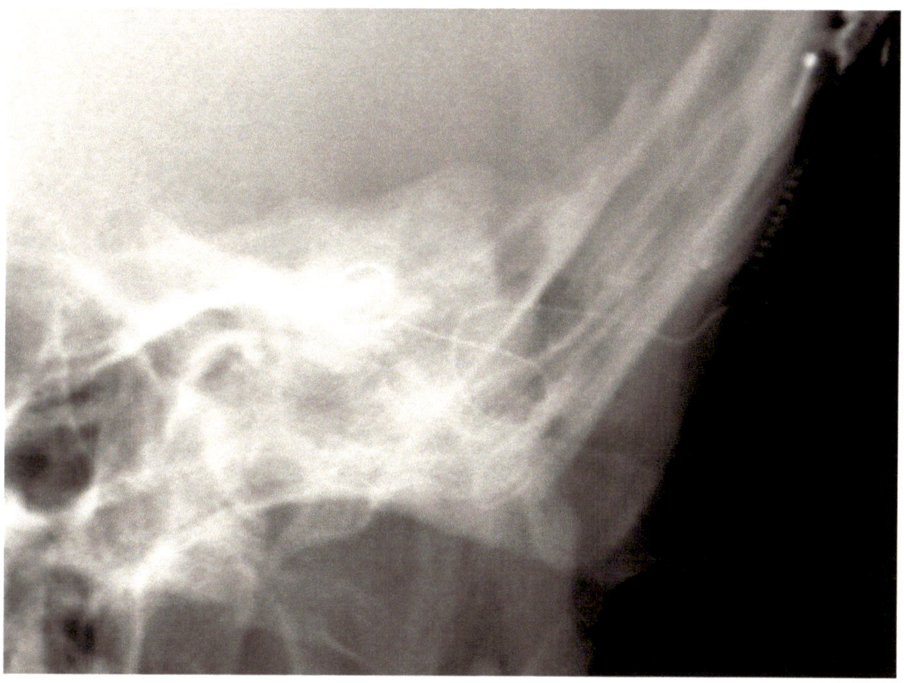

Fig. 13.5.14 Postoperative radiography shows a nicely curved electrode.

Comment

With partial ossification and difficult landmarks, the approach is easier in a canal wall down technique (subtotal petrosectomy).

Case 13.6 Otosclerosis Grade 2, Perioperative Placement of the Electrode into the Double Ring (Fig. 13.6.1–Fig. 13.6.7)

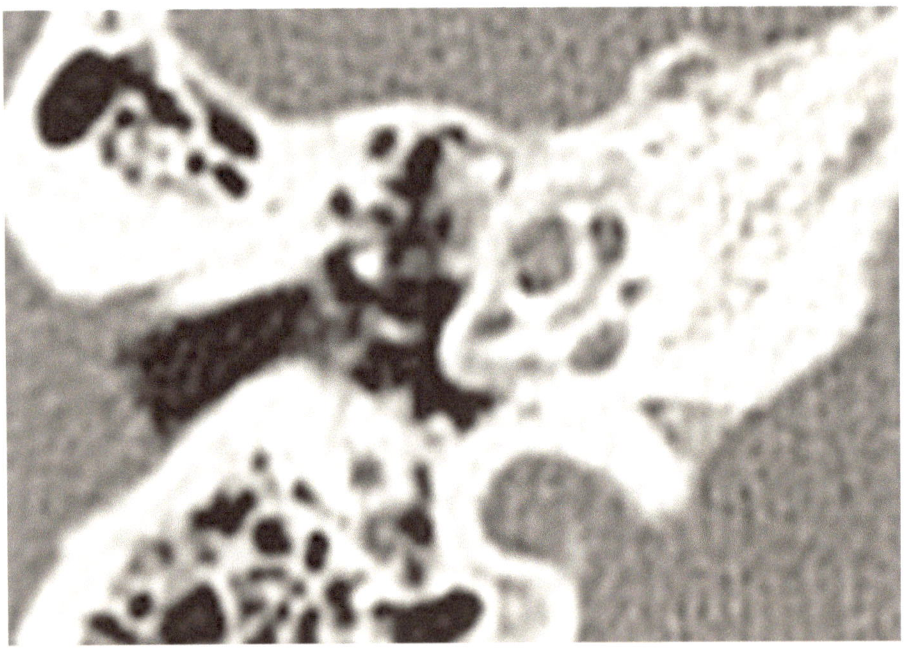

Fig. 13.6.1 A 51-year-old woman with profound deafness due to otosclerosis. On imaging she has clear retrofenestral otosclerosis with a double ring sign, an extra lumen just next to the basal turn and the apical cochlea. Seen here on the right side.

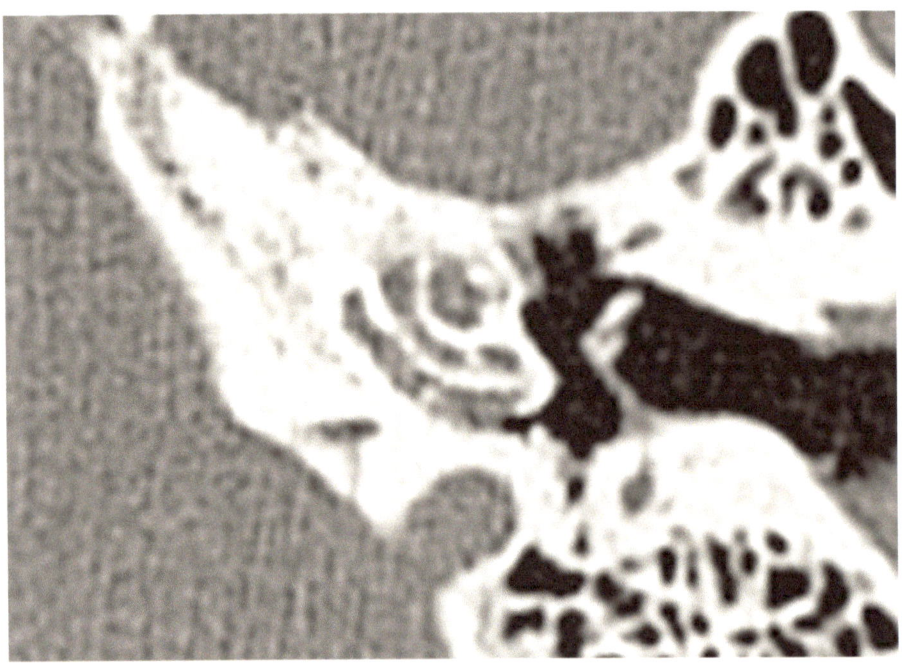

Fig. 13.6.2 On the left side, the same radiologic appearance with an apparent lumen just next to the round window and parallel to the basal turn. The round window is calcified and the basal turn partly ossified.

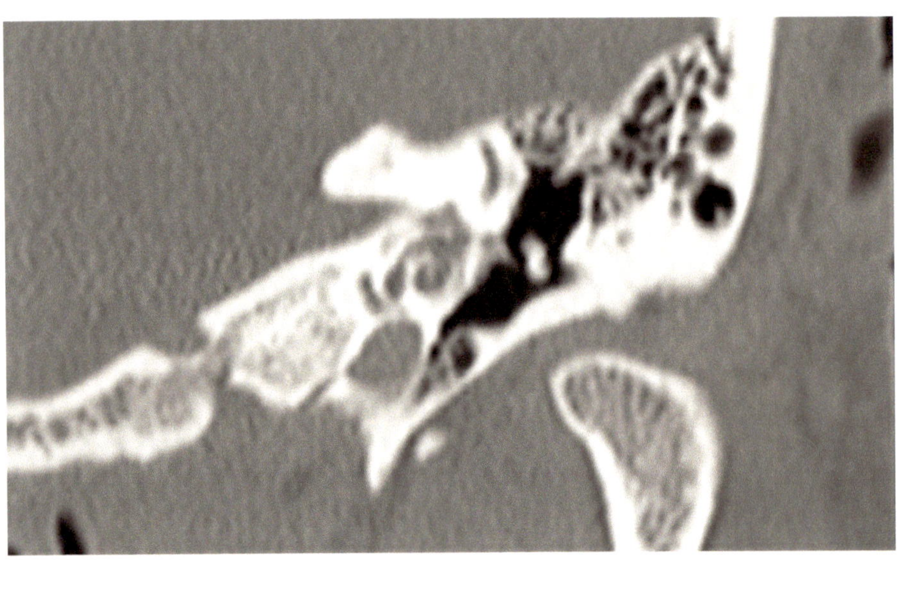

Fig. 13.6.3 The patient still had some benefit from her right hearing aid so her left ear was selected for cochlear implantation. The otospongiotic bone was all around the cochlea so a precurved electrode was chosen for insertion to avoid facial nerve stimulation at the apical electrodes.

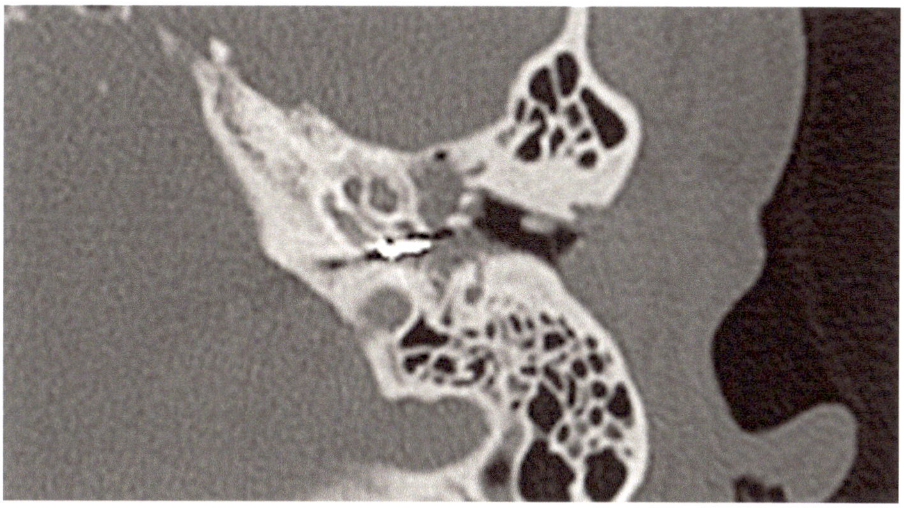

Fig. 13.6.4 The electrode was inserted through a posterior tympanotomy approach and the round window was exposed. A small lumen was found and partly enlarged. The electrode was inserted gently, as shown here.

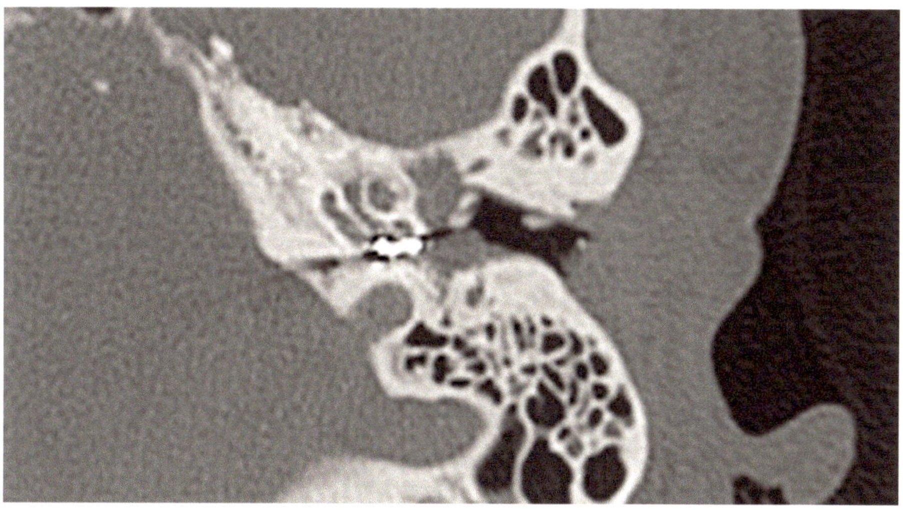

Fig. 13.6.5 After the insertion of several electrodes the resistance increased (a feeling of kinking) and the insertion was stopped before taking out the stylet. A perioperative CT scan showed that the electrode had entered the double ring. A false route had formed and the electrode was taken out.

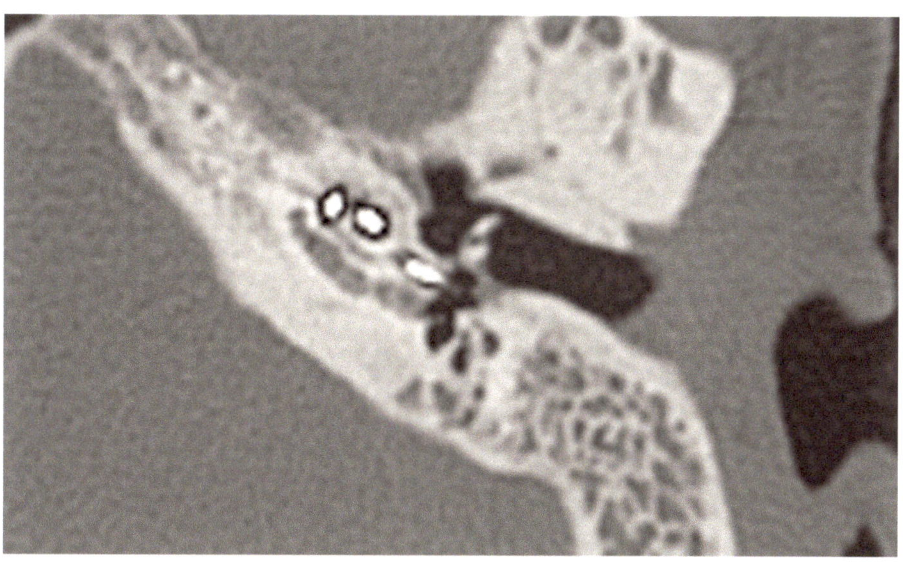

Fig. 13.6.6 After the CT imaging the next attempt was made more anteriorly. After drilling the space between the round window and anterior crus of the stapes, the scala vestibuli was opened.

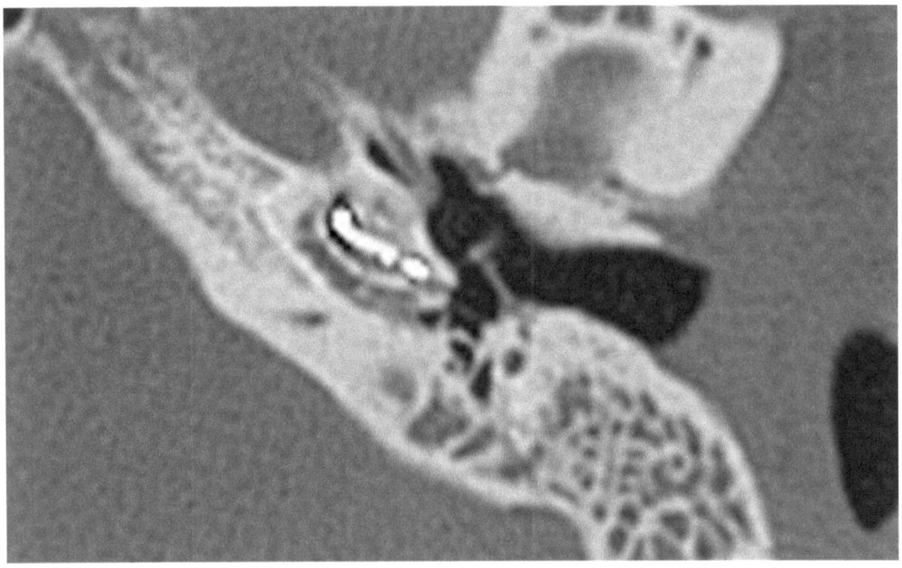

Fig. 13.6.7 This technique led to a proper insertion into the scala vestibuli as the scala tympani was calcified.

Comment

With a double ring, as a false lumen, immediately next to the basal turn of the cochlea, it is probably better to attempt a scala vestibuli insertion. An alternative is to use a canal wall down approach (subtotal petrosectomy) to obtain a better overview of and access to the right scala and avoid false lumen insertion.

Case 13.7 Severe Cochlear Otosclerosis (Grade 3). Sequential CI Placement with Unilateral Placement of the Electrode into the Internal Auditory Canal (Fig. 13.7.1–Fig. 13.7.19)

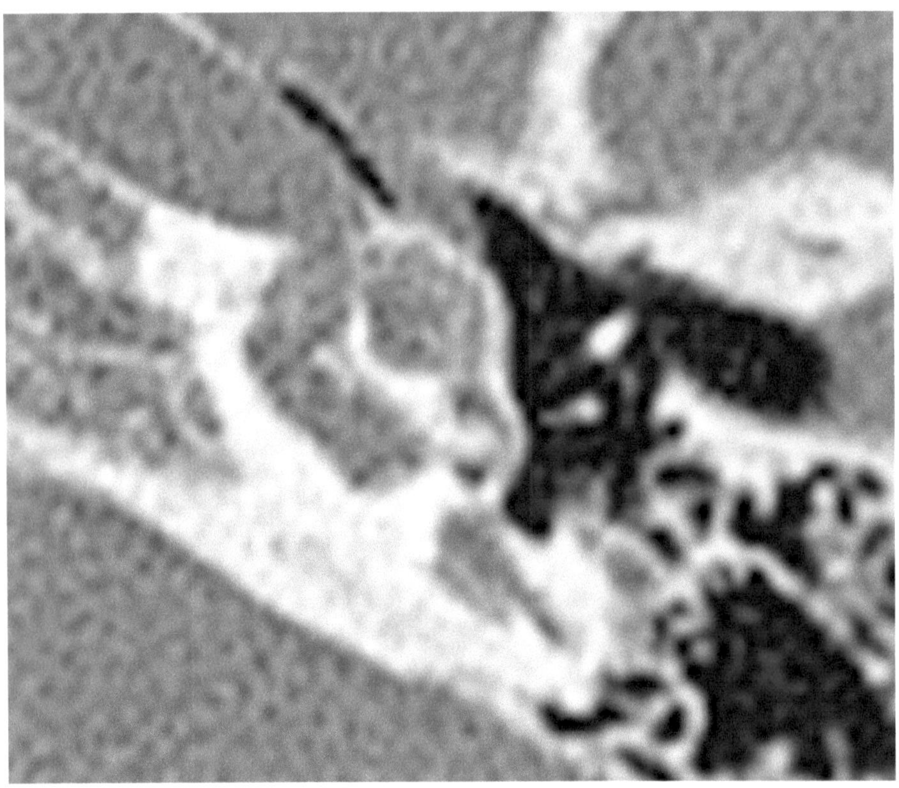

Fig. 13.7.1 In this 33-year-old man with severe hearing loss, we found severe cochlear otosclerosis on CT scanning. The contour of the left cochlea is hardly visible.

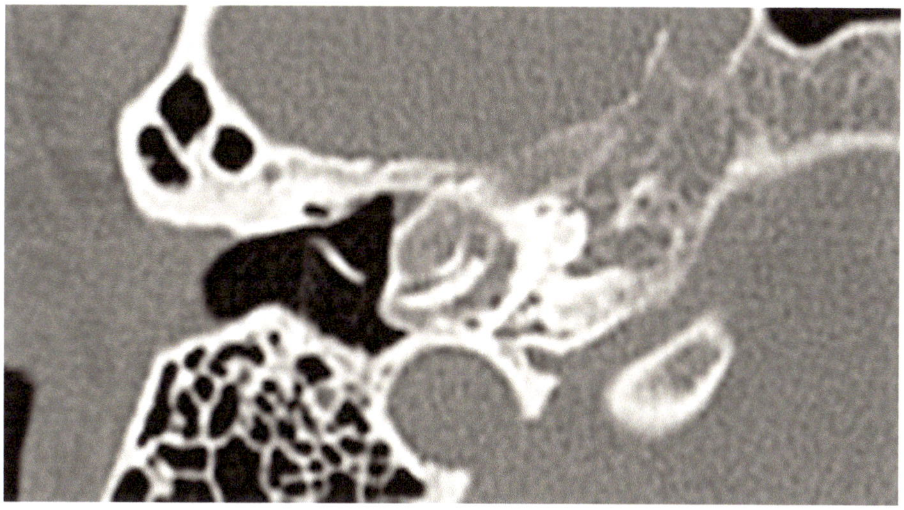

Fig. 13.7.2 The right ear had even worse hearing loss and a hearing aid did not add much to his hearing. Cochlear implantation on the right side was planned. For access, safety, and prevention of complications a subtotal petrosectomy should have been chosen; the standard procedure was chosen due to inexperience.

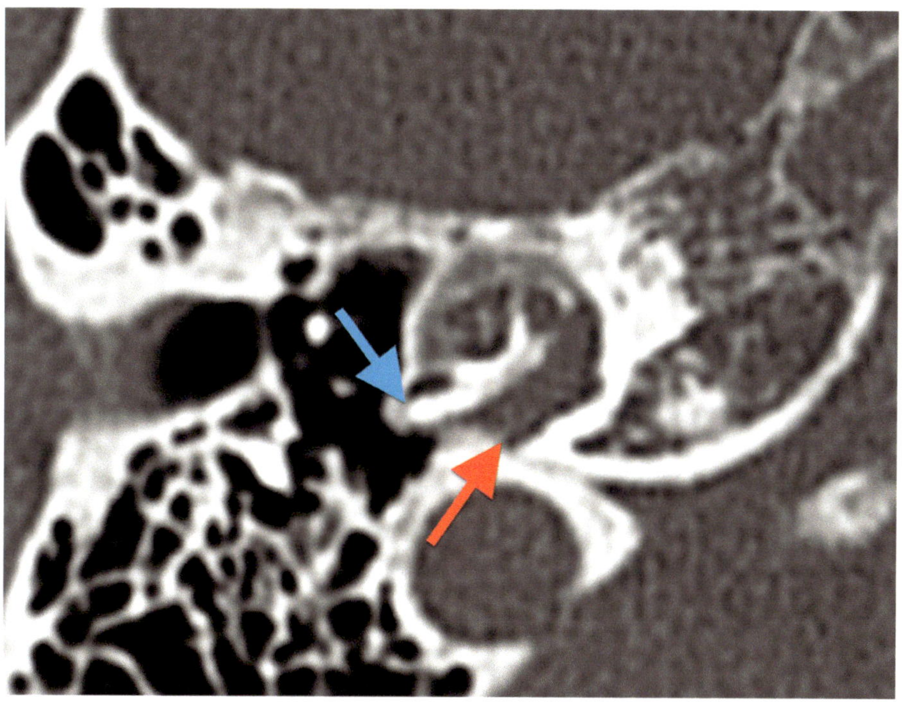

Fig. 13.7.3 The right cochlea is surrounded by a decalcified otospongiotic area (*red arrow*) parallel to the basal turn. The round window and scala tympani are calcified (*blue arrow*) and during surgery will be unrecognizable. A false route can easily complicate the insertion.

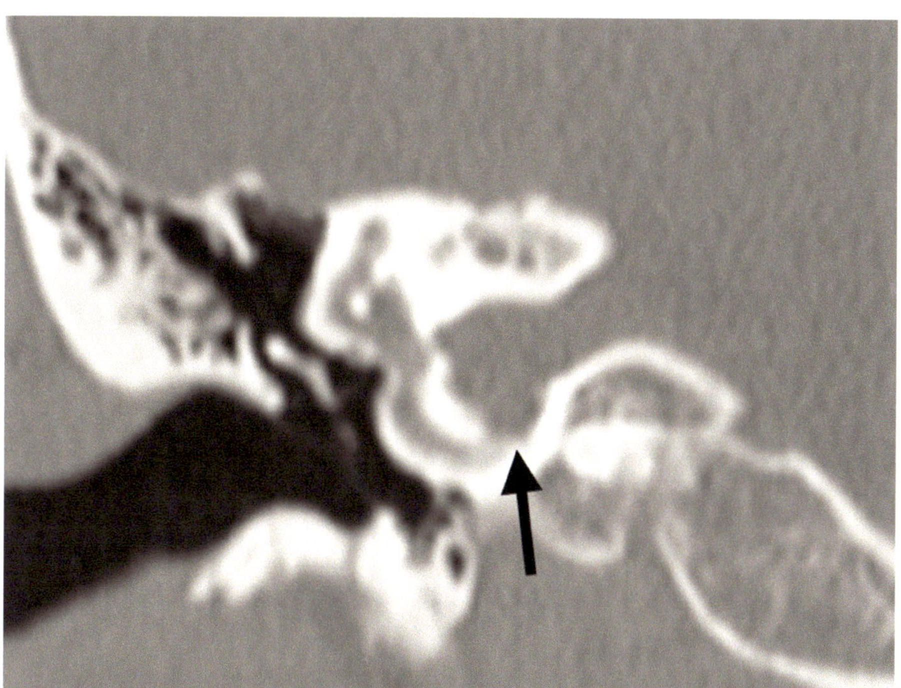

Fig. 13.7.4 On coronal CT scan the bony internal auditory canal is also decalcified (*black arrow*) making the natural bony border of the basal turn and internal auditory canal fragile.

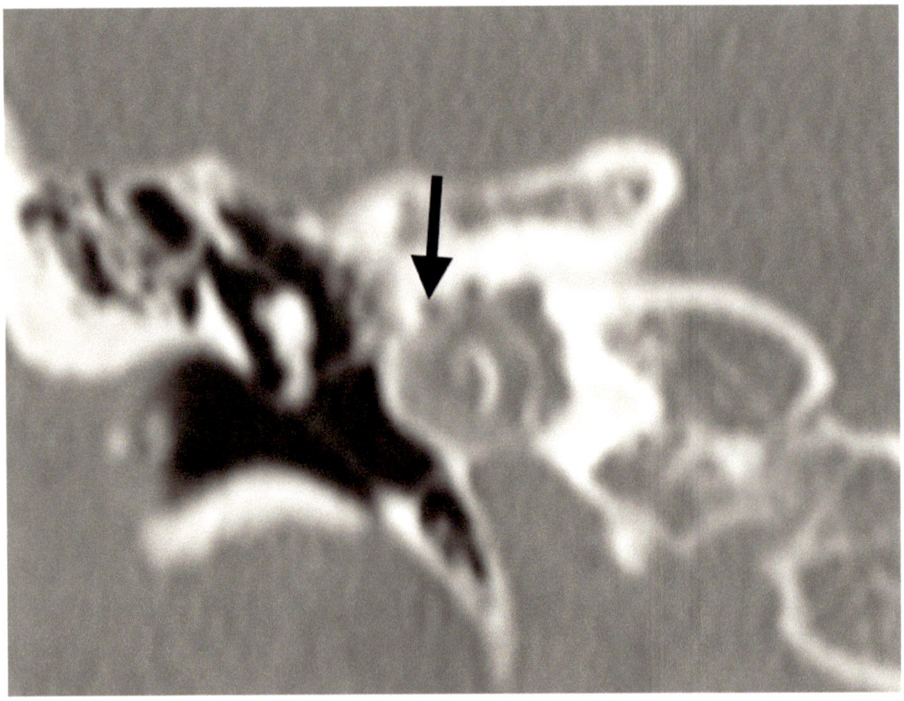

Fig. 13.7.5 The otic capsule is also decalcified on the superior border, which makes the electrical resistance much less toward the facial nerve (*black arrow*). Stimulation of the nerve could be a postoperative problem, as explained preoperatively to the patient.

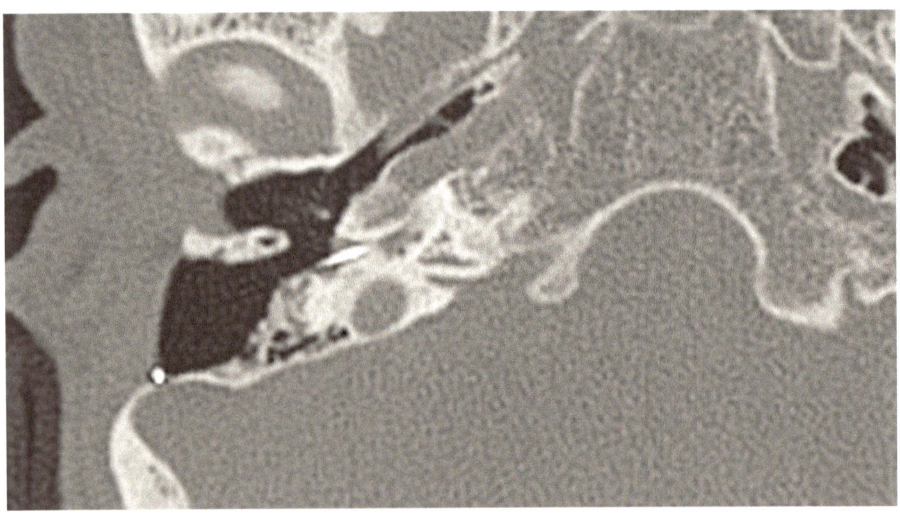

Fig. 13.7.6 The round window area was opened by a posterior tympanotomy approach and immediately a CSF gusher appeared. The gusher subsided after several minutes and the electrode was inserted into the lumen created at the round window. The insertion was accomplished without any problem or resistance. Halfway NRT measurements were done to verify position. Then the insertion was completed in an advanced-off-stylet manner.

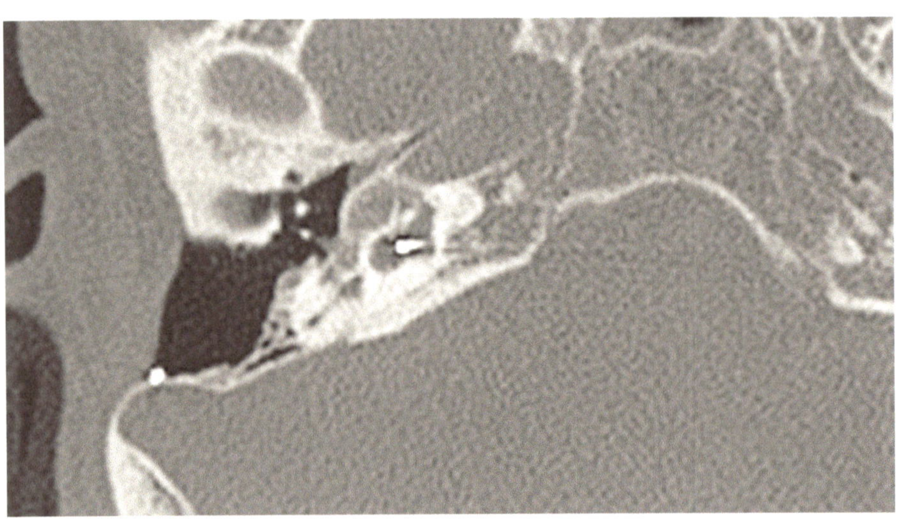

Fig. 13.7.7 A perioperative CT scan was done to confirm position. The electrode, as shown here, was beyond the cochlea and into the internal auditory canal. Many electrodes produced facial stimulation in neural response measurement.

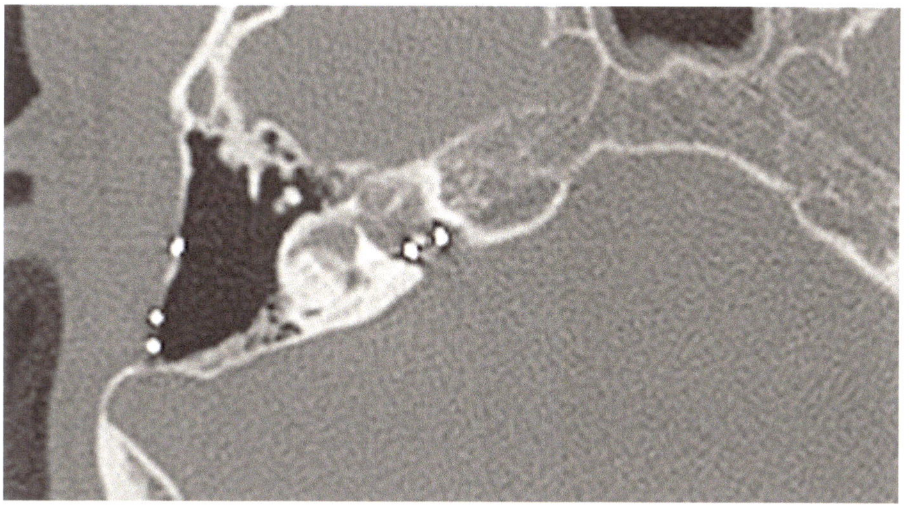

Fig. 13.7.8 The basal electrodes (8 out of 21) gave auditory responses. The electrode was kept in (with the curl in the internal auditory canal as shown here) and not pulled out because of the potential risk. The cochleostomy was packed securely. As mentioned before, a subtotal petrosectomy would have been the second line of defense with the risk of meningitis in this case with a CSF gusher.

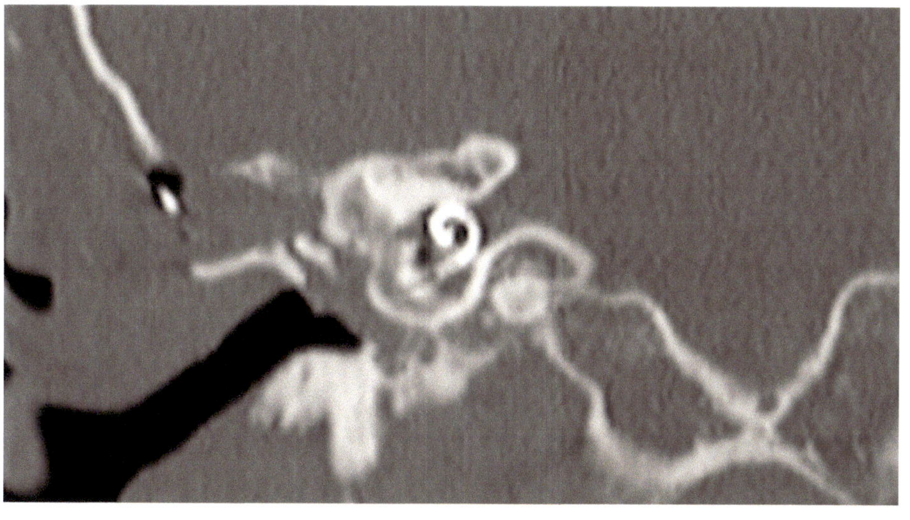

Fig. 13.7.9 With the electrode in the internal auditory canal but with 8 electrodes working properly, the patient was rehabilitated and scored 100% open-set speech performance. This good result lasted for a year and then diminished to 85%. The other ear was evaluated for implantation.

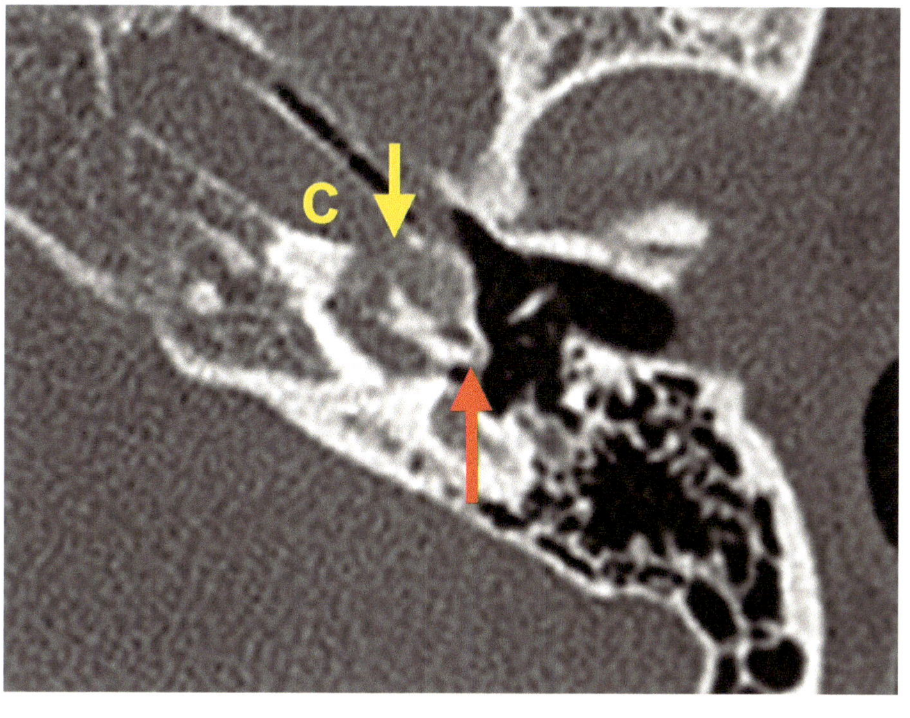

Fig. 13.7.10 The left ear CT scan showed a similar aspect to the right ear prior implantation. The round window was fully calcified (*red arrow*) and the otic capsule was severely decalcified *(yellow arrow)*. Not mentioned at the right ear (as less visible in **Fig. 13.7.7**) but the natural bony border to the carotid artery (C) has been diminished at both sides.

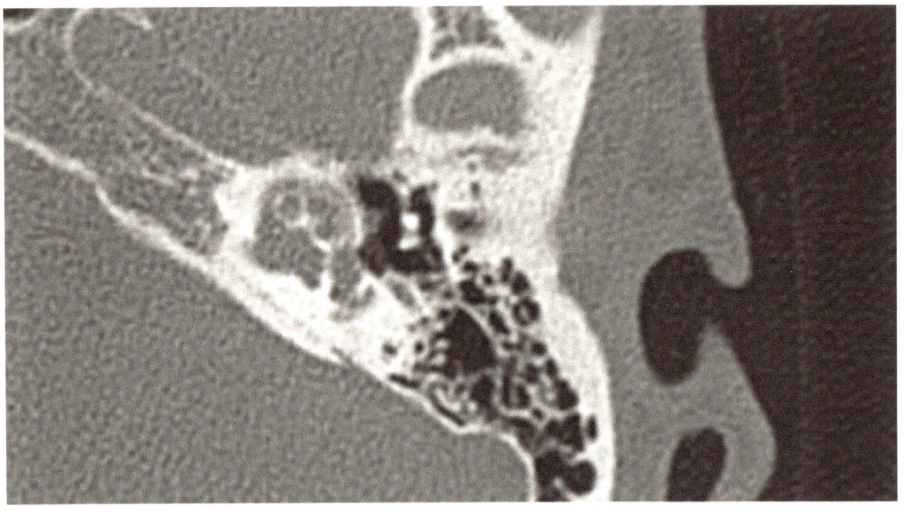

Fig. 13.7.11 Similar to the right ear, the internal auditory canal was decalcified at the border of the cochlea. Again there is a risk of insertion via a false route.

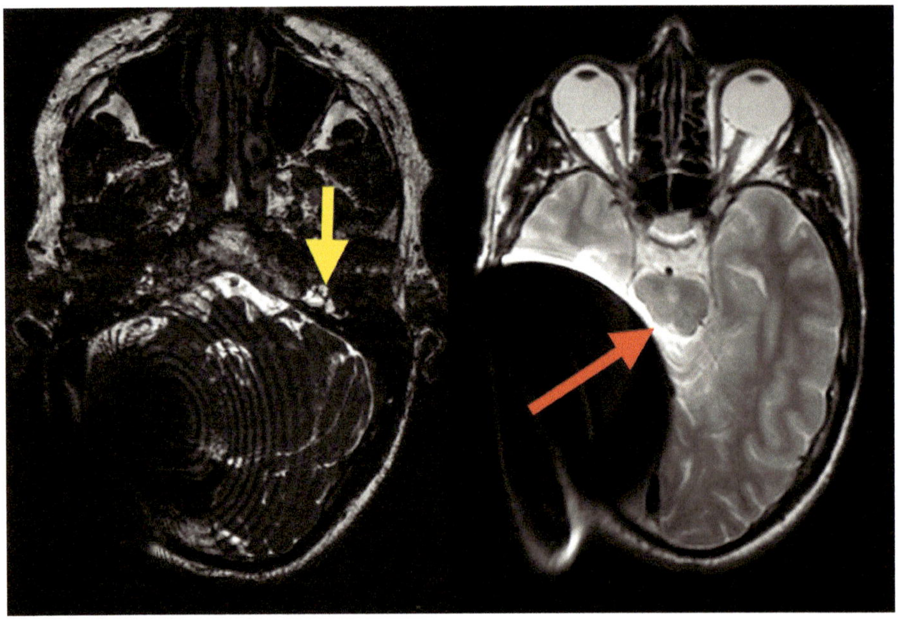

Fig. 13.7.12 The obliteration of the scala tympani was also assessed with MRI. A 1.5 T MRI scan was performed with a firm head bandage. This was painful but no harm to the CI was noted. A clear artifact due to the magnet is seen at the implanted ear (T2 sequence, *red arrow*). The contralateral inner ear is still visible (CISS sequence, *yellow arrow*).

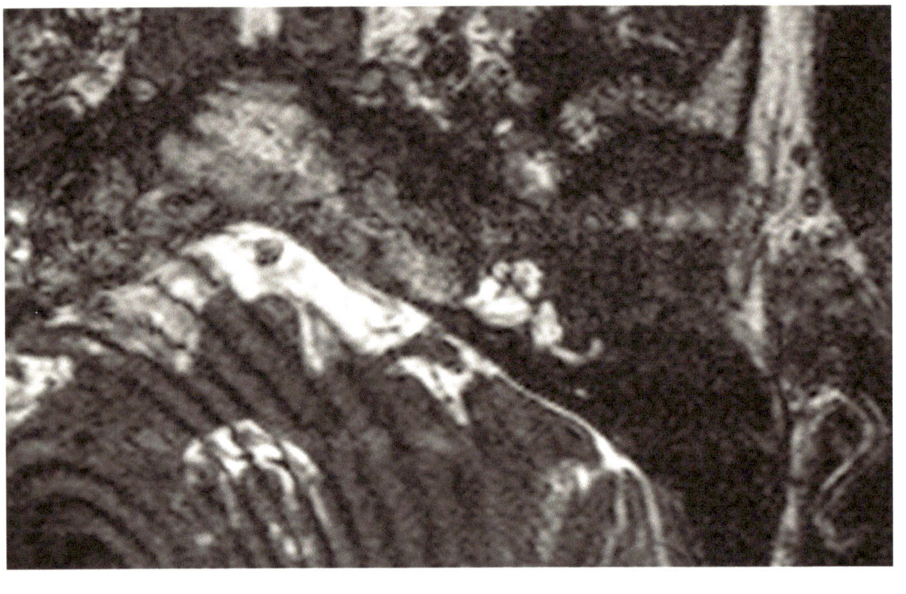

Fig. 13.7.13 A widening of the internal auditory canal is also appreciated on MRI. Furthermore, the middle and apical turn appear well filled with fluid with no obliteration.

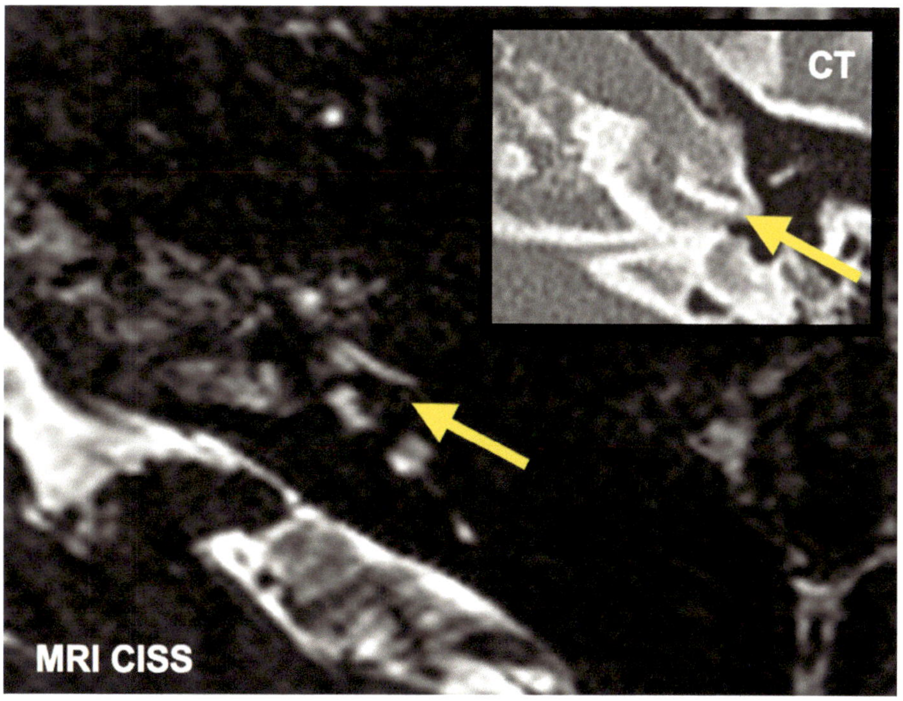

Fig. 13.7.14 Scala tympani ossification. The basal turn is different. It is obliterated within the scala tympani, as shown here on a MRI CISS sequence image and the corresponding CT image as insert (*yellow arrows* point to the obliteration/fluid loss). A scala vestibuli approach is the planned procedure in this case.

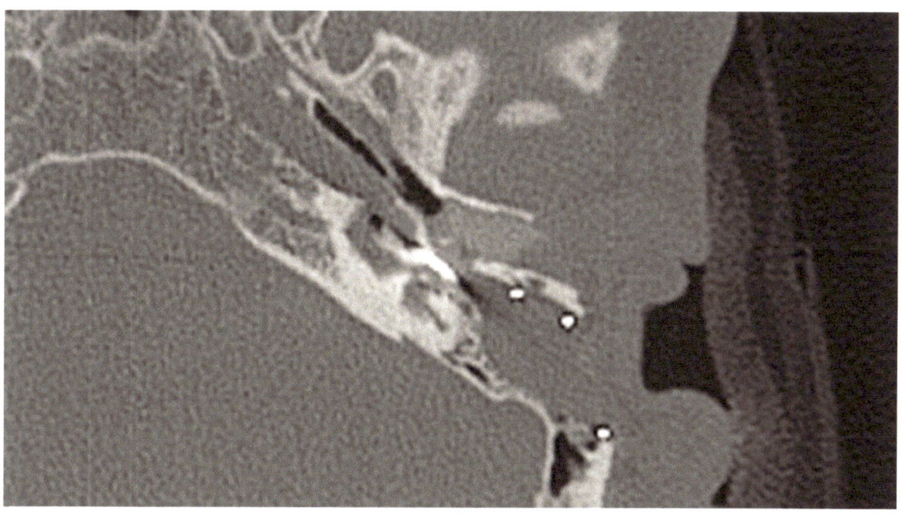

Fig. 13.7.15 The surgery was planned with the option of a CT scan during surgery. A perioperative CT was done after opening of the scala vestibuli and insertion of the first part of the electrode. Perioperative blood collection is seen in the mastoid and ear canal. The more hyperintense part in the external auditory canal is probably iodine. Neural response was positive and the scan shows good positioning into the cochlea.

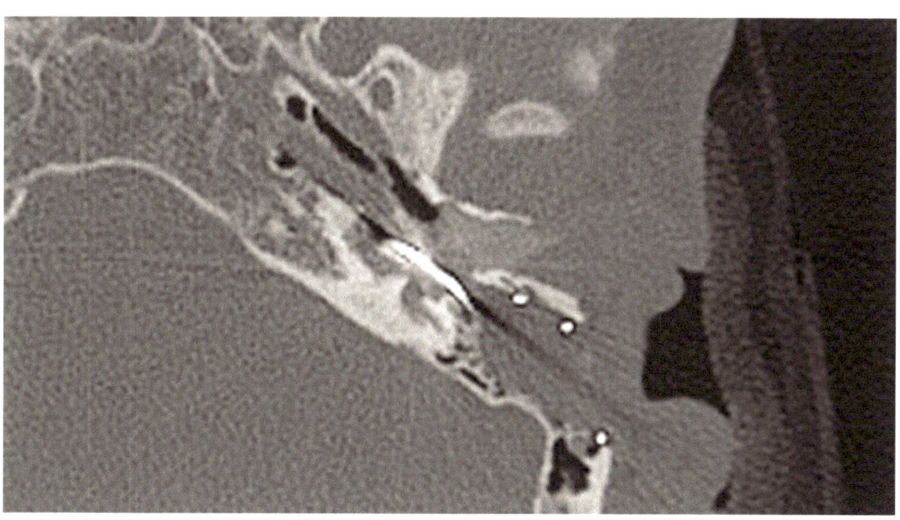

Fig. 13.7.16 Another perioperative CT image. The electrode is anterior of the calcified scala tympani. There was no gusher during this surgery.

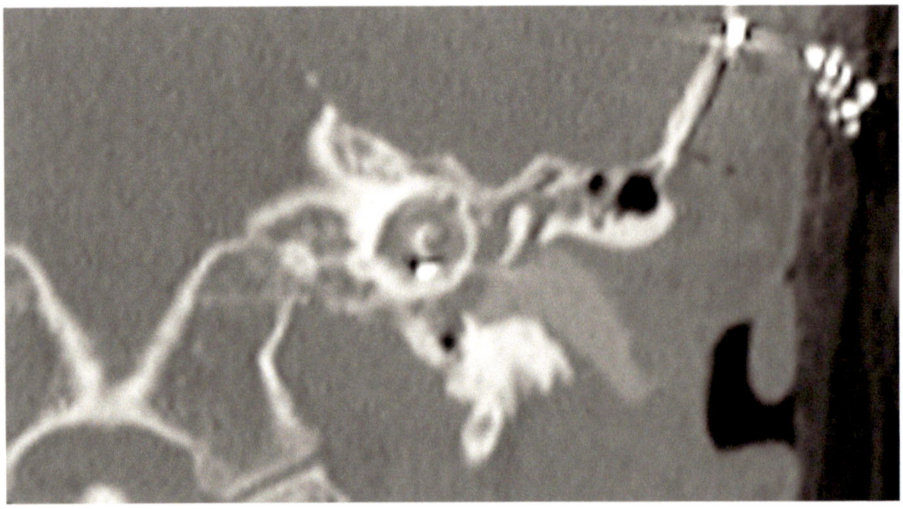

Fig. 13.7.17 A perioperative coronal CT image is less informative as the border toward the internal auditory canal is hard to see in these images. The electrode was gently advanced off the stylet and secured in the cochleostomy.

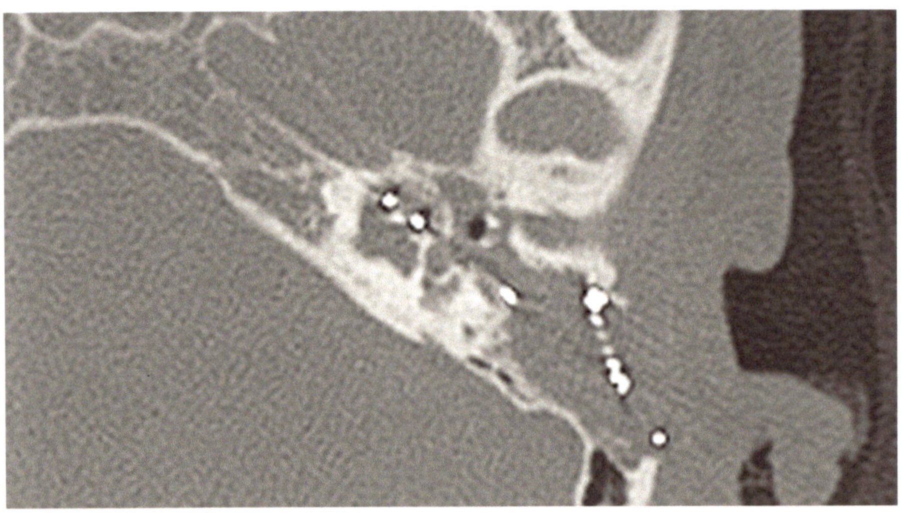

Fig. 13.7.18 After surgery the CT shows the curl of the electrode within the cochlea and not within the internal auditory canal.

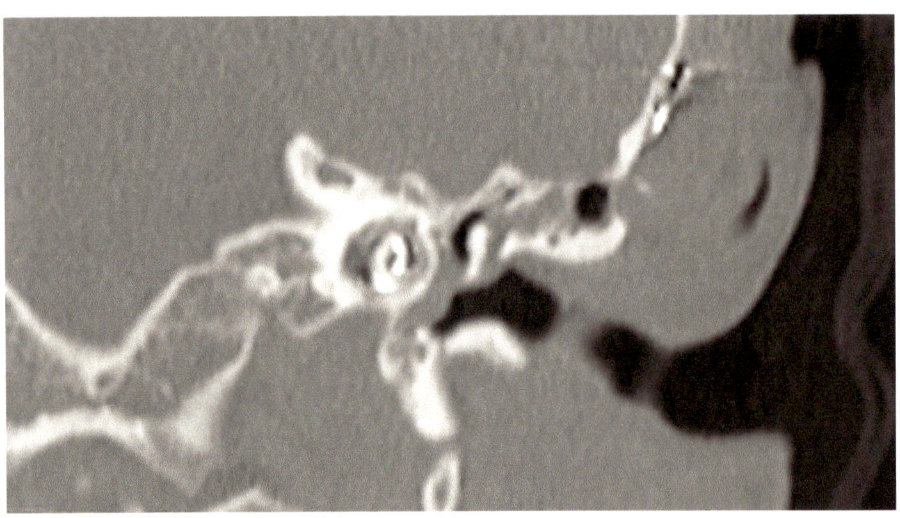

Fig. 13.7.19 The coronal scan shows the complete curved electrode within the cochlea postoperatively. Within a couple of months the patient had 100% speech performance and now uses his telephone again.

Comment

Severe otosclerosis with the chance of a false lumen insertion, or insertion into the carotid artery of the internal auditory canal, can present various lessons. First, the electrode should be inserted with no force and preferably using a straight/flexible electrode. Second, the occurrence of a CSF gusher is better controllable and this improves prevention of meningitis. Third, placement of a CI is possible, even in severe otosclerosis; an ABI does not seem indicated.

Case 13.8 Revision Surgery with Cochlear Ossification after Stapedotomy (Fig. 13.8.1–Fig. 13.8.8)

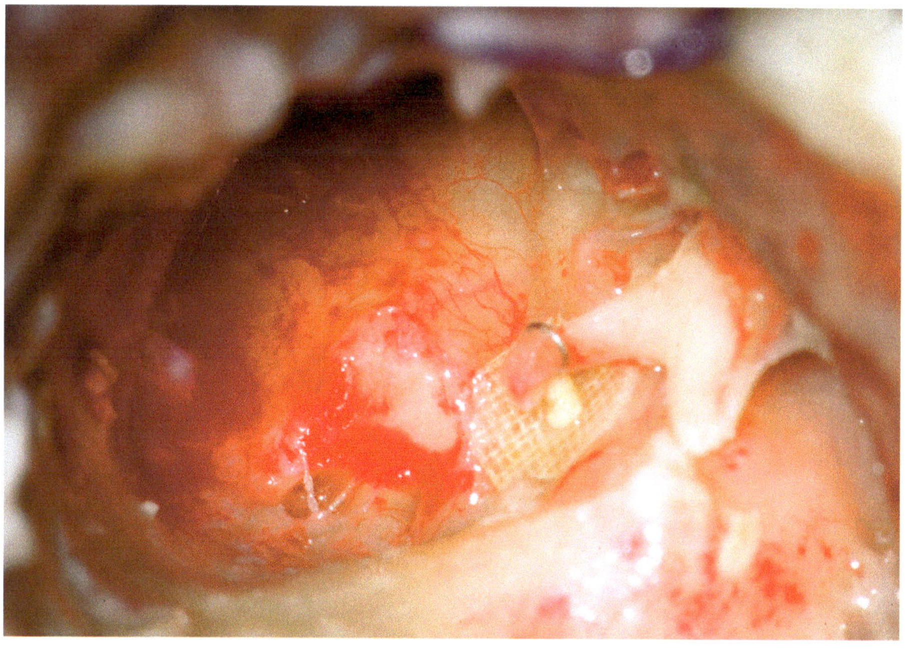

Fig. 13.8.1 This patient underwent surgery for advanced otosclerosis in another department but without result, and this was followed by progressive profound hearing loss. The posterior canal wall has been removed, and the malleus is taken out. Arrangement of the prosthesis with respect to the incus is shown. Silicon sheeting covers the oval window.

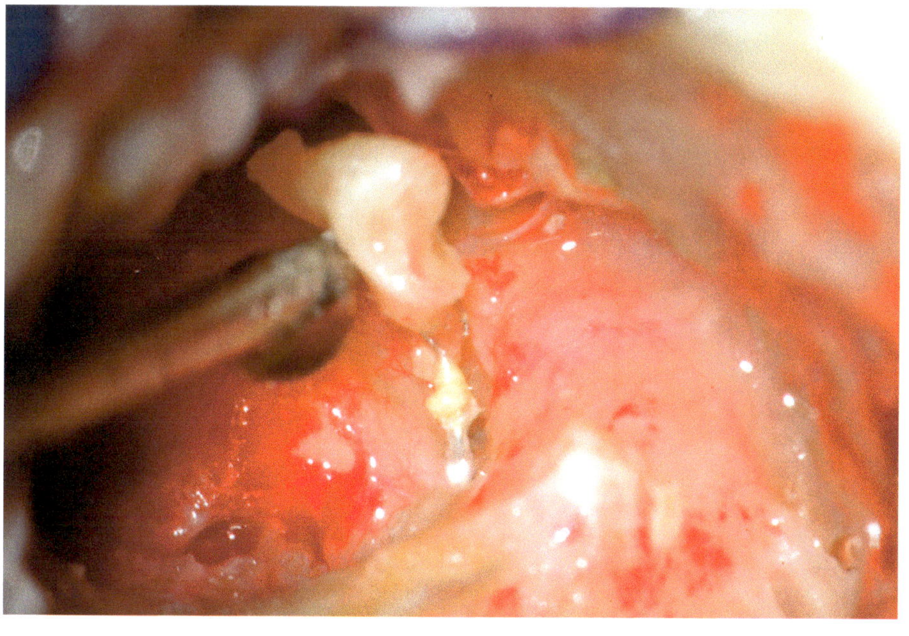

Fig. 13.8.2 The incus is removed, and the prosthesis is taken out.

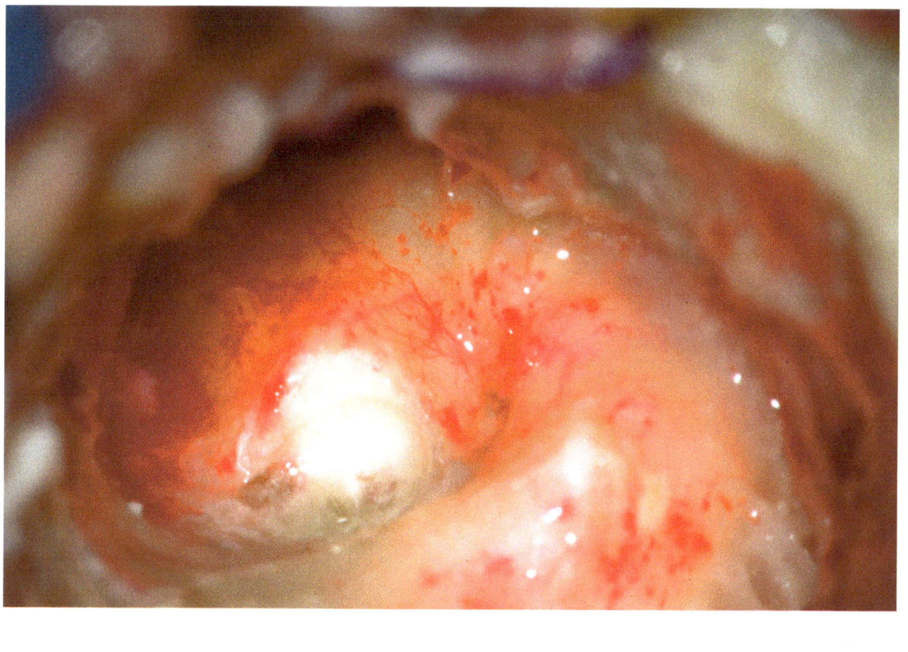

Fig. 13.8.3 The promontory is drilled to open the cochlea. As seen, the basal turn of the cochlea is ossified.

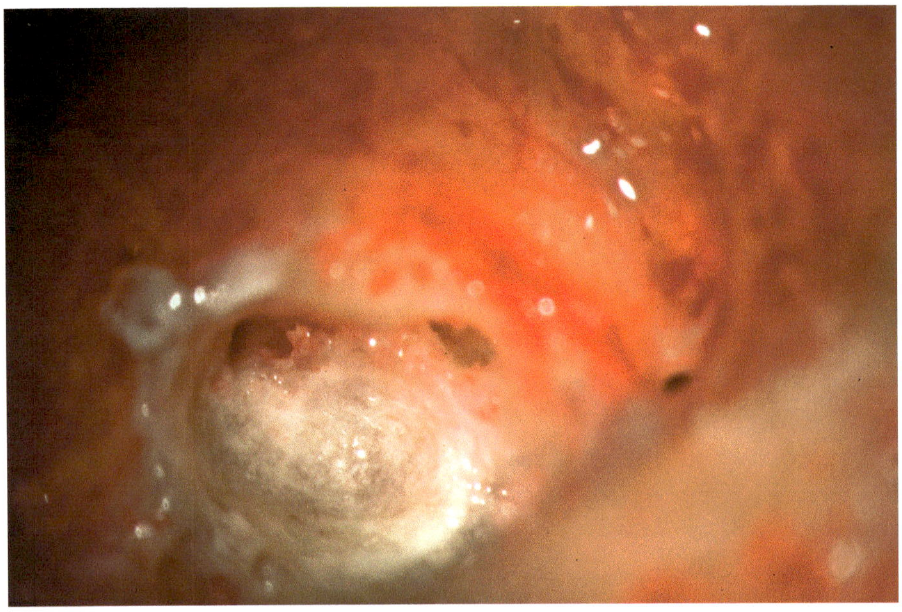

Fig. 13.8.4 The ossified basal turn is opened near the area of the round window.

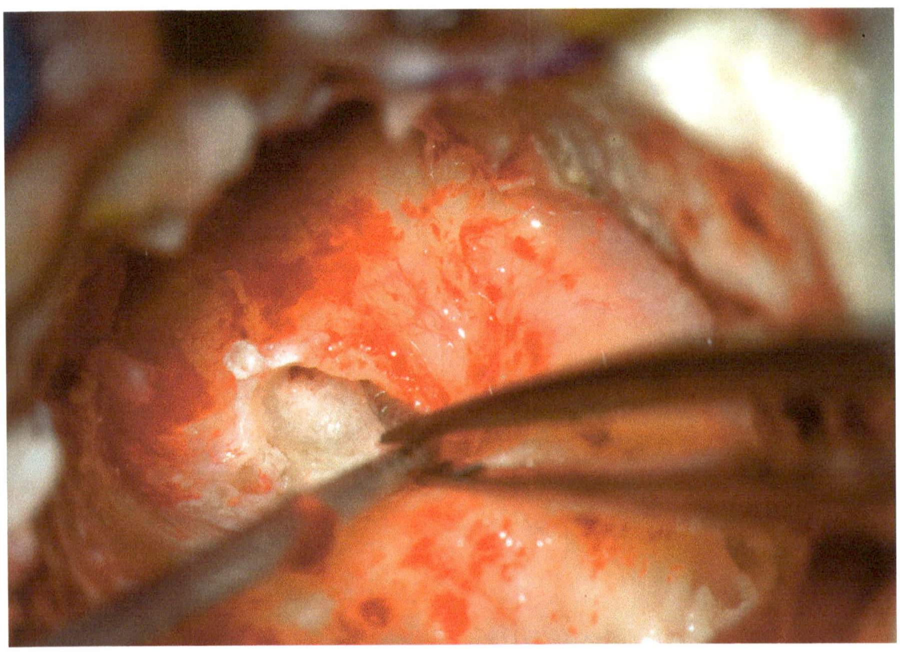

Fig. 13.8.5 The array is introduced into the cochlea with watchmaker's forceps.

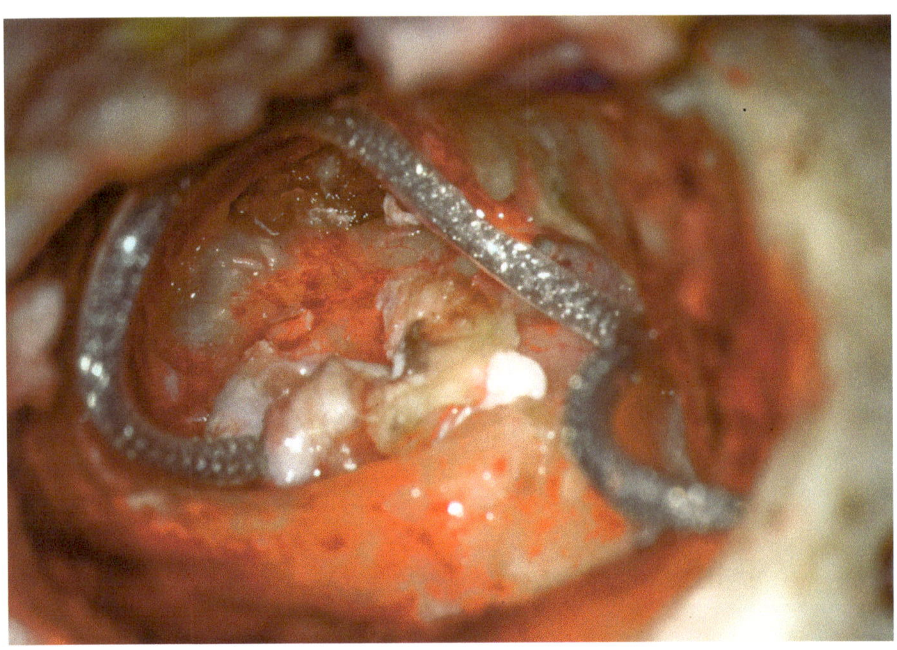

Fig. 13.8.6 After completion of the insertion, the opening is closed with pieces of periosteum.

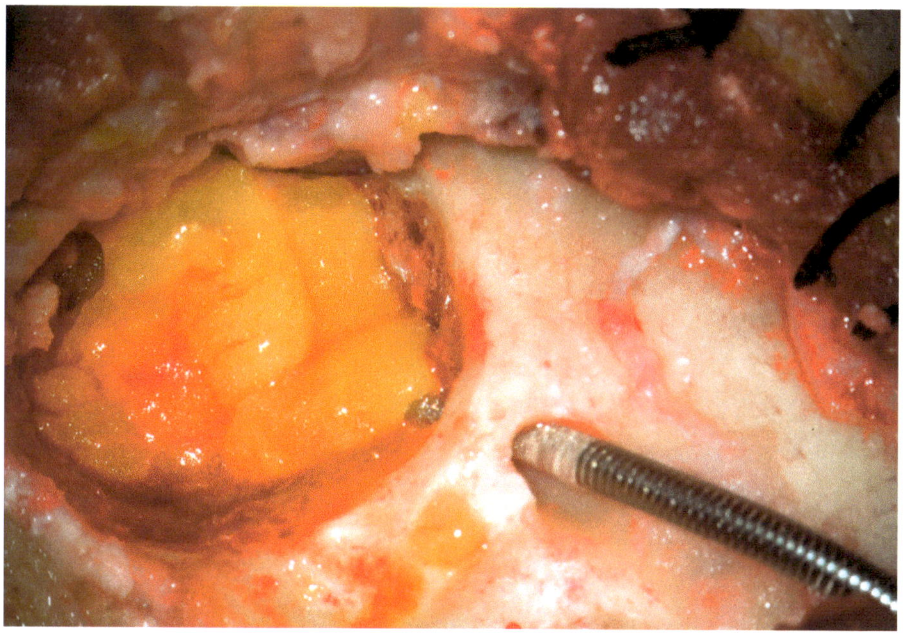

Fig. 13.8.7 The cavity is packed with abdominal fat. Note that the electrode array is passed through a hole for optimal anchorage without ligation.

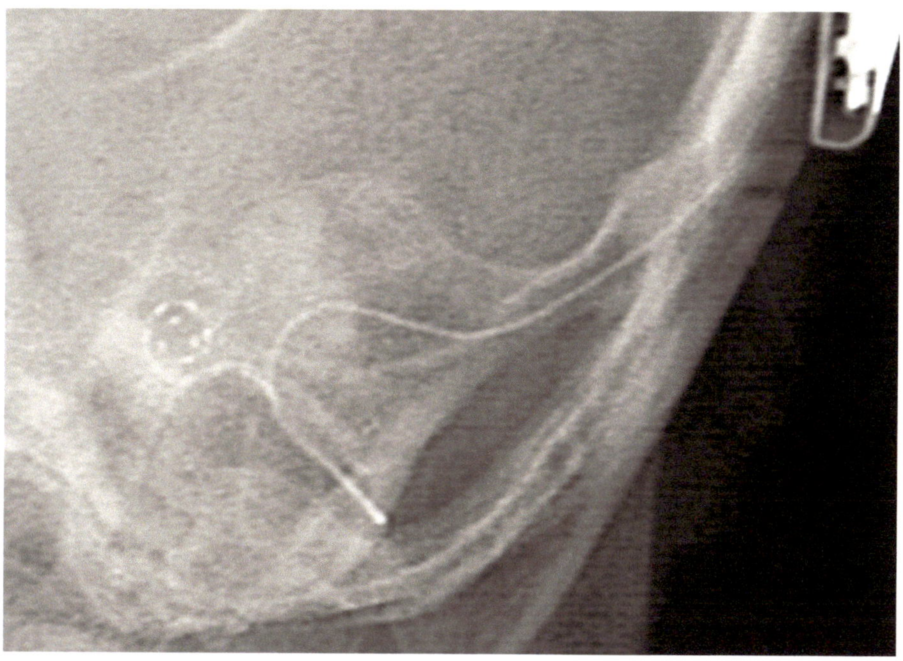

Fig. 13.8.8 Postoperative radiography shows a good arrangement of the electrode array.

Pearls and Pitfalls in Otosclerosis

Assessment

- Many otosclerosis patients have mixed hearing loss, which is unmeasurable once they have severe to profound hearing loss. Try to find older audiograms to confirm the conductive status.
- In case of conductive hearing loss consider stapedotomy as a rehabilitation option before considering a CI.
- Thoroughly examine the CT scan to plan the correct approach.
- On CT scan: watch for calcification of the round window and scala tympani. Watch for otospongiotic changes around the cochlea (double ring), especially next to the round window. Watch for previous chain reconstruction.
- When a CT scan shows multiple otospongiotic (decalcified) lesions around the cochlea, beware of the fragile bony border toward the internal auditory canal, facial nerve, and carotid artery.
- Counsel the patient according to the lesions seen on the scan. Mention if appropriate: CSF gusher, postoperative facial nerve stimulation, misplacement of the electrode, longer surgery time, and fitting problems.
- In case of prominent calcification of the scala tympani, especially in combination with an otospongiotic double ring, consider a subtotal petrosectomy. It will give better access, a better overview, and a direct solution in case of CSF leakage. It will also diminish the chance of postoperative cochleitis or meningitis.
- If possible, consider a perioperative CT scan and/or perioperative neural response measurements to ensure the correct placement before proceeding with the surgery/implantation.

Surgery

- Make sure that you choose the correct approach (posterior tympanotomy or subtotal petrosectomy, scala tympani, or scala vestibuli) in case of expected difficulties.
- Beware of changed landmarks. Often the round window is not visible because of calcification.
- Beware of CSF gushers and make a large enough cochleostomy opening to seal firmly with periosteum pieces.
- During surgery stimulate all electrodes to reveal facial nerve stimulation (FNS). This is often seen in the middle electrodes as they are in the superior part of the cochlea.

Postoperative

- If FNS is present, start the fitting by shutting off the electrode with FNS. Then try electrode-by-electrode to switch these electrodes on again.
- Sometimes high voltages are needed in otospongiotic cochleae because of the low resistance of the decalcified otic capsule. The current will spread easily.

References

1. Rotteveel LJ, Proops DW, Ramsden RT, Saeed SR, van Olphen AF, Mylanus EA. Cochlear implantation in 53 patients with otosclerosis: demographics, computed tomographic scanning, surgery, and complications. Otol Neurotol 2004;25(6):943–952
2. House HP, Sheehy JL. Stapes surgery: selection of the patient. Ann Otol Rhinol Laryngol 1961;70:1062–1068
3. Rama-López J, Cervera-Paz FJ, Manrique M. Cochlear implantation of patients with far-advanced otosclerosis. Otol Neurotol 2006;27(2):153–158
4. Fayad J, Moloy P, Linthicum FH Jr. Cochlear otosclerosis: does bone formation affect cochlear implant surgery? Am J Otol 1990;11(3):196–200
5. Marshall AH, Fanning N, Symons S, Shipp D, Chen JM, Nedzelski JM. Cochlear implantation in cochlear otosclerosis. Laryngoscope 2005;115(10):1728–1733
6. Ramsden R, Rotteveel L, Proops D, Saeed S, van Olphen A, Mylanus E. Cochlear implantation in otosclerotic deafness. Adv Otorhinolaryngol 2007;65:328–334
7. Lee TC, Aviv RI, Chen JM, Nedzelski JM, Fox AJ, Symons SP. CT grading of otosclerosis. AJNR Am J Neuroradiol 2009;30(7):1435–1439
8. Psillas G, Kyriafinis G, Constantinidis J, Vital V. Far-advanced otosclerosis and cochlear implantation. B-ENT 2007;3(2):67–71
9. Ramsden R, Bance M, Giles E, Mawman D. Cochlear implantation in otosclerosis: a unique positioning and programming problem. J Laryngol Otol 1997;111(3):262–265
10. Berrettini S, Burdo S, Forli F, et al. Far advanced otosclerosis: stapes surgery or cochlear implantation? J Otolaryngol 2004;33(3):165–171
11. Calmels MN, Viana C, Wanna G, et al. Very far-advanced otosclerosis: stapedotomy or cochlear implantation. Acta Otolaryngol 2007;127(6):574–578
12. Quaranta N, Bartoli R, Lopriore A, Fernandez-Vega S, Giagnotti F, Quaranta A. Cochlear implantation in otosclerosis. Otol Neurotol 2005;26(5):983–987
13. Sainz M, Garcia-Valdecasas J, Ballesteros JM. Complications and pitfalls of cochlear implantation in otosclerosis: a 6-year follow-up cohort study. Otol Neurotol 2009;30(8):1044–1048
14. Toung JS, Zwolan T, Spooner TR, Telian SA. Late failure of cochlear implantation resulting from advanced cochlear otosclerosis: surgical and programming challenges. Otol Neurotol 2004;25(5):723–726
15. Merkus P, van Loon MC, Smit CF, Smits C, de Cock AFC, Hensen EF. Decision making in advanced otosclerosis: an evidence-based strategy. Laryngoscope 2011;121(9):1935–1941
16. van Loon MC, Merkus P, Smit CF, Smits C, Witte BI, Hensen EF. Stapedotomy in cochlear implant candidates with far advanced otosclerosis: a systematic review of the literature and meta-analysis. Otol Neurotol 2014;35(10):1707–1714
17. Bosman AJ, Smoorenburg GF. Intelligibility of Dutch CVC syllables and sentences for listeners with normal hearing and with three types of hearing impairment. Audiology 1995;34(5):260–284
18. Ruckenstein MJ, Rafter KO, Montes M, Bigelow DC. Management of far advanced otosclerosis in the era of cochlear implantation. Otol Neurotol 2001;22(4):471–474
19. Merkus P, Di Lella F, Di Trapani G, et al. Indications and contraindications of auditory brainstem implants: systematic review and illustrative cases. Eur Arch Otorhinolaryngol 2014;271(1):3–13
20. Bigelow DC, Kay DJ, Rafter KO, Montes M, Knox GW, Yousem DM. Facial nerve stimulation from cochlear implants. Am J Otol 1998;19(2):163–169
21. Muckle RP, Levine SC. Facial nerve stimulation produced by cochlear implants in patients with cochlear otosclerosis. Am J Otol 1994;15(3):394–398
22. Rayner MG, King T, Djalilian HR, Smith S, Levine SC. Resolution of facial stimulation in otosclerotic cochlear implants. Otolaryngol Head Neck Surg 2003;129(5):475–480
23. Frijns JH, Kalkman RK, Briaire JJ. Stimulation of the facial nerve by intracochlear electrodes in otosclerosis: a computer modeling study. Otol Neurotol 2009;30(8):1168–1174

Further Reading

Frattali MA, Sataloff RT. Far-advanced otosclerosis. Ann Otol Rhinol Laryngol 1993;102(6):433–437

Ghonim MR, el-Degwy AA, el-Sharabasy AE. Far-advanced otosclerosis. ORL J Otorhinolaryngol Relat Spec 1997;59(6):332–335

Glasscock ME, Storper IS, Haynes DS, Bohrer PS. Stapedectomy in profound cochlear loss. Laryngoscope 1996;106(7):831–833

House WF. Oval window and round window surgery in extensive otosclerosis; a preliminary report. Laryngoscope 1959;69(6):693–701

Iurato S, Ettorre GC, Onofri M, Davidson C. Very far-advanced otosclerosis. Am J Otol 1992;13(5):482–487

Khalifa A, el-Guindy A, Erfan F. Stapedectomy for far-advanced otosclerosis. J Laryngol Otol 1998;112(2):158–160

Lippy WH, Battista RA, Schuring AG, Rizer FM. Far-advanced otosclerosis. Am J Otol 1994;15(2):225–228

Lippy WH, Burkey JM, Arkis PN. Word recognition score changes after stapedectomy for far advanced otosclerosis. Am J Otol 1998;19(1):56–58

Mosnier I, Bouccara D, Ambert-Dahan E, Ferrary E, Sterkers O. Cochlear implantation and far-advanced otosclerosis. Adv Otorhinolaryngol 2007;65:323–327

Myers D, Wolfson RJ, Tibbels EW Jr, Winchester RA. Apparent total deafness due to advanced otosclerosis. Arch Otolaryngol 1963;78:52–58

Shea PF, Ge X, Shea JJ Jr. Stapedectomy for far-advanced otosclerosis. Am J Otol 1999;20(4):425–429

Sheehy JL. Far-advanced otosclerosis; diagnostic criteria and results of treatment; report of 67 cases. Arch Otolaryngol 1964;80:244–249

Wiet RJ, Morgenstein SA, Zwolan TA, Pircon SM. Far-advanced otosclerosis. Cochlear implantation vs stapedectomy. Arch Otolaryngol Head Neck Surg 1987;113(3):299–302

14 Otomastoiditis and Cochlear Implantation

Several types of middle ear and mastoid infections, as well as the presence of a previous canal wall down cavity, can hamper cochlear implantation. This chapter deals with the preoperative management of the following diseases combined with cochlear implantation:

- **Chronic suppurative otitis media**
  - Without cholesteatoma
  - With middle ear atelectasis
  - With cholesteatoma
  - Presence of a radical cavity/canal wall down
- **Otitis media with effusion in children and adults**

Postimplantation chronic and acute middle ear and mastoid disease is dealt with in Chapter 7 and is only briefly mentioned here.

14.1 Chronic Suppurative Otitis Media

Patients with chronic suppurative otitis media (CSOM) might also become candidates for cochlear implantation after losing their sensorineural hearing due to the chronic middle ear infection, cavity infection, or cholesteatoma destruction or due to previous surgery. At the same time some CI candidates may suffer a chronic middle ear infection coincidentally without relation to the cause of their deafness. For both groups cochlear implantation would lead to hearing restoration, but the presence of the infection has been regarded as a (relative) contraindication.[1–5]

The most important risk for cochlear implantation in this group is recurrence of the infection, which could lead to labyrinthitis, meningitis, or extrusion of the implant.[6,7] The latter can be either extrusion of the electrode array out of the cochlea or through the tympanic membrane, or breakdown of the retroauricular skin covering the receiver-stimulator.[3,6–10]

14.1.1 Preoperative Evaluation

The presence of active or inactive chronic middle ear disease is one of the items that has to be queried during the history-taking with each new CI candidate. Special attention should be paid to earlier ear surgery, eustachian tube dysfunction/presence of cleft palate, perforations of the eardrum or frequent use of ventilation tubes, and presence of cholesteatoma or atelectasis during ENT examination. CT images will give additional information such as poor pneumatization of the mastoid, opacified mastoid cells, confirmation of cholesteatoma, or other signs of CSOM. The presence of nasal pathology or allergy has to be checked and treated when required. Patients with higher risks of infection or wound healing problems have to be identified (previous radiotherapy, immune deficiencies).

As the different forms of CSOM can be considered as a continuum, several different options in treatment exist. Which to choose depends on the type of pathology, the patient, and the surgeon's experience and choice. As limited treatment of chronic middle ear disease will very often have only a temporary effect, safer more radical options are favored. This should preferably be decided on before implantation, because revision surgery with radical removal of all pathology in the presence of a CI is difficult if not impossible and carries a serious risk of accidently sacrificing the CI during the procedure. Also, adequate pharmaceutical treatment is difficult once an infection is present, due to biofilm formation on the surface of the cochlear implant.[11–13] For these reasons subtotal petrosectomy (SP) may be considered as the primary surgical solution because it represents the safer option, allowing CI insertion in the same stage in the majority of cases. In presence of a severe preoperative infection, even in SP the CI insertion may be delayed to a second stage to be performed after a few months. More information on SP can be found in Chapter 10.

14.1.2 Surgical Treatment

Simple **perforations** in the tympanic membrane with a dry, inactive middle ear can be closed using a staged procedure, starting with a tympanomastoidectomy or myringoplasty. Three months later, when the drum has proven to be still intact without signs of CSOM or otitis media with effusion (OME) the cochlear implantation can be performed using posterior tympanotomy approach.[14] However, in some cases, the perforation functions as a physiologic grommet, preventing active disease (CSOM/OME). The myringoplasty (with or without mastoidectomy) could cause the CSOM to reappear and interfere with the cochlear implantation. Simple failure of the myringoplasty should also be considered. For these reasons subtotal petrosectomy and cochlear implantation (SP + CI) in one stage can be the preferred option.[15]

In **CSOM without cholesteatoma** the infection has to be eradicated. Staged surgery can be performed, with at least 3 months between tympanomastoidectomy and cochlear implantation.[14] The perioperative treatment with antibiotics can be extended into these months. A preoperative culture of the external ear canal can reveal colonization with multidrug-resistant pathogens that can cause lasting infections. Good antibiotic prophylaxis based on such a culture will lower the risk of postoperative infection. In case of an active persistent infection with *Pseudomonas aeruginosa* or multiple resistant *Staphylococcus aureus*, a canal wall up tympanomastoidectomy performed under antibiotic coverage and a longer waiting time before implantation can be necessary. Alternatively, subtotal petrosectomy and CI placement can be performed in these cases, either in one stage or in a two-stage procedure.

In presence of **middle ear atelectasis**, staged canal wall up surgery with strengthening of the tympanic membrane using cartilage can be performed. In these cases, postoperatively a wait and watch policy is advised to allow diagnosis of any recurrence. However, in severe atelectasis, SP is the better option to prevent later development of cholesteatoma or electrode extrusion.[8] This is even more important to consider in patients with a cleft palate, eustachian tube dysfunction, or atelectasis.[7]

In **CSOM with cholesteatoma** either staged canal wall up surgery, staged SP, or SP combined with CI (in one stage) can be performed.

After canal wall up surgery in a cholesteatoma case, however, a longer waiting time of 9 to 12 months is advised. Still, there is never an absolute guarantee of total eradication of disease. Residual or recurrent cholesteatoma can develop long after the 9 to 12 months waiting time. We therefore prefer SP combined with CI. An advantage of SP is the fact that it allows more radical removal of disease and thus lowers the risk of recurrence. A meticulous surgical technique may reduce the risk of residual/entrapped cholesteatoma to almost zero.[15–17] A disadvantage of SP is that the cavity becomes hidden from external inspection, with a need for radiologic follow-up to check for entrapment of cholesteatoma. SP in cholesteatoma cases can be performed in two stages when the ear is actively infected or when the surgeon is not sure of total removal of the disease.

Finally, the presence of a **previous radical cavity** also demands special care. Early attempts to insert a cochlear implant in an existing radical cavity (canal wall down) resulted in a high rate of complications, mainly extrusion of the array through the very thin epithelial lining of the cavity.[4,6,10,18] Also, cavities are in direct contact with the external environment and can easily and repeatedly become infected. Regular cleaning of the cavity once or twice a year at the outpatient clinic can produce damage to the epithelial lining, with a potential risk for the implant. Infections of the cavity confer a higher risk of developing labyrinthitis, meningitis, and implant extrusion. Although there are different techniques for covering the array described (using muscle or cartilage), we feel that SP with abdominal fat is the safest and most permanent solution in cases with a previous radical cavity. Alternatively, a technique with closure of the external ear canal and eustachian tube without abdominal fat obliteration is described, which can be useful in children without much fat.[19] In a dry, inactive cavity SP can be performed in a single stage; in an infected cavity a staged procedure may be considered.

14.1.3 Postoperative Imaging

Follow-up with imaging might be required when there is risk of residual or recurrent cholesteatoma. The presence of a cochlear implant impedes the routine use of MRI for follow-up of cholesteatoma cases, although MRI up to 1.5 T can be used safely after application of a head bandage to fixate the implant.[20,21] However, the visibility of a possible cholesteatoma on MRI will be compromised because of the presence of an 8-cm artifact (see Chapter 3). Removal of the magnet requires only two small procedures (removal and replacement) performed under local anesthesia and in sterile circumstances (in adults), but artifacts from the cochlear implant (up to 3 cm) will still be present. Moreover, both procedures may lead to infection of the surgical site and weakening of the pocket carrying the magnet, giving more risk of displacement.[21]

CT imaging is a good option for follow-up, following the patient at 1, 3, 5, and 10 years postoperatively, even though it is not the gold standard for detecting residual cholesteatoma. The capacity of CT in this situation is improved by the presence of air (in combined approach, staged surgery) or abdominal fat (in SP), both of which create an ideal interface for differentiation. Also repeated CT examinations might demonstrate the lesion to be growing and thus more suspect for cholesteatoma (see Chapter 10, **Fig. 10.1** and **Fig. 10.2**).

14.1.4 Special Populations

Not all patients are equally vulnerable to middle ear infections. There are several groups that need more attention before planning a cochlear implantation. These groups also have a higher risk for complications or loss of the CI postoperatively. The prolonged use of antibiotics (local application using ear drops or systemically applied) can lead to fungal biofilm formation that might also need treatment.[12]

Risk factors for infection or extrusion

- Children under 3 years of age
- Otitis due to multiple resistant bacteria such as *Staphylococcus aureus* or *Pseudomonas aeruginosa*
- Tuberculous otitis media
- Cleft palate/eustachian tube dysfunction
- Immune deficiencies (e.g., AIDS/HIV, diabetes mellitus, chemotherapy, other)
- Radiotherapy
- Osteoradionecrosis
- Multiple skin incisions or previous wound healing problem

Multidrug-Resistant *Staphylococcus aureus/Pseudomonas aeruginosa*/Other

In patients with a history of chronic otomastoiditis/otitis media or in patients with continuous use of a hearing aid, the external ear canal can be permanently colonized with these bacteria. Postoperative infections may be prevented by taking a culture of the external ear canal preoperatively and treating accordingly, starting antibiotics 1 week preoperatively.[22,23]

Tuberculous Otitis Media

Tuberculous otitis media (TOM) presents a rare form of chronic otitis media and is usually only recognized late.[24,25] Specific tests for tuberculosis are not routinely performed. Although the incidence is low, only 0.05 to 0.9% of all chronic middle ear infections in developed countries, worldwide it is rising. Classic symptoms are refractory otorrhea, necrotic eardrums with granulation tissue, white exudate, and single or multiple perforations. Complications can comprise sensorineural hearing loss, fistulas, facial paralysis, labyrinthitis, osteomyelitis, and spread of infection to the central nervous system (CNS). When no reaction to antibacterial or antifungal therapy is seen, TOM has to be considered. Intensive treatment with antituberculosis therapy should be started and continued for at least 6 months.[24–27] It is wise to perform cochlear implantation only after adequate treatment. Cochlear fibrosis or ossification in TOM has been reported[26] and seems likely to occur in part of the TOM population due to the long-lasting inflammation. Loss of sensorineural hearing in TOM patients could also be the result of the antituberculosis therapy (aminoglycosides). Interactions occur between HIV infection and tuberculosis and therefore HIV testing is recommended in patients with TOM.

Cleft Palate/Eustachian Tube Dysfunction

Due to eustachian tube dysfunction in patients with a cleft palate (or in patients with middle ear atelectasis), there is a higher risk for CSOM with development of cholesteatoma or OME. SP technique is advised.[7]

Radiotherapy

Previous radiotherapy can lead to sensorineural hearing loss but can also hamper implantation. Pathologic changes could lead to middle ear effusion, eustachian tube fibrosis, and chronic suppurative otitis media. Radiotherapy can also lead to intracochlear fibrosis and ossification,[28] to fibrosis and scarring of tissues in the internal auditory canal, and to obliterative endarteritis that has an influence on the vessels in the radiation field.[29] As the skin too can be affected (radiation dermatitis), thought should be given to a minimal incision and skin flap design.[29] Management of irradiated cases can be challenging, but an irradiated ear without any infection and rehabilitated with a cochlear implant should still be possible.[29] An SP in combination with a cochlear implant seems a reasonable solution in these rare cases, although some suggest muscle flap obliteration instead of obliteration with fat.[29]

Osteoradionecrosis

In osteoradionecrosis the blood supply to the temporal bone is compromised, with necrosis of bone as a result. Osteoradionecrosis has been reported as a lasting source of infection,[30] possibly with softening of the temporal bone making facial nerve damage more likely. This pathology can be treated with local débridement, local antibiotics and hyperbaric oxygen, and sometimes surgical removal of bone sequesters is necessary. Staged surgery is advised.[30]

14.2 Otitis Media with Effusion

A second group of patients presenting with preoperative middle ear infections are children (and some adults) who present with otitis media with effusion (OME) intermingled with episodes of acute otitis media (AOM). This entity is related to upper airway disease, hypertrophy of the adenoid and tonsils, immature anatomy, eustachian tube dysfunction, and the still developing immune system. In adults OME is seen in the presence of allergy or sinus disease, eustachian tube dysfunction, or atelectasis; or in nasopharyngeal pathology.

In OME cases, pre as well as post cochlear implantation, ventilation tubes can be inserted. Ventilation tubes do not represent a contraindication to cochlear implantation once they are present in a dry, trouble-free ear.[14,31] Checking on adenoid and tonsil hypertrophy, performing a preventive adenoidectomy, and treating allergy or chronic sinus disease are recommended in this population. The management of ventilation tubes in CI patients is not much different than in any other patient with ventilation tubes. Sometimes the tubes have been inserted in combination with ABR measurement for better diagnostics on hearing loss before the cochlear implantation.

It is advised to perform the insertion at least 2 to 6 weeks before CI surgery.[31] Counseling of the patient or parents of a child patient needs to include the higher risk of otitis media and thus meningitis because of the presence of ventilation tubes. Also recommended is counseling of the general practitioner on these higher risks with the need for prescription of systemic antibiotics in case of middle ear disease. Children under 3 years of age are known to have a high incidence of acute otitis media: 50% have three episodes of AOM by 3 years of age and the peak occurs around 1 year.[14] In patients (often children) with middle ear infections, an outpatient check 1 week before surgery is an extra safeguard for adequate preoperative management with better chances of successful surgery. Recent otorrhea, the presence of mucosal edema, and mucopurulent fluid found during surgery are considered contraindications for cochlear implantation. In pediatric CI candidates some surgeons proceed with implantation in the least affected ear to create access to hearing/speech language development, and place a ventilation tube in the contralateral ear that receives a delayed second-side implantation later. This possibility of placing only one implant, because of inflammation in the other ear, has to be included in preoperative counseling of the parents.[31] Further counseling on the delayed second implant might be necessary; not all parents will agree with proceeding with the second implant.

Table 14.1 shows the different middle ear and mastoid infections with their management.

14.3 Postoperative Chronic Middle Ear and Mastoid Disease

Postimplantation infections can be directly related to the surgery or can represent the ongoing middle ear disease that was already present before implantation. Surgeons have to recognize the cases with preexisting pathology before cochlear implant surgery and need to adjust the work-up and surgical strategy.

In postimplantation inactive infection with progression of **atelectasis**, toward development of cholesteatoma or extrusion of the cochlear electrode array through the eardrum, a tympanoplasty with strengthening of the membrane by using cartilage can be performed. Also a postoperative tympanic membrane **perforation** should be closed. Both procedures represent a threat to the cochlear implant or could induce entrapped cholesteatoma. Antibiotic coverage during the procedure is advised. Conversion to an SP may represent a more definitive treatment, but poses more risks for the CI.

In an **active CSOM** without presence of cholesteatoma, treatment with intravenous antibiotics is sometimes sufficient to resolve the infection, even with a CI present. In the presence of fluctuation (of fluid) around the receiver-stimulator, the site needs to be punctured and the fluid needs to be cultured, using either a needle for aspiration or a small incision in the retroauric-

Table 14.1 Preimplantation middle ear and mastoid pathology: management and treatment

Preoperative middle ear disease	Management	Treatment
Otitis media with effusion	In *children*: check adenoid and tonsil hypertrophy, allergy	Ventilation tubes combined with adenoidectomy ± tonsillectomy on indication, 2–6 weeks prior to CI
	In *adults*: check nasopharynx for tumor, allergy, chronic sinus disease	Ventilation tubes Treat nasal disease
Chronic suppurative otitis media	Inactive disease with presence of perforation	Staged surgery with CT and myringoplasty and CI 3 months later or one stage SP + CI
	Inactive disease with atelectasis	Staged CT combined with cartilage strengthening of membrane and CI 3 months later or one-stage SP + CI
	Active infection	Staged surgery with CT under antibiotic coverage with myringoplasty, followed 6 months later by second stage with CI or one stage SP + CI
	Active infection suppurative	Staged surgery: SP and CI 6 months later
	Check allergy, chronic sinus disease	Treat nasal disease
Chronic suppurative otitis media with cholesteatoma	Limited cholesteatoma	Staged surgery, starting with CT with cartilage, 9 months later second look + CI *or*
	Extensive cholesteatoma	SP approach in 1 or 2 stages; second stage after at least 6 months
Radical cavity	Active infection	Staged SP, 6 months later CI
	Stable, dry cavity	One-stage SP + CI
Presence of retracted or perforated eardrum	Cleft palate? Eustachian tube dysfunction? Check adenoid, tonsils, allergy, chronic sinus disease, nasopharynx	Consider one stage SP + CI

Abbreviations: CT, combined approach technique: tympanotomy and mastoidectomy; SP, subtotal petrosectomy.

Table 14.2 Postimplantation middle ear and mastoid pathology: management and treatment

Postimplantation middle ear disease	Examination	Treatment
Otitis media with effusion	Otoscopy, tympanogram	Ventilation tube insertion
Chronic suppurative otitis media Active	Otoscopy, culture CT mastoid: check for cholesteatoma	Intensive treatment with intravenous antibiotics for 10 days, puncture and culture. Repetitive check-ups at outpatient clinic afterward If no result: explantation and IV antibiotics
Inactive		Myringoplasty under antibiotic prophylaxis Repetitive check-ups
Chronic suppurative otitis media with cholesteatoma		Indication for explantation and removal of cholesteatoma, either in one-stage SP + CI, or two-stage SP
Middle ear atelectasis		*Active form:* IV antibiotics Consider tympanoplasty in inactive phase to strengthen membrane under AB coverage *Inactive form:* watchful waiting, regular check of membrane

ular scar. Caution should be taken not to damage the receiver-stimulator or the electrode arrays. An additional head bandage is necessary when a void is present. In limited infections this usually solves the problem, but in more extended infections this may not be sufficient. Biofilm formation could already have started, making pharmaceutical treatment more difficult if not impossible.[11] Then only explantation and reimplantation after settling of the infection (after 3–6 months) remain as a viable option.

In cases with **cholesteatoma** and an implant, explantation of the device seems inevitable. Removal of the cholesteatoma is advised through an SP approach with reimplantation simultaneously or staged after several months.

The rate of explantation for medical reasons, including postoperative infection and implant extrusion, is around 1 to 3% for adults and 2 to 8% for children.[23] Likelihoods for explantation mentioned are 1:3 in the presence of a postauricular abscess and 1:10 in otitis media.[23] Thus these postimplantation infections have to be taken very seriously. Chapter 7 presents some examples of postoperative infections and their management.

Table 14.2 shows the different postoperative middle ear infections with their management.

14.4 Acute Postoperative Middle Ear and Mastoid Infection

Finally, postimplantation acute middle ear infections with/without intratemporal or intracranial complications can also develop in a CI patient. These are also not necessarily related to the CI, but do form a serious threat for the patient and the implant. Treatment needs to be prompt and vigorous, and usually leads to explantation. See **Table 14.2** and Chapter 7.

14.5 Removal of Cochlear Electrode and Use of Dummy Electrode

When a cochlear implant has to be explanted and the cochlea itself is not involved by the infection, it is best to leave the distal, intracochlear part of the electrode array in the cochlea and remove the rest of the implant. In this way the lumen of the cochlea remains patent for future re-implantation but also remains sealed off from the infection. In case of a purulent infection with extension around the electrode array or invasion of the cochlea by the infection, the electrode array needs to be removed. A dummy electrode can be inserted in the cochlea to keep the lumen patent.[32] A higher risk of meningitis is present in the last situation. Antibiotic treatment is necessary perioperatively.

14.5.1 Dummy Electrode

In sporadic cases a dummy electrode is needed to keep the cochlear lumen patent, without placement of an actual cochlear implant. This could be necessary, for example, in active otomastoiditis with meningitis, where the infection is still too active for implantation, but with the need to safeguard the lumen in the cochlea for future insertion (after 3–6 months). Also in revision surgery during which the cochlear implant needs to be removed, the cochlear electrode array should be cut off and left in the cochlea. Only when there is ongoing infection in the cochlea (cochleitis) should the array be replaced with a dummy electrode to keep the lumen accessible for future insertion of a new electrode array (see Case 7.6 in Chapter 7).

A dummy electrode could also be of help in countries where the insurance and reimbursement relating to cochlear implantation takes time to organize, especially in the more acute cases.[32]

Dummy electrodes (sterile nonfunctional electrodes) can be provided on request by the companies supplying the CIs: the diameter needs to be the same size as the electrode of the intended eventual cochlear implant. During the replacement, the fibrous sheath surrounding the dummy electrode can easily be recognized and the real electrode can be inserted using this same sheath to give proper access.

Case 14.1 Cochlear Implantation in a Patient with Radical Cavity Right Ear (Fig. 14.1.1–Fig. 14.1.16)

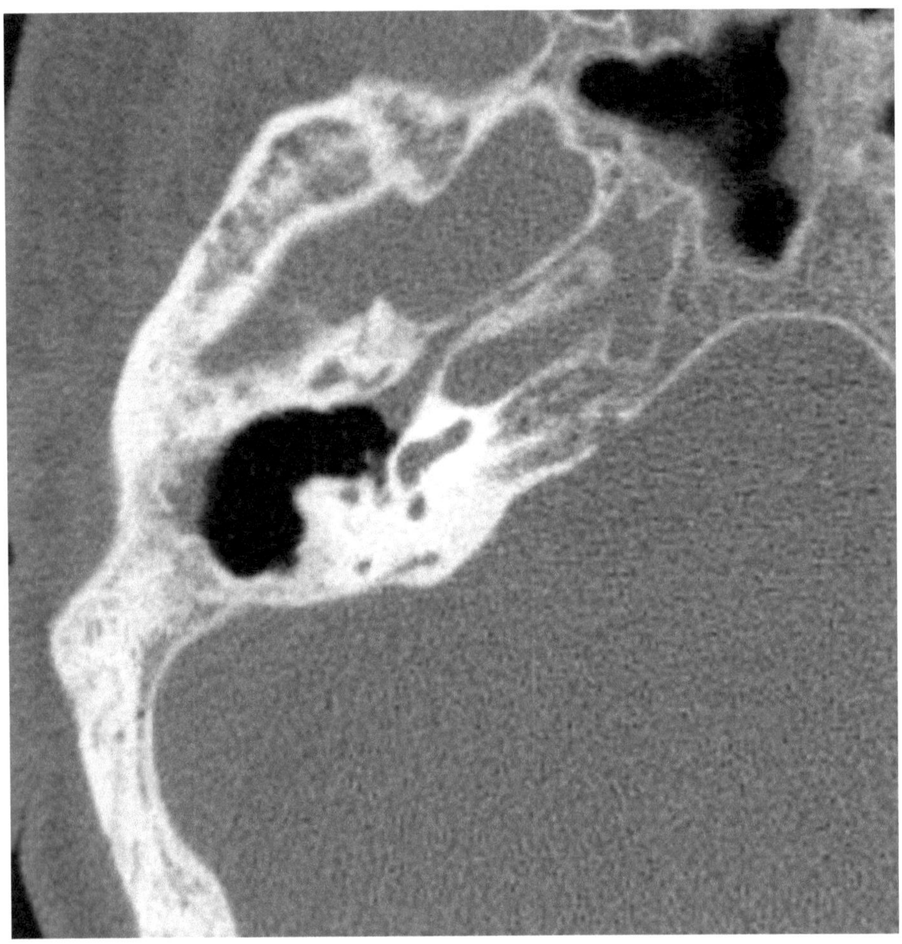

Fig. 14.1.1 This case represents an example of subtotal petrosectomy combined with CI in a chronic infected cavity. A 70-year-old man had had a right radical cavity for 17 years with anacusis. On the other side he had residual hearing with minimal benefit from a hearing aid. On CT there were no signs of ossification of the cochlea.

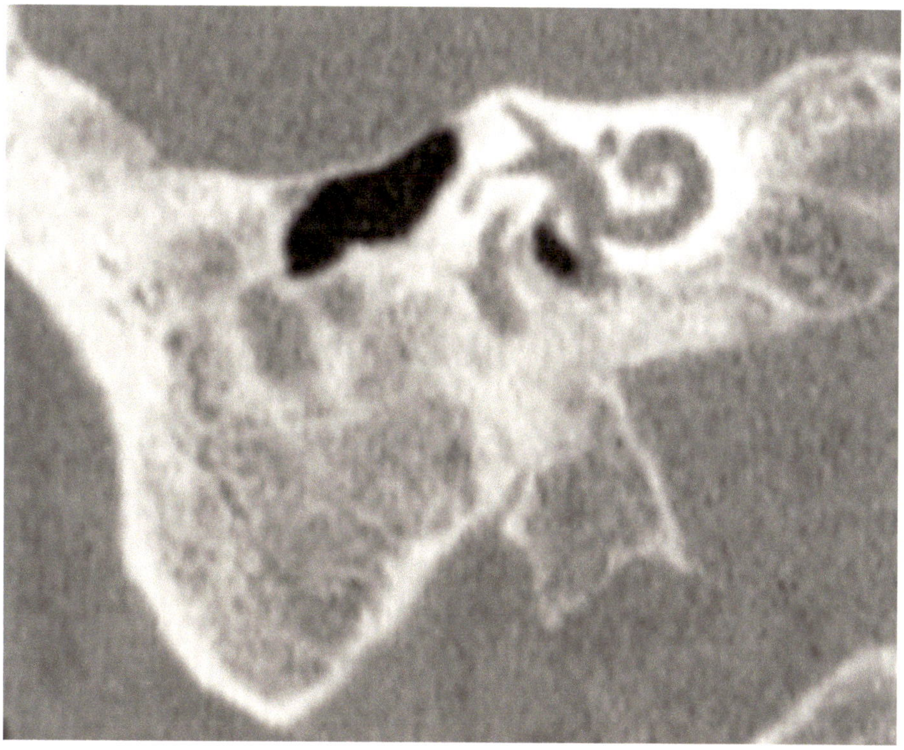

Fig. 14.1.2 Note the sclerotized mastoid tip, the sign of a chronic infection or badly aerated ear. No cochlear ossification is present, however.

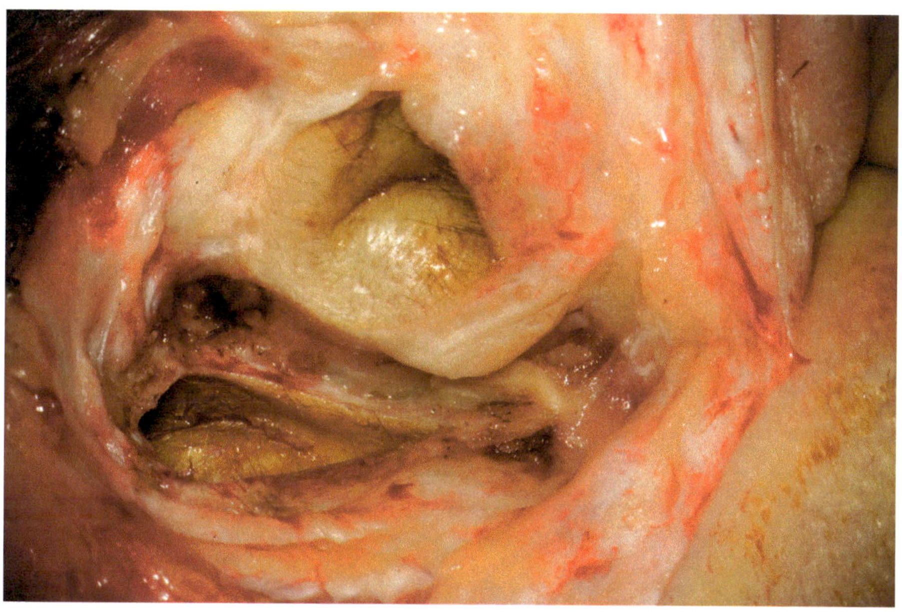

Fig. 14.1.3 Transection of the external auditory canal of the previously enlarged meatus.

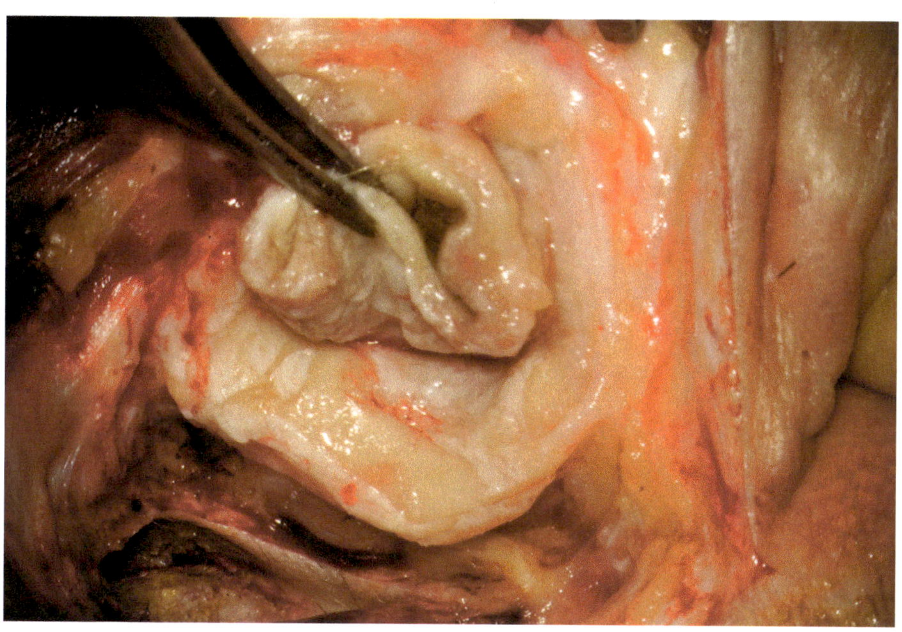

Fig. 14.1.4 Dissection of the meatal skin from the cartilage.

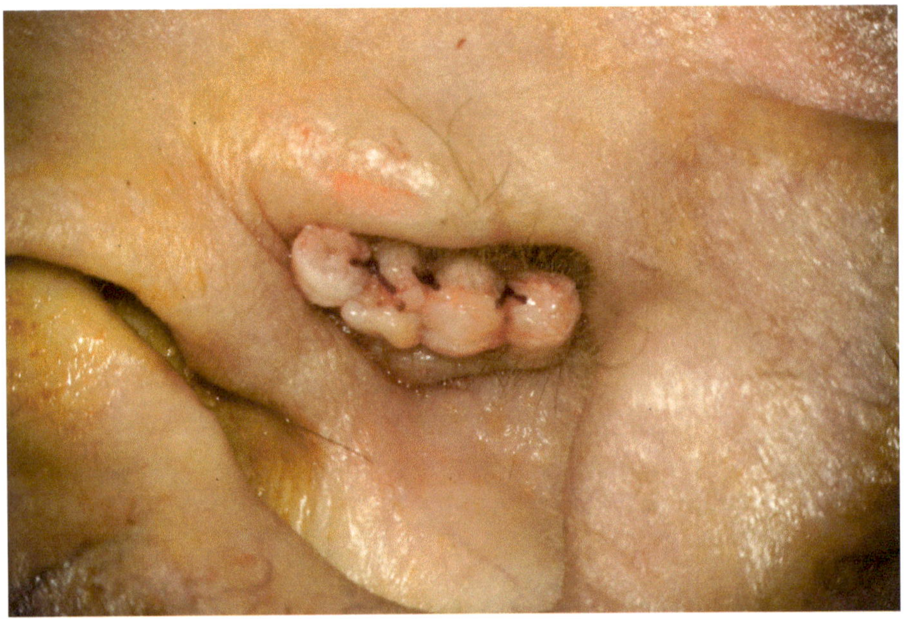

Fig. 14.1.5 The skin is everted and sutured using resorbable material.

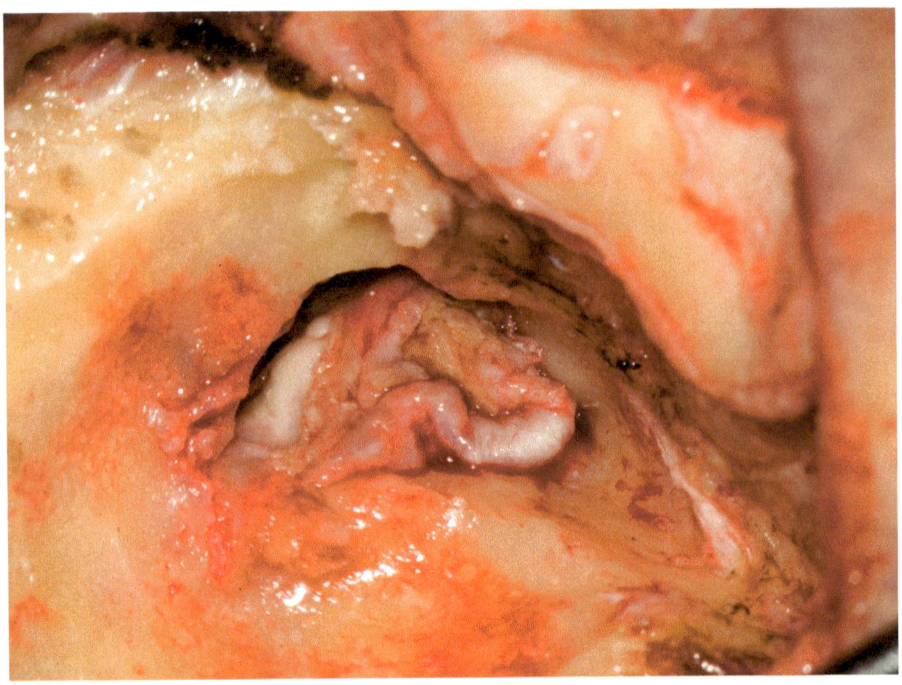

Fig. 14.1.6 The skin lining of the cavity has to be removed meticulously. This is to prevent entrapment of skin that can develop into cholesteatoma once the cavity is closed off.

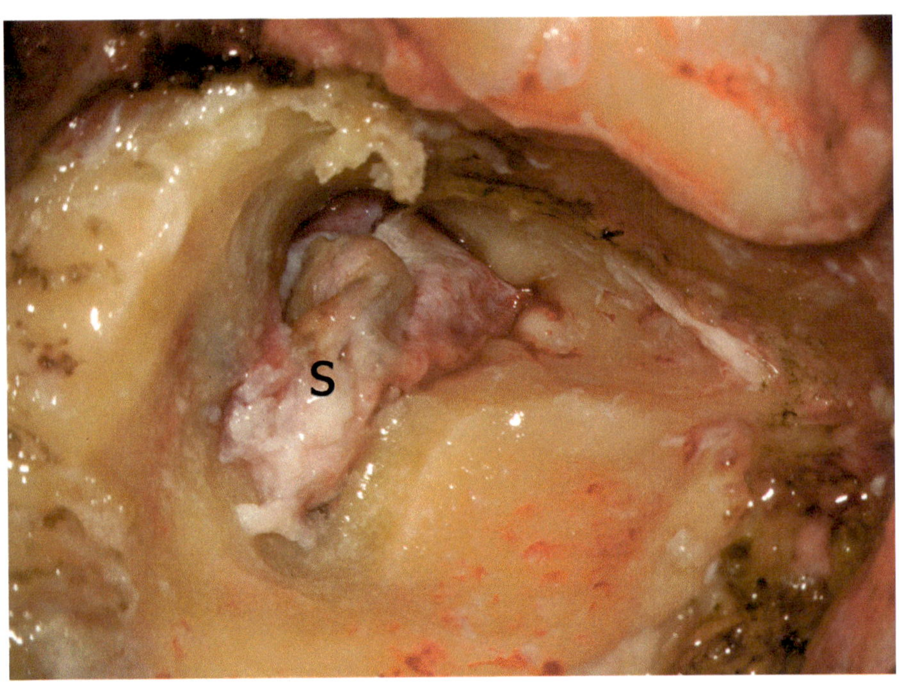

Fig. 14.1.7 Mobilizing the skin (S) lining.

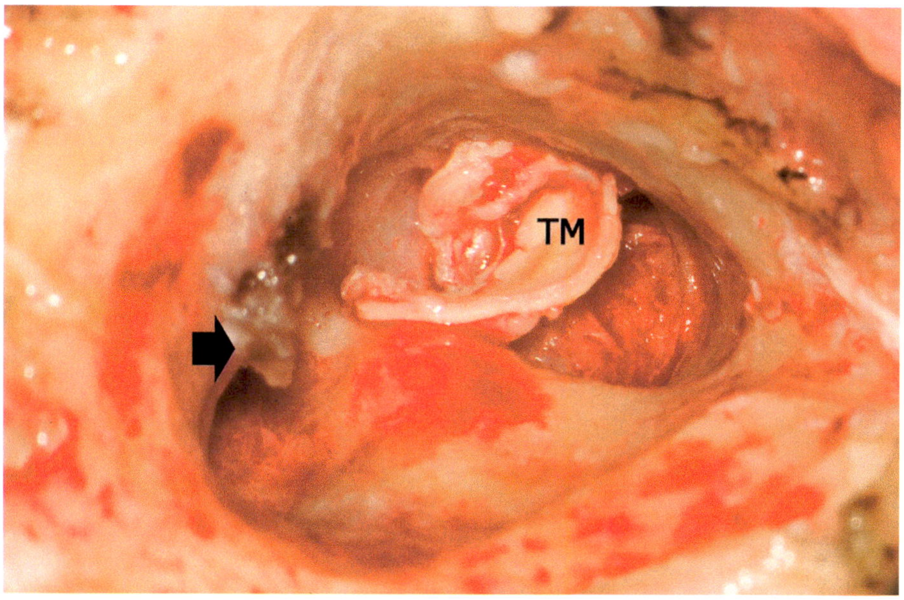

Fig. 14.1.8 The tympanic membrane (TM), incus, and malleus are removed in one piece. A small brain herniation has been coagulated (*arrow*).

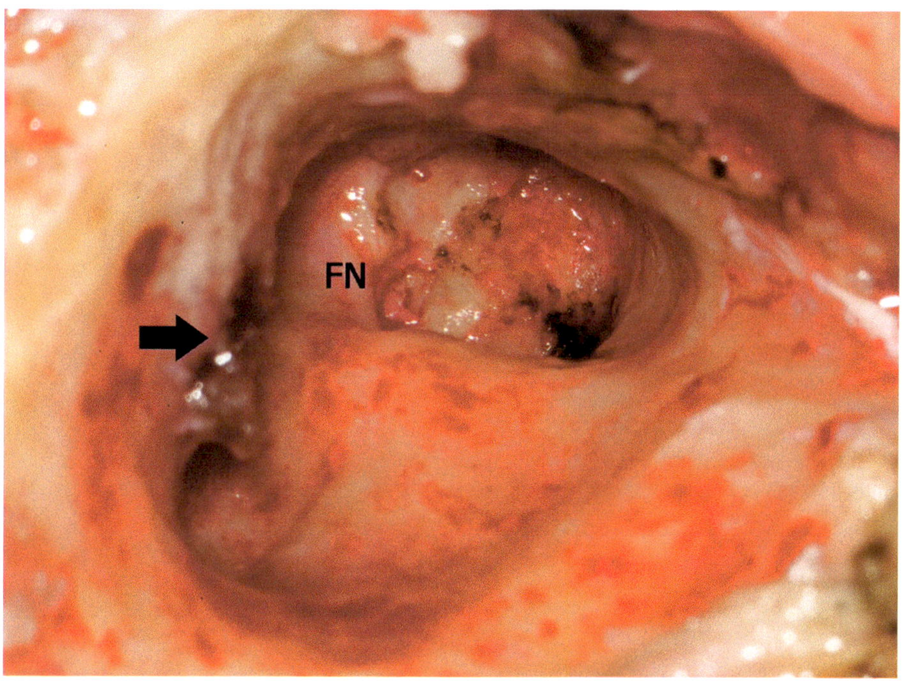

Fig. 14.1.9 Removal of the skin and the eardrum with ossicles has been completed. FN, facial nerve; *arrow*, herniation.

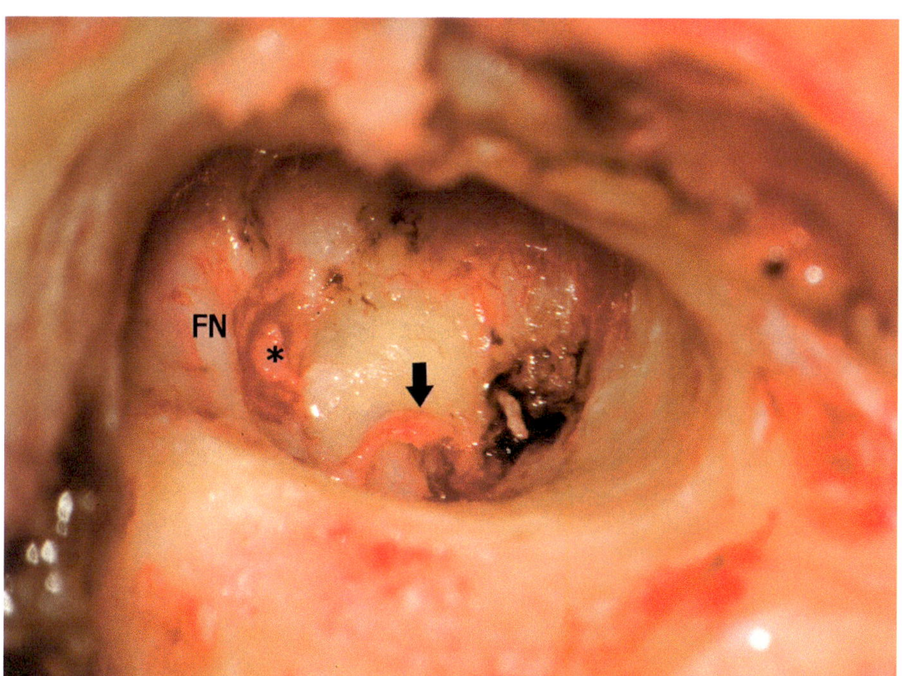

Fig. 14.1.10 Locations of both the oval window (*) and round window (*arrow*) are identified. FN, facial nerve.

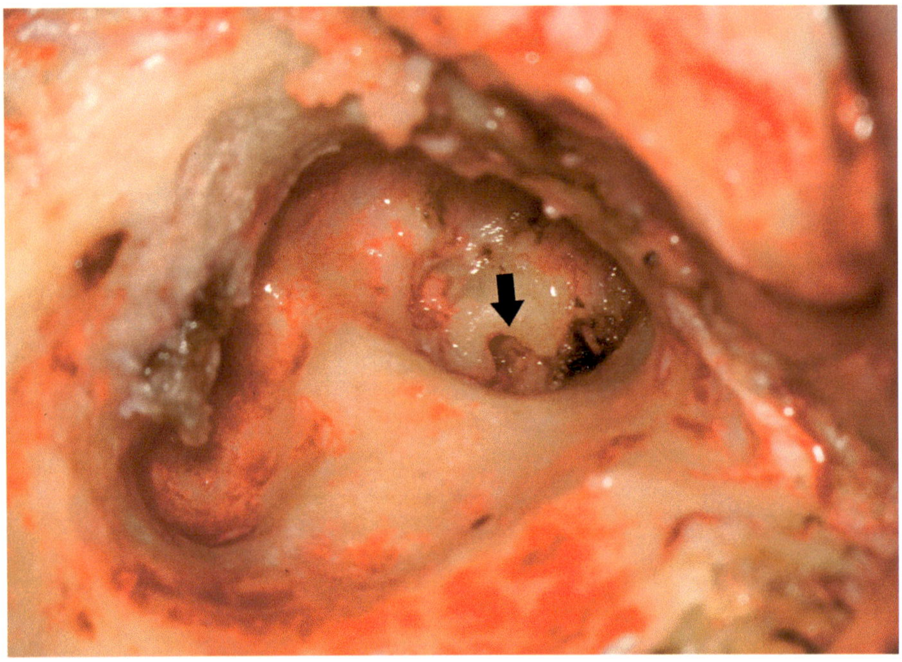

Fig. 14.1.11 The area of the round window niche (*arrow*) is cleaned.

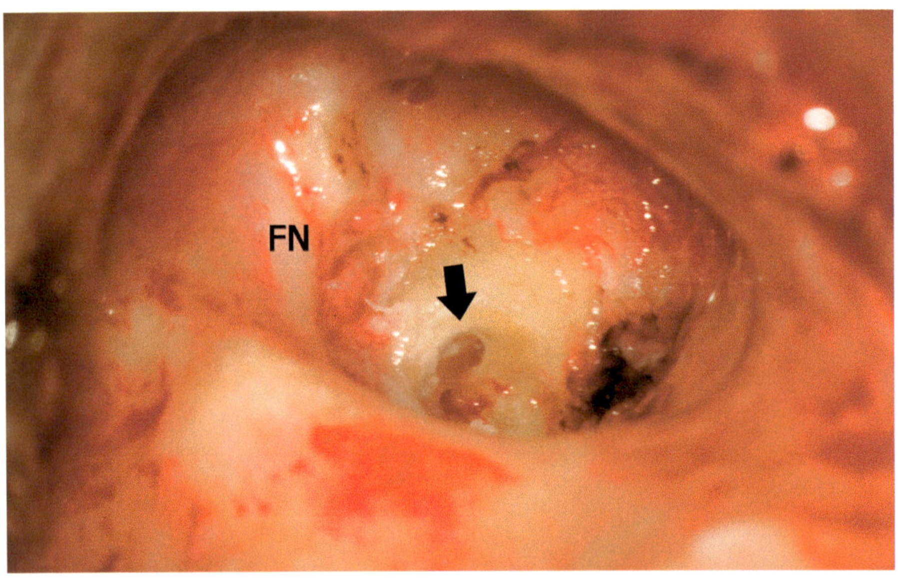

Fig. 14.1.12 The bony borders of the round window niche are drilled (*arrow*); allowing visualization and exposure of the round window membrane. FN, facial nerve.

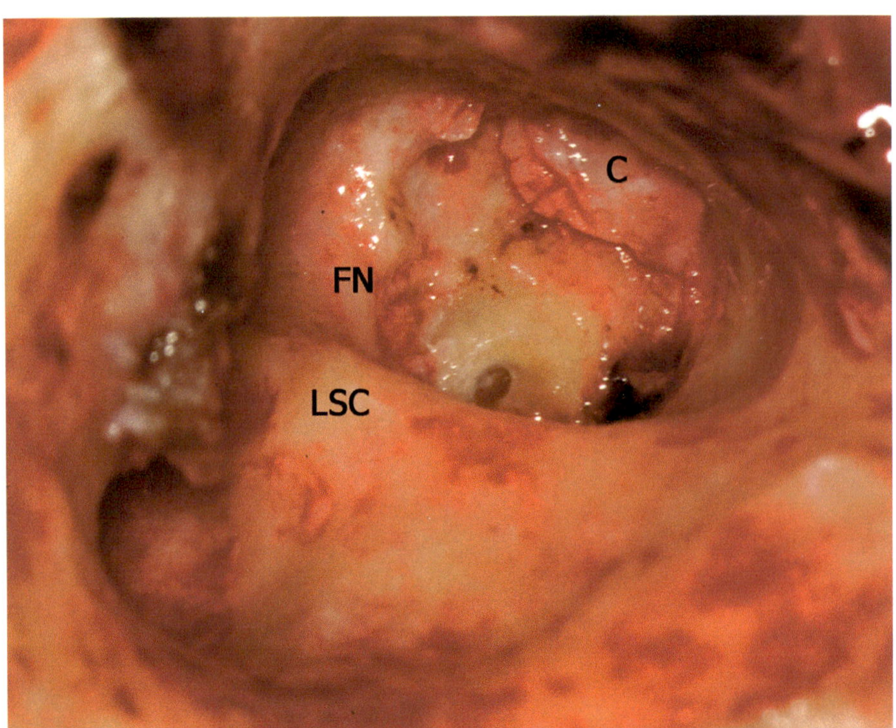

Fig. 14.1.13 The eustachian tube has been obliterated with cartilage (C) to exclude the cavity from the nasopharynx. FN, facial nerve; LSC, lateral semicircular canal.

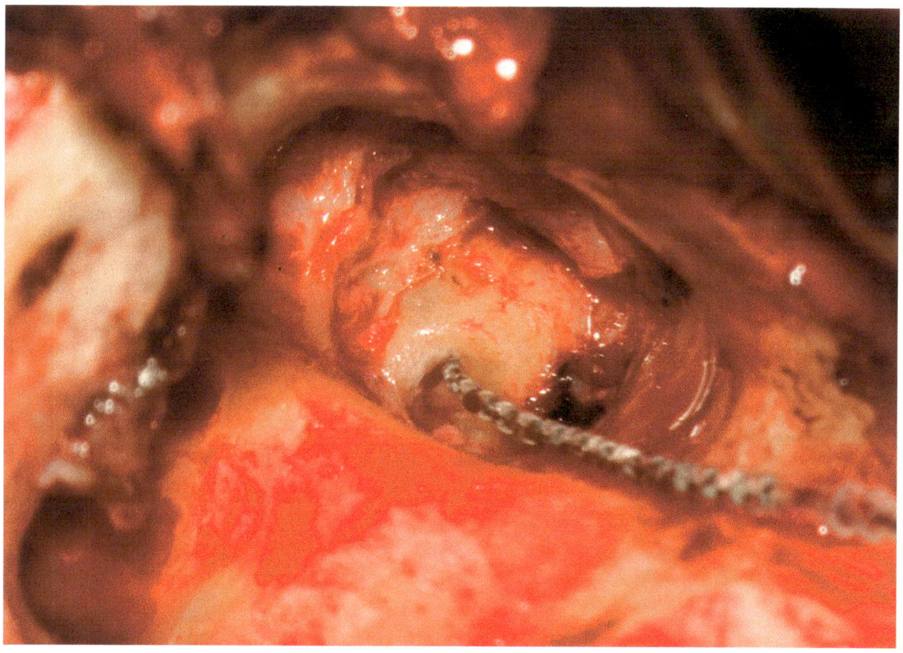

Fig. 14.1.14 The electrode array is inserted through the round window.

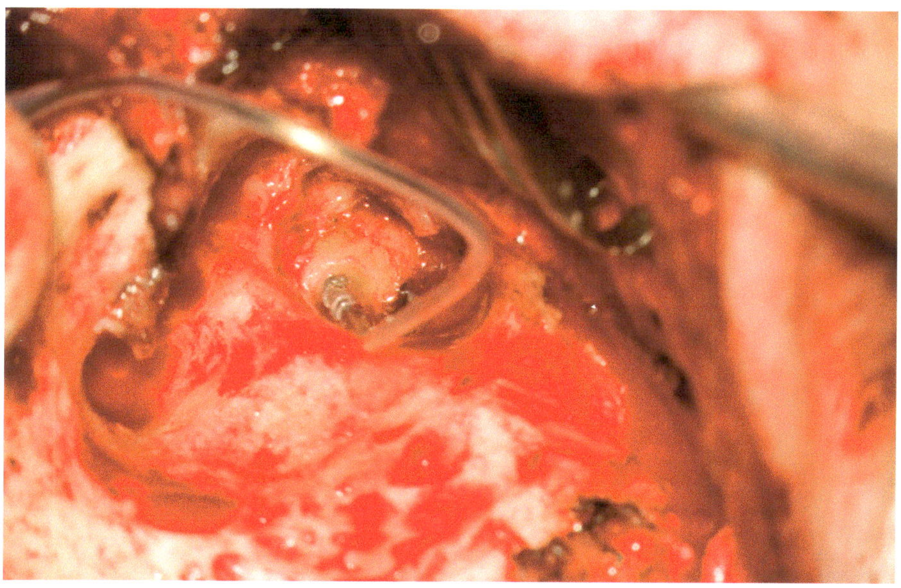

Fig. 14.1.15 A full array insertion has been accomplished.

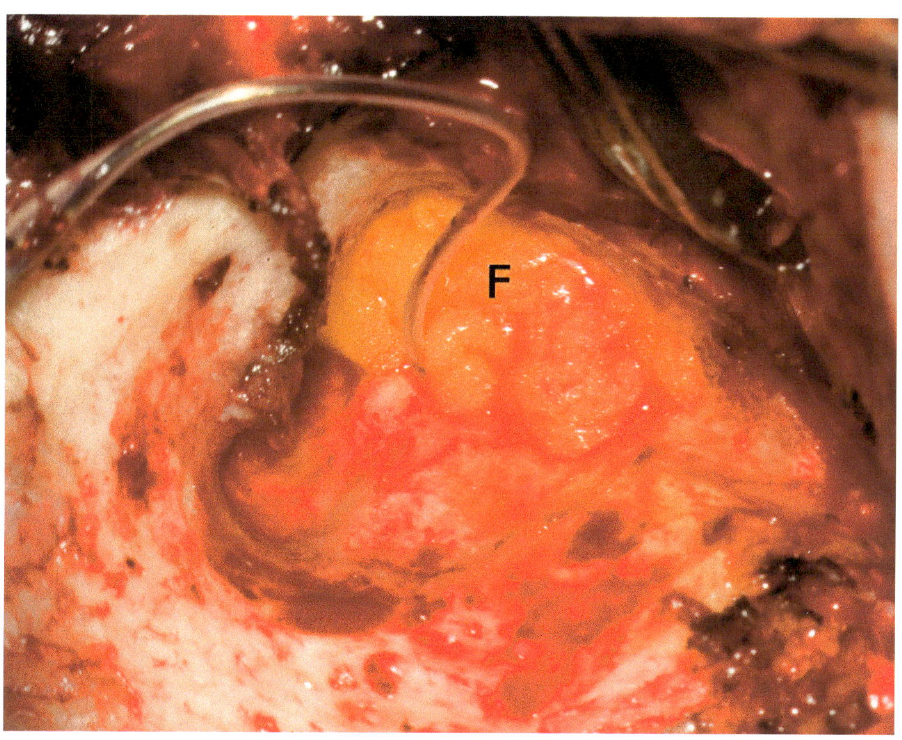

Fig. 14.1.16 After electrophysiologic tests the cavity is obliterated with abdominal fat (F).

Case 14.2 Cochlear Implantation in Patient with Chronic Otitis Media Right Ear with Presence of Perforation (Fig. 14.2.1 and Fig. 14.2.2)

(Complete surgical Case 10.1 in Chapter 10)

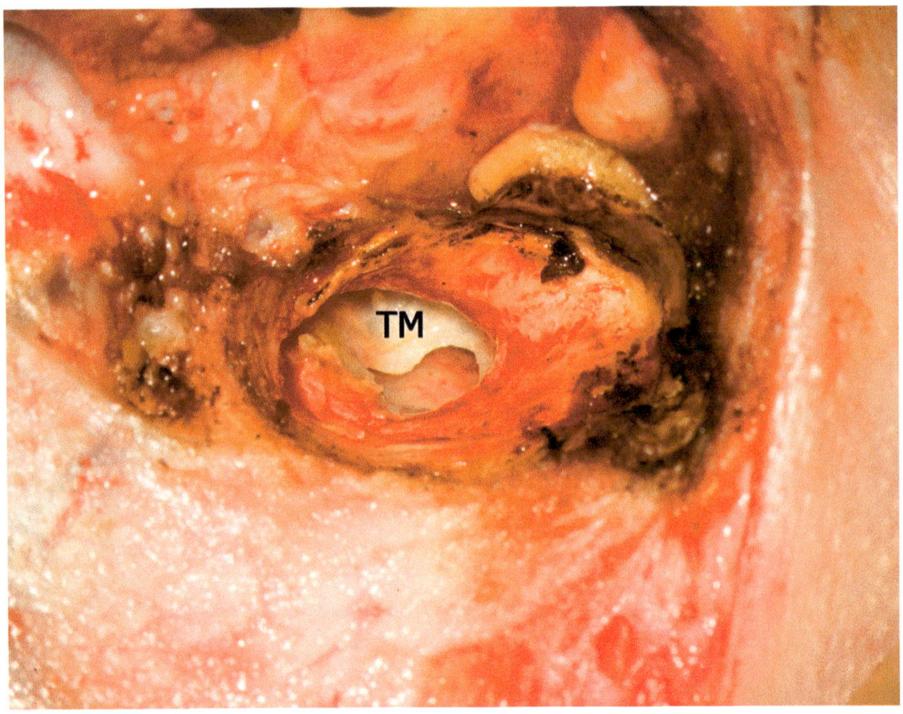

Fig. 14.2.1 After removal of the lateral part of the skin of the external ear canal, the perforation in the tympanic membrane (TM) can be well observed. The mucosa of the middle ear seems not to be inflamed.

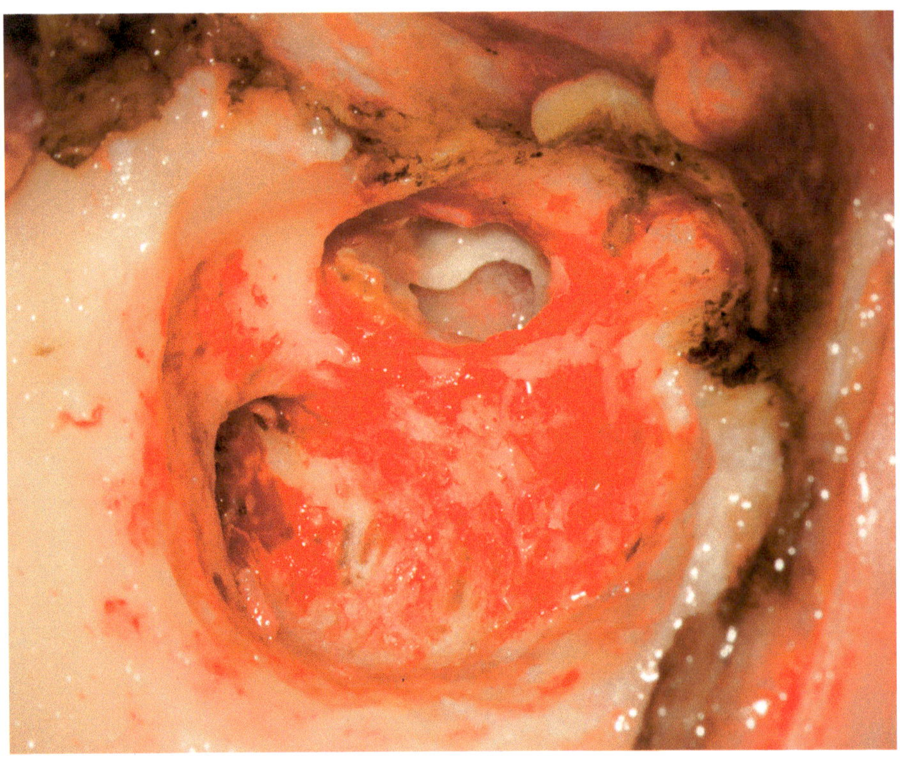

Fig. 14.2.2 Start with the canal wall down approach in preparation for subtotal petrosectomy to create a safe environment for the cochlear implant. This case is suitable for performing SP + CI in a single-stage procedure because the ear is not infected.

Case 14.3 Cochlear Implantation in a Patient with a Radical Cavity Left Ear (Fig. 14.3.1–Fig. 14.3.3)

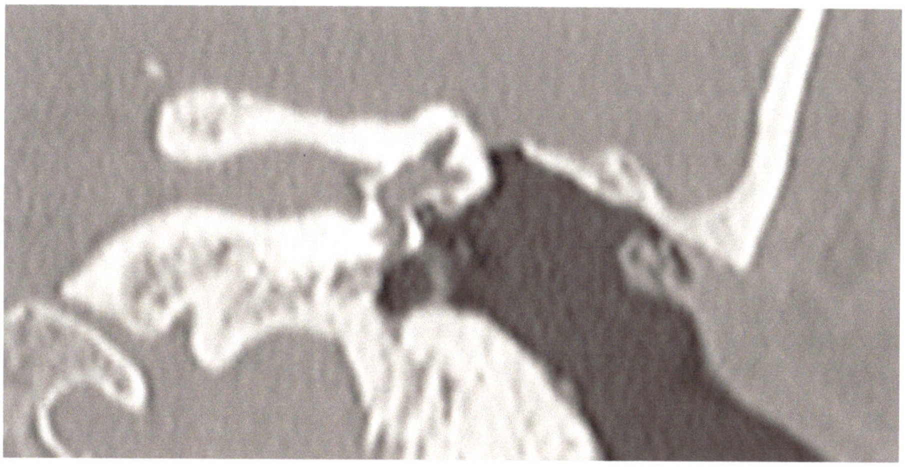

Fig. 14.3.1 A male patient who is suffering vertigo spells has had a dead ear since previous canal wall down surgery. Coronal CT shows a radical cavity. The cavity appears dry, there is no sign of infection, and the mucosal lining is thin.

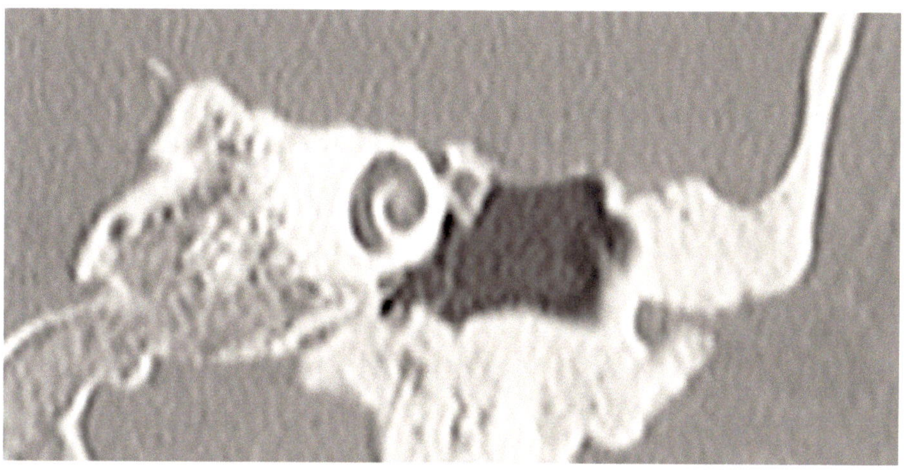

Fig. 14.3.2 No residual cells can be seen.

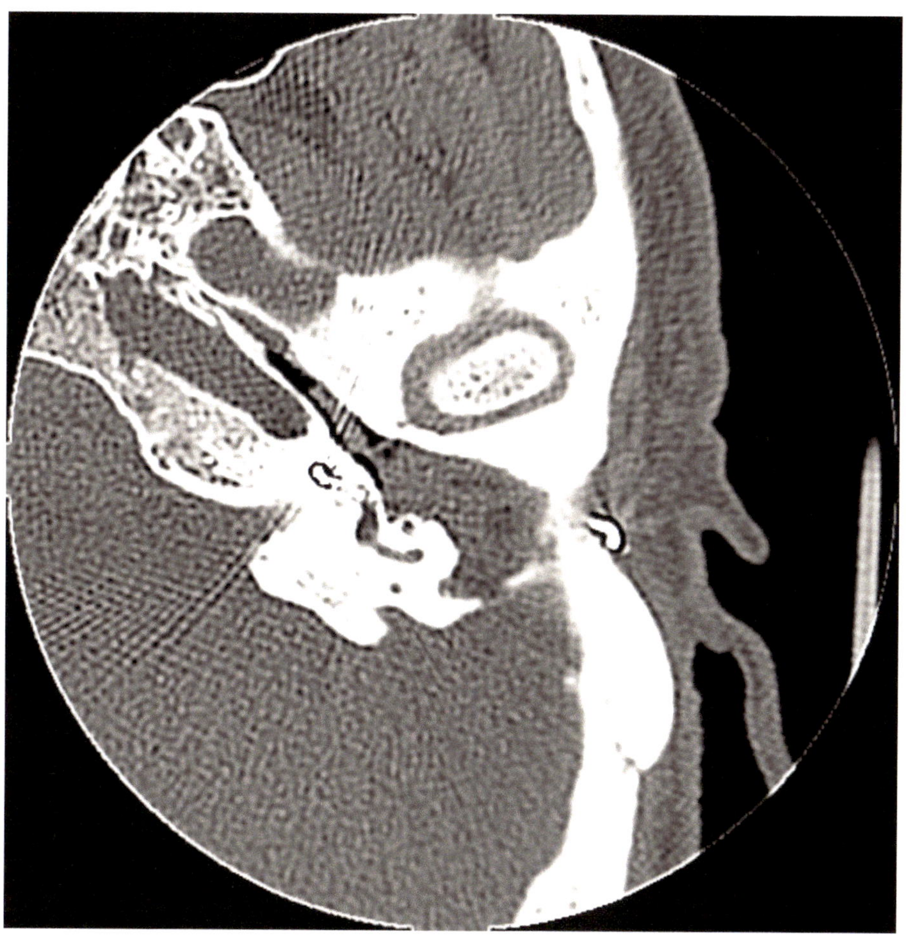

Fig. 14.3.3 Postoperative CT image shows the obliteration of the cavity and the eustachian tube (with some air left). The cochlear array can be seen in the basal turn.

Pearls and Pitfalls

- Presence of OME is not considered a contraindication for implantation, nor is the presence of ventilation tubes.
- Insertion of ventilation tubes is advised 2 to 6 weeks before cochlear implantation.
- Consider SP in all cases of CSOM, in particular in presence of cholesteatoma, atelectasis, or a cleft palate.
- In presence of purulent infection, staged surgery may be a safer option, whatever approach is planned.
- Especially in children, a shorter period between sequential implantations, resulting in implantation at a younger age, is better for outcome.[33–36]
- To prevent migration of a middle ear infection intracranially along the electrode array, most surgeons use soft tissue to seal around the cochleostomy (and posterior tympanotomy).[37,38] Additionally, fibrous tissue sheets are formed around the electrode within a few weeks, sealing the cochleostomy and providing some defense against spread of infection.

Reference Video

See Video 14.1.

References

1. Axon PR, Mawman DJ, Upile T, Ramsden RT. Cochlear implantation in the presence of chronic suppurative otitis media. J Laryngol Otol 1997;111(3):228–232
2. Gray RF, Irving RM. Cochlear implants in chronic suppurative otitis media. Am J Otol 1995;16(5):682–686
3. Incesulu A, Kocaturk S, Vural M. Cochlear implantation in chronic otitis media. J Laryngol Otol 2004;118(1):3–7
4. Issing PR, Schönermark MP, Winkelmann S, Kempf HG, Ernst A. Cochlear implantation in patients with chronic otitis: indications for subtotal petrosectomy and obliteration of the middle ear. Skull Base Surg 1998;8(3):127–131
5. Kim CS, Chang SO, Oh SH, Lee HJ, Choi BY, Park YH. Cochlear implantation in chronic ear disease. Cochlear Implants Int 2004;5 Suppl 1:156–157. doi: 10.1002/cii.212
6. Leung R, Briggs RJS. Indications for and outcomes of mastoid obliteration in cochlear implantation. Otol Neurotol 2007;28(3):330–334
7. Roehm PC, Gantz BJ. Cochlear implant explantation as a sequela of severe chronic otitis media: case report and review of the literature. Otol Neurotol 2006;27(3):332–336
8. Xenellis J, Nikolopoulos TP, Marangoudakis P, Vlastarakos PV, Tsangaroulakis A, Ferekidis E. Cochlear implantation in atelectasis and chronic otitis media: long-term follow-up. Otol Neurotol 2008;29(4):499–501
9. Hellingman CA, Dunnebier EA. Cochlear implantation in patients with acute or chronic middle ear infectious disease: a review of the literature. Eur Arch Otorhinolaryngol 2009;266(2):171–176
10. Postelmans JTF, Stokroos RJ, Linmans JJ, Kremer B. Cochlear implantation in patients with chronic otitis media: 7 years' experience in Maastricht. Eur Arch Otorhinolaryngol 2009;266(8):1159–1165
11. Antonelli PJ, Lee JC, Burne RA. Bacterial biofilms may contribute to persistent cochlear implant infection. Otol Neurotol 2004;25(6):953–957
12. Cristobal R, Edmiston CE Jr, Runge-Samuelson CL, Owen HA, Firszt JB, Wackym PA. Fungal biofilm formation on cochlear implant hardware after antibiotic-induced fungal overgrowth within the middle ear. Pediatr Infect Dis J 2004;23(8):774–778
13. Pawlowski KS, Wawro D, Roland PS. Bacterial biofilm formation on a human cochlear implant. Otol Neurotol 2005;26(5):972–975
14. Barañano CF, Sweitzer RS, Mahalak ML, Alexander NS, Woolley AL. The management of myringotomy tubes in pediatric cochlear implant recipients. Arch Otolaryngol Head Neck Surg 2010;136(6):557–560
15. Free RH, Falcioni M, Di Trapani G, Giannuzzi AL, Russo A, Sanna M. The role of subtotal petrosectomy in cochlear implant surgery—a report of 32 cases and review on indications. Otol Neurotol 2013;34(6):1033–1040. doi: 10.1097/MAO.0b013e318289841b
16. Vercruysse JP, De Foer B, Somers T, Casselman JW, Offeciers E. Mastoid and epitympanic bony obliteration in pediatric cholesteatoma. Otol Neurotol 2008;29(7):953–960
17. De Foer B, Vercruysse JP, Pouillon M, Somers T, Casselman JW, Offeciers E. Value of high-resolution computed tomography and magnetic resonance imaging in the detection of residual cholesteatomas in primary bony obliterated mastoids. Am J Otolaryngol 2007;28(4):230–234
18. Pasanisi E, Vincenti V, Bacciu A, et al. Multichannel cochlear implantation in radical mastoidectomy cavities. Otolaryngol Head Neck Surg 2002;127(5):432–436
19. El-Kashlan HK, Arts HA, Telian SA. External auditory canal closure in cochlear implant surgery. Otol Neurotol 2003;24(3):404–408
20. Wackym PA, Michel MA, Prost RW, Banks KL, Runge-Samuelson CL, Firszt JB. Effect of magnetic resonance imaging on internal magnet strength in Med-El Combi 40+ cochlear implants. Laryngoscope 2004;114(8):1355–1361
21. Crane BT, Gottschalk B, Kraut M, Aygun N, Niparko JK. Magnetic resonance imaging at 1.5 T after cochlear implantation. Otol Neurotol 2010;31(8):1215–1220
22. Hoep LS, Merkus P, van Schie A, Rinkel RN, Smit CF. The value of nuclear scans in cochlear implant infections. Eur Arch Otorhinolaryngol 2006;263(10):895–899
23. Masterson L, Kumar S, Kong JH, et al. Cochlear implant failures: lessons learned from a UK centre. J Laryngol Otol 2012;126(1):15–21
24. Abes GT, Abes FL, Jamir JC. The variable clinical presentation of tuberculosis otitis media and the importance of early detection. Otol Neurotol 2011;32(4):539–543
25. Chirch LM, Ahmad K, Spinner W, Jimenez VE, Donelan SV, Smouha E. Tuberculous otitis media: report of 2 cases on Long Island, N.Y., and a review of all cases reported in the United States from 1990 through 2003. Ear Nose Throat J 2005;84(8):488–497, 490, 492 passim
26. Chen CF, Liu ZH, Xie J, Ma XB, Li Y, Gong SS. Cochlear implant challenges encountered in tuberculous otitis media. Asian Pac J Trop Med 2012;5(5):416–419
27. Vaamonde P, Castro C, García-Soto N, Labella T, Lozano A. Tuberculous otitis media: a significant diagnostic challenge. Otolaryngol Head Neck Surg 2004;130(6):759–766
28. Hoistad DL, Ondrey FG, Mutlu C, Schachern PA, Paparella MM, Adams GL. Histopathology of human temporal bone after cis-platinum, radiation, or both. Otolaryngol Head Neck Surg 1998;118(6):825–832
29. Adunka OF, Buchman CA. Cochlear implantation in the irradiated temporal bone. J Laryngol Otol 2007;121(1):83–86
30. Leonetti JP, Marzo SJ, Zender CA, Porter RG, Melian E. Temporal bone osteoradionecrosis after surgery and radiotherapy for malignant parotid tumors. Otol Neurotol 2010;31(4):656–659
31. Holland JF, Galvin KL, Briggs RJ. Planned simultaneous bilateral cochlear implant operations: how often do children receive only one implant? Int J Pediatr Otorhinolaryngol 2012;76(3):396–399. doi: 10.1016/j.ijporl.2011.12.019. Epub 2012
32. Kirtane MV, More YI, Mankekar G. Cochlear stenting: how I do it. Eur Arch Otorhinolaryngol 2010;267(6):985–987
33. Gordon KA, Valero J, Papsin BC. Auditory brainstem activity in children with 9–30 months of bilateral cochlear implant use. Hear Res 2007;233(1–2):97–107. Epub 2007
34. Sharma A, Gilley PM, Dorman MF, Baldwin R. Deprivation-induced cortical reorganization in children with cochlear implants. Int J Audiol 2007;46(9):494–499
35. Galvin KL, Hughes KC, Mok M. Can adolescents and young adults with prelingual hearing loss benefit from a second, sequential cochlear implant? Int J Audiol 2010;49(5):368–377. doi: 10.3109/14992020903470767
36. Scherf F, van Deun L, van Wieringen A, et al. Hearing benefits of second-side cochlear implantation in two groups of children. Int J Pediatr Otorhinolaryngol 2007;71(12):1855–1863. Epub 2007

37. Hoffman RA. Cochlear implant in the child under two years of age: skull growth, otitis media, and selection. Otolaryngol Head Neck Surg 1997;117(3 Pt 1):217–219
38. Clark GM, Blamey PJ, Busby PA, et al. A multiple-electrode intracochlear implant for children. Arch Otolaryngol Head Neck Surg 1987;113(8):825–828

Further Reading

Achiques MT, Morant A, Muñoz N, et al. [Cochlear implant complications and failures]. [Article in Spanish]. Acta Otorrinolaringol Esp 2010;61(6):412–417

Basavaraj S, Shanks M, Sivaji N, Allen AA. Cochlear implantation and management of chronic suppurative otitis media: single stage procedure? Eur Arch Otorhinolaryngol 2005;262(10):852–855

Bendet E, Cerenko D, Linder TE, Fisch U. Cochlear implantation after subtotal petrosectomies. Eur Arch Otorhinolaryngol 1998;255(4):169–174

Brown KD, Connell SS, Balkany TJ, Eshraghi AE, Telischi FF, Angeli SA. Incidence and indications for revision cochlear implant surgery in adults and children. Laryngoscope 2009;119(1):152–157

Fayad JN, Eisenberg LS, Gillinger M, Winter M, Martinez AS, Luxford WM. Clinical performance of children following revision surgery for a cochlear implant. Otolaryngol Head Neck Surg 2006;134(3):379–384

Nadol JB Jr, Eddington DK. Histologic evaluation of the tissue seal and biologic response around cochlear implant electrodes in the human. Otol Neurotol 2004;25(3):257–262

Parnes LS, Gagne JP, Hassan R. Cochlear implants and otitis media: considerations in two cleft palate patients. J Otolaryngol 1993;22(5):345–348

Pasanisi E, Vincenti V, Bacciu A, et al. Multichannel cochlear implantation in radical mastoidectomy cavities. Otolaryngol Head Neck Surg 2002;127(5):432–436

Roland JT Jr, Alexiades G, Jackman AH, Hillman D, Shapiro W. Cochlear implantation in human immunodeficiency virus-infected patients. Otol Neurotol 2003;24(6):892–895

Rubin LG. Prevention and treatment of meningitis and acute otitis media in children with cochlear implants. Otol Neurotol 2010;31(8):1331–1333

Sanna M, Dispenza F, Flanagan S, De Stefano A, Falcioni M. Management of chronic otitis by middle ear obliteration with blind sac closure of the external auditory canal. Otol Neurotol 2008;29(1):19–22

Valencia DM, Rimell FL, Friedman BJ, Oblander MR, Helmbrecht J. Cochlear implantation in infants less than 12 months of age. Int J Pediatr Otorhinolaryngol 2008;72(6):767–773

van der Putten L, de Bree R, Plukker JT, et al. Permanent unilateral hearing loss after radiotherapy for parotid gland tumors. Head Neck 2006;28(10):902–908

Vincenti V, Pasanisi E, Bacciu A, et al. Cochlear implantation in a human immunodeficiency virus-infected patient. Laryngoscope 2005;115(6):1079–1081

Weiner GM, O'Connell JE, Pahor AL. The role of surgery in tuberculous mastoiditis: appropriate chemotherapy is not always enough. J Laryngol Otol 1997;111(8):752–753

15 Inner Ear Malformations and Implantation

15.1 Introduction

Implantation in patients with a malformation of the inner ear or cochlear nerve abnormality is challenging. Generally speaking, the more severe and less common the malformation the more challenging the case is. In addition, the outcome becomes less predictable and the risks of the surgery increase. In rare but severe malformations, the discussion is ongoing about how to rehabilitate: with a cochlear implant (CI) or auditory brainstem implant (ABI)? Some knowledge of the embryology is needed to understand the classification of the malformations, but more important is knowledge of the radiologic differences.

15.2 Embryology

The inner ear develops in the third to the tenth week of gestation. In the third week, two otocysts, on either side of the hindbrain, subdivide in two pouches. The ventral portion develops into the cochlear duct and the saccule. The dorsal segment is transformed into the endolymphatic sac and duct, the utricle, and the semicircular canals. By the tenth week the morphology of the adult inner ear can already be fully recognized. Ossification of the cartilage capsule of the cochlea and labyrinth begins in week 14 and is completed in week 23.[1]

15.3 Classification of Malformations

Congenital inner ear malformations can be variable, and are often classified according to a suggested arrest during the development of the membranous and bony labyrinth.[2–5] Cochleovestibular malformations are related to malformations of the bony internal auditory canal and/or the cochlear nerve, but also with isolated cases of cochlear nerve hypoplasia or aplasia, a narrowed internal auditory canal (IAC), or an isolated malformation of the vestibular part of the inner ear. Rare malformations, as in CHARGE syndrome or X-linked incomplete partition type 3, do not match the "arrest in development" classification, but they cannot be left out of this overview. The classification is a tool to define different groups of pathology, but in reality there seems to be gradual transition between the different groups.

Classification of Malformations of the Labyrinth, the IAC, and the Cochlear Nerves

Malformation of the membranous labyrinth

- Complete: membranous labyrinthine dysplasia
- Partial: cochleosaccular dysplasia, cochlear basal turn dysplasia

Malformations of the membranous and osseous labyrinth

- Incomplete partition type 2 (including enlarged vestibular aqueduct [EVA])
- Large vestibular aqueduct syndrome (LVAS)
- Cochlear (vestibular) hypoplasia
- Incomplete partition type 1 (cystic cochleovestibular anomaly)
- Common cavity
- Cochlear aplasia
- Cochleovestibular aplasia (Michel deformity)
- Incomplete partition type 3 (X-linked)
- Labyrinthine dysplasia (isolated)
- CHARGE syndrome–associated malformations

Malformations of the cochlear nerve and inner ear canal

- Cochlear nerve hypoplasia or deficiency
- Cochlear nerve aplasia
- Inner ear canal hypoplasia

In this chapter we discuss and present the auditory rehabilitation options in malformations of the cochleovestibular structures, the IAC, and the cochlear nerve.

To define the malformations we use the terms:

- *Aplasia*: complete lack of development
- *Hypoplasia*: incomplete development
- *Dysplasia*: aberrant development

The *labyrinth* refers to the complete inner ear, consisting of the cochlea and the vestibular system.

15.3.1 Malformation of the Membranous Labyrinth

In the era of cochlear implantation patients with isolated membranous malformations will often be implanted even though the patient and the surgeon are not familiar with this entity because it is not visible on imaging.

There are no key features in the radiologic work-up and the surgical approach is not different from that in standard cases. Perhaps in the future higher-resolution imaging will show the membranous dysplasias.

Complete Membranous Labyrinthine Dysplasia

Complete membranous labyrinthine dysplasia is extremely rare and has been described with Jervell–Lange-Nielsen syndrome and Usher syndrome.[6]

Partial Membranous Labyrinthine Dysplasia

There are two forms of partial membranous labyrinthine dysplasia: (1) cochleosaccular dysplasia in which the organ of Corti is partially or completely missing,[7] and (2) cochlear basal turn dysplasia, in which the dysplasia is limited to the basal turn of the cochlea. The latter may be related to familial high-frequency sensorineural hearing loss (SNHL) in patients who would be candidates for electroacoustic stimulation, which is addressed in Chapter 9.

15.3.2 Malformations of the Membranous and Osseous Labyrinth

(See **Table 15.1**.)

In the Jackler classification the incomplete partition was divided into severe and mild types and enlarged vestibular aqueduct (EVA) was not strictly associated with either type of malformation. In the newer classification of Sennaroglu and Saatci the incomplete partition type 2 (IP-2) is strictly associated with an EVA while IP-1 is not. Furthermore, the distinction between mild and severe cochlear hypoplasia is abandoned, and a more clearly defined new entity, the incomplete partition type 1 (IP-1), is proposed.[2,4] Subtypes of a certain malformation can also be classified[8] and will be mentioned in the following overview.

Incomplete Partition Type 2 (Including LVAS)

This is the most common malformation: it is thought of as an arrest in development in the seventh week of gestation.

Classification

Incomplete partition type 2 (IP-2)

IP-2 consists of three components: a cystic cochlear apex with a normal basal turn, a dilated vestibule, and an enlarged vestibular aqueduct. The cochlea consists of 1.5 turns, in which the middle and apical turns unite to form a cystic apex. There is no interscalar septum between the middle and apical turns. Combined with a dilated vestibule and an enlarged vestibular aqueduct, this is known as the classical Mondini deformity,[9,10] but is better referred to nowadays as incomplete partition type 2.

Enlarged vestibular aqueduct (EVA)

EVA is defined as an enlargement of the aqueduct exceeding the diameter of the posterior semicircular canal on an axial image in which both structures are shown.[5] Other definitions are those of Valvassori,[11] Phelps,[12] and Zheng,[13] and the most often used definition is the measurement of the vestibular aqueduct at its broadest diameter in the middle of the long axis of the aqueduct, exceeding 1.5 mm (**Fig. 15.1** and **Fig. 15.2**).

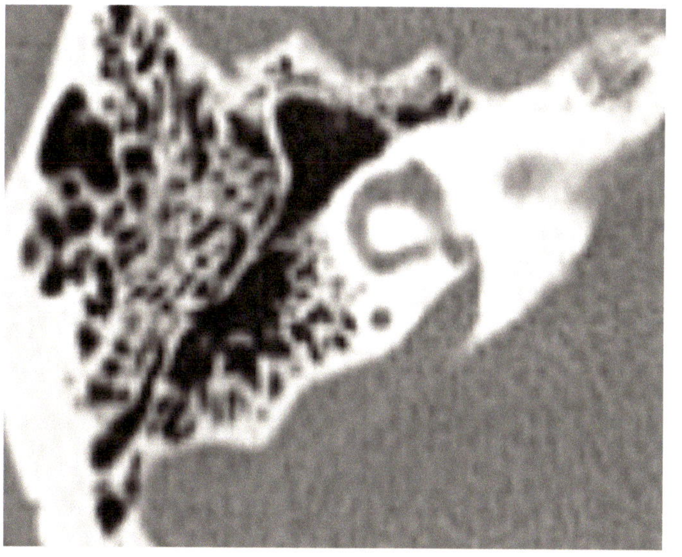

Fig. 15.1 An enlarged vestibular aqueduct seen on CT in an axial view.

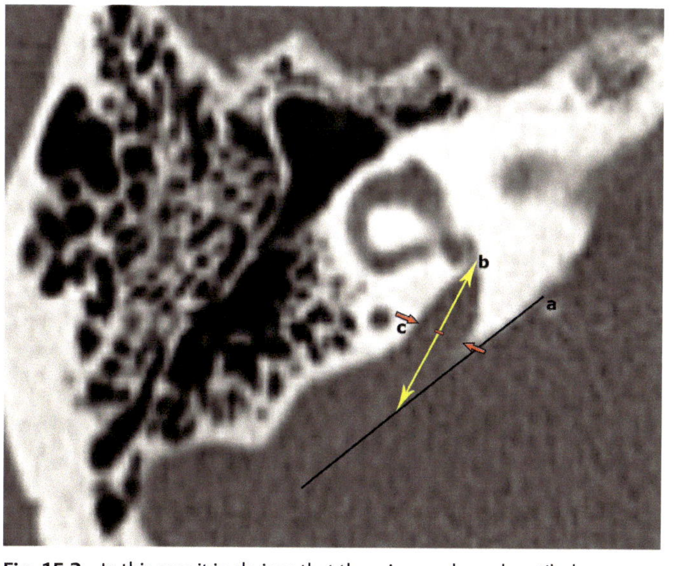

Fig. 15.2 In this case it is obvious that there is an enlarged vestibular aqueduct, but it is a good example to explain how to measure the mid duct diameter: (a) Create a "virtual" line (black line) along the posterior cranial fossa dura, the duct cannot be seen/measured beyond this point. (b) Create in the middle of the duct a line between the most anteromedial point and the posterolateral point (*yellow arrow*). (c) The middle of this line (*red cross mark*) is the best position to measure the diameter of the vestibular aqueduct in millimeters: in this case between the two *red arrows*.

Table 15.1 Malformations of the membranous and osseous labyrinth: The two most commonly used classifications and their differences

Jackler 1987[2]	Sennaroglu 2002[4]
Incomplete partition (mild)/Mondini deformity	Incomplete partition type 2 (IP-2)
Cochlear hypoplasia (mild)	
Incomplete partition (severe)	Cochlear hypoplasia
Cochlear hypoplasia (severe)	Incomplete partition type I (IP-1)
Common cavity	Common cavity
Cochlear aplasia	Cochlear aplasia
Michel deformity	Michel deformity

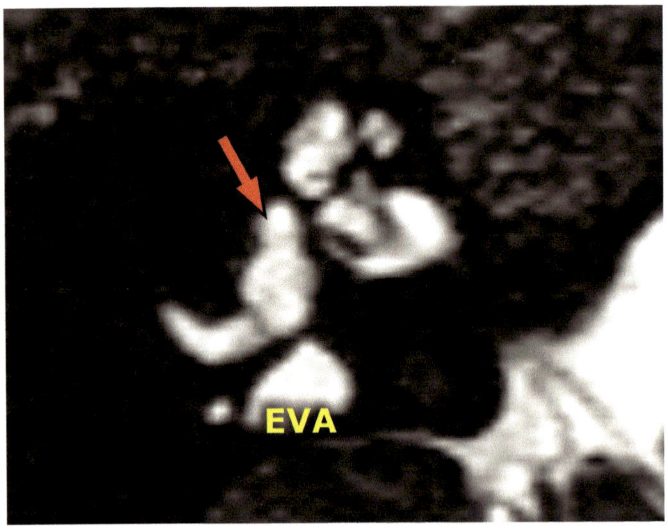

Fig. 15.3 An enlarged vestibular aqueduct (EVA) shown on T2W MRI (CISS). An enlarged vestibule (*red arrow*) together with the EVA and cochlear cystic apex (see next image) make the classic incomplete partition type 2 (as described by Mondini in 1791).

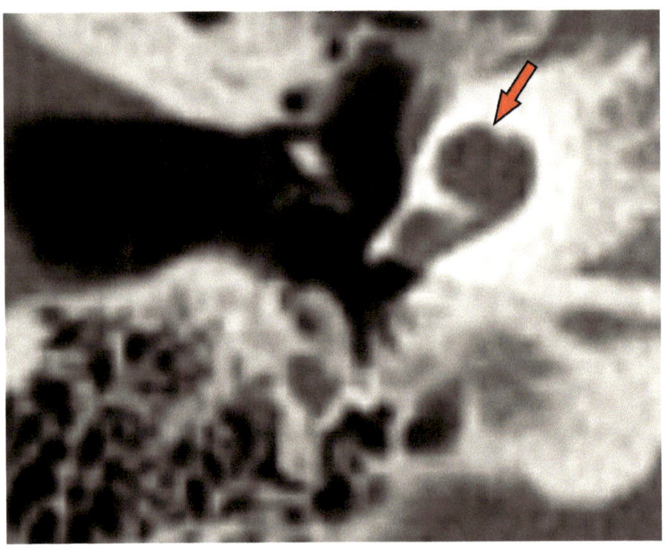

Fig. 15.4 Incomplete separation of the cochlear turns; the middle and apical turns form a cystic structure without an interscalar septum between the middle and apical turns (the normal location of this septum would have been at the *red arrow*).

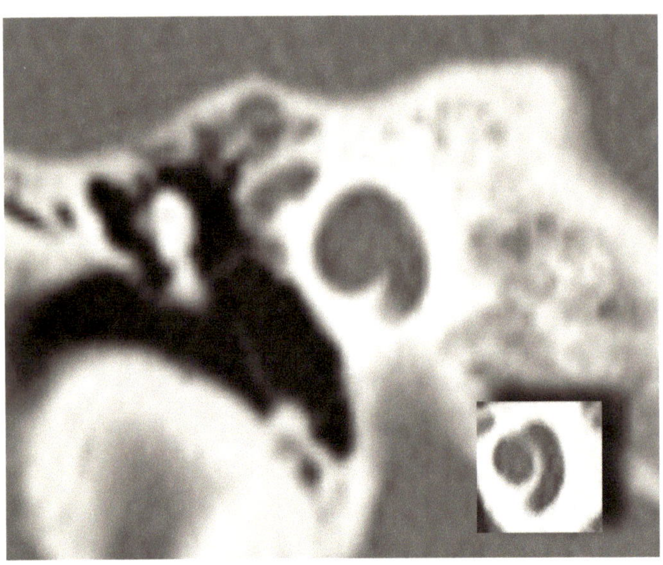

Fig. 15.5 An incomplete partition of the cochlea in a coronal view: the middle and apical turns form a cystic structure. The insert shows the normal aspect of cochlear partition.

Large vestibular aqueduct syndrome (LVAS)

The enlarged vestibular aqueduct is also suggested to occur as a solitary malformation, without a concurrent cochlear dysplasia.[14] This would then be a patient with SNHL and an EVA, which is referred to as the large vestibular aqueduct syndrome. It remains doubtful whether this is a separate entity as more recent research has shown that the modiolus is abnormal in almost all cases with an EVA.[15] Most likely there is a gradual dysplasia of the apical modiolus and interscalar septation in association with an EVA.

Clinical Features

The classical presentation is progressive or fluctuating sensorineural hearing loss, beginning in childhood. Sudden deafness can be present after minor head trauma, but is not present in all cases with IP-2.[16]

Incomplete partition type 2 is associated with Pendred syndrome: all patients with Pendred syndrome have an IP-2 .

IP-2, or at least the EVA, can also be associated with BOR (branchio-oto-renal) syndrome, Waardenburg syndrome, and several other syndromes.[17] Patients with IP-2 and hearing loss, without a proven genetic cause, are considered to have the LVAS, and thus an EVA and hearing loss.

(See **Fig. 15.1, Fig. 15.3–Fig. 15.5.**)

Cochlear (Cochleovestibular) Hypoplasia

It is thought that this is due to an arrest in development in the sixth week of gestation.

Classification

In cochlear (cochleovestibular) hypoplasia the cochlea and vestibule and vestibular structures are separated but less developed than in IP-2. All structures seem smaller (hypoplastic) than in a normal labyrinth. The cochlea is less than 4 mm in height or has fewer than 2.5 turns. The intracochlear organization can be normal or dysplastic. No EVA is seen in these malformations, the IAC is normal or has a hypoplastic diameter, and the semicircular system is hypoplastic or aplastic.[18] Hypoplastic cochleae are sometimes subclassified as type I, budlike; type II, cystic hypoplasia; and type III, cochlea with fewer than 2 turns.

Clinical Features

These patients mostly present with a congenital severe to profound sensorineural hearing loss.

(See **Fig. 15.6–Fig. 15.10.**)

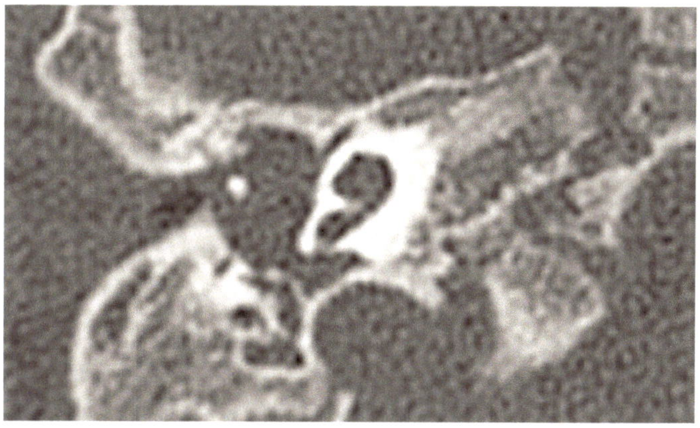

Fig. 15.6 In this CT scan of a child with a cochlear hypoplasia, the apical and middle turns are confluent and the basal turn is visible.

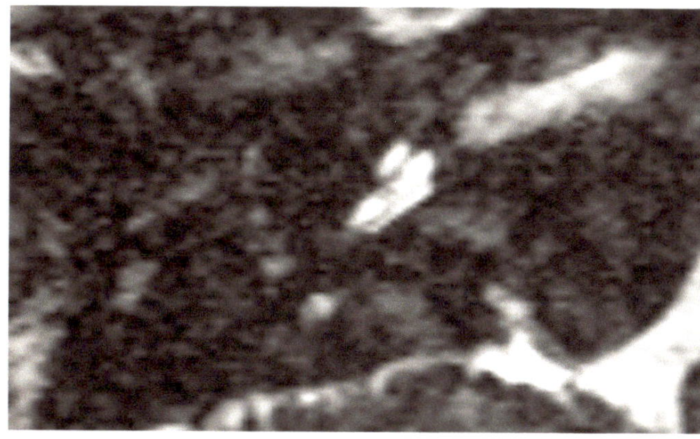

Fig. 15.7 The MRI CISS sequence shows a clear partition of the basal turn, which makes the difference from an IP-1.

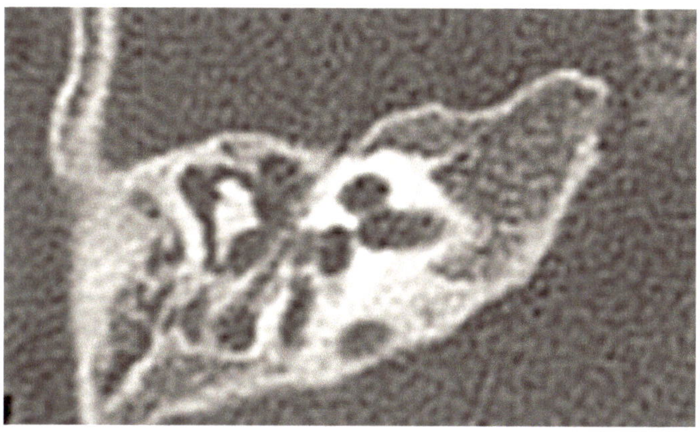

Fig. 15.8 The CT images show the cochlear apical malformation as a rounded lumen instead of a more flattened middle and apical turn. This example would still be classified as type III: "less than two turns" cochlear hypoplasia.

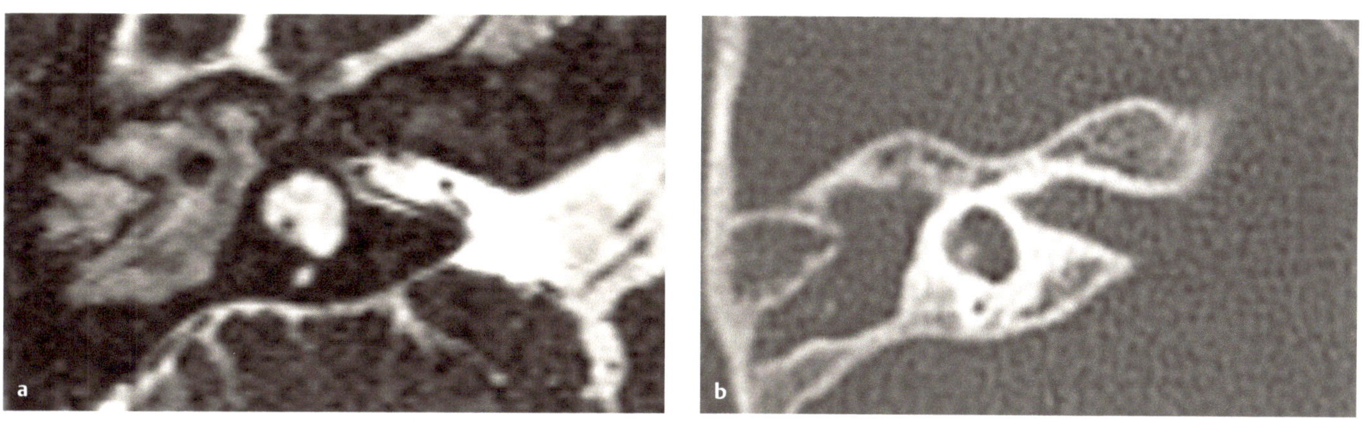

Fig. 15.9a, b In the MRI CISS **(a)** and the CT image **(b)**, the labyrinth malformation is seen with a small bony island within the dysmorphic small lateral semicircular canal. This type of labyrinth is not specific for cochlear hypoplasia and could exist in IP-1 or in cochlear hypoplasia.

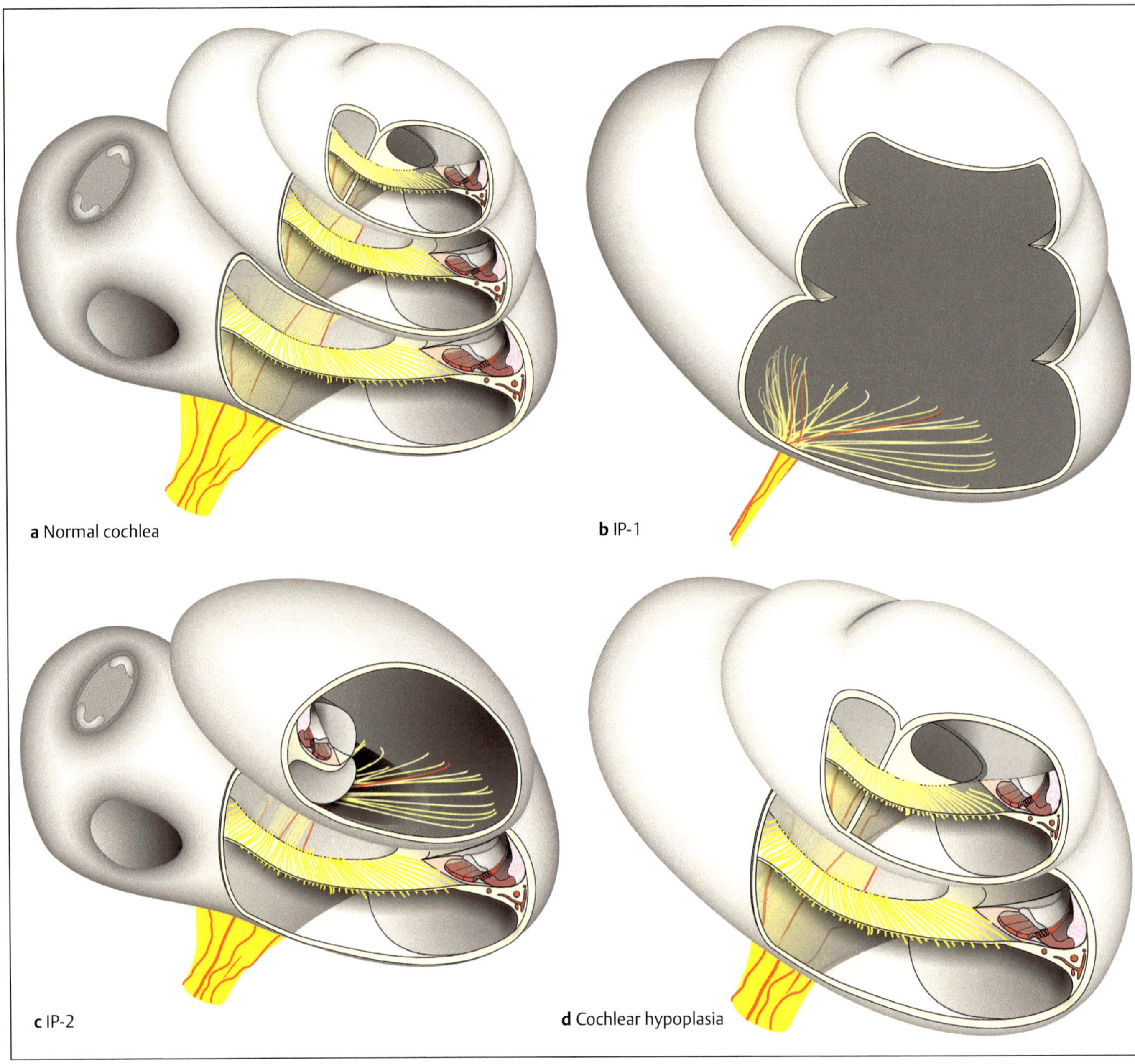

Fig. 15.10a–d Schematic representation of the normal cochlea (**a**), IP type 1 (**b**), IP type 2 (**c**), and cochlear hypoplasia (**d**). The differences between IP-1, IP-2, and cochlear hypoplasia are the size and the inner structures (modiolus and septi) of the cochlea. In an IP-1 the cochlea is cystic and no interscalar septi are visible. Also the modiolus is absent. In a cochlear (vestibular) hypoplasia and IP-2 the cochlea is smaller but still has interscalar septi and a modiolus is present. The best way to distinguish the differences between these entities is on MRI.

Incomplete Partition Type 1 (Cystic Cochleovestibular Anomaly)

It is thought that this is due to an arrest in development in the fifth week of gestation.

Classification

In this malformation (IP-1) a cystic cochlea is connected to a cystic vestibule. The cochlea does not have interscalar septi and the modiolus appears to be completely absent. In fact it is an unpartitioned cochlea despite the name given to this type of malformation. The cochlea looks like an empty cystic space. This is accompanied by grossly dilated vestibule. Separate structures of the cochlea and the vestibule are still recognizable (this in contrast to the common cavity malformation). The lateral canal is mostly cystic, while the other semicircular canals can also be malformed. The cribriform area between the cochlea and the IAC can be open, with a direct connection of the empty vestibule to the cerebrospinal fluid in the IAC.

(See **Fig. 15.11–Fig. 15.13.**)

Common Cavity

The common cavity malformation is thought of as an arrest in development in the fourth week of gestation.

Classification

In a common cavity there is one single cavity, representing cochlea and vestibule, without any differentiation between cochlear and vestibular structures. If the cavity is located at the posterior side of the IAC there is no distinction between common cavity and a cochlear aplasia. It seems that all common cavities

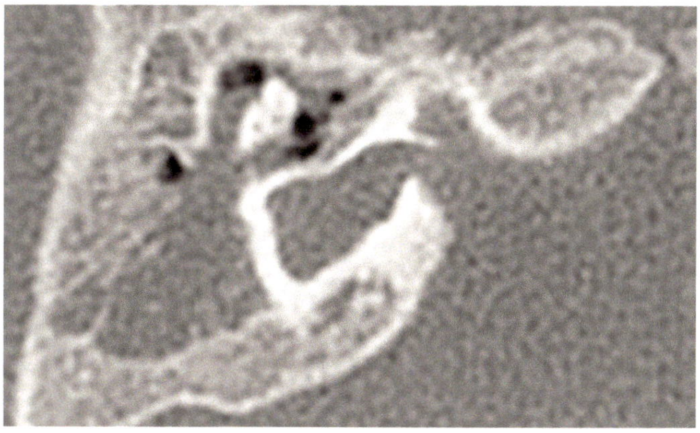

Fig.15.11 The cystic cochleovestibular anomaly of the labyrinth can be distinguished as two separated but dysplastic structures (this image and **Fig. 15.12**). It differs from a common cavity malformation, which consists of only one cystic structure.

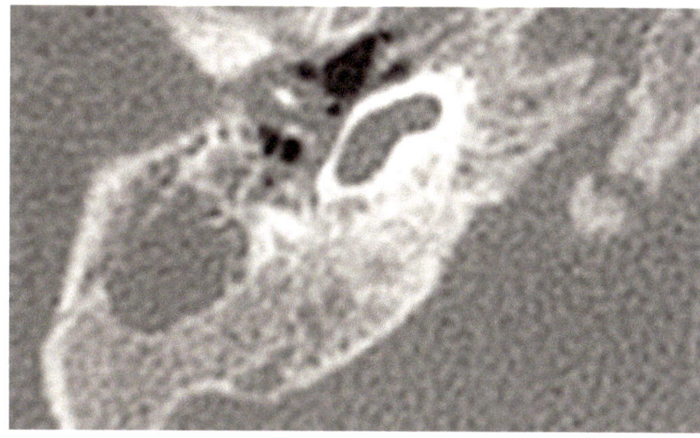

Fig. 15.12 If the cystic cochlea contains some form of partition it is a cochlear hypoplasia, but if it is unstructured, without intracochlear separation or modiolus, it is an IP-1. The best way of analyzing the partition and the scalar organization is on MRI. (See **Fig. 15.13**, MRI of the same cochlea.)

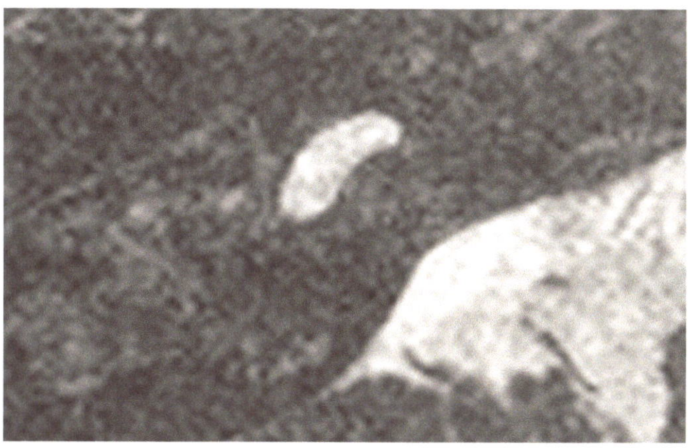

Fig. 15.13 In the cochlea of an IP-1 case there is no partition, only a cystic cavity. This can best be seen on MRI. (See **Fig. 15.10b**.)

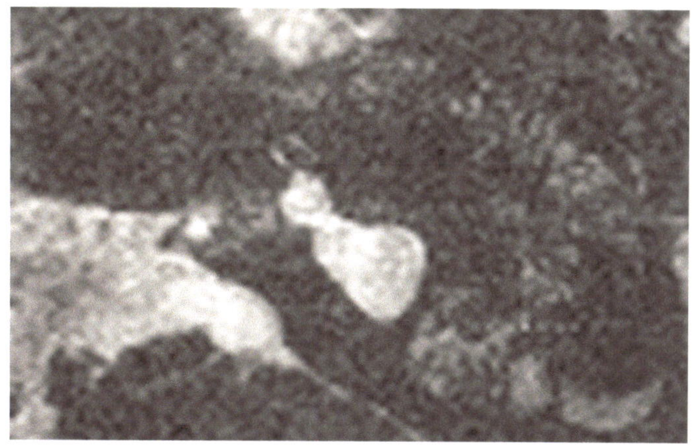

Fig. 15.14 Sometimes it is hard to distinguish a cochlear aplasia from a common cavity. On this MRI image of another patient, the IAC is not very clear and either a cochlear aplasia or a common cavity can be seen. Only the connection and the size of the internal auditory canal will divide the cochlear aplasia case from a common cavity case. There is no "gray area" in this definition.

have an abnormal diameter of the IAC, directly correlated with the size of the common cavity.[4,19,20] Furthermore, the cavity has an open connection with the IAC, but a membranous separation may be apparent. A bulging stapes footplate can also be associated with a common cavity.[21]

It is important in these cases to look for the neural structures connecting to the cavity on MR imaging. This will provide essential information in case of candidacy for a CI. If the neural connection is not clearly visible on MRI, a connection can still be possible.

(See **Fig. 15.14** and **Table 15.2**.)

Table 15.2 Classification of inner ear anomalies and their definitions

Structure	Malformation	Definition
Cochlea	Michel deformity	Complete absence of all cochlear and vestibular structures
	Cochlear aplasia	Complete absence of the cochlea
	Common cavity deformity	Cystic cavity representing the cochlea and vestibule without showing any differentiation into cochlea and vestibule
	IP-1	Cochlea of normal size but cystic appearance with no internal structures identified
	Cochlear hypoplasia	Small cochlea with either intact or incomplete partition.
	IP-2	Cochlea of normal size is shortened to 1.5 turns with an intact basal turn
Vestibule	Dilated vestibule	Axial width is larger than 4.7 mm and coronal width is larger than 3.8 mm
	Vestibular hypoplasia	Axial width is smaller than 3.6 mm and coronal width is smaller than 2.6 mm
SCC	Isolated lateral SCC dysplasia	Bony island width (axial) is smaller than 2.7 mm and bony island width (coronal) is smaller than 2.3 mm or bony island of the LSC is fused to the vestibular wall on coronal section
	Other SCC dysplasia	All SCC anomalies except for the above two deformities
IAC	Narrow IAC	Simultaneous smaller measurements at the opening; IAC at the posterior cranial fossa (PCF) (axial) <4.7 mm, coronal opening <3 2 mm, and midpoint width coronal <3.2 mm
	Shortened IAC	IAC length shorter than 7.1 mm
Fundus	Opened fundus	Absence of bony septum between the IAC and cochlea or vestibule (cochlear aperture)
	Enlarged vestibular aqueduct	The vestibular aqueduct orifice is wider than the diameter of PSC lumen on the axial slice, displaying both structures simultaneously; or the vestibular aqueduct is wider than 1.5 mm at midpoint

Source: modified from Shim et al 2006[20] and Purcell 2003[22].

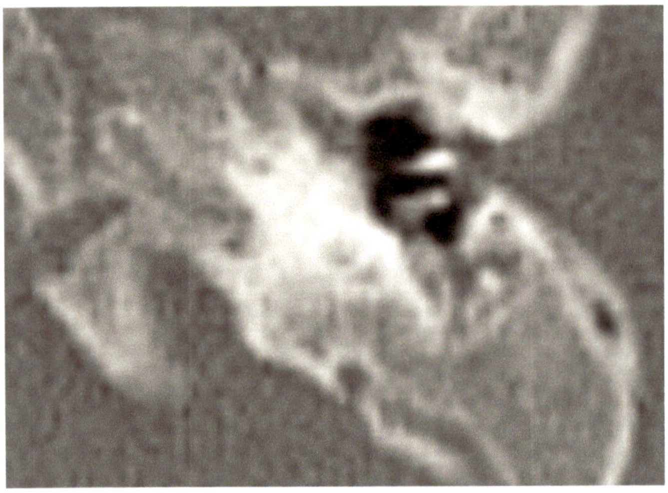

Fig. 15.15 The first of five images of the same patient with a left-sided cochlear aplasia **(Fig. 15.15–Fig. 15.19)**. In this axial CT image, at the position of the cochlea, there is no promontory, no oval window niche, and no cochlea visible. The first visible structure in the anterior labyrinthine bone is mostly the facial nerve or the internal auditory canal.

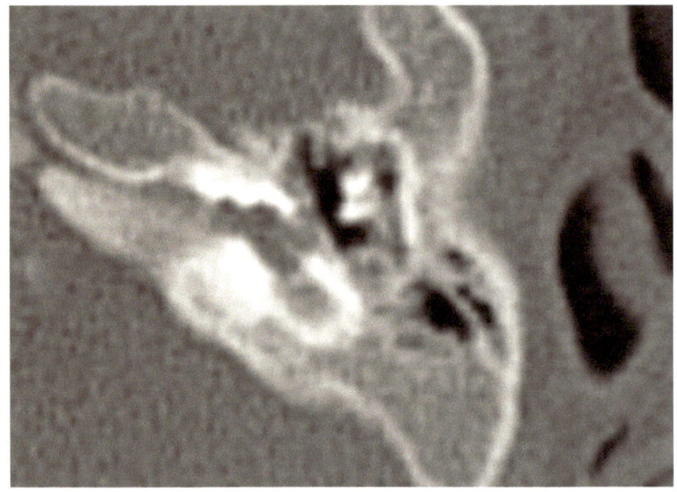

Fig. 15.16 In this axial image the IAC can be seen as a narrow hypoplastic canal in a more posterior direction. Anterior to the lateral end of the IAC no cochlear structure is visible. The incus and malleus seem to have normal dimensions but the course of the facial nerve is often aberrant.

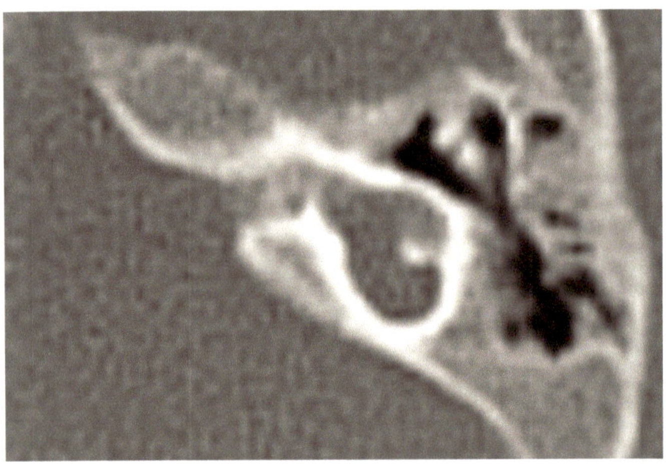

Fig. 15.17 The lateral canal seen on this axial CT image is dysplastic with a tiny bony island.

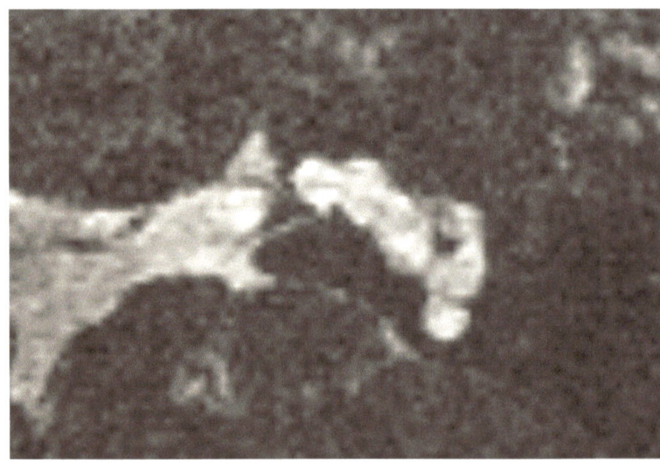

Fig. 15.18 In this axial MRI image a slightly different axial angle (compared with the CT scan, **Fig. 15.17**) of the labyrinth is seen. There is no cochlea seen anterior to the internal auditory canal. It may be that the rudimentary cochlea is embedded within the complete malformation, which makes differentiation from a common cavity difficult.

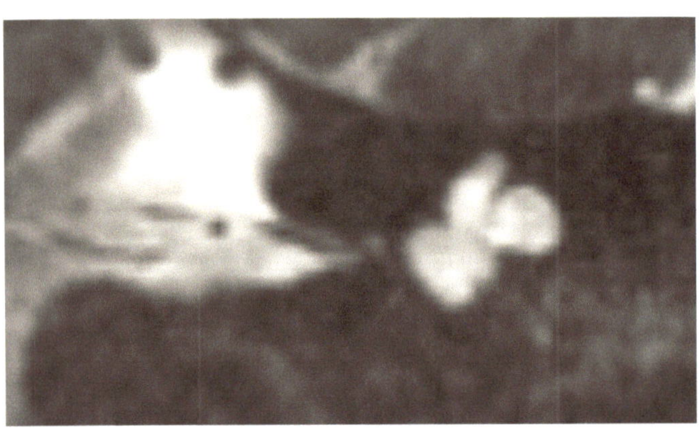

Fig. 15.19 A coronal image showing a dysplastic lateral semicircular canal (LSC) and a dysplastic superior semicircular canal (SSC). In cochlear aplasia the vestibular part can be dysplastic or partly hypoplastic. The facial nerve is well visible on this image; the vestibulocochlear nerve is less visible on other images.

Cochlear Aplasia

Cochlear aplasia is thought as an arrest in development at the fourth week of gestation.

Classification

Cochlear aplasia is only slightly different from the common cavity, and one could debate whether it is a separate entity. Anterior to the lateral part of the IAC there is no structure that could be distinguished as a (rudimentary) cochlea. A vestibular structure is present, but is mostly a dysplastic vestibule or lateral semicircular canal.

One has to be sure that it is not a completely ossified cochlea, in which the bony area would be of normal dimensions and a promontory would be present. The promontory would be absent in a malformation and the labyrinthine part of the facial nerve would be at the position of the cochlea.

(See **Fig. 15.15–Fig. 15.19**.)

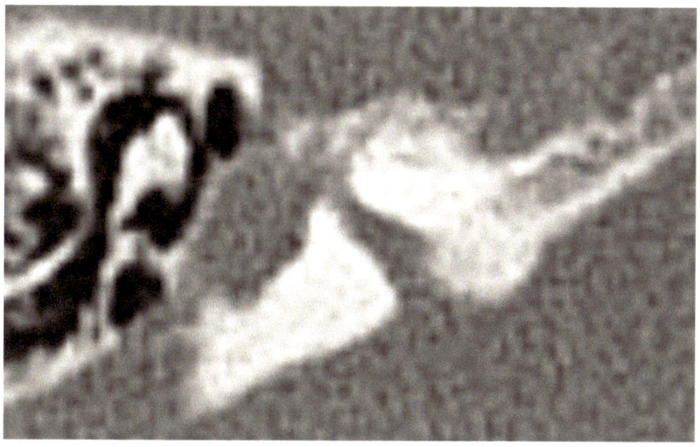

Fig. 15.20 Example of a cochleovestibular aplasia. Although there appears to be some spongy bone formation adjacent to the middle ear, the small internal auditory canal does not end in a "labyrinth-like" structure. Note that the "ice cream cone" ossicles are normally shaped.

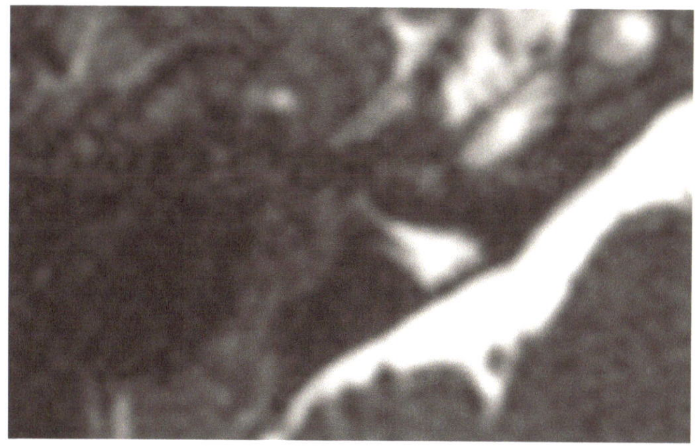

Fig. 15.21 MRI image of the same patient as in **Fig. 15.21**. There seems to be only one nerve in the IAC and the spongy bone formation does not incorporate any open fluid-filled structure.

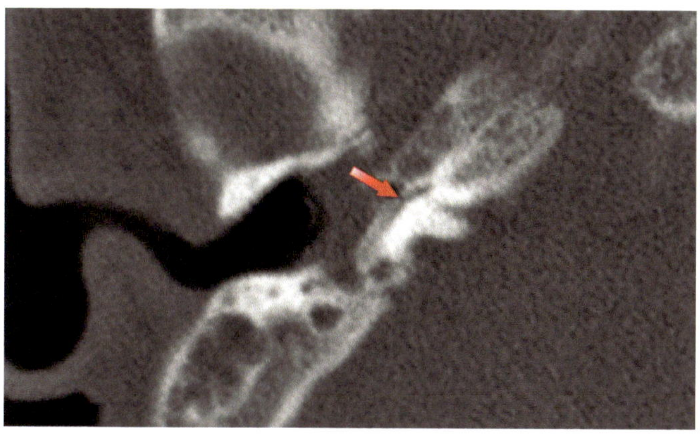

Fig. 15.22 Another example of a cochleovestibular aplasia. The only structure recognizable at the location of the inner ear is the horizontal tympanic part of the facial nerve (*red arrow*).

Cochleovestibular Aplasia (Michel)

It is thought that this is due to an arrest in development before or at the third week of gestation.

Classification

There is complete absence of all cochlear and vestibular elements. It can be associated with absence of the IAC. A normal middle ear and ossicles can be present.

(See **Fig. 15.20–Fig. 15.22.**)

Incomplete Partition Type 3 (X-linked)

This malformation is also known as X-linked deformity.[23,24]

Classification

The most important aspect of the deformity is deficiency of bone between the lateral end of the bulbous IAC and basal turn of the cochlea.

Clinical Features

There is an association of X-linked mixed deafness with a stapes gusher (a profuse flow of cerebrospinal fluid if the stapes is disturbed). This distinct type of deformity differs between male and female subjects. Most predominantly a typical IP-3 malformation is seen in some severely deaf males.[24] In females with IP-3 there is a slight hearing loss and the anomaly has a milder form.

The absence of the bony cochlear aperture would make the insertion of a multichannel electrode risky, as the deficient bone would almost certainly mean that the electrode would enter the IAC rather than staying in the cochlear coils.

Genetic studies have shown that there are at least two types of X-linked deafness,[24,25] some of which have normal inner ears as shown by CT.

(See **Fig. 15.23–Fig. 15.25.**)

Labyrinthine Dysplasia (Isolated)

Classification

A true classification of this type of malformation does not exist. The simplest definition would be a malformed labyrinth with a radiologically normal cochlea. Measurements can be used to define a normal and a malformed labyrinth. Most prominent in commonly malformed is the lateral semicircular canal (LSC). (See **Fig. 15.26.**)

CHARGE Syndrome–Associated Malformations

Classification

CHARGE is an acronym for *coloboma of the eye, heart defects, atresia of the nasal choanae, retardation of growth and/or development, genital and/or urinary abnormalities, and ear abnormalities and deafness.* These features are no longer used in making a diagnosis of CHARGE syndrome, but the name persists. CHARGE syndrome is the leading cause of congenital deaf-blindness. Very few people with CHARGE will have all of its recognized features.

Genetically, ~60% of those tested have a mutation of the *CHD7* gene.

Clinical Features

Hearing loss is mostly profound sensorineural, but conductive hearing loss, mixed hearing loss, or mild to moderate SNHL are also seen. Aside from deafness, the most common ear anomaly

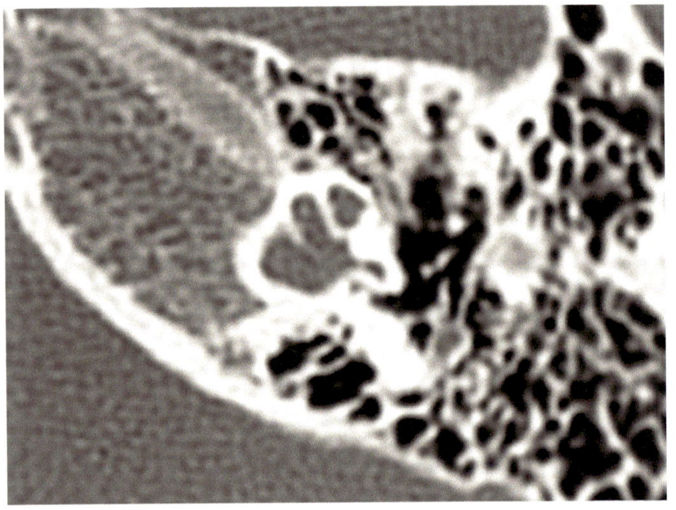

Fig. 15.23 The cochlear aperture is open with a direct connection between the cochlea and the IAC. This increases the intralabyrinthine pressure and also the pressure on the ossicular chain resulting in mixed hearing loss. During implantation it is common to experience a CSF gusher.

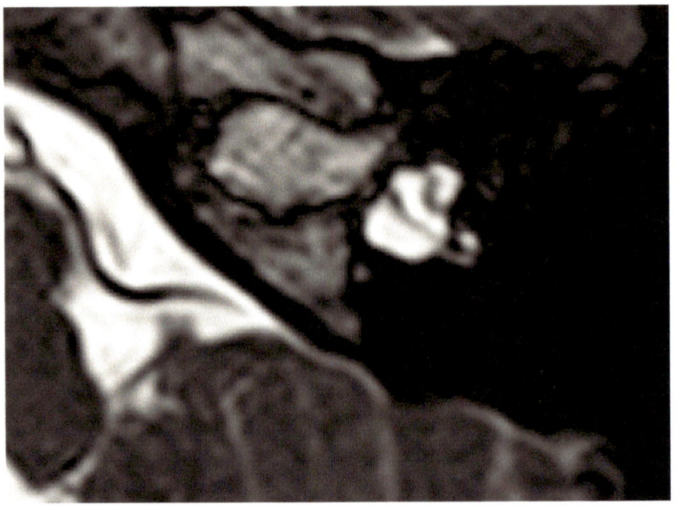

Fig. 15.24 The same section as in **Fig. 15.23** on MRI.

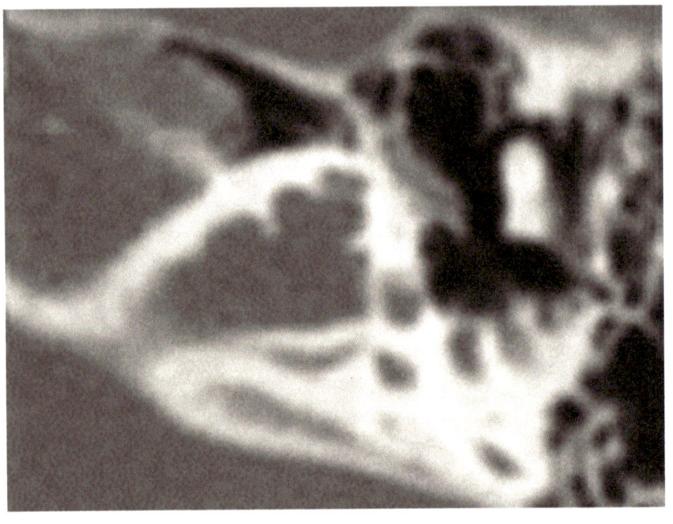

Fig. 15.25 A CT scan of a patient with an X linked IP-3 malformation. The wide cochlear aperture makes a CSF gusher during implantation inevitable.

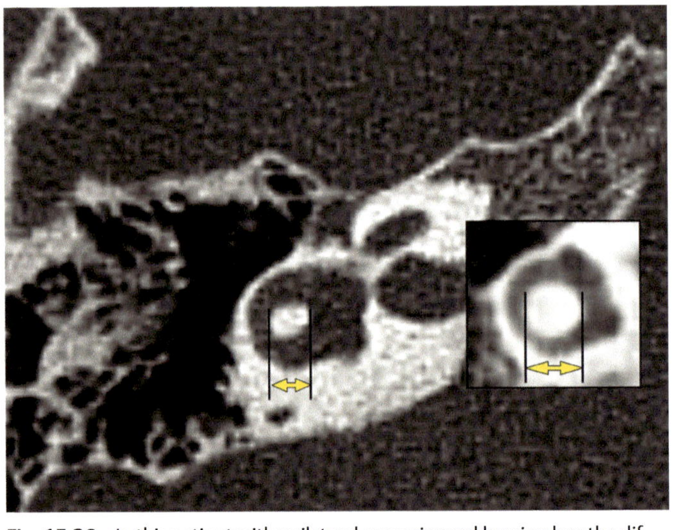

Fig. 15.26 In this patient with unilateral sensorineural hearing loss the difference between the left and right lateral semicircular canal (LSC) was obvious. In the insert one can appreciate the rotated left LSC, compared with the right LSC. The diameter of "the bony island" within the LSC (*yellow arrows*) is a good measure for defining malformed or not malformed.

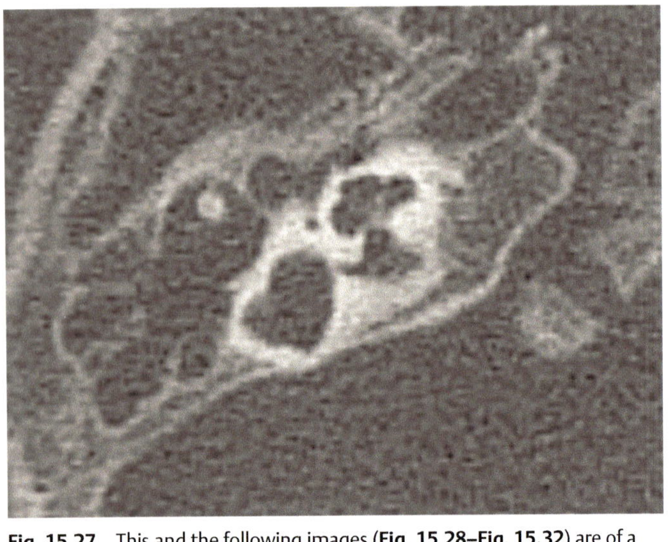

Fig. 15.27 This and the following images (**Fig. 15.28–Fig. 15.32**) are of a girl with CHARGE syndrome. On this CT image of the right side, the hypoplastic LSC and the narrow cochlear aperture are visible. The cochlea itself appears to be normal in size.

seen in CHARGE syndrome is the abnormal appearance of bowl-shaped and concave ears, known as "lop ears." On imaging, substantial abnormalities of the inner ear including hypoplasia or aplasia of the semicircular canals and abnormalities of the cochlea and vestibule are seen. Abnormalities are frequent and multiple, mostly of the facial nerve, the venous system, the cochlear aperture, and the cochlear nerve.

The facial nerve is more commonly affected in children with CHARGE syndrome (and VACTERL association), displaced anteriorly adjacent to or within the round window niche.[26] Also frequently described are venous displacement or malformations within the temporal bone.[27] Cochlear aperture narrowing or atresia is seen on CT, but even with profound SNHL some have normal cochlear apertures. Absent or deficient cochlear nerves have been associated with CHARGE syndrome.[28,29] Often the mastoid and middle ear is hypoplastic and also the round window can be hypoplastic or even aplastic.[29]

(See **Fig. 15.27–Fig. 15.32**.)

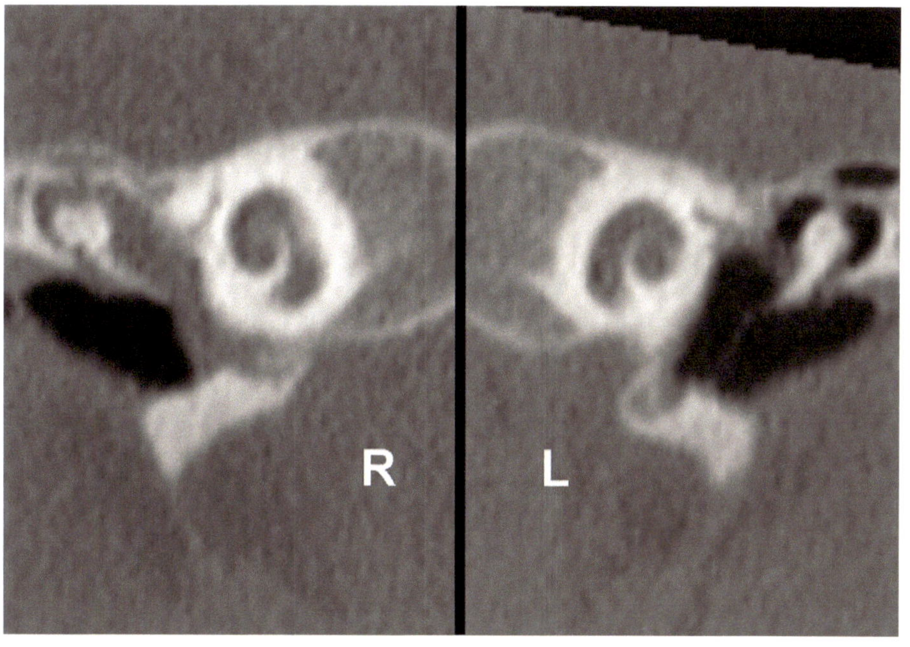

Fig. 15.28 The cochleae are of normal size on both sides.

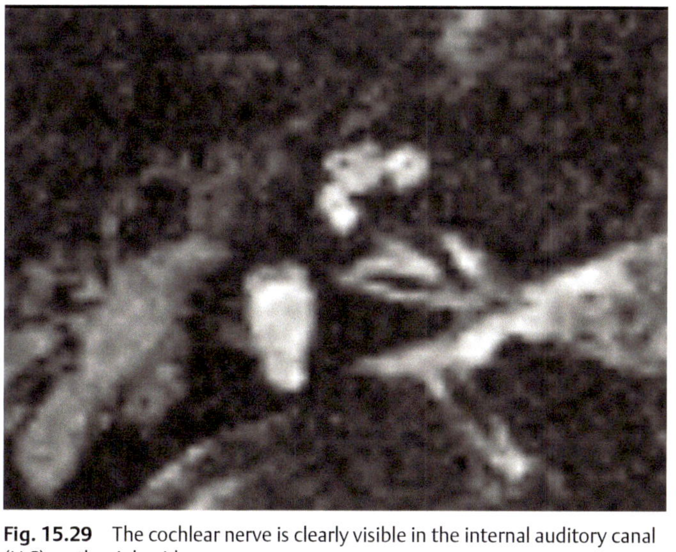

Fig. 15.29 The cochlear nerve is clearly visible in the internal auditory canal (IAC) on the right side.

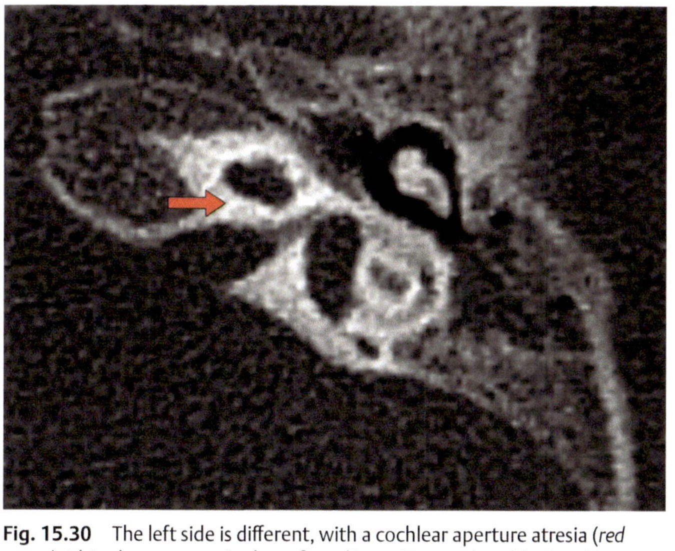

Fig. 15.30 The left side is different, with a cochlear aperture atresia (*red arrow*). This phenomenon is also referred to as "trapped cochlea" and is strongly associated with CHARGE syndrome. There appears to be no connection between the IAC and the cochlea on CT.

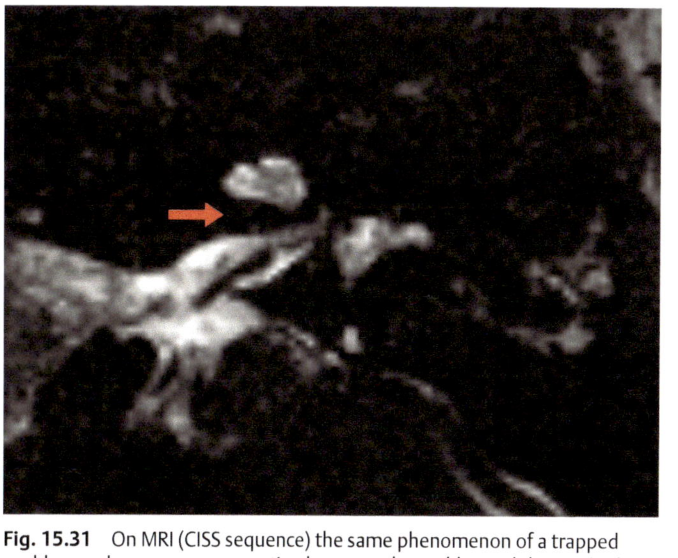

Fig. 15.31 On MRI (CISS sequence) the same phenomenon of a trapped cochlea can be seen: no connection between the cochlea and the IAC (*red arrow*). The cochlear nerve is not visible, although some gray lines are present.

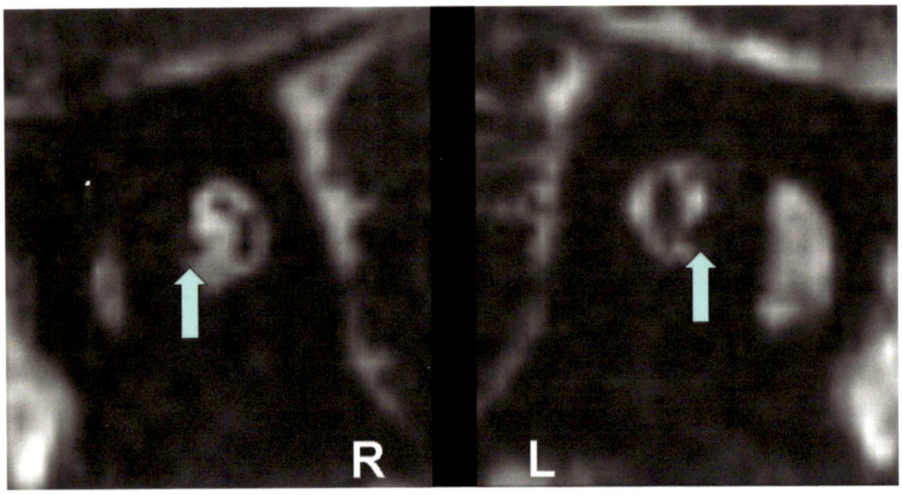

Fig. 15.32 MRI sagittal view perpendicular to the IAC of the right and left side, just at the level of the cochlea/fundus. On the right side (R) a cochlear nerve is visible (*arrow*); on the left side a nerve also appears to be present (*arrow*), although it is wholly at the anterior wall of the IAC.

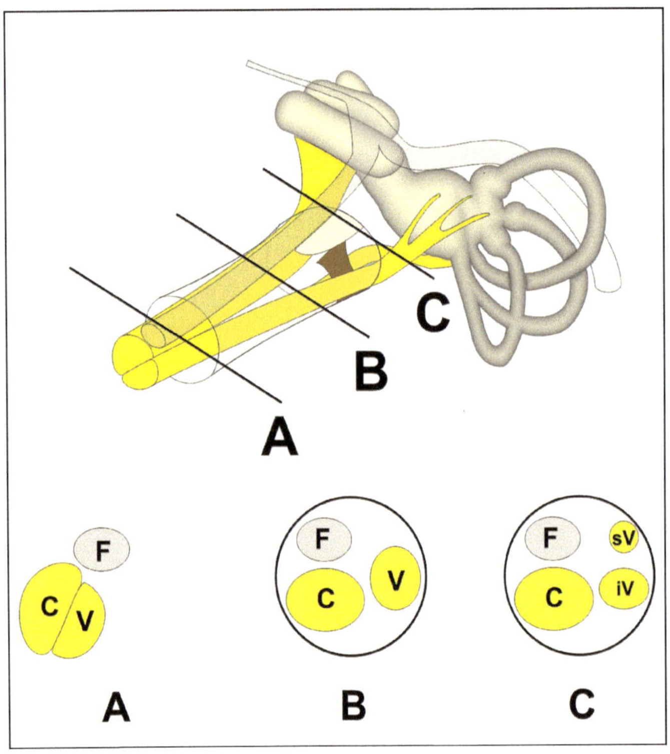

Fig. 15.33 Normal anatomy of the internal auditory canal and inner ear. The nervous elements are represented at three different levels (**A, B, C**) of the internal auditory canal. C, cochlear nerve fibers of the vestibulocochlear nerve; V, vestibular nerve fibers of the vestibulocochlear nerve; F, facial nerve; sV, superior vestibular nerve; iV= inferior vestibular nerve.

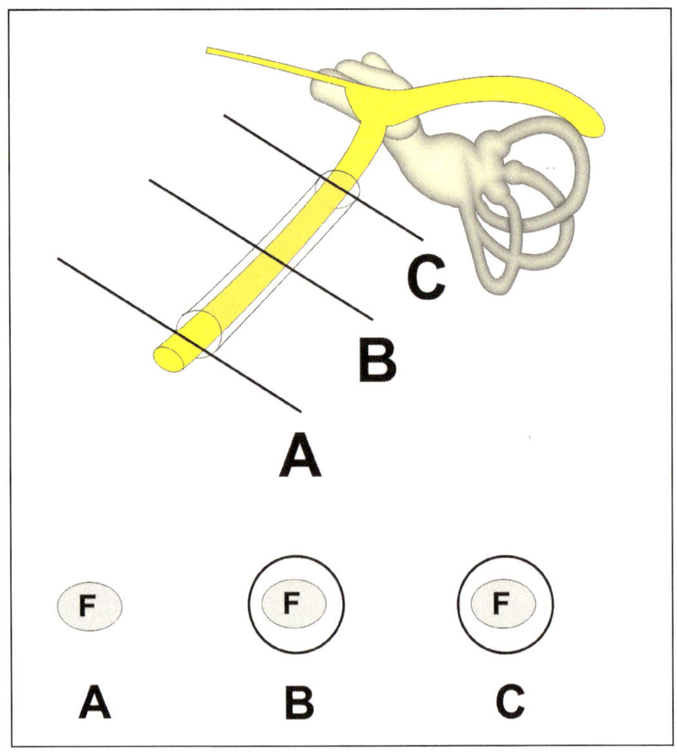

Fig. 15.34 Type I vestibulocochlear nerve (VCN) hypoplasia/aplasia. *Nerve:* complete VCN affected. *Labyrinth:* the labyrinth may be normal or dysplastic. *IAC:* stenotic IAC and only the facial nerve (F) seems to be present in the IAC. Contents of the internal auditory canal are represented at three different levels (**A, B, C**).

15.3.3 Malformation of the Cochlear Nerve and Inner Ear Canal

(Vestibulo) Cochlear Nerve Hypoplasia and Aplasia

The radiologic entity of vestibulocochlear nerve (VCN) aplasia was first reported in 1997.[30] It was shown that the 3D Fourier transformation-CISS (3DFT-CISS) MRI with parasagittal reconstruction on the course of the VCN allowed identification of the facial nerve and of the VCN with its cochlear and inferior and superior vestibular branches. See Chapter 3, **Fig. 3.38** and **Fig. 3.39**.

The existence of a VCN deficiency can be strongly suspected in combination with certain types of malformations, especially in IAC malformations, cochlear aplasia, common cavity, IP-1, and rarely in cochlear hypoplasia. In these cases an additional MRI scan is absolutely necessary before implantation to ensure the status of the VCN. No VCN deficiency is associated with the following malformations: LVAS, IP-2, isolated dysplasia of the semicircular canals, and X-linked deafness. In all of these cases the VCN is expected to be thicker than the facial nerve.[31]

Classification

In deciding whether the VCN is hypoplastic it is common to compare the diameter of the facial nerve with that of the cochlear nerve in a sagittal plane (oblique) through the IAC. VCN aplasia is radiologically classified as the nerve not being visible on appropriate sagittal MR images.

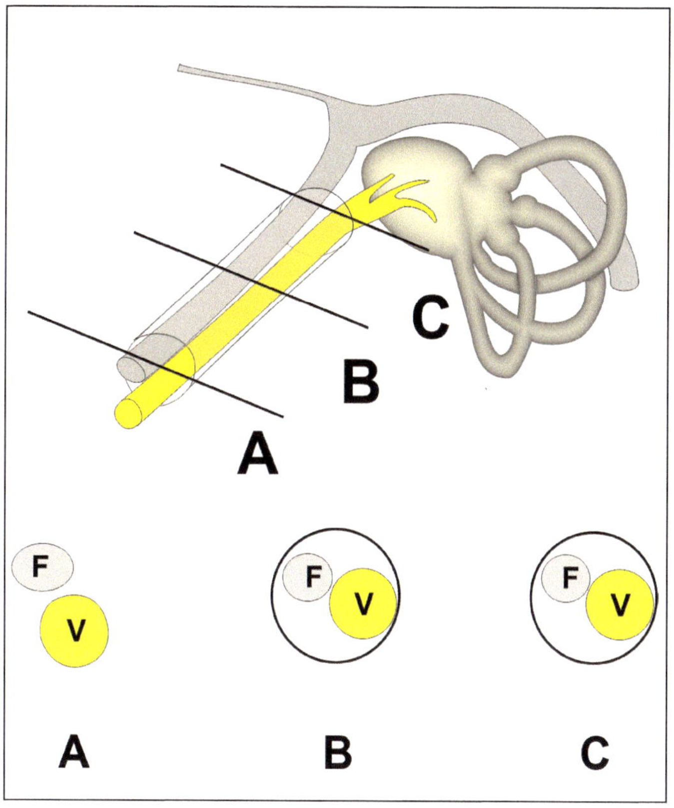

Fig. 15.35 Type IIa VCN hypoplasia/aplasia. *Nerve:* cochlear branch of VCN affected. *Labyrinth:* dysplasia, even common cavity. Contents of the internal auditory canal are represented at three different levels (**A, B, C**). F, facial nerve; V, vestibular nerve.

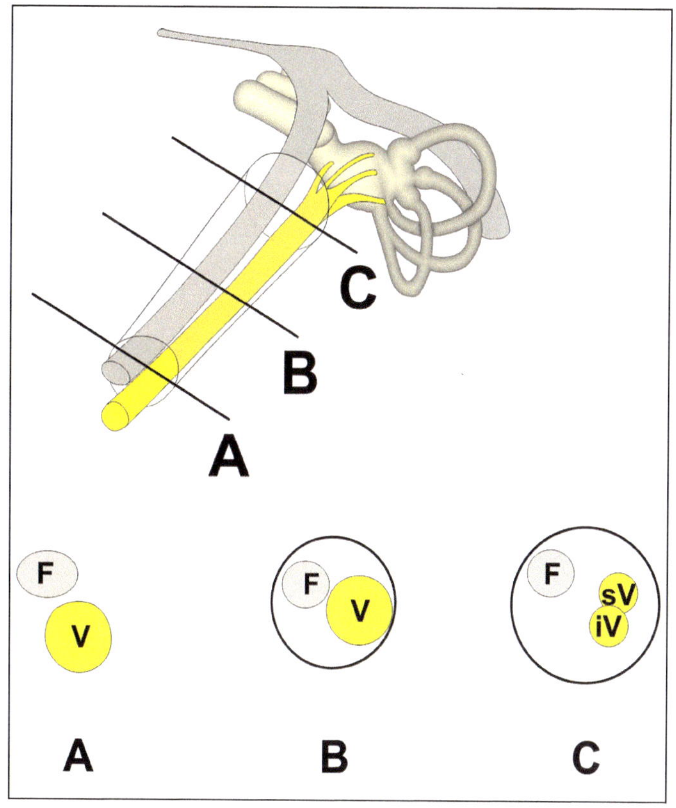

Fig. 15.36 Type IIb VCN hypoplasia/aplasia. *Nerve:* cochlear branch of VCN affected. *Labyrinth:* normal morphology. Contents of the internal auditory canal are represented at three different levels (**A, B, C**).

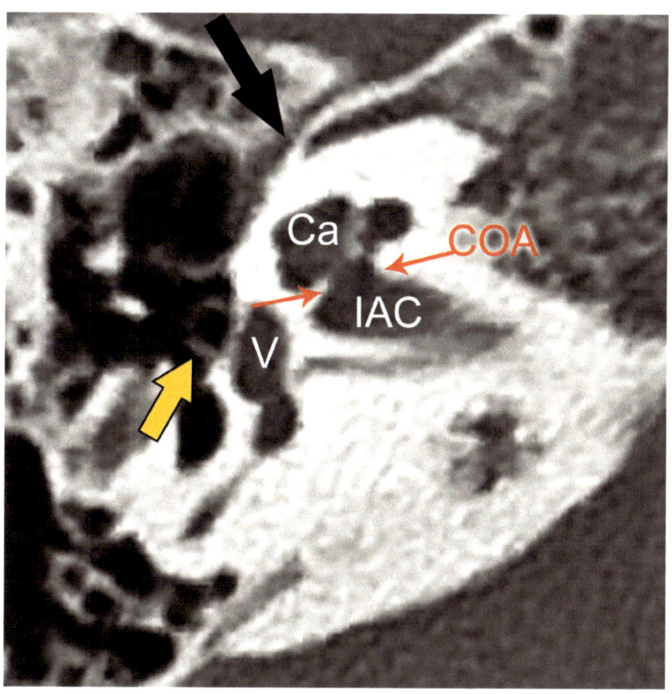

Fig. 15.37 The diameter of the cochlear nerve canal, also known as cochlear aperture (COA, between the *red arrows*), was measured along the inner margin of its bony walls at its middle portion on an axial image of the base of the modiolus. Other structures in this picture are explained in Chapter 3, **Fig. 3.5**. Ca, cochlear apex; IAC, internal auditory canal; V, vestibule.

According to the first report there are four types (I, IIa, IIb, III) of hypoplasia/aplasia of the VCN. Type III (only the vestibular branch affected) has actually never been reported and will therefore not be mentioned further.[30]

(See **Fig. 15.33–Fig. 15.36**.)

Internal Auditory Canal Malformation

A narrow internal auditory canal is associated with hypoplasia or aplasia of the cochlear nerve (CN) on imaging,[32,33] though not all cases with a narrow IAC have absent nerves or nerve fibers.[31,33] Internal auditory canal stenosis is often associated with malformation of the labyrinth.[31]

Classification

A cochlear nerve canal, also known as cochlear aperture, of diameter less than 1.5 mm is most often associated with CN hypoplasia[33,34] and therefore often considered as an IAC stenosis. This borderline is essentially arbitrary as other diameters are also suggested in the literature and the diameter of the IAC can be small without any pathology. (See **Fig. 15.37**.)

Table 15.3 Overview of the most prominent anatomical features of the most common malformations and implant tips according to these abnormalities

Malformation	Anatomy	Special feature	Implant tips
Incomplete partition 2 (IP-2)	Cochlea and vestibular normal size, cochlea 1.5 turns	EVA	Normal implant
Incomplete partition 3 (IP-3) (X-linked)	Normal cochlea but absent cochlear aperture, bulbous IAC	Open IAC	Expect CSF gusher, STP, normal electrode
Cochlear hypoplasia	Cochlea and vestibule are separate	Vestibule normal or hypoplastic, IAC normal or small	Shorter electrode
Incomplete partition 1 (IP-1)	Cystic cochleovestibular malformation	Enlarged IAC, no EVA	Full banded electrode, shorter electrode
Common cavity	One large cochleovestibular cyst	IAC size with respect to cyst	Full band, precurved electrode, LSC Beware of gusher, STP
Cochlear aplasia	No cochlea, only a vestibule/canal	No bulging of the promontory	No CI, possibly ABI
Michel deformity	No cochlea or vestibular elements		No CI, ABI

Abbreviations: IP, incomplete partition; EVA, enlarged vestibular aqueduct; IAC, internal auditory canal; CI, cochlear implant; ABI, auditory brainstem implant; STP, subtotal petrosectomy; LSC, lateral semicircular canal insertion.

15.4 Cochlear and Auditory Brainstem Implantation in Malformations

(See **Table 15.3**.)

15.4.1 Cochlear Implantation in IP-2

Suggested approach: normal transmastoidal posterior tympanotomy approach.
Implant advice: normal implant.
Special care: other than some oozing of the perilymph and special attention to the tight closure of the cochleostomy, there is no difference from a normal implantation.
Outcome/counseling: the expectations with a CI in a patient with IP-2 are overall good and open-set speech perception can be expected.[26]

15.4.2 Cochlear Implantation in IP-3

Suggested approach: subtotal petrosectomy because of CSF leak.
Implant advice: normal implant; preferably a precurved electrode; normal or wider cochleostomy with good periosteal strip packing.
Special care: CSF gusher very likely; tight closure of the cochleostomy; fat obliteration of the subtotal petrosectomy cavity. Beware of facial nerve stimulation when programming.
Outcome/counseling: the expectations with a CI in a patient with IP-3 is overall good, even comparable to non-malformed CI users, but counsel about possible perioperative and postoperative risks (facial nerve stimulation, CSF leak, meningitis).[35,36]

15.4.3 Cochlear Implantation in Cochlear Hypoplasia

Suggested approach: transmastoidal.
Implant advice: normal or shorter electrode.
Special care: the round window can be difficult to localize and the facial nerve can have an aberrant course.
Outcome/counseling: outcomes are dependent on (1) how many electrodes are inserted correctly; (2) how complete the innervation of the hypoplastic cochlea is. The expectations should therefore be tempered accordingly.

15.4.4 Cochlear Implantation in IP-1

Suggested approach: transmastoidal, anticipate subtotal petrosectomy.
Implant advice: electrode, depending on the size and shape of the cochlear cavity. A lateral wall electrode has better chances of successful stimulation.
Special care: the cochlear aperture should be assessed with scanning and, if there is an open connection with the IAC, a gusher and a subtotal petrosectomy should be anticipated. Also a small cochlear aperture can be present, then a hypoplasia or even aplasia of the VCN may be present.
Outcome/counseling: insufficient data are available in the literature, but it seems that the unpartitioned cystic cochlea will not do much better than in a common cavity. Also a hypoplastic VCN could diminish functional outcomes.

15.4.5 Cochlear Implantation in Common Cavity

Suggested approach: an electrode insertion via a transmastoid labyrinthotomy is suggested. Take into consideration a subtotal petrosectomy, because of the apparent connection with the IAC and an aberrant facial nerve.

Implant advice: outer wall "uncoiled" electrode, as histologic studies have shown that neural elements can be present at the outer wall of the cavity.[3]

Special care: often an aberrant course of the facial nerve is encountered. Good imaging and surgical planning are required.

Outcome/counseling: from none to 40% open-set speech perception can be expected. Counsel accordingly.[26,37] Especially in combination with cochlear nerve deficiency, the results are poor.

15.4.6 Cochlear Implantation or ABI in CHARGE

Suggested approach: subtotal petrosectomy is advised for facial nerve and vascular anomalies. Because of the often small anatomy, conversion to a canal wall down approach should be anticipated. Good facial nerve monitoring is extremely important.

Implant advice: cochlear anomalies are not common, thus any CI electrode would be feasible. ABI in selected cases, often after a CI attempt.

Special care: note the possibility of a "trapped cochlea" with atresia of the cochlear aperture. Good imaging (CT and MRI) is essential. An attempt at CI placement and testing is preferred if connection of nerve fibers toward the cochlea is doubtful. ABI in cases with no reaction or no connection of the cochlea to the cochlear nerve.

Outcome/counseling: the results after CI surgery vary due to the differing extents of additional disabilities such as developmental delay, intellectual delay, and visual impairment. Age at implantation and extent of malformation (e.g., cochlear nerve hypoplasia/ aplasia) also play a role.[38]

15.4.7 ABI or CI in Common Cavity or Aplasia of the Cochlea?

When there is no cochlear lumen, it would appear impossible to place a cochlear implant. But if there is a rudimentary cavity or some kind of lumen that seems connected with the brainstem, a cochlear implant could be attempted. At least a promontory test should be done to exclude the possibility of auditory nerve fibers running to the labyrinthine malformation. Imaging alone is not sufficient proof of a disconnection between the labyrinth and brainstem.[39–41]

Only in a complete lack of labyrinthine lumen, as in Michel deformity, is there a direct indication for an ABI.

15.4.8 ABI or CI in Cochlear Nerve Aplasia or a Small IAC?

Cases with apparent cochlear nerve aplasia on imaging are often associated with a small internal auditory canal.[32] Nonetheless, several recent publications point out that the absence of a visible cochlear nerve on imaging or a hypoplastic IAC does not preclude auditory innervation of the cochlea.[39–41] Cochlear implantation can be a valuable option for patients with apparent cochlear nerve aplasia as long as they have undergone appropriate testing.[40] Electrically evoked ABR is critical in the evaluation of this patient group.[40,42,43] The outcomes with cochlear implantation can be unsatisfactory[44] and clear counseling advice should be given not to overestimate the results of cochlear implantation. In the literature, patients with type IIa aplasia had some audiological outcome but no open set speech understanding.

If there is proof of a bilateral absent cochlear nerve or nerve fibers after sufficient stimulation, or if there is a complete cochlear aplasia or a bilateral Michel deformity, an ABI could be a solution to create some chance of hearing development.[26,32]

15.4.9 Auditory Brainstem Implantation in Labyrinthine Aplasia (Michel Deformity)

Suggested approach: translabyrinthine approach. In a retrosigmoid approach more traction on the cerebellum is needed. See Chapter 8.

Implant advice: there seems no difference in outcome between the current ABIs in the market. Note that the ABI from Cochlear is the only implant with a removable magnet.

Special care: often an aberrant course of the facial nerve is encountered. Good imaging and surgical planning are required.

Outcome/counseling: with the Cochlear ABI the outcomes can be varied. Sound identification, or poor closed-set word recognition, seem the highest achievable.[32,45]

15.5 Risks in Malformation CI Surgery

15.5.1 Facial Nerve Injury

An aberrant facial nerve is frequently seen in the group of inner ear malformations.[32,37,46] Accurate imaging, secure planning of the surgical approach, and perioperative facial nerve monitoring are crucial to avoid this complication. Subtotal petrosectomy is often helpful to visualize the nerve.

15.5.2 Facial Nerve Stimulation

Two situations have been presented in which the facial nerve can be stimulated during fitting or use of the CI[32]: an aberrant course of the facial nerve or a close relation between facial nerve and cochlea in the IAC in combination with an open cochlear aperture (IP-3/common cavity). The choice of electrode can be very important in this issue. Sometimes reimplantation is necessary[47] or implantation of the other ear can be evaluated.[35]

15.5.3 CSF Gusher

With a direct connection from the cochlea to the IAC, a CSF gusher is inevitable.[26,35,37] Sometimes a bulging stapes footplate can be distinguished as a predictor for CSF pressure.[22] Elevating the head of the operating table and waiting for a while is generally sufficient to obtain a clear surgical field. In this step, the size of the cochleostomy is also important. Although some authors have suggested the possible smallest cochleostomy in such cases,[48] nowadays the tendency of experienced surgeons is to create a relatively large cochleostomy and to place the pieces of muscles around the electrode array and put bone dust over them.[3,19,49] More important points are to secure any CSF leak in the middle ear by closing the eustachian tube and to close the ear canal and the wound in several layers, as described in Chapter 10 on subtotal petrosectomy.

A corklike electrode (**Fig. 15.38**) has been designed for this type of complication. This electrode will help to create "a first line of defense" but will probably not prevent meningitis. We believe that the corklike electrode in combination with a subtotal petrosectomy (second line of defense) will minimize the chances of a CSF leak and more importantly of meningitis.

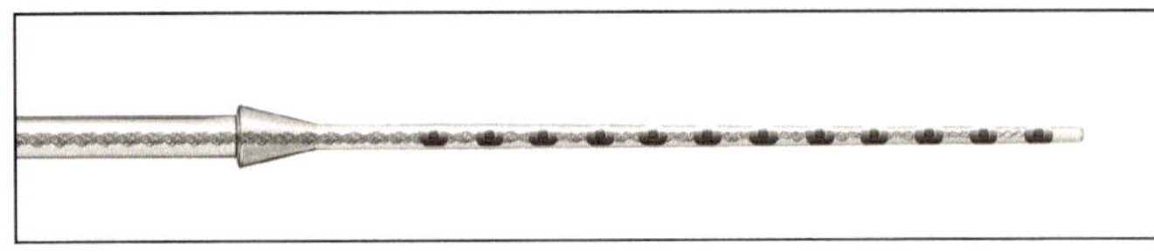

Fig. 15.38 The corklike stopper FORM electrode by Med El designed especially for malformed cochleae. This electrode is available in 24-mm and 19-mm versions.

15.5.4 Meningitis

Meningitis is associated with an easy pathway between the middle ear or mastoid and the inner ear. In malformations the barrier that resists bacterial intrusion is much more feeble than in a patient with normal inner ear morphology. Therefore, meningitis can occur prior to implantation and, more strikingly, the malformation is sometimes revealed for the first time as a result of the diagnostic work-up for meningitis.[21] Standard cochlear implant surgery alone will not change this anatomical weak barrier. To avoid meningitis after implantation it is of utmost importance to secure the surgical cavity during subtotal petrosectomy meticulously, as in the translabyrinthine approach.[50] Without surgical eradication of the mucosa and closure of the middle ear and mastoid cavity, postoperative meningitis can occur.[21]

15.5.5 Complications

Major and minor complications (for discussion see Chapter 7) in patients with malformations are reported in relatively small series, with various malformations. The range of reported complications is therefore greatly variable. It seems that overall the percentage of minor complications is higher because of the anatomical differences mentioned above, but the reimplantation rate in malformation cases may not be different than in "normal" CI patients. (See **Table 15.4**.)

15.5.6 No Auditory Effect/Nonuse

Minor or no auditory effect and subsequent nonuse can be expected in severe malformations, but especially in case of cochlear nerve deficiency.[26]

Reprogramming, reimplantation, other-side implantation, or auditory brainstem implantation are other options. All of these should be considered as well as or compared with sign language.

15.6 Summary

15.6.1 Inner Ear Malformations

The current classification of inner ear malformations, in order from *most to least* dysplastic cochlea, consists of

- Cochleovestibular aplasia (Michel deformity)
- Cochlear aplasia
- Common cavity
- Incomplete partition type 1 (cystic cochleovestibular anomaly)
- Incomplete partition type 2
- Incomplete partition type 3 (X-linked)
- Cochlear hypoplasia
- Labyrinthine dysplasia (isolated)

Not included in this consecutive list are the CHARGE syndrome–associated malformations.

Table 15.4 Reported percentage of complications in children with cochlear implant and cochlear malformations

Report	Complications	
	Major (%)	Minor (%)
Hoffman et al (1997)[51]	–	33
Eisenman et al (2001)[52]	0	11.7
Buchman et al (2004)[53]	14.2	7.1
Mylanus et al (2004)[36]	–	7.6
Loundon et al (2005)[54]	0	5.5
Papsin (2005)[5]	3	2
Kim et al (2006)[55]	2.1	–
Sennaroglu et al (2006)[19]	0	15
Lee et al (2011)[56]	0	17

Note: The number of patients is overall low, and the malformations and complications reported are variable.

15.6.2 Internal Auditory Canal and Vestibulocochlear Nerve Malformations

The existence of a VCN deficiency can be strongly suspected in combination with IAC malformations, cochlear aplasia, common cavity, IP-1, and rarely in cochlear hypoplasia.

15.6.3 CI or ABI

It seems that in the majority of labyrinth malformations with bilateral severe to profound hearing loss there is an indication for a CI. An ABI is indicated when there is no labyrinthine lumen; if imaging indicates an absent cochlear nerve, testing still has to be done to prove an absence of nerve fibers running along with other nerves in the internal auditory meatus.

15.6.4 Results of Implantation

The outcomes in malformations can be various: whereas the IP-2 patient is expected to achieve an open-set speech performance, patients with severe malformations will only attain sound detection. The best results with cochlear implantation are seen in the least malformed cochleae. In the most severe malformations, ABI is indicated.

Pearls and Pitfalls in Malformations of the Labyrinth and Cochlear Nerve Hypoplasia/Aplasia

- The difference between IP-1 and a cochlear (vestibular) hypoplasia is the inner structure of the cochlea. In IP-1 the cochlea is cystic and no interscalar septi are visible. Also the modiolus is absent. In a cochlear (vestibular) hypoplasia the cochlea is smaller but still has interscalar septi and a modiolus.
- In IP-3, which is rarely encountered, the wide cochlear aperture makes a CSF gusher during implantation inevitable. A wider cochleostomy with good packing and a subtotal petrosectomy are advised.
- Michel deformity is a cochleovestibular aplasia that can be associated with absence of the IAC. The middle ear and ossicles can be completely normal. ABI is the only solution.
- VCN deficiency is be strongly suspected in combination with IAC malformations, cochlear aplasia, common cavity, IP-1, and rarely in cochlear hypoplasia.
- MRI is absolutely necessary before implantation in case of IAC malformations, cochlear aplasia, common cavity, IP-1, and cochlear hypoplasia to ensure the status of the VCN and rule out VCN hypoplasia or aplasia.
- CT is useful to show anomalies of the middle ear and facial nerve that may necessitate the use of a subtotal petrosectomy in cochlear implant surgery.

Case 15.1 Incomplete Partition Type 2 and Bilateral CI Implantation (Fig. 15.1.1–Fig. 15.1.4)

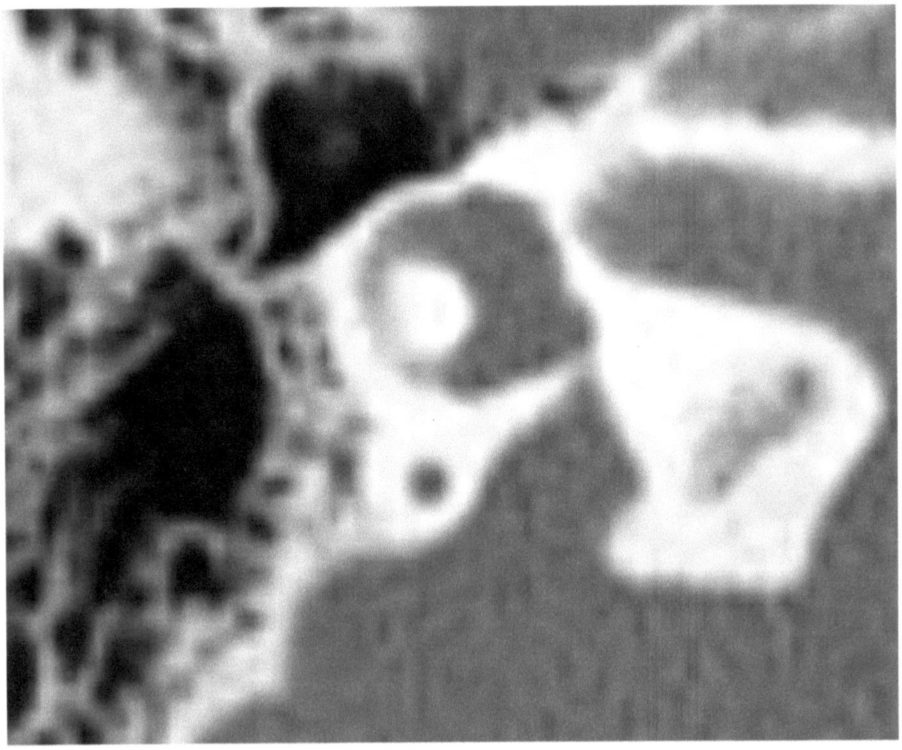

Fig. 15.1.1 Enlarged vestibular aqueduct (EVA) and a more dilated vestibule in a woman who had progressive hearing loss. Her hearing declined over time to preoperative levels of less than 20% speech performance.

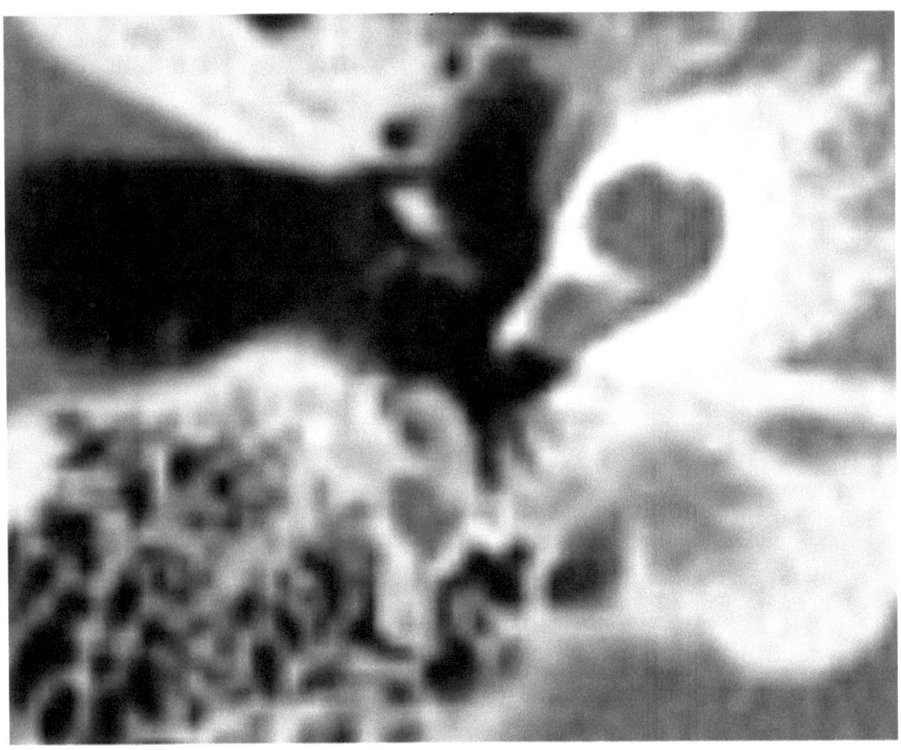

Fig. 15.1.2 On this CT image the cochlea has an incompletely partitioned apical turn. The basal turn is normally developed but the apical and middle turns are unseparated. The triad of Mondini is complete: cochlear unpartitioned apical-middle turn, dilated vestibule, and EVA.

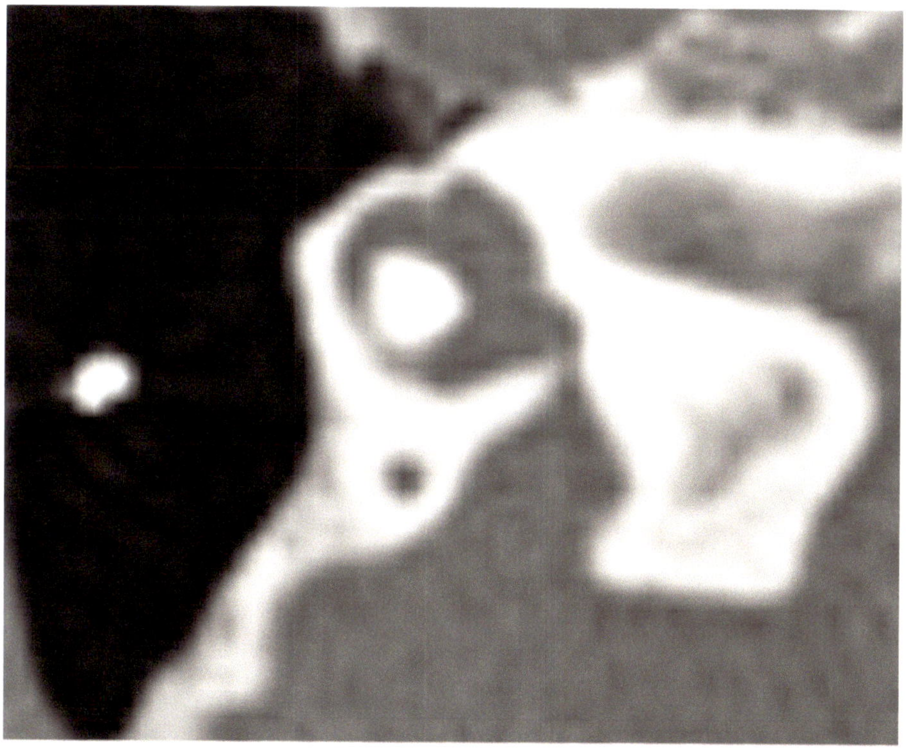

Fig. 15.1.3 No different approach is necessary for the surgery of a patient with an EVA. CSF gushers are not an issue, but perilymph oozing is possible. With a good cochleostomy closure this should not be a problem. In this postoperative axial CT image the mastoidectomy is completely air-filled and the electrode is visible (as a hyperintense dot) before it enters the cochlea.

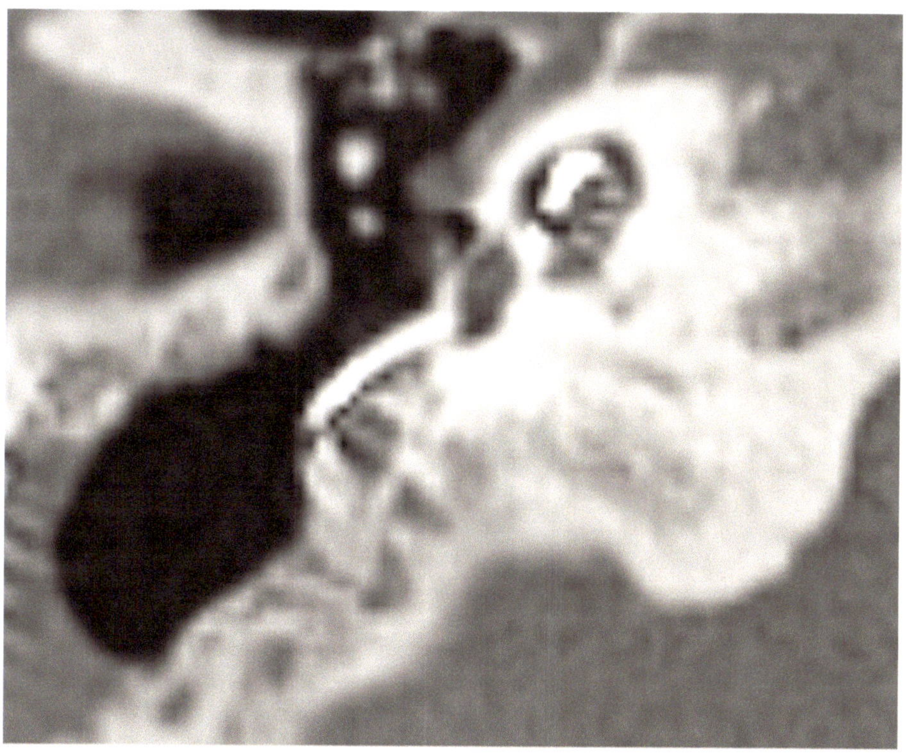

Fig. 15.1.4 The intracochlear electrode is visible on this postoperative axial CT image. The tip of the electrode is visible within the cystic apical part of the cochlea. A fairly air-filled middle ear can be appreciated. The patient had uneventful rehabilitation training and can hold a conversation with relatives on the telephone.

Comment

The rehabilitation (surgery and outcome) in patients with an IP-2 malformation does not differ from that for the average CI implantee.

Case 15.2 CI and Subtotal Petrosectomy in Patient with CHARGE Syndrome (Fig. 15.2.1–Fig. 15.2.14)

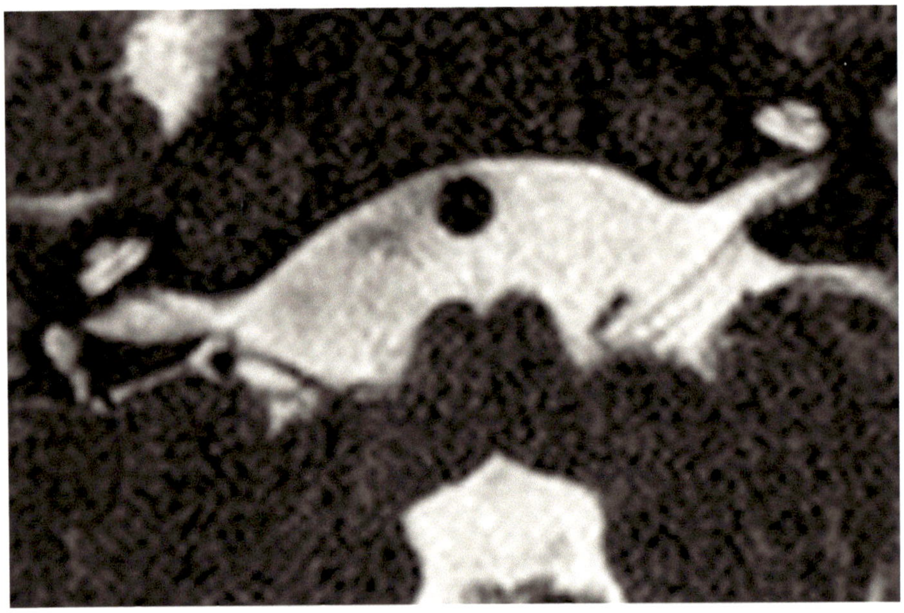

Fig. 15.2.1 In CHARGE syndrome different kinds of malformations can occur. On this MR image of a 3-year-old boy with CHARGE syndrome, the connection of the vestibulocochlear nerve is doubtful on the left side, whereas the right-sided cochlea seems to be connected with a nerve in the IAC. The boy was almost blind and bilaterally deaf and was in need of urgent hearing rehabilitation.

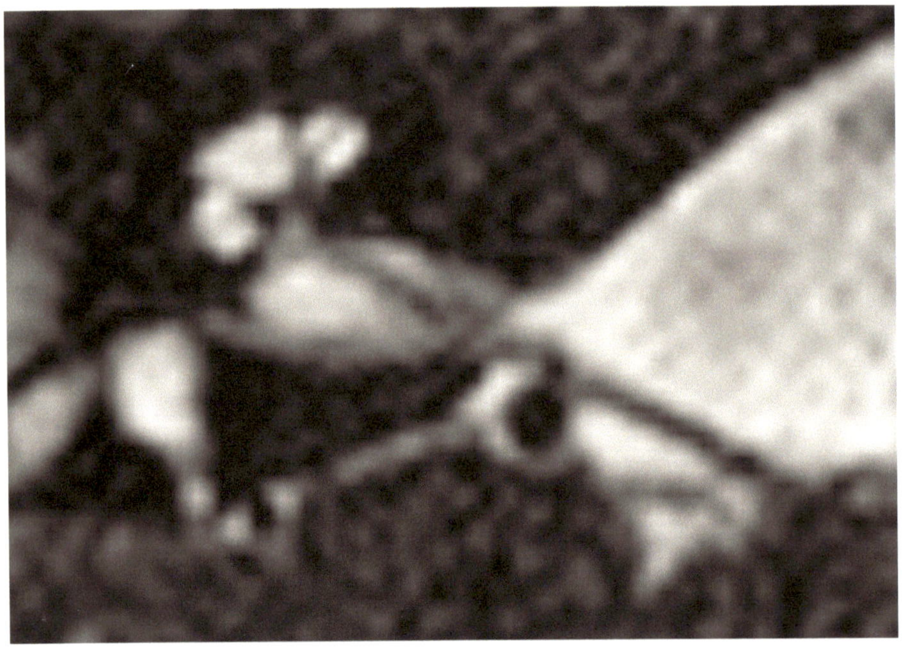

Fig. 15.2.2 In the assessment of this boy MRI showed a well-developed cochlea and a visible cochlear nerve. The vestibular part of the labyrinth was partly absent, with only a rudimentary LSC/vestibule. FN is not visible; clinical function was grade IV.

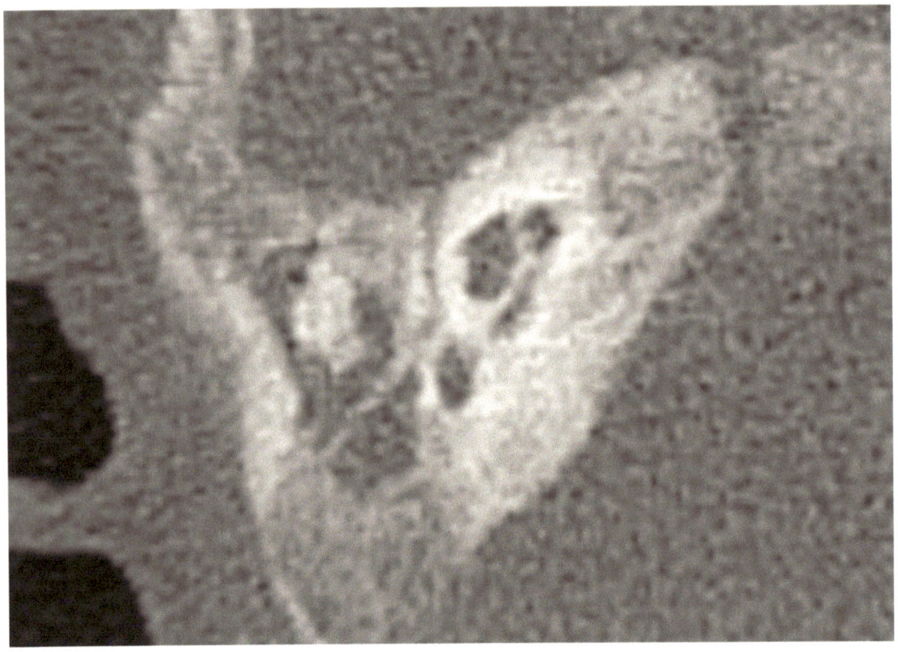

Fig. 15.2.3 A thin tympanic portion of the facial nerve is recognizable in a sclerotic middle ear.

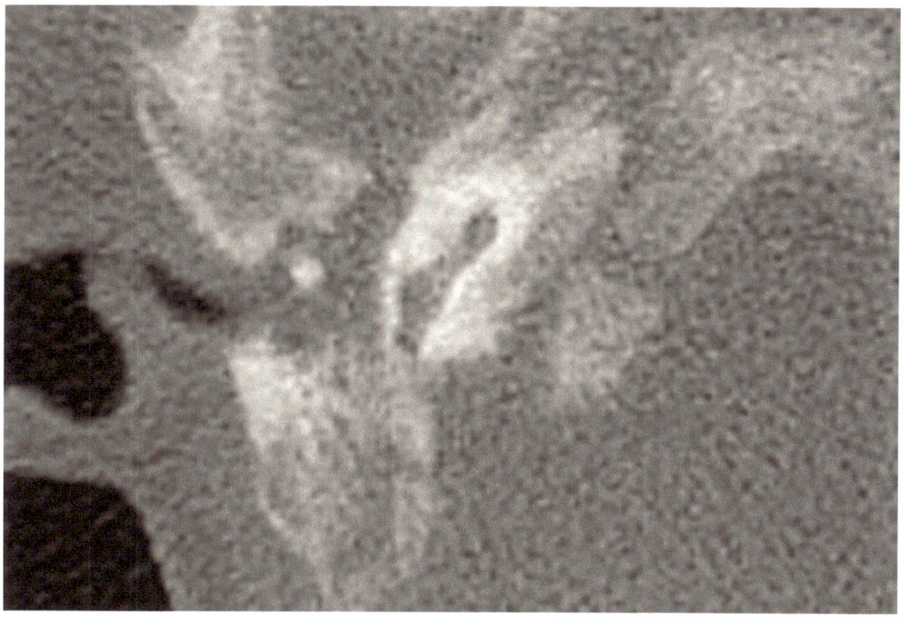

Fig. 15.2.4 The basal turn appears patent and a small lumen around the round window is apparent. However, from these CT images it is not clear whether the round window would be easily visible as a landmark during surgery. In the planning we considered making a wide access (subtotal petrosectomy) to provide the best opportunities.

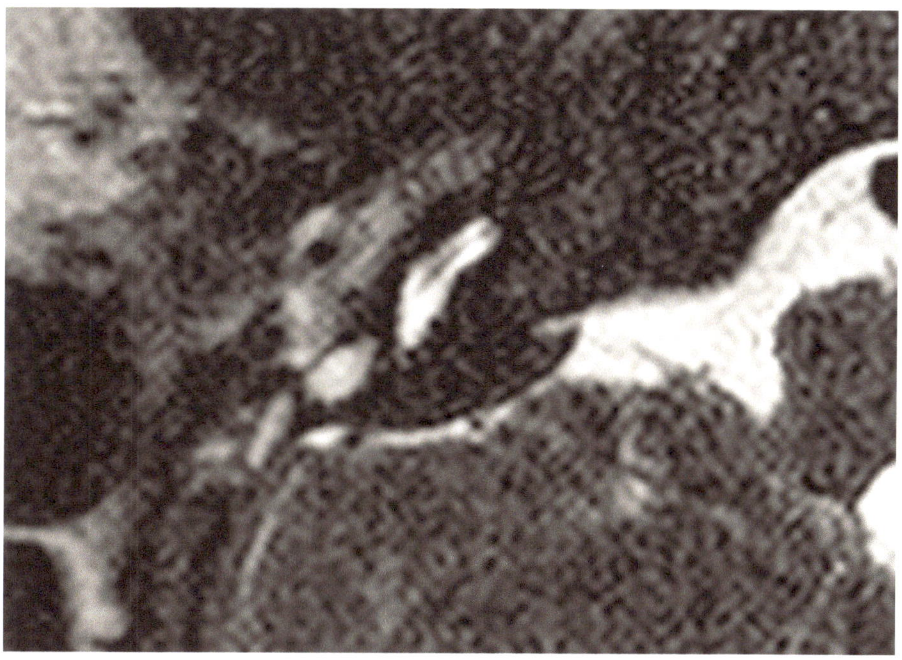

Fig. 15.2.5 MRI confirmed normal patency of the basal turn and two scalae.

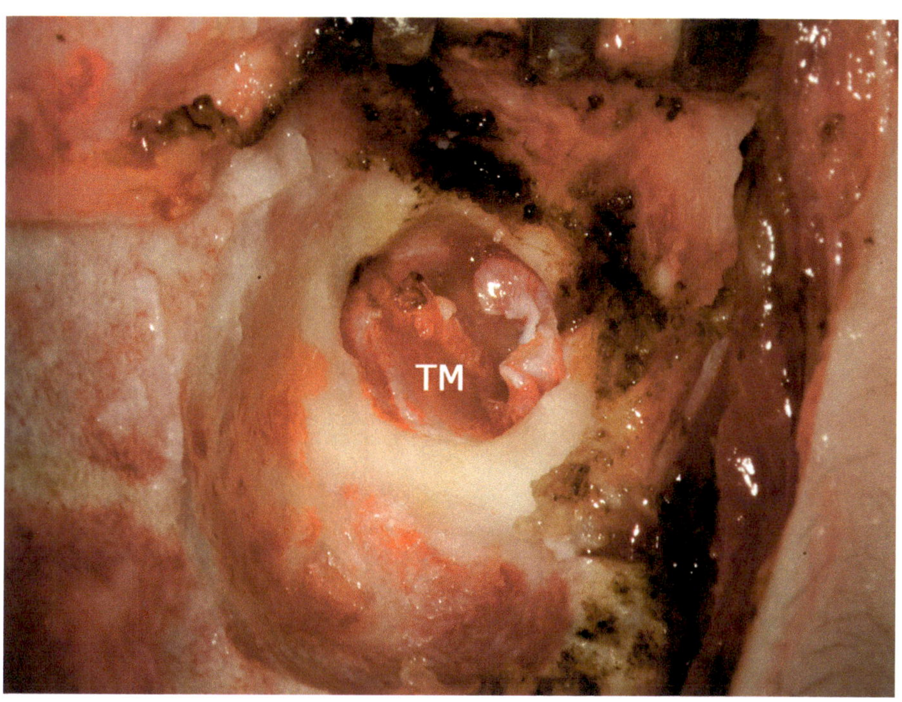

Fig. 15.2.6 After blind-sac closure of the external auditory canal a subtotal petrosectomy is performed. Only few air cells are present. The tympanic membrane (TM) can be appreciated at this stage.

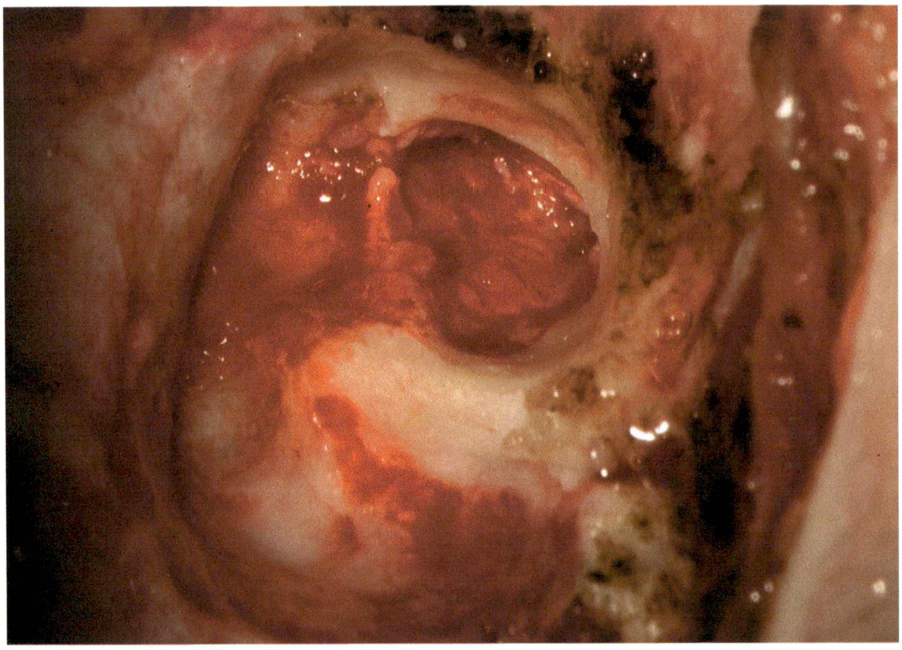

Fig. 15.2.7 Once the canal wall down procedure was almost completed the anatomical landmarks were difficult to find. Most important is the course of the facial nerve, which is often aberrant in CHARGE syndrome.

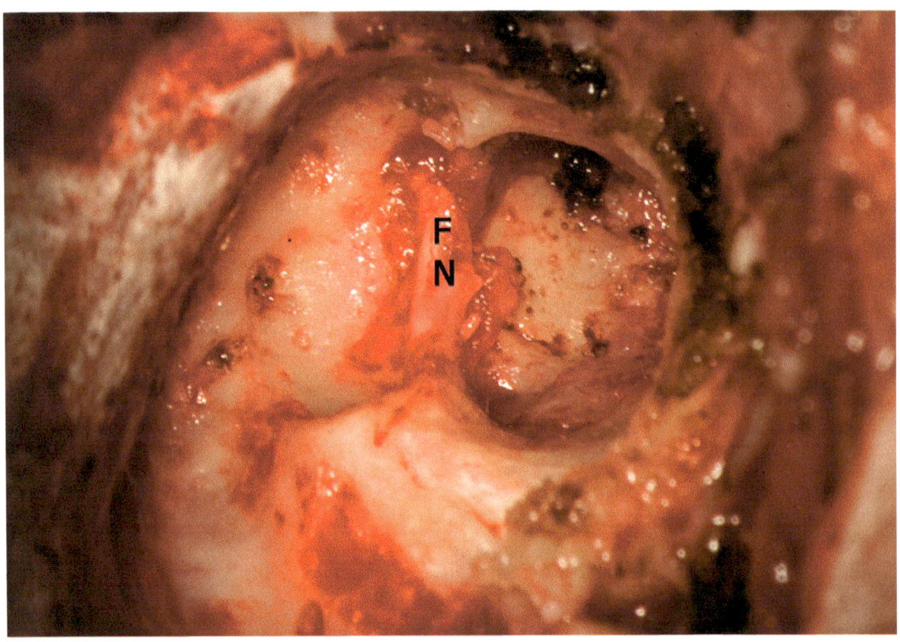

Fig. 15.2.8 Here the facial nerve (FN) is uncovered in its tympanic segment. Much hypertrophic mucosa was removed with caution. A clear view of the oval and round windows is still not possible. The open access via subtotal petrosectomy facilitated a safe and satisfactory overview in this case.

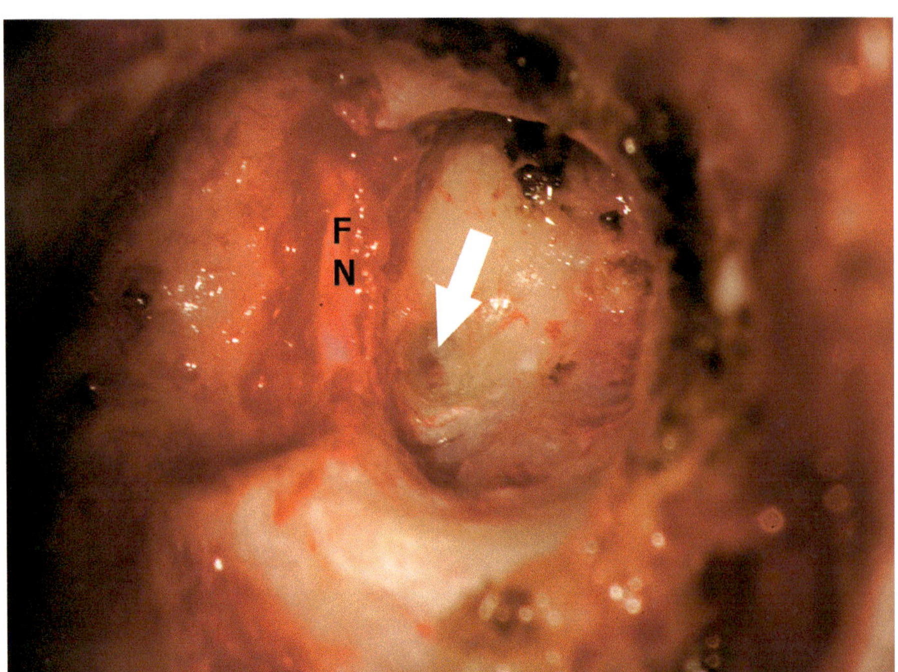

Fig. 15.2.9 Gentle drilling at the best location for the round window, according to the scan and experience, does not reveal a lumen. Drilling is stopped at the appearance of a "dark" area (*arrow*). FN, facial nerve.

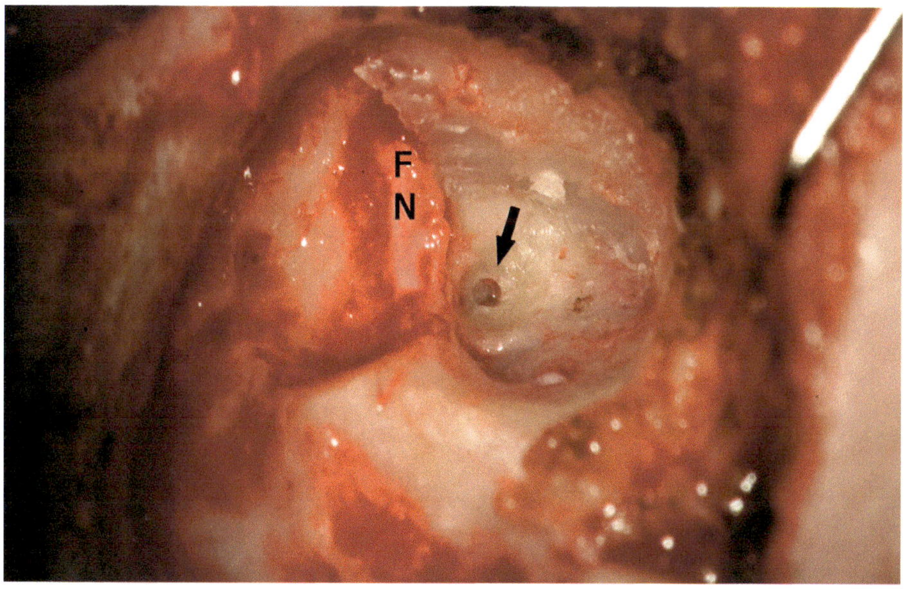

Fig. 15.2.10 Once the eustachian tube is sealed off with muscle and bone wax (see the anterior part of the image), the previously identified "dark area" is drilled and a lumen is found (*arrow*). FN, facial nerve.

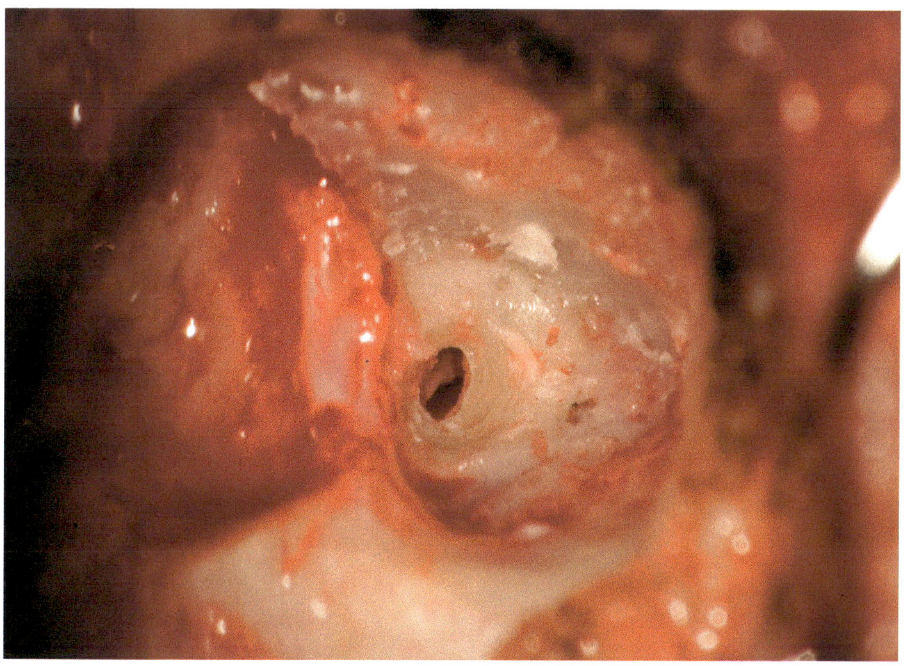

Fig. 15.2.11 The lumen is slowly enlarged with a drill and hooks.

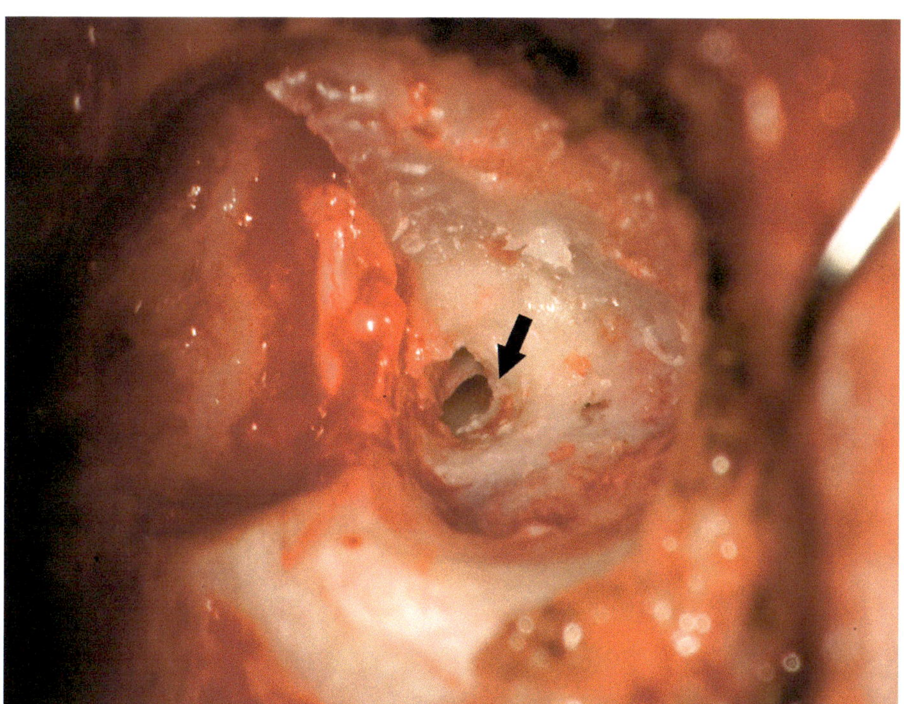

Fig. 15.2.12 The osseous spiral lamina is distinguished and the insertion into the scala tympani, the lowest scala in this image (*arrow*), is prepared.

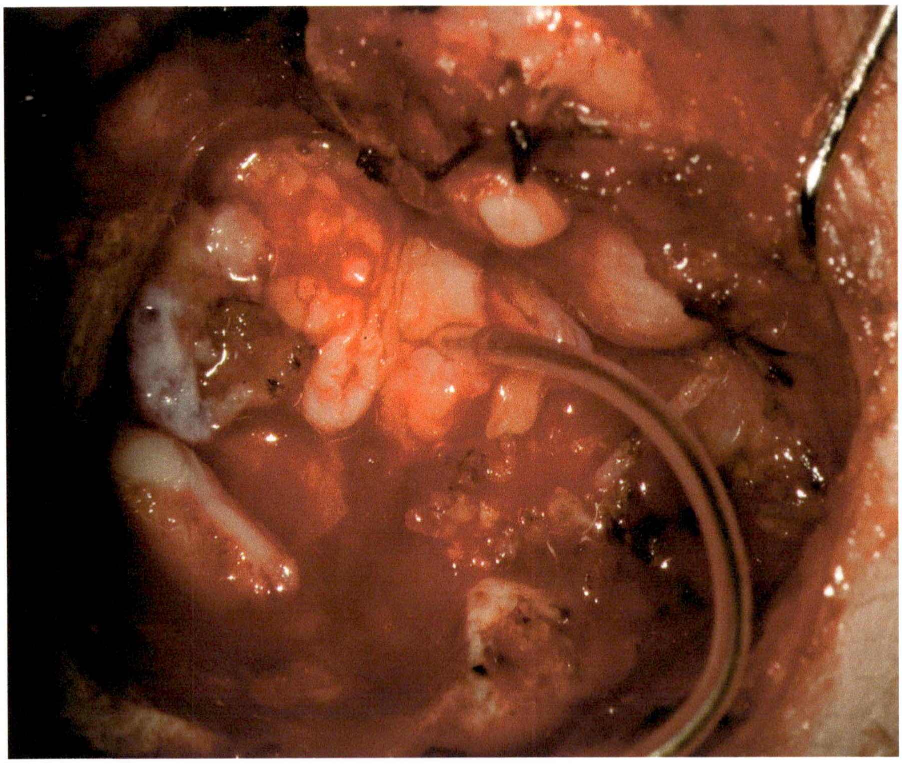

Fig. 15.2.13 After insertion, the cavity is obliterated with fat and closed in layers.

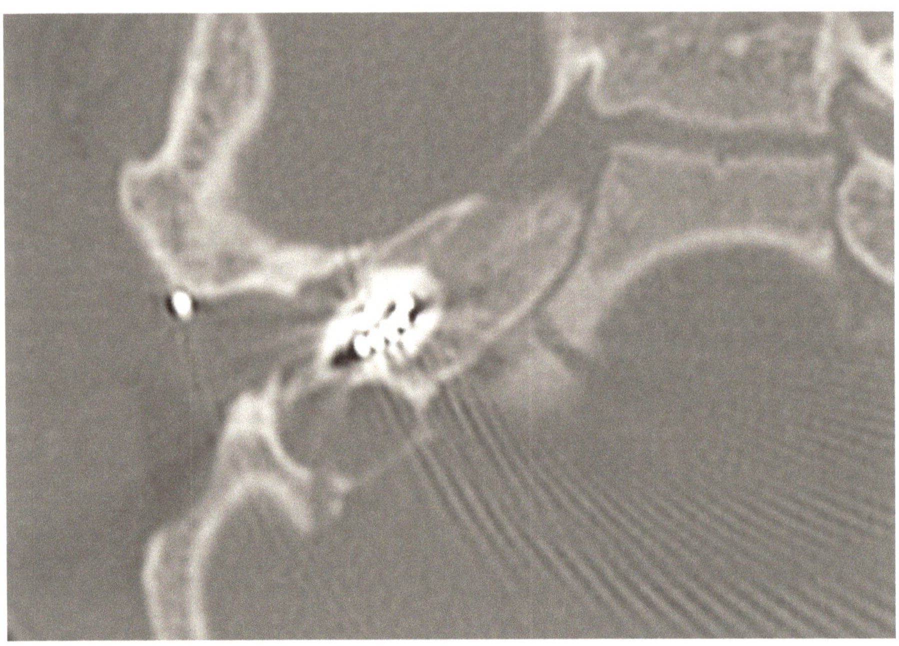

Fig. 15.2.14 On postoperative CT the electrode within the cochlea can be seen. The boy has sound identification and some verbalization, but is still far behind in speech and language development.

Comment

In CHARGE malformation the surgery can be difficult and the anatomical landmarks hard to find: a wide access surgery is preferable.

Case 15.3 CI in a Patient with Cochlear Hypoplasia (Fig. 15.3.1–Fig. 15.3.3)

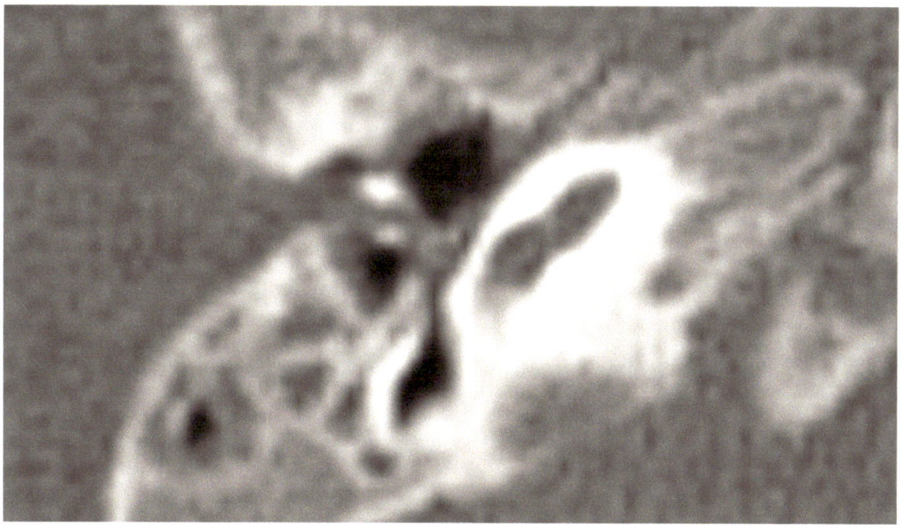

Fig. 15.3.1 This congenitally deaf girl of 12 months was seen to assess her CI candidacy. During scanning we found a hypoplastic cochlea. Further assessment with MRI was needed to assess the intracochlear structure.

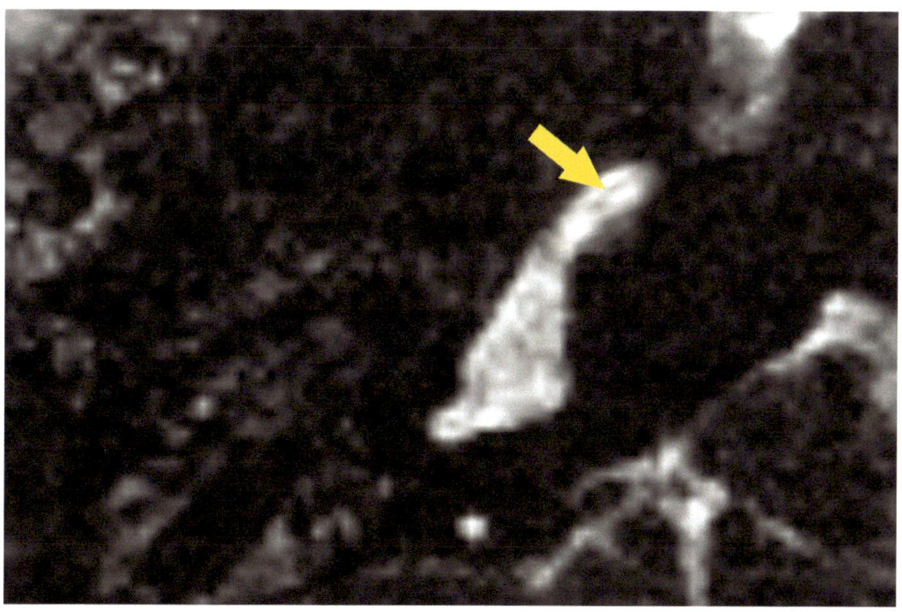

Fig. 15.3.2 On MRI the hypoplastic cochlea still showed separation of the scalae of the basal turn (*yellow arrow*). The malformation is therefore a cochlear hypoplasia (instead of IP-1, with an "empty" cystic cochlea). The IAC contained two nerves all the way up to the labyrinth (not shown here).

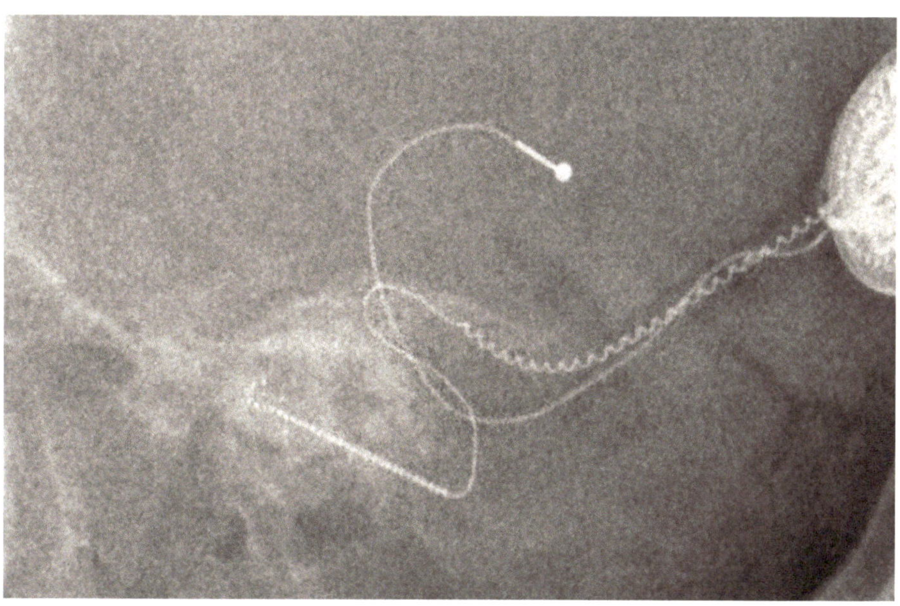

Fig. 15.3.3 On this postoperative radiograph one can see the electrode in the basal turn. We opted for a full band lateral wall electrode because of the minor curve of the cochlea and the full band spread of the signal. The girl, now 4 years old, has a 100% closed-set digits score, simple speech understanding without signs, and good speech understanding with sign language (CAP 5).

Comment

The distinction between IP-1 and cochlear hypoplasia is only made on MRI images.

Case 15.4 CI and Subtotal Petrosectomy in Patient with IP-1 (Fig. 15.4.1–Fig. 15.4.11)

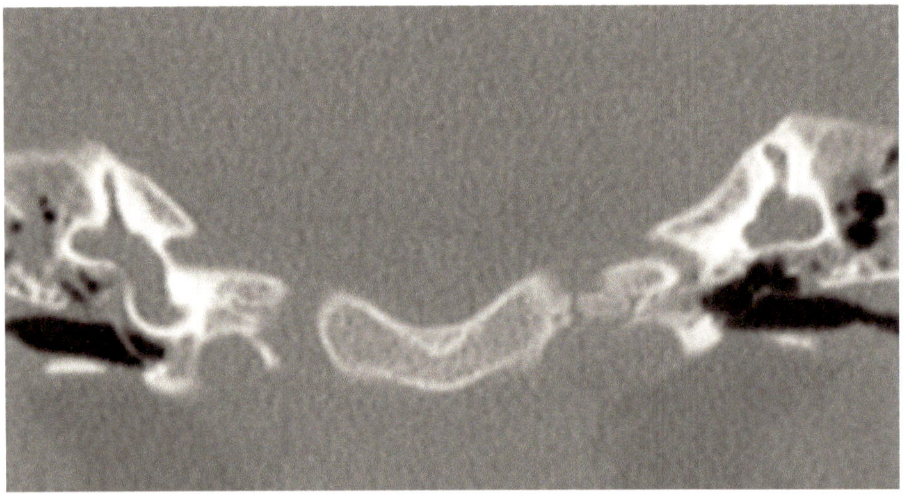

Fig. 15.4.1 During general anesthesia, a CT scan (and MRI) was made in the assessment of a 9-month-old boy. Bilateral malformed labyrinth was seen, with a dilated LSC.

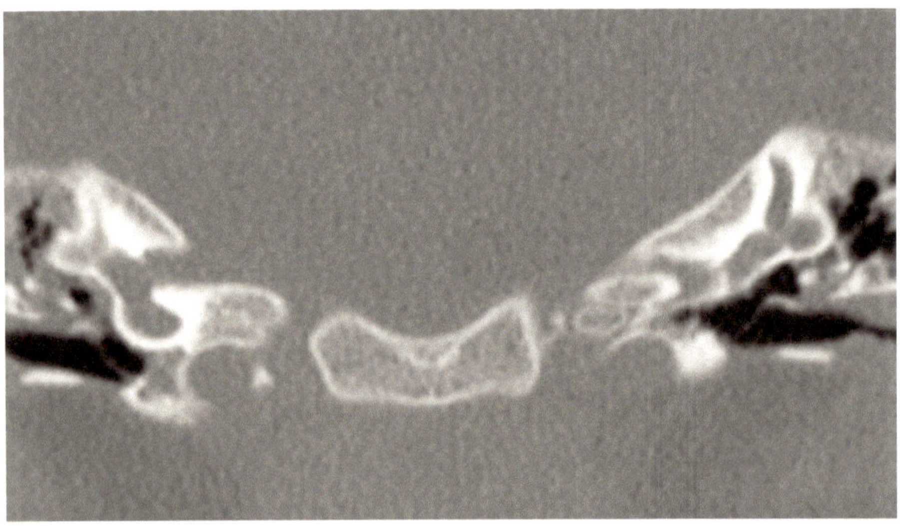

Fig. 15.4.2 The curve of the cochlea was not visible and the right cochlea had a cystic appearance. The left cochlea is not clearly visible on this coronal image.

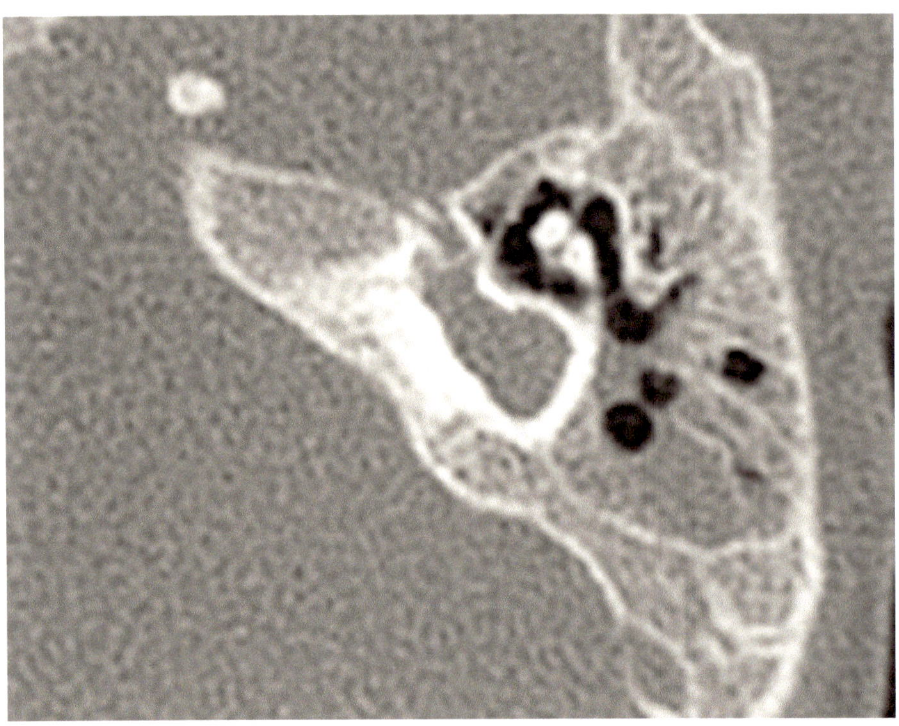

Fig. 15.4.3 The left labyrinth, in axial view, only showed a cochleovestibular cystic lesion without any differentiation between cochlea and semicircular canals. A common cavity or a cochlear aplasia is suggested.

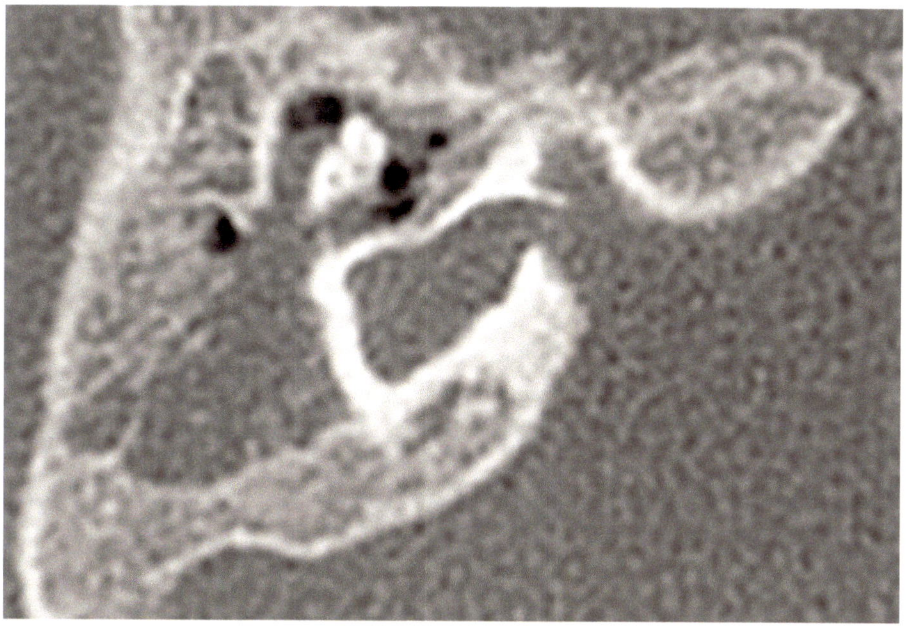

Fig. 15.4.4 On the right side a similar cystic lesion was seen at the location of the labyrinth, but in contrast to the left side the anterior end of the lesion was confluent with a cochlear-like "tail" (see the next image).

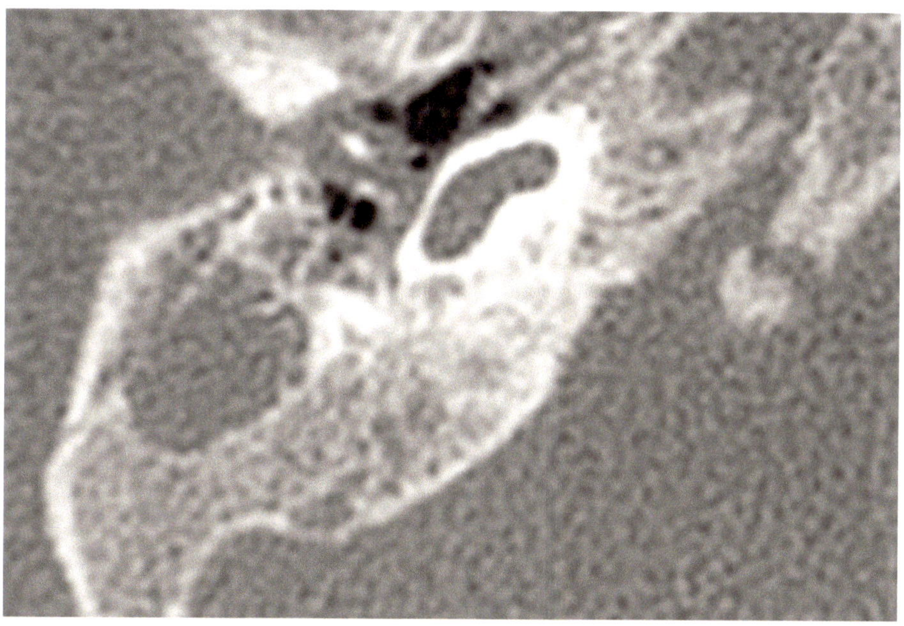

Fig. 15.4.5 A smaller but cochlear-shaped "tail" is connected to the cystic labyrinth. MRI images were analyzed for intracochlear septation and the connection to the brainstem.

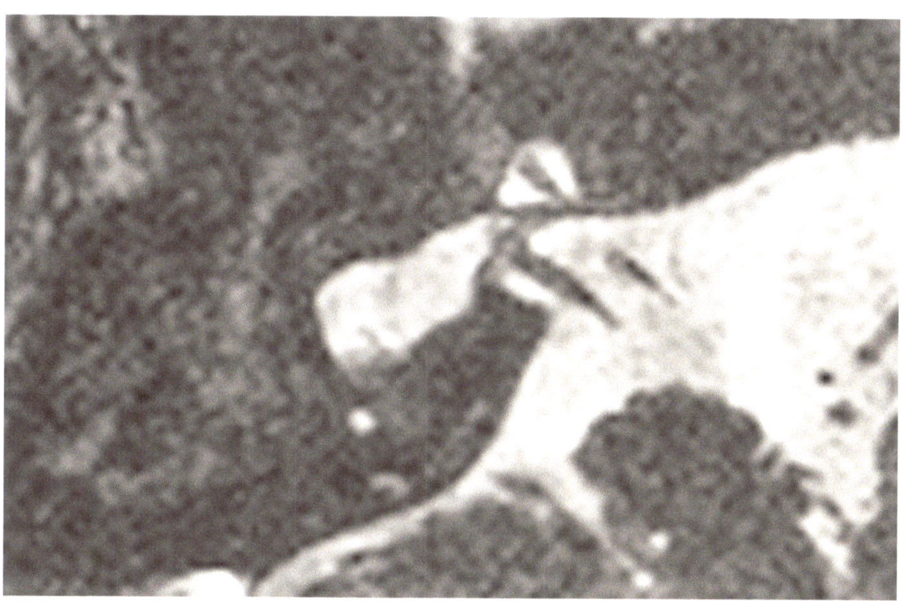

Fig. 15.4.6 In the right-side IAC two nerves were seen with strange straight endings at the cystic labyrinth. None of the nerves split into a more cochlear or a more vestibular part.

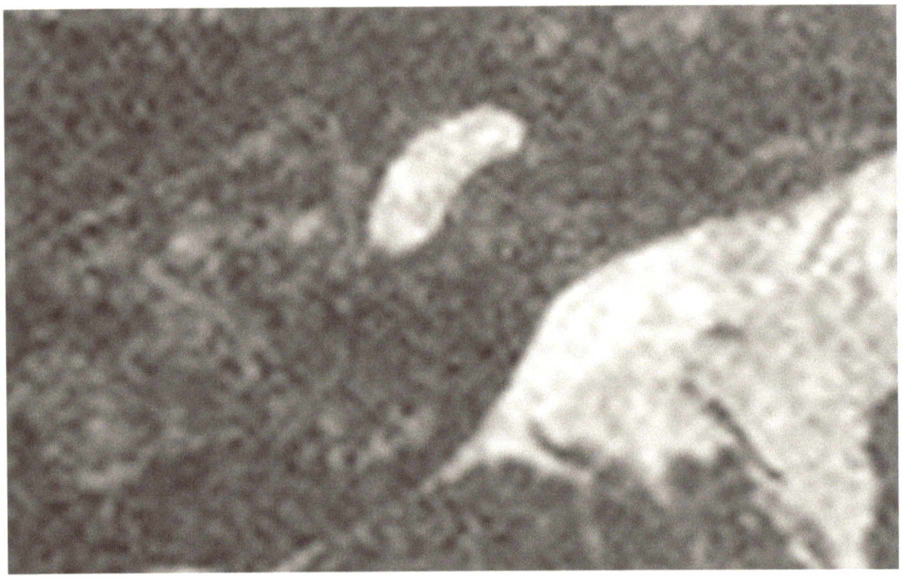

Fig. 15.4.7 At the level of the cochlear part of the malformation only a cystic cochlea was visible; connection with a nerve could not be distinguished in these images. In IP-1, also called the cystic cochleovestibular anomaly, only a cystic cochlea is seen.

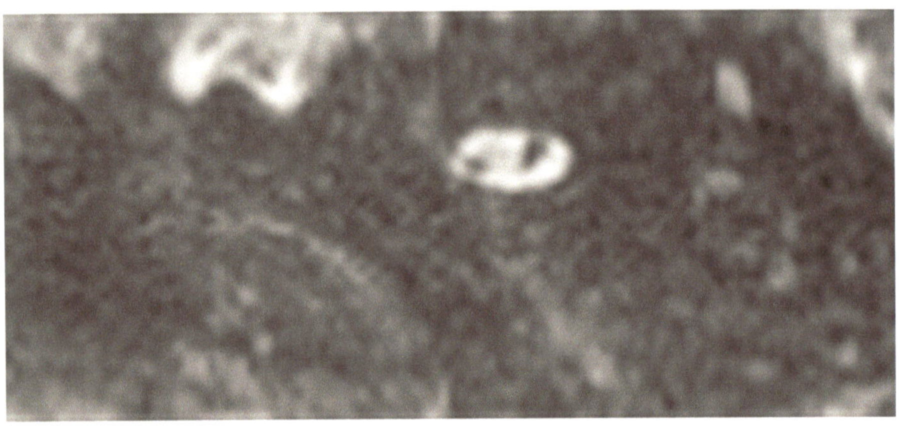

Fig. 15.4.8 In a sagittally reconstructed 3D CISS MR image perpendicular to the internal auditory canal (see Chapter 3) the nerve coming from the brainstem can be followed. Here we appreciate both the seventh and eighth nerves.

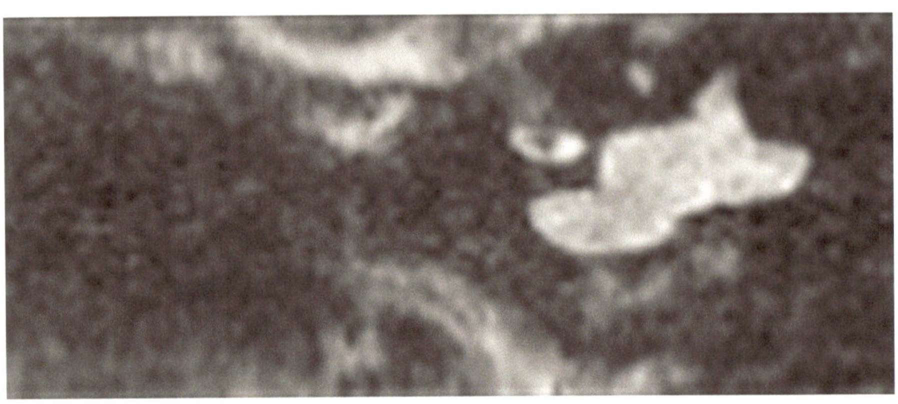

Fig. 15.4.9 At the level of the malformed labyrinth the vestibulocochlear (most posterior) nerve can be seen in close proximity to the malformed labyrinth.

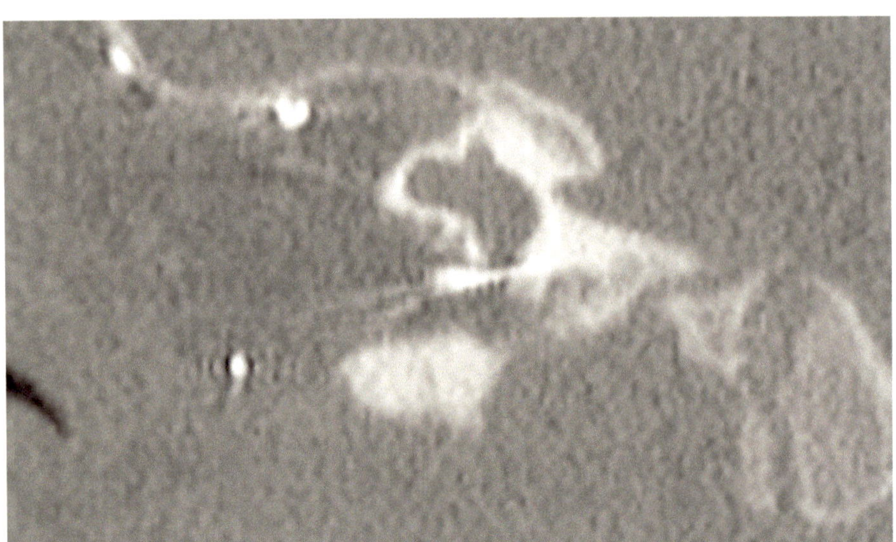

Fig. 15.4.10 A subtotal petrosectomy approach was chosen to provide good access and good control in case of a CSF gusher. No CSF gusher occurred, and a straight electrode was inserted. The cavity was closed with fat and muscle. (Postoperative coronal image.)

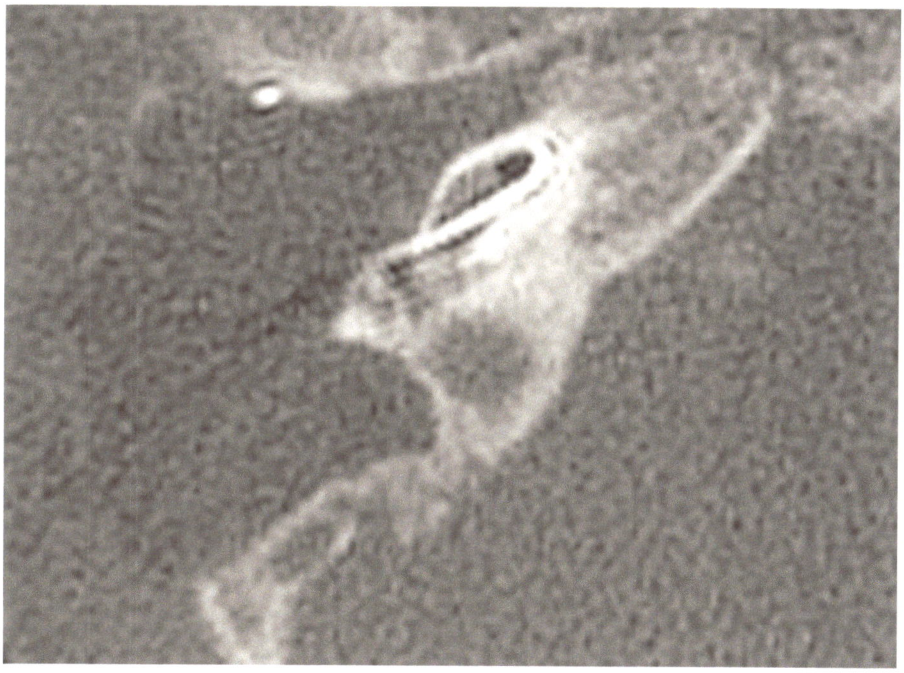

Fig. 15.4.11 During surgery a planned partial insertion was performed: 10 electrodes inserted with a straight full band electrode. Good impedances were measured, no NRT reactions or stapedial tendon reflex at any electrode. After 2 years of rehabilitation the patient has reactions in free field from 40 dB and recognizes environmental sounds (CAP 3).

Comment

Clear MRI images are needed to define the status of the nerve in the internal auditory canal.

Case 15.5 Unilateral IP-1 Malformation with CI Implantation in Two Attempts (Fig. 15.5.1–Fig. 15.5.19)

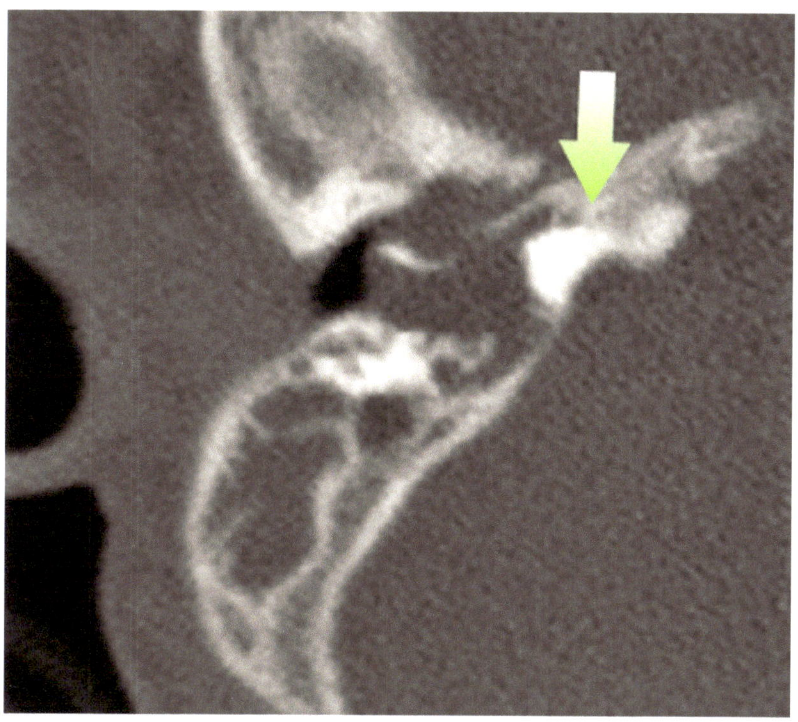

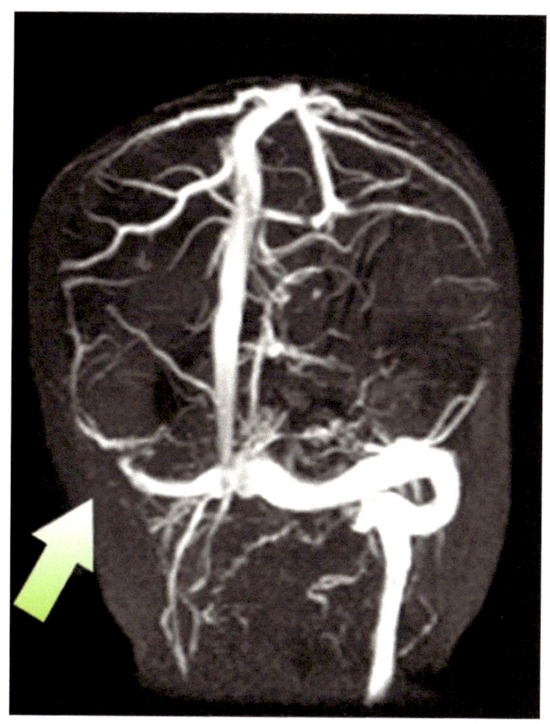

Fig. 15.5.1 This 3-year-old boy had a ventriculoperitoneal shunt because of an insufficient and malformed venous drainage of the brain. He was profoundly deaf and during radiologic assessment a cochlear aplasia (left, CT image, *arrow*) and malformed transverse and sigmoid sinuses (right, venous-phase MRI, *arrow*) were found on the right side.

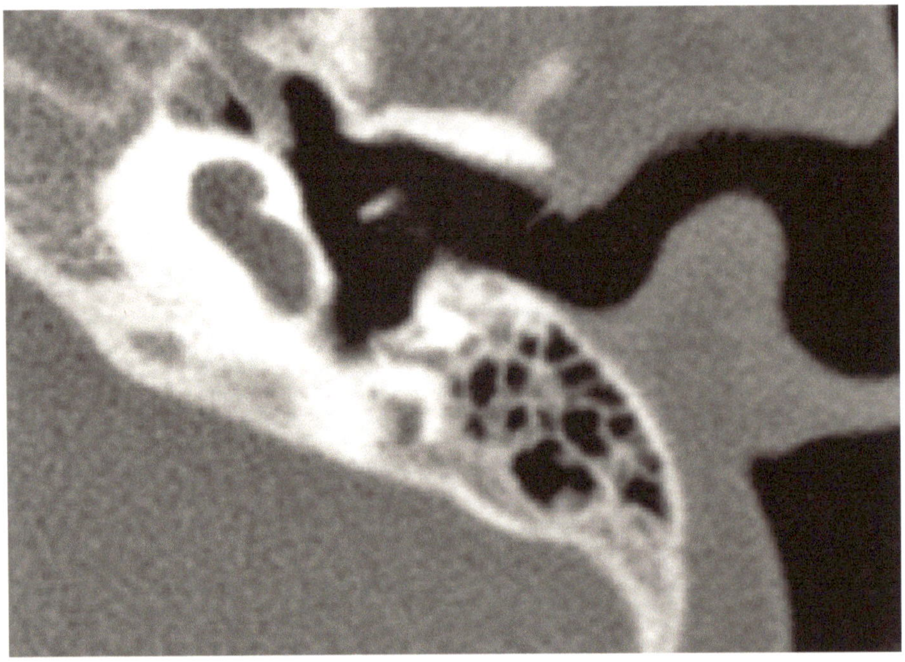

Fig. 15.5.2 In the left ear, shown here on CT, he had a hypoplastic cochlea.

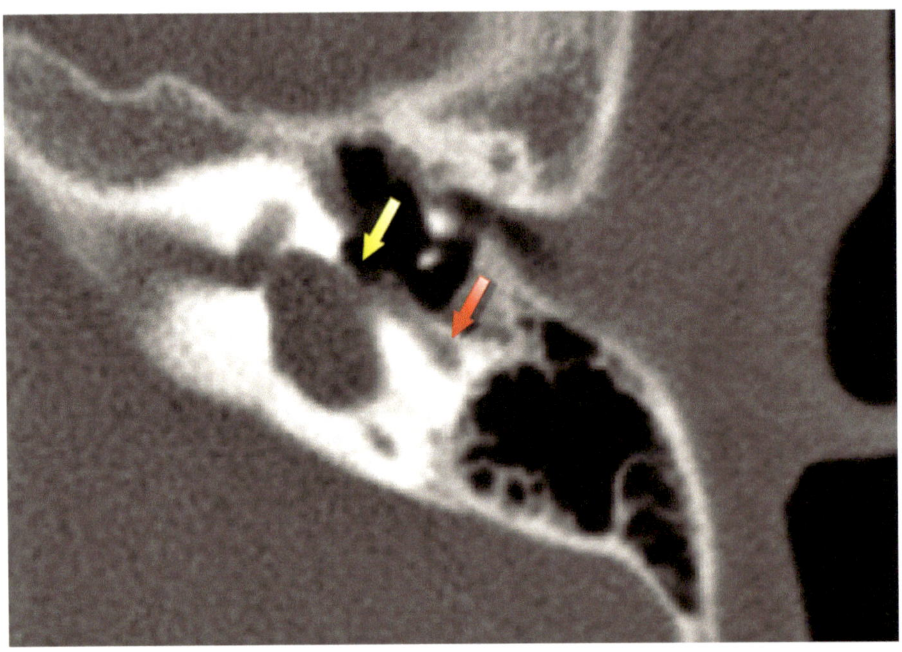

Fig. 15.5.3 The hypoplastic cochlea was connected to a dysmorphic labyrinth. But the oval window niche (*yellow arrow*) and facial nerve (*red arrow*) appeared normal.

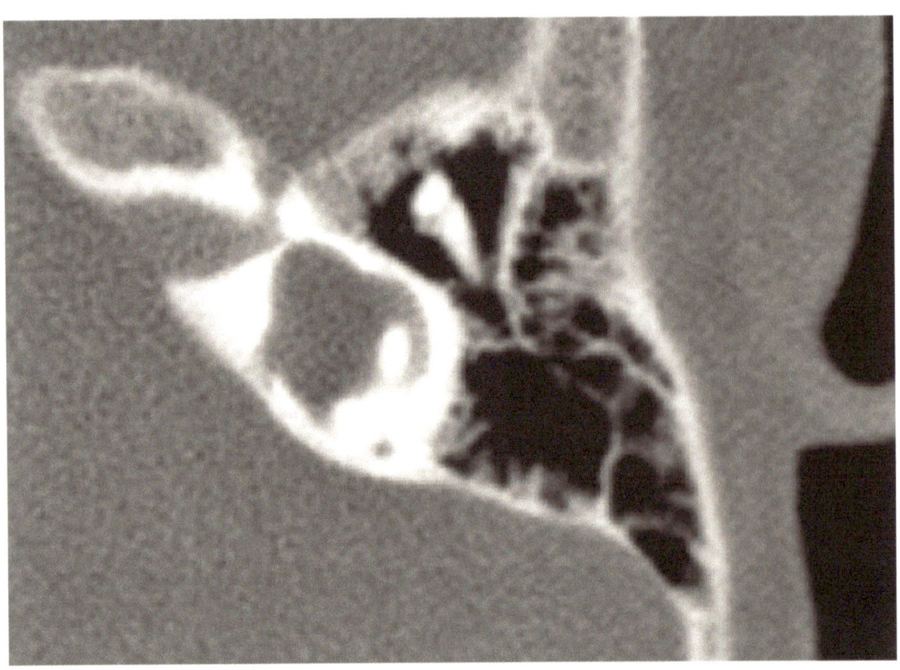

Fig. 15.5.4 The connection to the IAC was not enlarged and the ossicles are normally formed. The vestibule/LSC is vastly dilated.

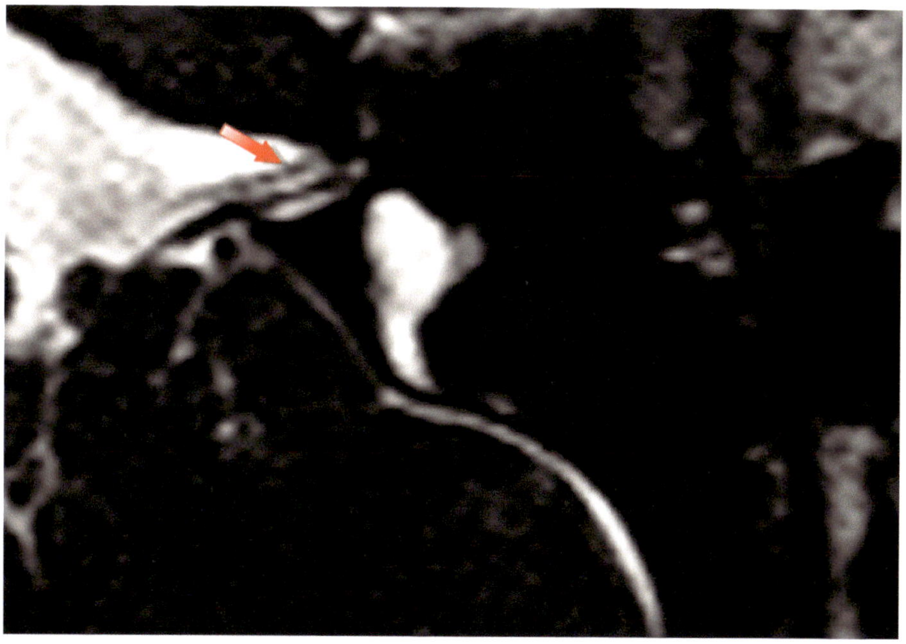

Fig. 15.5.5 The MR images were used to analyze the intracochlear septation and the presence of a vestibulocochlear nerve. In this image two nerves are visible within the IAC (*red arrow*).

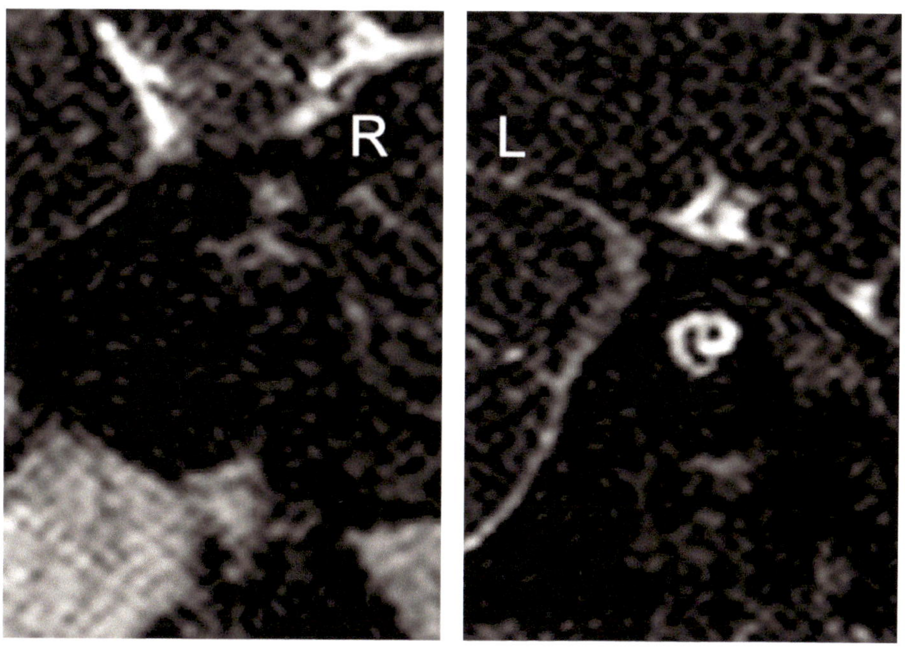

Fig. 15.5.6 The nerves in the IAC were analyzed with sagittal images perpendicular to the IAC. In this image the right side (R) "empty" cerebellopontine angle is compared with the left side (L) IAC with at least three nerves.

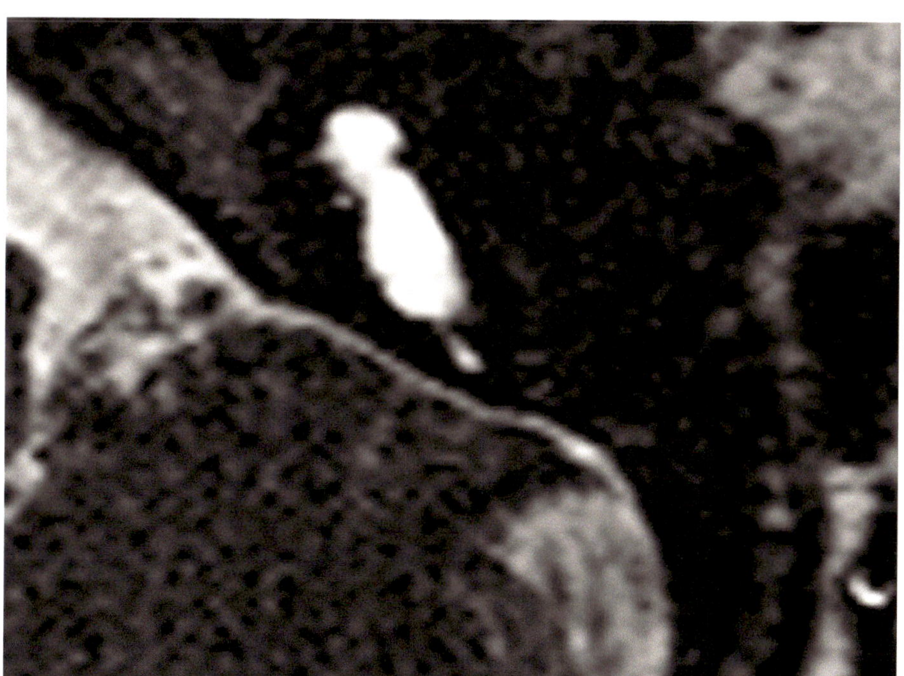

Fig. 15.5.7 The cochlea is cystic and does not contain any septation. The diagnosis of cystic cochleovestibular anomaly or IP-1 with neural connection to the brainstem was clear and CI implantation was scheduled.

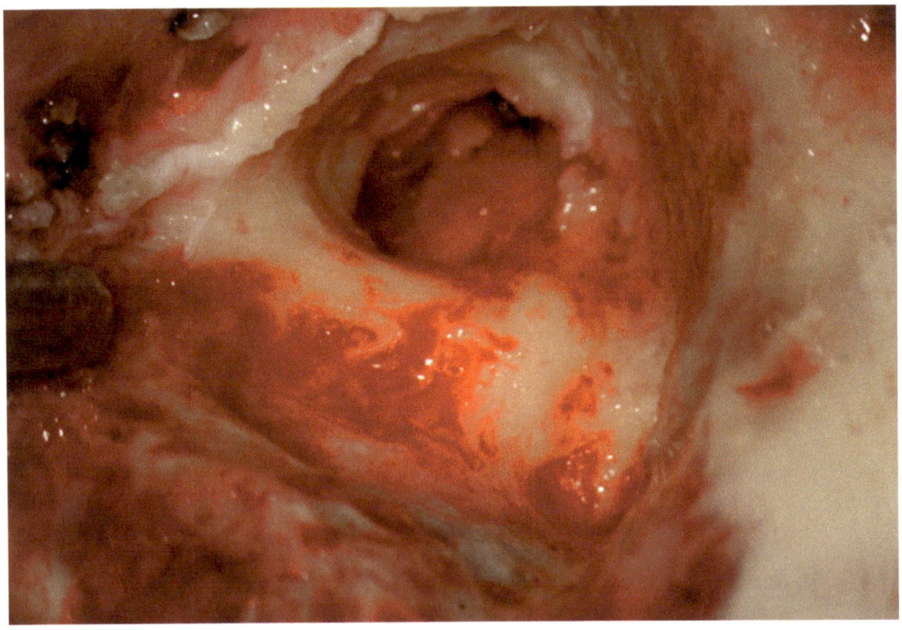

Fig. 15.5.8 After blind-sac closure of the ear canal, the posterior canal wall was lowered to provide a wide access to the middle ear.

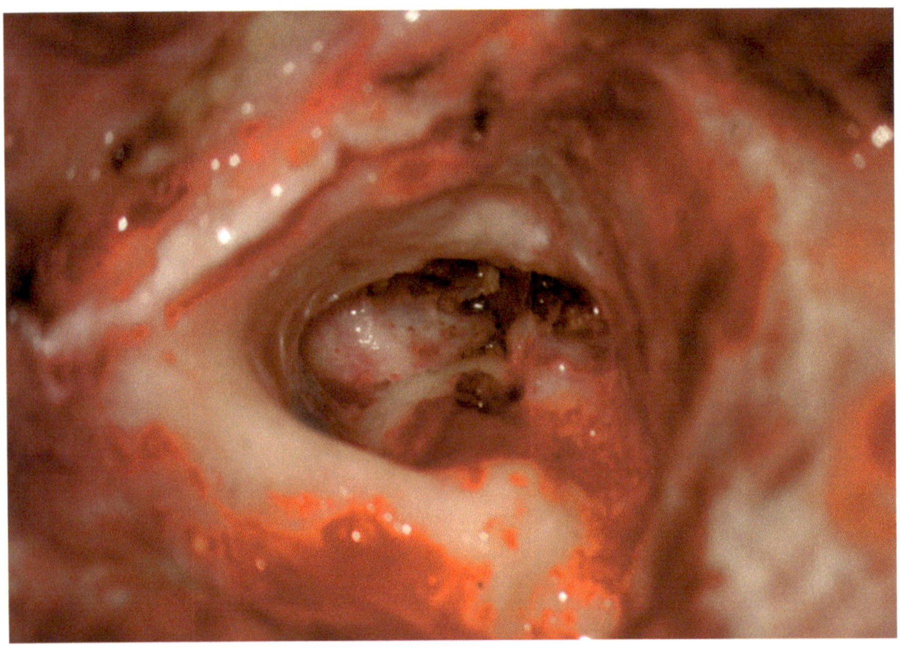

Fig. 15.5.9 The mucosa at the entrance of the eustachian tube was coagulated before closing the tube with the tensor tympani muscle obliteration, which is an alternative for a free muscle flap. The final closure is done with bone wax. Everything was then ready for the implantation phase.

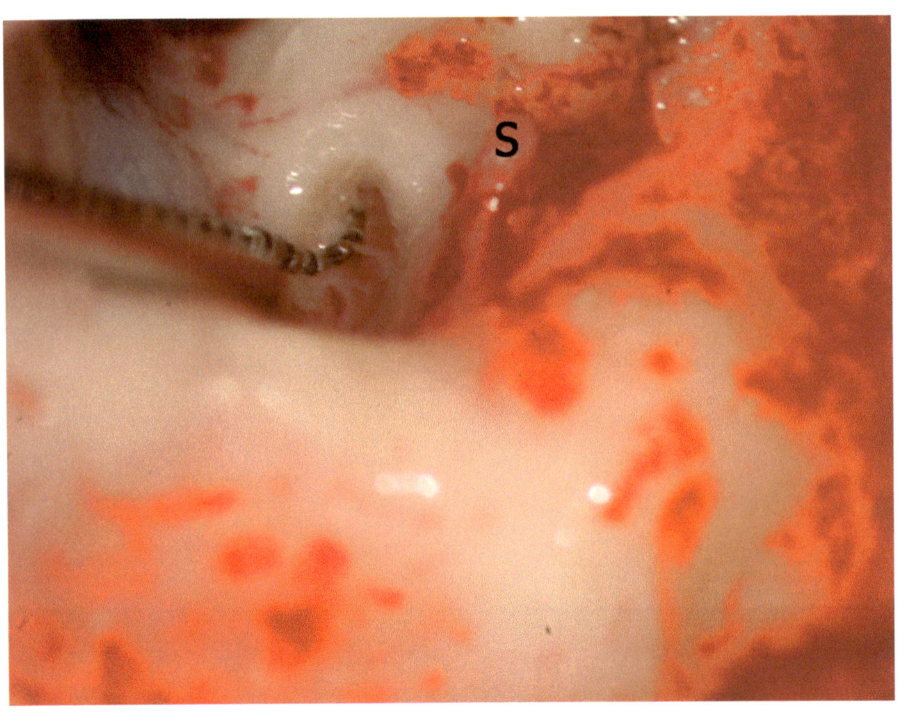

Fig. 15.5.10 The round window niche was drilled for a better view of the window before opening it. A lateral wall electrode was used for insertion. More cranially, the head of the stapes is still visible. S, stapes.

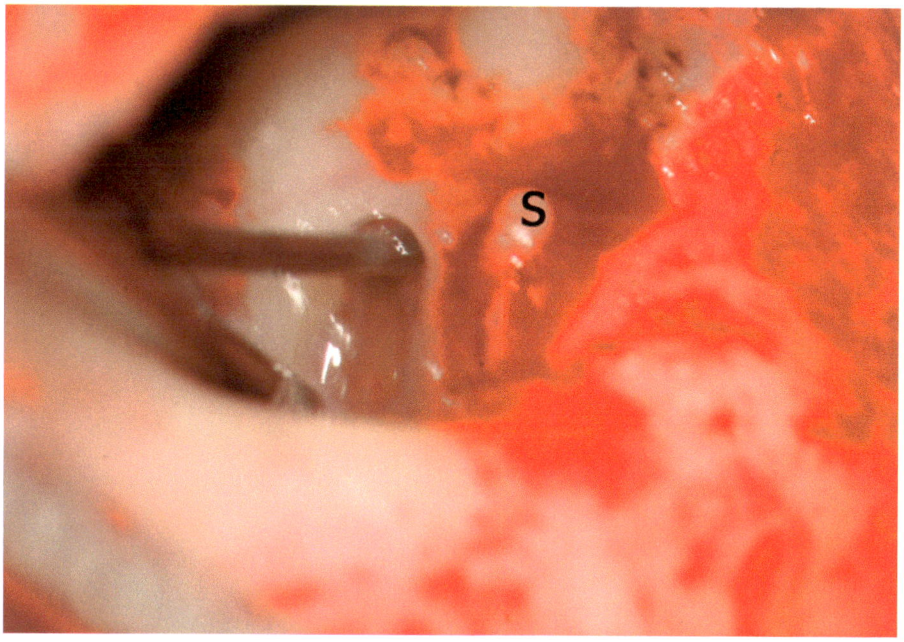

Fig. 15.5.11 The electrode was easily inserted. On measurement, neural responses were only partly present. S, stapes.

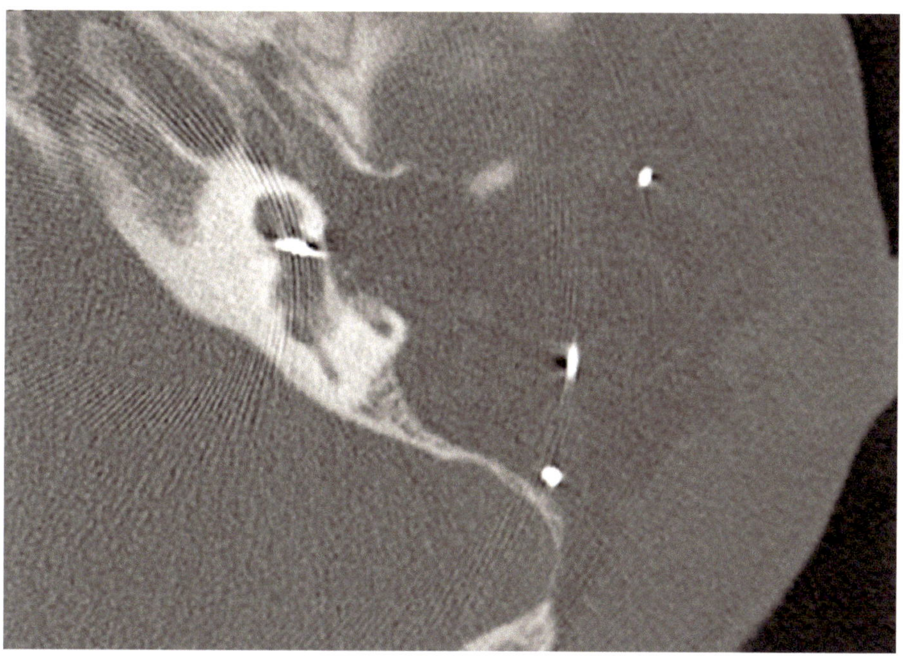

Fig. 15.5.12 Postoperative CT showed insertion at the correct location.

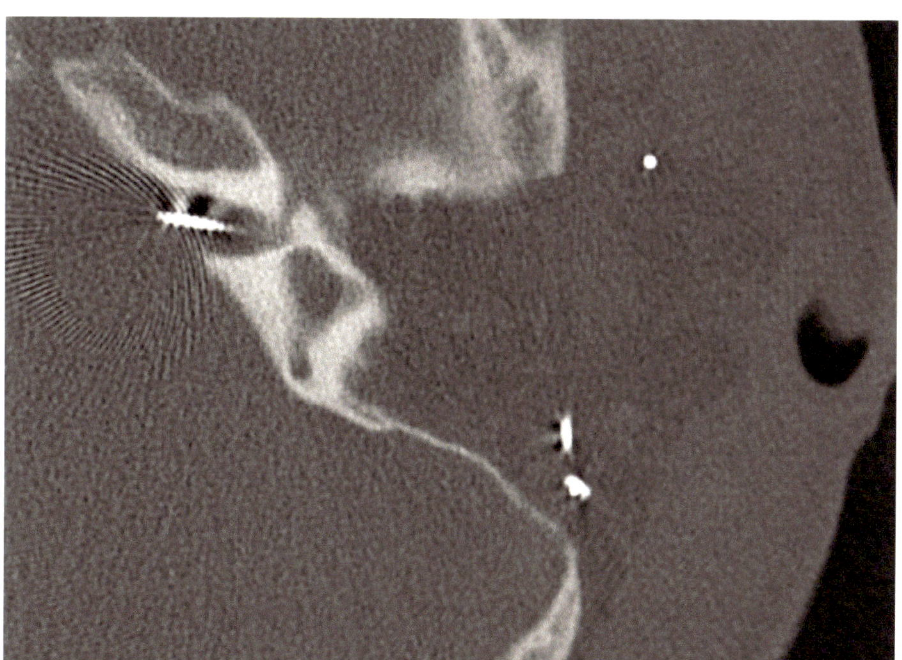

Fig. 15.5.13 The electrode actually went straight into the IAC.

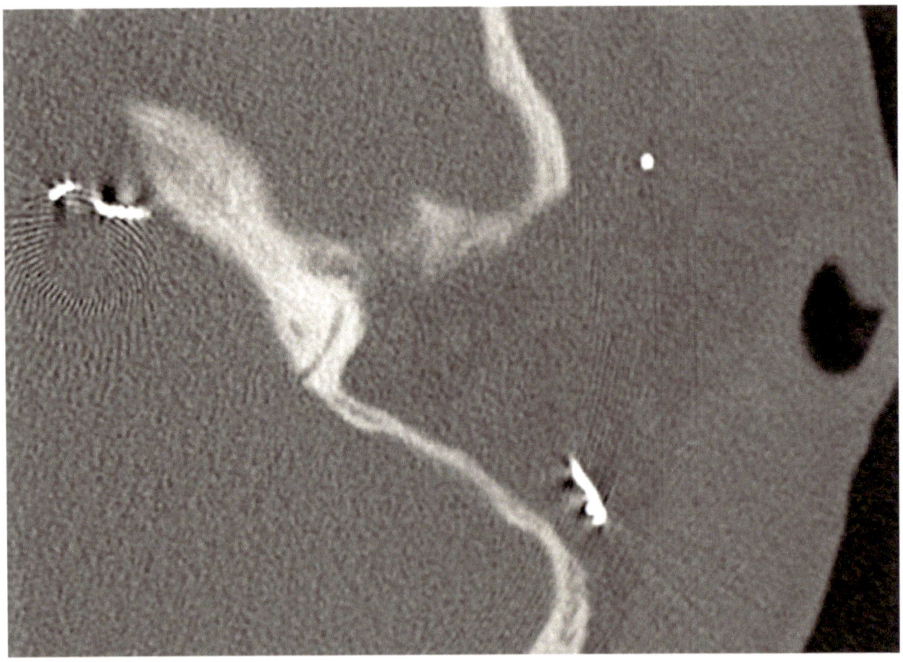

Fig. 15.5.14 The tip of the electrode was in the CPA. Revision surgery was planned during the same admission.

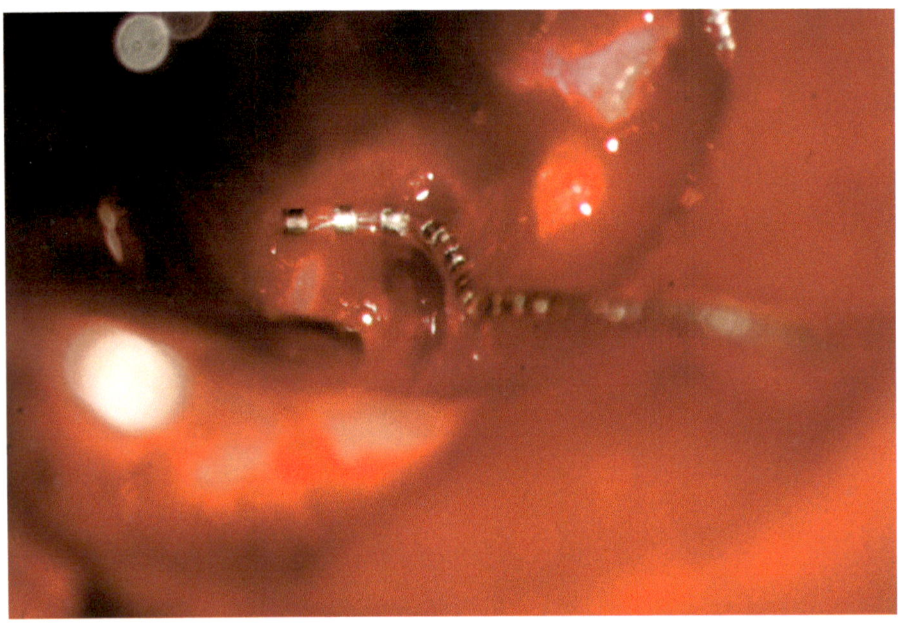

Fig. 15.5.15 During the second surgery the electrode was slowly removed. Some CSF came with it but no gusher was seen.

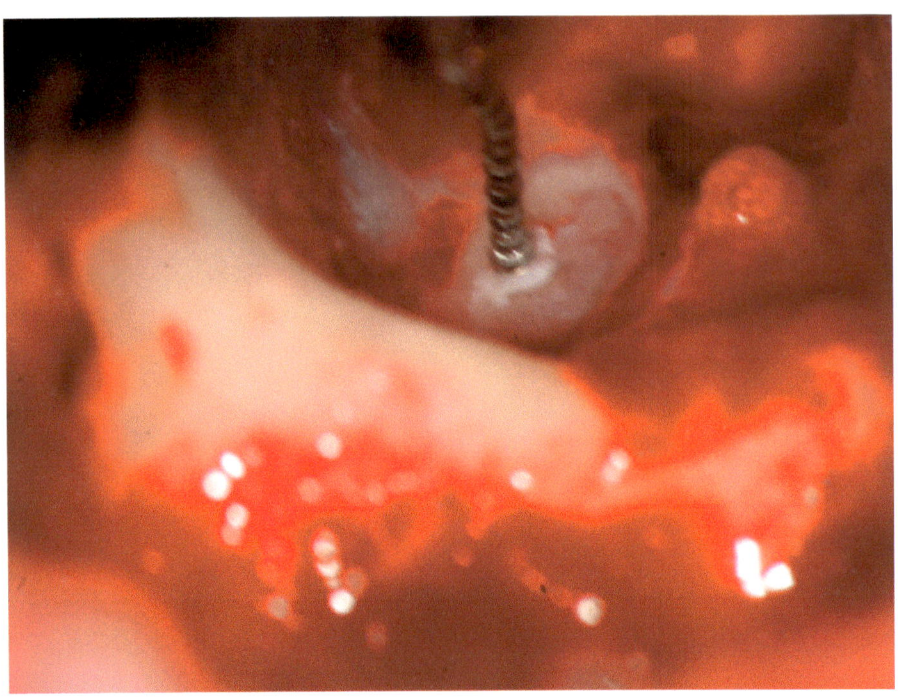

Fig. 15.5.16 A new full-band electrode was inserted through the same cochleostomy, but directed more anterocaudally.

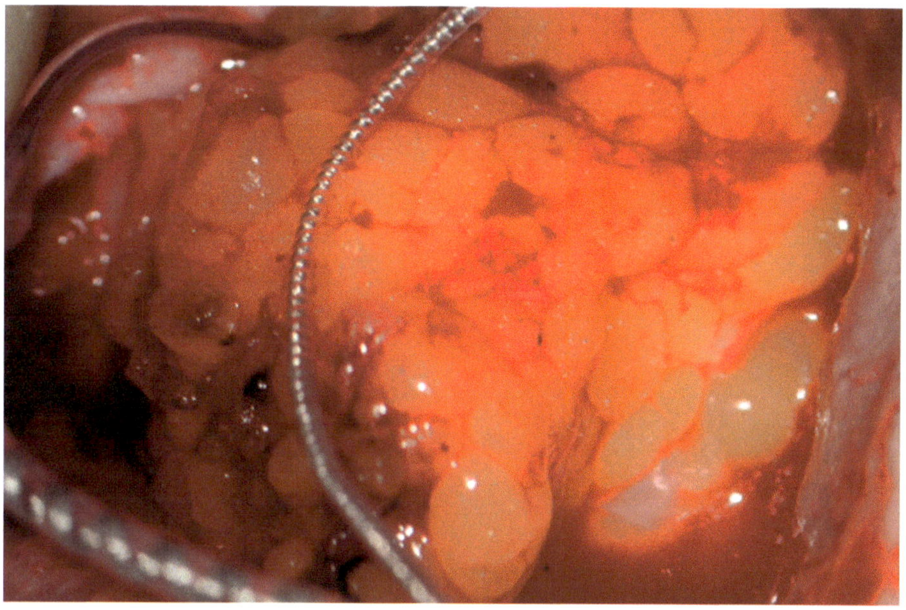

Fig. 15.5.17 The cavity was closed off with abdominal fat.

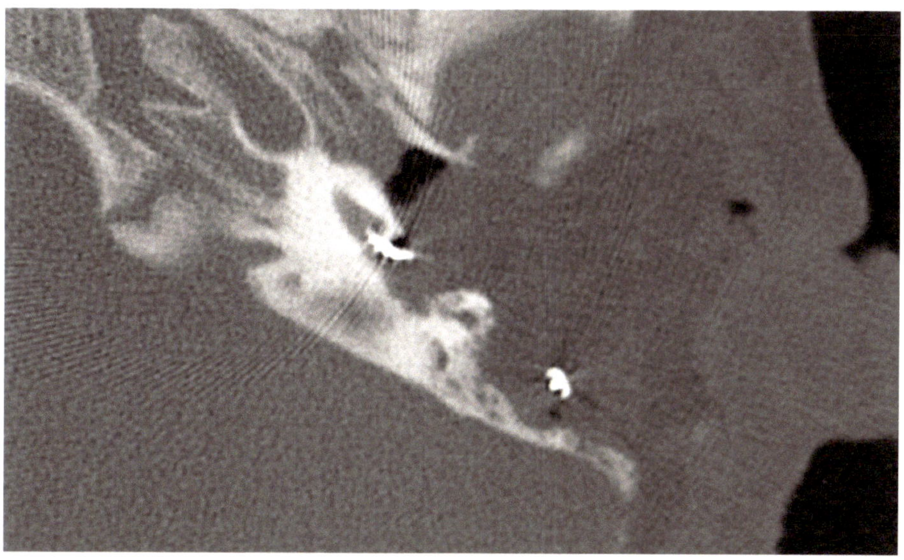

Fig. 15.5.18 The new postoperative CT image showed the electrode making the curve toward anterior.

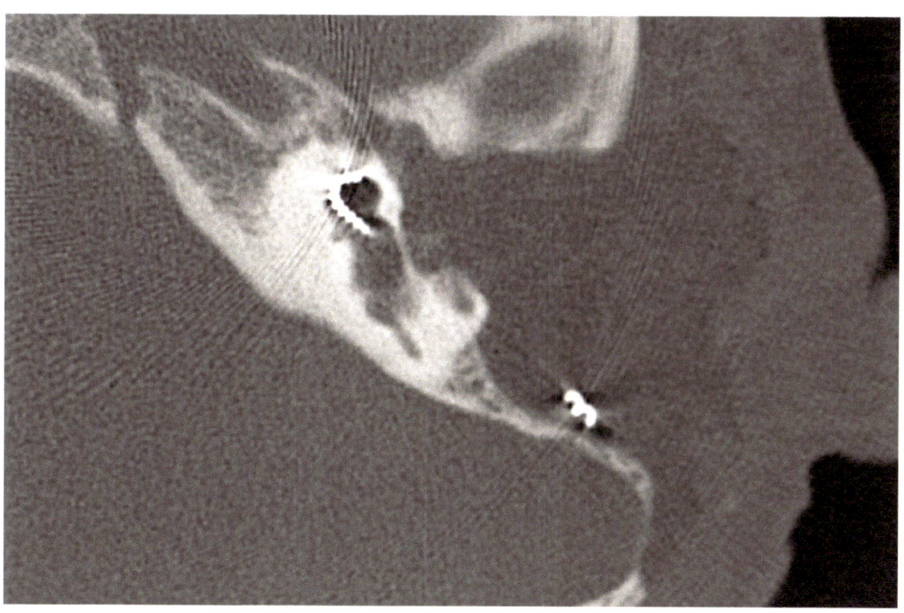

Fig. 15.5.19 The full electrode could not be inserted because of the cystic hypoplastic cochlea. There was a neural response during surgery, especially in the low frequencies. The same responses were obtained postoperatively. The child wants to use the implant. His hearing and speech performance will be followed closely.

Comment

Even in a canal wall down approach it is sometimes hard to insert correctly into the malformed cochlea. CSF gusher should be expected and pre- and postsurgery radiology is essential.

Case 15.6 X-linked IP-3 Malformation; CI with Subtotal Petrosectomy Because of CSF Gusher
(Fig. 15.6.1–Fig. 15.6.13)

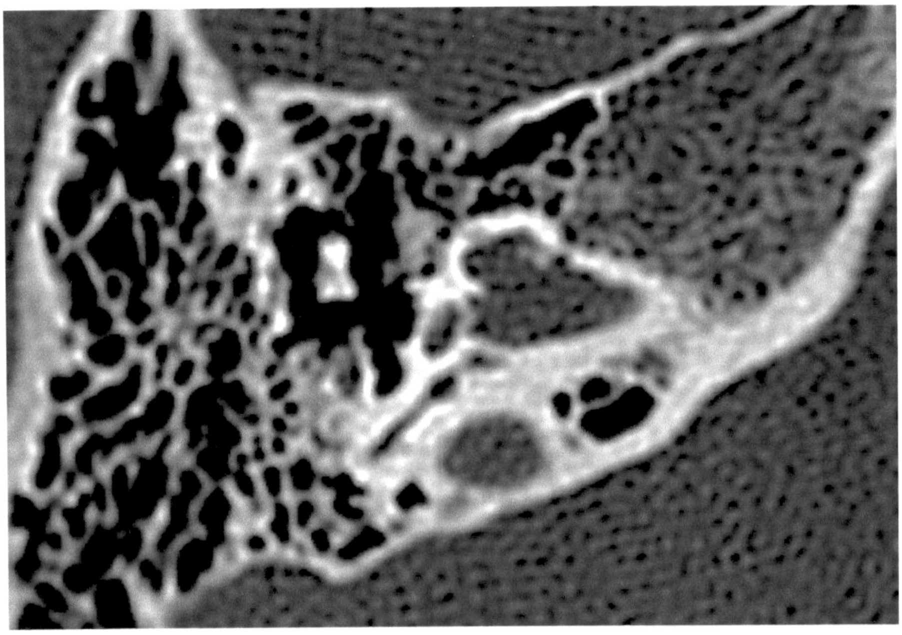

Fig. 15.6.1 A male youth of 13 years of age with bilateral profound SNHL was assessed for implantation. Only on the right side was there some reaction at 85 dB. There was no improvement of hearing with hearing aids. Otoscopy and tympanometry were normal. CT scan of the right ear showed a wide connection between the IAC and the cochlea.

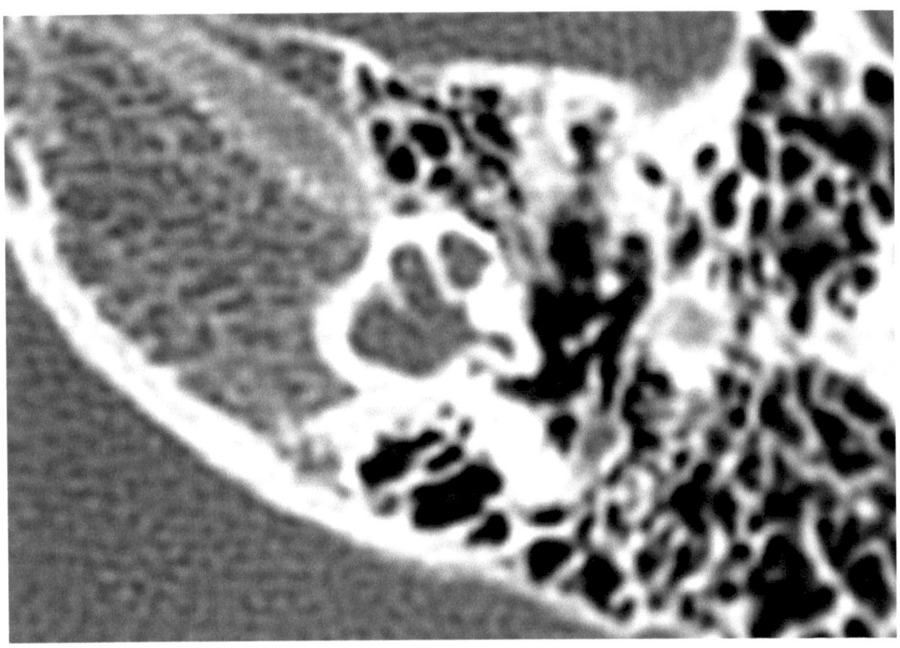

Fig. 15.6.2 On the left side we encounter a similar malformation which is typical for a IP-3. The cochlear aperture is widened and the modiolus seems absent.

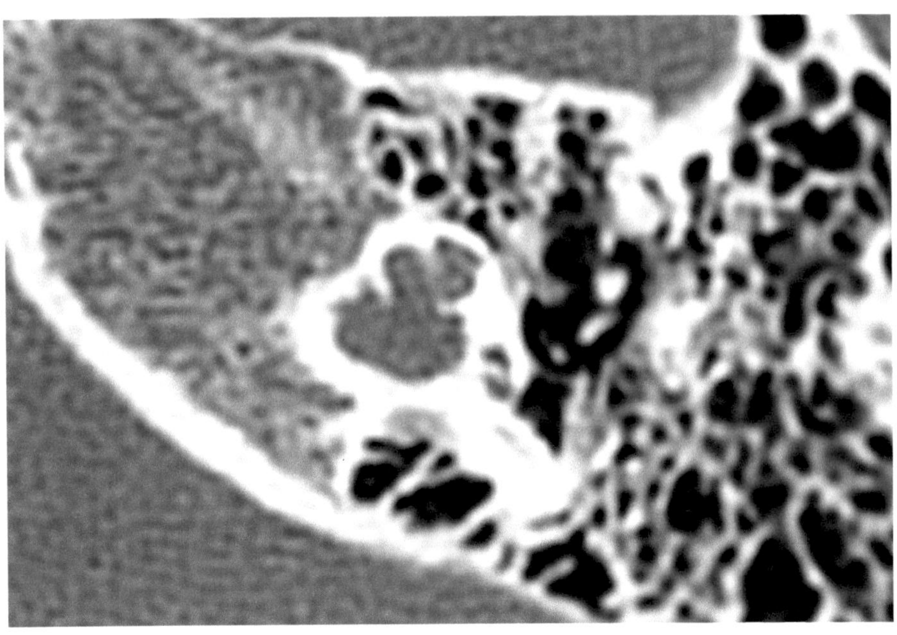

Fig. 15.6.3 There are still 2.5 turns of the cochlea but the modiolus is absent and the separation between the basal turn and the IAC is not visible.

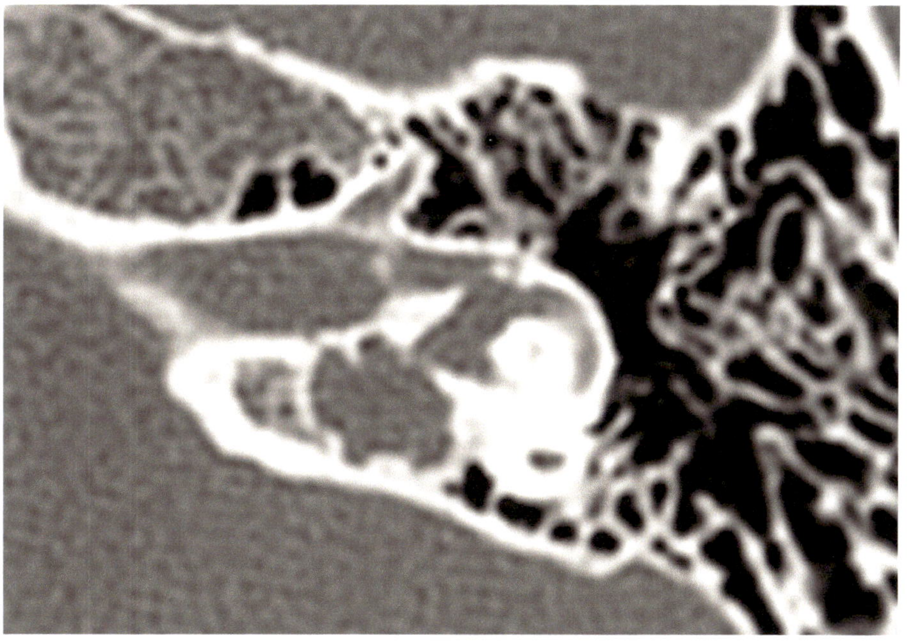

Fig. 15.6.4 The separation of the IAC between the facial nerve and the more posterior vestibular part of the IAC is prominent. The image is symmetrical as it is in all cases of IP-3.

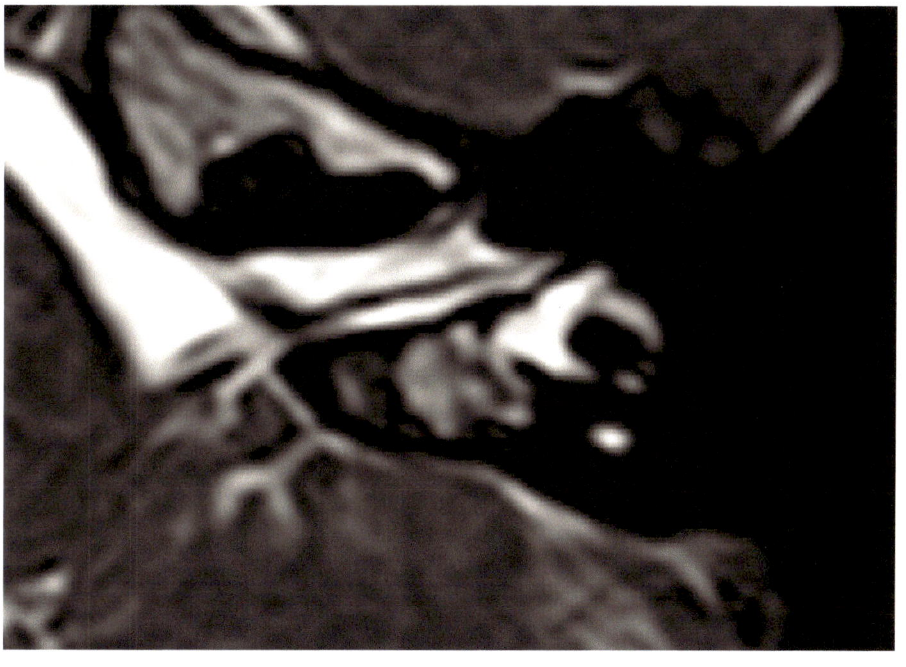

Fig. 15.6.5 There are two nerves running from the brainstem toward the labyrinth (best seen at the fundus).

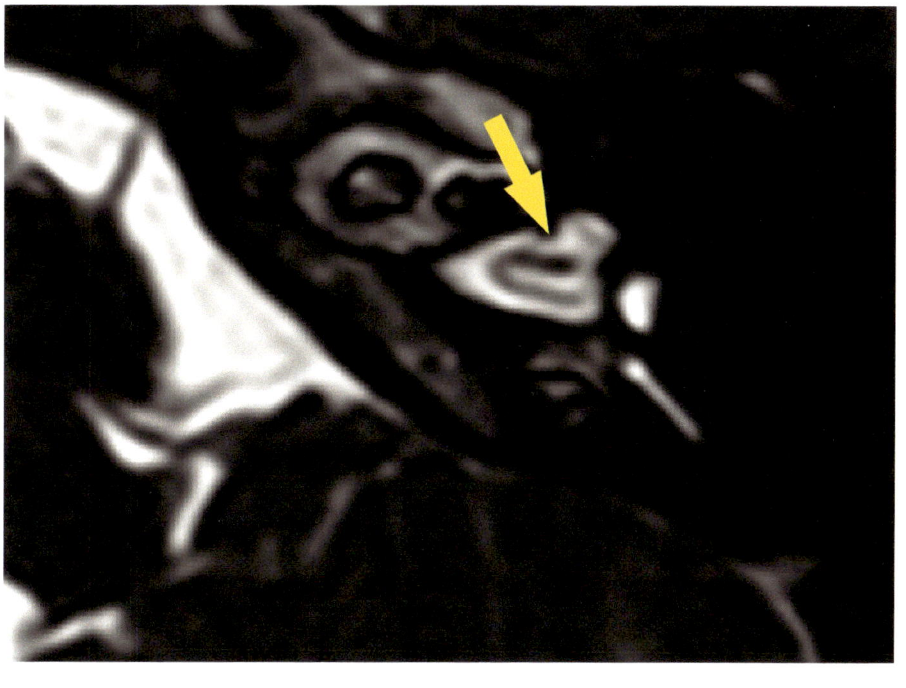

Fig. 15.6.6 Here the opening between cochlea and the IAC is visible (*yellow arrow*). The nerves run in an "open space."

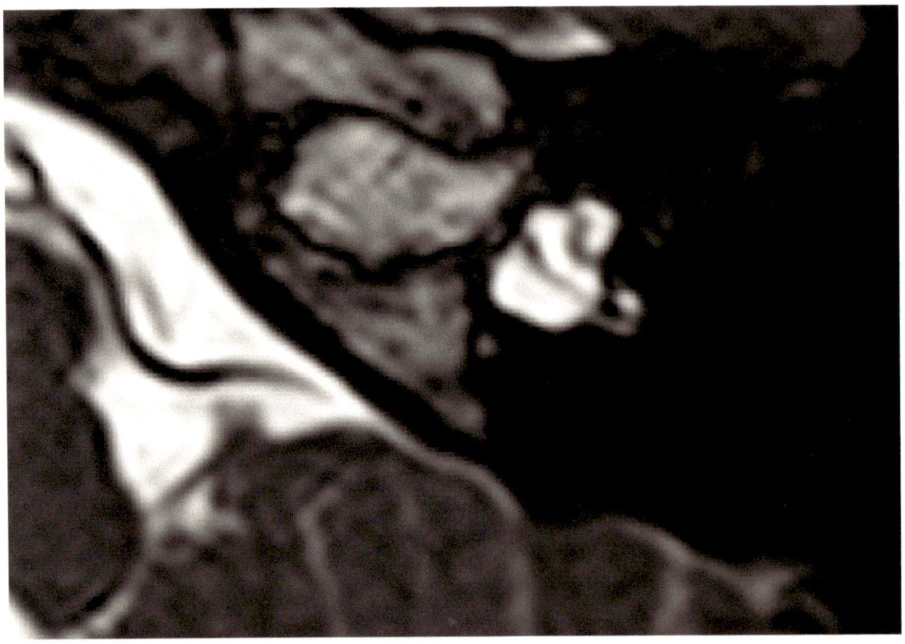

Fig. 15.6.7 The cochlea does not have clear separation between scalae, but still at least two turns are visible.

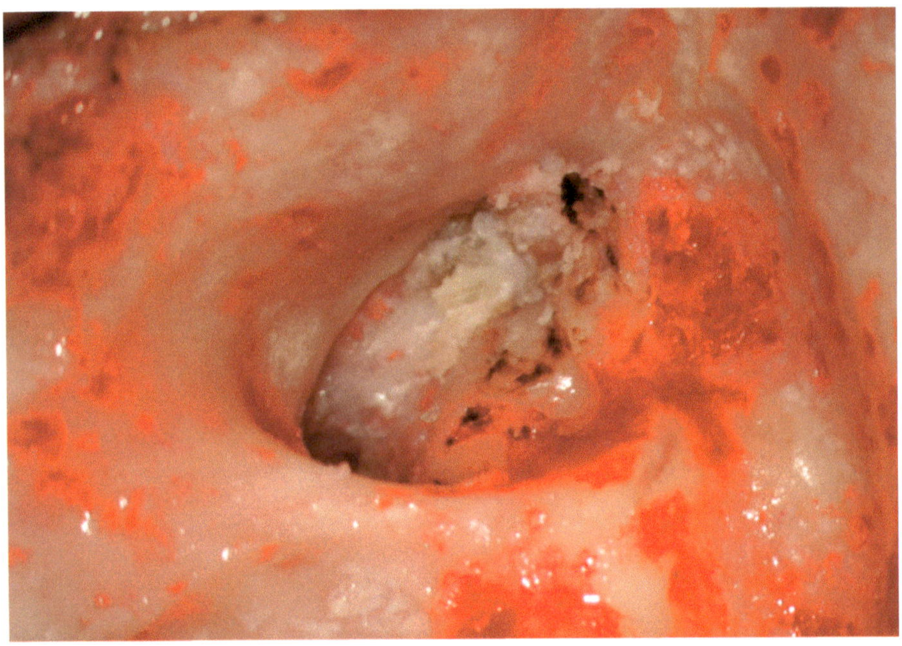

Fig. 15.6.8 Cochlear implantation was done through a subtotal petrosectomy. Here the eustachian tube has been closed with bone wax.

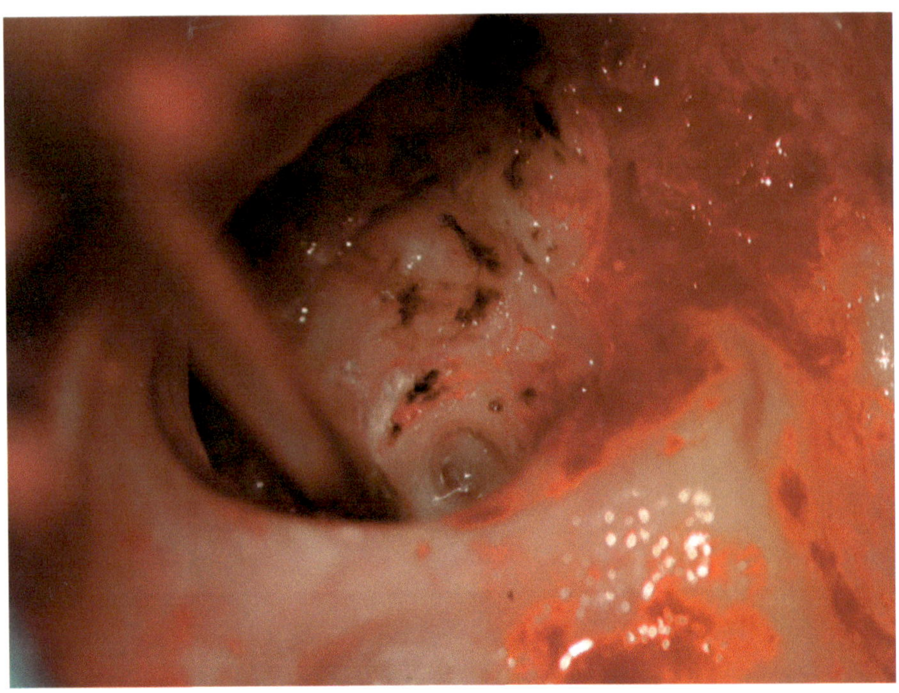

Fig. 15.6.9 The round window niche is uncovered and is slowly drilled to reveal the window. As soon as the window was opened large amounts of CSF appeared. This is the reason for the suction in this picture.

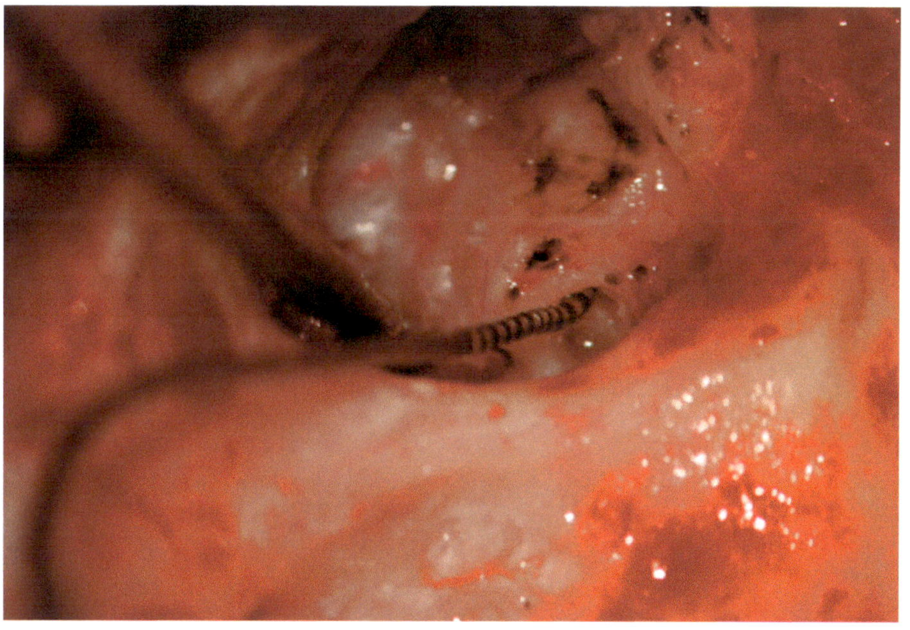

Fig. 15.6.10 Once the window and part of the basal turn was recognizable the electrode was inserted. CSF drainage had to be managed with constant suction.

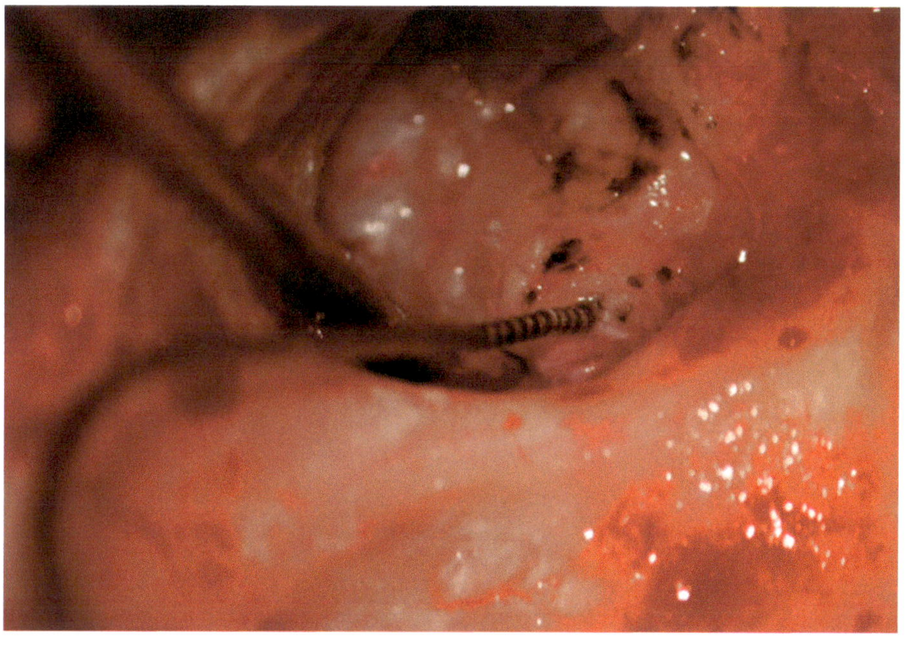

Fig. 15.6.11 The cochleostomy was well packed as a CSF gusher is a potential risk for a recurrent CSF leak or meningitis. The "second layer" of defense was the subtotal petrosectomy, with eradication of the mucosal layer and sealing off the middle ear from the nasal cavity and the external environment.

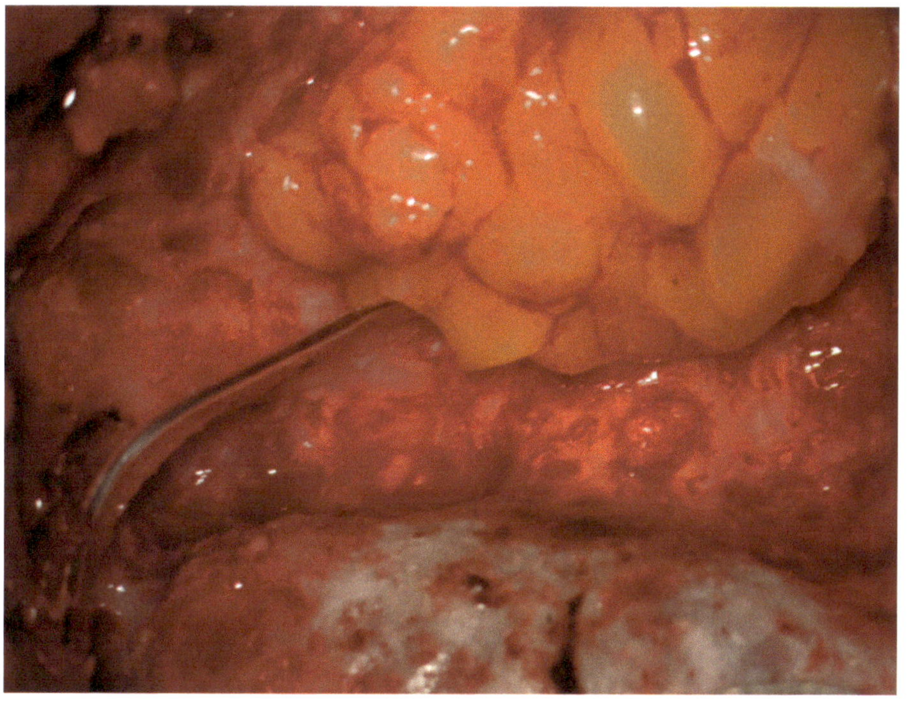

Fig. 15.6.12 Abdominal fat was used to give a stable and safe ear and a good cosmetic result.

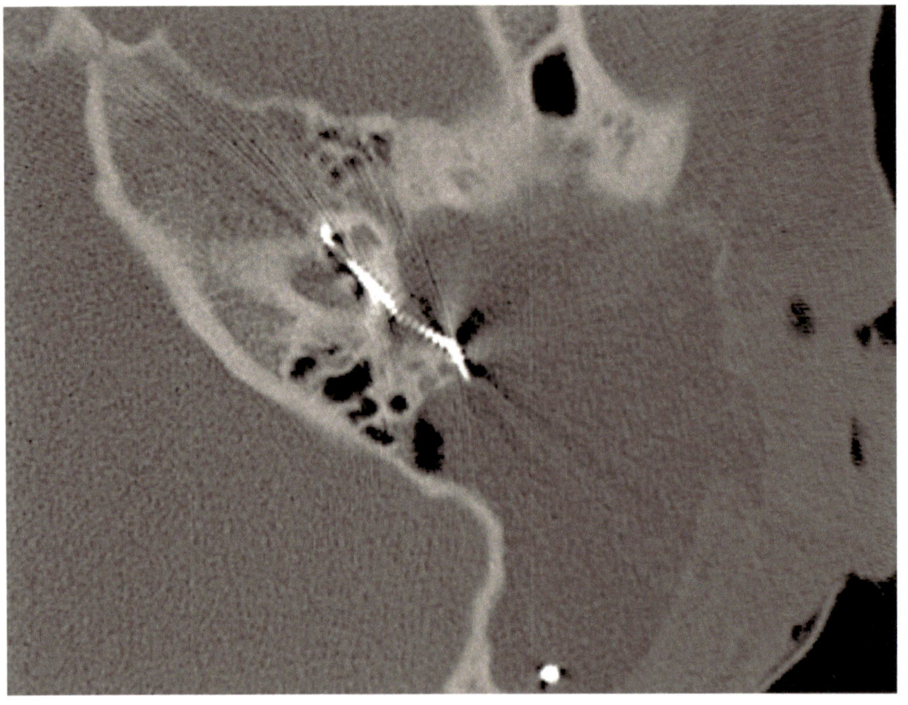

Fig. 15.6.13 Postoperative CT showed a good position of the electrode and firm sealing of the cavity.

Comment

In IP-3 a CSF gusher is inevitable and precautions should be taken beforehand to control the situation.

Case 15.7 A Patient with Cochlear Nerve Aplasia; CI Implantation Converted to ABI Placement (Fig. 15.7.1–Fig. 15.7.20)

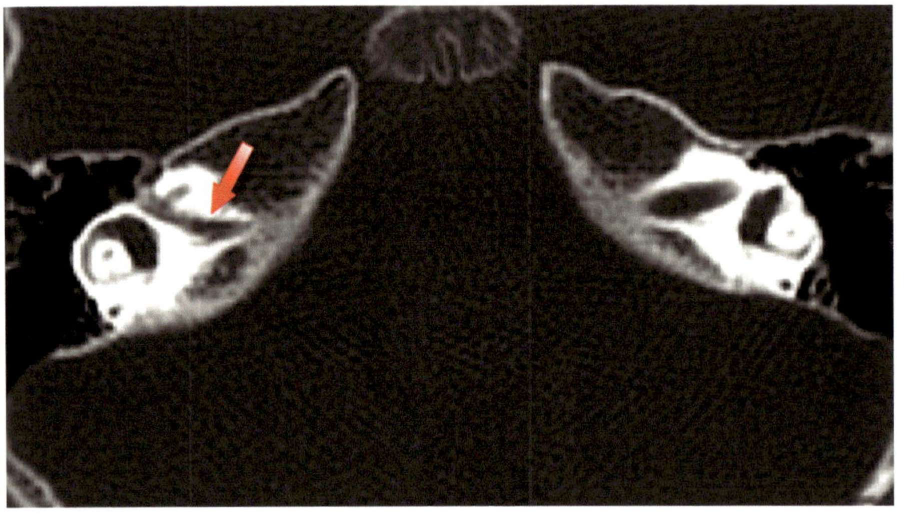

Fig. 15.7.1 A 2-year-old girl was seen because of bilateral profound hearing loss. On CT there was bilaterally a small IAC with a normal inner ear. The right side had the smaller IAC size (*red arrow*).

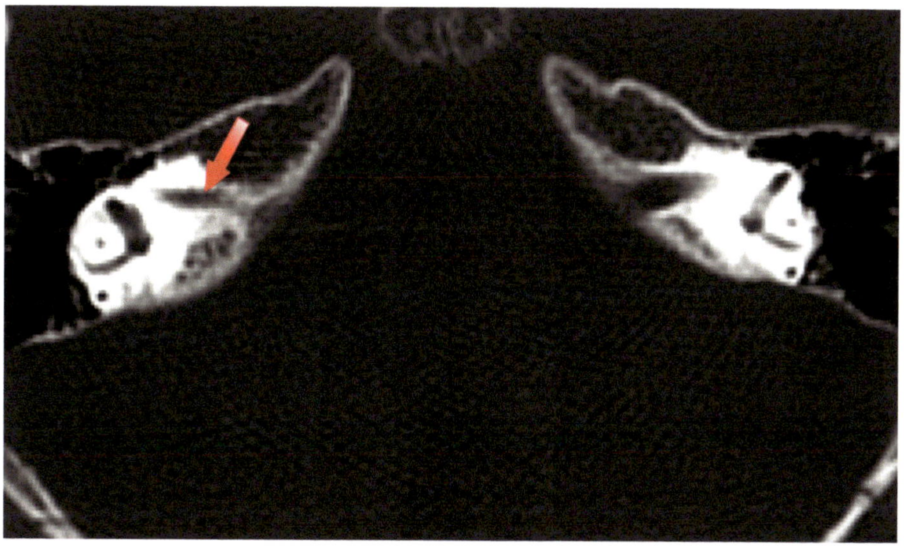

Fig. 15.7.2 The right IAC was a straighter line, as seen on this CT image (*red arrow*). Normally the IAC shape is more tapered from wide to smaller at the fundus.

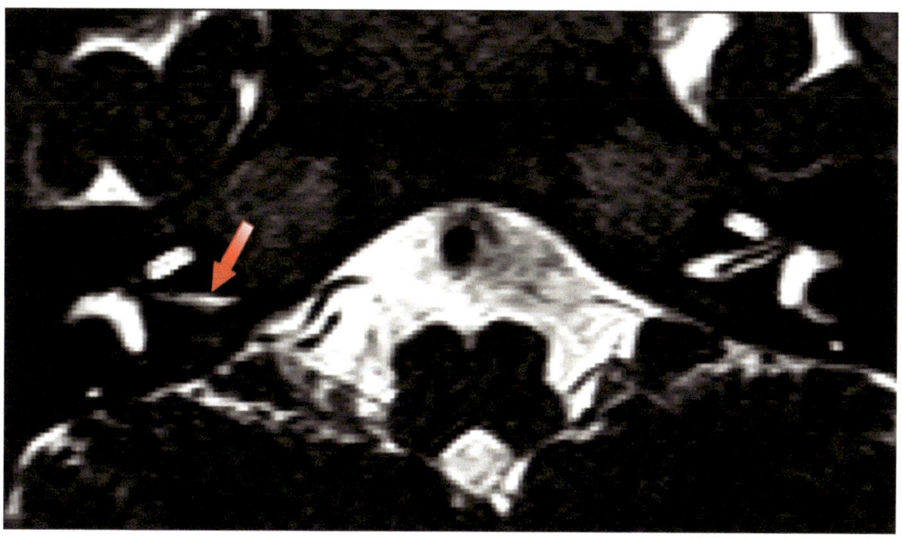

Fig. 15.7.3 On axial MRI the small right-side IAC (*red arrow*) does not show any nerve, whereas the other side shows one prominent nerve.

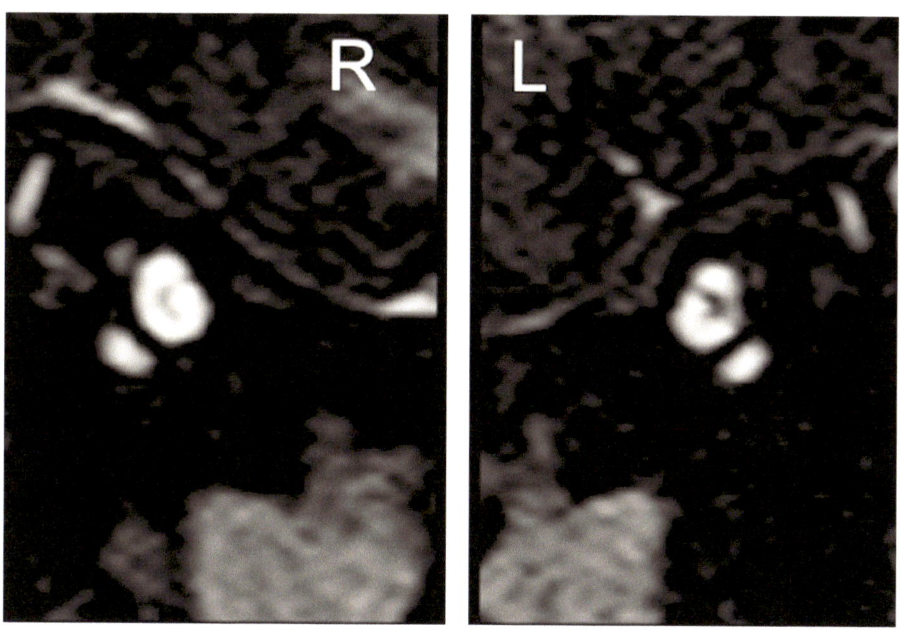

Fig. 15.7.4 On reconstructed sagittal images through the IAC, the right side vaguely shows three nerves. The left IAC contains more detailed nerves. The existence of a cochlear nerve is doubtful on these images. The right ear, with the better neural image, was chosen for an attempted CI placement.

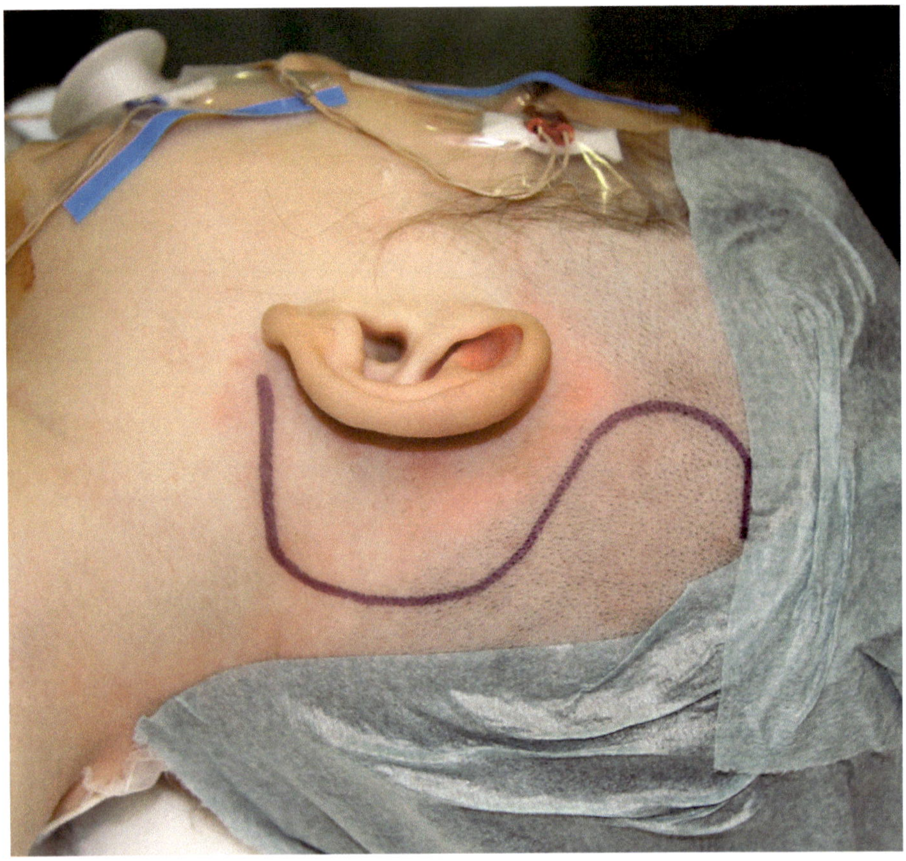

Fig. 15.7.5 Left ear. A wide approach was chosen to allow switching to a translabyrinthine approach (TLA) in case of an ABI conversion. The S-shaped incision line (as shown here) starts just on the mastoid tip and at least 5 cm above the pinna. If previous ear surgery has taken place, enlargement of the old incision should be attempted, to avoid skin necrosis due to insufficient blood supply.

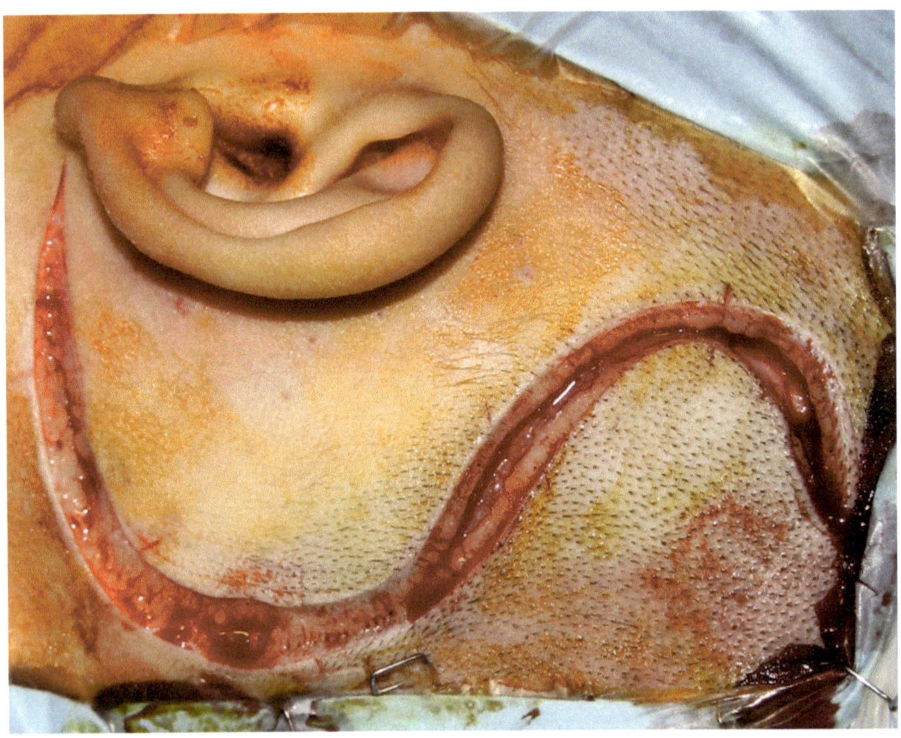

Fig. 15.7.6 Incision of the skin. First, small skin cuts perpendicular to the incision were marked at different locations along the incision line. Then the cutaneous and subcutaneous layer was cut, just onto the fascia of the temporal muscle.

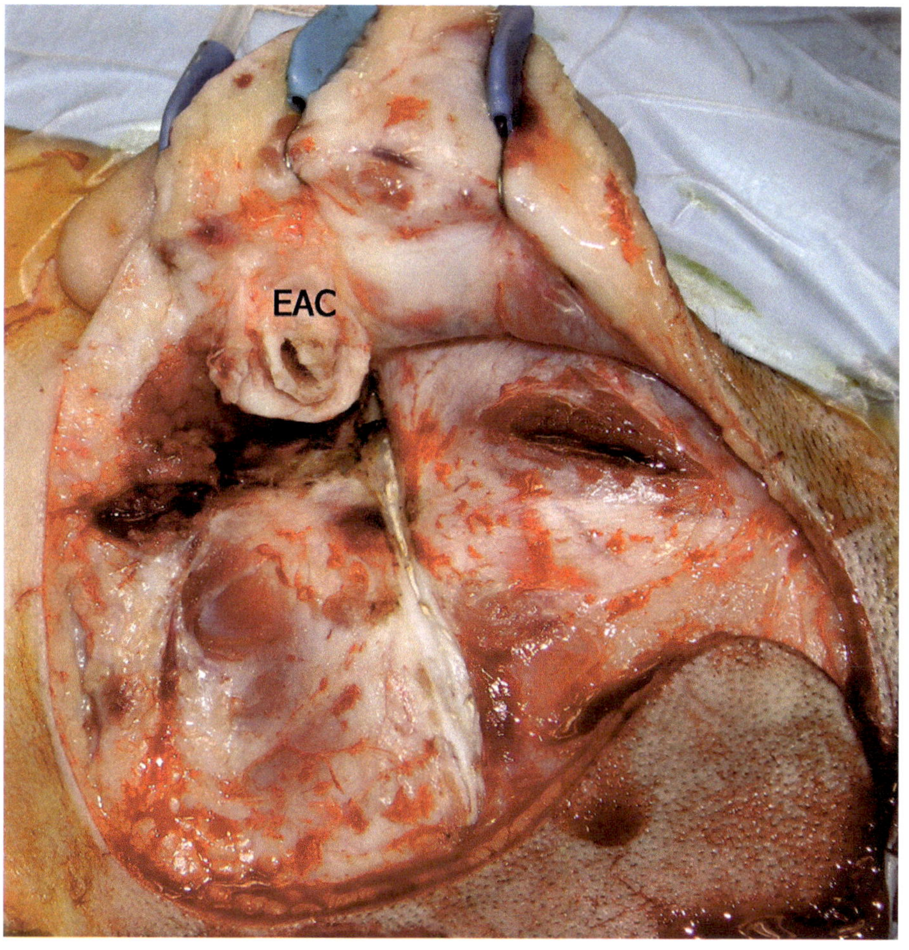

Fig. 15.7.7 The skin flap was deflected and fixated with "surgical fish hooks." The external auditory canal (EAC) was cut and an extra flap was created just behind the EAC (cartilage or subcutaneous flap) to form an extra layer of closure.

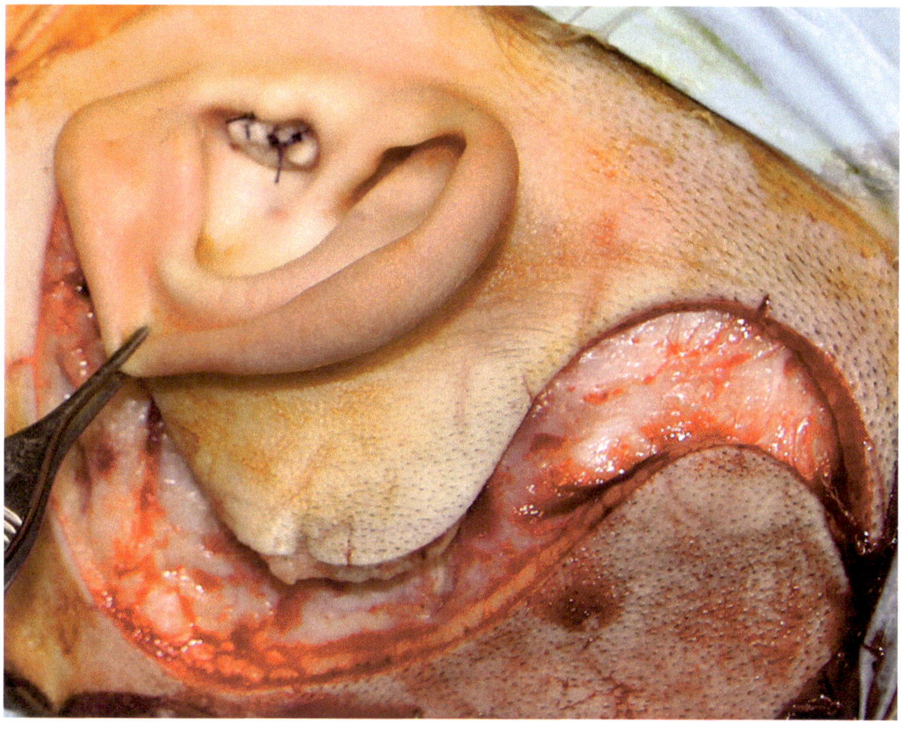

Fig. 15.7.8 Here we see the closed-off ear canal.

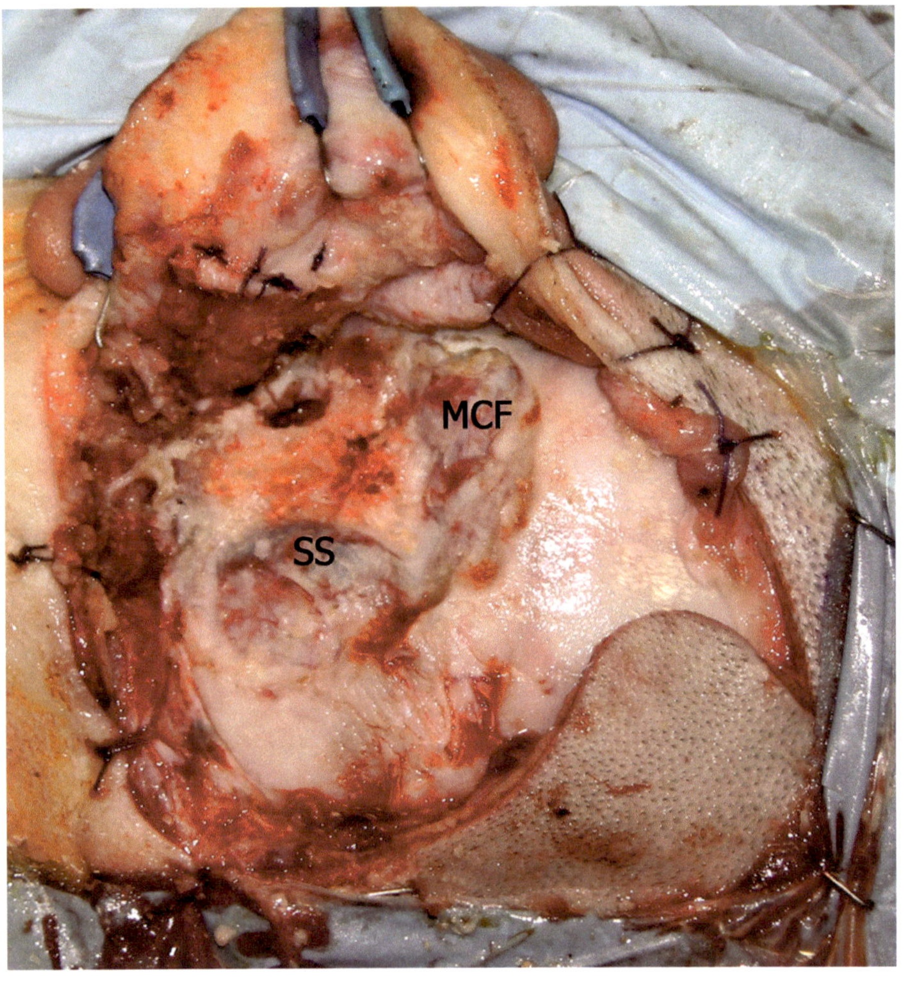

Fig. 15.7.9 The wide mastoidectomy was then performed, and the muscle flap was temporarily sutured cranially for protection of the flap, diminishing bleeding, and improving exposure. SS, sigmoid sinus; MCF, middle cranial fossa.

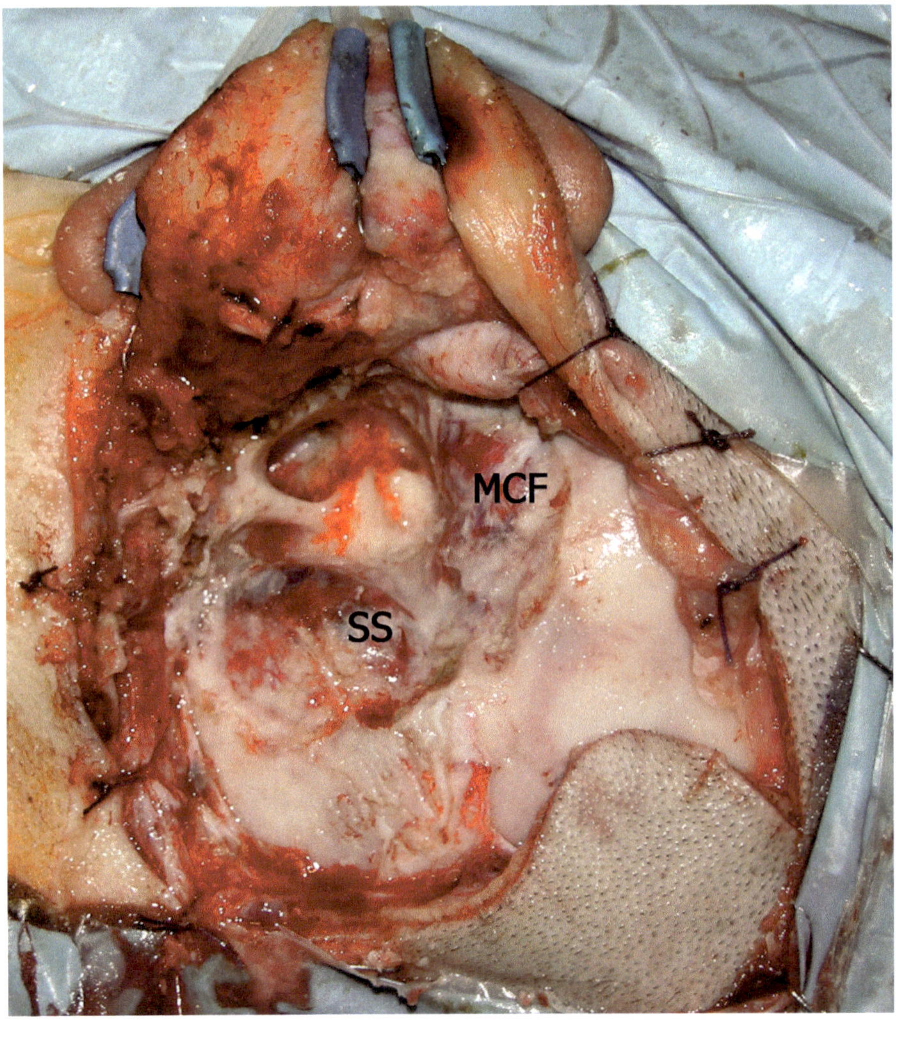

Fig. 15.7.10 The canal wall was lowered to the level of the facial nerve, and the cochlea could be fully appreciated. At this stage the scrub nurse and surgeon prepared for CI implantation. SS, sigmoid sinus; MCF, middle cranial fossa.

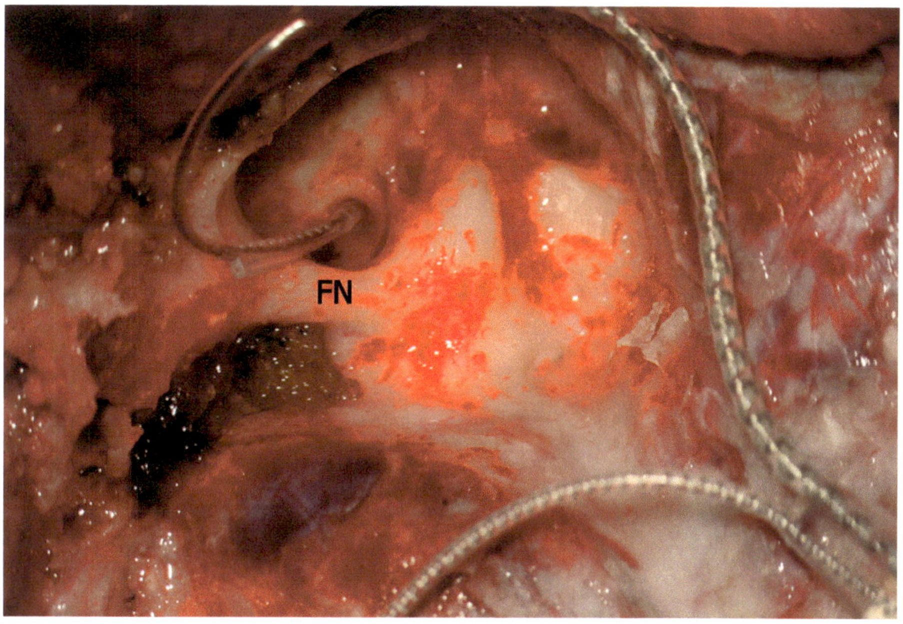

Fig. 15.7.11 The cochlear implant was inserted and the implantation was uneventful, but the EABR showed no response. The approach was then extended to a translabyrinthine approach for ABI insertion as preoperatively planned. FN, facial nerve.

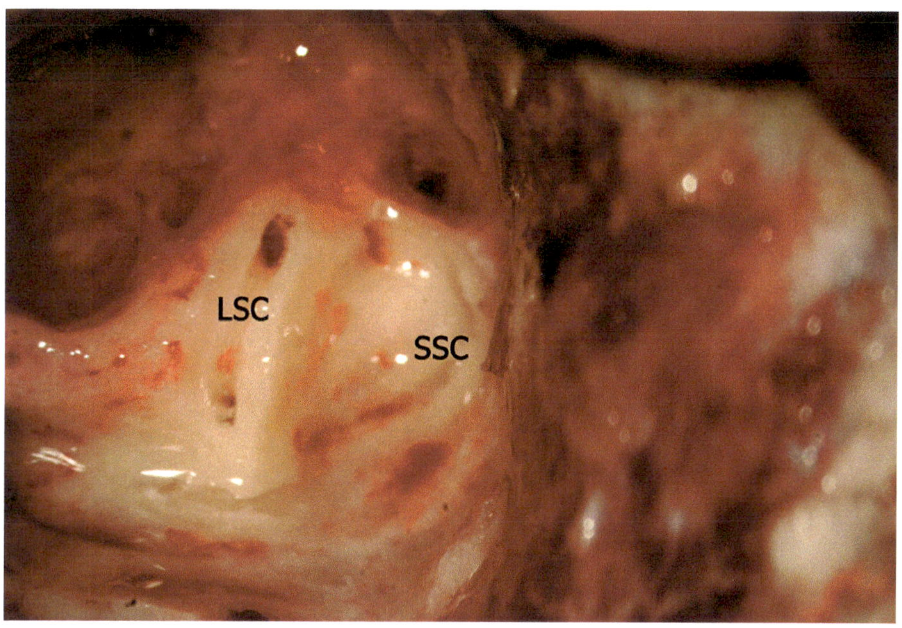

Fig. 15.7.12 The cochlear implant was removed and a labyrinthectomy was started. LSC, lateral semicircular canal; SSC, superior semicircular canal.

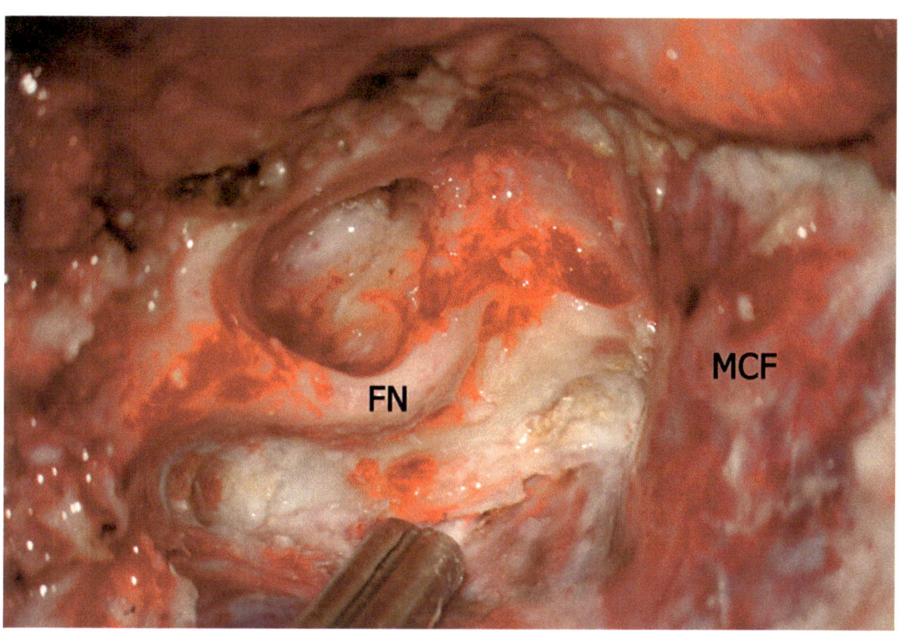

Fig. 15.7.13 A labyrinthectomy, removal of the EAC and middle ear, and closure of the eustachian tube were performed. FN, facial nerve; MCF, middle cranial fossa.

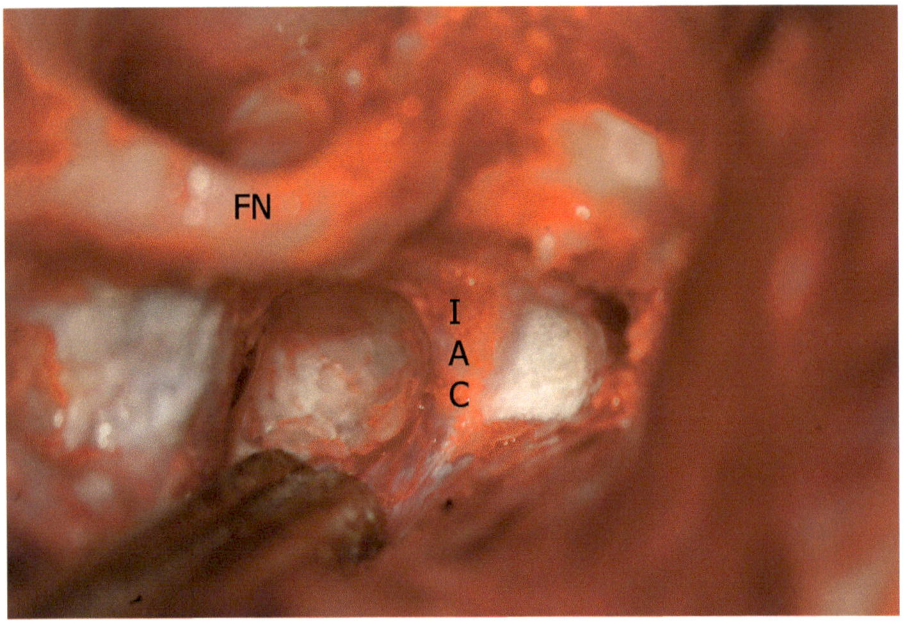

Fig. 15.7.14 The internal auditory canal (IAC) was skeletonized and a large circumference of bone removal was performed around the IAC, before opening the dura and IAC. FN, facial nerve.

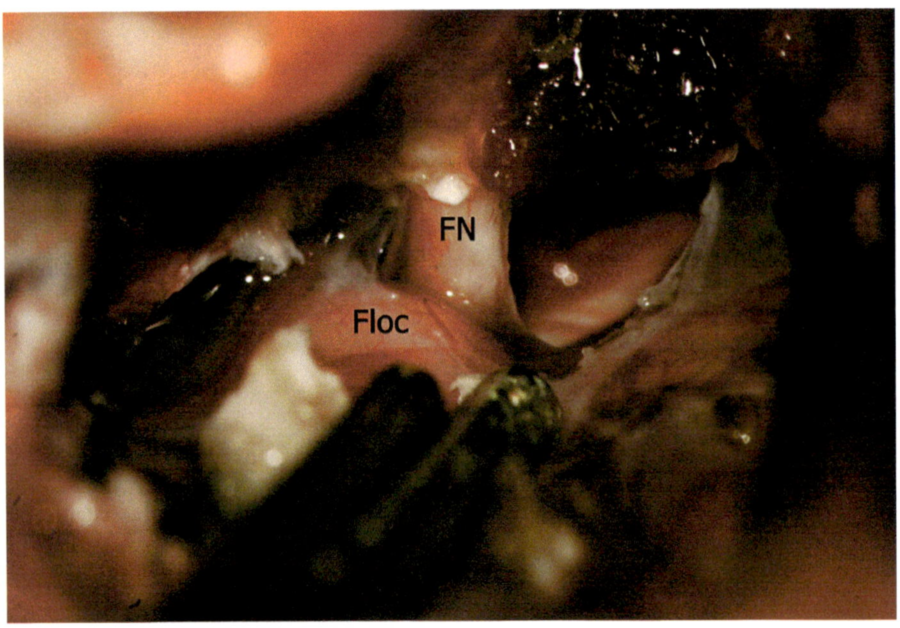

Fig. 15.7.15 The nerve(s) in the CPA may be appreciated after opening of the dura. In this case only the facial nerve is present. FN, facial nerve; Floc, flocculus.

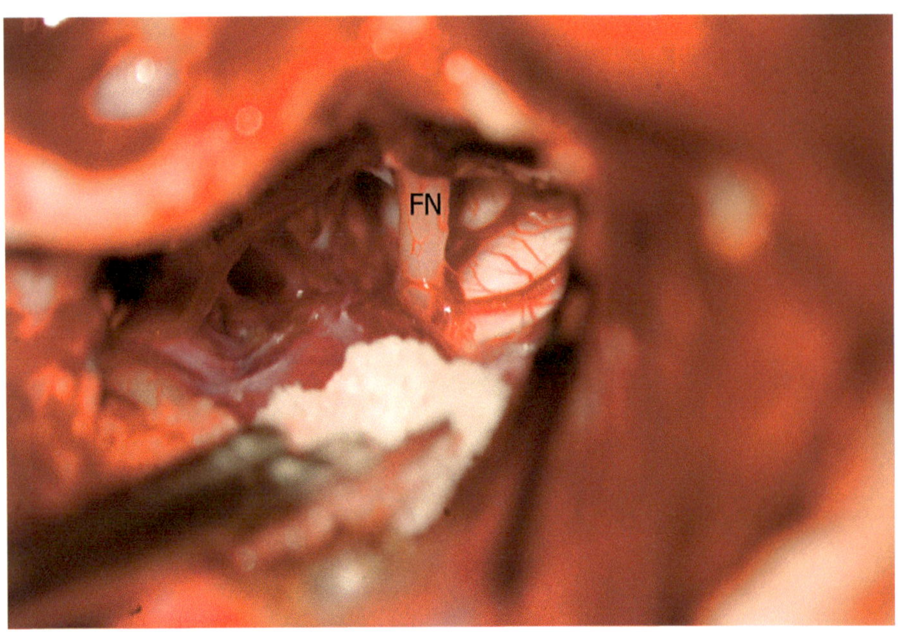

Fig. 15.7.16 Even at the brainstem only the facial nerve is present. FN, facial nerve.

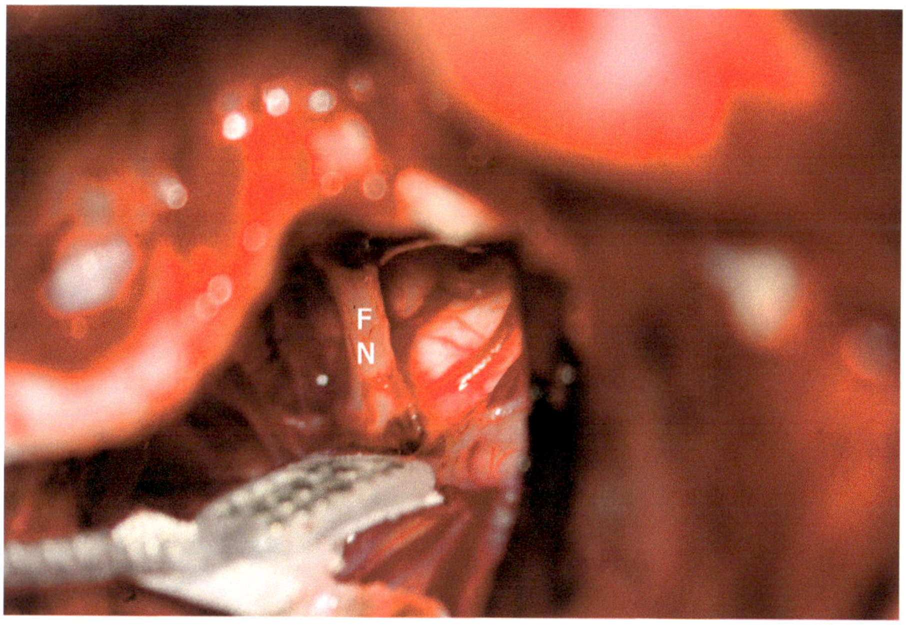

Fig. 15.7.17 The ABI electrode array is ready to be slowly inserted. FN, facial nerve.

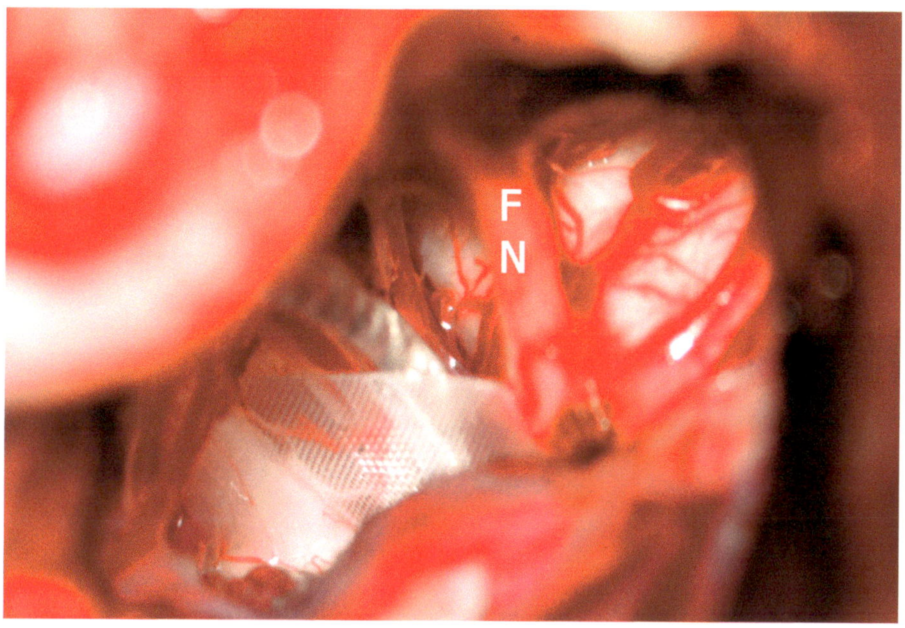

Fig. 15.7.18 The facial nerve was one of the landmarks in this case and the foramen of Luschka was opened to insert the ABI. FN, facial nerve.

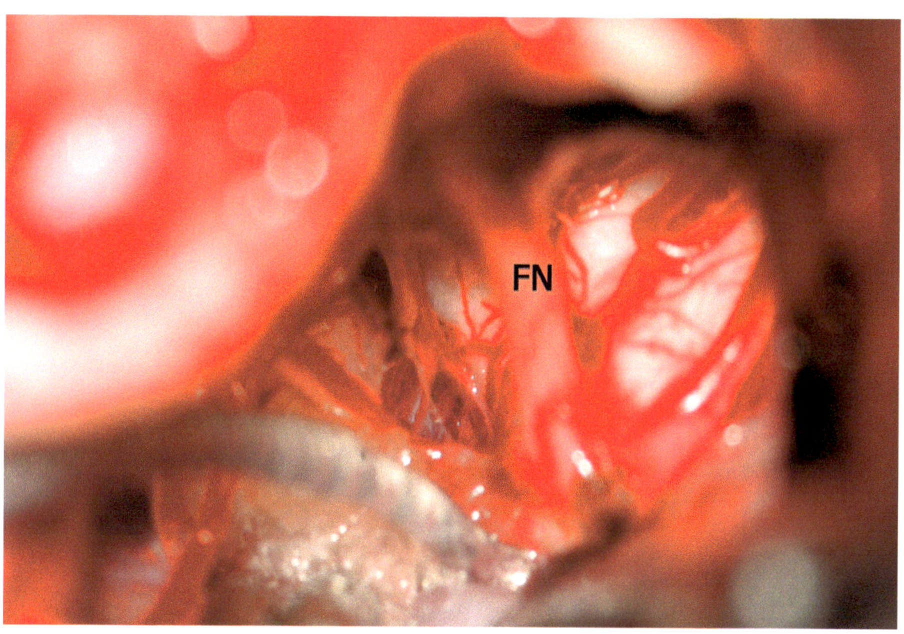

Fig. 15.7.19 The ABI is then in the correct position and the audiologist should test all electrodes for EABR reactions. This is a time-consuming but important part of the procedure. The ABI can be moved slightly if necessary to improve the number of electrodes giving auditory stimulation. In this case it was possible to record intraoperative auditory responses. FN, facial nerve.

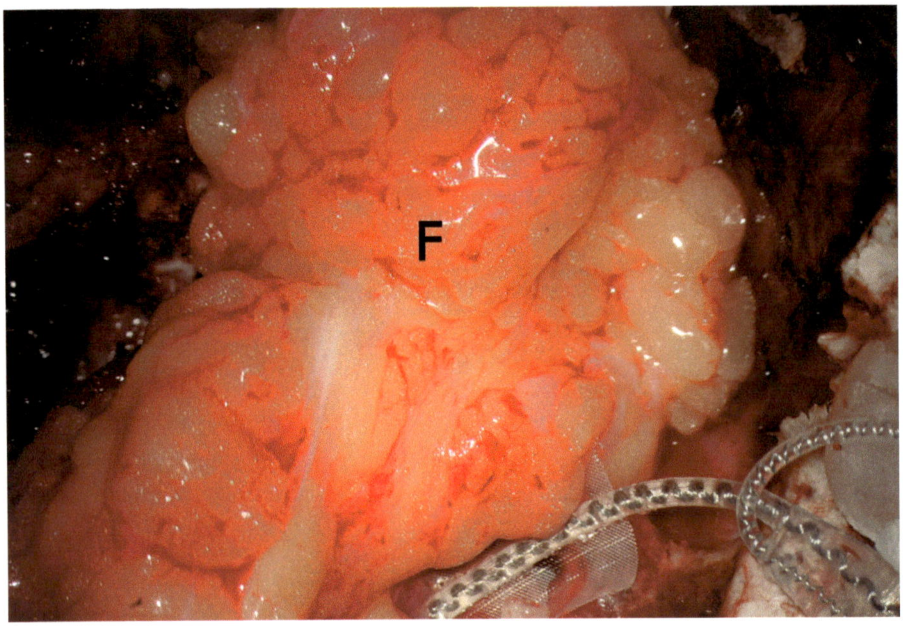

Fig. 15.7.20 The cavity was finally filled with abdominal fat (F), for protection and also to fixate the electrodes. Initial results were encouraging. The young patient uses the implant and recognizes different sounds. She has also started to say simple words.

Comment

In some case of malformation, imaging and testing are necessary to discover who will be a good CI candidate and who cannot benefit from a CI. ABI is only indicated as the first choice in the case of no cochlear structure. In a case like this, very likely with vestibulocochlear nerve agenesis, surgery was needed to confirm whether there was an ABI indication.

Reference Video

See Video 15.1.

References

1. Baino T, Fayad JN. Malformations of the ear. In: Kirtane MV, Brackmann D, Borkar DM, De Souza C, eds. Comprehensive Textbook of Otology. Diagnosis, Management and Operative Techniques. Mumbai: Bhalani Publishing House; 2010:194–211
2. Jackler RK, Luxford WM, House WF. Congenital malformations of the inner ear: a classification based on embryogenesis. Laryngoscope 1987;97(3 Pt 2, Suppl 40)2–14
3. Graham JM, Phelps PD, Michaels L. Congenital malformations of the ear and cochlear implantation in children: review and temporal bone report of common cavity. J Laryngol Otol Suppl 2000;25:1–14
4. Sennaroglu L, Saatci I. A new classification for cochleovestibular malformations. Laryngoscope 2002;112(12):2230–2241
5. Papsin BC. Cochlear implantation in children with anomalous cochleovestibular anatomy. Laryngoscope 2005;115(1 Pt 2, Suppl 106)1–26
6. Friedmann I, Fraser GR, Froggatt P. Pathology of the ear in the cardioauditory syndrome of Jervell and Lange-Nielsen (recessive deafness with electrocardiographic abnormalities). J Laryngol Otol 1966;80(5):451–470
7. Nomura Y, Kawabata I. Scheibe dysgenesis of the inner ear. J Laryngol Otol 1980;94(12):1345–1352
8. Sennaroglu L. Cochlear implantation in inner ear malformations—a review article. Cochlear Implants Int 2010;11(1):4–41
9. Paparella MM. Mondini's deafness. A review of histopathology. Ann Otol Rhinol Laryngol Suppl 1980;89(2 Pt 3):1–10
10. Mondini C. Anatomica surdi nati sectio. De Bononiesi Scientarium et Artium Instituto atque Academia Commenarii. Banoniae 1791;7:419
11. Valvassori GE, Clemis JD. The large vestibular aqueduct syndrome. Laryngoscope 1978;88(5):723–728
12. Phelps PD. Dilatation of the vestibular aqueduct/the association with congenital deafness. Clin Otolaryngol Allied Sci 1994;19(2):93–94
13. Zheng Y, Schachern PA, Cureoglu S, Mutlu C, Dijalilian H, Paparella MM. The shortened cochlea: its classification and histopathologic features. Int J Pediatr Otorhinolaryngol 2002;63(1):29–39
14. Phelps PD, Lloyd GAS. Diagnostic Imaging of the Ear. Berlin: Springer; 1990:43
15. Lemmerling MM, Mancuso AA, Antonelli PJ, Kubilis PS. Normal modiolus: CT appearance in patients with a large vestibular aqueduct. Radiology 1997;204(1):213–219
16. Colvin IB, Beale T, Harrop-Griffiths K. Long-term follow-up of hearing loss in children and young adults with enlarged vestibular aqueducts: relationship to radiologic findings and Pendred syndrome diagnosis. Laryngoscope 2006;116(11):2027–2036
17. Chen A, Francis M, Ni L, et al. Phenotypic manifestations of branchio-oto-renal syndrome. Am J Med Genet 1995;58(4):365–370
18. Sennaroglu L, Saatci I. Unpartitioned versus incompletely partitioned cochleae: radiologic differentiation. Otol Neurotol 2004;25(4):520–529
19. Sennaroglu L, Sarac S, Ergin T. Surgical results of cochlear implantation in malformed cochlea. Otol Neurotol 2006;27(5):615–623
20. Shim HJ, Shin JE, Chung JW, Lee KS. Inner ear anomalies in cochlear implantees: importance of radiologic measurements in the classification. Otol Neurotol 2006;27(6):831–837
21. Ehmer DR Jr, Booth T, Kutz JW Jr, Roland PS. Radiographic diagnosis of trans-stapedial cerebrospinal fluid fistula. Otolaryngol Head Neck Surg 2010;142(5):694–698
22. Purcell DD, Fischbein N, Lalwani AK. Identification of previously "undetectable" abnormalities of the bony labyrinth with computed tomography measurement. Laryngoscope 2003;113(11):1908–1911
23. Nance WE, Setleff R, McLeod A, Sweeney A, Cooper C, McConnell F. X-linked mixed deafness with congenital fixation of the stapedial

footplate and perilymphatic gusher. Birth Defects Orig Artic Ser 1971;07(4):64–69

24. Phelps PD, Reardon W, Pembrey M, Bellman S, Luxom L. X-linked deafness, stapes gushers and a distinctive defect of the inner ear. Neuroradiology 1991;33(4):326–330
25. Reardon W, Middleton-Price HR, Malcolm S, et al. Clinical and genetic heterogeneity in X-linked deafness. Br J Audiol 1992;26(2):109–114
26. Buchman CA, Teagle HF, Roush PA, et al. Cochlear implantation in children with labyrinthine anomalies and cochlear nerve deficiency: implications for auditory brainstem implantation. Laryngoscope 2011;121(9):1979–1988
27. Friedmann DR, Amoils M, Germiller JA, et al. Venous malformations of the temporal bone are a common feature in CHARGE syndrome. Laryngoscope 2012;122(4):895–900
28. Holcomb MA, Rumboldt Z, White DR. Cochlear nerve deficiency in children with CHARGE syndrome. Laryngoscope 2013;123(3):793–796
29. Morimoto AK, Wiggins RH III, Hudgins PA, et al. Absent semicircular canals in CHARGE syndrome: radiologic spectrum of findings. AJNR Am J Neuroradiol 2006;27(8):1663–1671
30. Casselman JW, Offeciers FE, Govaerts PJ, et al. Aplasia and hypoplasia of the vestibulocochlear nerve: diagnosis with MR imaging. Radiology 1997;202(3):773–781
31. Giesemann AM, Kontorinis G, Jan Z, Lenarz T, Lanfermann H, Goetz F. The vestibulocochlear nerve: aplasia and hypoplasia in combination with inner ear malformations. Eur Radiol 2012;22(3):519–524
32. Sennaroglu L, Ziyal I, Atas A, et al. Preliminary results of auditory brainstem implantation in prelingually deaf children with inner ear malformations including severe stenosis of the cochlear aperture and aplasia of the cochlear nerve. Otol Neurotol 2009;30(6):708–715
33. Miyasaka M, Nosaka S, Morimoto N, Taiji H, Masaki H. CT and MR imaging for pediatric cochlear implantation: emphasis on the relationship between the cochlear nerve canal and the cochlear nerve. Pediatr Radiol 2010;40(9):1509–1516
34. Komatsubara S, Haruta A, Nagano Y, Kodama T. Evaluation of cochlear nerve imaging in severe congenital sensorineural hearing loss. ORL J Otorhinolaryngol Relat Spec 2007;69(3):198–202
35. Incesulu A, Adapinar B, Kecik C. Cochlear implantation in cases with incomplete partition type III (X-linked anomaly). Eur Arch Otorhinolaryngol 2008;265(11):1425–1430
36. Kang WS, Shim BS, Lee KS. Audiologic performance after cochlear implantation in children with X-linked deafness: comparison with deaf children with a normal inner ear structure. Otol Neurotol 2013;34(3):544–548
37. Mylanus EA, Rotteveel LJ, Leeuw RL. Congenital malformation of the inner ear and pediatric cochlear implantation. Otol Neurotol 2004;25(3):308–317
38. Arndt S, Laszig R, Beck R, et al. Spectrum of hearing disorders and their management in children with CHARGE syndrome. Otol Neurotol 2010;31(1):67–73
39. Acker T, Mathur NN, Savy L, Graham JM. Is there a functioning vestibulocochlear nerve? Cochlear implantation in a child with symmetrical auditory findings but asymmetric imaging. Int J Pediatr Otorhinolaryngol 2001;57(2):171–176
40. Warren FM III, Wiggins RH III, Pitt C, Harnsberger HR, Shelton C. Apparent cochlear nerve aplasia: to implant or not to implant? Otol Neurotol 2010;31(7):1088–1094
41. Song MH, Kim SC, Kim J, Chang JW, Lee WS, Choi JY. The cochleovestibular nerve identified during auditory brainstem implantation in patients with narrow internal auditory canals: can preoperative evaluation predict cochleovestibular nerve deficiency? Laryngoscope 2011;121(8):1773–1779
42. Colletti V, Shannon RV, Carner M, Veronese S, Colletti L. Complications in auditory brainstem implant surgery in adults and children. Otol Neurotol 2010;31(4):558–564
43. Beltrame MA, Bonfioli F, Frau GN. Cochlear implant in inner ear malformation: double posterior labyrinthotomy approach to common cavity. Adv Otorhinolaryngol 2000;57:113–119
44. Govaerts PJ, Casselman J, Daemers K, De Beukelaer C, Yperman M, De Ceulaer G. Cochlear implants in aplasia and hypoplasia of the cochleovestibular nerve. Otol Neurotol 2003;24(6):887–891
45. Eisenberg LS, Johnson KC, Martinez AS, et al. Comprehensive evaluation of a child with an auditory brainstem implant. Otol Neurotol 2008;29(2):251–257
46. Song JJ, Park JH, Jang JH, et al. Facial nerve aberrations encountered during cochlear implantation. Acta Otolaryngol 2012;132(7):788–794
47. Battmer R, Pesch J, Stöver T, Lesinski-Schiedat A, Lenarz M, Lenarz T. Elimination of facial nerve stimulation by reimplantation in cochlear implant subjects. Otol Neurotol 2006;27(7):918–922
48. Weber BP, Dillo W, Dietrich B, Maneke I, Bertram B, Lenarz T. Pediatric cochlear implantation in cochlear malformations. Am J Otol 1998;19(6):747–753
49. Gstoettner WK, Hamzavi J, Baumgartner WD, Czerny CC. Fixation of the electrode array with bone paté in cochlear implant surgery. Acta Otolaryngol 2000;120(3):369–374
50. Merkus P, Taibah A, Sequino G, Sanna M. Less than 1% cerebrospinal fluid leakage in 1,803 translabyrinthine vestibular schwannoma surgery cases. Otol Neurotol 2010;31(2):276–283
51. Hoffman RA, Downey LL, Waltzman SB, Cohen NL. Cochlear implantation in children with cochlear malformations. Am J Otol 1997;18(2):184–187
52. Eisenman DJ, Ashbaugh C, Zwolan TA, Arts HA, Telian SA. Implantation of the malformed cochlea. Otol Neurotol 2001;22(6):834–841
53. Buchman CA, Copeland BJ, Yu KK, Brown CJ, Carrasco VN, Pillsbury HC III. Cochlear implantation in children with congenital inner ear malformations. Laryngoscope 2004;114(2):309–316
54. Loundon N, Rouillon I, Munier N, Marlin S, Roger G, Garabedian EN. Cochlear implantation in children with internal ear malformations. Otol Neurotol 2005;26(4):668–673
55. Kim LS, Jeong SW, Huh MJ, Park YD. Cochlear implantation in children with inner ear malformations. Ann Otol Rhinol Laryngol 2006;115(3):205–214
56. Lee KH, Lee J, Isaacson B, Kutz JW, Roland PS. Cochlear implantation in children with enlarged vestibular aqueduct. Laryngoscope 2010;120(8):1675–1681

Further Reading

Morera C, De-Paula C, Mas F, Cavallé L. Cochleo-vestibular nerve (CVN) malformations with normal or dysplastic cochlea – cochlear or brain stem implantation? Int J Pediatr Otorhinolaryngol 2011;75(Suppl 1):11

Pakdaman MN, Herrmann BS, Curtin HD, Van Beek-King J, Lee DJ. Cochlear implantation in children with anomalous cochleovestibular anatomy: a systematic review. Otolaryngol Head Neck Surg 2012;146(2):180–190

Phelps PD, Coffey RA, Trembath RC, et al. Radiological malformations of the ear in Pendred syndrome. Clin Radiol 1998;53(4):268–273

Sennaroglu L, Colletti V, Manrique M, et al. Auditory brainstem implantation in children and non-neurofibromatosis type 2 patients: a consensus statement. Otol Neurotol 2011;32(2):187–191

Acknowledgment

We thank Professor Miguel Arístegui, ENT surgeon, Madrid, Spain, for sharing some of his cases and radiology images.

16 Neurofibromatosis Type 2 and Auditory Implantation

Neurofibromatosis type 2 (NF2) is an autosomal dominant disease with a gene penetrance of over 95%. This disease has a propensity to produce tumors deriving from neural crest elements and is therefore characterized by bilateral vestibular schwannomas, with other presentations including schwannomas of the other cranial and peripheral nerves, meningiomas, and juvenile posterior subcapsular cataract. Rarely, ependymomas and astrocytomas develop. Almost all affected persons develop bilateral vestibular schwannomas by the age of 30 years and the average age of onset of such findings in individuals with NF2 is 18 to 24 years.

Variable expressivity of NF2 among individuals results in varying size, location, and number of tumors. Although these tumors are not malignant, their anatomical location and multiplicity generally lead to high morbidity and early mortality. The average life expectancy is 36 years and actuarial survival from the time of establishment of the correct diagnosis is 15 years. An earlier diagnosis and better-organized treatment in tertiary centers can provide a better chance of survival.

NF2 is not related genetically or phenotypically to neurofibromatosis type 1 (NF1). Individuals with NF2 are unlikely to have the cognitive problems (mental retardation and learning disability) that are usually seen in those with NF1. Patients with NF2 may have "café au lait" spots and cutaneous neurofibromas, but they are fewer and less severe than in NF1 patients; they are not the key features of the condition. Schwannomas almost never undergo malignant transformation to neurofibrosarcoma.

16.1 Difference in Comparison with Sporadic Vestibular Schwannoma

- Tumor growth in patients with NF2 generally presents much earlier in life than in sporadic vestibular schwannoma.
- The growth rate of the schwannomas is usually faster and the tumor may reach a remarkable size and cause severe distortion of the brainstem in NF2. The internal auditory canals are more markedly enlarged and their bony wall can be irregularly eroded. The tumor may even erode through the roof of the internal auditory canal and/or extend into the middle cranial fossa. Additionally, the tumor may invade the cochlear modiolus and extend into the basal turn of the cochlea.
- In many cases, there can be simultaneous schwannomas of other cranial nerves, often at the level of jugular foramen, as well as meningiomas. In some instances, all branches and end organs of the vestibular nerve, selected bundles of the cochlear nerve, the facial nerve, and other cranial and peripheral nerves within the temporal bone are affected by a proliferation of Schwann cells. They can be localized, diffuse, or both, so that decision making and surgical procedures are made extra difficult. Clinically, spinal involvement by the tumor may occasionally make positioning of the patient difficult. Cervical spine involvement may also pose a problem for intubation.
- Histologically, tumors in NF2 are indistinguishable from the conventional vestibular schwannoma. However, in some instances, they may display a conspicuously whorled pattern strongly resembling that of certain meningiomas.

16.2 Clinical Diagnosis

Clinical diagnosis of NF2 is typically determined by the presence of bilateral vestibular schwannomas. However, NF2 can also be diagnosed in the presence of more rare combinations of different pathologies (**Fig. 16.1**).

The molecular genetics of NF2 is summarized in **Table 16.1**. Molecular genetic testing of the NF2 gene is available clinically. The main role of molecular genetic testing is in early detection of at-risk individuals (primarily children of affected individuals) for surveillance and medical management. It can also be used to confirm the diagnosis of NF2. Genetic confirmation of NF2 is important because patients identified with NF2 need genetic counseling, which has a pivotal role with regard to expectation and family planning. Prenatal screening for NF2 is possible by analysis of DNA extracted from fetal cells obtained by amniocentesis at ~15 to 18 weeks' gestation or by chorionic villus sampling at ~10 to 12 weeks' gestation.

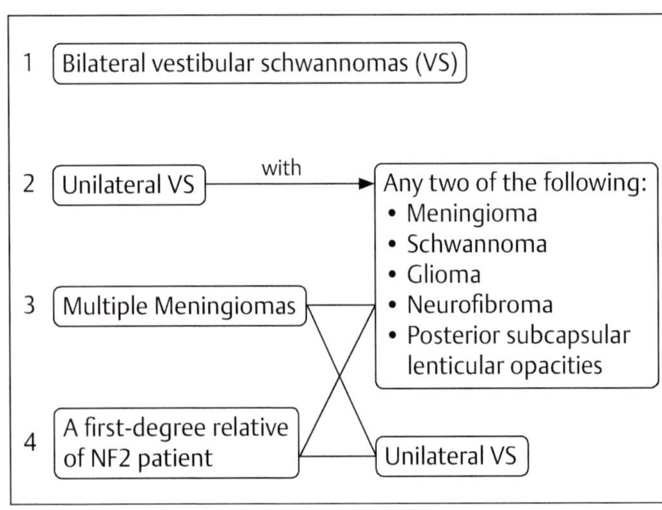

Fig. 16.1 Clinical diagnosis of NF2 is obtained in the case of bilateral vestibular schwannomas (1) or in the case of one of the combinations (2–4) of various pathologies shown in this figure.

Table 16.1 Molecular genetics of neurofibromatosis 2

Gene symbol	Chromosomal locus	Protein name
NF2	22q12.2	Merlin

16.3 Clinical Manifestations of Disease

Schwannoma usually affects vestibular nerves bilaterally, although only one side can be affected in certain individuals (mosaicism). Vestibular schwannomas are likely to present simultaneously. More rarely schwannomas can present only unilaterally, with the second tumor revealing itself at a later time. Schwannomas may also develop on other cranial and peripheral nerves. Generally, sensory nerves are more frequently affected than motor nerves.

Spinal tumors are observed in at least two-thirds of individuals with NF2. They often pose the most devastating and difficult aspects of this disease to manage. The most common spinal tumors are schwannomas, which usually originate within the intravertebral canal on the dorsal root and extend both medially and laterally, taking the shape of a "dumbbell." Intramedullary tumors of the spinal cord such as astrocytoma and ependymoma occur in 5 to 33% of individuals with NF2. Most individuals with spinal cord involvement have multiple tumors, but they tend not to develop corresponding symptoms.

Meningioma develops in approximately half of individuals with NF2. Most are intracranial lesions, though spinal meningiomas can occur. NF2 meningiomas tend to occur less frequently in the skull base and are usually of the fibroblastic variety. Meningiomas in the orbit may compress the optic nerve and result in visual loss. Those at the skull base may cause cranial neuropathy, brainstem compression, and hydrocephalus. Meningioma may be the presenting feature of NF2, particularly in childhood.

Ocular involvement is present in one-third of individuals with NF2. They lose visual acuity in one or both eyes. Posterior subcapsular lens opacity, rarely progressing to a visually significant cataract, is the most common ocular finding. Lens opacities may appear prior to the onset of symptoms from vestibular schwannoma. Retinal hamartoma and epiretinal membrane are seen in up to one-third of individuals. Intracranial and intraorbital tumors may result in diminished visual acuity and diplopia.

Mono/polyneuropathy is an increasingly recognized feature of NF2, occurring particularly in childhood. This is frequently presented as a facial palsy, usually with only partial recovery, a squint (third nerve palsy), or foot or hand drop.

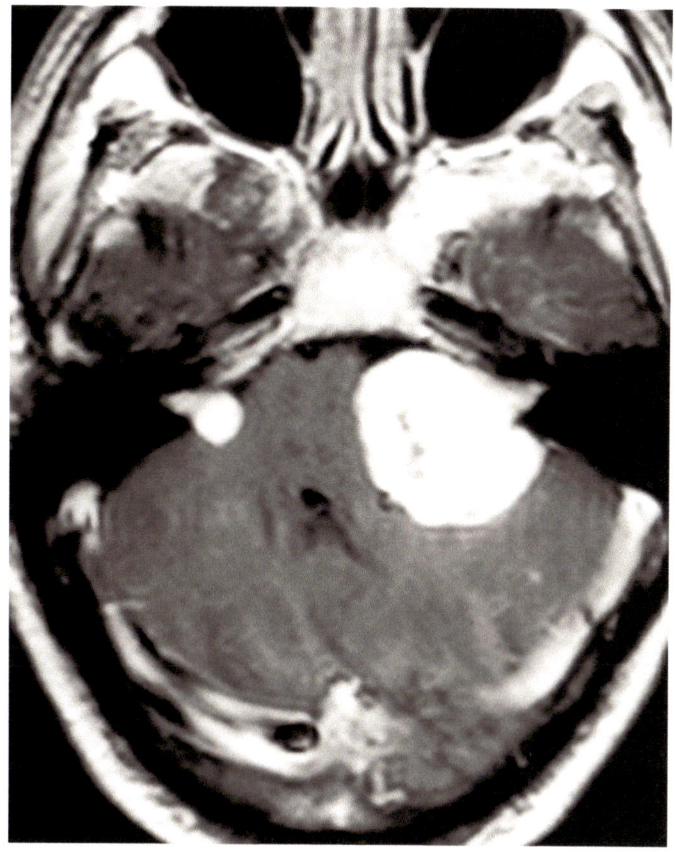

Fig. 16.2 Asymmetrical bilateral vestibular schwannomas with compression of the brainstem by the left tumor. This marked difference in size is the most common presentation.

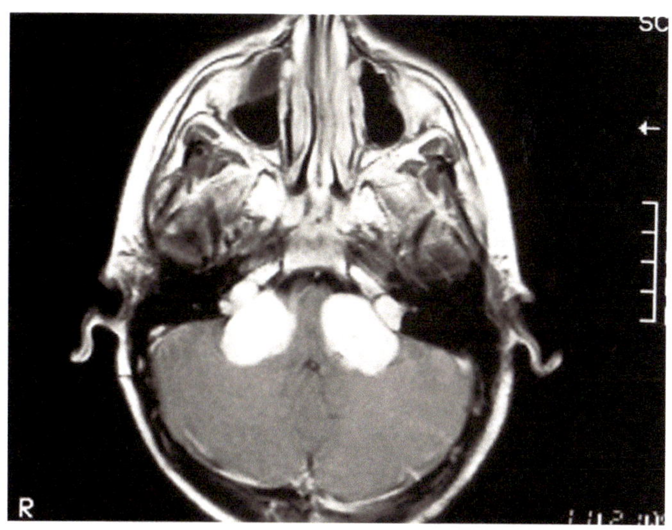

Fig. 16.3 Bilateral vestibular schwannomas. Note how the tumors are squeezing the brainstem.

16.4 Management

Diagnosis, evaluation, treatment, follow-up, and genetic counseling of patients with NF2 can best be performed in multidisciplinary clinics. The full management is beyond the scope of this book and only the management of intracranial lesions and follow-up are discussed here.

16.5 Vestibular Schwannoma (Fig. 16.2–Fig. 16.6)

Hearing preservation is very important in the management of individuals with NF2. All patients will have regular hearing evaluation, including auditory brainstem response (ABR), pure tone audiometry, and speech discrimination testing. The assessment of these parameters has dual roles. First, it gives an idea of tumor progression; and second, it significantly influences the management of these patients, including the timing and the type of surgery.

Therapy remains primarily surgical. Small vestibular tumors that are localized completely intracanalicularly can often be totally resected with preservation of both hearing and facial nerve function. Larger tumors should be surgically removed. If we can succeed in preserving the cochlear nerve, a cochlear implant (CI) is feasible. In cases where the cochlear nerve is sacrificed, an auditory brainstem implant (ABI) is indicated. We believe that there is no role for stereotactic radiotherapy in the management of NF2 patients, because the outcomes from radiation treatment for individuals with NF2 are not as good as for individuals with

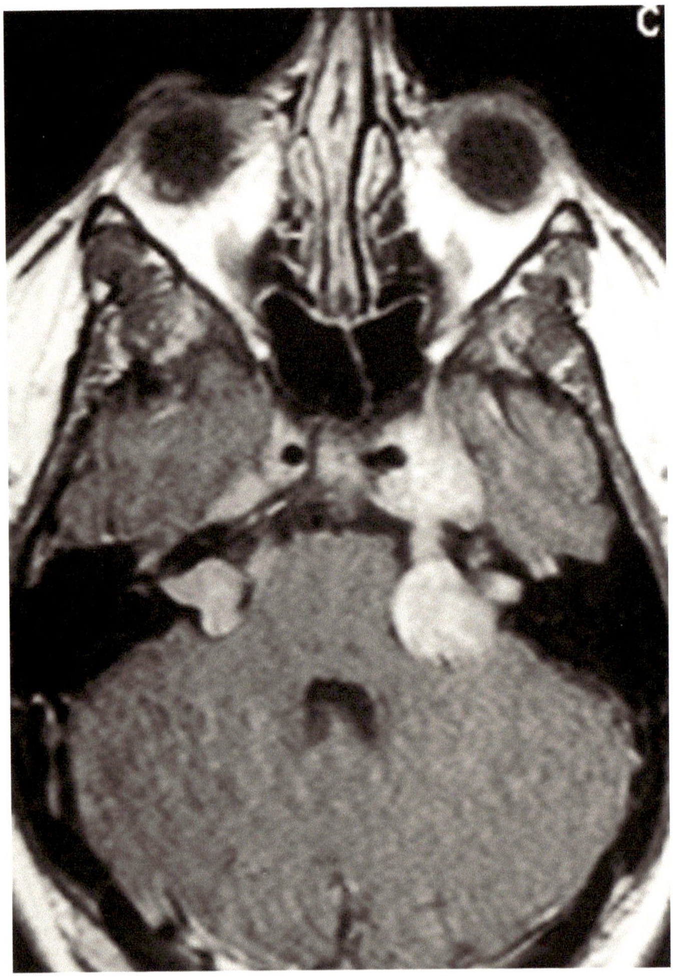

Fig. 16.4 Bilateral vestibular schwannomas and trigeminal nerve schwannomas are present.

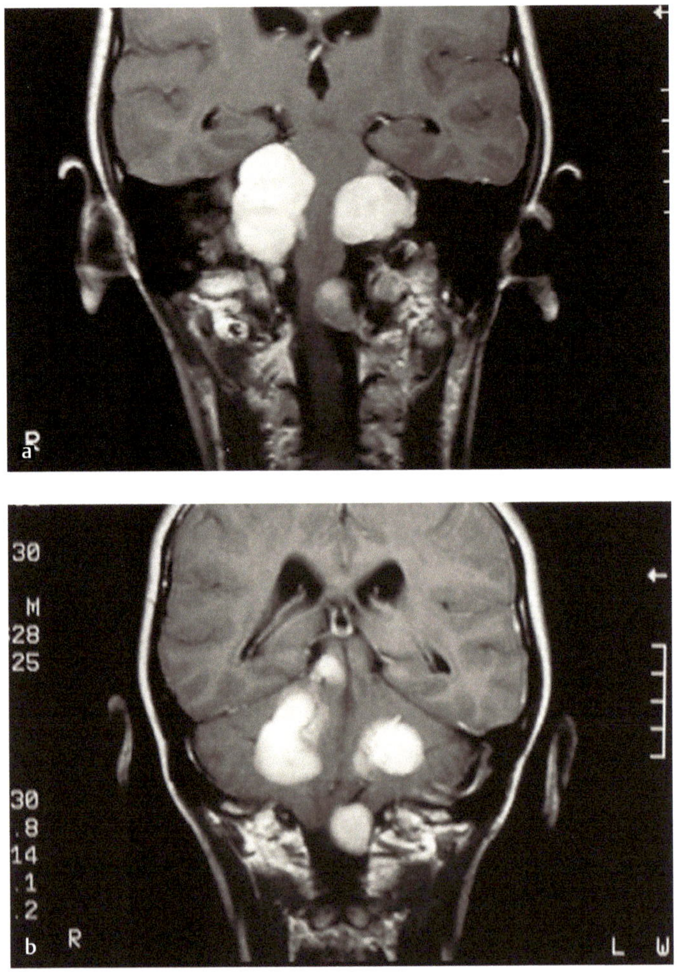

Fig. 16.5a, b Presentation of multiple schwannomas.

a Note that a piece of tumor is wedged into the brainstem. In such cases, the patient must be informed of the possibility of subtotal resection of the tumor.

b Note also the lower cranial nerve schwannoma.

sporadic unilateral vestibular schwannoma, demonstrating only ~60% long-term tumor control. Malignant transformation is a possible, but probably not common, sequela.

16.6 Other Tumors

The other intracranial, cranial nerve, or spinal nerve tumors are very slow growing and surgical intervention for these tumors may cause disability years before it would occur naturally. Radiation therapy of NF2-associated tumors should be considered carefully because radiation exposure may induce, accelerate, or transform tumors in an individual with an inactive tumor-suppressor gene.

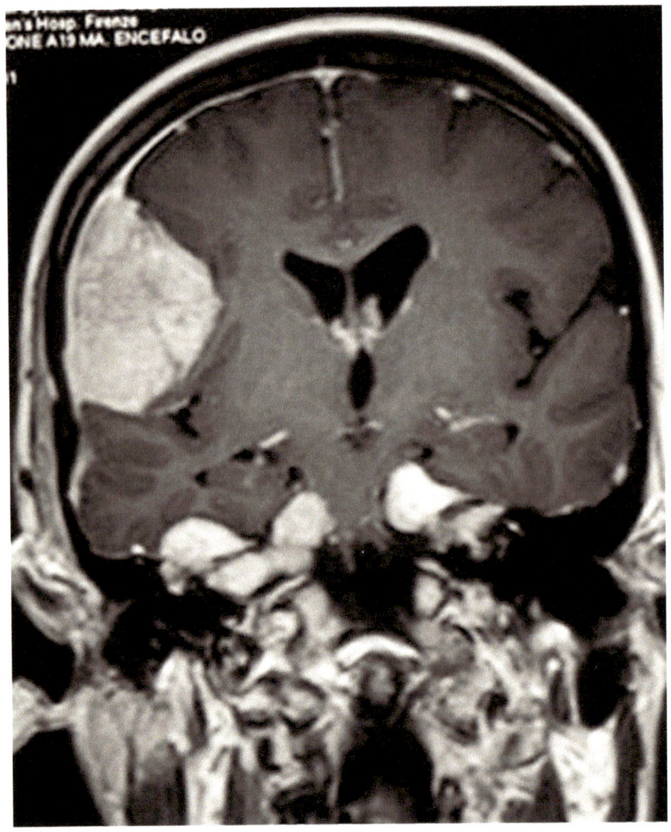

◀ **Fig. 16.6** Bilateral vestibular schwannomas, temporal meningioma, and lower cranial nerve schwannoma are present.

16.7 Surveillance

- **At-risk asymptomatic individuals.** Individuals, especially children who are at risk of developing NF2, are closely monitored. Early recognition of NF2 may allow for earlier intervention and consequently better final outcome. This can be done with DNA-based testing.
- **At-risk asymptomatic individuals testing positive for the mutant genes.** Individuals belonging to this category need regular annual MRI scanning from the teenage years until at least the fifth decade because some individuals with NF2 do not have any symptoms until they reach their sixth decade.
- **Individuals with tumor.** Patients in this group need follow-up and regular annual (at least) MRI scanning for life. Even patients who have undergone complete surgical removal of bilateral vestibular schwannoma still need long follow-up, because vestibular schwannomas still have a chance of regrowing and, more importantly, existing or new occurrences of meningiomas and/or other cranial nerve schwannomas should be monitored.

16.8 Decision Making

Fig. 16.7 and **Fig. 16.8** schematize decision making on surgery for NF2 patients at Gruppo Otologico. The surgical approach depends on the presence of hearing and tumor size. If hearing is preserved, the same plan would be applied to the other side. In the case with hearing loss, a CI or auditory brainstem implant would be placed concomitantly according to the status of the cochlear nerve.

16.8.1 Tumor Size

- When the tumor is larger than 1.5 cm, with contralateral hearing present, we will attempt surgical removal by the enlarged translabyrinthine approach with concomitant cochlear or ABI implantation.
- If the tumor is less than 1.5 cm or is positioned intracanalicularly, the options are dependent on hearing.

16.8.2 Preoperative Hearing

- **No hearing:** surgery with intention of cochlear nerve preservation and concomitant CI placement if applicable.
- **Hearing present:** an attempt at hearing preservation technique with auditory implant (CI or ABI) in the same stage if unsuccessful, or close observation with regular MRI scans and hearing evaluation.

If the ear is the only hearing ear, there are two possible options. One is to monitor the hearing closely and to offer surgical treatment when the hearing starts to deteriorate. The second option is to attempt a hearing preservation approach with possible cochlear implantation if necessary. Counseling of the patient plays a role in which decision is taken.

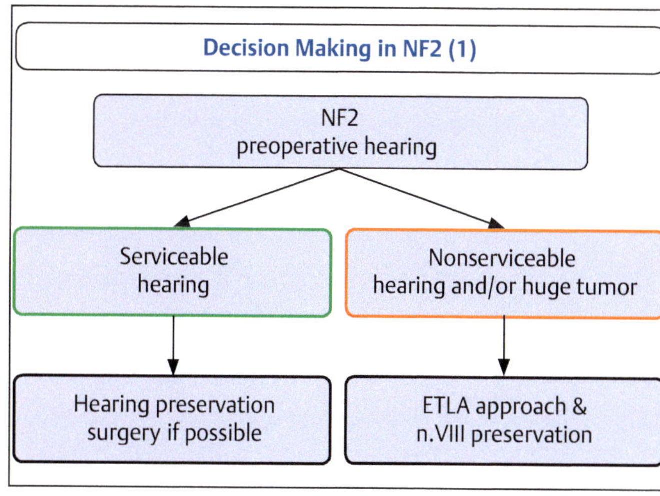

Fig. 16.7 NF2 flow 1. Scheme for decision making on surgery for NF2 patients at Gruppo Otologico.

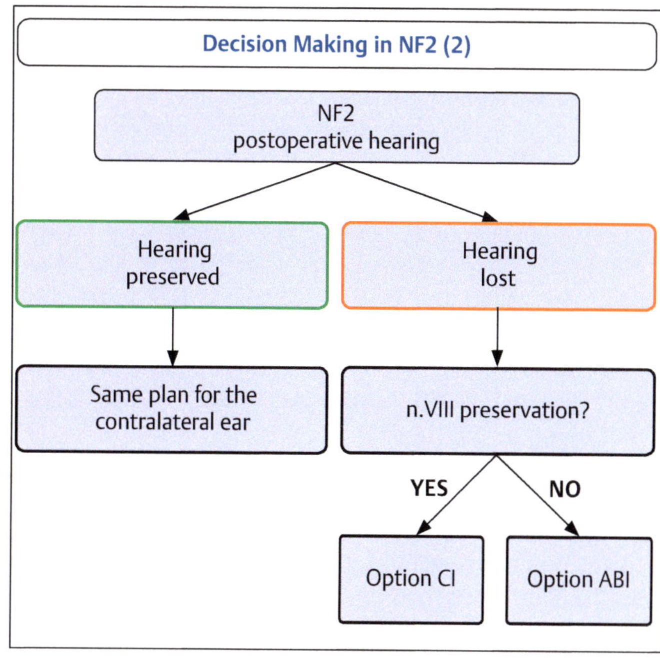

Fig. 16.8 NF2 flow 2. Scheme for decision making on surgery for NF2 patients at Gruppo Otologico.

16.8.3 Complications of the Tumor

Any patient with neurological complications related to the vestibular schwannoma may also need surgical intervention, regardless of the size of tumor.

16.9 Type of Operation

Having decided to perform the surgery (see **Fig. 16.8**), usually the first aim is to remove the tumor completely and safely. The approach chosen should allow us to achieve this primary aim. Preservation of hearing (or of the cochlear nerve) is a secondary aim.

There is no fixed rule. Each patient has a different situation and the management is individualized accordingly. However, as a rule of thumb, with a tumor less than 1.5 cm we would be likely to try the hearing preservation approach (if hearing is still worth preserving), which is either the middle cranial fossa approach or a combined retrosigmoid–retrolabyrinthine approach. If the hearing is lost but the cochlear nerve is preserved, a CI may be inserted, usually in the same stage. If the cochlear nerve has to be sacrificed, the only remaining possibility is an ABI, to be inserted during the same stage to avoid a new surgical procedure in the cerebellopontine angle. This is impossible to achieve via the middle cranial fossa approach because there is no access to the Luschka foramen.

If the tumor is greater than 1.5 cm, we tend to approach the tumor via the extended translabyrinthine transapical approach with concomitant placement of a hearing implant. We may place either a CI or an ABI depending on the cochlear nerve viability.

Unfortunately, at the time of writing, no reliable test is available to gain information intraoperatively on the functionality of a preserved cochlear nerve to guide the choice between a CI or an ABI. The ideal tool to provide this information would be a temporary intracochlear electrode, but no such tool or implant is on the market at present.

16.10 Operation Side

If the patient presents with bilateral vestibular schwannomas, the convention is always to remove the larger tumor. This decision is usually made easier because the larger tumor very often corresponds to the worse-hearing ear. If the tumors are of similar size, the tumor on the side with the worse-hearing ear should be removed first.

If the larger tumor corresponds to the better-hearing ear, careful individualized management is necessary. We could remove the larger tumor, taking care to preserve the cochlear nerve for the coming CI. In case of failure, an ABI can be placed. One could also argue that we should take out the smaller tumor on the worse-hearing ear, because the risk of injuring the cochlear and facial nerves during removal of smaller tumors is usually lower. In this case a CI may be more strongly indicated. Both arguments are legitimate and should be explored with the patient and family at length. Ultimately, in such situations, the patient may have to decide.

16.11 ABI in Neurofibromatosis Type 2

Auditory brainstem implants (ABIs) can provide patients deafened by NF2 with a chance to regain meaningful hearing. These devices are similar in design and function to cochlear implants (CIs). Current multichannel ABI technology affords a level of performance in aiding speech comprehension. After programming, ~85% of patients experience auditory perception with their ABI. Many patients can achieve limited open-set speech discrimination, and a small but significant number of patients are able to attain sound-only open-set speech comprehension such as telephone use.[1,2] The majority will develop the ability to recognize environmental sounds and obtain marked improvement in lip reading.

16.12 Indications and Contraindications for Auditory Brainstem Implants

Patients with NF2 who are 12 years old or older and who also have reasonable expectations and motivation and strong family support are indicated for ABIs. They may have or will have profound bilateral hearing loss after a natural history of tumors or unsuccessful preservation of the cochlear nerve during tumor removal.

The only absolute contraindication to the placement of an ABI is in a patient with an active purulent infection in the middle ear or a very short life expectancy. Relative contraindications may include patients who meet the formal criteria but who lack adequate support or motivation, as outlined above. Additionally, when the cochlear nerve can be preserved intact after resection of the vestibular schwannoma, placement of a CI is indicated.

16.13 Removable Magnet in ABI Implants

The Nucleus ABI24M auditory brainstem device (Cochlear, Sydney, Australia) has a flat silicone plate electrode carrier (3 × 8.5 mm) with 21 plate electrodes (each 0.7 mm) and a removable magnet in the receiver-stimulator. The two other ABI implants currently on the market are *without* a removable magnet: the Digisonic SP ABI (Neurelec MXM, France) has 15 electrodes (0.7 mm) on an electrode carrier (3 × 8mm); and the Concerto ABI (MED-EL, Innsbruck, Austria) has 12 electrodes (each 0.55 mm) and 1 reference contact (0.75 mm) on a flat electrode carrier (diameter 5.5 × 3.0 mm). For further details see Chapter 4.

In patients with NF2 the removability of the magnet can be important as continuous follow-up with MRI is necessary. All ABIs (all three devices mentioned) are MRI compatible (at 1.5 T) without removal of the magnet from the receiver–stimulator, but with special precautions (head bandage and information about the pulling sensation) and creation of an artifact on the MR scan (see Chapter 3). An MRI scan with a higher magnetic field or less artifact can only be achieved by removal of the magnet. In the United States the rules about scanning with the magnet in place are more strict and have led in NF2 patients to removal of the magnet and use of an adhesional disk on the scalp.[2] Inability to remove the magnet in an ABI makes it less favorable in NF2 patients.

16.14 First-side Versus Second-side Surgery

The aims of first-side surgery in our institution are absolutely complete tumor removal and preservation of the facial nerve, and possibly preservation of the cochlear nerve. We attempt to place the ABI after tumor removal on the first side if the cochlear nerve cannot be preserved, which is in concordance with most centers' practice.[2–5] Even if the device does not give the patient optimal benefit after this surgery, the opportunity remains to implant on the contralateral side when surgery is required. The patient thereby has a second chance to obtain a functioning implant. Conversely, if the first-side surgery is successfully accomplished and the device is functioning, the user can become accustomed to the device while they are still able to hear with the other ear. This situation may help the patient to acclimatize to ABI sounds.

16.15 Promontory Testing

Promontory testing is the direct stimulation of the cochlear promontory via an electrode placed surgically in the middle ear. A negative result of promontory testing—when pitch is not perceived—implies a retrocochlear cause of deafness. A positive result—when pitch is perceived in response to stimulation—indicates that the cochlear nerve is capable of transmitting tonal information centrally, thus making the patient an ideal candidate for cochlear implantation. Hence, in certain situations, when the anatomical integrity of the cochlear nerve has been preserved after tumor removal performed years before, promontory testing is used to assess whether the patient is a good candidate for a cochlear implant. Newer strategies/devices are being developed to provide more reliable measurements during surgery to test the functionality and feasibility of a cochlear implant after removal of the tumor.

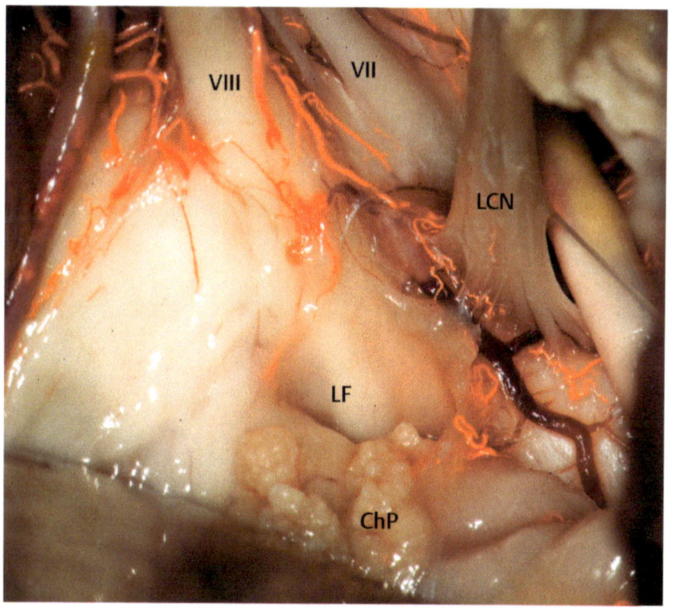

Fig. 16.9 Microscopic view of the foramen of Luschka on an injected specimen. ChP, choroid plexus; VII, facial nerve; VIII, vestibulocochlear nerve; LCN, lower cranial nerves; LF, foramen of Luschka.

16.16 Surgical Considerations (Fig. 16.9 and Fig. 16.10)

16.16.1 Intraoperative Monitoring

For a more complete overview of monitoring, see Chapter 4. The highlights will be discussed here.

Intraoperative monitoring of electrically evoked auditory potentials and monitoring of other cranial nerves that may be stimulated (mainly the facial and vagus nerves) is crucial during placement of ABIs on several grounds. Monitoring of ABR can corroborate accurate electrode placement, whereas monitoring of neighboring cranial nerves may detect inadvertent stimulation of regional structures.

In intraoperative electrical ABR, the first wave of the ABR observed will be wave III, which represents the cochlear nuclei. Ideally, three waves would be expected: those of the cochlear nuclei (III), the olivary nuclei (IV), and the nuclei of the lateral lemniscus (V). In practice, one to three responses, termed P1–P3, are usually seen. The presence of one or more responses helps corroborate proper electrode placement. No correlations have been found between the number or quality of waveform responses (i.e., P1, P2, and P3) and the efficacy of ABI, but the number of electrodes functioning is related to the accuracy of array location as well as to hearing outcome.

It should also be noted here that electrical ABR monitoring is understood more as an adjunct to anatomical means for localizing the cochlear nuclei. Its role is rather to confirm that the ABI stimulates the auditory brainstem with minimal or no stimulation of other structures. Insofar as the surgeon is confident of adequate electrode placement on the basis of reliable anatomical landmarks, even the complete absence of ABR waves does not necessarily predict that the ABI will fail to impart useful hearing.

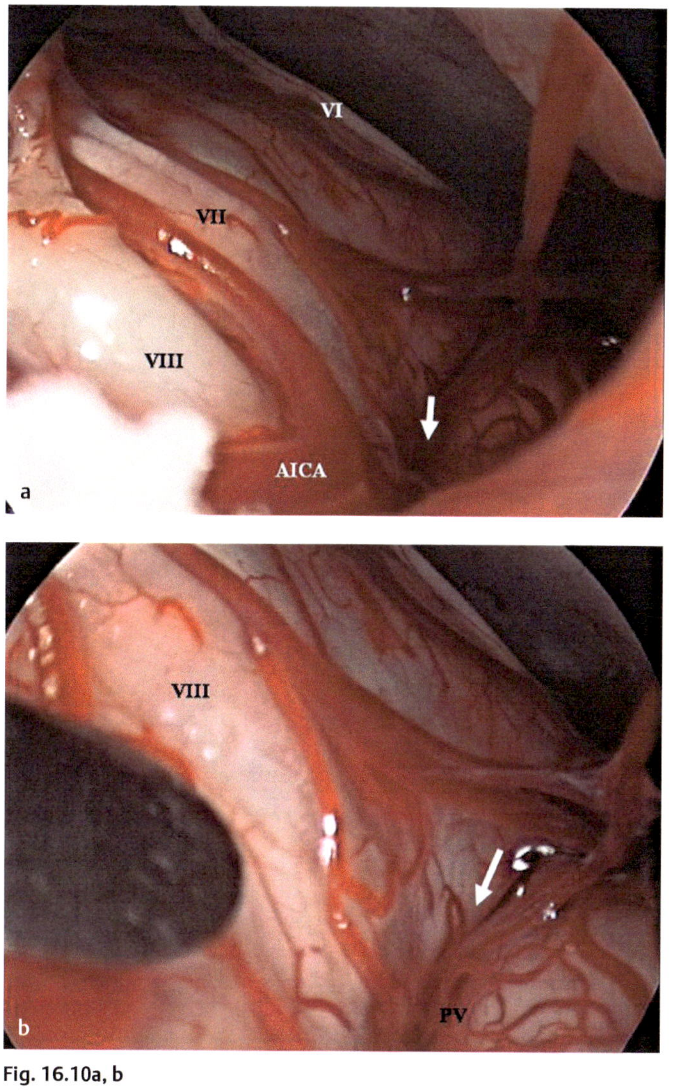

Fig. 16.10a, b

a Microscopic view of the foramen of Luschka (*arrow*).

b At higher magnification, the bulbopontine junction is clearly appreciated. AICA, anterior inferior cerebellar artery; PV, plexus of veins; VI, abducens nerve; VII, facial nerve; VIII, vestibulocochlear nerve.

Case 16.1 Cochlear Implantation in NF2 Patient with Small VS (Fig. 16.1.1 and Fig. 16.1.2)

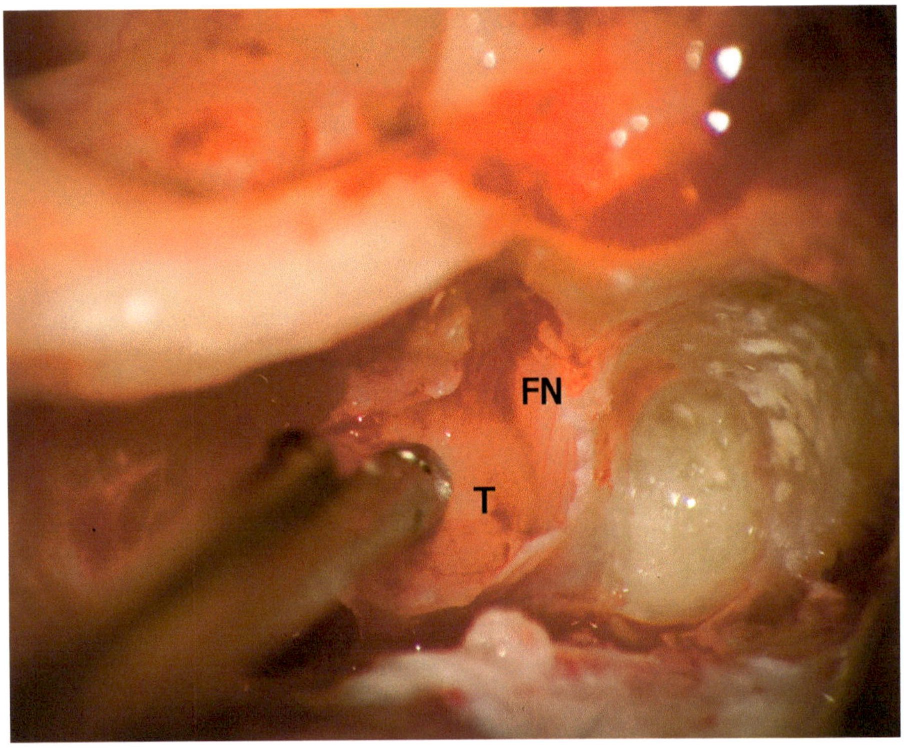

Fig. 16.1.1 In NF2 a small tumor gives the option of tumor removal and CI placement in the same surgery. In this case, with nonserviceable hearing at this ear, the vestibular schwannoma was removed via a translabyrinthine approach. Pictures are of a comparable case with unilateral vestibular schwannoma (no NF2) and cochlear implantation during the same surgery, but represent the same surgical steps (see Case 17.1, Chapter 17). FN, facial nerve; T, tumor.

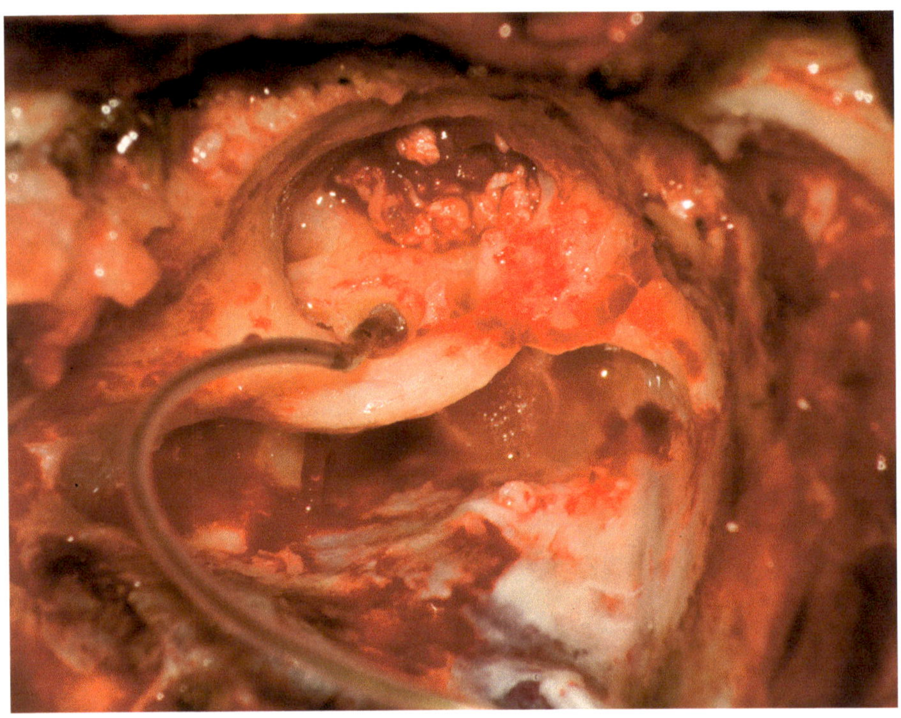

Fig. 16.1.2 If the cochlear nerve is preserved during tumor removal in a NF2 patient, cochlear implantation can be undertaken. This surgical approach provides a direct rehabilitation option in combination with tumor removal. One has to be aware that sometimes the function of the cochlear nerve can be distorted, even though the anatomical integrity is intact.

Comment

Cochlear implantation should not be ruled out as an option in NF2 patients.

Case 16.2 Right-sided (Second) Tumor Removal with ABI Placement in a Bilaterally Deaf NF2 Patient (Fig. 16.2.1–Fig. 16.2.23)

A patient with NF2 presented with bilateral hearing loss and bilateral large vestibular schwannomas among other intracranial tumors. The larger tumor (left side) had already been removed 4 years before through an enlarged translabyrinthine approach. The plan for the right side was to remove the tumor through an enlarged translabyrinthine approach, trying to preserve the cochlear nerve for a potential CI. If the preservation of the cochlear nerve appeared difficult, the plan was to shift to brainstem implantation.

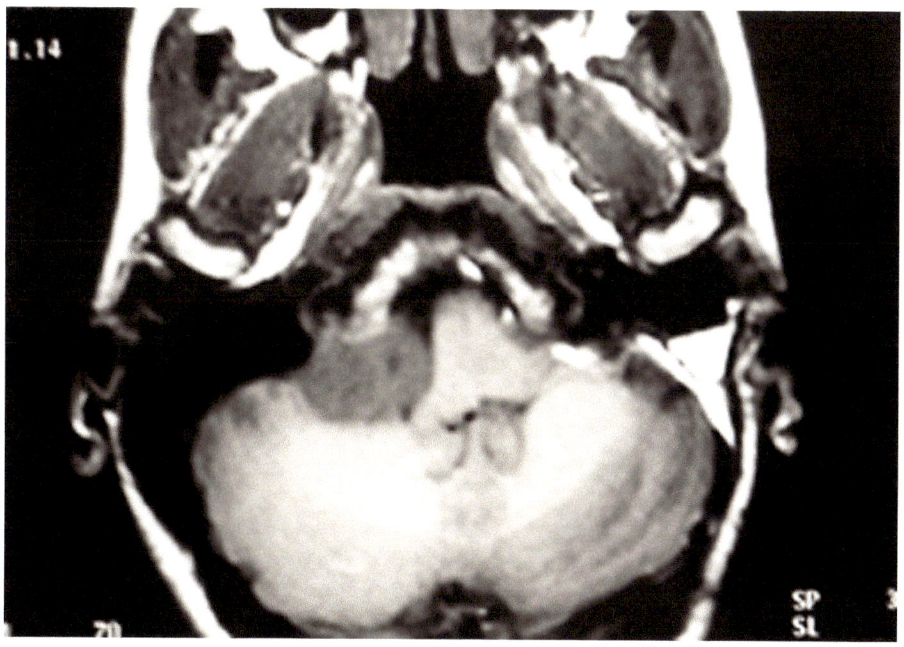

Fig. 16.2.1 MRI in 1999 shows a large right-sided vestibular schwannoma, with residual hearing remaining in an NF2 patient. The fat used to obliterate the mastoid cavity of the contralateral ear is also visible. A "wait and scan" policy was adopted for the right vestibular schwannoma.

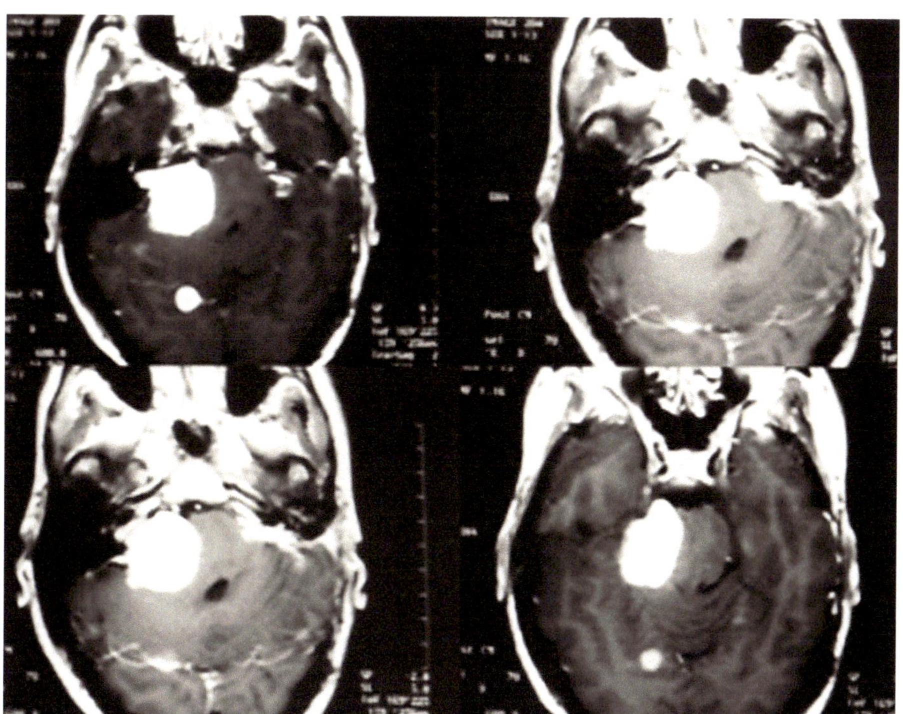

Fig. 16.2.2 After 4 years of follow-up the tumor grew and hearing was lost. Surgical removal was planned through a translabyrinthine approach with a concomitant ABI for the restoration of hearing.

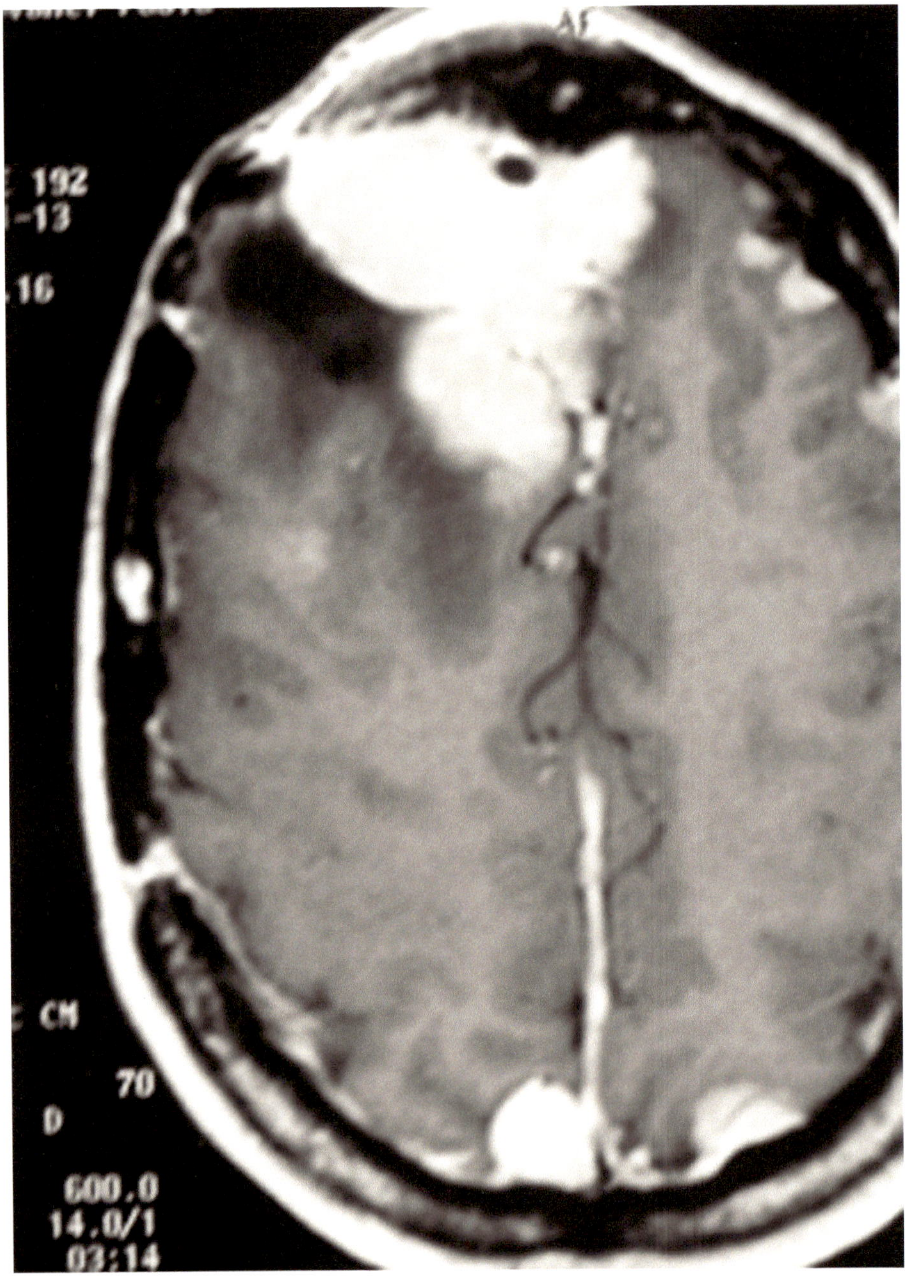

Fig. 16.2.3 This patient also has multiple falx and sagittal meningiomas.

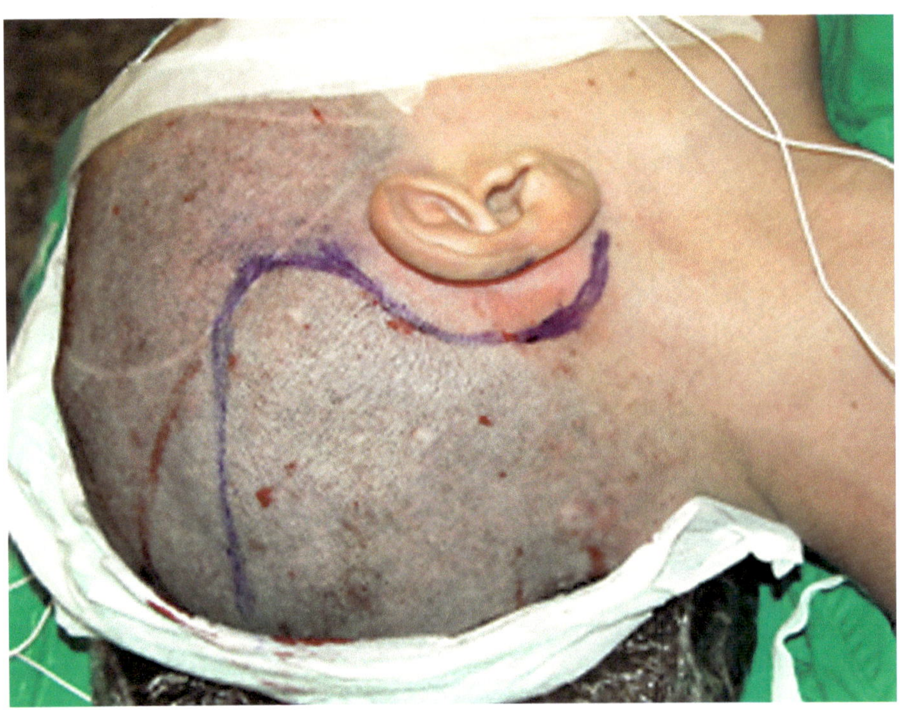

Fig. 16.2.4 The surgical incision utilized in this case is an inverted S-shape, larger than the conventional incision for a CI. This is also different from the regular incision for solitary vestibular schwannoma.

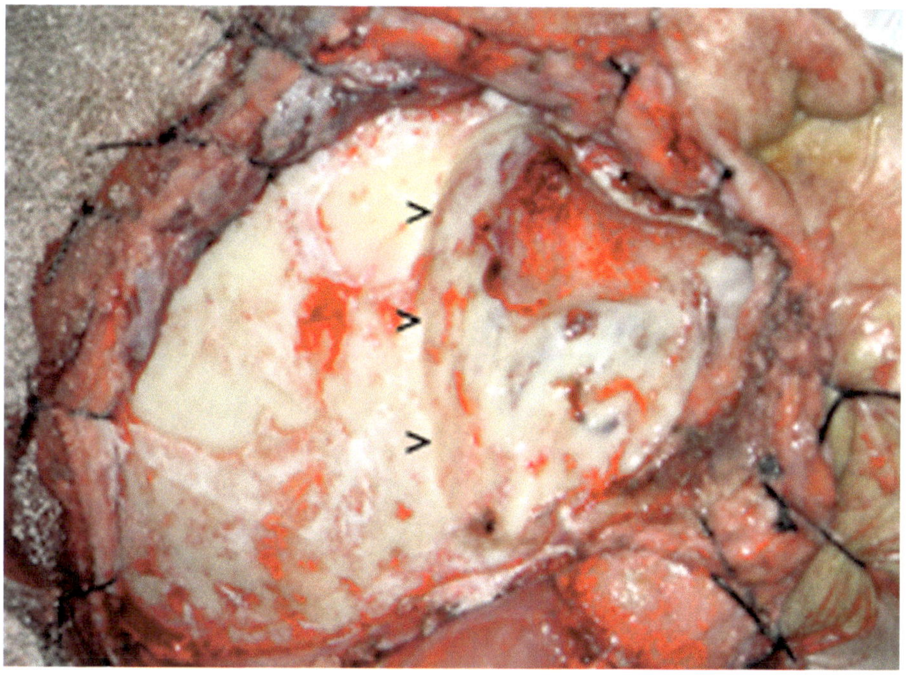

Fig. 16.2.5 An extended mastoidectomy has been performed. The only difference from the enlarged translabyrinthine approach is that bone removal over the middle cranial fossa is somewhat limited (*arrowheads*) to allow for the space necessary for the creation of the bed of the implant.

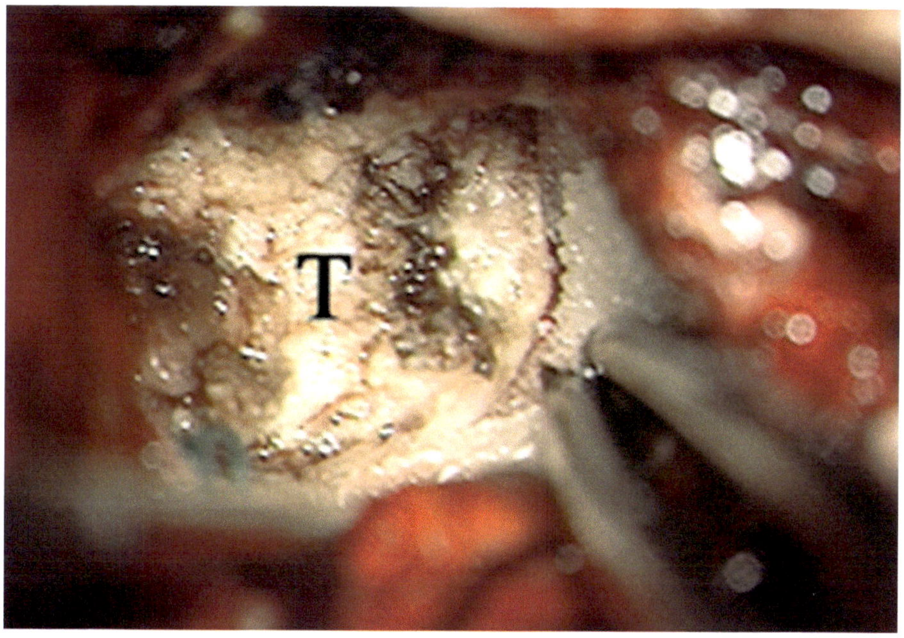

Fig. 16.2.6 Bloodless removal of the tumor (T) is started.

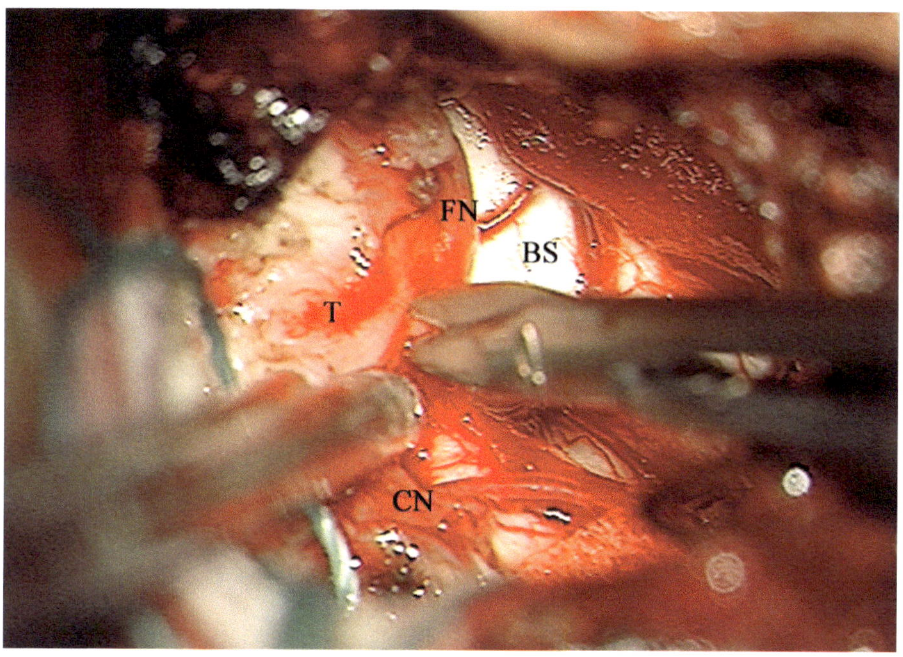

Fig. 16.2.7 The last part of the tumor (T) is here being dissected from the facial (FN) and cochlear nerves (CN). BS, brainstem.

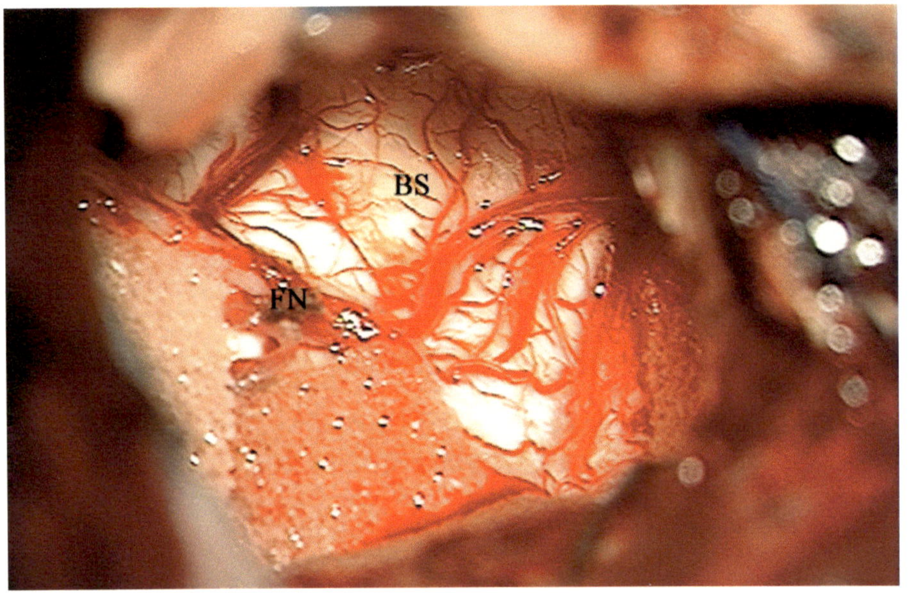

Fig. 16.2.8 Total tumor removal has been achieved, preserving the facial nerve (FN). Unfortunately, the cochlear nerve was interrupted in this case. BS, brainstem.

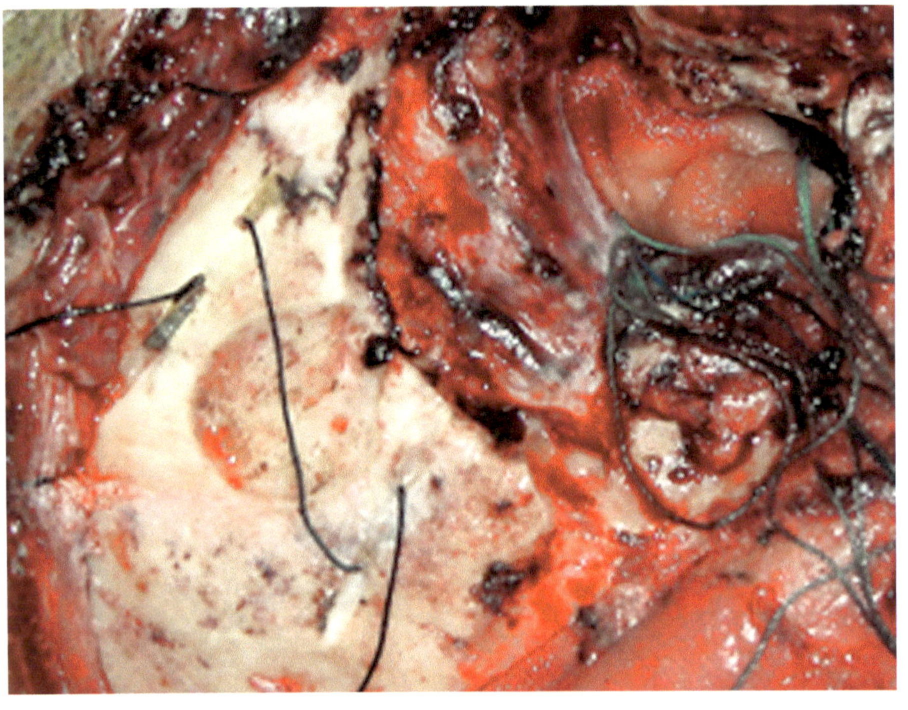

Fig. 16.2.9 After tumor removal, the bed for the implant is created in the posterior superior angle of the approach. While the drilling for this step is being done, the dural opening is obliterated temporarily to prevent bone dust from entering the intradural space.

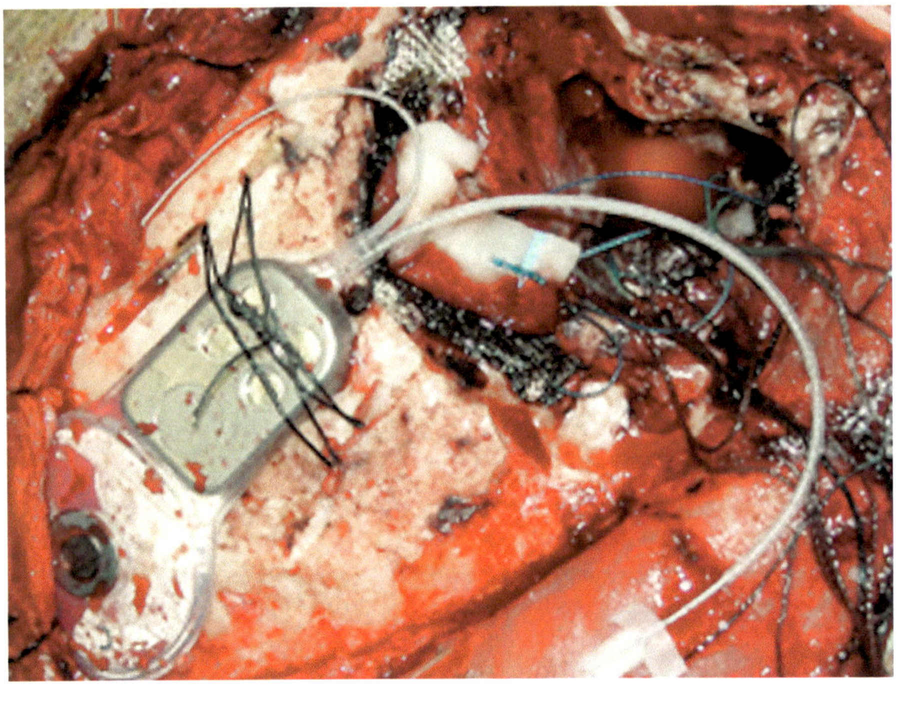

Fig. 16.2.10 The receiver-stimulator complex of the implant is fixated in its bed.

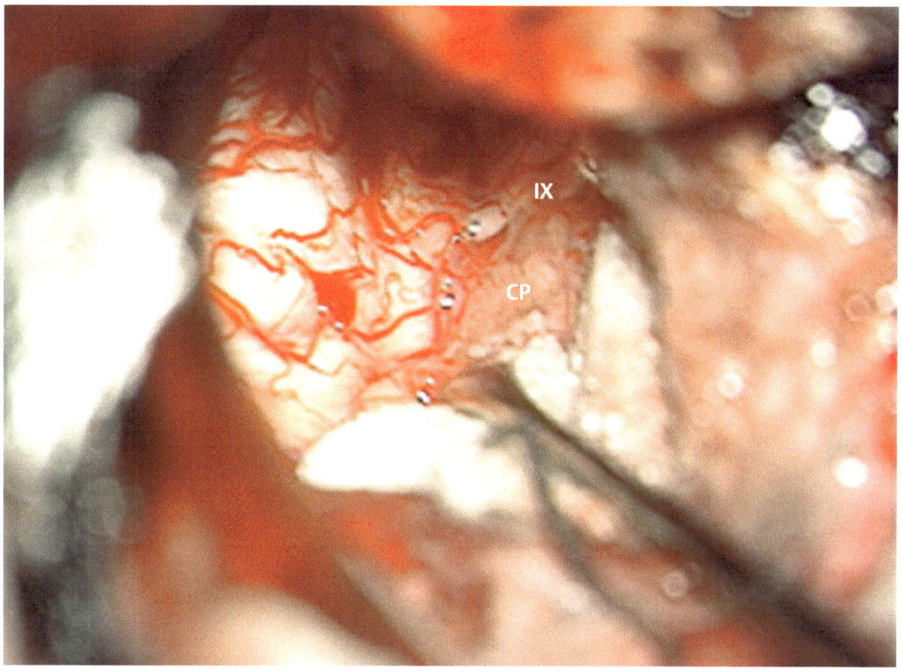

Fig. 16.2.11 Identification of the foramen of Luschka is started at the level of the root of the glossopharyngeal nerve (IX) by mild and gentle retraction of the flocculus together with the choroid plexus (CP).

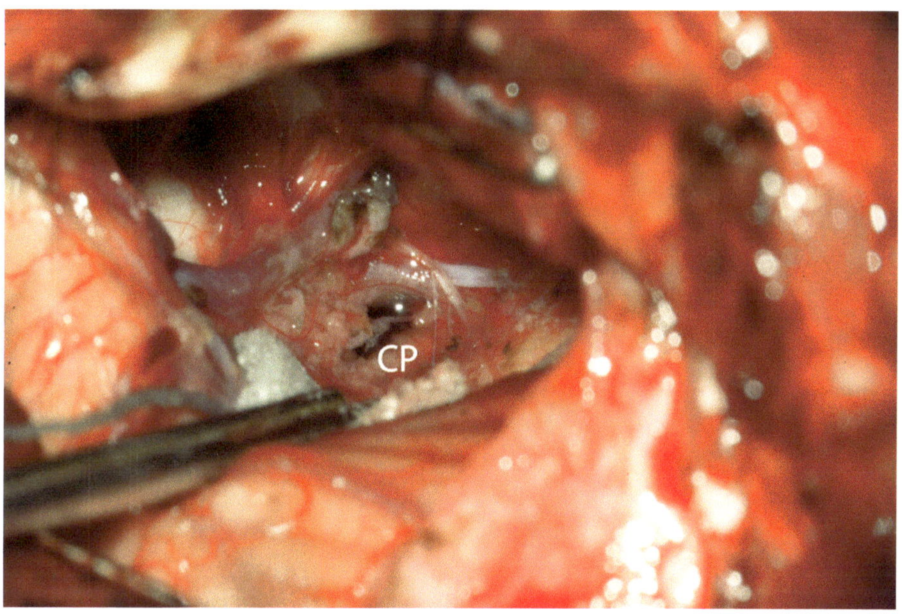

Fig. 16.2.12 Anatomical variations make identification of the foramen of Luschka more or less difficult; in this case the opening of the foramen was larger than usual and much easier to find. CP, choroid plexus.

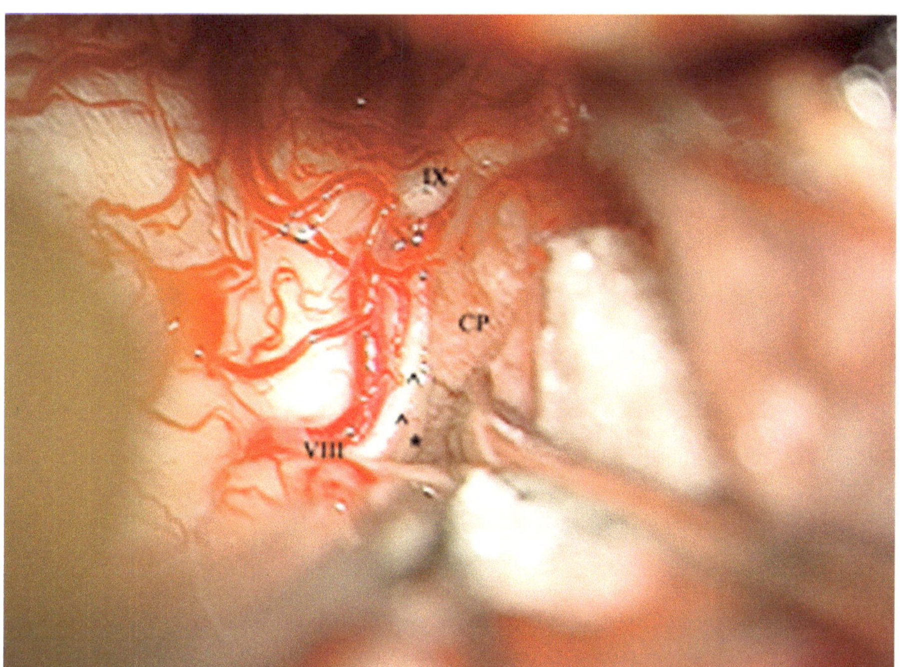

Fig. 16.2.13 Retracting the choroid plexus (CP) posterolaterally reveals the foramen of Luschka. Note that the tenia (*arrowheads*) forms the boundary of the lateral recess and the division line between the cochlear nerve (VIII) and the ventral cochlear nucleus. Note also the smooth glistening surface of the ventral cochlear nucleus (✱). IX, glossopharyngeal nerve.

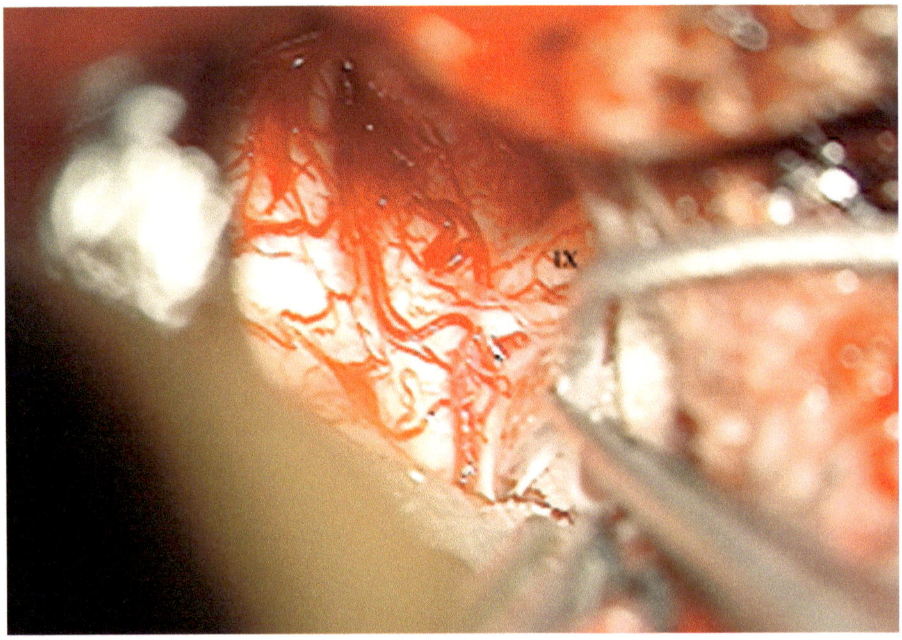

Fig. 16.2.14 The array of the brainstem implant is held gently using nontoothed forceps. IX, glossopharyngeal nerve.

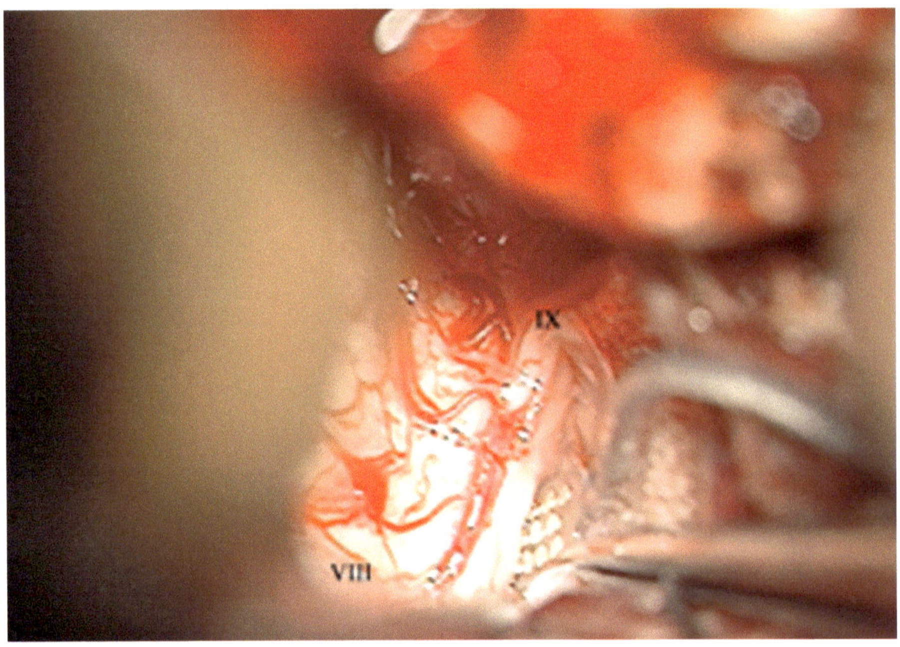

Fig. 16.2.15 The array is partially inserted. Note that the surface of the electrodes should be directed anterior-superiorly to lie in contact with the uncovered posterior surface of the ventral cochlear nucleus. VIII, vestibulocochlear nerve; IX, glossopharyngeal nerve.

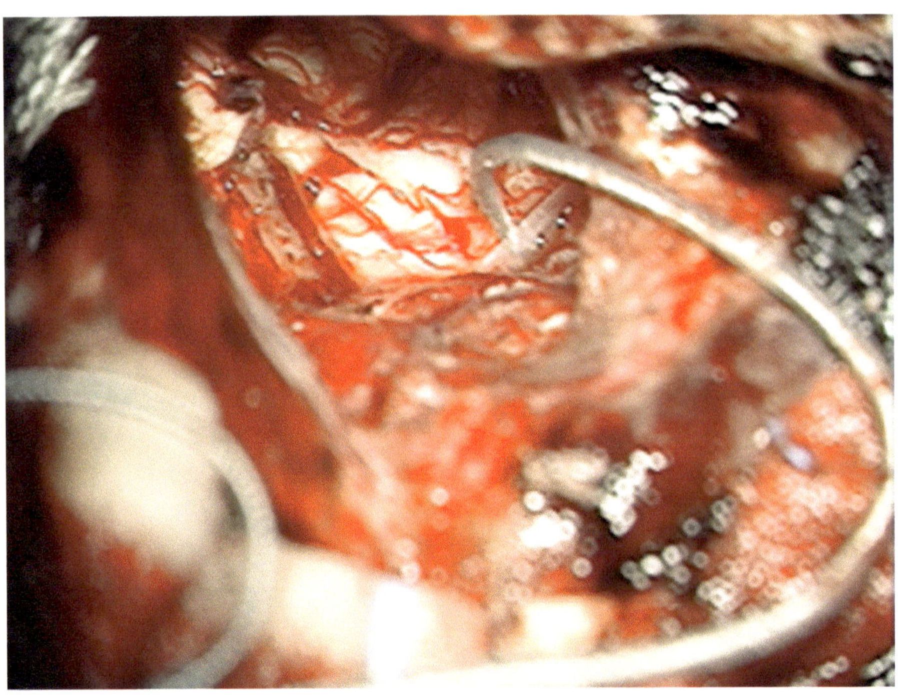

Fig. 16.2.16 The electrode array is fully inserted.

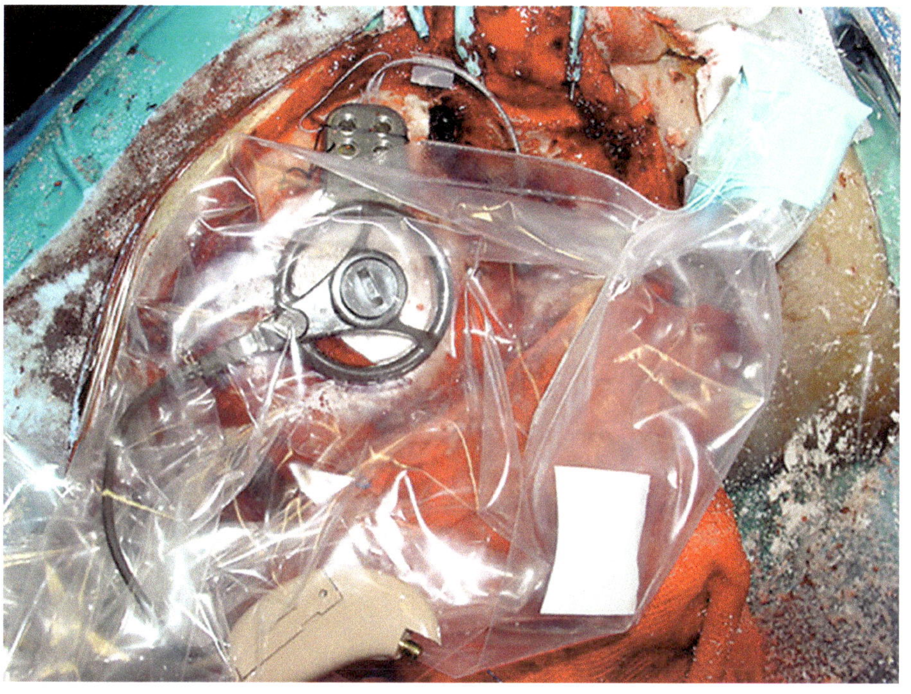

Fig. 16.2.17 Electrical auditory brainstem response monitoring is performed to check the positioning of the array.

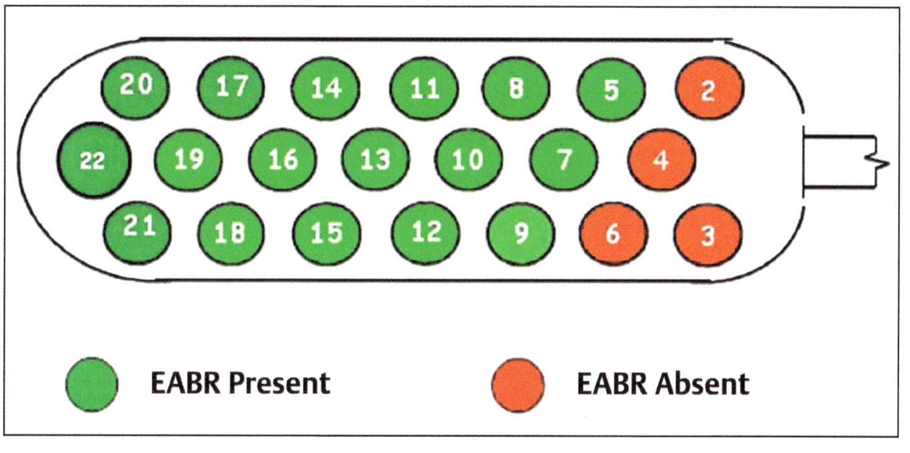

Fig. 16.2.18 N24 electrode intraoperative mapping indicating that most channels are functioning apart from 2, 3, 4, and 6. In this case, the array may be inserted more medially.

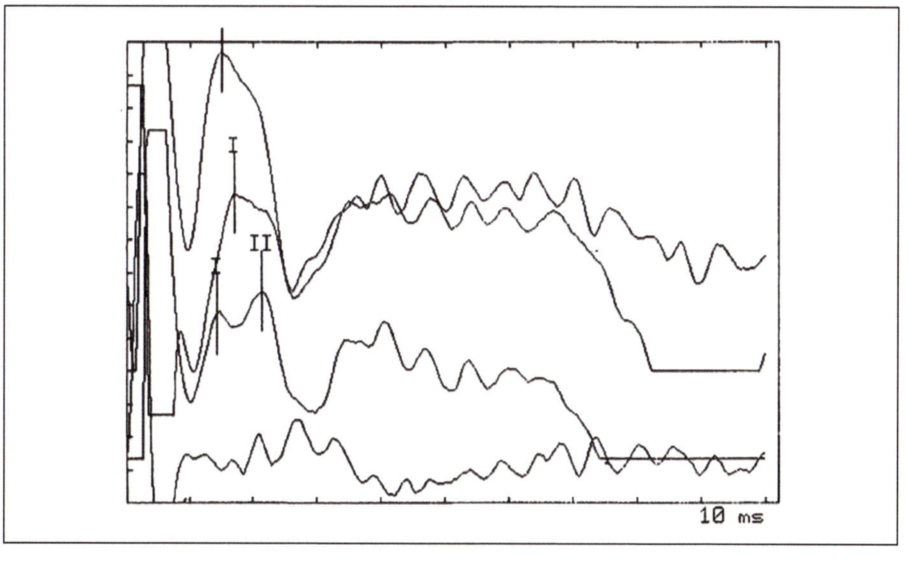

Fig. 16.2.19 Sample intraoperative recording of electrical auditory brainstem response. This shows PI and PII waves indicating hearing stimulation.

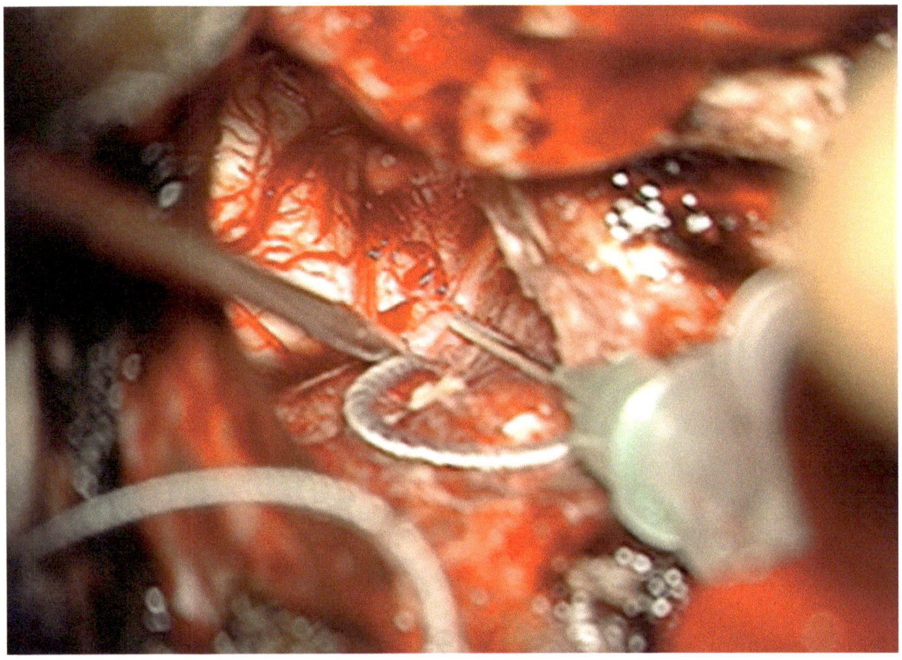

Fig. 16.2.20 After checking the correct positioning of the electrode array, fibrin glue and a piece of fascia are used to further secure the array in position.

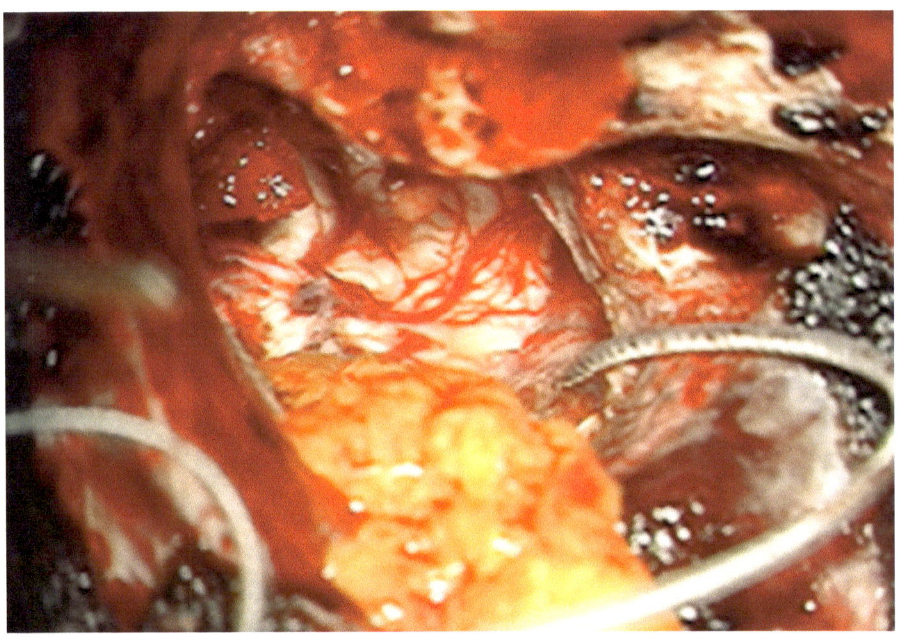

Fig. 16.2.21 Obliteration of the cavity is started using long strips of abdominal fat.

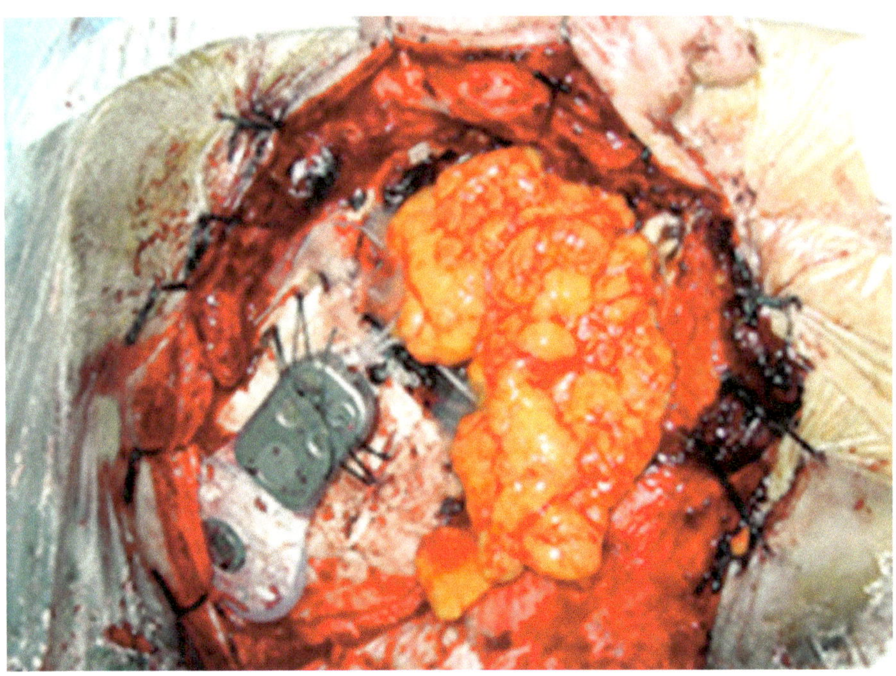

Fig. 16.2.22 The implant in place with surrounding fat. The surgical defect is now closed in layers.

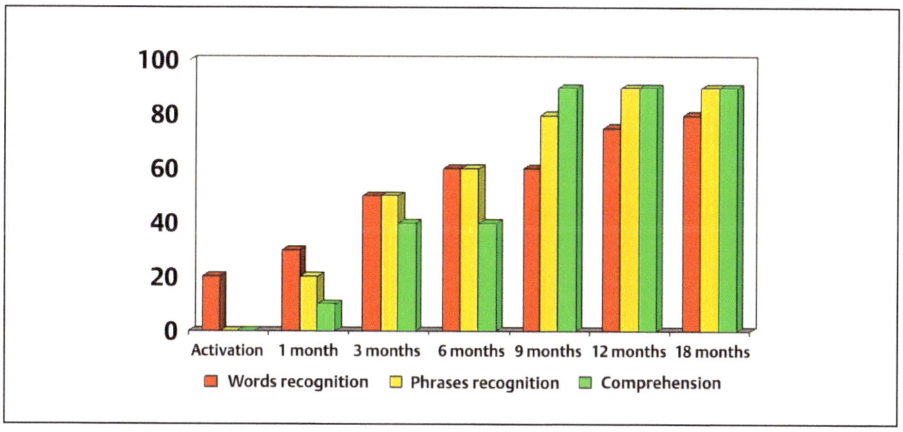

Fig. 16.2.23 Hearing outcome of this patient, demonstrating progressive comprehension.

Comment

In some NF2 cases, ABI placement can restore hearing to a reasonable level.

Case 16.3 Left ABI in NF2 Case with Deaf Left Ear and Normal Hearing on the Right (Fig. 16.3.1–Fig. 16.3.5)

An NF2 patient with bilateral vestibular schwannomas presented with left hearing loss (normal hearing in the right ear). The translabyrinthine tumor removal was performed in the left side with a concomitant ABI.

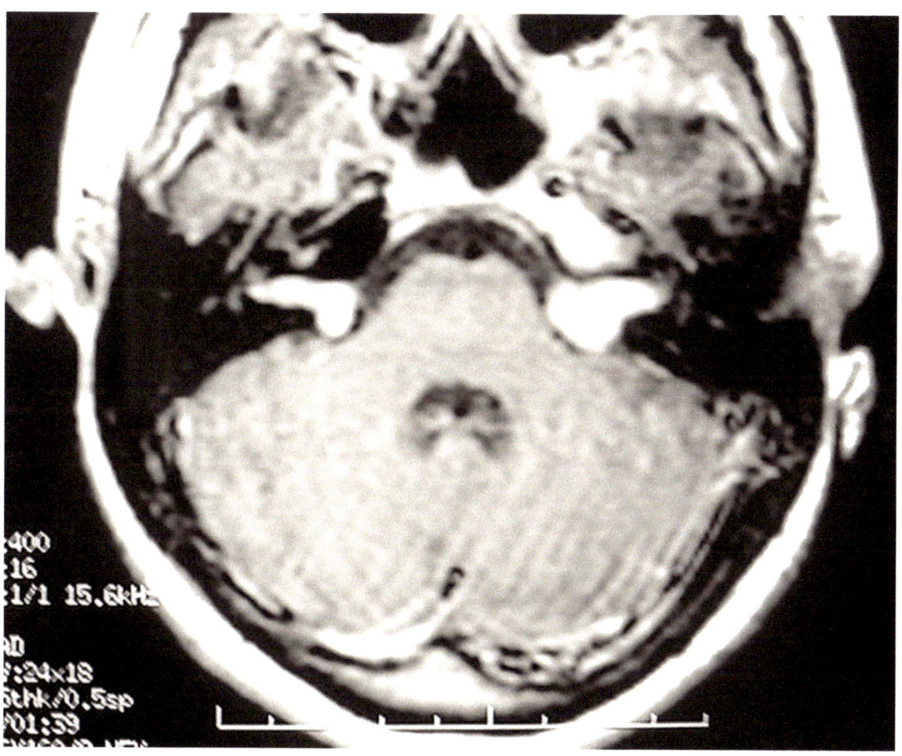

Fig. 16.3.1 MRI of bilateral vestibular schwannomas. The left-sided tumor was larger than the right-sided one.

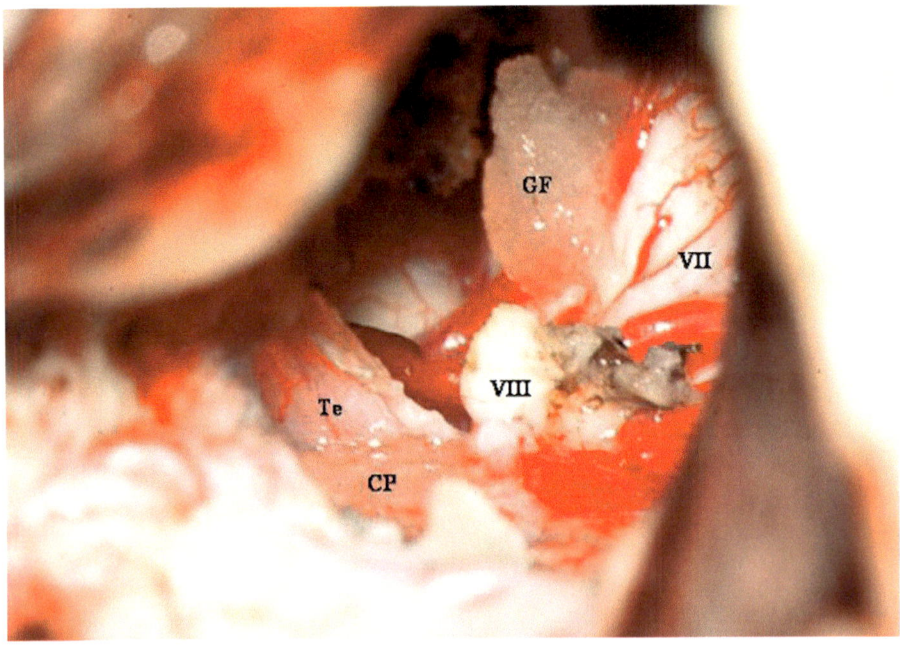

Fig. 16.3.2 The cochlear nerve was transected during tumor removal. CP, choroid plexus; GF, Gelfoam; Te, tenia; VII, facial nerve; VIII, vestibulocochlear nerve.

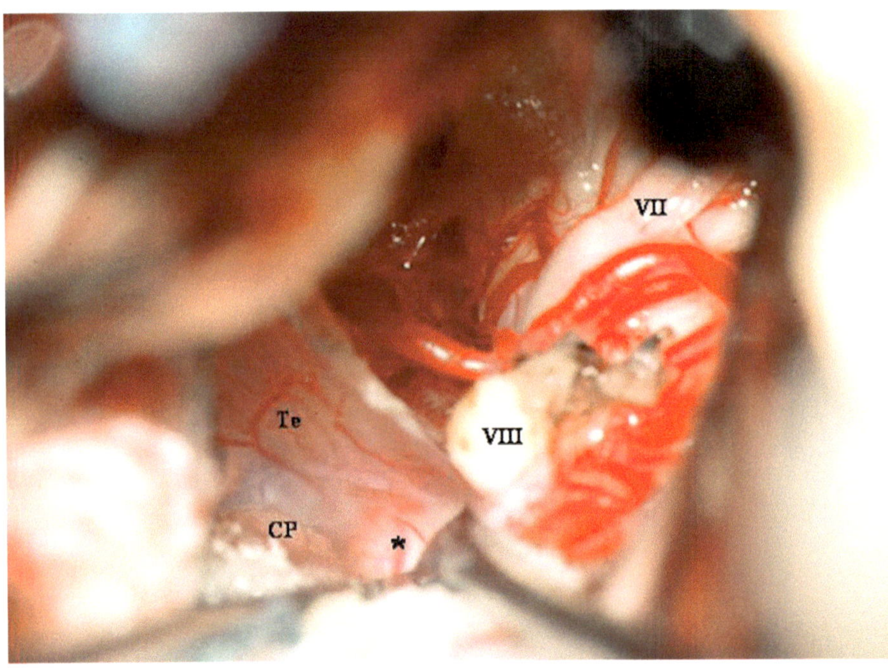

Fig. 16.3.3 The foramen of Luschka is identified beyond the choroid plexus near the cochlear nerve stump after gentle retraction. CSF is observed exiting upon a Valsalva maneuver. ∗, cochlear nucleus complex; CP, choroid plexus; Te, tenia; VII, facial nerve; VIII, vestibulocochlear nerve.

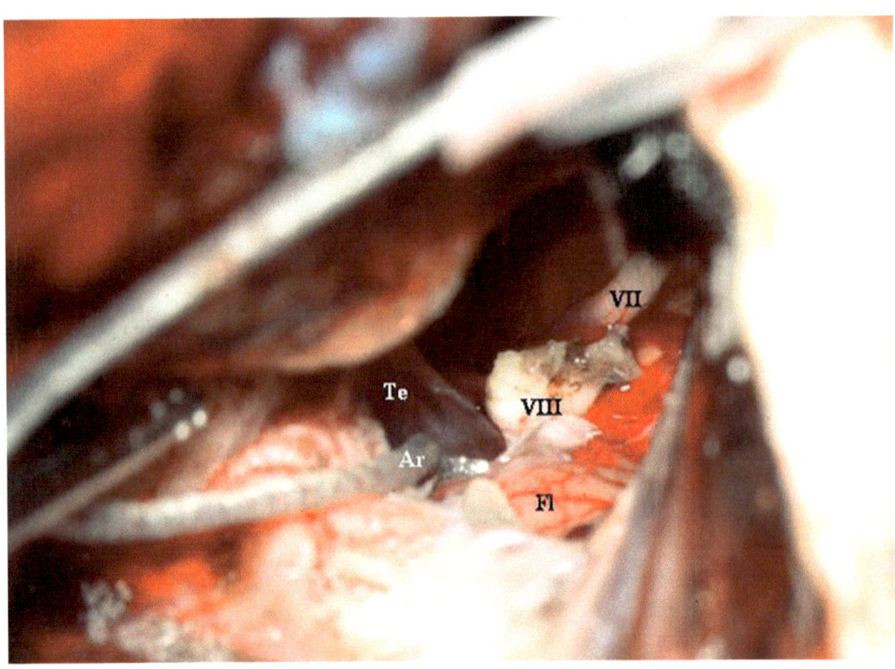

Fig. 16.3.4 The electrode array is inserted into the lateral recess. Ar, electrode array; Fl, flocculus; Te, tenia; VII, facial nerve; VIII, vestibulocochlear nerve.

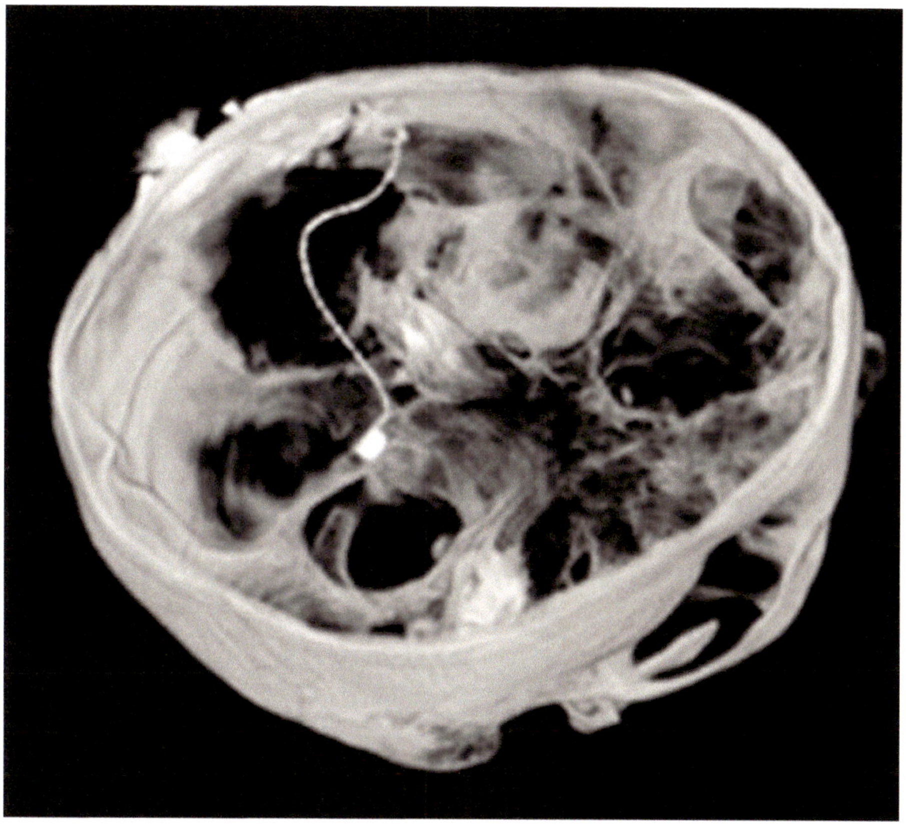

Fig. 16.3.5 3D reconstruction of postoperative CT images is helpful in verifying the correct location of electrode and lead.

Comment

In NF2 the hearing always deteriorates bilaterally. Implantation on the first side, even with normal hearing contralaterally, is therefore the consensus.

Case 16.4 Right-sided (First) Tumor Removal and ABI Placement in an NF2 Patient (Fig. 16.4.1–Fig. 16.4.3)

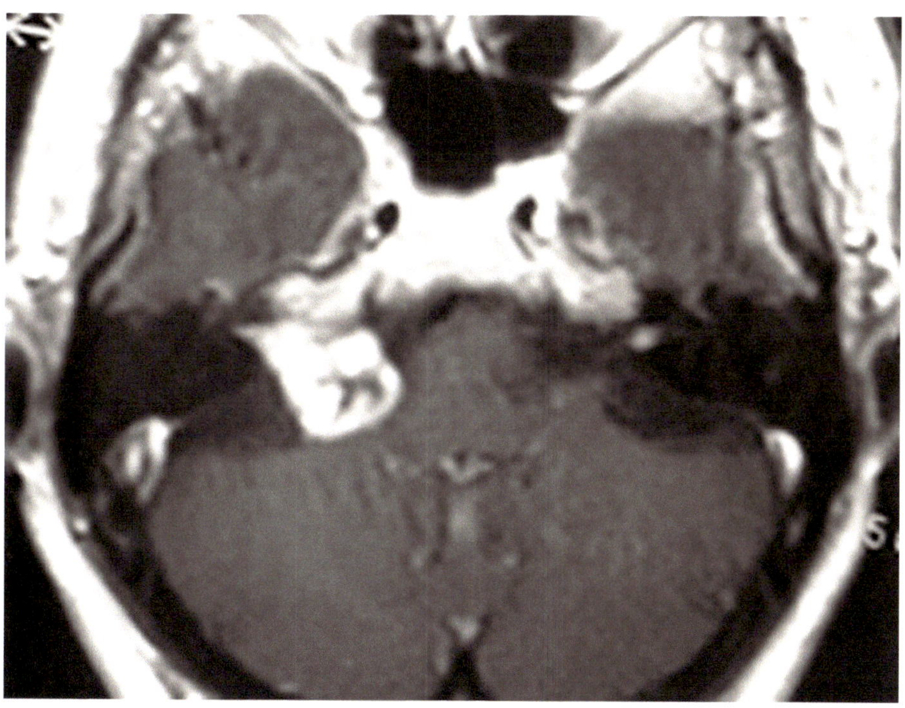

Fig. 16.4.1 An NF2 patient with bilateral schwannomas had symmetrical bilateral hearing loss. MRI showing a marked difference in size between the two sides. Right-sided tumor removal via translabyrinthine approach and concomitant auditory brainstem implant were planned.

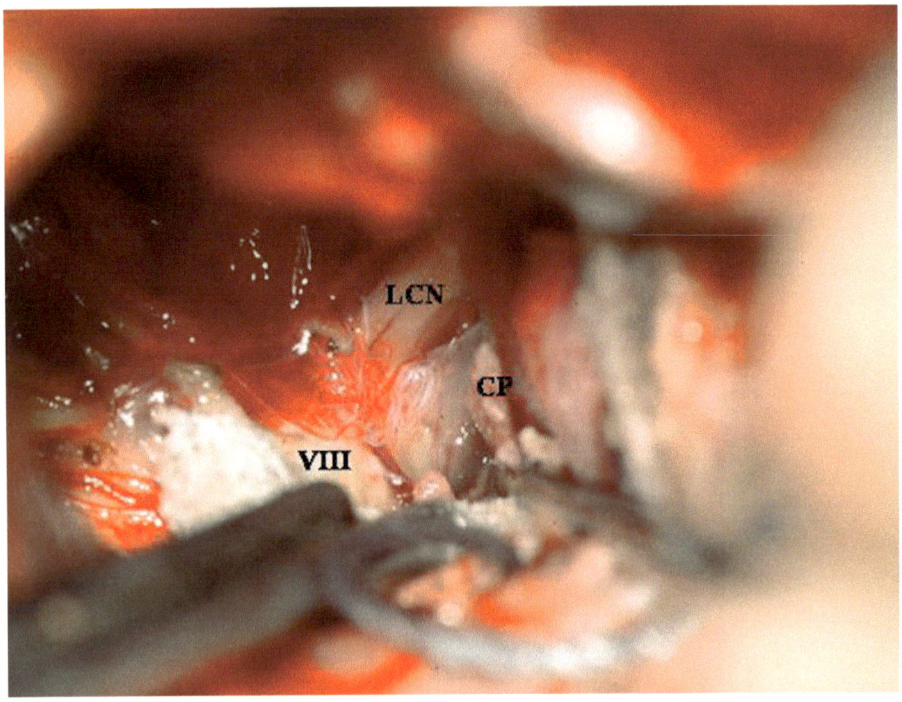

Fig. 16.4.2 The cochlear nerve could not be preserved in this case, so that concomitantly an auditory brainstem implant was placed. CP, choroid plexus; LCN, lower cranial nerves; VIII, stump of the cochlear nerve.

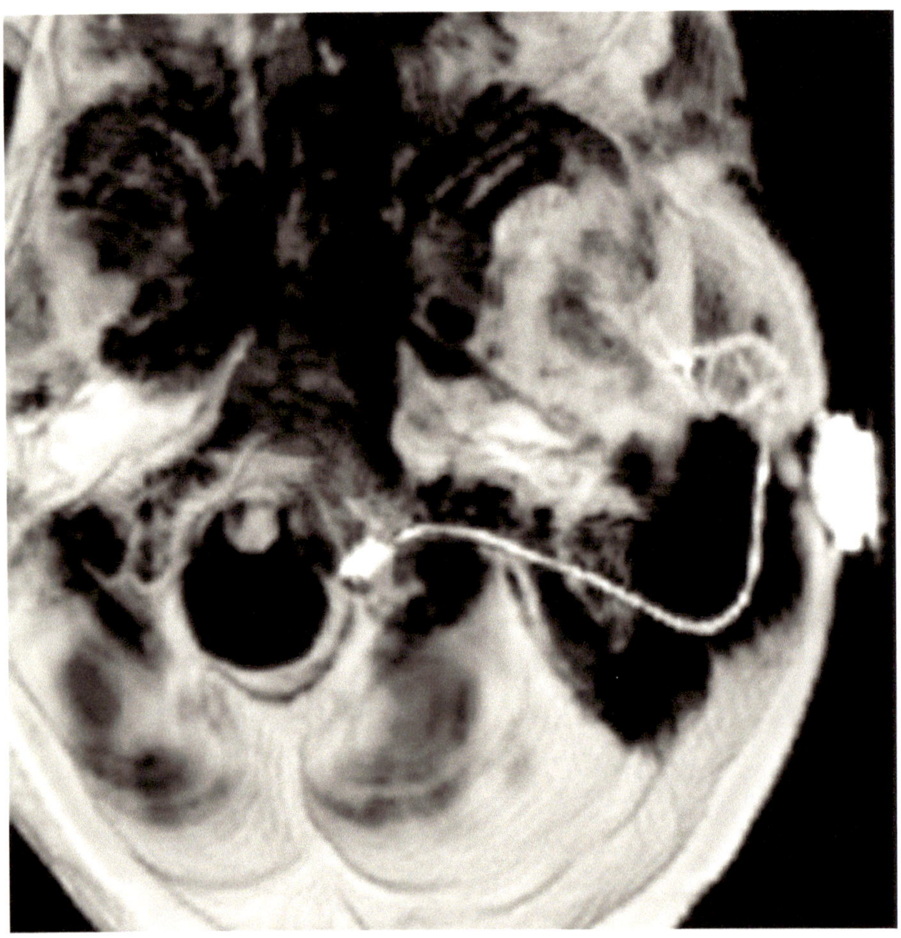

Fig. 16.4.3 Postoperative 3D CT image shows the correct placement of the auditory brainstem implant.

Comment

Cochlear nerve preservation should be attempted, but if it is not achieved an ABI insertion can be performed sequentially.

Case 16.5 CI Placement and Meningioma Removal via Translabyrinthine Approach in an NF2 Patient (Fig. 16.5.1 and Fig. 16.5.2)

An NF2 patient with a right-sided meningioma and a left-sided vestibular schwannoma. This patient had total deafness in the right ear and gradually progressive hearing loss in the left ear. The meningioma was removed through a translabyrinthine approach in combination with a subtotal petrosectomy and cochlear implant (CI) insertion.

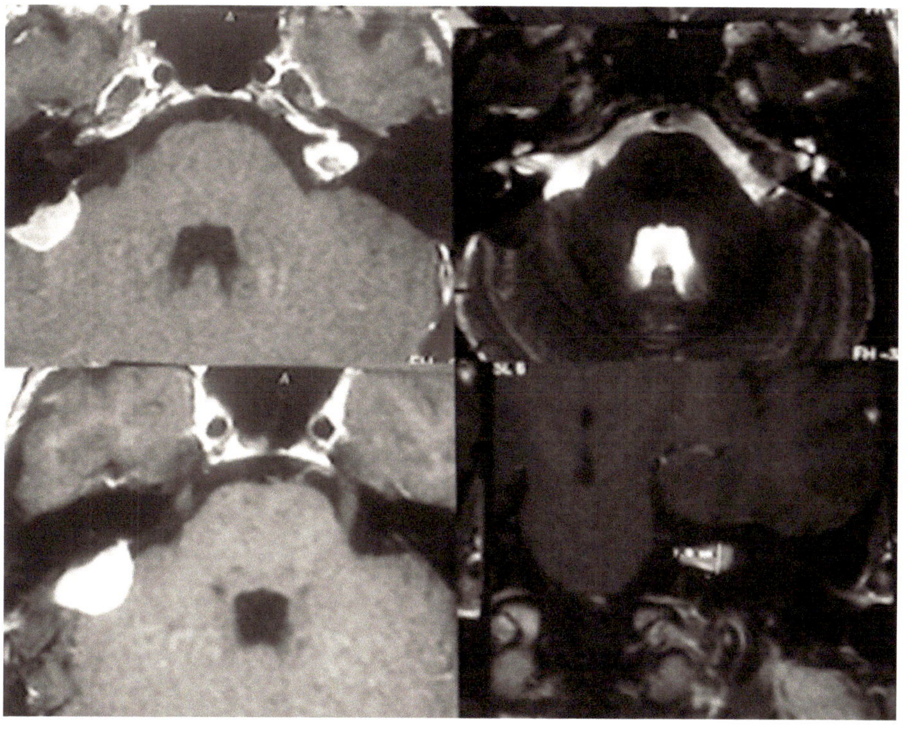

Fig. 16.5.1 MR images showing a right-sided posterior fossa meningioma and a left-sided small vestibular schwannoma.

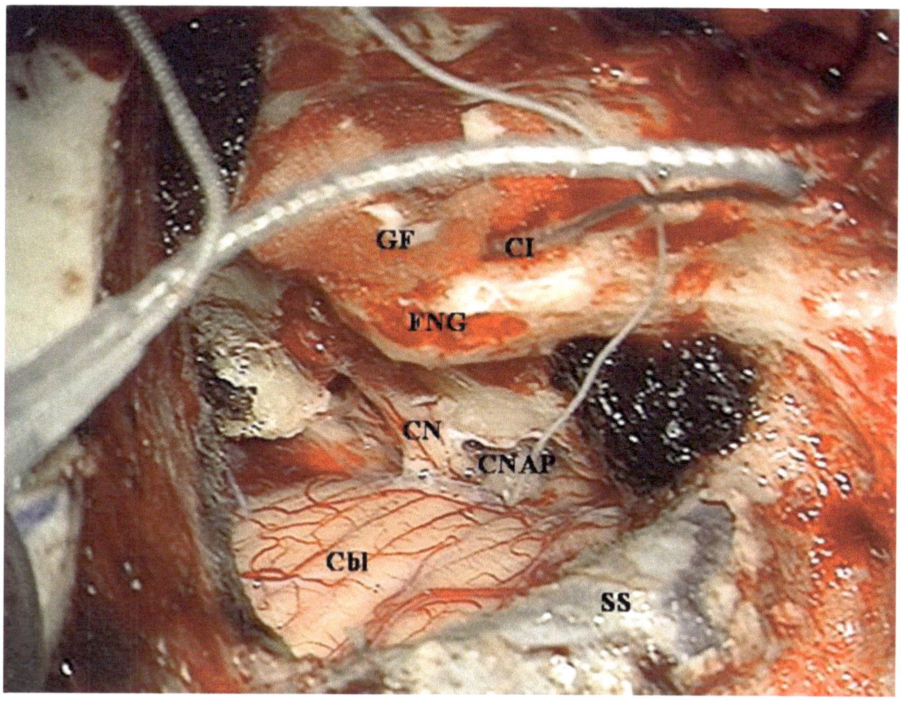

Fig. 16.5.2 In this case, the translabyrinthine approach was used for removal of a posterior fossa meningioma. The cochlear nerve was successfully preserved and so a cochlear implant was placed. Cbl, cerebellum; CI, cochlear implant; CN, cochlear nerve; CNAP, cochlear nerve action potential lead; FNG, facial nerve genu; GF, Gelfoam; SS, sigmoid sinus.

Comment

Meningiomas can cause sensorineural hearing loss (SNHL) in NF2 patients and can be treated in the same fashion when they appear at the same location as a vestibular schwannoma.

16.17 Summary of NF2 and Implantation

- Auditory brainstem implants (ABIs) can restore meaningful hearing in patients deafened by NF2. In a minority of NF2 patients it is possible to restore the hearing with a cochlear implant (CI).
- Multichannel ABIs can be implanted at the time of first- or second-side surgery for tumors involving the auditory nerve. We favor a translabyrinthine approach for ABI and in the first surgery.
- Appropriate expectations and motivation on the part of the patient are essential. Many ABI patients are initially discouraged by the quality of the sound heard with an ABI. They must understand that active participation in their auditory rehabilitation program is crucial to continue to improve their proficiency with the device.
- Almost all patients can expect to obtain some auditory perception and awareness of environmental sounds (level I: signal function). Only a minority of patients are able to achieve sufficient open-set speech comprehension to use the telephone (level III: open-set speech perception). Most experience a significant improvement in open-set speech comprehension when the implant is used as an adjunct to lip reading (level II).
- Speech comprehension continues to improve for as long as 8 years after implantation. More than 90% of recipients use their ABI daily. The majority of patients are satisfied with their decision to receive an ABI and would recommend the device to others.

Pearls and Pitfalls

- Cochlear implants can be used when the cochlear nerve is preserved.
- The enlarged translabyrinthine approach is best suited for total removal of a tumor of any size and the concomitant placement of ABI. This approach enables access to the lateral recess more easily.
- Drilling of the bone over the middle cranial fossa dura should be limited to what is needed to create a receiver well.
- The electrode carrier of the ABI must be positioned correctly in the lateral recess, facing the dorsal cochlear nucleus as well as the intraventricular part of the ventral cochlear nucleus. Intraoperative electrical ABR measurements are necessary and a larger number of functioning electrodes may indicate the positioning to be better, with probably better hearing results. The position of the electrode carrier needs to be adjusted (during surgery) if not enough electrodes are functioning.
- Monitoring of other cranial nerves is important to check on the correct position of the ABI because they could also be stimulated by the electrodes. This would demonstrate the position of the ABI to be incorrect.

Reference Video

See Video 16.1.

References

1. Sanna M, Di Lella F, Guida M, Merkus P. Auditory brainstem implants in NF2 patients: results and review of the literature. Otol Neurotol 2012;33(2):154–164
2. Schwartz MS, Otto SR, Brackmann DE, Hitselberger WE, Shannon RV. Use of a multichannel auditory brainstem implant for neurofibromatosis type 2. Stereotact Funct Neurosurg 2003;81(1-4):110–114
3. Nevison B, Laszig R, Sollmann WP, et al. Results from a European clinical investigation of the Nucleus multichannel auditory brainstem implant. Ear Hear 2002;23(3):170–183
4. Behr R, Müller J, Shehata-Dieler W, et al. The high rate CIS auditory brainstem implant for restoration of hearing in NF-2 patients. Skull Base 2007;17(2):91–107
5. Grayeli AB, Kalamarides M, Bouccara D, Ambert-Dahan E, Sterkers O. Auditory brainstem implant in neurofibromatosis type 2 and non-neurofibromatosis type 2 patients. Otol Neurotol 2008;29(8):1140–1146

Further Reading

Ahsan S, Telischi F, Hodges A, Balkany T. Cochlear implantation concurrent with translabyrinthine acoustic neuroma resection. Laryngoscope 2003;113(3):472–474

Angeli RD, Piccirillo E, Di Trapani G, Sequino G, Taibah A, Sanna M. Enlarged translabyrinthine approach with transapical extension in the management of giant vestibular schwannomas: personal experience and review of literature. Otol Neurotol 2011;32(1):125–131

Arístegui M, Denia A. Simultaneous cochlear implantation and translabyrinthine removal of vestibular schwannoma in an only hearing ear: report of two cases (neurofibromatosis type 2 and unilateral vestibular schwannoma). Otol Neurotol 2005;26(2):205–210

Arriaga MA, Marks S. Simultaneous cochlear implantation and acoustic neuroma resection: imaging considerations, technique, and functional outcome. Otolaryngol Head Neck Surg 1995;112(2):325–328

Di Lella F, Merkus P, Di Trapani G, Taibah A, Guida M, Sanna M. Vestibular schwannoma in the only hearing ear: role of cochlear implants. Ann Otol Rhinol Laryngol 2013;122(2):91–99

Ebinger K, Otto S, Arcaroli J, Staller S, Arndt P. Multichannel auditory brainstem implant: US clinical trial results. J Laryngol Otol Suppl 2000;(27):50–53

Edgerton BJ, House WF, Hitselberger W. Hearing by cochlear nucleus stimulation in humans. Ann Otol Rhinol Laryngol Suppl 1982;91(2 Pt 3):117–124

Graham J, Lynch C, Weber B, Stollwerck L, Wei J, Brookes G. The magnetless Clarion cochlear implant in a patient with neurofibromatosis 2. J Laryngol Otol 1999;113(5):458–463

Grayeli AB, Bouccara D, Kalamarides M, et al. Auditory brainstem implant in bilateral and completely ossified cochleae. Otol Neurotol 2003;24(1):79–82

Grayeli AB, Kalamarides M, Bouccara D, Ben Gamra L, Ambert-Dahan E, Sterkers O. Auditory brainstem implantation to rehabilitate profound hearing loss with totally ossified cochleae induced by pneumococcal meningitis. Audiol Neurootol 2007;12(1):27–30

Hitselberger WE, House WF, Edgerton BJ, Whitaker S. Cochlear nucleus implants. Otolaryngol Head Neck Surg 1984;92(1):52–54

Hoffman RA, Kohan D, Cohen NL. Cochlear implants in the management of bilateral acoustic neuromas. Am J Otol 1992;13(6):525–528

Hulka GF, Bernard EJ, Pillsbury HC. Cochlear implantation in a patient after removal of an acoustic neuroma. The implications of magnetic resonance imaging with gadolinium on patient management. Arch Otolaryngol Head Neck Surg 1995;121(4):465–468

Kanowitz SJ, Shapiro WH, Golfinos JG, Cohen NL, Roland JT Jr. Auditory brainstem implantation in patients with neurofibromatosis type 2. Laryngoscope 2004;114(12):2135–2146

Laszig R, Kuzma J, Seifert V, Lehnhardt E. The Hannover auditory brainstem implant: a multiple-electrode prosthesis. Eur Arch Otorhinolaryngol 1991;248(7):420–421

Laszig R, Marangos N, Sollmann P, et al. Initial results from the clinical trial of the nucleus 21-channel auditory brain stem implant. Am J Otol 1997;18(6, Suppl)S160

Laszig R, Sollmann WP, Marangos N. The restoration of hearing in neurofibromatosis type 2. J Laryngol Otol 1995;109(5):385–389

Lenarz M, Matthies C, Lesinski-Schiedat A, et al. Auditory brainstem implant part II: subjective assessment of functional outcome. Otol Neurotol 2002;23(5):694–697

Lenarz T, Lim HH, Reuter G, Patrick JF, Lenarz M. The auditory midbrain implant: a new auditory prosthesis for neural deafness-concept and device description. Otol Neurotol 2006;27(6):838–843

Lenarz T, Moshrefi M, Matthies C, et al. Auditory brainstem implant: part I. Auditory performance and its evolution over time. Otol Neurotol 2001;22(6):823–833

Lesinski-Schiedat A, Frohne C, Illg A, et al. Auditory brainstem implant in auditory rehabilitation of patients with neurofibromatosis type 2: Hannover programme. J Laryngol Otol Suppl 2000;(27):15–17

Lustig LR, Yeagle J, Driscoll CL, Blevins N, Francis H, Niparko JK. Cochlear implantation in patients with neurofibromatosis type 2 and bilateral vestibular schwannoma. Otol Neurotol 2006;27(4):512–518

Maini S, Cohen MA, Hollow R, Briggs R. Update on long-term results with auditory brainstem implants in NF2 patients. Cochlear Implants Int 2009;10(Suppl 1):33–37

Marangos N, Stecker M, Laszig R. Topodiagnosis of deafness: strategy for treatment of neurofibromatosis type 2. J Laryngol Otol Suppl 2000;(27):3–7

Marangos N, Stecker M, Sollmann WP, Laszig R. Stimulation of the cochlear nucleus with multichannel auditory brainstem implants and long-term results: Freiburg patients. J Laryngol Otol Suppl 2000;(27):27–31

Merkus P, Di Lella F, Di Trapani G, et al. Indications and contraindications of auditory brainstem implants: systematic review and illustrative cases. Eur Arch Otorhinolaryngol 2014;271(1):3–13

Merkus P, Taibah A, Sequino G, Sanna M. Less than 1% cerebrospinal fluid leakage in 1,803 translabyrinthine vestibular schwannoma surgery cases. Otol Neurotol 2010;31(2):276–283

Neff BA, Wiet RM, Lasak JM, et al. Cochlear implantation in the neurofibromatosis type 2 patient: long-term follow-up. Laryngoscope 2007;117(6):1069–1072

Odat HA, Piccirillo E, Sequino G, Taibah A, Sanna M. Management strategy of vestibular schwannoma in neurofibromatosis type 2. Otol Neurotol 2011;32(7):1163–1170

Otto SR, Brackmann DE, Hitselberger WE, Shannon RV, Kuchta J. Multichannel auditory brainstem implant: update on performance in 61 patients. J Neurosurg 2002;96(6):1063–1071

Otto SR, Shannon RV, Wilkinson EP, et al. Audiologic outcomes with the penetrating electrode auditory brainstem implant. Otol Neurotol 2008;29(8):1147–1154

Piccirillo E, Guida M, Flanagan S, Lauda L, Fois P, Sanna M. CNAP To predict functional cochlear nerve preservation in NF-2: cochlear implant or auditory brainstem implant. Skull Base 2008;18(4):281–287

Piccirillo E, Hiraumi H, Hamada M, Russo A, De Stefano A, Sanna M. Intraoperative cochlear nerve monitoring in vestibular schwannoma surgery—does it really affect hearing outcome? Audiol Neurootol 2008;13(1):58–64

Ramsden R, Khwaja S, Green K, O'Driscoll M, Mawman D. Vestibular schwannoma in the only hearing ear: cochlear implant or auditory brainstem implant? Otol Neurotol 2005;26(2):261–264

Sanna M, Khrais T, Guida M, Falcioni M. Auditory brainstem implant in a child with severely ossified cochlea. Laryngoscope 2006;116(9):1700–1703

Sanna M, Russo A, Taibah A, Falcioni M, Agarwal M. Enlarged translabyrinthine approach for the management of large and giant acoustic neuromas: a report of 175 consecutive cases. Ann Otol Rhinol Laryngol 2004;113(4):319–328

Simmons FB, Mongeon CJ, Lewis WR, Huntington DA. Electrical stimulation of acoustical nerve and inferior colliculus (results in man). Arch Otolaryngol 1964;79:559–568

Sollmann WP, Laszig R, Marangos N. Surgical experiences in 58 cases using the Nucleus 22 multichannel auditory brainstem implant. J Laryngol Otol Suppl 2000;(27):23–26

Temple RH, Axon PR, Ramsden RT, Keles N, Deger K, Yücel E. Auditory rehabilitation in neurofibromatosis type 2: a case for cochlear implantation. J Laryngol Otol 1999;113(2):161–163

Thedinger BA, Cueva RA, Glasscock ME III. Treatment of an acoustic neuroma in an only-hearing ear: case reports and considerations for the future. Laryngoscope 1993;103(9):976–980

Tono T, Ushisako Y, Morimitsu T. Cochlear implantation in an intralabyrinthine acoustic neuroma patient after resection of an intracanalicular tumour. J Laryngol Otol 1996;110(6):570–573

Vincent C, Zini C, Gandolfi A, et al. Results of the MXM Digisonic auditory brainstem implant clinical trials in Europe. Otol Neurotol 2002;23(1):56–60

Vincenti V, Pasanisi E, Guida M, Di Trapani G, Sanna M. Hearing rehabilitation in neurofibromatosis type 2 patients: cochlear versus auditory brainstem implantation. Audiol Neurootol 2008;13(4):273–280

Yamakami I, Yoshinori H, Saeki N, Wada M, Oka N. Hearing preservation and intraoperative auditory brainstem response and cochlear nerve compound action potential monitoring in the removal of small acoustic neurinoma via the retrosigmoid approach. J Neurol Neurosurg Psychiatry 2009;80(2):218–227

17 Implantation in Skull Base and Temporal Bone Lesions

In this chapter additional indications for auditory implantation using a cochlear implant or an auditory brainstem implant are discussed; this group is miscellaneous and contains various skull base lesions and some more exceptional neurotologic pathology not discussed in the previous chapters.

In general this group of extended indications is small and concerns a limited subset of patients who are severely bilaterally hearing deprived because of miscellaneous disorders. The group includes patients with a skull base lesion in one ear and a deaf contralateral ear not available for implantation (which otherwise would have been the first option), as well as rare bilateral pathology such as temporal bone fractures and Meniere disease.

While the same pathology in just a single ear would not lead to cochlear implantation, in this group of patients an individualized, well considered, and sometimes experimental decision is made in the quest for hearing restoration. The outcomes cannot always be predicted in advance; only afterward does the result become clear.

The pathology in this group can be divided into

1. Skull base lesions: tumor or expansive lesions of the skull base and petrous bone
2. Nontumor lesions violating the integrity of the otic capsule (petrous bone fractures or labyrinthectomy)

Neurofibromatosis type 2 (NF2) would fall in the first category and presents the largest group of patients in whom experience with both types of auditory implants (cochlear implant [CI] and auditory brainstem implant [ABI]) has been gained. NF2 cannot be considered as an "additional" indication for auditory implantation; the ABI was invented for this type of pathology, but in management and decision making basically the same principles apply. Auditory implantation in NF2 is dealt with separately in Chapter 16.

17.1 CI versus ABI

There is growing evidence that better results in speech perception are achieved with a CI (whenever feasible) than with an ABI.[1–5] This appears to be related to easier access, better stabilization of the implant, and use of the tonotopy in the cochlea as opposed to that of the cochlear nucleus. Cochlear implantation should therefore always be considered as a first choice in this category of patients, when possible. Additionally the surgical risks in cochlear implantation are smaller than those in auditory brainstem implantation (see Chapters 5 and 8).

17.2 Preoperative Conditions

The feasibility of cochlear implantation depends crucially on two important anatomical conditions in CI decision making:

1. Preservation and integrity of the cochlear nerve
2. Patency and integrity of the cochlea

These are especially important for the pathology dealt with in this chapter, because the cochlear nerve or the cochlea itself could be deranged by the pathology, making deployment of a CI less practical or even impossible, and resulting in an ABI as the only possible option.

In tumor or expansive lesions of the skull base and petrous bone, both factors could be distorted, depending on location and type of pathology. In skull base lesions it is possible that the decision for CI or ABI can only be made intraoperatively, after the anatomical situation has become clear. Preoperative audiologic measurements can give useful but not prognostic information (pure tone audiogram, auditory brainstem response [ABR] electric promontory stimulation). The loss of vascular supply to the labyrinth can lead to labyrinthitis ossificans affecting the patency of the cochlea and leading to loss of spiral neurons in the long term.[6,7] This makes it preferable, if not mandatory, to perform cochlear implantation in the same surgery before the occurrence of the ossification due to the vascular damage.

In the nontumor lesions especially, the patency and integrity of the cochlea is an important factor. In fractures due to trauma or due to active labyrinthitis ossificans the cochlear patency might be lost. The risk of the cochlear nerve being torn off the modiolus as a result of the trauma is in our opinion infinitesimal: the forces necessary to create this kind of lesion are not compatible with survival[1]; moreover, not one case with bilateral cochlear nerve rupture has been published. Therefore, the first factor is of minor concern in fractures of the otic capsule.[5] After labyrinthectomy the presence of labyrinthitis ossificans is usually limited to only the round window area[7] because the vascularization of the internal auditory canal (IAC) is left intact during the labyrinthectomy, which is different from the case in surgery for removal of an IAC tumor. Also, the cochlear nerve is preserved.

In cases with preoperative or intraoperative violation of the otic capsule there is also a risk of cochlear ossification due to labyrinthitis ossificans. Because of this risk, it is best to perform cochlear implantation during the same procedure (even though delayed implantation up to a maximum of 18 months is mentioned in the literature[8,9]).

More information on cochlear ossification and labyrinthitis ossificans can be found in Chapter 11.

17.3 Intraoperative Audiometric Testing

Electrical stapedial reflex (ESR) measurements, electrically evoked compound action potential (ECAP) measurements using neural response testing (NRT or NRI), and electrically evoked auditory brainstem response (EABR) testing can only be performed after insertion of the electrode array. Thus, in some cases, the cochlear implant functions as a diagnostic tool in addition to the surgeon's intraoperative findings. Although the cochlear nerve and nucleus may be anatomically intact, their functionality could be hampered by compression due to the skull base lesion. At present no reliable test is available to gain information on this issue, although electrical promontory stimulation (EPS) seems to be useful to assess the survival of neural elements preoperatively.[10–12] However, when EPS results are negative it does not necessarily mean that the cochlear implant will not function (it could be a false negative). Its value is therefore limited.[13,14]

Tysome et al suggested that a temporary intracochlear electrode would be the ideal tool for gaining this information.[13] A brainstem electrode array and cochlear electrode array combined in one implant, allowing one to use whichever delivers the best result, would also be a valuable tool. Such a tool or implant has only been used in a research project and is not commercially available.

17.4 Indications

17.4.1 Skull Base Lesions

Sporadic reports have appeared in the literature regarding these particular cases; they include cochlear implantation in isolated vestibular schwannoma (VS) in the only hearing ear (and in NF2),[4,7,13,15–19] in petrous bone cholesteatoma,[20] and in a paraganglioma case.[21]

Cochlear implantation in pediatric medulloblastoma[22] and in Langerhans cell histiocytosis (LCH)[23,24] has also been described. The combination of surgical excision of the local pathology, chemotherapy, and radiotherapy as well as cochlear implantation makes these indications challenging.

The outcome can be affected by the finding that the cochlear nerve or nucleus has been compressed by the tumor, or can be influenced by loss of vascularization or spasm of the internal auditory artery.[8] These factors can lead to a temporary or long-term disappointing outcome of the cochlear implantation, which cannot be predicted preoperatively. Previous radiotherapy can also negatively affect the CI/ABI outcome.[25–28]

Recurrence of pathology or postsurgical scarring around the cochlear nerve can also negatively influence the outcome in the long term.[2,8,29] Neff et al in their long-term study on cochlear implantation in VS patients reported that neither of these effects was found with a minimum follow-up of 5 years.[2] Roehm et al reported a patient with a recurrence of VS only after 22 years, showing that cochlear implantation is sometimes a valuable and long-lasting interim step (as in this case lasting 22 years) in treatment to achieve hearing restoration.[29] When the cochlea or the cochlear nerve cannot be preserved, ABI remains the only available option.

Unfortunately, anatomical preservation of the cochlea and cochlear nerve does not guarantee their functionality and presently no intraoperative test is available to evaluate this functionality. Such an evaluation is extremely important because, in the case of a nonfunctioning CI, revision surgery for ABI insertion in a cerebellopontine angle already operated on and filled with fat is particularly demanding if not actually impossible due to fibrosis in the presence of delicate structures.

In these skull base cases surgery is often performed through translabyrinthine approach. In this approach the hearing is sacrificed but the cochlea is preserved; this keeps both the CI and the ABI option available during the surgery. During the translabyrinthine approach the vascularization of the IAC is usually sacrificed: this can lead to labyrinthitis ossificans.[7]

When a CI is planned the approach is usually combined with a subtotal petrosectomy to reduce the risk of a postoperative CSF rhinorrhea by plugging the eustachian tube and obliterating the residual cavity (Chapter 10). In this situation the possibility of a subcutaneous CSF collection is actually increased somewhat, because after transection of the EAC the musculoperiosteal layer is incomplete.

Radiologic follow-up remains necessary to identify recurrence of the primary pathology but also to identify possible inclusion cholesteatoma in the occluded cavity. CT follow-up is performed at 1, 3, 5, and 10 years after surgery. The presence of the CI impedes the routine use of MRI because the magnet and implant create artifacts (see also Chapter 3).

17.4.2 Previous Radiotherapy

When the sensorineural hearing loss is caused by radiotherapy treatment, the results of cochlear implantation show reasonable to good responses, as reported in several studies.[25,28,30–32] Radiotherapy has been proven to affect the stria vascularis and the organ of Corti with its hair cells, while the higher auditory pathways (brainstem, cochlear nerve) generally remain functionally intact, even in the longer term as shown by Low et al.[27] Counseling on the likelihood of a modest outcome after radiotherapy seems wise.

Other side effects of radiotherapy can hamper implantation: pathologic changes leading to middle ear effusion, eustachian tube fibrosis, and chronic suppurative otitis media. Osteoradionecrosis has been reported as a lasting source of infection[33] and softening of the temporal bone, making facial nerve damage more likely. Radiotherapy can also lead to intracochlear fibrosis and ossification,[26] fibrosis and scarring of tissues in the internal auditory canal, and obliterative endarteritis that has an influence on vessels throughout the radiation field.[32] As also the skin can be affected (radiation dermatitis), thought should be given to a minimal incision and skin flap design.[32] Long-term hearing outcomes of cochlear implantation in irradiated patients may deteriorate because of recurrence of pathology or the causes mentioned above. This should be discussed with the patient, whose expectations should not run too high.

17.4.3 Non-Skull Base Lesions

Non-Skull Base Indications for Auditory Implantation

- CI combined with labyrinthectomy in Meniere disease
- CI in fracture of the otic capsule

Labyrinthectomy in Meniere Disease

Performing a labyrinthectomy in Meniere disease can be considered one of the last steps in gaining control of vestibular function. This surgical step should only be considered when several pharmaceutical, dietary, and lifestyle options, as well as intratympanic gentamicin have been attempted.[34–37] Also endolymphatic sac decompression and selective vestibular nerve sectioning have been suggested as surgical methods.

The anatomical destruction of the vestibular system via transmastoid three-canal labyrinthectomy (drilling of all three semicircular canals with removal of all neuroepithelial tissues in vestibulum and ampullae) allows resolution of the vertigo spells in 93 to 100% of cases.[36] The nonresponsive cases usually suffer bilateral Meniere disease. However, the direct consequence of a labyrinthectomy is the loss of residual hearing. Therefore usually only severely hearing deprived patients are elected for this approach. This is not a large group as only 10% of Meniere cases drop below 61 dB on average pure tone audiometry, and fewer than 5% drop below 81 dB.[38] Bilateral Meniere disease develops in 10 to 15% to 15 to 40% of cases and usually presents within 5 years after the unilateral onset. In these cases the sensorineural hearing loss in the first affected ear is usually worse.[17] In presence of contralateral severe hearing loss, simultaneous labyrinthectomy and cochlear implantation may be considered.[35] In addition, patients affected by bilateral Meniere disease fitted with common hearing aids usually do not attain good performance due to the hearing fluctuation and the minimal compliance between detection and complaint threshold.

Simple transmastoid labyrinthectomy, because of the preservation of the vascularization of the cochlea, often does not produce extended ossification/fibrosis.[7] Therefore, theoretically, implantation may also be delayed to a second step. Combining the two surgeries (transmastoid labyrinthectomy and cochlear implantation through a standard facial recess approach), however, is relatively easy and the procedure is safe to carry out in the same stage. Although loss of any residual hearing after labyrinthectomy is a fact, quality of life measurements made after labyrinthectomy in Meniere disease show 98% of patients to be positive.[34]

Late cochlear implantations, years after the labyrinthectomy, show improvement in auditory gain, but the results in general are worse than with simultaneous implantation.[39]

Another consideration in Meniere disease regarding cochlear implantation is the fact that the spiral ganglion cell count and function of the cochlear nerve might be lower because of the primary disease. Histologic study of postlabyrinthectomy bones demonstrated survival of around 10,000 spiral ganglion cells: only 10% of cases drop to around 3,000. Both these amounts have been proven to be enough for proper CI functioning.[6,36,39] Based on the explanations above, hearing results of cochlear implantation combined with labyrinthectomy are usually good.

Fracture of the Otic Capsule

Temporal bone trauma can lead to fracture lines that damage the facial nerve (palsy), labyrinth (vertigo), skull base (CSF leakage), ossicles (conductive hearing loss), and cochlea (sensorineural hearing loss) in various combinations.[40–42] Damage to the otic capsule can be found especially in transverse fractures (mostly due to occipital trauma). There are several causes for this sensorineural hearing loss: disruption of the membranous labyrinth with mixture of perilymphatic and endolymphatic fluids, loss of the integrity of the membranous cochlea with loss of the cochlear transducer function, and vascular compromise or hemorrhage. The presence of a persistent perilymph fistula or secondary endolymphatic hydrops can also be of influence.[43] The spiral ganglion cells and modiolus usually remain intact and also the cochlear nerve itself usually remains intact and in connection with the cochlea.[1]

Cochlear implantation in patients with otic capsule–damaging fractures usually leads to good results in hearing rehabilitation,[5] although some patients do not perceive this outcome as successful because of the sudden loss of their normal hearing after the trauma.[41] In spite of this psychological drawback, the risk of labyrinthine ossification triggered by the trauma (not by loss of vascularization in the IAC) makes urgent implantation necessary, and might lead to a less than perfect outcome due to the development of fibrous intracochlear tissue surrounding the electrode array.[44–46] When implantation is performed late (after months) the risk of ossification or loss of spiral ganglion cells might also compromise the outcome[45]; transverse fractures may lead to loss of spiral ganglion cells over time[47] and can lead to progressive decrease of CI results. Another reported drawback is that cochlear implantation may be challenging because of a displaced fracture line that can impede electrode insertion.[48]

Several histopathologic studies show that in fractures the enchondral part of the cochlear capsule heals with fibrous tissue instead of with new bone, thus presenting a lasting risk for meningitis.[46,49] Another complication described is a higher incidence of facial nerve stimulation (especially at the level of the geniculate ganglion) caused by the low resistance of the fracture line.[44] The inner endosteal layer and the outer periosteal layer do heal, but only with very thin layers and often incompletely.[49] This necessitates isolation from the external environment by means of subtotal petrosectomy with closure of the eustachian tube and external ear canal and obliteration with fat, to minimize the risk of otitis media leading to meningitis and also in cases without cochlear implantation.[50]

17.5 Contraindications and Risks of Implantation in Skull Base Surgery/ Neurotology

In general, the risks related to these procedures are a combination of the risks of both surgeries: the risks of implantation and the risks during surgery for the primary pathology. The presence of the implant may increase risks of infection, CSF leak, and meningitis, but the limited number of reported cases hinders statistical confirmation.

In these exceptional cases, CI and ABI placement are good treatment options and we should take into consideration that the CI or ABI is sometimes the only option available for these patients if they are not to remain completely deaf. There seem to be no absolute contraindications, but the higher risks involved in some of the skull base procedures must be considered carefully in the counseling. The risk–benefit ratio needs to be discussed with the patient before the definitive decision is made.

Case 17.1 Cochlear Implantation Combined with Removal of Small Vestibular Schwannoma Left Ear (Fig. 17.1.1–Fig. 17.1.13)

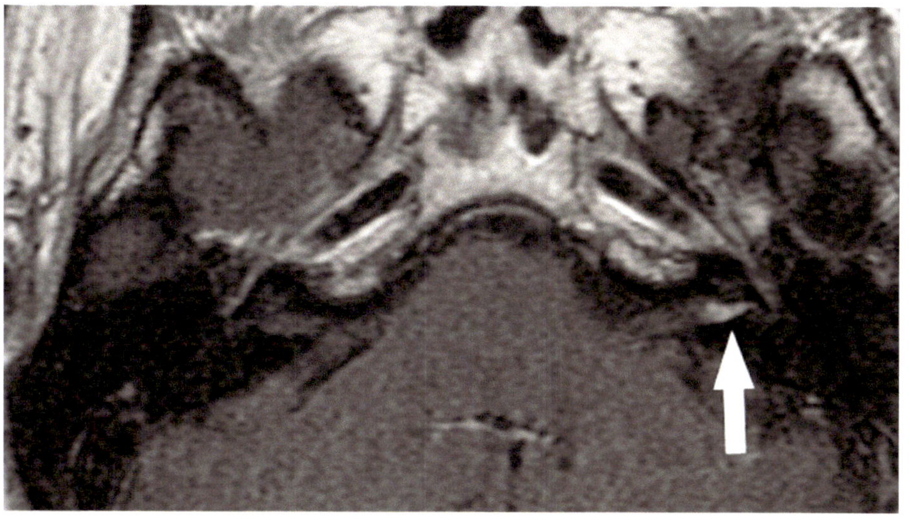

Fig. 17.1.1 Preoperative MRI showing a intracanalicular vestibular schwannoma on the left side (*arrow*).

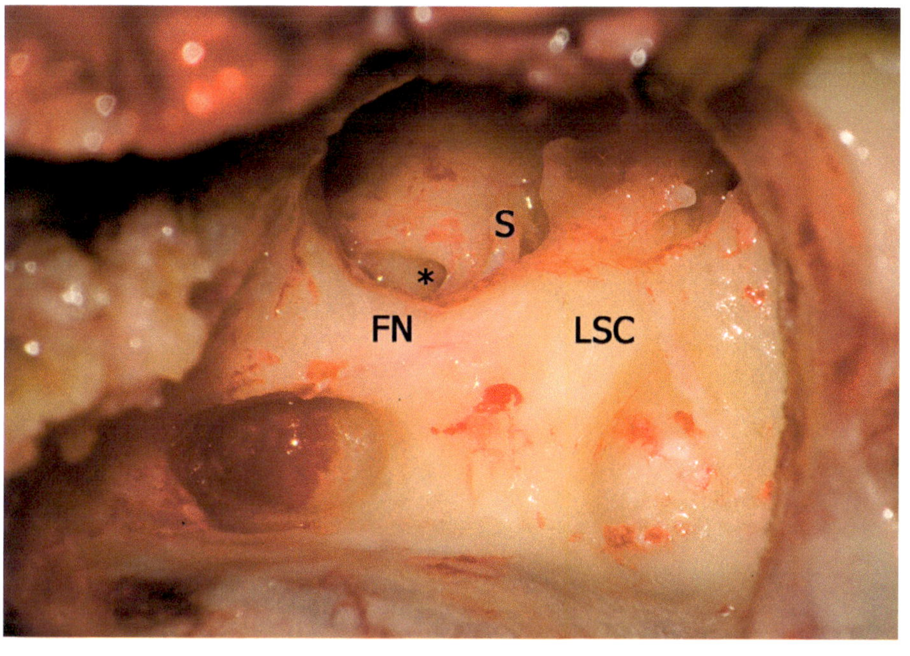

Fig. 17.1.2 The canal wall down cavity procedure is performed. The horizontal semicircular canal (LSC) and facial nerve canal (FN) can clearly be seen, as well as the stapes (S) and round window niche (*).

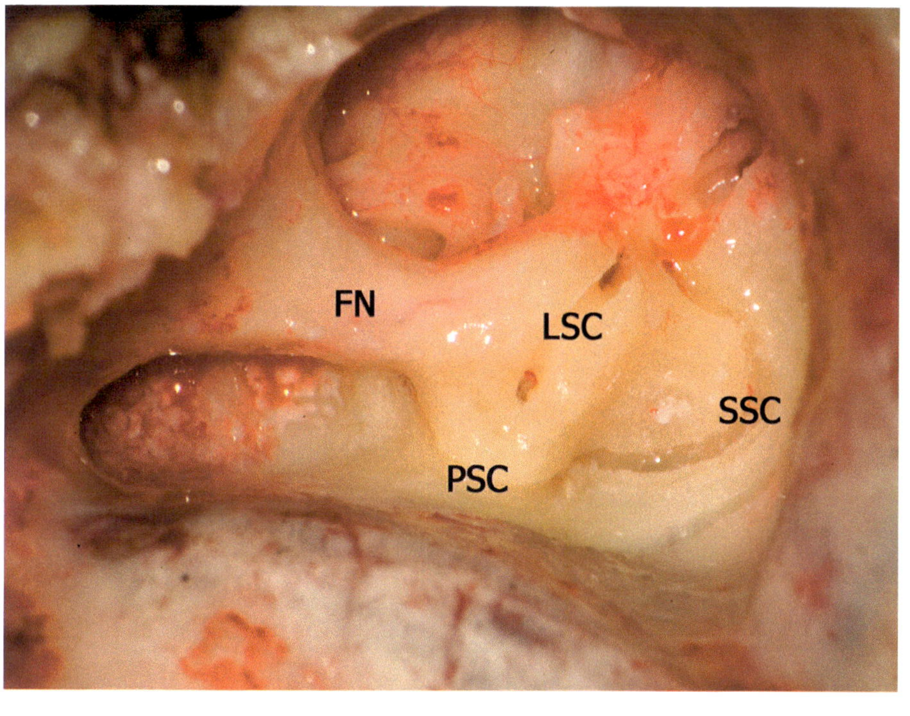

Fig. 17.1.3 Start of the translabyrinthine procedure with opening of semicircular canals. LSC, lateral semicircular canal; PSC, posterior semicircular canal; SSC, superior semicircular canal; FN, facial nerve.

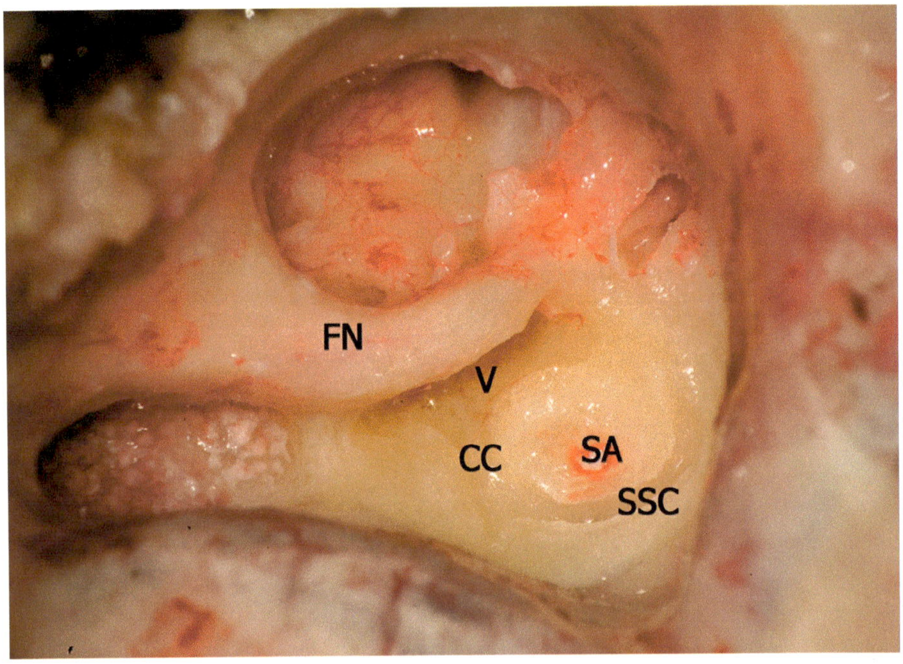

Fig. 17.1.4 Removal of labyrinth block and opening of the vestibule (V). Note the subarcuate artery (SA) central in the plane of the superior semicircular canal (SSC). CC, common crus; FN, facial nerve.

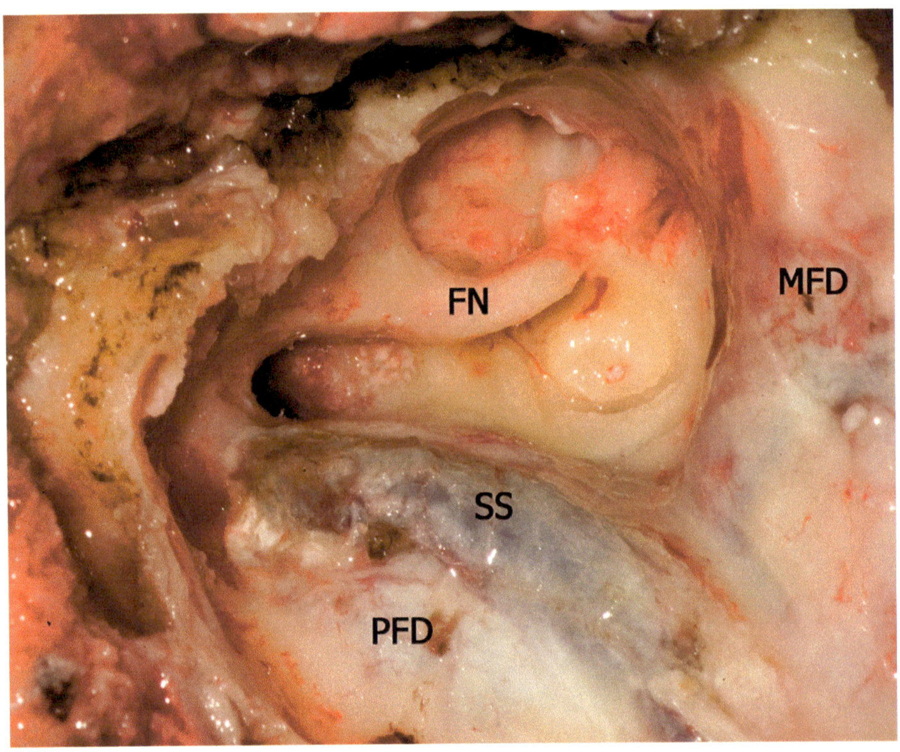

Fig. 17.1.5 The middle (MFD) and posterior fossa dura (PFD) are exposed for better access. SS, sigmoid sinus; FN, facial nerve.

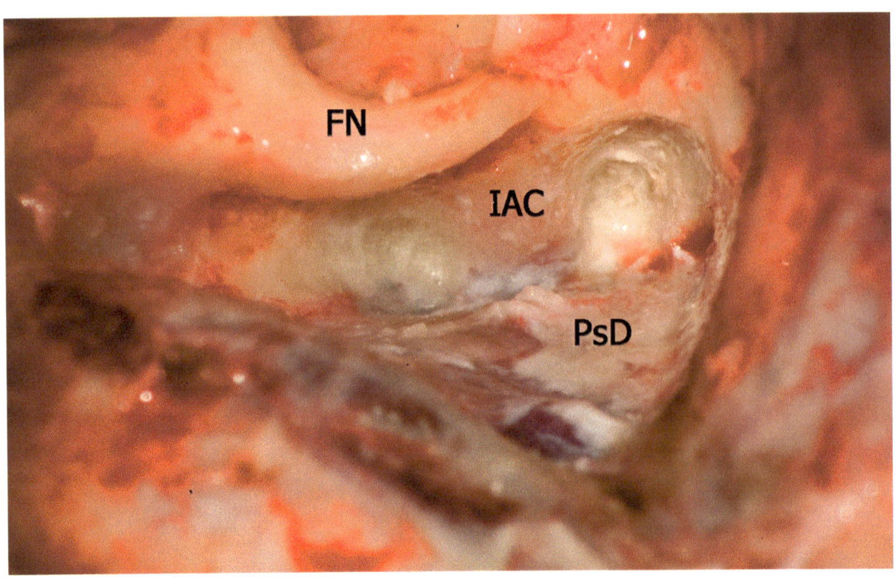

Fig. 17.1.6 Identification and skeletonization of the internal auditory canal (IAC). PsD, presigmoid dura; FN, facial nerve.

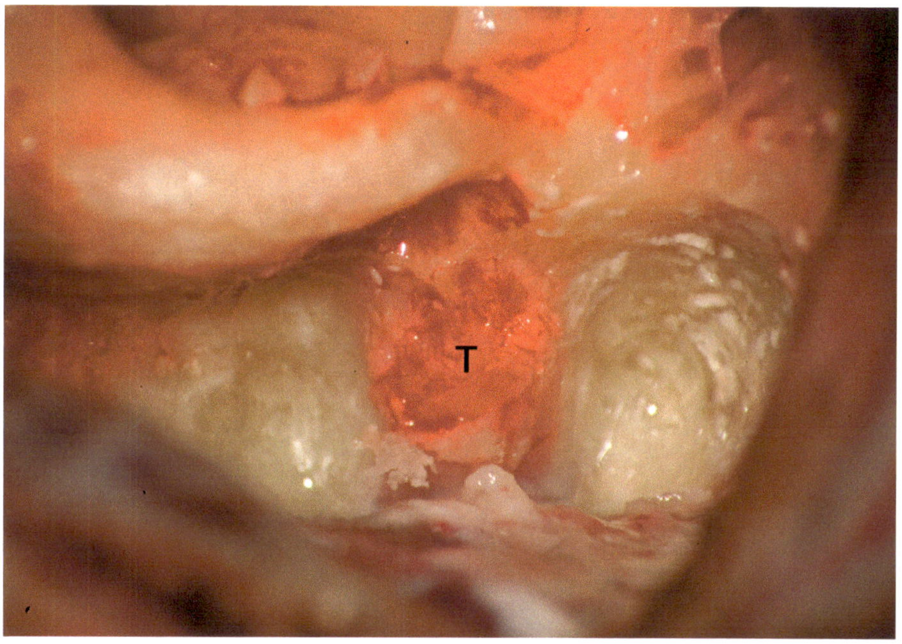

Fig. 17.1.7 All bone is removed over the internal auditory canal: the intracanalicular schwannoma (T) now becomes visible.

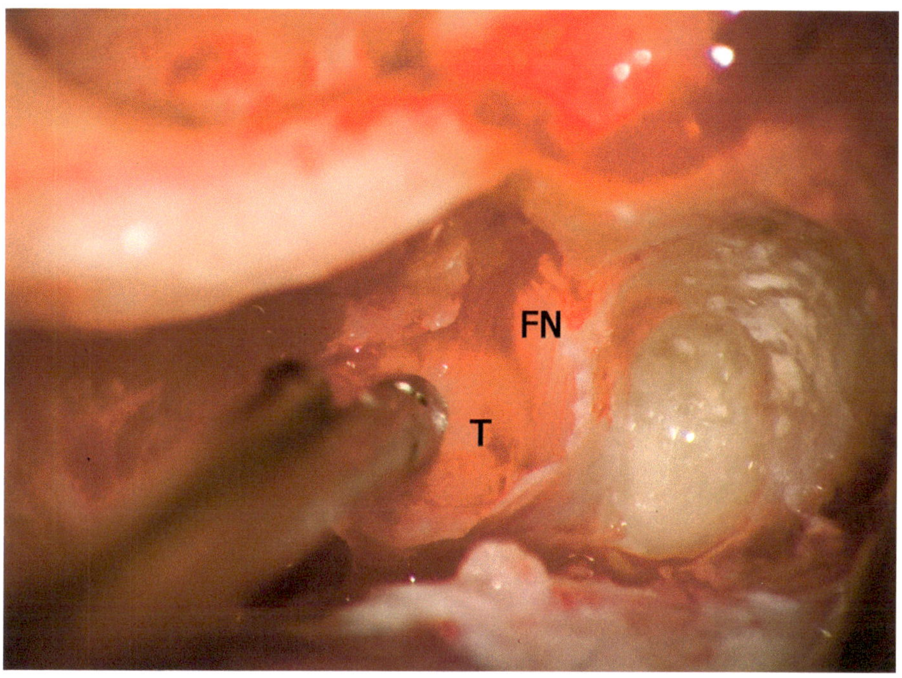

Fig. 17.1.8 With posterior-inferior displacement of the tumor (T), the facial nerve (FN) is identified at the fundus of the internal auditory canal.

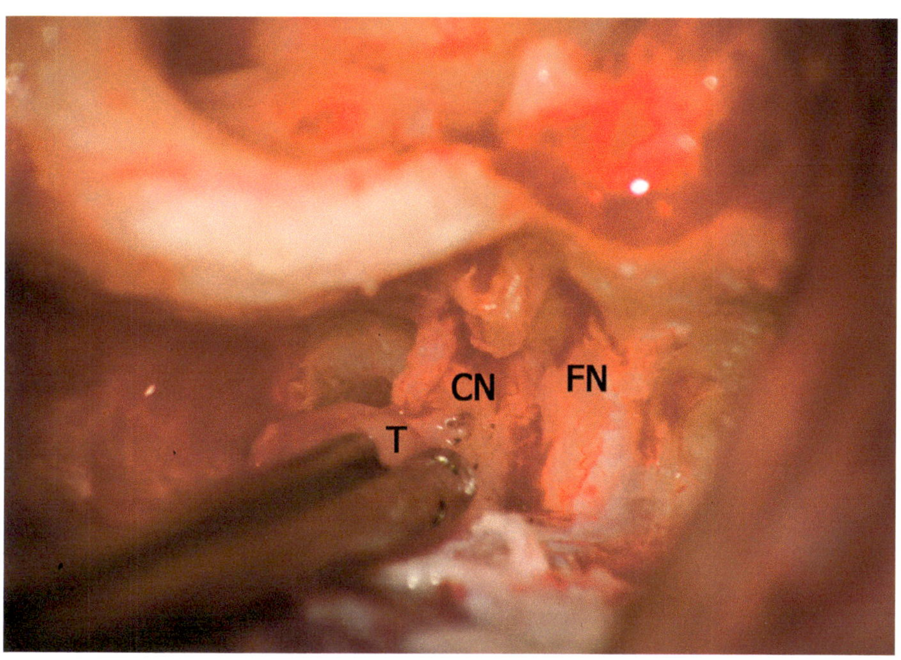

Fig. 17.1.9 Inferior-anteriorly the cochlear nerve (CN) also becomes visible. FN, facial nerve; T, tumor.

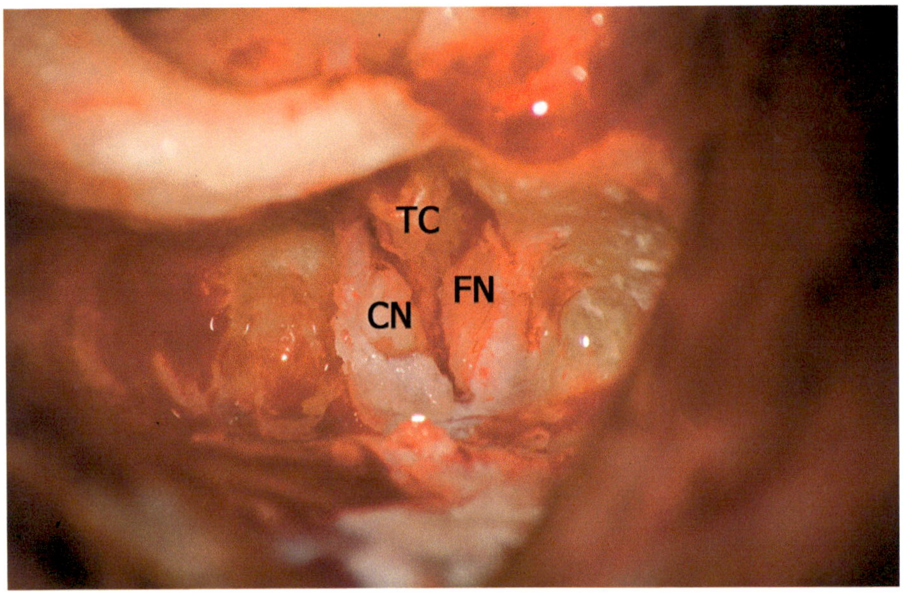

Fig. 17.1.10 After removal of the entire schwannoma the transverse crest (TC) becomes visible with cranially the facial nerve (FN) and caudally the cochlear nerve (CN).

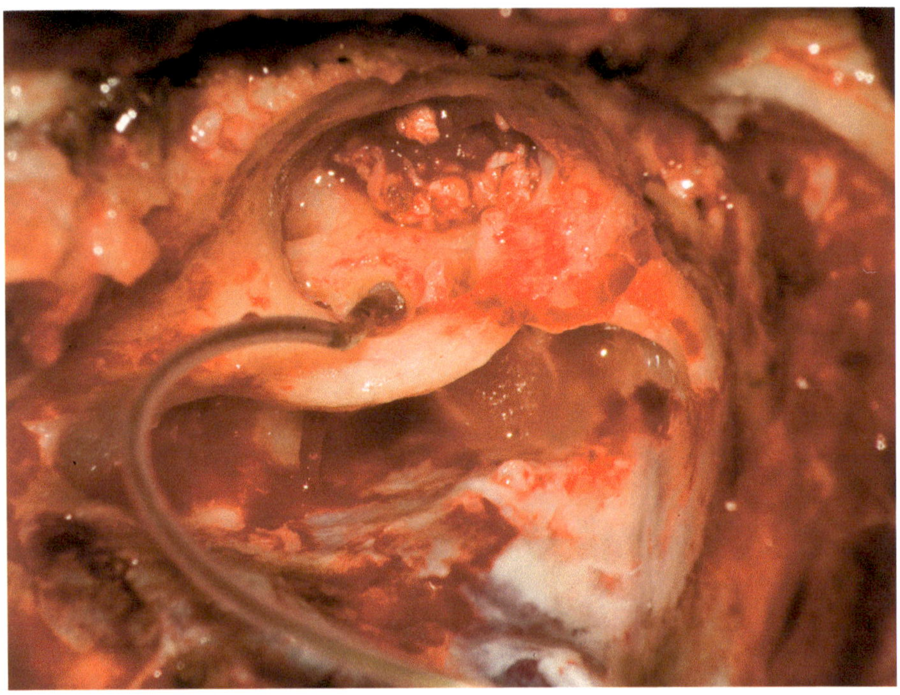

Fig. 17.1.11 Cochlear implantation is now carried out using the round window approach. Spongostan covers the IAC.

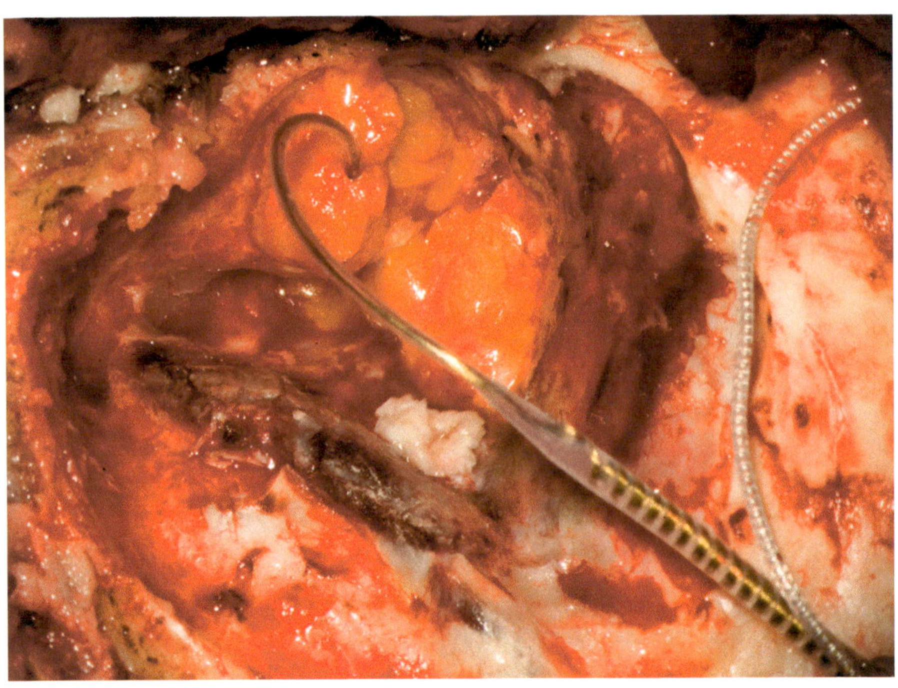

Fig. 17.1.12 First, the eustachian tube is obliterated (not shown here; see Chapter 10). Then the cavity is obliterated with abdominal fat impregnated in rifampicin, after fixating the electrode array in the round window niche with small pieces of fascia and fibrin glue.

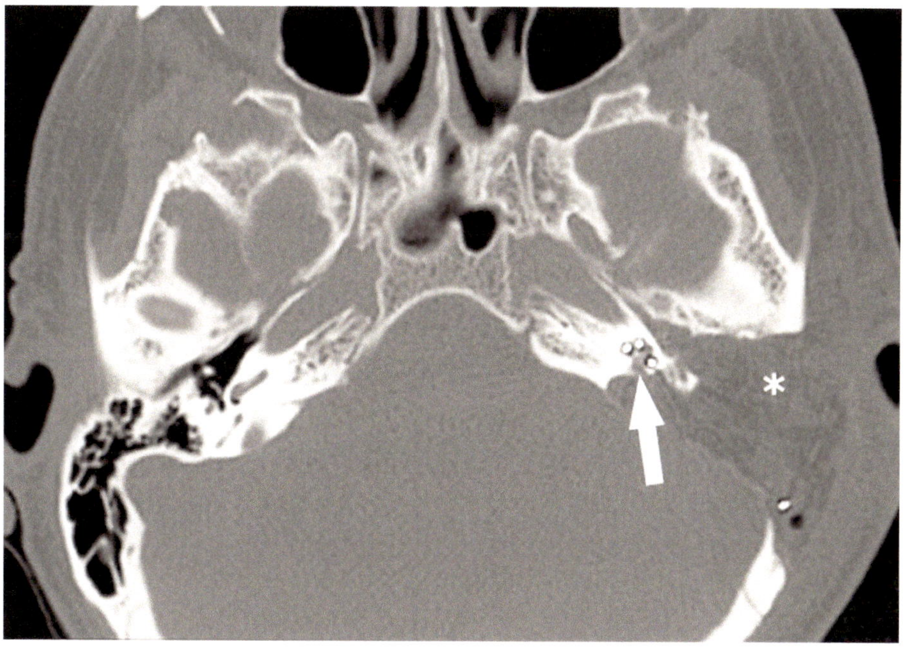

Fig. 17.1.13 Postoperative CT image, showing the obliterated cavity (*) with the cochlear electrode array inserted in the cochlea (*arrow*).

Case 17.2 Cochlear Implantation Combined with Labyrinthectomy in Meniere Disease (Left Ear) (Fig. 17.2.1–Fig. 17.2.9)

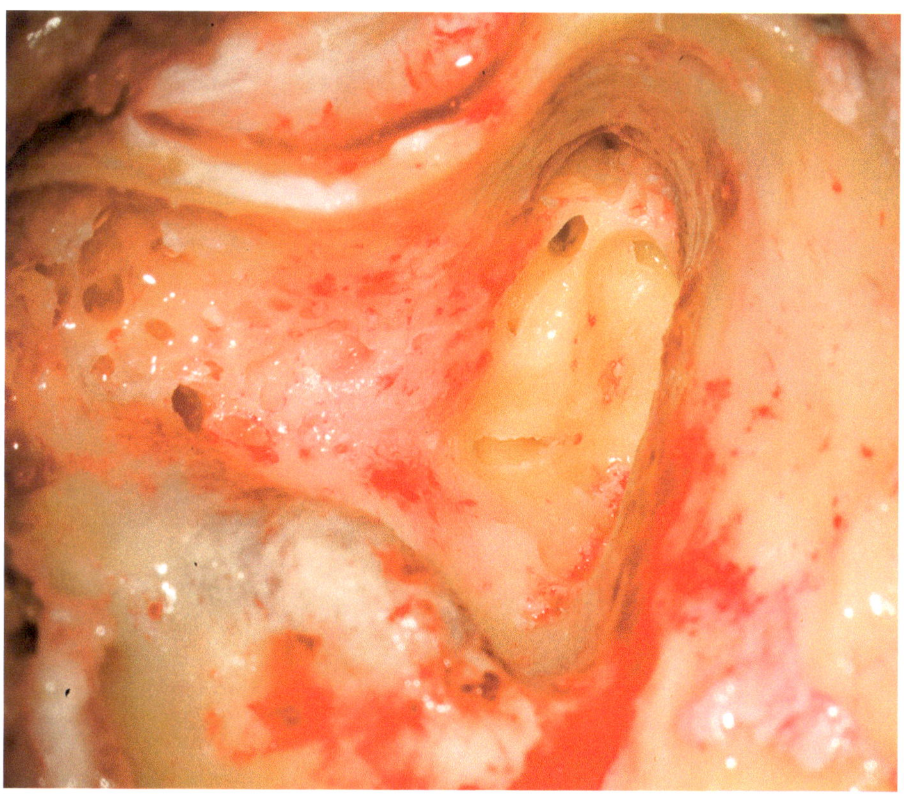

Fig. 17.2.1 A canal wall up approach is used: the semicircular canals have been opened.

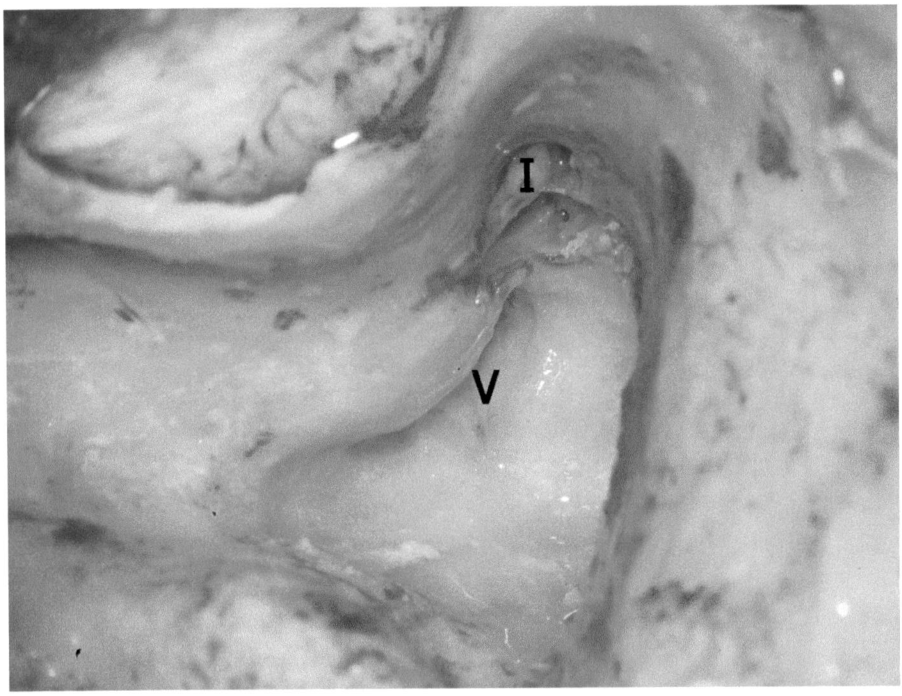

Fig. 17.2.2 The vestibule (V) is opened as treatment against Meniere vertigo attacks. The incus (I) is visible anteriorly in the epitympanum.

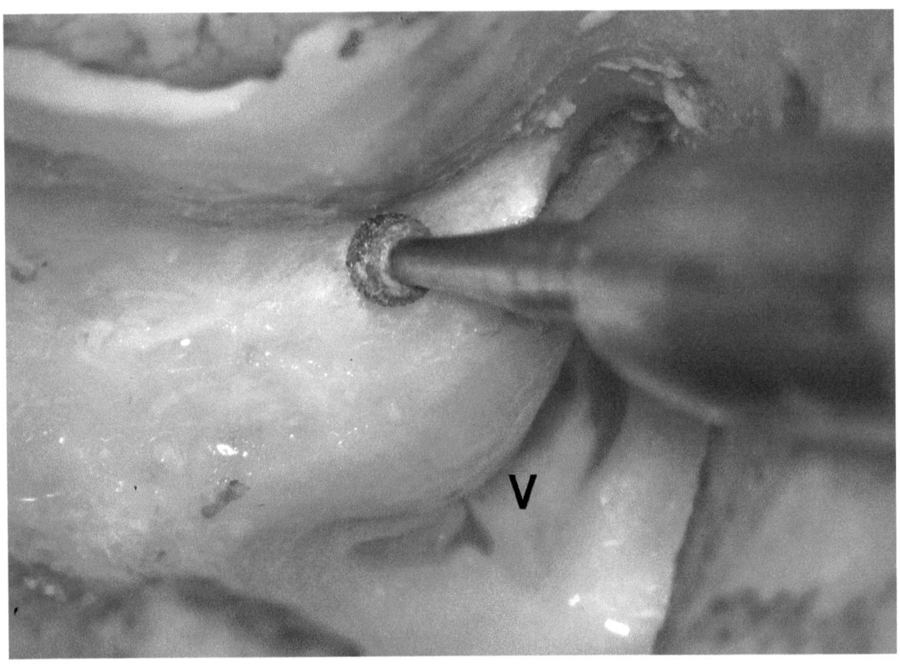

Fig. 17.2.3 Drilling of the posterior tympanotomy is started. V, vestibule.

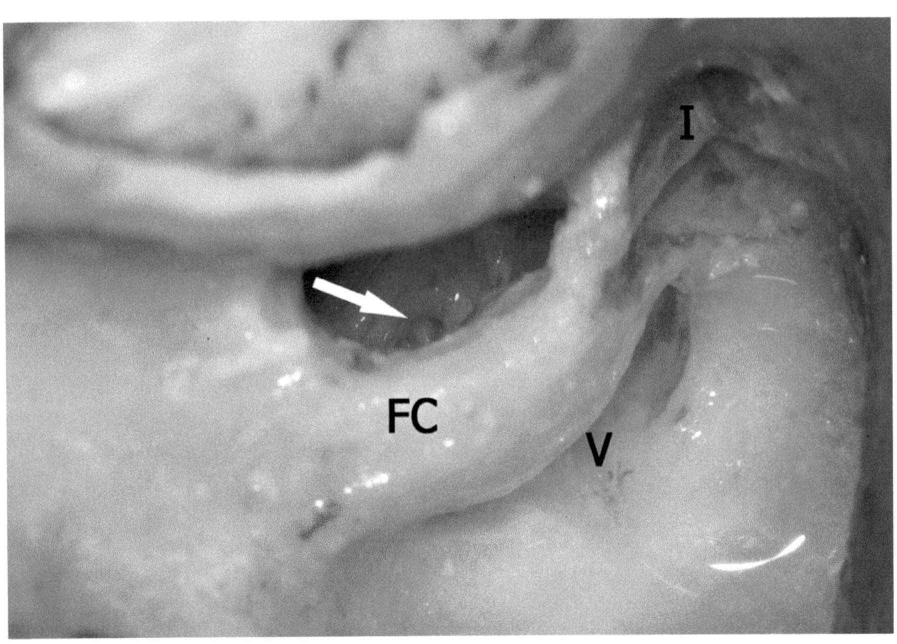

Fig. 17.2.4 With the vertical part of the facial nerve, buttress, and chorda tympani as landmarks, the facial recess is opened, giving access to the middle ear and round window niche (*arrow*). V, vestibule; I, incus; FC, fallopian canal.

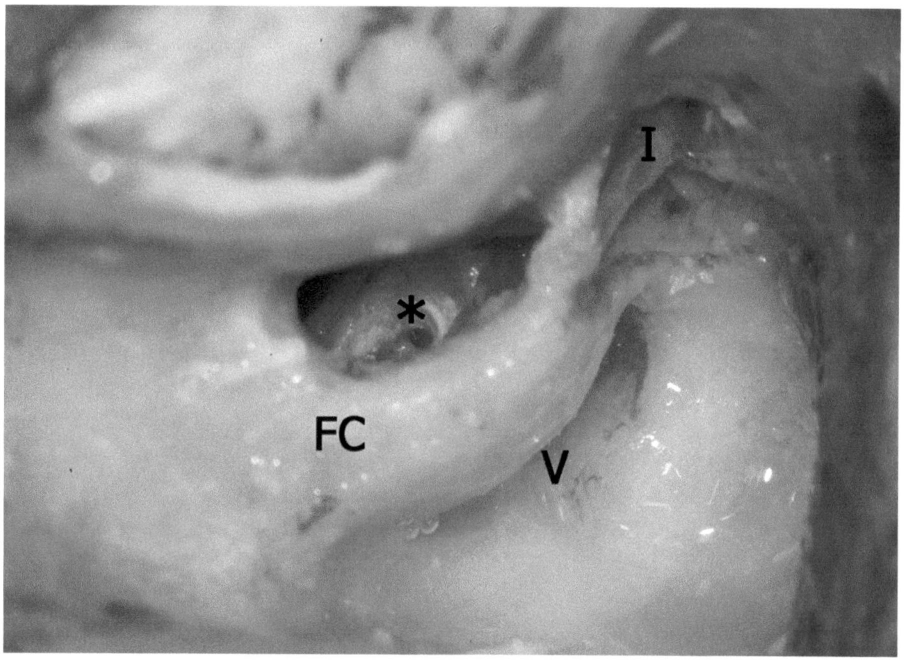

Fig. 17.2.5 The bony overhang over the round window niche (*) is removed. V, vestibule; I, incus; FC, fallopian canal.

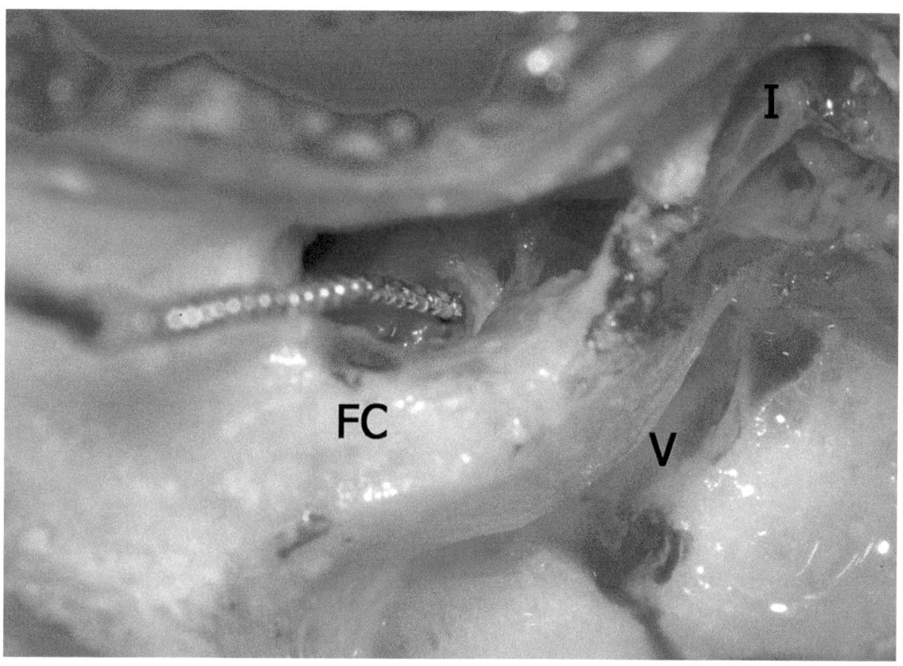

Fig. 17.2.6 The electrode array is introduced into the cochlea via the round window. V, vestibule; I, incus; FC, fallopian canal.

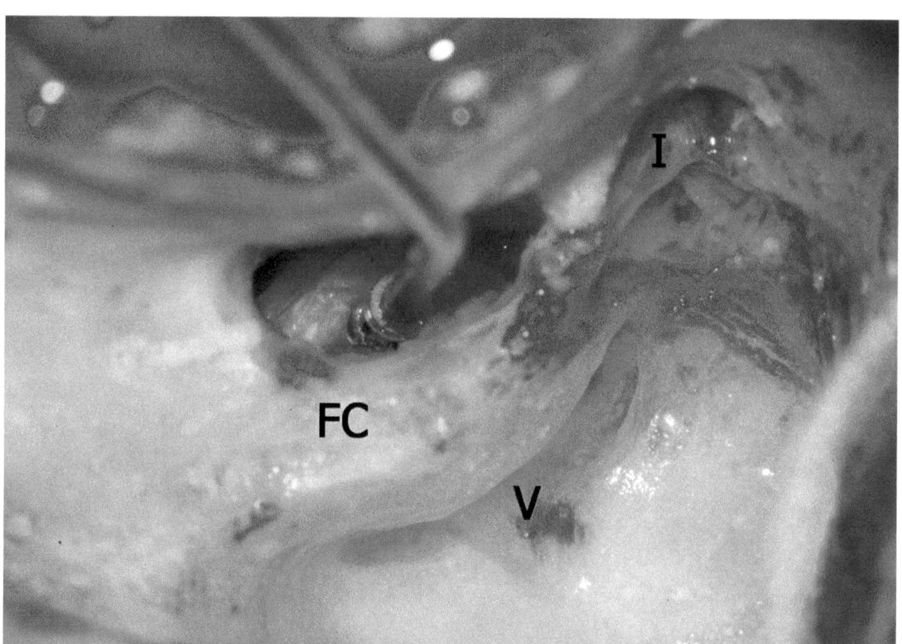

Fig. 17.2.7 The electrode array is inserted fully into the cochlea. Note the direction of the electrode array; it points in the direction of the basal turn, anterior-inferiorly. No resistance was met during this insertion. V, vestibule; I, incus; FC, fallopian canal.

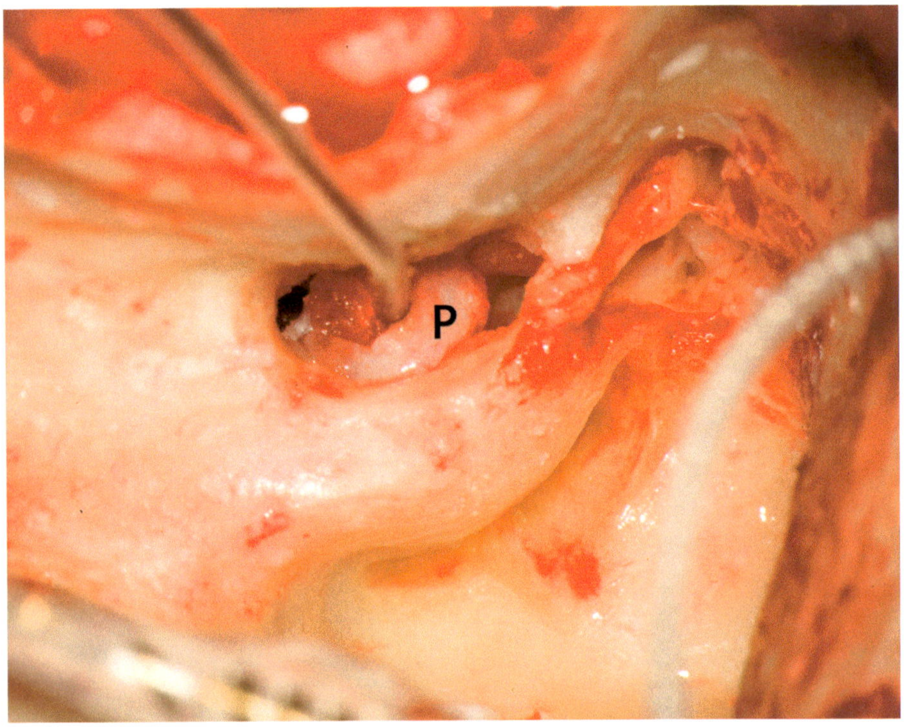

Fig. 17.2.8 The implant is fixated with fascia at the round window niche and in the posterior tympanotomy. Subsequently the epitympanum is sealed off with periosteum (P) and the cavity and the vestibule are filled with abdominal fat.

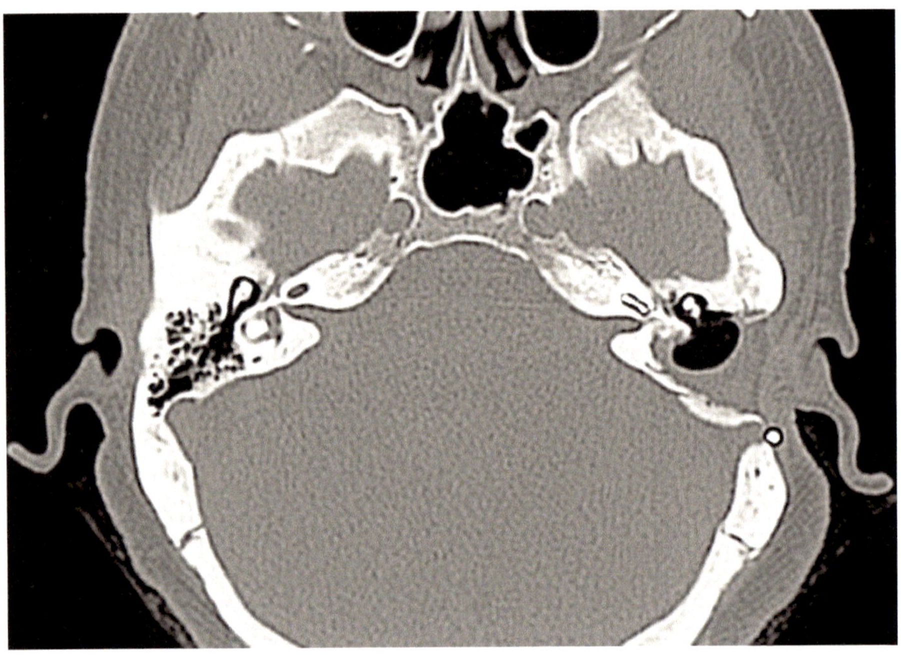

Fig. 17.2.9 The postoperative CT image (1 year) shows the electrode array in the left ear. Note the partial resorption of fat from the occluded cavity.

Case 17.3 Bilateral Fracture of Otic Capsule with Bilateral Deafness (Fig. 17.3.1 and Fig. 17.3.2)

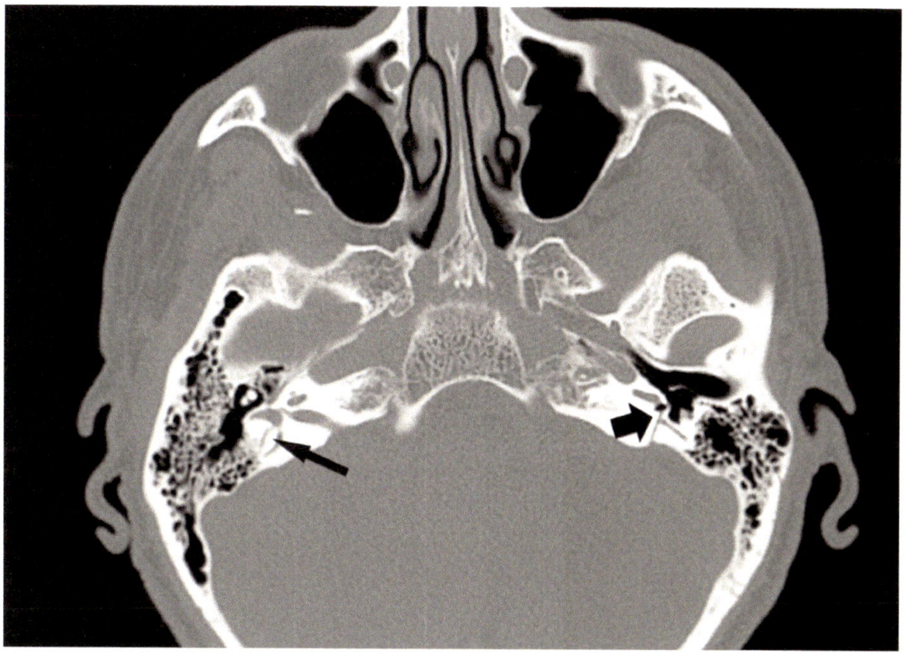

Fig. 17.3.1 CT imaging of patient with bilateral petrous bone fracture. Preoperative image: the fracture lines traverse the vestibule on the right side (*long arrow*) and the cochlea on the left side (*short arrow*).

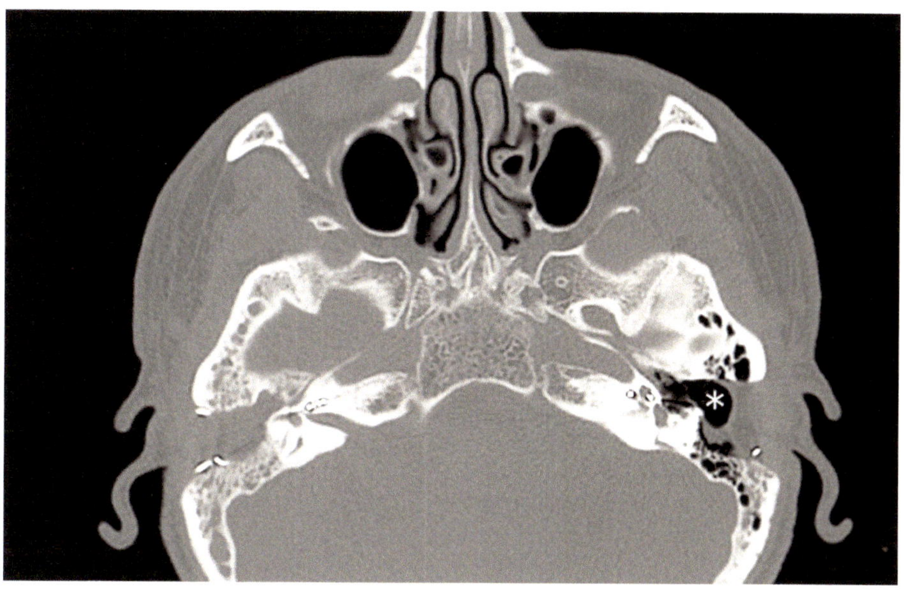

Fig. 17.3.2 Postoperative CT scan after bilateral cochlear implantation. Note the fat resorption in the left ear (*). Possibly the closure of the eustachian tube has been insufficient in the left ear.

Case 17.4 Supralabyrinthine Petrous Bone Cholesteatoma: Simultaneous Removal of the Cholesteatoma Right Ear and Cochlear Implantation (Fig. 17.4.1–Fig. 17.4.6)

Male patient, born 1946, suffering vertigo spells.

Right ear: petrous bone cholesteatoma with erosion of the superior semicircular canal and roof of the internal auditory canal. He had mixed hearing loss and is using a hearing aid.
Left ear: dead ear since previous canal wall down surgery.

Surgery.

Right ear: translabyrinthine approach + subtotal petrosectomy + CI.
Left ear: SP + CI.

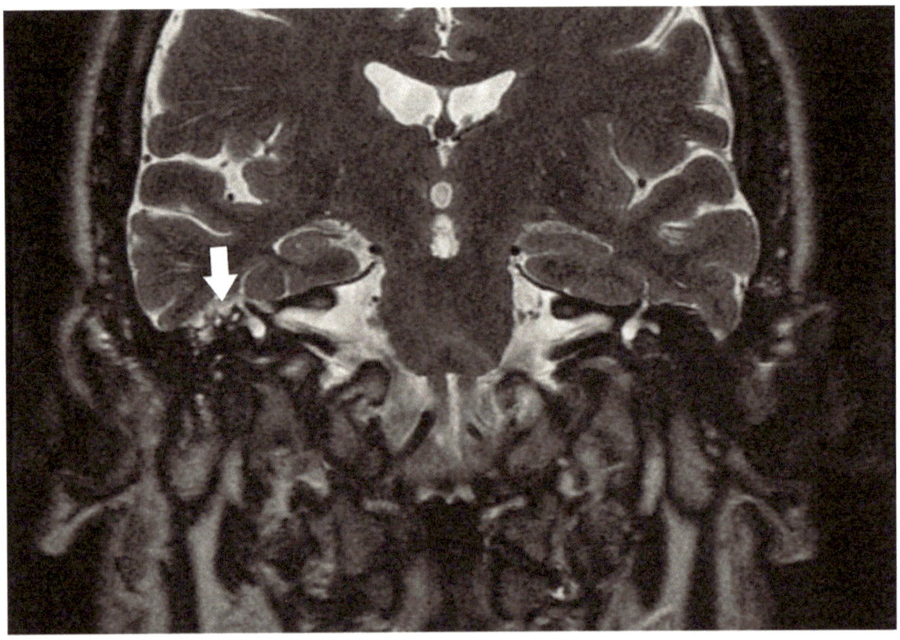

Fig. 17.4.1 Coronal T2W MRI showing hyperintense tissue along the middle fossa dura on the right side (*arrow*). There is no visible border between temporal lobe and hyperintense tissue and the affected superior semicircular canal can be seen.

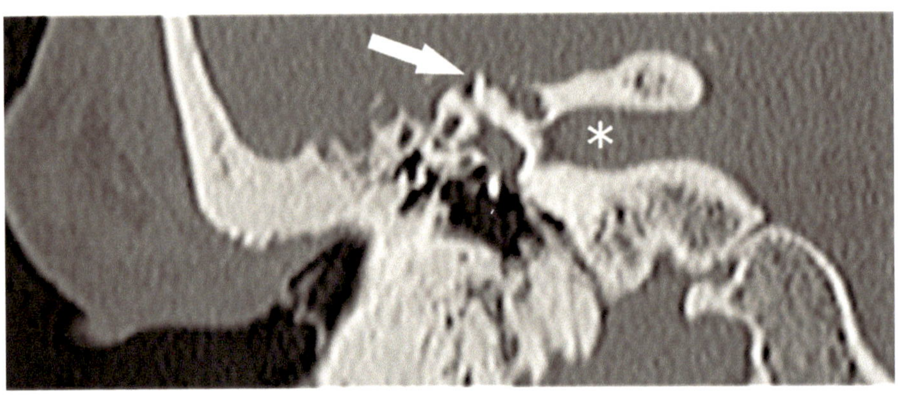

Fig. 17.4.2 On coronal CT an erosive lesion is visible that extends medially toward the internal auditory canal (✱). The tegmen is partially eroded and the superior semicircular canal (*arrow*) is affected cranially.

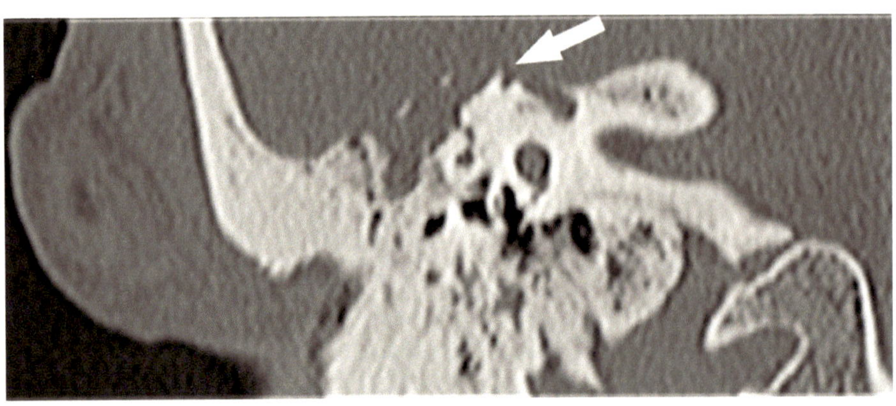

Fig. 17.4.3 More anteriorly, the same aspect is visible. Clear erosion of the SSC (*arrow*).

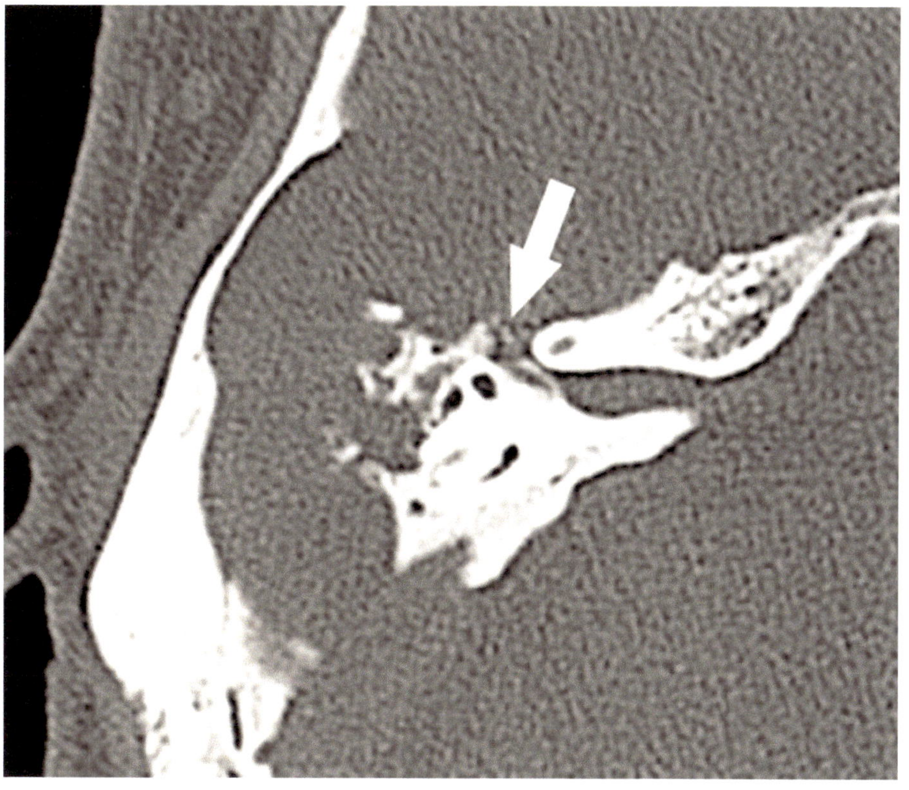

Fig. 17.4.4 The labyrinthine portion of the facial nerve (*arrow*) is also in close relation with the lesion.

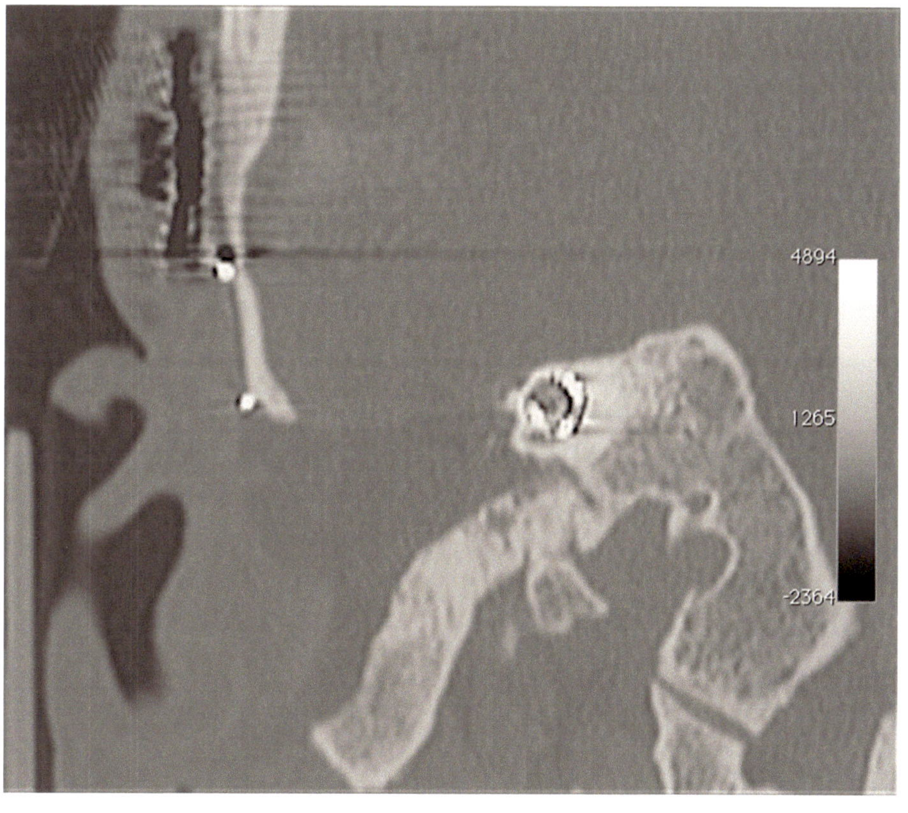

Fig. 17.4.5 After removal of the petrous bone cholesteatoma, using a combination of SP and translabyrinthine approach, the cochlea was found to be intact. Cochlear implantation was performed during the same procedure. The cavity was closed off from the external environment and filled with abdominal fat. This postoperative coronal CT scan shows the correct location of the array in the cochlea.

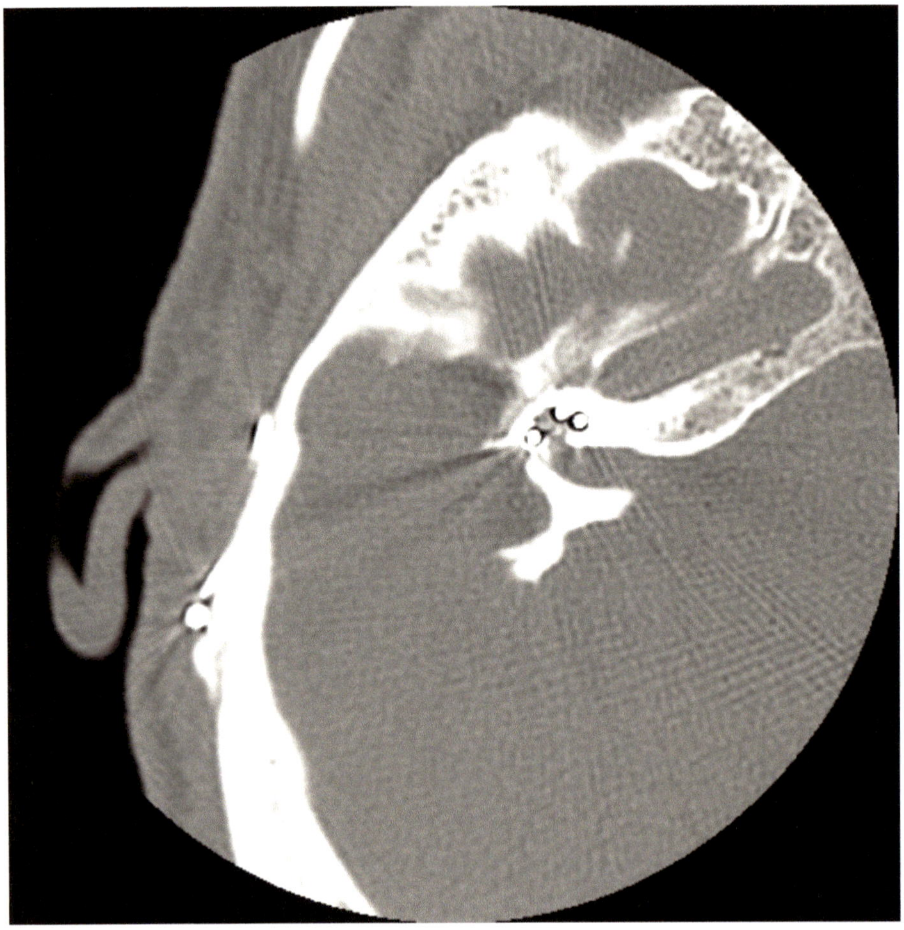

Fig. 17.4.6 Same postoperative CT scan in axial plane. Note the absence of the posterior labyrinth removed during the surgery.

Pearls and Pitfalls

- Cochlear implants and ABI can play a role in the revalidation of hearing in patients with skull base lesions and expansive lesions of the temporal bone, as well as in some more exceptional neurotologic pathology (Meniere disease, fracture).
- It is not unusual that a step-wise plan has to be made for each individual patient with a nonstandard auditory implant indication.
- In general the risks are the combination of the risks of the two surgeries (risks of skull base approach and CI/ABI).
- In the presence of significant alteration of the anatomy there can be a higher risk of a false route and nonauditory stimulation of the internal auditory canal or dehiscent facial nerve.
- Preoperative radiotherapy, chemotherapy, or embolization, if applicable, could lead to higher risks of infection, or could affect the outcome of cochlear implantation.
- In fractures of the temporal bone a risk of false route is present.
- Auditory implantation with CI or MRI will limit the possibility of MRI follow-up (due to artifacts), which might be necessary in this group of pathology. CT imaging will show contrast with the abdominal fat placed in the cavity and can be used for follow-up of the cavity (see Chapter 10).

Reference Video

See Video 17.1.

References

1. Merkus P, Di Lella F, Di Trapani G, et al. Indications and contraindications of auditory brainstem implants: systematic review and illustrative cases. Eur Arch Otorhinolaryngol 2014;271(1):3–13
2. Neff BA, Wiet RM, Lasak JM, et al. Cochlear implantation in the neurofibromatosis type 2 patient: long-term follow-up. Laryngoscope 2007;117(6):1069–1072
3. Ramsden R, Khwaja S, Green K, O'Driscoll M, Mawman D. Vestibular schwannoma in the only hearing ear: cochlear implant or auditory brainstem implant? Otol Neurotol 2005;26(2):261–264
4. Vincenti V, Pasanisi E, Guida M, Di Trapani G, Sanna M. Hearing rehabilitation in neurofibromatosis type 2 patients: cochlear versus auditory brainstem implantation. Audiol Neurootol 2008;13(4):273–280
5. Medina M, Di Lella F, Di Trapani G, et al. Cochlear implantation versus auditory brainstem implantation in bilateral total deafness after head trauma: personal experience and review of the literature. Otol Neurotol 2014;35(2):260–270
6. Chen DA, Linthicum FH Jr, Rizer FM. Cochlear histopathology in the labyrinthectomized ear: implications for cochlear implantation. Laryngoscope 1988;98(11):1170–1172
7. Belal A. Is cochlear implantation possible after acoustic tumor removal? Otol Neurotol 2001;22(4):497–500
8. Kveton JF, Abbot C, April M, Drumheller G, Cohen N, Poe DS. *Cochlear implanting after transmastoid labyrinthectomy.* Laryngoscope 1989;99:610–613
9. Facer GW, Facer ML, Fowler CM, Brey RH, Peterson AM. Cochlear implantation after labyrinthectomy. Am J Otol 2000;21(3):336–340
10. Friedman RA, Brackmann DE, Mills D. Auditory-nerve integrity after middle-fossa acoustic-tumor removal. Otolaryngol Head Neck Surg 1998;119(6):588–592
11. Marangos N, Stecker M, Laszig R. Topodiagnosis of deafness: strategy for treatment of neurofibromatosis type 2. J Laryngol Otol Suppl 2000;(27):3–7
12. Ramsden RT, Timms MS. Promontory stimulation following labyrinthectomy. J Laryngol Otol 1991;105(9):729–731

13. Tysome JR, Macfarlane R, Durie-Gair J, et al. Surgical management of vestibular schwannomas and hearing rehabilitation in neurofibromatosis type 2. Otol Neurotol 2012;33(3):466–472
14. Brown CJ. Clinical uses of electrically evoked auditory nerve and brainstem responses. Curr Opin Otolaryngol Head Neck Surg 2003;11(5):383–387
15. Arístegui M, Denia A. Simultaneous cochlear implantation and translabyrinthine removal of vestibular schwannoma in an only hearing ear: report of two cases (neurofibromatosis type 2 and unilateral vestibular schwannoma). Otol Neurotol 2005;26(2):205–210
16. Di Lella F, Merkus P, Di Trapani G, Taibah A, Guida M, Sanna M. Vestibular schwannoma in the only hearing ear: role of cochlear implants. Ann Otol Rhinol Laryngol 2013;122(2):91–99
17. Lustig LR, Yeagle J, Driscoll CLW, Blevins N, Francis H, Niparko JK. Cochlear implantation in patients with neurofibromatosis type 2 and bilateral vestibular schwannoma. Otol Neurotol 2006;27(4):512–518
18. Sanna M, Di Lella F, Guida M, Merkus P. Auditory brainstem implants in NF2 patients: results and review of the literature. Otol Neurotol 2012;33(2):154–164
19. Zanetti D, Campovecchi CB, Pasini S, Nassif N. Simultaneous translabyrinthine removal of acoustic neuroma and cochlear implantation. Auris Nasus Larynx 2008;35(4):562–568
20. Husseini ST, Guida M, Negri M, Falcioni M. Bilateral cochlear implantation in a patient with petrous bone cholesteatoma in the only hearing ear: case report. J Laryngol Otol 2011;125(12):1272–1274
21. Selivanova O, Gouveris H, Mann W. Cochlear implantation after surgery for bilateral jugular foramen paragangliomas: a case report. Eur Arch Otorhinolaryngol 2009;266(3):463–464
22. Roland JT Jr, Cosetti M, Liebman T, Waltzman S, Allen JC. Cochlear implantation following treatment for medulloblastoma. Laryngoscope 2010;120(1):139–143
23. Segel JM, McKinnon BJ. Bilateral cochlear implantation in bilateral Langerhans cell histiocytosis. Cochlear Implants Int 2013;14(3):178–180
24. Torkos A, Czigner J, Kiss JG, Tóth F, Szamosközi A, Jóri J. Cochlear implantation for treatment-induced ototoxic deafness in Langerhans cell histiocytosis. A case report. Eur Arch Otorhinolaryngol 2005;262(6):496–500
25. Formanek M, Czerny C, Gstoettner W, Kornfehl J. Cochlear implantation as a successful rehabilitation for radiation-induced deafness. Eur Arch Otorhinolaryngol 1998;255(4):175–178
26. Hoistad DL, Ondrey FG, Mutlu C, Schachern PA, Paparella MM, Adams GL. Histopathology of human temporal bone after cis-platinum, radiation, or both. Otolaryngol Head Neck Surg 1998;118(6):825–832
27. Low WK, Burgess R, Fong KW, Wang DY. Effect of radiotherapy on retro-cochlear auditory pathways. Laryngoscope 2005;115(10):1823–1826
28. Soh JM, D'Souza VD, Sarepaka GK, Ng WN, Ong CS, Low WK. Cochlear implant outcomes: a comparison between irradiated and non-irradiated ears. Clin Exp Otorhinolaryngol 2012;5(Suppl 1):S93–S98
29. Roehm PC, Mallen-St Clair J, Jethanamest D, et al. Auditory rehabilitation of patients with neurofibromatosis Type 2 by using cochlear implants. J Neurosurg 2011;115(4):827–834
30. Trotter MI, Briggs RJS. Cochlear implantation in neurofibromatosis type 2 after radiation therapy. Otol Neurotol 2010;31(2):216–219
31. Chua DY, Tan HK. Successful rehabilitation with cochlear implant in post-irradiation induced hearing loss in nasopharyngeal carcinoma patient. Ann Acad Med Singapore 2007;36(1):74–77
32. Adunka OF, Buchman CA. Cochlear implantation in the irradiated temporal bone. J Laryngol Otol 2007;121(1):83–86
33. Leonetti JP, Marzo SJ, Zender CA, Porter RG, Melian E. Temporal bone osteoradionecrosis after surgery and radiotherapy for malignant parotid tumors. Otol Neurotol 2010;31(4):656–659
34. Diaz RC, LaRouere MJ, Bojrab DI, Zappia JJ, Sargent EW, Shaia WT. Quality-of-life assessment of Ménière's disease patients after surgical labyrinthectomy. Otol Neurotol 2007;28(1):74–86
35. Morgan M, Flood L, Hawthorne M, Raje S. Chemical labyrinthectomy and cochlear implantation for Menière's disease—an effective treatment or a last resort? J Laryngol Otol 1999;113(7):666–669
36. Wareing MJ, O'Connor AF. The role of labyrinthectomy and cochlear implantation in Menière's disease. Ear Nose Throat J 1997;76(9):664–666, 668, 671–672
37. Zwolan TA, Shepard NT, Niparko JK. Labyrinthectomy with cochlear implantation. Am J Otol 1993;14(3):220–223
38. Watanabe I, Imai S, Ikeda M, Ishida A. Time series analysis of the course of Menière's disease. Acta Otolaryngol Suppl 1997;528:97–102
39. Osborn HA, Yeung R, Lin VYW. Delayed cochlear implantation after surgical labyrinthectomy. J Laryngol Otol 2012;126(1):63–65
40. Chung JH, Shin MC, Min HJ, Park CW, Lee SH. Bilateral cochlear implantation in a patient with bilateral temporal bone fractures. Am J Otolaryngol 2011;32(3):256–258
41. Vermeire K, Brokx JPL, Dhooge I, Van de Heyning PH. Cochlear implantation in posttraumatic bilateral temporal bone fracture. ORL J Otorhinolaryngol Relat Spec 2012;74(1):52–56
42. Zanetti D, Campovecchi CB, Pasini S. Binaural cochlear implantation after bilateral temporal bone fractures. Int J Audiol 2010;49(10):788–793
43. Lyos AT, Marsh MA, Jenkins HA, Coker NJ. Progressive hearing loss after transverse temporal bone fracture. Arch Otolaryngol Head Neck Surg 1995;121(7):795–799
44. Camilleri AE, Toner JG, Howarth KL, Hampton S, Ramsden RT. Cochlear implantation following temporal bone fracture. J Laryngol Otol 1999;113(5):454–457
45. Shin JH, Park S, Baek SH, Kim S. Cochlear implantation after bilateral transverse temporal bone fractures. Clin Exp Otorhinolaryngol 2008;1(3):171–173
46. Sudhoff H, Linthicum FH Jr. Temporal bone fracture and latent meningitis: temporal bone histopathology study of the month. Otol Neurotol 2003;24(3):521–522
47. Morgan WE, Coker NJ, Jenkins HA. Histopathology of temporal bone fractures: implications for cochlear implantation. Laryngoscope 1994;104(4):426–432
48. Chen ZN, Yin SK. Cochlear implantation in a patient with bilateral temporal bone fractures resulting from temporomandibular joint surgery. Chin Med J (Engl) 2012;125(22):4160
49. Pollak AM, Pauw BK, Marion MS. Temporal bone histopathology: residents' quiz. Otogenic pneumococci meningitis after transverse temporal bone fracture during childhood. Am J Otolaryngol 1991;12(1):56–58
50. Free RH, Falcioni M, Di Trapani G, Giannuzzi AL, Russo A, Sanna M. The role of subtotal petrosectomy in cochlear implant surgery—a report of 32 cases and review on indications. Otol Neurotol 2013;34(6):1033–1040

Further Reading

Bendet E, Cerenko D, Linder TE, Fisch U. Cochlear implantation after subtotal petrosectomies. Eur Arch Otorhinolaryngol 1998;255(4):169–174

Berryhill WE, Graham MD. Chemical and physical labyrinthectomy for Meniere's disease. Otolaryngol Clin North Am 2002;35(3):675–682

Colletti V, Carner M, Miorelli V, Guida M, Colletti L, Fiorino F. Cochlear implant failure: is an auditory brainstem implant the answer? Acta Otolaryngol 2004;124(4):353–357

Fisch U, Mattox D. Microsurgery of the Skull Base. Stuttgart: Thieme; 1988

Helbig S, Rader T, Bahmer A, Baumann U. A case of bilateral cochlear implantation in single-sided untreated acoustic neurinoma. Acta Otolaryngol 2009;129(6):694–696

Kveton JF, Tarlov EC, Drumheller G, Katcher P, Abbott C. Cochlear nerve conduction block: an explanation for spontaneous hearing return after acoustic tumor surgery. Otolaryngol Head Neck Surg 1989;100(6):594–601

Linthicum FH Jr, Brackmann DE. Bilateral acoustic tumors. A diagnostic and surgical challenge. Arch Otolaryngol 1980;106(12):729–733

Linthicum FH Jr, Fayad J, Otto S, Galey FR, House WF. Inner ear morphologic changes resulting from cochlear implantation. Am J Otol 1991;12(Suppl):8–10, discussion 18–21

Lustig LR, Yeagle J, Niparko JK, Minor LB. Cochlear implantation in patients with bilateral Ménière's syndrome. Otol Neurotol 2003;24(3):397–403

Merkus P, Taibah A, Sequino G, Sanna M. Less than 1% cerebrospinal fluid leakage in 1,803 translabyrinthine vestibular schwannoma surgery cases. Otol Neurotol 2010;31(2):276–283

Ransom ER, Judy KD, Bigelow DC. Concurrent cochlear implantation with resection of skull base hemangiopericytoma following sudden deafness in an only hearing ear. Skull Base 2010;20(4):279–284

Shin YJ, Fraysse B, Sterkers O, Bouccara D, Rey A, Lazorthes Y. Hearing restoration in posterior fossa tumors. Am J Otol 1998;19(5):649–653

Toh EH, Luxford WM. Cochlear and brainstem implantation. 2002. Neurosurg Clin N Am 2008;19(2):317–329, vii

Wiet RJ, Harvey SA, O'Connor CA. Recent advances in surgery of the temporal bone and skull base. South Med J 1993;86(1):5–12

18 Bone Conduction Implants

Bone conduction implants deliver the acoustic stimulus directly through the skull bones to the inner ear, bypassing the outer and middle ear structures. They can be divided in two main groups:

- **Implantable devices with a transcutaneous abutment**, properly called bone anchored hearing aids (BAHAs), in which sound vibrations are received and amplified by a sound processor that is connected to an osteointegrated transcutaneous fixture. The sound processor and the fixture work like an active unit transmitting the sound to the bone.
- **Implantable devices without transcutaneous abutment**, in which the sound processor is magnetically coupled to the osteointegrated bone anchored implant and the sound is transmitted through the skin to the magnetic implant that is thus passively stimulated.

Implantable bone conduction devices have been developed to restore hearing in patients with disease affecting the external or middle ear in whom conventional surgery has been performed with poor functional results or in whom surgical rehabilitation is contraindicated (e.g., otosclerosis in the only hearing ear. Due to the good results and the relative ease of the surgical procedures, the implantable bone conduction systems have rapidly gained favor since their introduction and indications have expanded to include many other conditions such as single-sided deafness.

18.1 Indications

Indications for implantable bone conduction devices can be divided into audiologic and otologic subgroups.

18.1.1 Audiologic Indications

CHL and MHL

Conductive hearing loss (CHL) and mixed hearing loss (MHL): with a bone conduction pure-tone average (PTA) between 0 and 45 or 55 dB HL (depending on the speech processor) and a speech discrimination score (SDS) of more than 60%. Bone conduction implants require less signal amplification than conventional hearing aids as the conductive loss is completely bypassed; this is particularly relevant in patients with a mean conductive loss of 30 dB or more.[1]

SSD

Single-sided deafness (SSD): bone conduction implantable devices are also indicated in the audiologic rehabilitation of patients suffering from severe to profound hearing loss or anacusis on one side and with a contralateral bone conduction PTA not exceeding 20 dB with an SDS better than 60%. Implantation on the deaf side allows for decrease in the head shadow effect and improves sound discrimination in noise.[2]

Generally speaking, implantable devices with transcutaneous abutment are considered more powerful than the analog devices without transcutaneous fixtures as sound vibrations are directly transmitted into the bone.

18.1.2 Otologic Indications

Otologic indications include deaf patients affected by congenital or acquired middle or external ear pathologies in whom surgical hearing rehabilitation is not indicated or has already been performed with poor functional results.

Chronic Otitis Media and Sequelae

- Chronic otitis media (COM) and cholesteatoma surgery sequelae with failure to restore a normally aerated middle ear and reduce/close the air–bone gap after properly performed tympanoplasty and ossiculoplasty.
- Radical cavities

Implantable bone conduction devices avoid the need for conventional endaural or retroauricular hearing aids, reducing the risk of infection and otorrhea in chronic ear patients. Patients with radical cavities or canal wall down tympanoplasties usually have a large external auditory meatus; they often require high amplification and a custom-made mold, with the accompanying risk of acoustic feedback.

Otosclerosis and Tympanosclerosis

Implantable bone conduction devices represent an option in patients with otosclerosis for whom surgery is not an option because of (multiple) previous unsuccessful surgeries or anatomical anomalies. The implantable systems are valid alternatives to the air conduction device if the air–bone gap exceeds 30 dB, due to their better performance and the absence of feedback.

Chronic External Auditory Canal Disease

Chronic external auditory canal disease (i.e., dermatitis, recurrent infections) and/or poor compliance with conventional hearing aids (because of itching or the occlusion effect) may be considered indications for implantable bone conduction devices.[2]

Aural Atresia

In the pediatric age group, the most common indication for a BAHA is bilateral congenital malformations represented by congenital aural atresia, in which functional surgery is known to achieve poor hearing results and may have significant complications.[2]

Middle Ear Obliteration/Subtotal Petrosectomy

Patients who have undergone middle ear obliteration or subtotal petrosectomy with blind-sac closure of the external auditory canal obtain significant benefit from the implantable bone conduction devices if there is a cochlear reserve according to the audiologic criteria.

18.2 Contraindications

Implantable bone conduction devices are contraindicated if the SDS is lower than 60% and the bone PTA (in the better hearing ear) exceeds 55 dB. Implantable devices, moreover, are contraindicated in patients with previously irradiated bone and psychiatric disease. Inability to maintain adequate hygiene represents a contraindication, as poor hygiene is a common reason for adverse skin reactions. Diabetic patients do not have an increased risk of implant loss or skin problems.

18.3 Implantable Devices with Transcutaneous Abutment

The BAHA and Ponto systems, developed by the Cochlear and Oticon companies, respectively, are defined as bone anchored hearing aids, being composed of an external sound processor and an implantable transcutaneous part. The implantable part is composed of a screw (the fixture) that is fastened to the bone and an abutment to which the sound processor is attached. Both the screw and the abutment length can be preoperatively decided according to each individual patient considering bone and skin thickness.

18.3.1 Preoperative Evaluation

In implantable devices such as the BAHA and Ponto systems, the external part (sound processor) actively transmits sound vibrations to the fixture screwed to the parietotemporal cortical bone; this allows for preoperative trials using cutaneous couplers.

Specific preoperative evaluation includes complete audiologic and otologic evaluation (i.e., otomicroscopy, tonal threshold, and speech discrimination score) and may be extended to include free field tonal audiometry and discrimination with and without the use of the device, allowing professionals and patients to objectively evaluate the change in auditory performances.

There are many cutaneous couplers available:

- **Rod-test:** a small rigid rod attached to the sound processor is kept in contact with the tip of the mastoid bone, the forehead, or the incisor teeth while using the device. This test allows the patients to have a quick estimation of possible benefits.
- **Test band/head band:** these are hairband-like steel springs attached to the sound processor. The test band is used for preoperative evaluation, while the softer head band may allow the use of the sound processor in patients who present temporary or permanent contraindications to the surgical implantation of the fixture (i.e., bone thickness less than 3 mm).
- **Soft band:** the sound processor may also be tested preoperatively mounted on a bandeaux-like band. The soft band may be used in children younger than 5 years of age who require auditory rehabilitation (i.e., in case of bilateral aural atresia).

The use of the soft band and head band or the test rod offers an easy, fast, and objective way of assessing bone conduction capacity that allows the patient to directly experience bone-conducted sound.

It should be made clear to the patients and parents that the subjective benefit obtained in these tests will be less than achieved by using the processor coupled to the osseointegrated fixture.

Preoperative temporoparietal bone thickness may be evaluated in young children (>5 years of age) and in adults undergoing revision surgery or surgery in a multioperated site by the means of a standard unenhanced temporal bone CT scan.

18.3.2 Key Features of the Devices

See **Fig. 18.1** and **Fig. 18.2**.

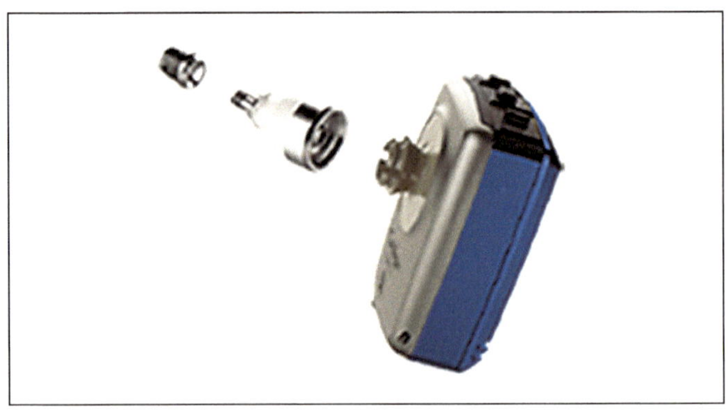

Fig. 18.1 Cochlear BAHA device: left to right, the fixture, the abutment, and the audioprocessor.

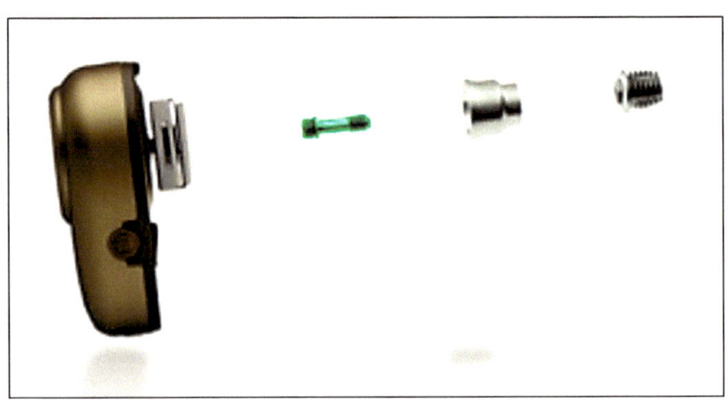

Fig. 18.2 Oticon PONTO device: right to left, the fixture, the abutment, the screw connecting the abutment and fixture, the audio processor.

18.3.3 Specific Indications

Audiologic indications for both devices include:

- Conductive hearing loss (CHL) or mixed hearing loss (MHL), with an average bone conduction threshold ≤45 dB (Ponto Pro and BAHA BP100) or 55 dB (Ponto Pro Power and BAHA BP110) and a speech discrimination score (SDS) of more than 60%. For bilateral fitting, the criterion is symmetric bone conduction thresholds (i.e., there is less than a 10 dB difference on average across 0.5, 1, 2, and 3 kHz, or less than 15 dB difference at individual frequencies).
- Single-sided deafness (SSD): bone conduction implantable devices are also indicated in the audiologic rehabilitation of patients suffering from severe to profound hearing loss or anacusis on one side. The contralateral average bone conduction threshold should not exceed 20 dB with a SDS better than 60%.

18.3.4 Contraindications

Implantable bone conduction devices with transcutaneous fixture are contraindicated in children younger than 5 years and in patients with a skull bone thickness of less than 3 mm.

18.3.5 Surgical Technique

Since Tjellstrom and colleagues first introduced the BAHA system in 1977,[3] the surgical procedure has been modified, with several teams reporting their adjustments. There are two major goals: osseointegration and prevention of soft tissue reactions. Currently two techniques are commonly used, one with skin (subcutaneous) thinning and the other without skin thinning. Thinning of the skin has been developed to prevent soft tissue movement around the implant, to reduce the amount of scar tissue formation, and to provide a thin hairless skin area directly in contact with the deeper bony layer.

The second technique is more straightforward as it does not require skin thinning; recent findings have demonstrated that patients treated without skin thinning showed favorable results in terms of skin reaction and implant integration after 2 years of follow-up.[4]

18.3.6 Postoperative Management and Follow-up

After surgery, standard care practices are adopted for the wound. If the postoperative period is uneventful, a manufacturer's technician activates the implant after 4 to 6 weeks.

18.3.7 Placement of an Implantable Device with Transcutaneous Abutment Using the Skin Thinning Technique: Surgical Steps

Marking the Implant Site

The implant should be located ~50 to 55 mm from the ear canal so that the sound processor will not touch the pinna in its final position. We usually mark the implant site on the temporal line. The skin incision is marked 10 mm anterior to the implant site, parallel to the hairline. An elliptical/rectangular area of 40 to 60 mm is then marked around the incision line for subsequent subcutaneous tissue reduction (see **Fig. 18.1.1**).

When planning the implant site one should be certain to consider anatomical variations due to congenital malformations or previous surgery, as well as the location of future reconstructive surgery. Patients with congenital microsomia may have a contracted mastoid process, low-lying middle fossa dura, and a sigmoid sinus closer than usual to the mastoid surface. However, sufficient bone for an implant is usually found.

Anesthesia

In adults the procedure is generally performed under local anesthesia. In children general anesthesia is preferred. The marked area is injected with a local anesthetic of lidocaine and epinephrine; usually 10 mL is used to infiltrate the skin and periosteum at the implant site.

Skin Incision and Soft Tissue Reduction

A 3- to 4-cm skin incision is made and carried to the periosteal layer, which is left intact, severing the skin and muscular layers (see **Fig. 18.1.2**).

Subcutaneous tissue around the skin incision is removed for an area of 40 to 60 mm marked out earlier. A large no. 22 knife blade is introduced into the dermis and moved parallel to the skin surface, removing the deep dermal and fat subcutaneous layers, and thus removing the hair follicles as well. The thickness of the skin around the incision should be less than 1 mm (see **Fig. 18.1.3**). The aim of the soft tissue reduction is to achieve a gradual tension-free edge sloping down toward the implant area.

Keeping the periosteum intact is extremely important for the blood supply required for the healing of the skin flap.

Periosteal Incision

A percutaneous needle is used through the skin at the implant site to identify the periosteal area to be addressed. A self-retaining retractor is placed to hold the edges of the incision and a cruciate incision is made in the periosteum. The four triangular periosteal flaps are raised using a microraspatory (see **Fig. 18.1.4**).

Bone Drilling

The implant site is prepared using the guide drill at high speed (2,000 rpm) under abundant irrigation to minimize bone heating. Bone drilling is initiated with the guide drill, keeping the spacer on 3 mm and the drill indicator attached (see **Fig. 18.1.5**). During drilling the bur is moved up and down and around to ensure that the cooling solution reaches the tip of the drill. While gradually deepening and widening the hole with the guide drill, it is important not to over-widen the section that will contain the implant as this may cause initial instability. The bottom of the hole is repeatedly checked visually and with a blunt dissector to check for bone at the base of the site. If there is adequate bone thickness, the spacer is removed, allowing drilling to continue to a depth of 4 mm (see **Fig. 18.1.6**). Drilling continues in the same manner, using the whole length of the drill to allow space for the countersink. In most adults there is sufficient bone thickness for a 4 mm implant.

During this step it is possible to penetrate the wall of the sigmoid sinus and open the dura mater; therefore, the surgeon should proceed with care.

Cooling is very important for all drilling procedures. Heat can damage the bone tissue and jeopardize osseointegration. It is important that the drilling is performed perpendicular to the skin surface, since this orientation will affect the orientation of the implant and the abutment. The drill indicator will facilitate correct drill orientation and should be used both with the guide drill and with the countersink drill.

Countersink Drilling

After preparation of the primary hole for the implant, the next step is to widen the hole to the exact diameter of the fixture.

This procedure is carried out with either a 3-mm or a 4-mm countersink drill, depending on the depth reached with the guide drill. The countersink is used at high speed (2,000 rpm) and should be moved up and down during drilling while ensuring that the cooling solution reaches the tip of the drill. Bone chips should be removed from the drill flutes frequently. When the surface is uneven, the countersink allows the flange of the titanium screw to have maximum contact with the bone surface.

The tip of the countersink is blunt to minimize the risk of damaging tissues (e.g., dura) at the bottom of the hole and a stop collar prevents excessive countersinking (see **Fig. 18.1.7**).

Implant Positioning

Implant insertion is performed using the same handpiece at a low speed setting. The torque limit on the motor panel should be adjusted according to the quality of the bone. In compact cortical bone a setting between 30 and 40 N-cm is recommended. In soft bone a lower torque setting of 10 to 20 N-cm should be used.

The self-tapping fixture with premounted abutment is delivered sterile and it is picked up with the abutment inserter (see **Fig. 18.1.8**). It is recommended that the drill indicator is also used during implant insertion.

The implant is installed without irrigation until the small grooves in the distal end of the implant are well within the canal so as to avoid distal contamination. After this step the implant placement continues under abundant irrigation. If the implant enters the hole on a wrong axis, the drill motor is put into reverse. The correct angle is then found and the implant is re-inserted. Here the drill indicator may be useful for setting the correct angle (see **Fig. 18.1.9**).

When the flange of the implant has reached the bone surface it stops automatically. The abutment inserter is then removed from the abutment. The periosteal flaps are then replaced near the implant base (see **Fig. 18.1.10**).

Skin Closure and Exteriorization of the Abutment

The skin is sutured in layers over the abutment. A hole is punched exactly over the abutment using a 4-mm-wide biopsy punch. The skin is carefully eased down over the abutment (see **Fig. 18.1.11**). If necessary, two small incisions are made to facilitate the process.

The healing cap is snapped onto the abutment and a long gauze soaked with antibiotic ointment, is loosely packed circumferentially around the implant. Alternatively, a custom-tailored foam dressing may be used (see **Fig. 18.1.12**). The healing cap should gently hold the dressing in place to compress the thinned skin in close contact with the bone. This prevents hematoma formation and allows direct apposition of the skin and periosteal layers.

A mastoid dressing is applied. The head bandage is usually not necessary.

Case 18.1 Bone Anchored Hearing Aid (Fig. 18.1.1–Fig. 18.1.12)

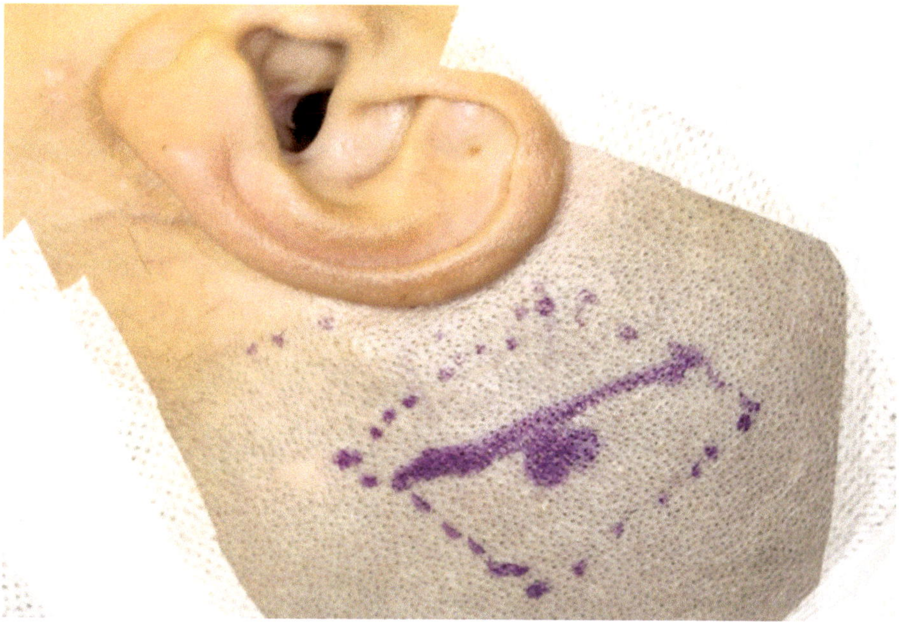

Fig. 18.1.1 Male patient. The skin incision is marked 10 mm anterior to the implant site, parallel to the hairline. An elliptical/rectangular area of 40 to 60 mm is then marked around the incision line for subsequent subcutaneous tissue reduction.

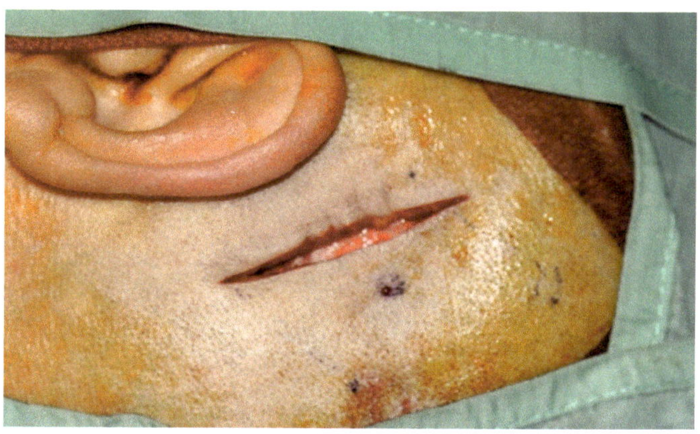

◀ **Fig. 18.1.2** A 3- to 4-cm-long skin incision is made and carried into the periosteal layer, which is left intact, severing the skin and muscular layers.

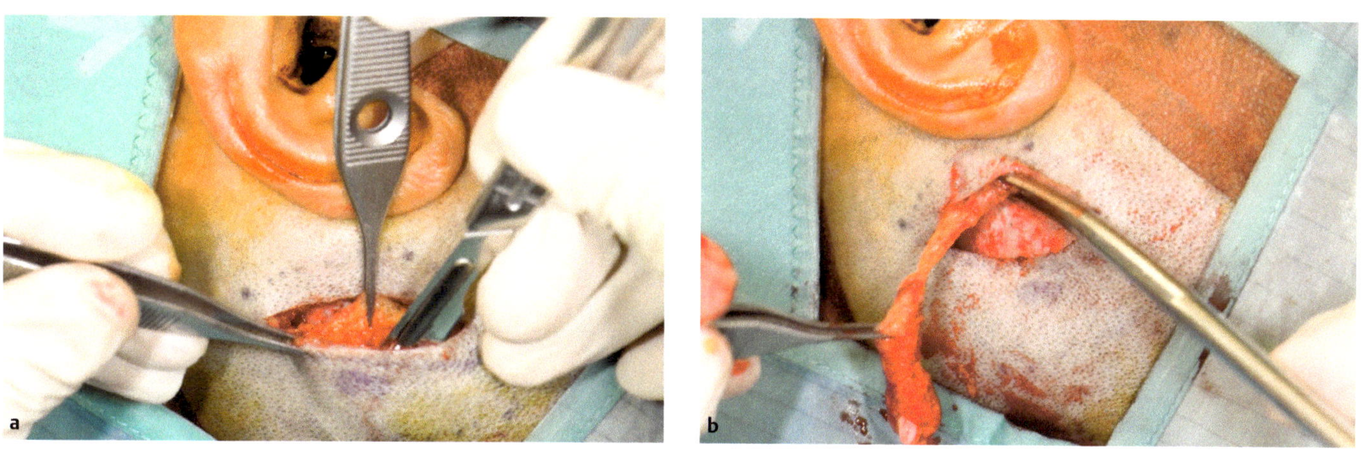

Fig. 18.1.3a, b

a A large no. 22 knife blade is introduced in the dermis and moved parallel to the skin surface, removing the deep dermal and fat subcutaneous layers up to the hair follicles.

b The subcutaneous tissue is then removed in the premarked area of 40 to 60 mm around the incision.

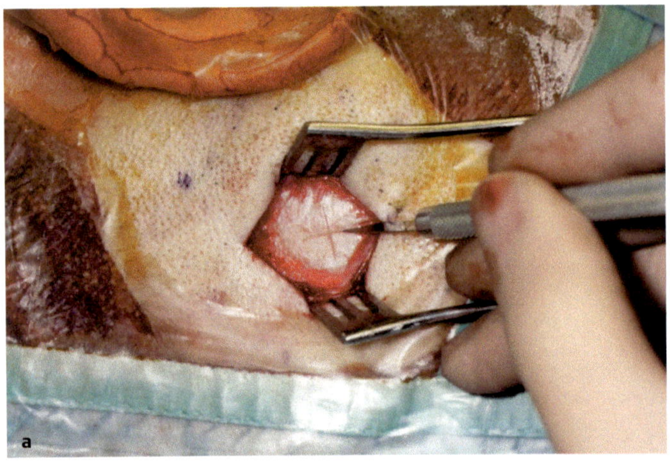

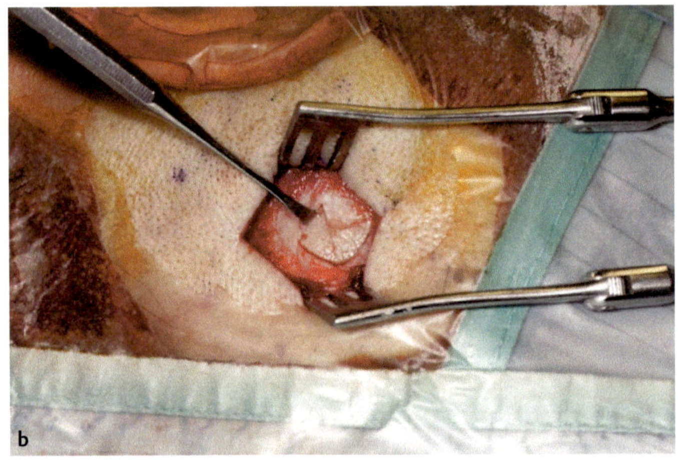

Fig. 18.1.4a, b A percutaneous needle is used through the skin at the implant site to identify the periosteal area to be addressed. A cruciate incision is then made in the periosteum (**a**) and the four flaps carefully elevated with a microraspatory (**b**).

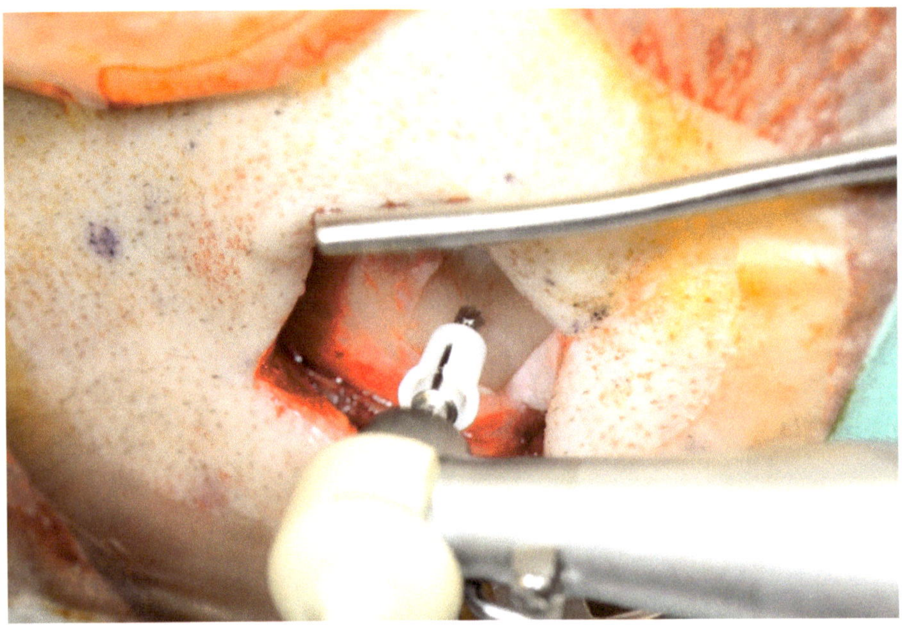

Fig. 18.1.5 Bone drilling is initiated with the guide drill, keeping the spacer on 3 mm and the drill indicator attached.

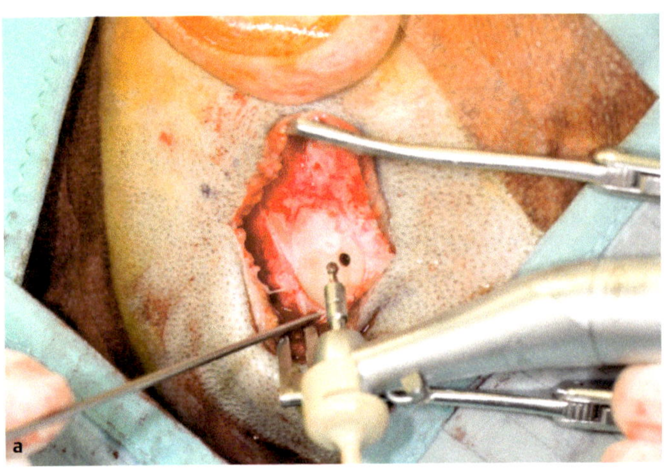

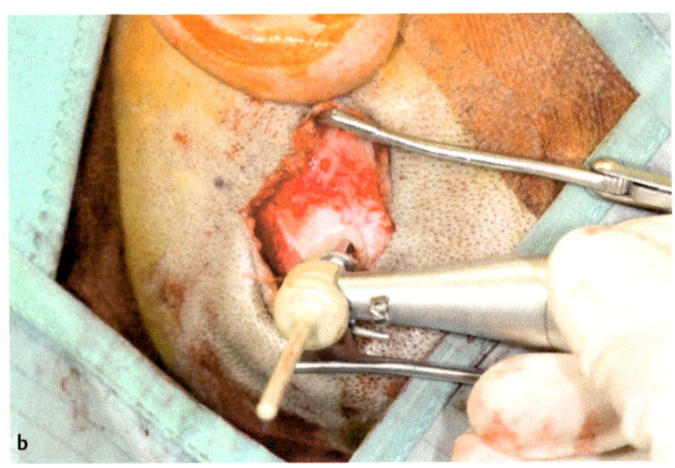

Fig. 18.1.6a, b If there is adequate bone thickness, the spacer is removed, allowing drilling to continue to a depth of 4 mm.

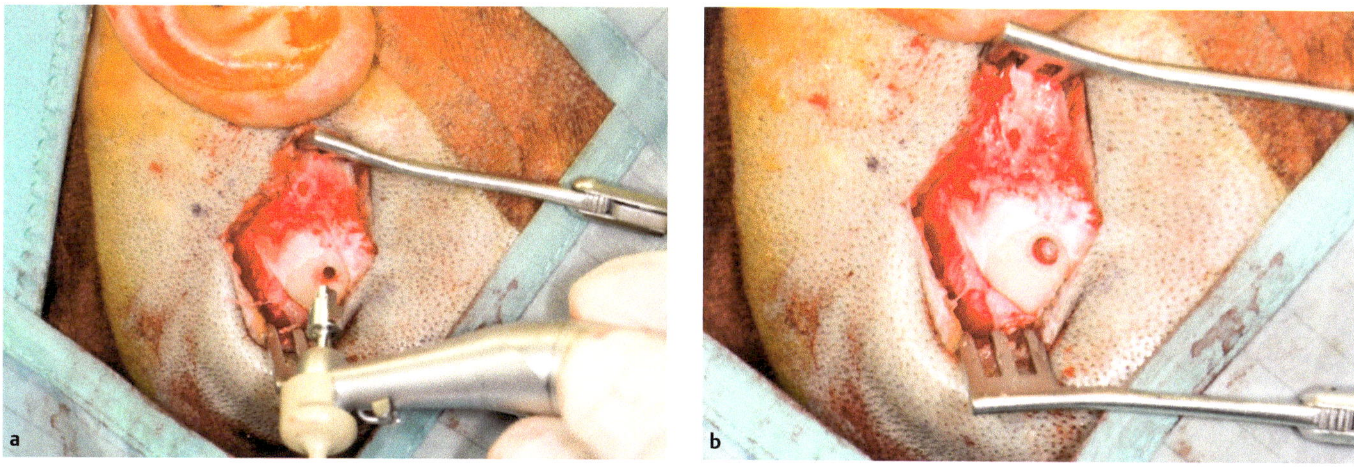

Fig. 18.1.7a, b Countersink drilling is used to widen the hole to the exact diameter of the fixture.

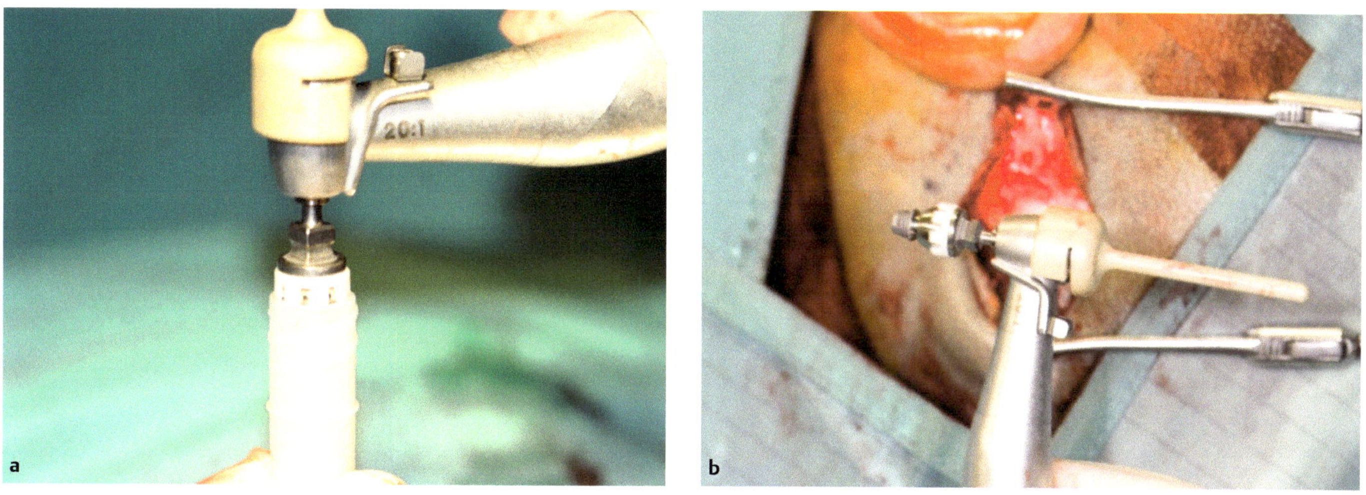

Fig. 18.1.8a, b The self-tapping fixture with premounted abutment is delivered sterile and it is picked up with the abutment inserter.

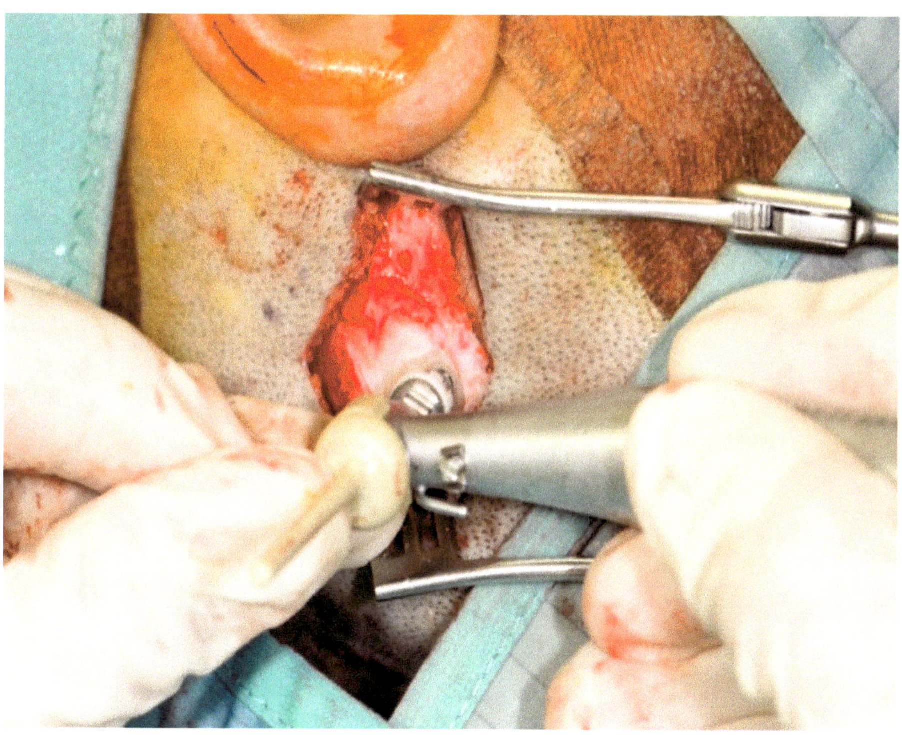

Fig. 18.1.9 The implant is installed without irrigation until the small grooves in the distal end of the implant are well within the canal so as to avoid distal contamination. The drill guide is used to achieve an optimal angle of insertion.

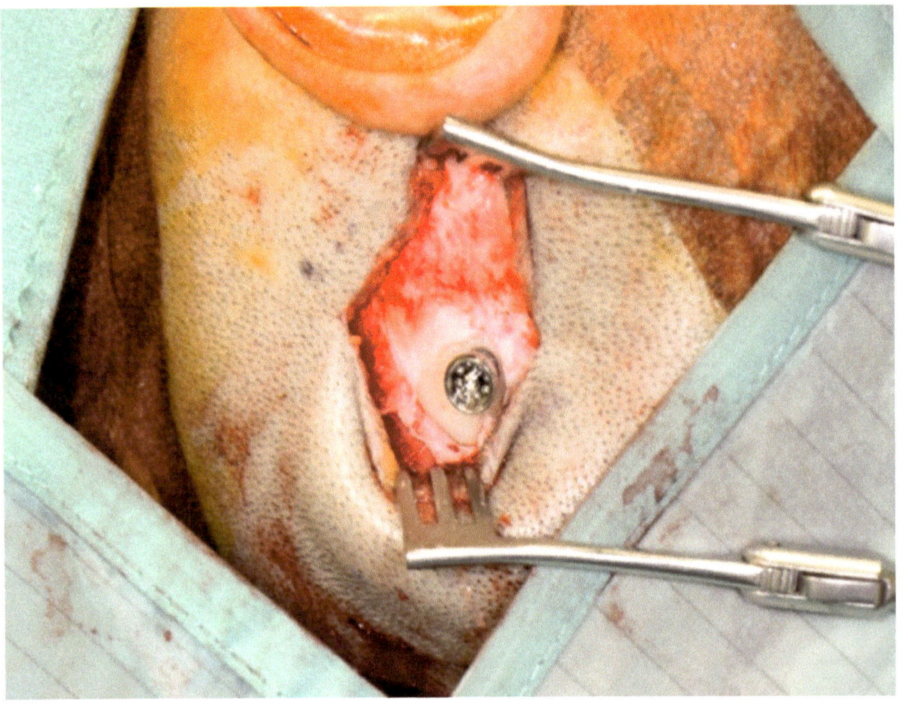

Fig. 18.1.10 The implant is inserted using the same drill handpiece at a low speed setting; it will automatically stops when the flanges of the implant reach the bone surface. The torque limit on the motor panel should be adjusted according to the quality of the bone. In compact cortical bone a setting between 30 and 40 N-cm is recommended. The periosteal flaps are then replaced near the implant base.

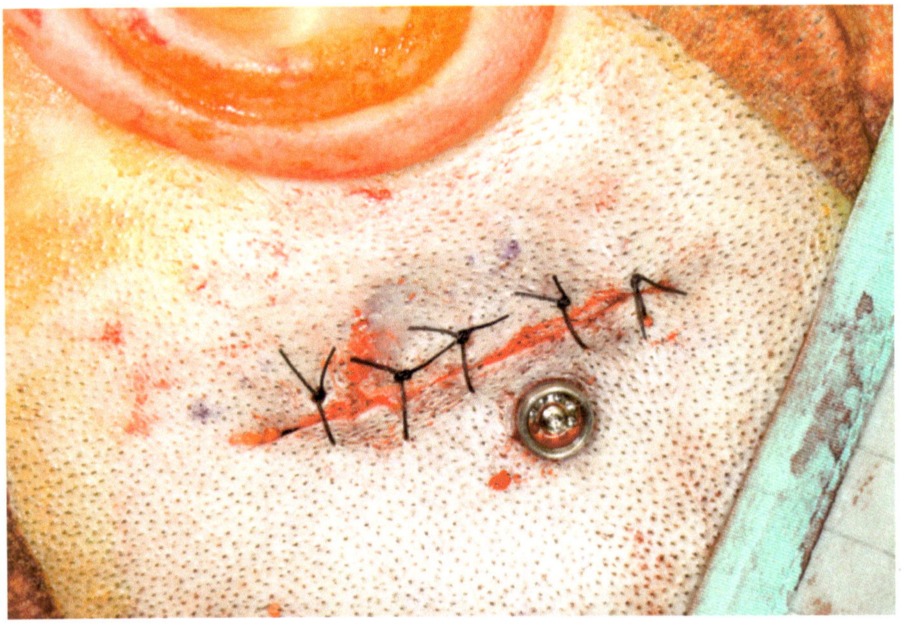

Fig. 18.1.11 The skin is sutured in layers over the abutment. A hole is then punched exactly over the abutment using a 4-mm-wide biopsy punch.

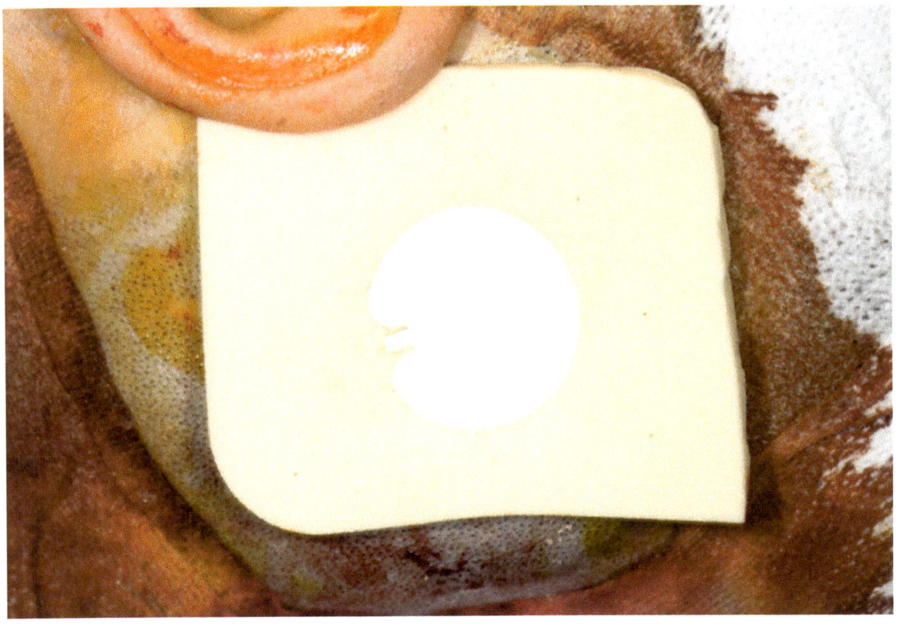

Fig. 18.1.12 The healing cap is snapped onto the abutment and a foam dressing is adapted to circumferentially enclose the implant.

Placement of an Implantable Device with Transcutaneous Abutment Using the Intact Skin Technique: Surgical Steps

Marking the Implant Site

As for the previously described technique with skin thinning, the implant should be located ~50 to 55 mm from the ear canal so that the sound processor will not touch the pinna in its final position. We usually mark the implant site on the temporal line. The skin incision is marked 10 mm anterior to the implant site, parallel to the hairline (see **Fig. 18.2.1**). In the intact skin technique, the implant can also be exteriorized through the incision. There is no need to mark the subcutaneous area to be thinned.

Measuring Skin Thickness

When using this technique, measurement of the skin thickness is a fundamental part of the procedure. It can be done with a thin needle *before* injection of local anesthetic (see **Fig. 18.2.2**). Compression of the skin should be avoided.

Choice of the Abutment Height

The choice of the height (length) of the abutment is based on skin thickness. With this technique, soft tissue reduction is only required for patients with a skin thicker than 10 mm. To obtain the ideal abutment height, 2 or 3 mm should be added to the measured skin thickness (see **Fig. 18.2.3**).

Anesthesia

The steps are the same as in the previous technique; in this case less anesthetic is required.

Skin Incision

The steps are the same as in the previous technique.

Periosteal Incision

A percutaneous needle is used through the skin at the implant site to identify the periosteal area to be addressed. A self-retaining retractor is placed to hold the edges of the incision and a cruciate incision is made in the periosteum. The four triangular periosteal flaps are raised using a microraspatory (see **Fig. 18.2.4**).

Bone Drilling

The steps are the same as in the previous technique (see **Fig. 18.2.5**).

Countersink Drilling

The hole for the implant is widened with the appropriate countersink drill (3 or 4 mm) using a speed of 2,000 rpm and cooling with saline irrigation. The drill should be kept free of bone deposits to avoid heat trauma to the surrounding tissues. The drill has a stop collar that helps prevent excessive countersinking (see **Fig. 18.2.6**).

Implant Positioning

The steps are the same as in the previous technique (see **Fig. 18.2.7** and **Fig. 18.2.8**).

Skin Closure and Exteriorization of the Abutment

The skin is closed in layers over the abutment. A hole is punched exactly over the abutment using a 4-mm-wide biopsy punch and a cylinder of skin is removed. The skin is gently eased over the abutment (see **Fig. 18.2.9**).

The healing cap is snapped onto the abutment and a long gauze, 1 cm wide and soaked with antibiotic ointment, is loosely packed circumferentially around the implant (see **Fig. 18.2.10**). A mastoid dressing is applied. The head bandage is usually not necessary.

Case 18.2 Bone Anchored Hearing Aid (Fig. 18.2.1–Fig. 18.2.10)

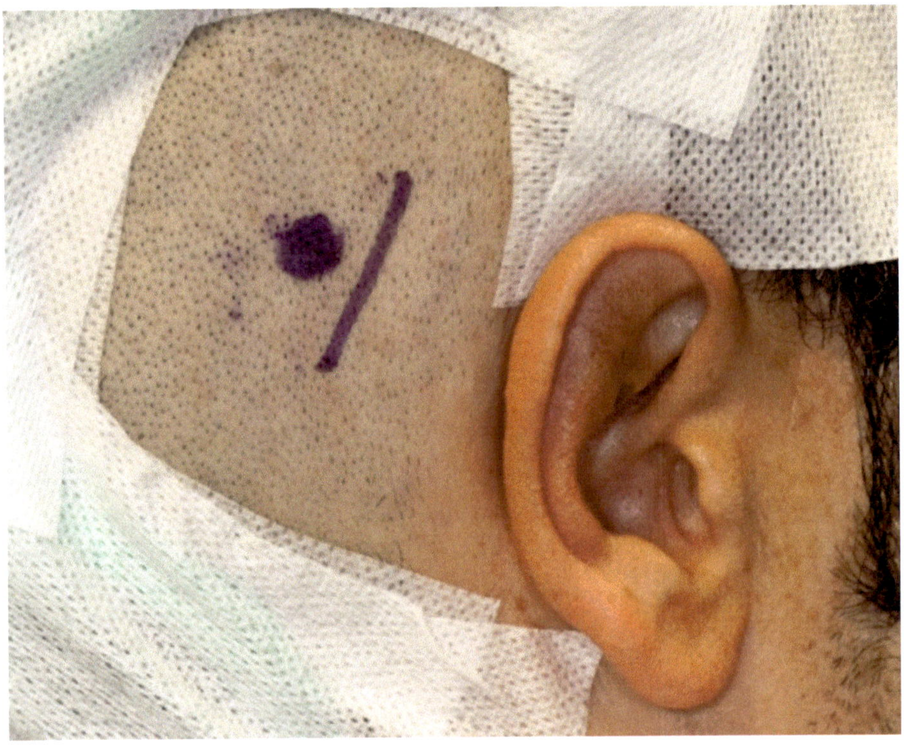

Fig. 18.2.1 Male patient. The implant should be located ~50 to 55 mm from the ear canal so that the sound processor will not touch the pinna in its final position. The implant site is usually marked on the temporal line. The skin incision is marked 10 mm anterior to the implant site, parallel to the hairline. In the intact skin technique, the implant can also be exteriorized through the incision. There is no need to mark the subcutaneous area to be thinned.

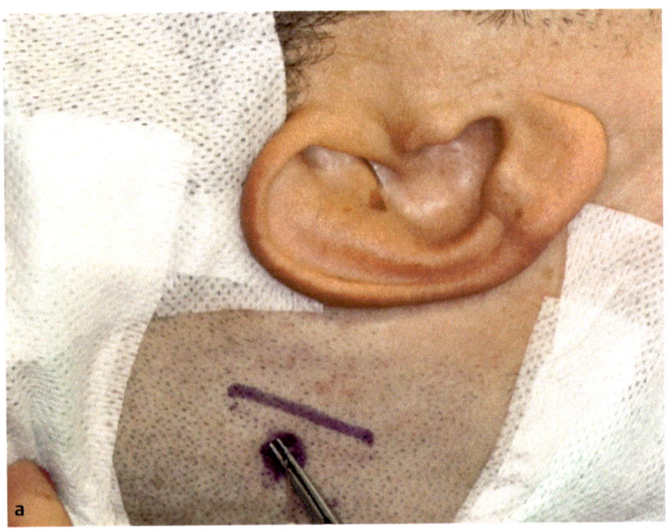

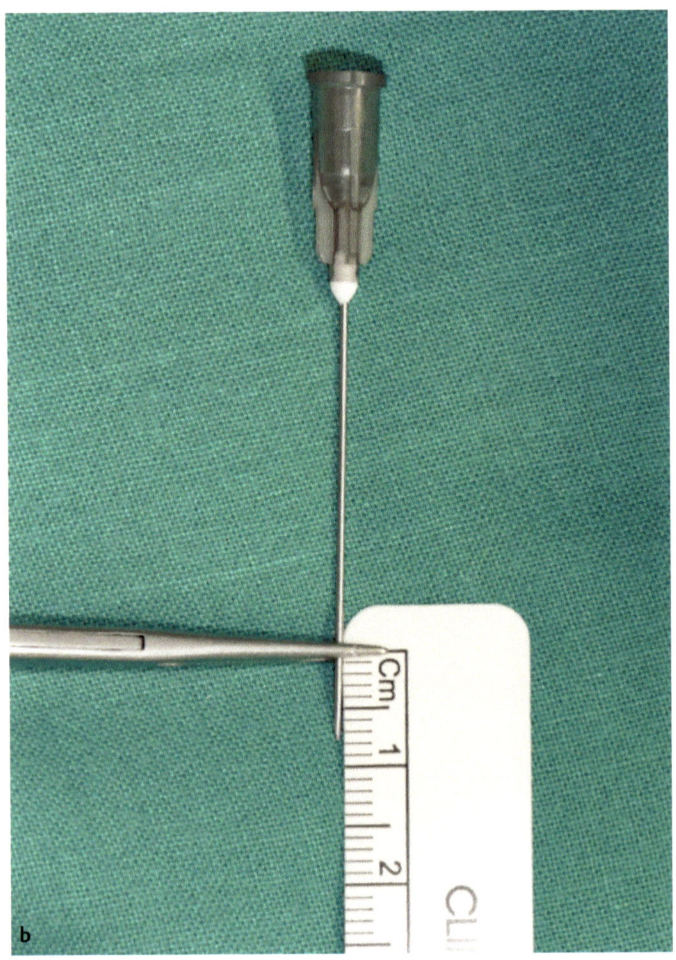

Fig. 18.2.2a, b Skin thickness is measured using a thin needle before injection of local anesthetic.

Approximate tissue thickness (mm)	Abutment length (mm)
3 or less	6
4-5	8
6-7	10
8-9	12
10 or more	12 with soft tissue reduction

◄ **Fig. 18.2.3** The choice of the height of the abutment is based on skin thickness. Soft tissue reduction is only required for patients with skin thicker than 10 mm. To obtain the ideal abutment height, 2 or 3 mm should be added to the measured skin thickness.

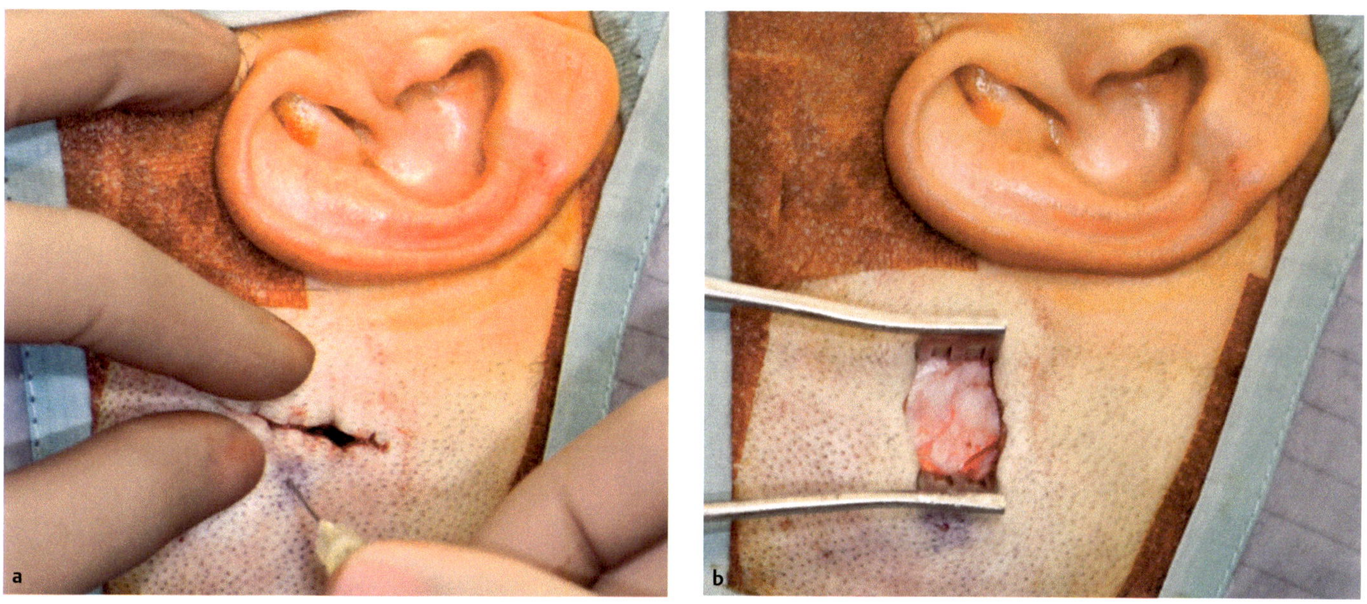

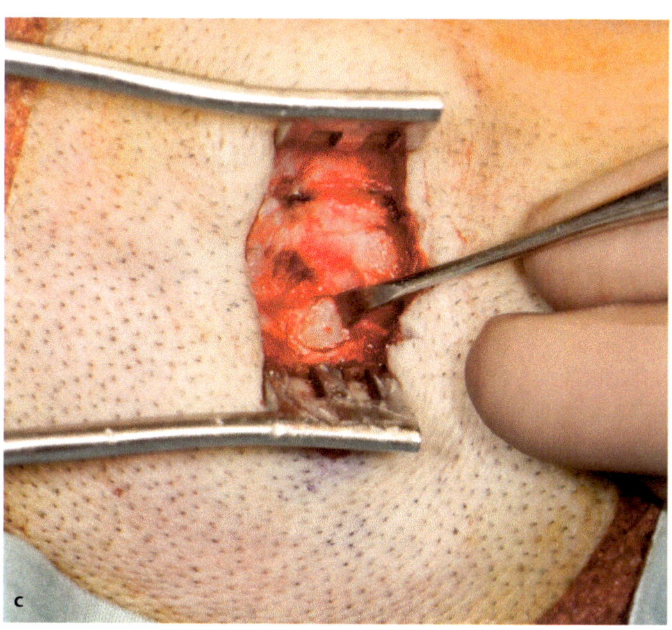

Fig. 18.2.4a–c The skin incision is carried through skin, subcutaneous tissue, and muscle to the periosteal plane, which is initially left intact. A percutaneous needle is used through the skin at the implant site to identify the periosteal area to be addressed (**a**). A self-retaining retractor is placed to hold the edges of the incision and a cruciate incision is made in the periosteum (**b**). The four triangular shaped periosteal flaps are carefully detached from bone using a microraspatory (**c**).

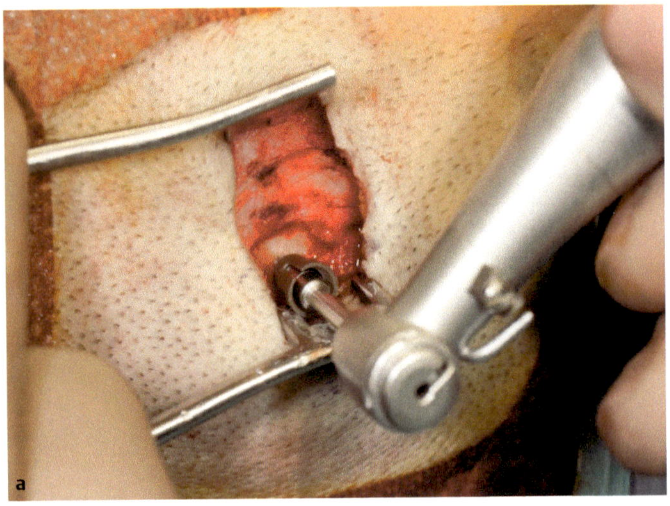

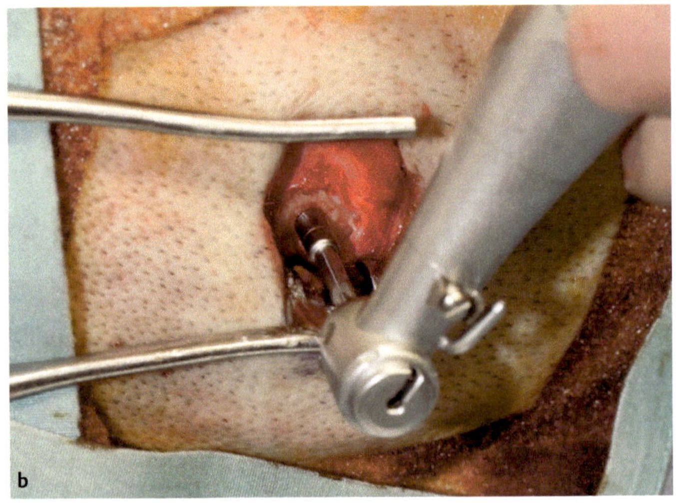

Fig. 18.2.5a, b
a Bone drilling is initiated with the guide drill, keeping the spacer on 3 mm.
b If there is enough bone, the spacer is removed and a 4-mm depth drill is used. The fundus is checked carefully with blunt instruments.

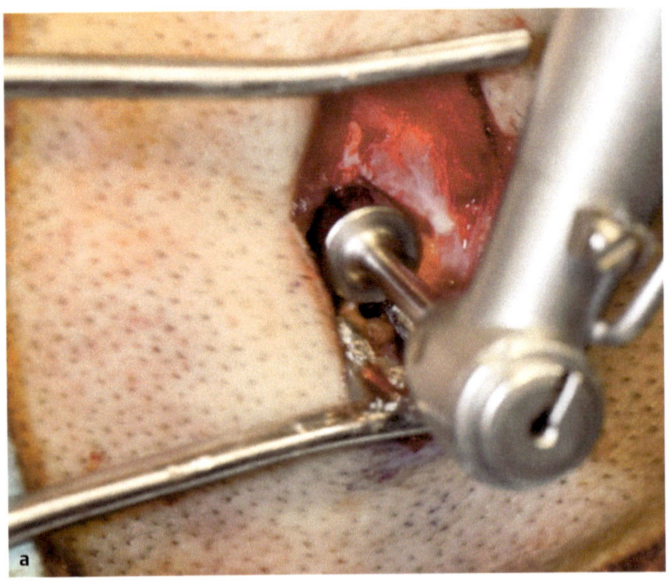

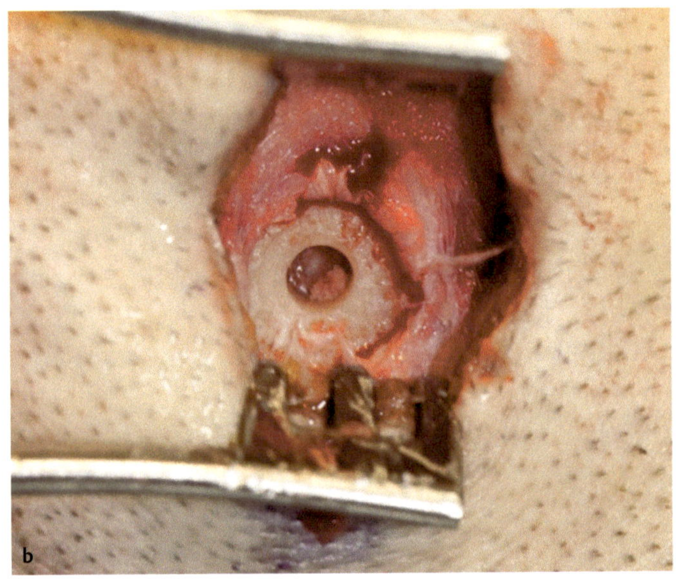

Fig. 18.2.6a, b The hole for the implant is widened with the appropriate countersink drill (3 or 4 mm) using a speed of 2,000 rpm and cooling with saline irrigation **(a)**. The drill has a stop collar that prevents excessive countersink and a double thread to create a double ring in the bone in order to better accommodate the abutment **(b)**.

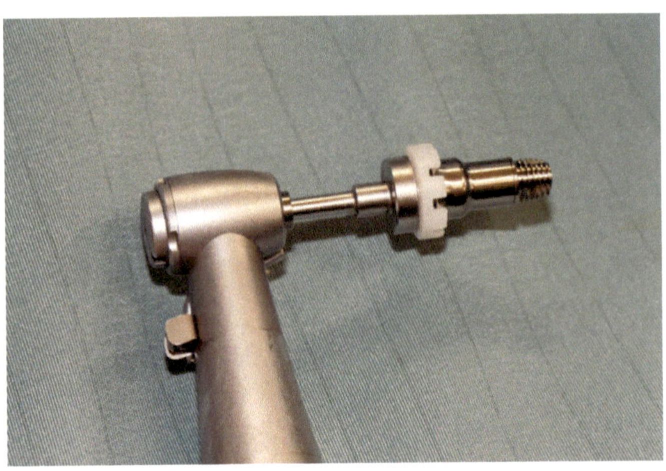

◀ **Fig. 18.2.7** The self-tapping fixture with premounted abutment is delivered sterile and it is picked up with the abutment inserter.

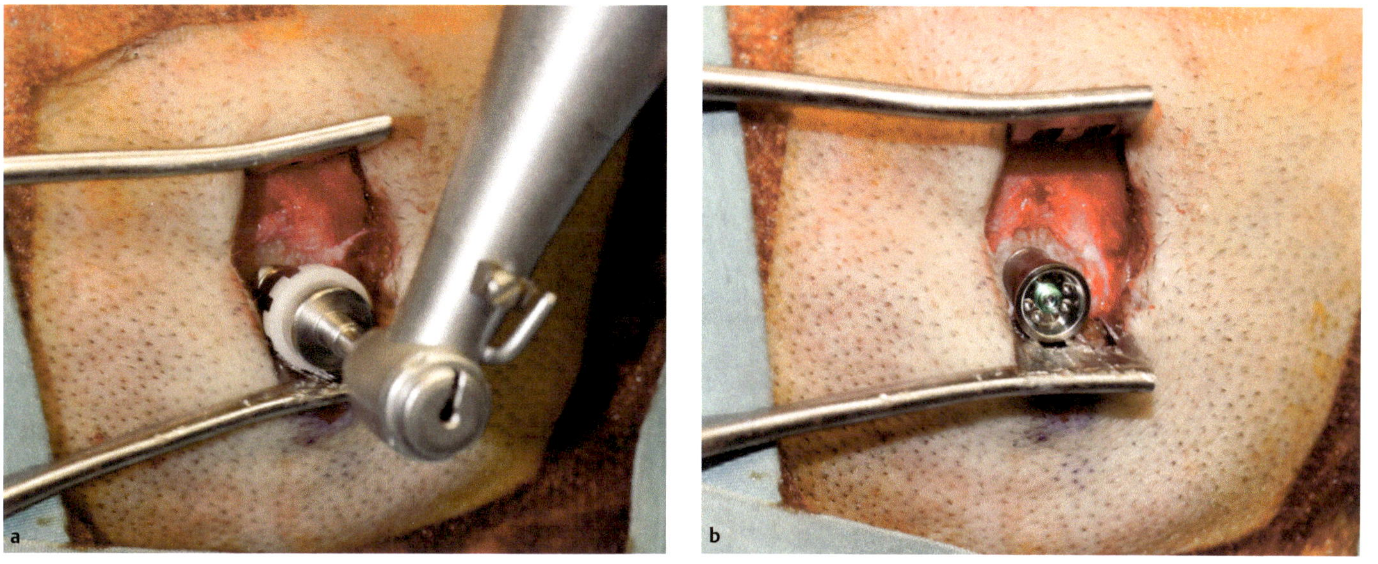

Fig. 18.2.8a, b The implant is installed without irrigation until the small grooves in the distal end of the implant are well within the canal, to avoid distal contamination. The implant is inserted using a low speed setting with the torque limit on the motor panel adjusted to between 30 and 40 N-cm. The periosteal flaps are then replaced near the implant base.

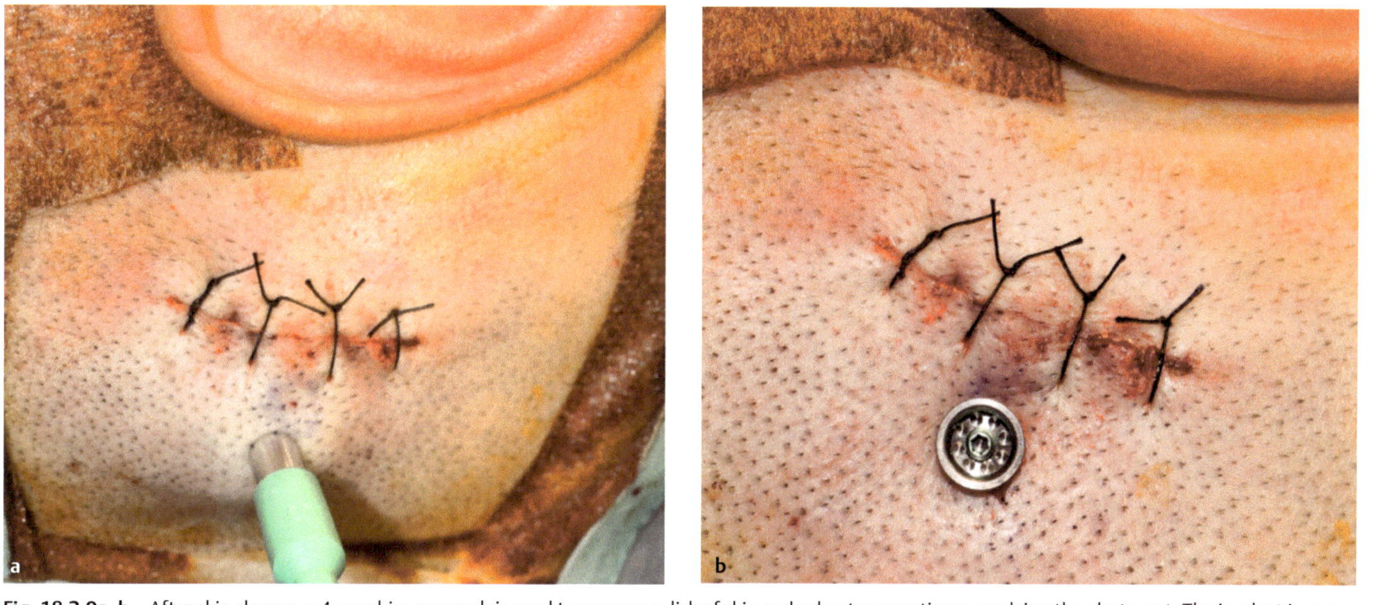

Fig. 18.2.9a, b After skin closure, a 4-mm biopsy punch is used to remove a disk of skin and subcutaneous tissue overlying the abutment. The implant is gently exteriorized through the hole.

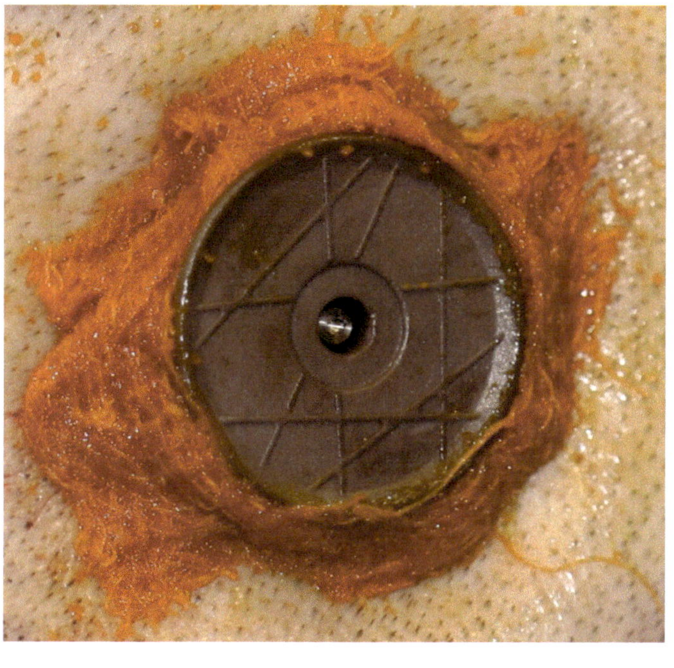

◀ **Fig. 18.2.10** The healing cap is snapped onto the abutment and a long gauze soaked with antibiotic ointment, is loosely packed circumferentially around the abutment.

18.4 Complications

Current techniques of fixture implantation and osseointegration are associated with minimal complications rates. However, the ultimate success of the bone anchored hearing aids depends heavily upon a meticulous surgical technique and correct postoperative hygiene maintenance of the abutment is also important.

Complications can be divided into two categories: intraoperative and postoperative complications.

18.4.1 Intraoperative Complications

Intraoperative complications are more common in children because most of these patients have craniofacial abnormalities. Despite this, the rates of implant survival and adverse skin reactions are comparable to those in adult patients.

Dural exposure without CSF leak does not constitutes a major complication. It is estimated that 70% of pediatric implant are installed in direct contact with either the dura mater or sigmoid sinus without any consequences. This complication may limit the length of the fixture that can be implanted but does not preclude the osseointegration.

Bleeding from a superficially located sigmoid sinus or a diploic vein can be managed when completing the procedure. The fixture itself will close the bleeding point. Rarely an alternative a bone wax plug may need to be used.

Epidural hematomas, although possible, are extremely rare.

These complications may limit the length of the fixture that can be implanted but do not preclude the osseointegration.

18.4.2 Postoperative Complications

The postoperative complications can be divided into two main categories: bone and soft tissue. The two categories are not completely separate, however, because extensive soft tissue complications can result in the loss of the implant. Bone complications essentially result in failure to osseointegrate.[5]

Loss of the osseointegrated fixture from the skull is a serious but rare complication. Fixture loss has been reported to be the result of trauma, especially in pediatric patients and those with poor hygiene. But the surgeon should not overlook possible causes of osseointegration failure represented by intraoperative thermal injury of bone due to inadequate irrigation with water during the drilling or by contact of the fixture with other tissue or gloves before it is implanted.

A possible alternative classification is in relation to severity, by dividing complications into major and minor.[6] **Major complications** have been defined as those requiring hospital care for patients or those with associated significant morbidity such as meningitis, brain abscess, or osteitis. **Minor complications** have been divided into complications requiring minimal office treatment and complications requiring revision ambulatory surgery. While the major complications are extremely rare, the minor complications, in particular skin reactions, may occur more frequently.

Holgher classified **skin reactions** into four grades: grade 1 corresponds to erythema of the skin around the abutment; grade 2 to skin with erythema and discharge; grade 3 to granulation tissue; and grade 4 to inflammation or infection that requires removal of the abutment.

18.5 Implantable Devices without Transcutaneous Abutment

The companies MED-EL and the Sophono have developed two different system of bone conduction implants: the Bonebridge and the Alpha systems, respectively. Both systems transmit the sound information through an intact skin layer.

The Bonebridge system includes an external part, the audio processor, and an implanted part, the bone conduction implant (BCI). The BCI is implanted in the mastoid and temporal region and is magnetically coupled to and stimulated by the audio processor through intact skin. The BCI vibrates transmitting the sound to the bone and the auditory system.

The Alpha hearing system comprises an external audio processor that contains a traditional bone conduction vibrator. Attached to the vibrator is a metal plate that is held to the head by a spacer shim. The magnetic spacer is in turn held to the head by a magnetic implant that is screwed to the skull with facial plating screws (Otomag, Belle, Germany). The implant consists of two magnets sealed in a titanium case. The implant is completely passive with no electronic or moving parts.[7]

Osseointegration is not needed in either system and patients can have their implants activated as soon as the wound has healed.

18.5.1 Preoperative Evaluation

Both systems may be preoperatively trialed using a soft band or head band in counseling of the patients; in both cases it again should be made clear to patients and parents that the subjective benefit obtained in these tests will be lower than achieved when using the processor coupled to the implants after their surgical placement.

A CT scan is done for all patients who will receive a Bonebridge to accurately determine where to place the device.

18.5.2 Key Features of the Devices

Bonebridge

See **Fig. 18.3**.

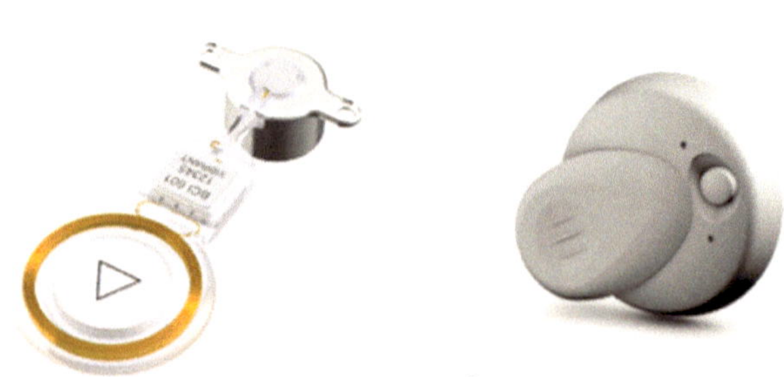

a b

Fig. 18.3a, b The BCI (bone conduction implant).
a The implantable component of the Bonebridge. The BCI is composed of the anteriorly placed bone conduction floating mass transducer (BC-FMT), which has a cylindrical shape and is the active vibrating part of the system, and of the posterior receiver coil.
b The Amadé audio processor, the externally worn component of the Bonebridge implant system.

Alpha 2 System

See **Fig. 18.4**.

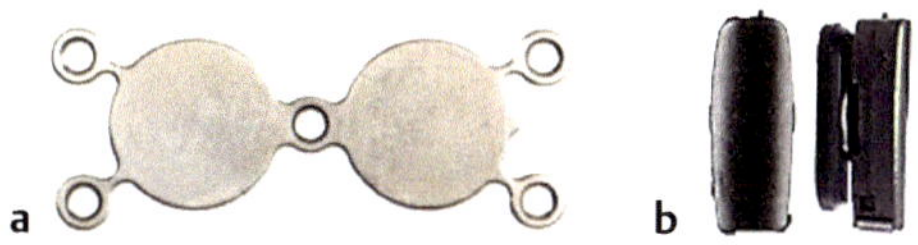

Fig. 18.4a, b Alpha system.
a The titanium covered magnets are the implantable part of the Alpha system, the Otomag.
b The active vibrating speech processor Alpha 2, magnetically coupled to the implant through intact skin.

18.5.3 Specific Indications

Audiologic indications for both devices include

- **Conductive (CHL) and mixed (MHL) hearing loss** with a mean bone conduction PTA between 0 and 45 dB (depending on the speech processor) and a speech discrimination score (SDS) of more than 60%.
- **Single-sided deafness (SSD):** bone conduction implantable devices are also indicated in the audiologic rehabilitation of patients suffering from severe to profound hearing loss or anacusis on one side and with a contralateral bone conduction PTA not exceeding 20 dB with an SDS better than 60%.

18.5.4 Contraindications

The Bonebridge and Alpha systems use magnetic transcutaneous coupling between the implant and the sound processor. In the Alpha system the bone implant may be responsible for the presence of artifacts on MR imaging but the device has been exposed safely to MRI fields up to 3 T. The Bonebridge on the other hand should not be exposed in MRI to fields >1.5 T as the implant could be damaged by magnetic interactions.

Both implants should be avoided in patients who need to undergo repeated brain MRI scanning because of the artifacts they generate.

The Alpha system is contraindicated in patients less than 5 years old, while the Bonebridge is contraindicated below 18 years.

18.5.5 Postoperative Management and Follow-up

After surgery, standard care practices are adopted for the retroauricular wound. If the postoperative period is uneventful, the implant is activated by a manufacturer's technician after 4 weeks.

18.5.6 Placement of the Bonebridge System: Surgical Steps

The bone conduction implant (BCI) is the implanted part of the Bonebridge system. It is usually planned to install the floating mass transducer (BC-FMT) at the level of the sinodural angle while the receiver coil will be placed under the skin of the retroauricular area.

Marking the Implant Site

When planning the implant site, the surgeon should use the shipped single-use templates (C-Sizer and T-Sizer) together with the CT images. The C-Sizer helps in determining the implant placement before incising the skin; it can be connected to the T-Sizer that reproduces the BC-FMT and helps to outline the exact size of the surgical seat and works as a drill guide to ensure correct orientation of the anchor holes.

After hair shaving and surgical preparation, the C- and T-sizers are connected and placed on the skin, with the T-Sizer lying over the sinodural angle and the C-Sizer angled approximatively 45° posterior-superiorly. A marking pen is used to outline the outer perimeter of the templates. The cutaneous incision is marked at least 2 cm from the anterior edge of the template at the level of the postauricular sulcus to minimize the risks of extrusion; it only needs to be large enough to drill the seat for the BC-FMT.

In atresia cases, the incision should be placed further posteriorly not impeding future auricle reconstruction procedures.

Anesthesia

The marked area is injected with a local anesthetic of lidocaine and epinephrine; usually less than 10 mL is used to infiltrate the skin and periosteum at the implant site.

Skin Incision

A 3- to 4-cm long postauricular skin incision is made to the level of the temporalis fascia. A second myoperiosteal layer is harvested and detached from the bone, incising the temporalis fascia (see **Fig. 18.3.1** and **Fig. 18.3.2**). The total thickness of the soft tissues should not exceed 7 mm as evaluated by the skin flap gauge provided with the device. If necessary, the posterior part of the myoperiosteal flap can be excised and the skin carefully thinned. The anterior portion of the myoperiosteal flap covering the BC-FMT must be preserved.

Bone Drilling

The position of the bed for the BC-FMT depends on the findings of the CT scan; soft tissues are elevated subperiosteally to expose the temporalis line and the posterior external auditory canal. A bone recess is created at the level of the sinodural angle at a depth of ~9 mm (see **Fig. 18.3.3**). An anteriorly placed sigmoid sinus or low middle fossa dura plate may be encountered; in these cases a diamond bur is used to thin as much bone as possible without damaging these structures. If a bed of 9 mm cannot be created, the surgeon may use titanium spacers.

Placement of the Implant and Fixation of the BCI

A periosteal pocket is developed posterior-superiorly to accommodate the coil and demodulator of the BCI (see **Fig. 18.3.4**). The bony bed and the subperiosteal pocket are checked using the T- and C-sizers. Fixation points are drilled with the 1.5-mm drill supplied using the T-Sizer as a guide; use of the T-Sizer prevents a drilling depth of more than 4 mm (see **Fig. 18.3.5**).

The surgeon then arranges the BCI in the surgical field, taking care not to touch surgical drapes, towels, or sponges. The monopolar electrocautery should be withdrawn from the field at this point, so it is recommended to establish complete hemostasis before unpacking the BCI.

The implant coil and demodulator are placed under the periosteum, bending the transition portion of the implant as required. The triangle shape on the magnet should face the skin. The BC-FMT should reside in the previously prepared bed (see **Fig. 18.3.6**). The screws are placed in each anchoring hole of the BC-FMT; the regular screws have a diameter of 2 mm and a length of 6 mm. The torque wrench provided is used to secure the screws in the mastoid bone; it is rotated clockwise until a secure fixation has been achieved; a torque of 10 N-cm is sufficient (see **Fig. 18.3.7**); a torque of more than 30 N-cm should not be applied.

The emergency screw provided (blue surface finish, 2.4 mm diameter and 6 mm long) is used if one of the screws has achieved less than optimal fixation.

Skin Closure

The whole BCI is visually and manually inspected to make certain it is secured in the desired position. The scalp is then closed in layers without touching the BC-FMT during the process (see **Fig. 18.3.8**). A light pressure dressing is applied.

Case 18.3 Bonebridge (Fig. 18.3.1–Fig. 18.3.8)

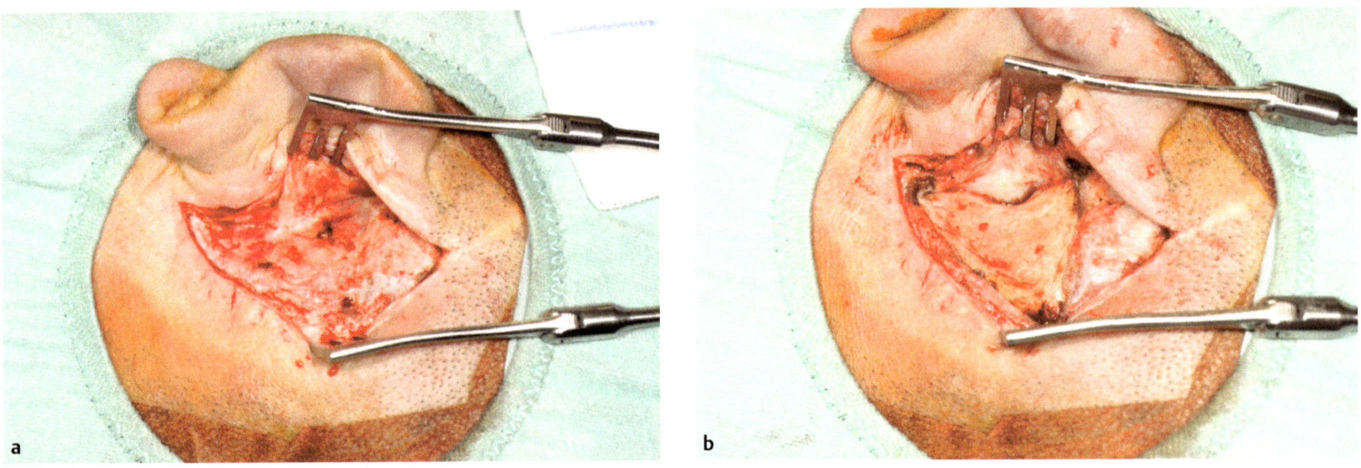

Fig. 18.3.1a, b Bonebridge system placement. Male patient.
a A postauricular skin incision is made to the level of the temporalis fascia.
b A second myoperiosteal layer is harvested and detached from the bone, incising the temporalis fascia. The posterior wall of the external auditory canal and the temporalis line are exposed. The total thickness of the soft tissues should not exceed 7 mm.

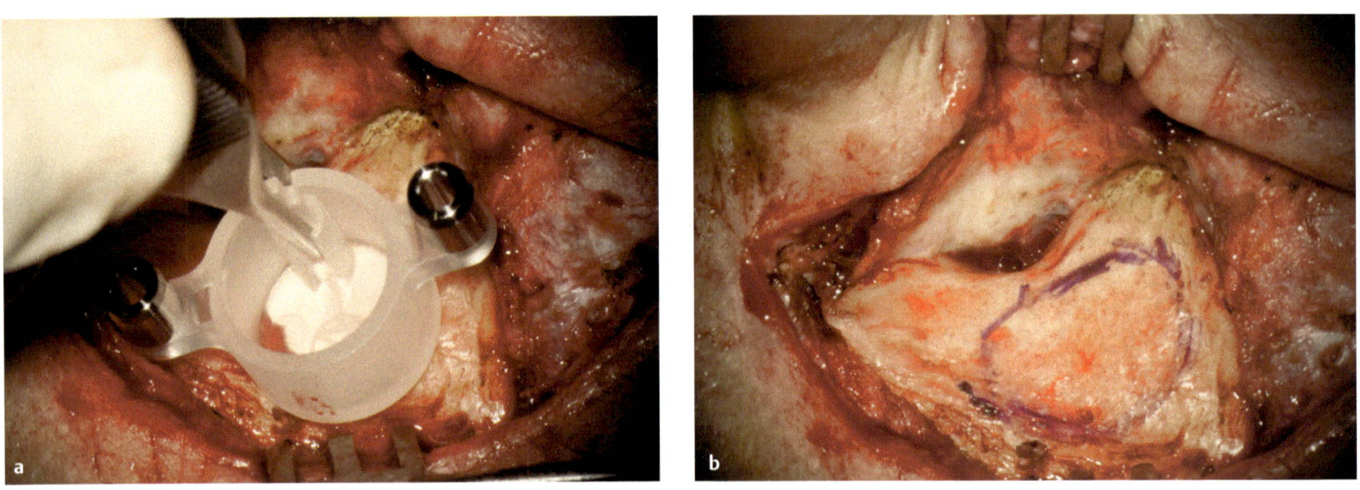

Fig. 18.3.2a, b The planned site of the bony bed is checked using the T-Sizer (**a**) and marked on the mastoid surface (**b**).

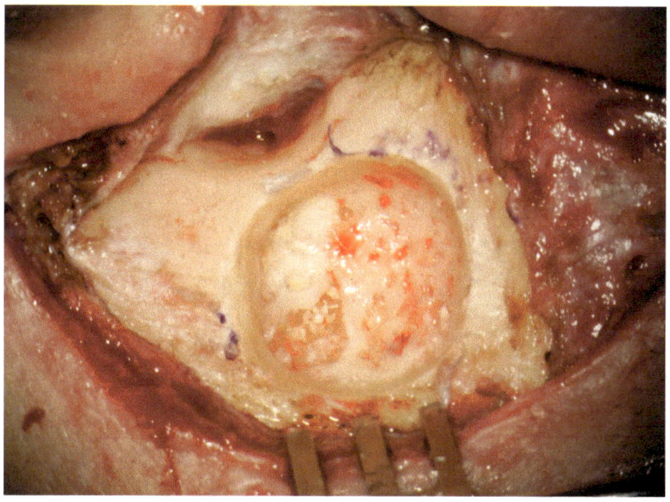

Fig. 18.3.3 A bone recess is created at the level of the sinodural angle at a depth of ~9 mm.

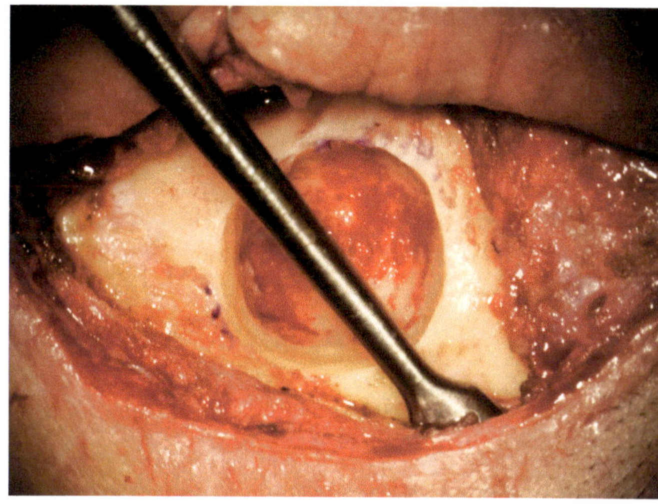

Fig. 18.3.4 A periosteal pocket is developed posterior-superiorly to accommodate the coil and demodulator of the BCI.

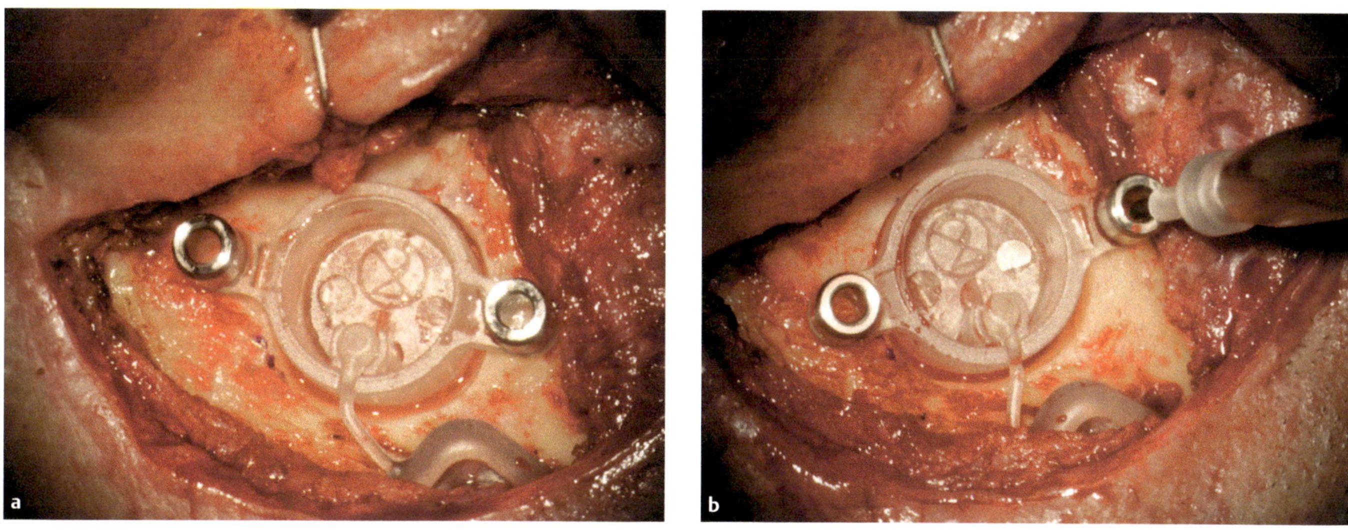

Fig. 18.3.5a, b Use of the T- and C-Sizer.

a The bony bed and the periosteal pocket are checked using the T- and C-sizers.

b Fixation points are drilled with the supplied 1.5-mm drill using the T-Sizer as a guide; using the T-Sizer prevents a drilling depth of more than 4 mm.

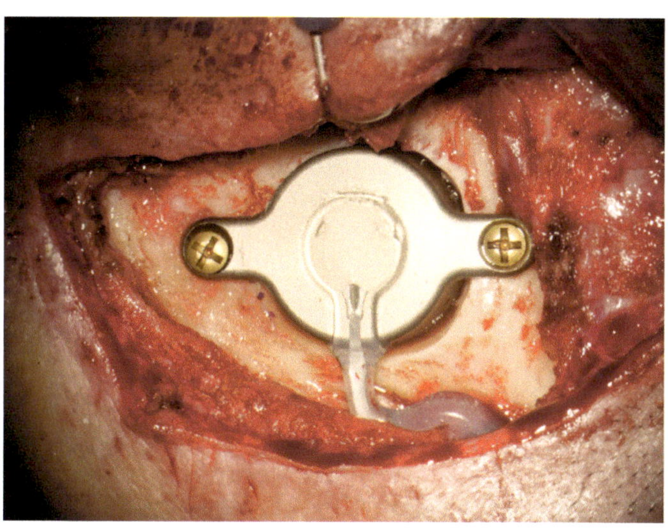

Fig. 18.3.6 The BC-FMT is placed in the previously prepared bed while the implant coil and demodulator are placed under the periosteum, bending the transition portion of the implant as required. The screws are placed in each anchoring hole.

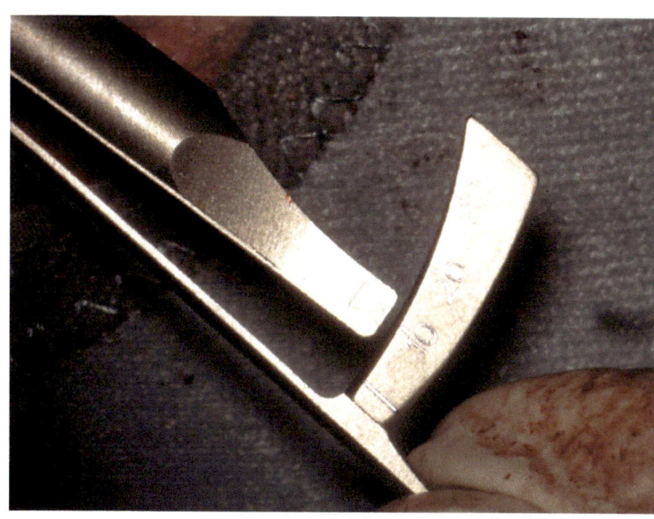

Fig. 18.3.7 The torque wrench provided is used to secure the screws in the mastoid bone; it is rotated clockwise until a secure fixation has been achieved; a force of 10 N-cm is usually enough.

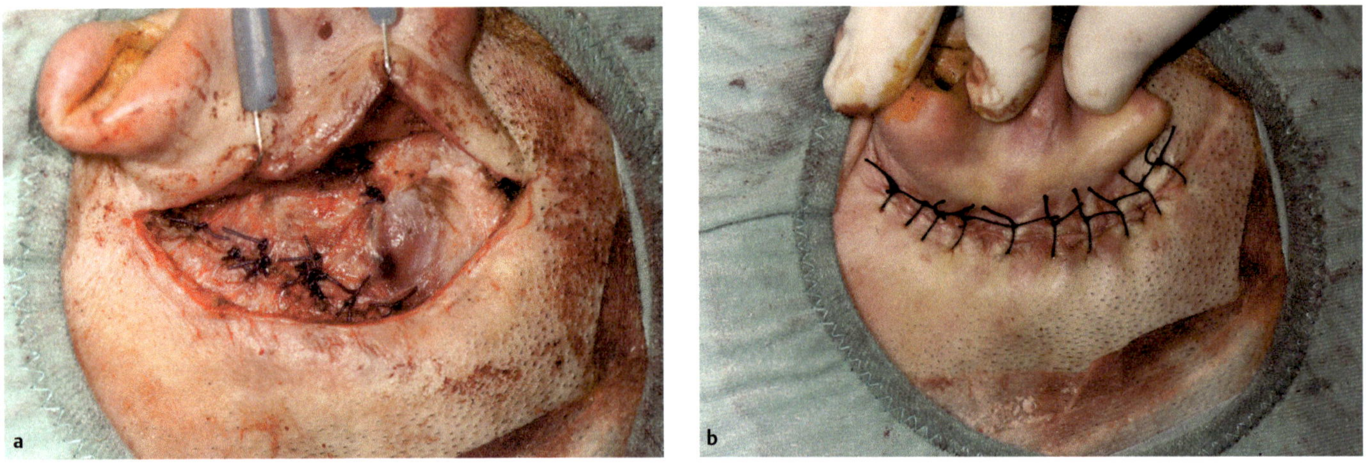

Fig. 18.3.8a, b The access is closed in layers.

18.5.7 Placement of the Alpha System: Surgical Steps

Marking the Implant Site

The hair should be clipped and the scalp shaved at the incision site immediately before surgery.

The proper position for the Otomag is 6 cm from the ear canal at a 45° angle posterior and superior to the ear canal (see **Fig. 18.4.1**). The incision should be made 7.5 to 8 cm from the external ear canal (1.5 to 2 cm from the location of the implant so that the incision is not directly over the implant) (see **Fig. 18.4.2**). The surgical template provided will aid the surgeon in ensuring proper placement by marking the skin with a surgical marking pen. A custom-prepared Silastic sheeting template may also be used.

Anesthesia

In adults the procedure is generally performed under local anesthesia. In children general anesthesia is preferred. The marked area is injected with a local anesthetic of lidocaine and epinephrine.

Skin and Soft Tissues Incision

The incision is performed on the skin markings and is carried through skin, subcutaneous, and myoperiosteal layers. The bone is exposed by elevating the flap in a subperiosteal plane (see **Fig. 18.4.3**).

Bone Drilling

The implant is ~2.6 mm thick and optimal tissue thickness over the implant is 4 to 5 mm. The surgical template is provided with 6-mm and 4-mm gauges for determining the appropriate skin flap thickness. Bone beds are recommended for the implant if the tissue thickness over the implant is less than 3 mm.

To create a bone bed, the position of the implant magnets on the bone are marked using the surgical template and the bone bed is drilled to a depth of ~3 mm (see **Fig. 18.4.4**). The implant template is useful in ensuring that the bone beds are of sufficient depth and diameter. A small amount of bone (0.5 mm) is also removed from the area where the brackets will lie, so that the implant smoothly follows the skull contour.

Placement and Fixation of the Otomag

After creation of the bone bed, the magnetic implant is installed using the specified screws such that the implant is oriented with the "This Side Up" label facing out. In addition, be sure to place the implant so that the small fiduciary mark is located in the most anterior and superior location. The screws are placed in each of the bracket holes to securely attach the implant to the skull. The first screw to be placed is the central one (see **Fig. 18.4.5**). The surface of the implant should be nearly flush with the surface of the mastoid (see **Fig. 18.4.6**).

Skin Checking and Closure

If the tissue flap is thicker than 6 mm, a 10-mm-wide strip of tissue is thinned down to 5 mm, directly over the implant magnets.

The wound is then closed in layers (see **Fig. 18.4.7a**) and a light dressing is applied after verifying the magnet strength (see **Fig. 18.4.7b**).

Case 18.4 Otomag (Alpha 2 System) (Fig. 18.4.1–Fig. 18.4.7)

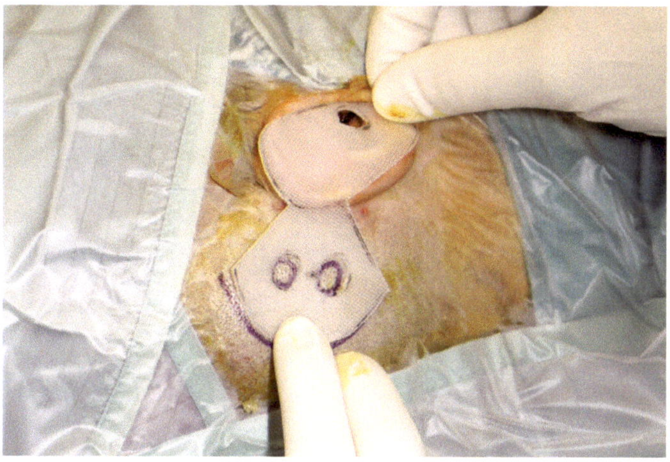

Fig. 18.4.1 Male patient. The proper position for the implant is 6 cm from the ear canal at a 45° angle posterior and superior to the ear canal. A custom-prepared Silastic sheet is used to mark the incision.

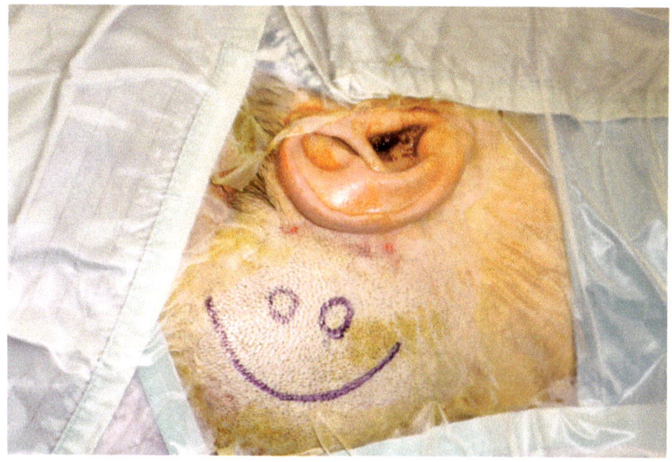

Fig. 18.4.2 The incision should be made 7.5 to 8 cm from the external ear canal (1.5 to 2 cm from the location of the implant so that the incision is not directly over the implant).

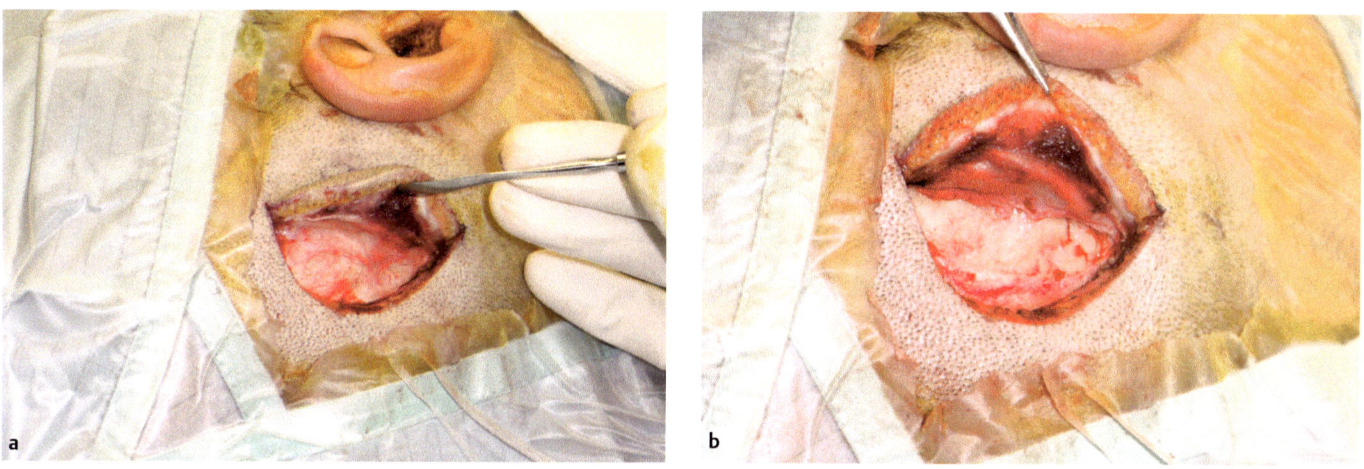

Fig. 18.4.3a, b The incision is performed on the skin markings and is carried through the skin, subcutaneous, and myoperiosteal layers **(a)**. The bone is exposed by elevating the flap in a subperiosteal plane **(b)**.

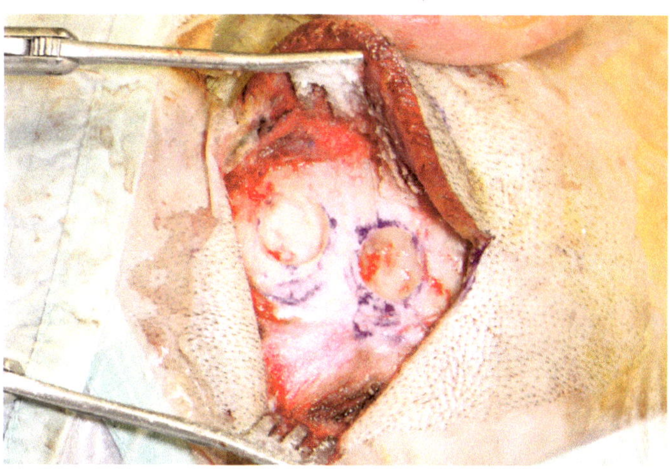

Fig. 18.4.4 To create a bone bed, the positions of the implant magnets on the bone are marked using the surgical template and the bone bed is drilled to a depth of ~3 mm.

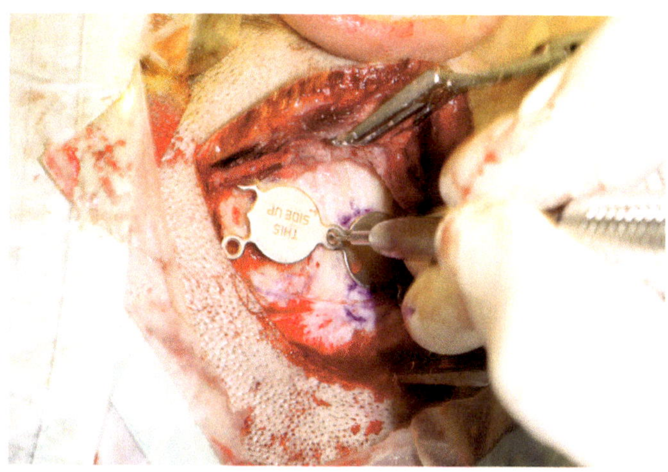

Fig. 18.4.5 After creation of the bone bed, the magnetic implant is installed using the specified screws such that the implant is oriented with the "This Side Up" label facing out. The first screw to be placed is the central one.

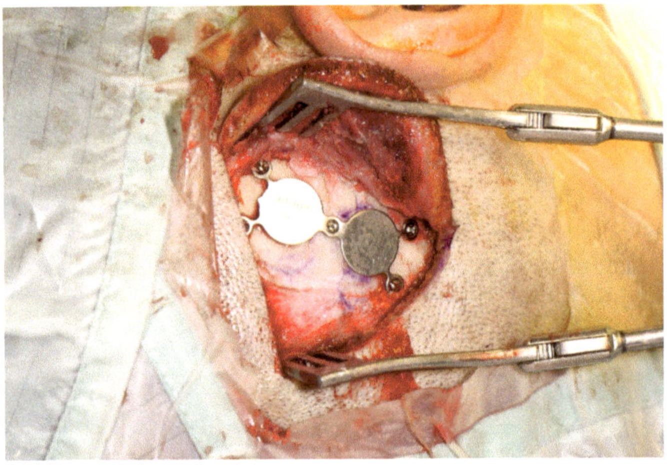

◀ **Fig. 18.4.6** At the end of the procedure the surface of the implant should be nearly flush with the surface of the mastoid.

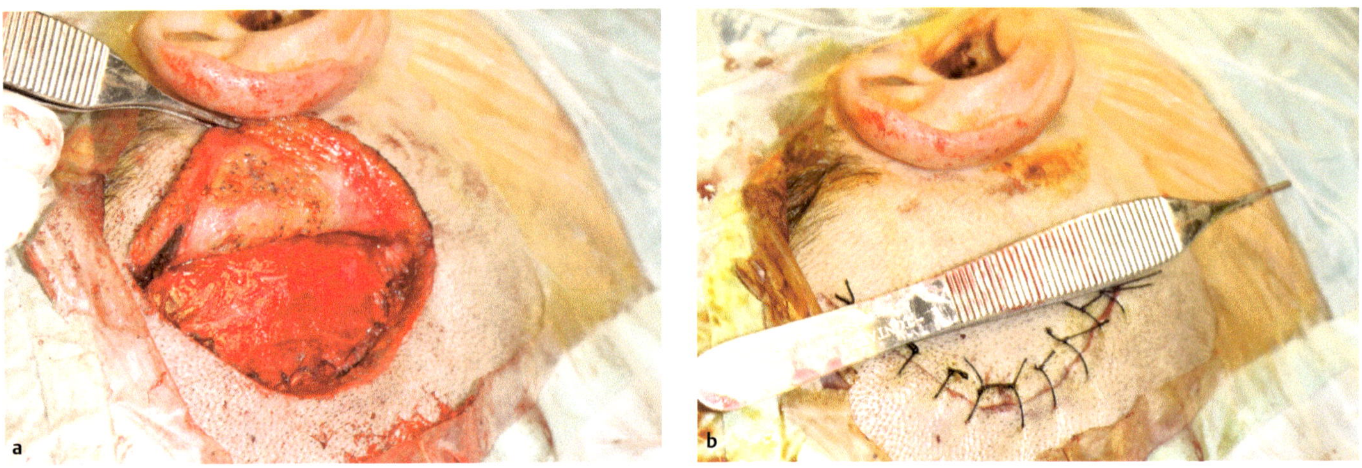

Fig. 18.4.7a, b The wound is closed in layers **(a)** and the strength of the magnet is tested at the end of the procedure **(b)**.

Reference Videos

See Video 18.1 and Video 18.2.

References

1. Snik AF, Mylanus EA, Proops DW, et al. Consensus statements on the BAHA system: where do we stand at present? Ann Otol Rhinol Laryngol Suppl 2005;195:2–12
2. McLarnon CM, Davison T, Johnson IJ. Bone-anchored hearing aid: comparison of benefit by patient subgroups. Laryngoscope 2004;114(5):942–944
3. Tjellström A, Håkansson B, Granström G. Bone-anchored hearing aids: current status in adults and children. Otolaryngol Clin North Am 2001;34(2):337–364
4. Hultcrantz M. Outcome of the bone-anchored hearing aid procedure without skin thinning: a prospective clinical trial. Otol Neurotol 2011;32(7):1134–1139
5. House JW, Kutz JW Jr. Bone-anchored hearing aids: incidence and management of postoperative complications. Otol Neurotol 2007;28(2):213–217
6. Wazen JJ, Young DL, Farrugia MC, et al. Successes and complications of the Baha system. Otol Neurotol 2008;29(8):1115–1119
7. de Wolf MJ, Hol MK, Huygen PL, Mylanus EA, Cremers CW. Clinical outcome of the simplified surgical technique for BAHA implantation. Otol Neurotol 2008;29(8):1100–1108

Further Reading

Alpha (S) & Alpha. (M) Physician Manual – REV B S0479-00 10/2013, download available on www.sophono.com

de Wolf MJ, Hol MK, Huygen PL, Mylanus EA, Cremers CW. Nijmegen results with application of a bone-anchored hearing aid in children: simplified surgical technique. Ann Otol Rhinol Laryngol 2008;117(11):805–814

Falcone MT, Kaylie DM, Labadie RF, Haynes DS. Bone-anchored hearing aid abutment skin overgrowth reduction with clobetasol. Otolaryngol Head Neck Surg 2008;139(6):829–832

Hobson JC, Roper AJ, Andrew R, Rothera MP, Hill P, Green KM. Complications of bone-anchored hearing aid implantation. J Laryngol Otol 2010;124(2):132–136

Hol MK, Bosman AJ, Snik AF, Mylanus EA, Cremers CW. Bone-anchored hearing aid in unilateral inner ear deafness: a study of 20 patients. Audiol Neurootol 2004;9(5):274–281

Kohan D, Morris LG, Romo T III. Single-stage BAHA implantation in adults and children: is it safe? Otolaryngol Head Neck Surg 2008;138(5):662–666

McDermott AL, Williams J, Kuo M, Reid A, Proops D. The Birmingham pediatric bone-anchored hearing aid program: a 15-year experience. Otol Neurotol 2009;30(2):178–183

Mylanus EA, van der Pouw KC, Snik AF, Cremers CW. Intraindividual comparison of the bone-anchored hearing aid and air-conduction hearing aids. Arch Otolaryngol Head Neck Surg 1998;124(3):271–276

19 Active Middle Ear Implants: Vibrant Soundbridge

The Vibrant Soundbridge (VSB): Symphonix/Med-El Vibrant Soundbridge is a middle ear auditory implant. It was originally designed for fixation to the incus with direct amplification of the natural ossicular movements, but it soon became clear that the vibratory stimulus produced by the implant could also be effectively delivered to the inner ear by direct stimulation of the round window (RW) membrane.

The VSB is composed of a surgically implantable part and an external component (**Fig. 19.1**). The external component is the audio processor (AP), which magnetically couples with the receiver-demodulator or VORP (vibrating ossicular prosthesis) implanted in the temporal region. The AP consists of a microphone, a microprocessor by which the incoming auditory stimulus is converted into an electrical signal, and a telemetry magnetic coil. The signal is amplified and modulated in the AP and transmitted across the skin to the VORP. The receiver coil of the VORP demodulates the signal and transfers it to the floating mass transducer (FMT) through the conduction cable. The FMT is responsible for transduction of signals into vibrations and directly stimulates the inner ear fluid through the ossicles. The FMT was originally developed to be secured to the long process of the incus through an incorporated titanium clip. Alternative coupling methods were subsequently developed; the FMT can be situated and fixated directly upon the round window membrane or, less frequently, to the stapes footplate or stapes remnants.

The FMT is an electromagnetic transducer containing a magnet of inertial mass within two electromagnetic coils; when the device is activated, the magnet mass vibrates, causing the entire unit to vibrate. The FMT has a cylindrical shape and measures ~2.3 mm in length and 1.6 mm in diameter, with a weight of 25 mg.[1]

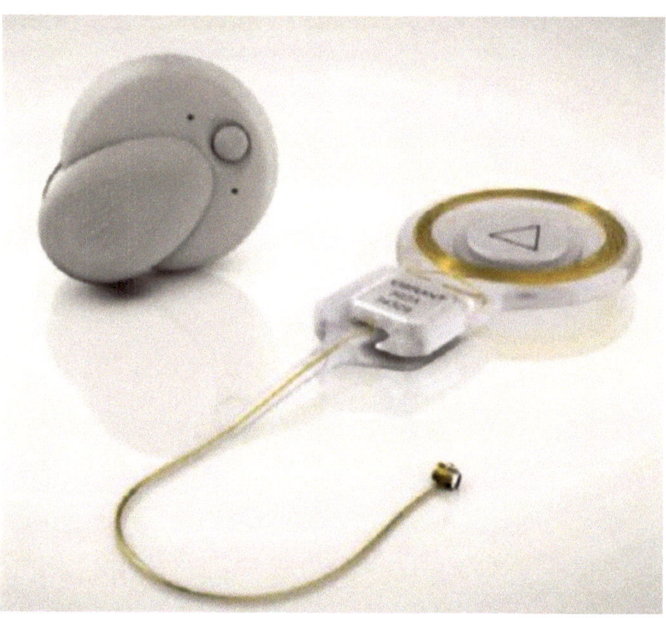

Fig. 19.1 The Vibrant Soundbridge system is depicted with the audio processor, and the VORP composed of the receiver coil, the connection link, and the floating mass transducer (FMT).

Positioning of the FMT depends mainly on the type of hearing loss and on the status of the ossicular chain.

19.1 Indications

There are three main indications for implanting a VSB, depending on the type and degree of hearing loss and on the status of the middle ear of the patient (**Fig. 19.2**).

- **Moderate to severe sensorineural hearing** loss especially in the high frequencies, with a speech discrimination threshold better than 50% at a comfortable listening or conversational speech level.[2,3] This audiologic indication overlaps with those of conventional hearing aids; the VSB should be offered to patients with stable sensorineural hearing loss (SNHL), normal middle ear function, absence of retrocochlear compromise, chronic external auditory canal disease, and/or poor compliance with hearing aids. Professionals in some fields may also need an open ear canal (e.g., physicians using stethoscopes, musicians, singers).

  In this category of patients the FMT is positioned on the long process of the incus through a posterior tympanotomy approach.
- **Mixed or conductive hearing loss**, secondary to[2,4]
  - Radical cavities
  - Middle ear obliteration/subtotal petrosectomy
  - Chronic otitis media and cholesteatoma surgery sequelae with failure to restore a normally aerated middle ear and reduce/close the air–bone gap after properly performed tympanoplasty and ossiculoplasty.
- **Mixed hearing loss (MHL) or conductive hearing loss** due to external auditory canal atresia and malformations of the external ear.[2,5] In these patients, most of whom are in the pediatric age group, a VSB can be implanted after plastic reconstruction of the pinna, or even before it if an appropriate and careful skin and soft tissue sparing technique is adopted to allow a later-stage aesthetic reconstruction. In malformation cases the FMT is placed on the round window membrane and a subtotal petrosectomy technique is adopted.

  In mixed hearing loss the tonal threshold for bone conduction should not be worse than 40 to 60 dB with a 30 to 40 dB air–bone gap and speech intelligibility results of at least 50%.

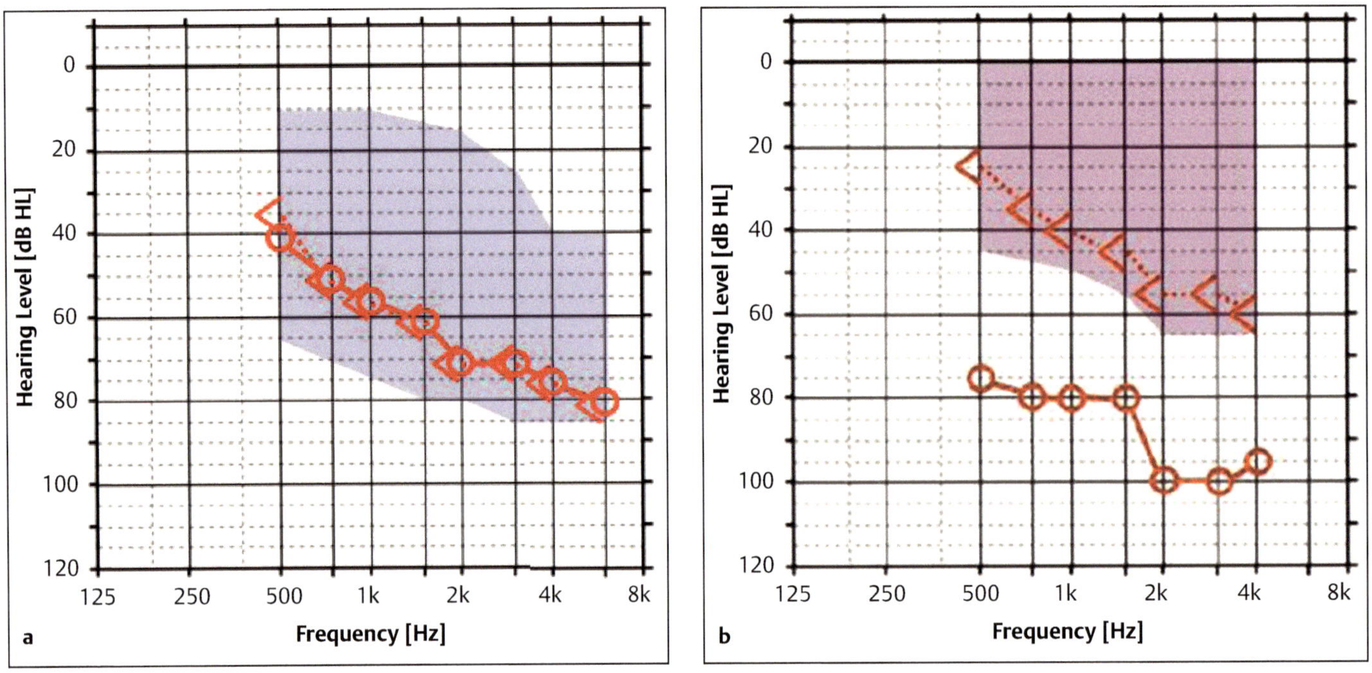

Fig. 19.2a, b Tonal threshold for VSB in SNHL (**a**) and mixed type hearing loss (**b**).

19.2 Contraindications

Patients offered or searching for a middle ear implant such as the Vibrant Soundbridge for SNHL with normal middle ear function should have undergone at least a trial period with conventional hearing aids. The role of the VSB in this category of patients is prominent in patients with chronic external ear disease and patients who do not tolerate the occlusion of the external canal.

Specific contraindications include:

- Fluctuating or rapidly progressive SNHL or decrease in bone conduction in MHL (i.e., autoimmune SNHL)
- Benefit from conventional hearing aids with no external canal disease
- Inner ear malformations
- Medical conditions requiring multiple MRI evaluations
- Failure of previously attempted auricle reconstruction, if a second attempt is planned

As MRI is becoming a common diagnostic procedure, all surgical candidates should be made aware of its possible effects on the implant. Possible side effects include loud noise, pain, and/or pressure in the ear region. The most serious complications are represented by FMT dislocation, involving surgical revision, implant demagnetization, and cochlear hearing loss. Moreover, MRI images are disturbed by the implant itself, with artifacts and consequent diagnostic difficulties.[6,7] MRI is thus not advised in patients undergoing VSB implantation.

19.3 Preoperative Evaluation

All patients should undergo clinical and radiologic assessment of their hearing loss, with special attention focused on excluding retrocochlear disease and on evaluating the status of the middle ear. In SNHL and MHL the bone conduction should be stable in the last 12 months. Complete audiologic testing should be performed, including threshold and speech discrimination audiometry, impedance measurement, and a CT scan of the temporal bones. MRI may be needed to rule out retrocochlear disease such as vestibular schwannomas.[2]

19.4 Postoperative Management and Follow Up

After surgery, standard care practices are adopted for the retroauricular wound. If the postoperative period is uneventful, the implant is activated by a manufacturer's technician after 6 to 8 weeks.

19.5 Surgical Steps: Incus Vibroplasty

The surgery requires proper positioning for mastoidectomy, hair shaving, and facial nerve monitoring. No special instruments are required for FMT positioning. Surgery is usually carried out under general anesthesia, allowing facial nerve monitoring and accommodating the patient's and the surgeon's comfort.

Surgical Steps

- Skin incision
- Creation of a musculoperiosteal layer
- Canal wall up mastoidectomy
- Posterior tympanotomy
- Exposure of the incudostapedial joint
- Drill out of the receiver well and implant fixation
- Positioning of the FMT on the incus
- Intraoperative testing
- Closure

19.5.1 Incision of Skin and Soft Tissues

The same principles described for skin incision in cochlear implantation are applied in VSB placement to prevent extrusion and to create adequate coverage of the receiver-demodulator. The positioning of the skin incision does not need to take into account a behind-the-ear speech processor as in cochlear implant surgery. A standard Lazy-S retroauricular incision is adopted and the lateral surface of the mastoid process is identified after incision of the musculoperiosteal layer. The receiver should be situated posterior to the skin incision to minimize the possibility of extrusion. Using the manufacturer's template, the area of the bony cradle for the receiver is marked posteriorly and superiorly to the mastoid process at the occipitoparietal junction and the size of the subperiosteal pocket is measured with a Freer elevator.

19.5.2 Mastoidectomy and Posterior Tympanotomy

A simple cortical mastoidectomy is performed. The approach should be limited but sufficient to identify the main surgical landmarks for posterior tympanotomy. The antrum is opened widely until the lateral canal is seen. Care should be taken when exposing the incus, moving the head of the bur from medial to lateral.

A small bony buttress is left inferior to the short process of the incus to protect it while drilling the facial recess approach.

The utmost attention should be paid to the ossicular chain as iatrogenic disruption will hamper implant positioning and possibly cause SNHL or even anacusis. The posterior canal wall is thinned out; aggressive drilling of the canal wall should be avoided as it may cause postoperative atrophy and skin retraction. The position of the third portion of facial nerve is inferred from the incus, the lateral canal, and visualization of the second tympanic portion. Exposure of the digastric ridge can be helpful but is rarely necessary. When the posterior wall is being thinned the chorda tympani can be identified, leaving the fallopian canal from inferior to superior and from medial to lateral. These surgical landmarks delineate a triangular area with the base on the incus and the apex pointing inferiorly. Drilling in this area will open the facial recess, allowing exposure of the middle ear and incudostapedial joint.

Correct placement of the FMT in the tympanic cavity may sometimes require widening of the facial recess approach, with transection of the chorda tympani nerve or skeletonization of the third portion of the facial nerve.

When widening the posterior tympanotomy one should take care not to injure the facial nerve medially or the tympanic annulus laterally.

19.5.3 Implant Positioning

After the opening of the facial recess with adequate exposure of the incus is achieved, the bony well for the receiver is drilled using a large cutting bur, taking care not to uncover the dural layer. A channel is drilled in the cortical bone toward the mastoid cavity to stabilize the implant while allowing passage for the connection wire and FMT. The subperiosteal pocket and the bony cradle should secure the implant in position tightly to avoid migration of the receiver. Fixation with nonresorbable sutures may further stabilize the implant.

The floating mass transducer (FMT) is then guided into the posterior tympanotomy and carefully clipped onto the incus. The FMT should move freely with the ossicular chain and the clip is secured and closed only after correct placement is achieved. In the correct positioning the long axis of the FMT is perpendicular to the footplate.

The positioning and crimping maneuvers should be performed carefully in order not to apply unnecessary force on the long process of the incus or the stapes. The crimping force should be uniform and steady to achieve the maximal coupling between the FMT and the long process of the incus.

19.5.4 Audiometric Testing

Intraoperative tests are performed after crimping of the FMT. There are two main types of tests when the ossicular chain is intact:

- Device integrity test
- Reversal transfer function test: this test measures the firmness/stability of the coupling between the FMT and the long process of the incus. A microphone is placed into the external auditory canal and measures the sound produced by the tympanic membrane moving in response to the stimulated FMT. Correct placement is indicated by a sound response identical to the stimulating sound in terms of frequency, intensity, and duration.

19.5.5 Closure

After intraoperative testing, the musculoperiosteal flaps, subcutaneous tissue, and skin are closed in layers. A head bandage is maintained for 24 hours. Before discharge, a bone conduction threshold tonal audiogram is obtained.

Case 19.1 Incus Vibroplasty (Fig. 19.1.1–Fig. 19.1.7)

Female patient, 50 years old. Audiologic evaluation showed bilateral moderate SNHL with a mean bone conduction PTA of 45 dB and an SDS of 85 at 60 dB. During a trial period of 6 months with conventional behind-the-ear hearing aids the patient presented recurrent episodes of external auditory canal infection, especially in the right ear. MRI was negative for retrocochlear disease.

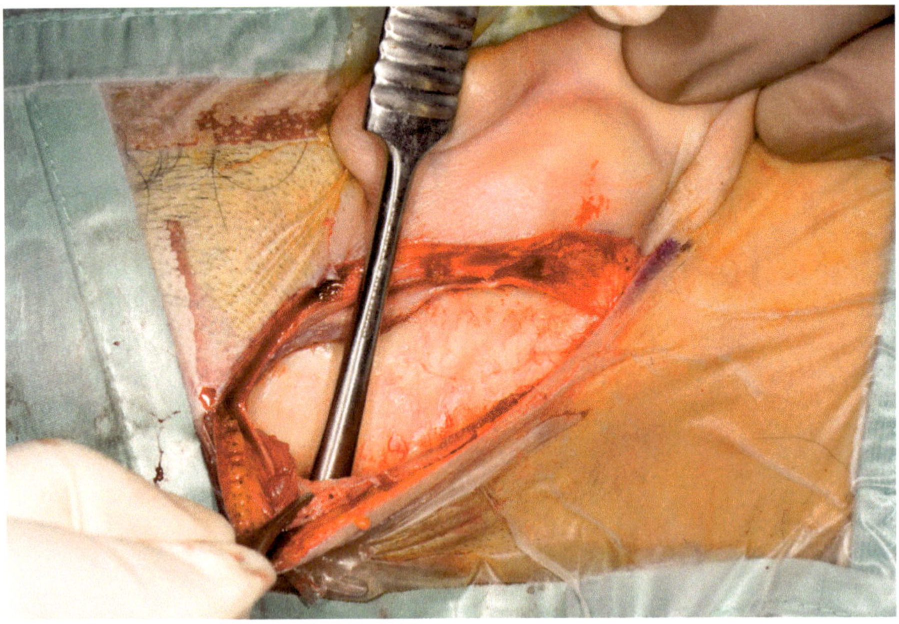

Fig. 19.1.1 After incision of the skin and myoperiosteal layer, the submuscular pocket for the receiver-demodulator is prepared with a round flat instrument.

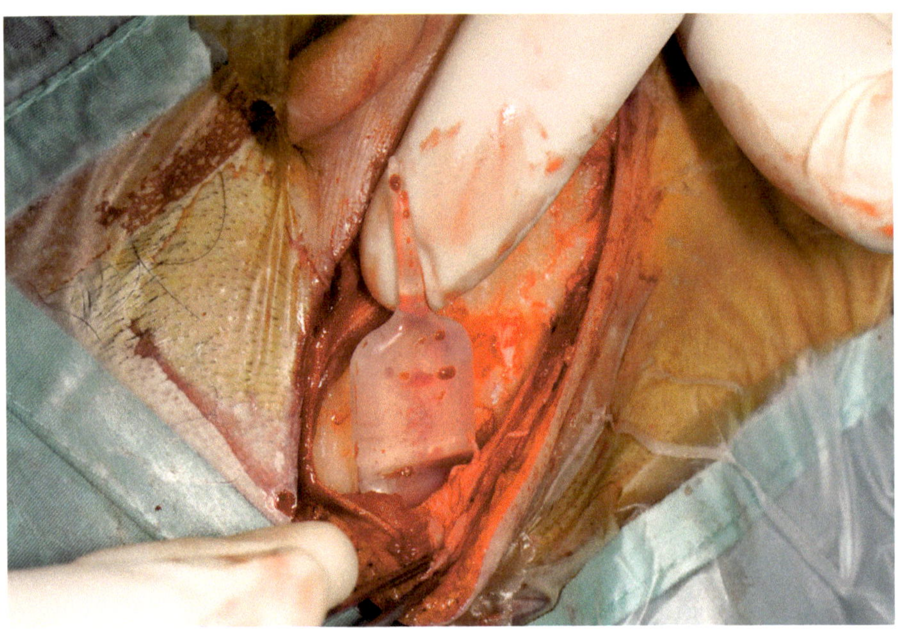

Fig. 19.1.2 The size of the submuscular pocket is assessed with a dummy implant.

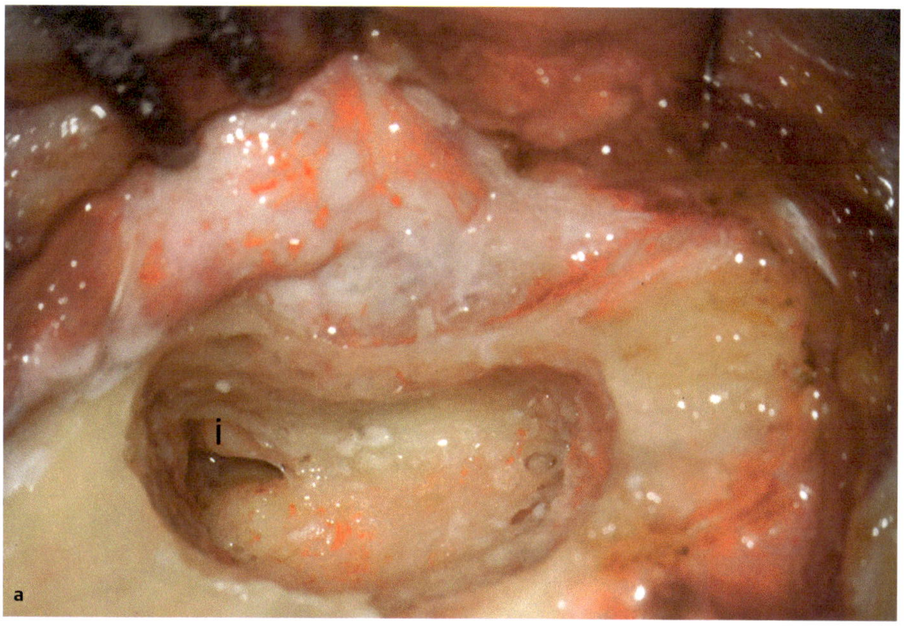

Fig. 19.1.3a, b

a A cortical mastoidectomy is performed, the antrum is opened, and the posterior canal wall is thinned enough to visualize the lateral canal and the short process of the incus ready to perform the posterior tympanotomy.

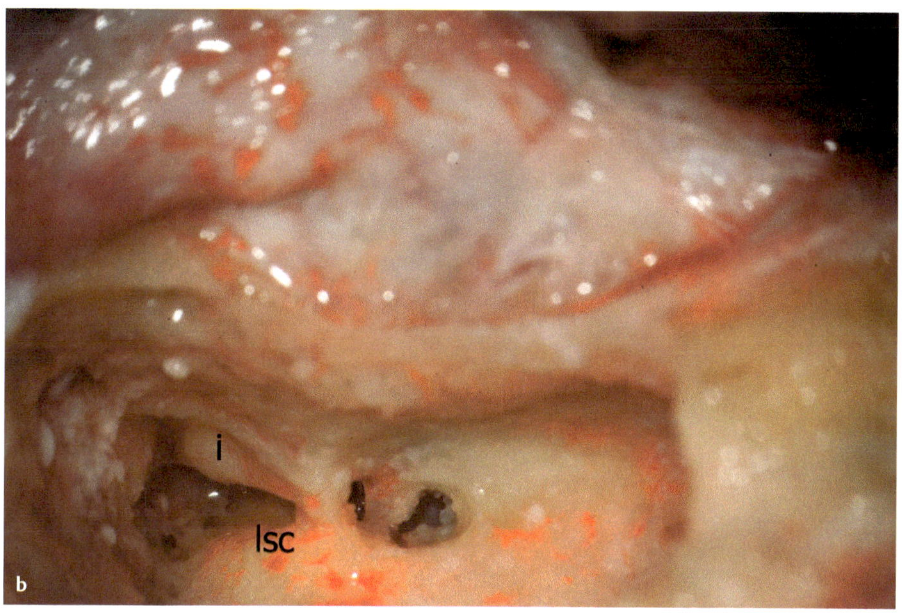

b The tympanotomy is started, leaving a bone buttress to protect the incus. The cordal crest is visible through the tympanotomy. I, incus; lsc, lateral semicircular canal.

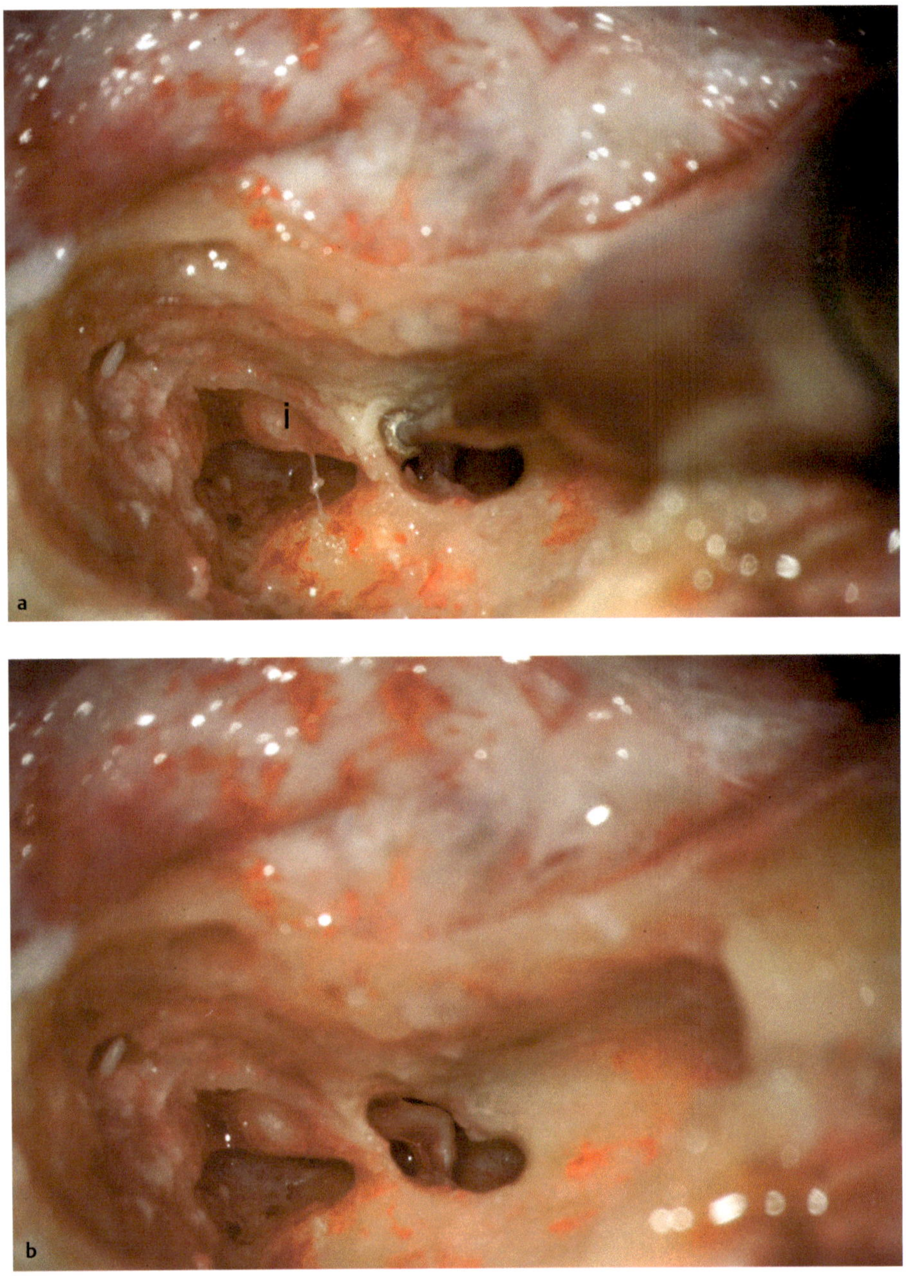

Fig. 19.1.4a, b

a The posterior tympanotomy is carefully enlarged with a 3-mm drill to completely visualize the long process of the incus and to create enough room for the FMT. I, incus.

b The tympanotomy at the end of the approach.

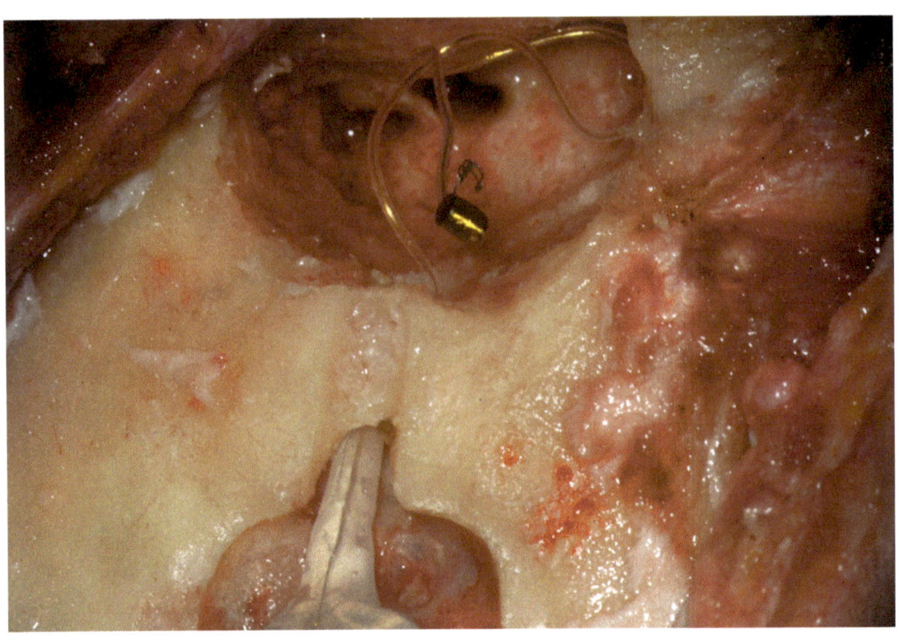

Fig. 19.1.5 After the bony cradle for the receiver has been drilled, a bony tunnel is created between it and the mastoid cavity, large enough to accommodate the connection cable and the FMT.

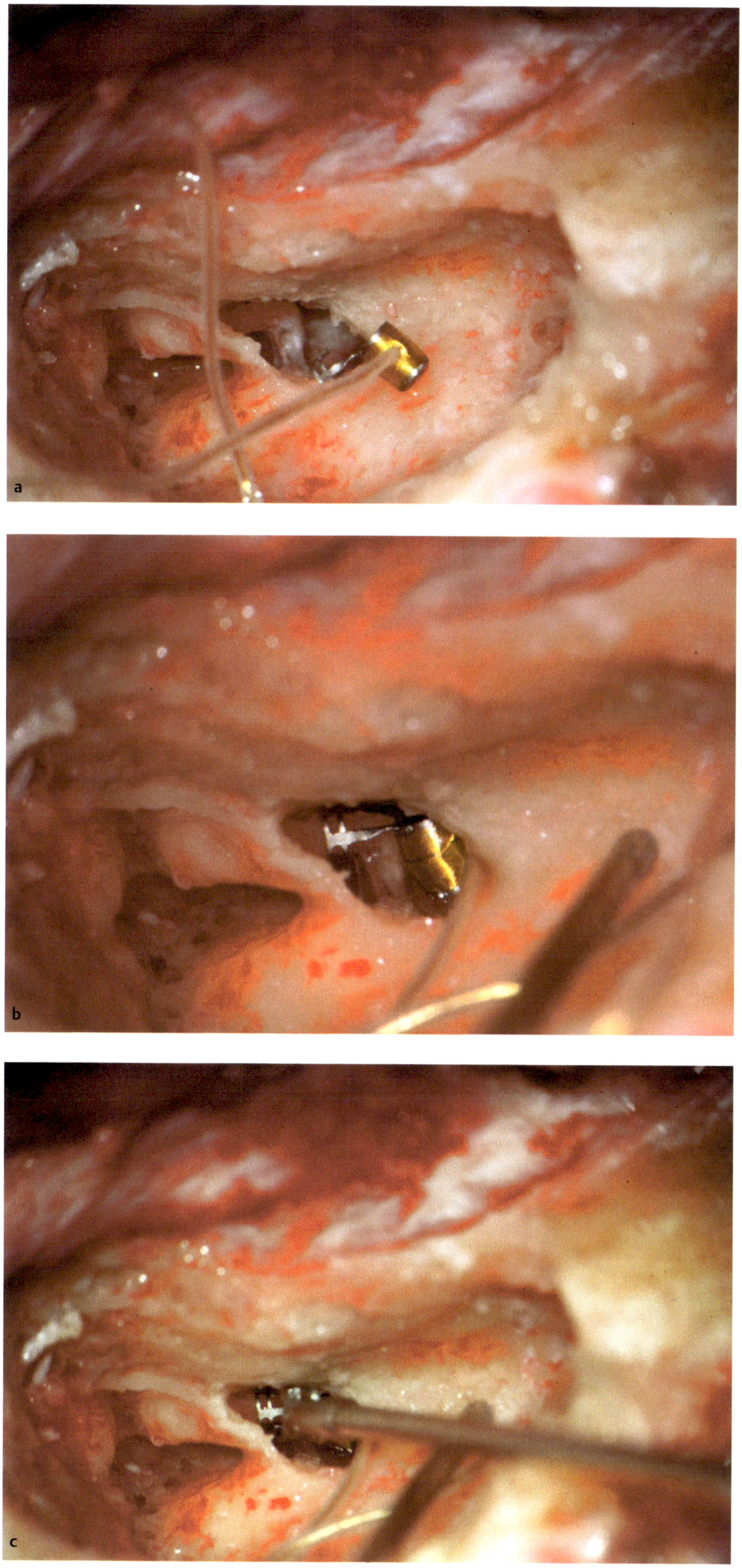

Fig. 19.1.6a–c

a The connection cable is housed in the mastoid cavity and the FMT is positioned near the posterior tympanotomy, checking whether further enlargement is needed to place it in the middle ear.

b The FMT has been inserted in the middle ear and the clip is secured to the incus. Care should be paid to the orientation of the FMT: its major axis should be perpendicular to the footplate.

c The FMT is crimped using an appropriate pair of forceps.

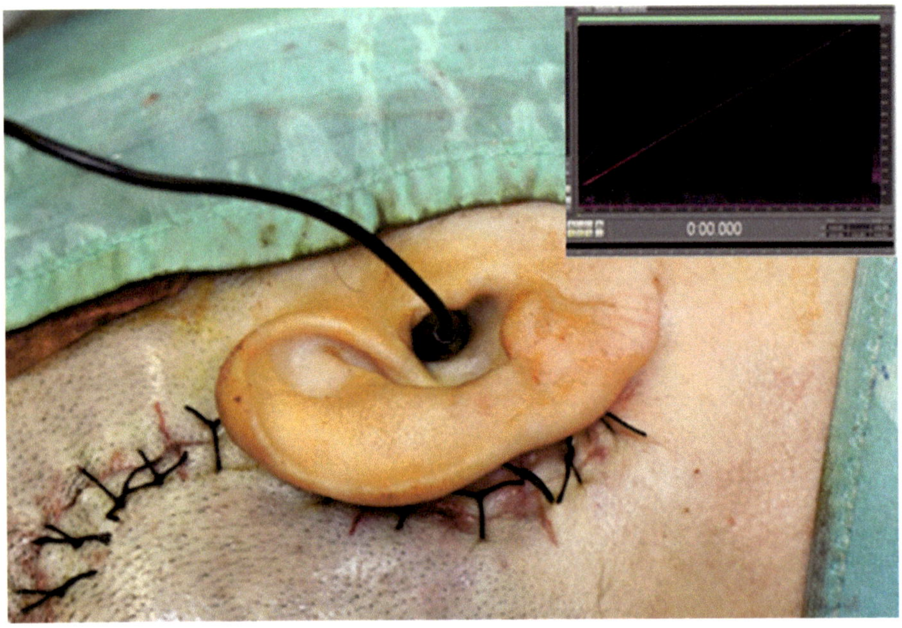

Fig. 19.1.7 After closure of the soft tissues and skin, the external auditory canal is cleaned of blood residue, the in-ear microphone is inserted, and a reversal transfer function test is performed (insert).

19.6 Surgical Steps: Round Window Vibroplasty

In case of previous unsuccessful middle ear surgeries (canal wall up and canal wall down mastoidectomies with persisting conductive or mixed hearing loss), radical cavities, lateral petrosectomy/middle ear obliteration, and in cases of aural atresia, the VSB can applied directly onto the round window membrane.

In these cases a subtotal petrosectomy is performed with blind sac closure of the external auditory canal. Persisting chronic disease (with or without cholesteatoma) is cleared either in a single stage or in a two-stage procedure. The subtotal petrosectomy approach aims to eliminate the middle ear cleft and allows regularization of the mastoidectomy cavity and clear identification of the surgical landmarks for safe and correct FMT positioning. At the end of surgery the cavity is obliterated with abdominal fat.

The surgery is carried under continuous facial nerve monitoring.

Cholesteatomatous otitis media is preferably treated in stages; the first stage consists of eradication of the pathology and preparation of the cavity for the future implant placement. The second surgical procedure with positioning of the implant is performed after at least 6 months.

Although it is technically feasible it is extremely rare to find good reasons and valid indications for a round window vibroplasty through a canal wall up technique.

Surgical Steps

- Skin incision
- Blind-sac closure of the external auditory canal in two layers
- Creation of musculoperiosteal layer
- Canal wall down mastoidectomy
- Disease clearing and cavity regularization
- Round window identification
- Drill-out of the receiver well and implant fixation
- Positioning of the FMT on the RW with fascia interposition and cartilage stabilization
- Intraoperative audiometric testing
- Closure

19.6.1 Incision of Skin and Soft Tissues

In revision after multiple surgeries, particular care must be taken when harvesting the cutaneous and myoperiosteal layers. A standard C or Lazy-S shaped retroauricular skin incision can be used on the previous scars or slightly posteriorly if wider exposure is required. A small piece of temporalis fascia or connective/scar tissue is harvested for later use when coupling the FMT to the round window membrane. The external auditory canal is transected and the lateral meatal skin is detached from the tragal cartilage and everted. After suturing of the skin from the outside, the tragal cartilage is transected and sutured with the posterior subcutaneous tissue flap. The same principles as described for skin incision in cochlear implantation are applied in VSB placement to prevent extrusion and to create adequate coverage of the receiver-demodulator. The positioning of the skin incision does not need to take into account a behind-the-ear speech processor as in cochlear implant surgery.

The receiver should be situated posterior to the skin incision to minimize the possibility of extrusion. Using the manufacturer's template the area of the bony cradle for the receiver is marked posterior and superior to the mastoid process at the occipitoparietal junction and the size of the subperiosteal pocket is checked with a Freer elevator.

19.6.2 Subtotal Petrosectomy

The surgical steps of subtotal petrosectomy were described by Fisch[8] and are the same presented in Chapter 10 (pages 158–178).

- After double-layer closure of the EAC, removal of the EAC skin, tympanic membrane, and ossicular remnants is carried out. The stapes, if present, is cleared of disease and left in place. Maximal care is taken not to leave skin remnants behind.
- The cavity is regularized, removing any bony overhang; diseased tissue corresponding to the primary pathology is removed. Pneumatic cell tracts are removed accordingly. Residual mucosa is completely removed from the tympanic cavity and the mastoid.

- The eustachian tube is packed with periosteum and bone wax.
- A small amount of fat (8–10 mL) is harvested from the abdomen.
- Depending on the underlying pathology, the implant can be placed at this stage or in a subsequent surgical procedure after 6 months.

19.6.3 Implant Positioning

A subperiosteal pocket is created with a Freer elevator posterior and superior to the mastoid process and the bony cradle from the implant is drilled at the occipitoparietal junction. The receiver-demodulator is placed in its cradle and fixated. The clip on the lateral aspect of the FMT is cut with straight scissors.

Particular care must be taken when positioning the FMT to obtain consistent contact between it and the round window membrane. The round window membrane should be adequately exposed and drilling of the bone surrounding its posterosuperior aspect may be required. The risk of cochlear trauma must be anticipated during this maneuver.

A small piece of temporalis fascia is interposed between the FMT and the round window membrane to prevent damage to the membrane itself[9] and to obtain optimal coupling. Further stabilization of the FMT may be obtained placing a small piece of cartilage and/or fascia on its inferior aspect toward the hypotympanum.

When the exposed surface of the round window membrane is smaller than the FMT diameter (i.e., less than 1.6 mm) or when drilling of the bony overhang significantly increases the risk of inner ear damage, a round window coupler may be used. It consists of a small hemispherical "cap" that has to be clipped onto the RW-facing surface of the FMT, reducing the active diameter of the transducer.

19.6.4 Audiometric Testing

Intraoperative tests of the coupling of the FMT with the round window membrane are represented by

- Device integrity test
- Electrocochleography: the stimulus is delivered using FMT. Intraoperative electrocochleography may help the surgeon to correctly place the FMT so as to obtain optimal coupling with the round window membrane.[10]

19.6.5 Closure

The myoperiosteal flaps, subcutaneous tissue, and skin are closed in layers. A head bandage is maintained for 24 hours. Before discharge a bone conduction threshold tonal audiogram is obtained.

Case 19.2 Round Window Vibroplasty (Fig. 19.2.1–Fig. 19.2.4)

Male patient, 62 years old with multiple surgeries for chronic otitis media in the left ear. Audiologic evaluation showed a moderate to severe mixed type hearing loss on the left with a mean bone conduction PTA of 30 dB and a mean air conduction PTA of 70 dB; the right ear had mild SNHL with a mean bone conduction PTA of 25 dB.

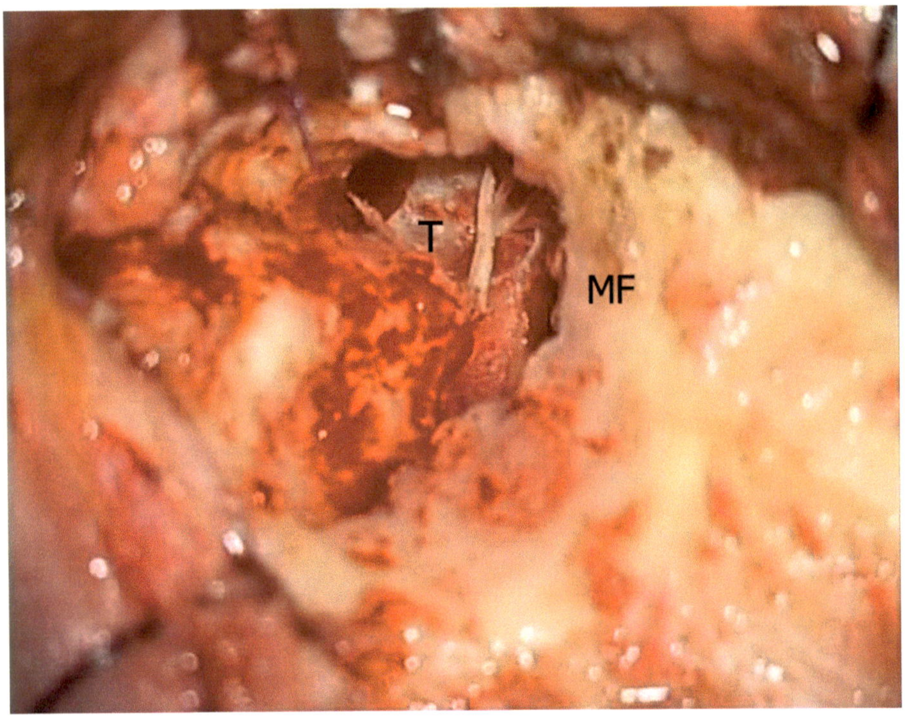

Fig. 19.2.1 After blind-sac closure of the external auditory canal, the residual cavity is regularized as in subtotal petrosectomy technique by removing any bony overhang from the middle fossa (MF) and facial ridge. The residual skin, tympanic membrane (T), and ossicles are removed.

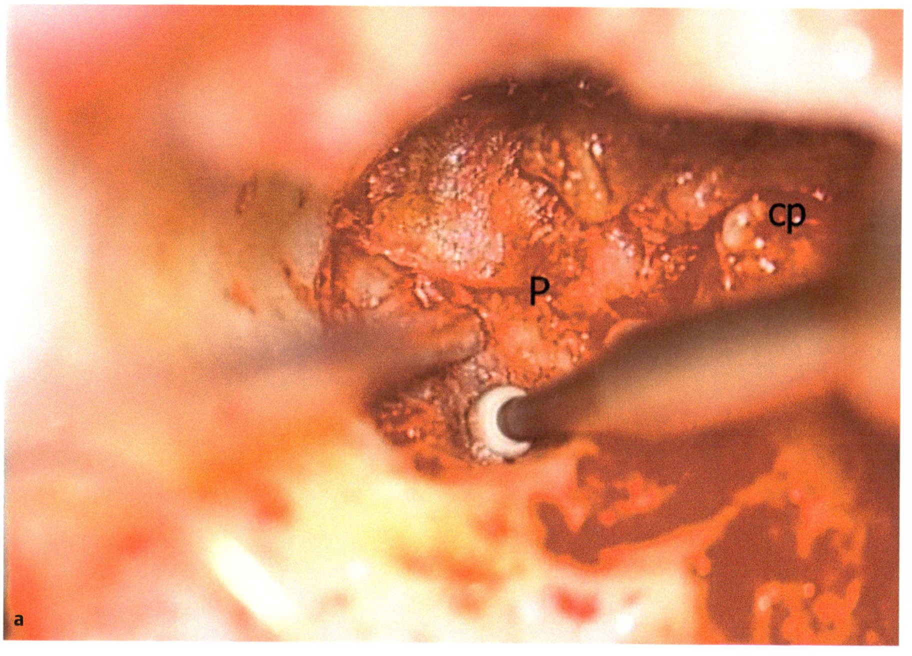

Fig. 19.2.2a, b The eustachian tube is plugged with periosteum and cartilage. The round window membrane is exposed by drilling the posterior and superior bony lip of the niche P, promontory; cp, cochleariform process.

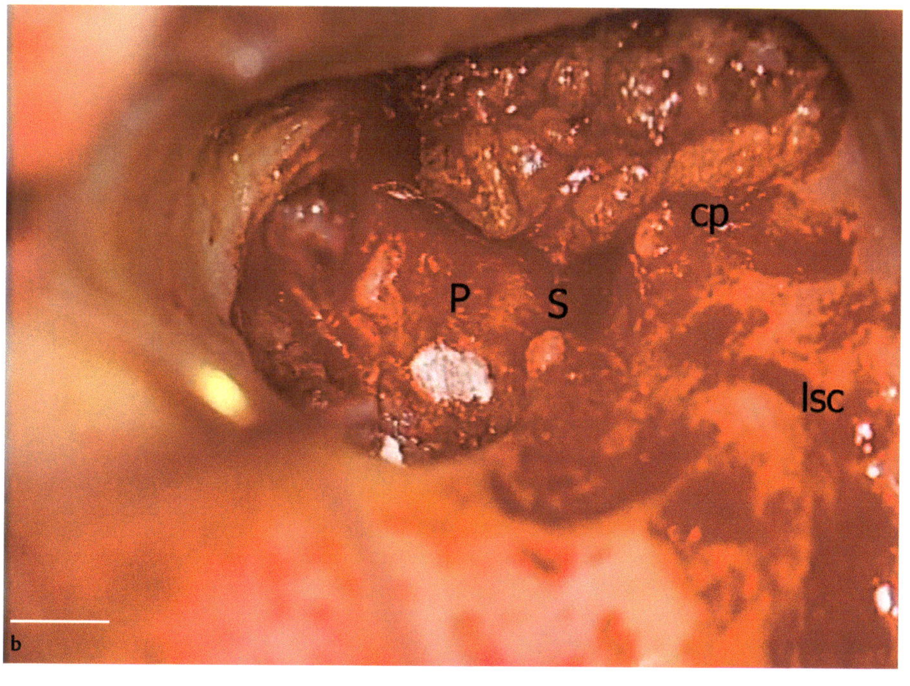

b The round window membrane is exposed and protected with fascia. P, promontory; cp, cochleariform process; lsc, lateral semicircular canal; s, stapes.

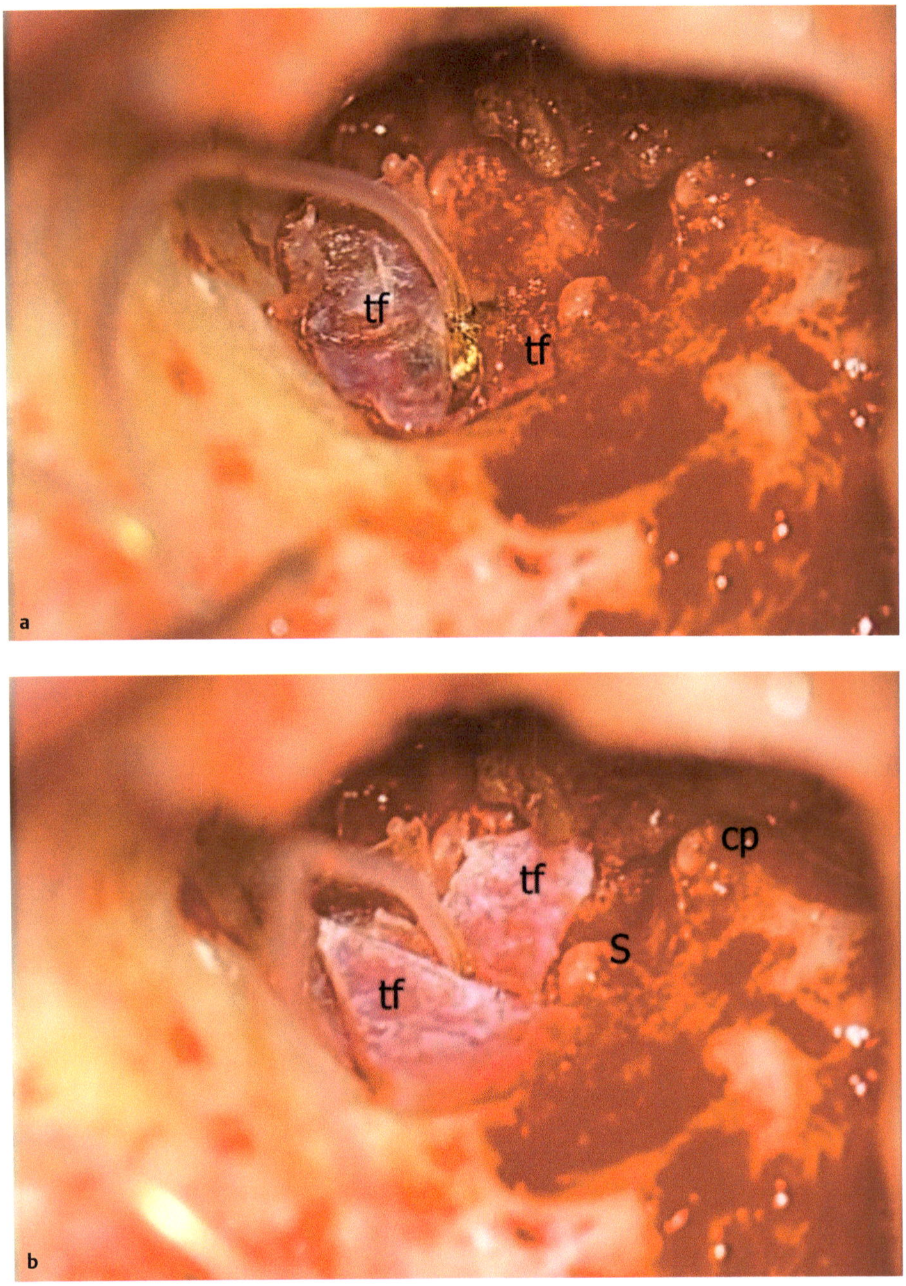

Fig. 19.2.3a, b The RW membrane is covered by a small piece of temporalis fascia. The fascia is also used to secure the FMT in place and stabilized with fibrin glue. Particular care must be paid to the lower aspect of the transducer as dislodgment is likely if it is not adequately supported. In some cases, fragments of tragal cartilage may be used to support the FMT. tf, temporalis fascia; cp, cochleariform process; s, stapes.

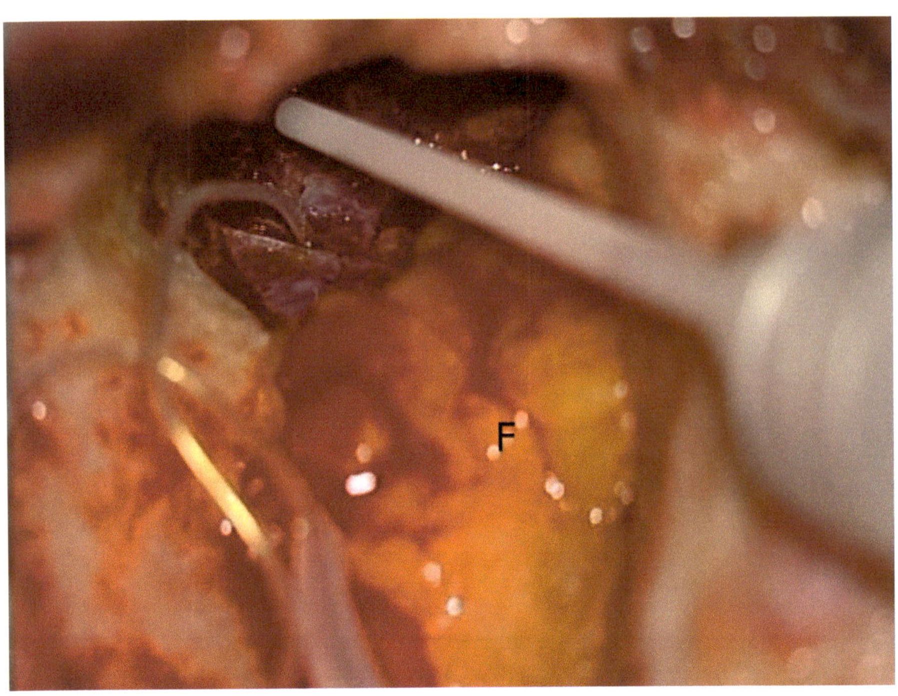

Fig. 19.2.4 After stabilization of the FMT, the cavity is filled with abdominal fat (F) and fibrin glue.

19.7 Results and Complications of VSB placement

Significant audiologic gain has been reported after VSB placement. Several studies have retrospectively confirmed the benefit in postoperative bone conduction and speech discrimination thresholds in SNHL cases[11] in the whole range of frequencies. The same holds true for both the bone and air conduction thresholds in mixed hearing loss cases, with a maximal gain in the midfrequencies.[12,13]

The main risk associated with VBS is decrease or loss of residual hearing; however, although possible, deterioration of preoperative tonal threshold is unlikely. Sudden loss of implant performance may be a rare consequence of FMT dislocation and may be due to insufficiently stable positioning of the FMT on the round window membrane; after CT imaging to confirm the diagnosis, dislocation is managed surgically. Other complications such as infection, extrusion of the implant, and hardware failure are rare instances.[14]

Caution must be used in patients who need to undergo MRI examinations; although studies have demonstrated the safety of the device up to 1.5 T, we advise that MRI should not be done unless it is of vital diagnostic significance.

Pearls and Pitfalls

- Active middle ear implants are indicated in patients with bilateral SNHL and medical contraindications and/or poor compliance with conventional hearing aids.
- When dealing with SNHL rehabilitation, a standard canal wall up approach is performed. Particular care is taken when performing the posterior tympanotomy; it should be sufficiently large to allow passage of the FMT without endangering the underlying facial nerve. Facial nerve monitoring is always used.
- When crimping the FMT to the incus, its major axis should be perpendicular to the footplate of the stapes. Care should be taken not to dislodge the incus while crimping the FMT.
- Active middle ear implantation may be used to rehabilitate mixed hearing loss in chronic ears after failure of traditional functional surgery or recurrence/persistence of disease. Surgery can be performed in a single stage or in two surgical steps depending on the primary pathology.
- Optimal coupling between the FMT and the round window membrane is necessary when performing a round window vibroplasty. This can be obtained by interposing a small piece of temporalis fascia between the FMT and the membrane and further stabilizing the transducer with conchal or tragal cartilage in its inferior aspect.

Reference Videos

See Video 19.1 and Video 19.2.

References

1. Ball GR. The Vibrant Soundbridge: design and development. Adv Otorhinolaryngol 2010;69:1–13
2. Wagner F, Todt I, Wagner J, Ernst A. Indications and candidacy for active middle ear implants. Adv Otorhinolaryngol 2010;69:20–26
3. Uziel A, Mondain M, Hagen P, Dejean F, Doucet G. Rehabilitation for high-frequency sensorineural hearing impairment in adults with the Symphonix Vibrant Soundbridge: a comparative study. Otol Neurotol 2003;24(5):775–783
4. Colletti V, Soli SD, Carner M, Colletti L. Treatment of mixed hearing losses via implantation of a vibratory transducer on the round window. Int J Audiol 2006;45(10):600–608
5. Frenzel H, Hanke F, Beltrame M, Steffen A, Schönweiler R, Wollenberg B. Application of the Vibrant Soundbridge to unilateral osseous atresia cases. Laryngoscope 2009;119(1):67–74
6. Todt I, Wagner J, Goetze R, Scholz S, Seidl R, Ernst A. MRI scanning in patients implanted with a Vibrant Soundbridge. Laryngoscope 2011;121(7):1532–1535
7. Cremers CW, O'Connor AF, Helms J, et al. International consensus on Vibrant Soundbridge® implantation in children and adolescents. Int J Pediatr Otorhinolaryngol 2010;74(11):1267–1269
8. Coker NJ, Jenkins HA, Fisch U. Obliteration of the middle ear and mastoid cleft in subtotal petrosectomy: indications, technique, and results. Ann Otol Rhinol Laryngol 1986;95(1 Pt 1):5–11
9. Nakajima HH, Dong W, Olson ES, Rosowski JJ, Ravicz ME, Merchant SN. Evaluation of round window stimulation using the floating mass transducer by intracochlear sound pressure measurements in human temporal bones. Otol Neurotol 2010;31(3):506–511
10. Colletti V, Mandalà M, Colletti L. Electrocochleography in round window Vibrant Soundbridge implantation. Otolaryngol Head Neck Surg 2012;146(4):633–640
11. Pok SM, Schlögel M, Böheim K. Clinical experience with the active middle ear implant Vibrant Soundbridge in sensorineural hearing loss. Adv Otorhinolaryngol 2010;69:51–58
12. Bernardeschi D, Hoffman C, Benchaa T, et al. Functional results of Vibrant Soundbridge middle ear implants in conductive and mixed hearing losses. Audiol Neurootol 2011;16(6):381–387
13. Foyt D, Carfrae M. Minimal access surgery for the Symphonix/Med-El Vibrant Soundbridge middle ear hearing implant. Otol Neurotol 2006;27(2):167–171
14. Skarzynski H, Olszewski L, Skarzynski PH, et al. Direct round window stimulation with the Med-El Vibrant Soundbridge: 5 years of experience using a technique without interposed fascia. Eur Arch Otorhinolaryngol 2014;271(3):477–482

Index

Note: Page numbers set **bold** indicate headings;
page numbers set *italic* indicate figures.